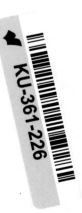

second edition

Principles and Practice of
Chiropractic

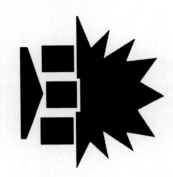

The first edition of this text was based on a conference sponsored by the International Chiropractors Association. This edition has been developed independent of but with the permission of the International Chiropractors Association.

second edition

Principles and Practice of Chiropractic

Edited by
Scott Haldeman, DC, PhD, MD, DSc (hon), FCCS(C), FRCP(C)
Associate Clinical Professor
Department of Neurology
University of California
Irvine, California
Adjunct Professor
Research Department
Los Angeles Chiropractic College
Whittier, California

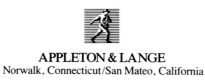

APPLETON & LANGE
Norwalk, Connecticut/San Mateo, California

0-8385-6360-0

Copyright © 1992 by Appleton & Lange
A Publishing Division of Prentice Hall
Copyright © 1980 by Appleton-Century-Crofts

93 94 95 96 / 10 9 8 7 6 5 4 3 2

Prentice-Hall International (UK) Limited, *London*
Prentice-Hall of Australia Pty. Limited, *Sydney*
Prentice-Hall Canada, Inc., *Toronto*
Prentice-Hall Hispanoamericana, S.A., *Mexico*
Prentice-Hall of India Private Limited, *New Delhi*
Prentice-Hall of Japan, Inc., *Tokyo*
Simon & Schuster Asia Pte. Ltd., *Singapore*
Editora Prentice-Hall do Brasil Ltda., *Rio de Janeiro*
Prentice-Hall, *Englewood Cliffs, New Jersey*

Library of Congress Cataloging-in-Publication Data

Principles and practice of chiropractic / edited by Scott Haldeman. –
  2nd ed.
     p.   cm.
  Rev. ed. of : Modern developments in the principles and practice of
chiropractic. c1980.
  Includes bibliographical references and index.
  ISBN 0-8385-6360—0
  1. Chiropractic. I. Haldeman, Scott. II. Modern developments in
the principles and practice of chiropractic.
  [DNLM: 1. Chiropractic. WB 905 P957]
RZ241.P75 1991
615.5'34—dc20
DNLM/DLC   91–33245
for Library of Congress   CIP

ISBN 0-8385-6360-0

9 780838 563601   90000

Production Editor: Eileen Burns and Sandra K. Huggard
Designer: S. M. Byrum

PRINTED IN THE UNITED STATES OF AMERICA

Contents

Contributors

Robert Anderson, MD, PhD, DC
Director of Manual Medicine
San Francisco Spine Institute at Seton Medical Center
Professor of Anthropology
Mills College
Oakland, California

Gary A. Auerbach, BS, DC
President
World Federation of Chiropractic
Tucson, Arizona

Paul B. Bishop, DC, PhD
Joint Injury and Disease Research Group of Calgary
University of Calgary
Calgary, Alberta
Canada

Alan Breen, DC
Director of Research
Anglo-European College of Chiropractic
Dorset, England
United Kingdom

Gert Bronfort, DC
Associate Professor
Division of Research
Northwestern College of Chiropractic
Bloomington, Minnesota

J. David Cassidy, DC, MSc (Orth), PhD, FCCS(C)
Research Fellow
Department of Orthopaedics
Royal University Hospital
University of Saskatchewan
Saskatchewan, Canada

Mary Ann Chance, DC
Editor
Journal of the Australian Chiropractors' Association
New South Wales, Australia

Carl S. Cleveland, III, DC
President
Cleveland Chiropractic College
Kansas City, Missouri

Ian Douglas Coulter, PhD
Past President
Canadian Memorial Chiropractic College
Ontario, Canada

James M. Cox, DC
Chiropractic Radiologist
Postgraduate Faculty
National College of Chiropractic
Lombard, Illinois

Lars B. Dahlin, MD, PhD
Laboratory of Experimental Biology
Department of Anatomy
University of Gothenberg
Gothenberg, Sweden
Department of Hand Surgery
University of Lund
Allmänna Sjukhuset
Malmö, Sweden

Kenneth F. DeBoer, PhD
Professor of Research
Palmer Research Institute
Davenport, Iowa

Muhammed Shahid Ilyas Dhami, PhD, DOHS
Professor of Toxicology and Biochemistry
Palmer College of Chiropractic–West
Sunnyvale, California
San Jose State University
San Jose, California

Jiri Dvorak, MD
Head of Neurology Department
Spine Unit
W. Schulthess Hospital
Zurich, Switzerland

Reginald V. Engelbrecht, DC
Past President
Chiropractic Association of South Africa
Bethlehem, South Africa

H. F. Farfan, BSc, MD, CM, FRCS(C)
Department of Orthopedic Surgery
St. Mary's Hospital and
Jewish General Hospital
Montreal, Canada

Leonard John Faye, DC
Department of Chiropractic Clinical Sciences
Los Angeles College of Chiropractic
Cleveland Chiropractic College
Los Angeles, California

Bruce Fligg, DC
Associate Professor
Postgraduate Studies
Clinical Biomechanics
Canadian Memorial Chiropractic College
Ontario, Canada

Stephen M. Foreman, DC, DABCO
Adjunct Assitant Professor,
Department of Diagnosis
Post Graduate Faculty
Los Angeles College of Chiropractic
Whittier, California

Pierre-Louis Gaucher-Pesleherbe, MA, DC, PhD
Diple. E.H.E.S.S.
Le Mans, France

Russell W. Gibbons
Editor
Chiropractic History
Pittsburgh, Pennsylvania

Lynton G.F. Giles, MSc, DC(C.), PhD
Senior Research Fellow
Division of Science and Technology
Griffith University
Queensland, Australia

Ronald Gitelman, DC
Professor
Postgraduate Studies
Chiropractic Sciences
Canadian Memorial Chiropractic College
Ontario, Canada

William V. Glenn, Jr., MD
Practice of Radiology
Carson, California

Adrian Grice, MSc, DC
Professor
Chiropractic Science Division
Canadian Memorial Chiropractic College
Ontario, Canada

Scott Haldeman, DC, PhD, MD, DSc.(hon.)
FCCS(C), FRCP(C)
Associate Clinical Professor
Department of Neurology
University of California
Irvine, California
Adjunct Professor
Research Department
Los Angeles Chiropractic College
Whittier, California

Sten H. Holm, PhD
Associate Professor
Department of Orthopaedics
University of Gothenberg

Sahlgren Hospital
Gothenberg, Sweden

Brian A. Howard, DC, MB, CHB, FRCP(C)
Assistant Professor
Department of Radiology
University of Toronto
Ontario, Canada

Joseph Howe, DC, DACBR, FICC
Professor, Department of Radiology
Post Graduate Faculty
Los Angeles College of Chiropractic
Whittier, California

Andries M. Kleynhans, OAM, B Sc, DC
Dean, School of Chiropractic and Osteopathy
Phillip Institute of Technology
Victoria, Australia

Matthew H. Kowalski, BS, DC
Chief Resident in Orthopedics
Research Associate
National College of Chiropractic
Lombard, Illinois

Peter Kranzlin, DC
Private Practice
Winterthur, Switzerland

Göran Lundborg, MD, PhD
Professor and Chairman
Department of Hand Surgery
University of Lund
Allmänna Sjukhuset
Malmö, Sweden

Tom Mayer, MD
Clinical Professor
Orthopedic Surgery
University of Texas
Southwestern Medical Center
Dallas, Texas

William C. Meeker, DC, MPH
Dean of Research
Palmer College of Chiropractic–West
Sunnyvale, California

Dale R. Mierau, BSPE, DC, FCCS(C)
Research Fellow
Department of Orthopaedics
Royal University Hospital
University of Saskatchewan
Saskatchewan, Canada

Timothy Mick, DC, DACBR
Acting Department Chair
Assistant Professor
Department of Radiology
Northwestern College of Chiropractic
Consulting Radiologist

Radiological Consultation Service
Bloomington, Minnesota

Robert D. Mootz, DC
Professor
Palmer College of Chiropractic–West
Sunnyvale, California
Director of Manual Medicine
San Leandro, California

Sean P. Moroney, DC, PhD
Former Associate Professor
Palmer College of Chiropractic
West Sunnyvale, Colorado

Daniel Muhlemann, PT, DC
Private Practice
Zurich, Switzerland

Reed B. Phillips, DC, PhD, DACBR
Professor and Interim Chairman
Department of Radiology
Los Angeles College of Chiropractic
Whittier, California

Peter Polatin, MD
Clinical Associate Professor of Psychiatry
Department of Psychiatry
University of Texas Southwest Medical Center
Dallas, Texas

Wolfgang Rauschning, MD, PhD
Associate Clinical and Research Professor
Swedish Medical Research Council
Department of Orthopaedic Surgery
University Hospital
Uppsala, Sweden

Lindsay J. Rowe, B.App.Sc. (Chiropractic), DACBR
New South Wales, Australia

Björn L. Rydevik, MD, PhD
Laboratory of Experimental Biology
Department of Anatomy
University of Gothenberg
Gothenberg, Sweden
Department of Orthopaedics
University of Gothenberg
Sahlgren Hospital
Gothenberg, Sweden

Akio Sato, MD, PhD
Director, Department of Physiology
Tokyo Metropolitan Institute of Gerontology
Tokyo, Japan

Dennis R. Skogsbergh, DC, DACBR
Assistant Clinical Professor of Orthopedics
Research Associate
National College of Chiropractic
Lombard, IL

Louis Sportelli, DC
Private Practice
Palmerton, Pennsylvania

Virgil Strang, DC
Dean of Philosophy
Palmer College of Chiropractic
Davenport, Iowa

Rand S. Swenson, DC, MD, PhD
Department of Neurology
Dartmouth-Hitchcock Medical Center
Hanover, New Hampshire

Kazuyoshi Takeyachi, DC
President
Japanese Association of Chiropractors
Tokyo, Japan

Christine M. Tamulaitis
Editor
Bulletin of the Foundation for the Advancement of
    Chiropractic Tenets

Gary A. Tarola, DC, DABCO
Fellow of the Academy of Chiropractic Orthopedics
Diplomate of the American Board of Chiropractic
    Orthopedics
Private Practice
Fogelsville, Pennsylvania

Allan G. J. Terrett
Lecturer
Department of Diagnostic Sciences
Phillip Institute of Technology
Victoria, Australia

John J. Triano, MA, DC, PhD(candidate)
Chief of Clinics Staff
Director, Ergonomics and Joint Laboratory
Clinics and Research
National College of Chiropractic
Lombard, Illinois

Howard Vernon, DC, FCCS (C)
Director of Research
Associate Professor
Canadian Memorial Chiropractic College
Ontario, Canada

Gerald Waagen, PhD, DC
Professor of Anatomy
Palmer College of Chiropractic–West
Sunnyvale, California

Beat Walchli, DC
Private Practice
Zurich, Switzerland

Michael R. Wiles, DC, FCCS (C)
Associate Professor and Director
Division of Chiropractic Science
Canadian Memorial Chiropractic College
Ontario, Canada

Preface

The past decade, since the publication of the first edition of this text, has seen the greatest change in chiropractic science, clinical approach, and acceptance in the almost 100 years of this profession's history. Chiropractors are no longer isolated in their private practice or excluded from government and privately funded health care institutions and facilities. Chiropractors are increasingly included within large multidisciplinary clinics with medical and osteopathic physicians, surgeons, and specialists. They are included in Medicare, Medicaid and other government-funded health care systems and participate in health maintenance organizations (HMOs) and preferred provider organizations (PPOs). Increasing numbers of chiropractors have hospital privileges and all now have access to medical specialist consultations.

This change in the status of chiropractic has made it necessary for chiropractors to understand and keep up with the scientific and clinical developments that influence their practice. Chiropractors must now be able to present their positions, theories, philosophy, and justification for treatment in terms that are understood and accepted by the other health care professionals.

Principles and Practice of Chiropractic (the second edition of *Modern Developments in the Principles and Practice of Chiropractic*) is designed to present the current status of chiropractic historical and philosophical thinking, the scientific and basic science research on which its theory is based, and to review the modern chiropractors armamentarium of diagnostic and treatment procedures. This book has been developed as a core text for the chiropractic student to use in a number of courses throughout his or her training.

In addition, this text has been developed as a reference for chiropractors who have graduated and are in practice who wish to keep up with the latest scientific and clinical developments in the profession without having to purchase a library of books. Furthermore, members of other health care professions who wish to develop a better understanding of chiropractic should be able to use this text to become aware of currently held views by the widest and most representative group of chiropractic educators, scientists, and clinicians ever to publish in a single book.

Organization

The text has been divided into four sections and two appendices. Before each section there is a brief introduction outlining the purpose of each chapter within the section. The sections follow, to some extent, the learning process of a chiropractic student as he or she progresses through their education. It is also the order in which a clinician who is unaware of chiropractic theories and practice can develop an understanding of the chiropractic approach to patients. Practicing chiropractors, on the other hand, will be able to rapidly find a chapter or section which he or she may wish to review without any difficulty.

The first section includes those topics which are commonly taught in the first year principle and philosophy courses at a chiropractic college. Many non-chiropractic readers may find it unusual to see a college teaching text with an entire section devoted to history and philosophy. This, however, has been an almost universal part of early chiropractic education and may be due to the youth of chiropractic as a profession and to its rapid development. There is a perceived need to establish in the student a sense of history and identity. Chiropractors also traditionally have an intense interest in philosophical concepts both materialistic/scientific and metaphysical/humanitarian. Without a firm understanding of prior theories and philosophical concepts students often have difficulty in placing the scientific and clinical materials in context.

The second section is dedicated to the major scientific and physiological principles which form the basis of chiropractic theory. These subjects are commonly taught at the same time as the basic science courses in the second year of a chiropractic student's education. Two fields are covered in depth: spinal biomechanics and neurophysiology. The biomechanical chapters are divided into the cervical and lumbar region and include the correlation of biomechanics with physiologic principles. The physiological chapters review nerve compression, reflex studies, the interaction between the somatic nervous system and the autonomic and hormonal control systems, and a review of physiological principles associated with spinal pain.

The third year of a chiropractic student's education is devoted to preclinical training. This includes the development of examination and diagnostic skills. The third section of this text reviews, in detail, the examination methods that a chiropractic student is expected to master. The radiologic chapters review the importance of x-rays and other imaging studies for pathology recognition and biomechanical analysis. In addition there are chapters on history taking, the physical, and orthopedic and neurologic examination as well as the use of laboratory studies and instruments to measure spinal function.

The fourth year of a chiropractic student's education is dedicated to mastering the clinical skills needed in his or her career. Although some basic manual skills are presented in the earlier years, it is the clinical internship year where the indications and contraindications for the various techniques must be studied and put into practice. The fourth section of this text is an in-depth presentation of the major chiropractic adjusting techniques with a review of the rationale behind each of the different methods of spinal adjusting and manipulation. There is, furthermore, discussion of the soft tissue techniques and rehabilitation that are becoming an integral part of chiropractic practice. The last two chapters review the potential complications of manipulation and the increasing importance of defined standards of care.

Appendix A is a review of the status of chiropractic in different countries of the world. Appendix B is a glossary of terms commonly used within the chiropractic profession. These appendixes are included as primary references for those individuals who would like to understand or study the international spread and development of chiropractic.

Development

When the second edition of this text was conceived a decision was made to expand the text from 16 independent chapters in the original text to 32 better organized and sequential chapters that would reflect a more traditional textbook format. The primary goal, however, remains the presentation of the most modern and current thinking, scientific research, and chi-

ropractic clinical practice methods. The text was also developed to reflect international as well as North American research and ideas and to include chiropractic thinking with as broad a base as possible.

With this in mind the search for authorities who would be invited to write chapters was not handicapped by professional, national, or theoretical barriers. Medical researchers such as Björn Rydevik, and Wolfgang Rauschning from Sweden, Akio Sato from Japan, and Tom Mayer from the United States are undisputed internationally recognized authorities. Chiropractors who have obtained their PhD in the basic sciences such as David Cassidy and Paul Bishop in Canada, Lynton Giles from Australia, and John Triano and Reed Phillips from the United States have become authorities in their specific fields of research. Other chapters have combined the expertise of medical and chiropractic specialists to give a more comprehensive approach with the combined knowledge of these two professions. The philosophical and sociological chapters combine the thinking of Palmer, Palmer West, Los Angeles, and Canadian Memorial Chiropractic Colleges. The clinical chapters, on the other hand, were drawn from the faculties of seven different chiropractic colleges from around the world. The contribution of authors from these diverse backgrounds has resulted in a text representative of a vast amount of knowledge, opinion, and expertise.

The Study Guide

To facilitate the teaching and learning of the material in this text by chiropractic faculty and their students a companion study guide has been developed by Mootz and Waagen. This study guide consists of 32 chapters representing the 32 chapters in this text. The study guide presents a brief synopsis of each chapter and the presentation of case studies and questions on the content of the text. Chiropractic instructors and students should find this study guide invaluable in understanding the details of *Principles and Practice of Chiropractic.*

Scott Haldeman

Acknowledgments

A text of this quality and magnitude requires a concerted effort by a large number of dedicated people. In a small young profession such as chiropractic, it requires a major time commitment by a significant percentage of its academic and intellectual leaders. The text could not, however, have been produced without the input from non-chiropractic scientists who, despite their busy schedules and unequaled prestige as scientific researchers, agreed to write chapters that could help change the thinking of a generation of chiropractic students.

This text is dedicated to those early chiropractic leaders who, despite minimal formal education in research methods, were responsible for setting the chiropractic profession on the path toward scientific exploration of their theories and practice. Such individuals as B. J. Palmer, Joe Janse, Henry Gillet, Fred Illi, Earl Homewood, and C. O. Watkins dedicated their entire lives to better understand the manner in which the spine functions. In addition, this text is dedicated to the numerous chiropractors in practice and, in particular, my father, Joshua Norman Haldeman, who encouraged a new generation of chiropractors to study beyond their clinic qualifications and to become active in scientific research.

The input of numerous other individuals is also acknowledged. The support of the International Chiropractic Association and Michael Pedigo, who was president at the time when the second edition was being negotiated, was essential to allow this text to be produced. The hard work and valuable advice by the editorial staff at Appleton & Lange insured the production of a high quality text.

Finally, there has to be special acknowledgment to the families of all the authors and especially my wife, Joan, for their patience and often personal assistance and support during the many hours of work, often at night and on weekends, which was necessary to produce this text.

Scott Haldeman

History, Philosophy, and Sociology

Not many professional textbooks devote an entire section and almost 20% of the chapters to the history, philosophy, and sociology of practice. The necessity of such inclusion and the intense interest in these topics by chiropractors are due perhaps to the youth of the chiropractic profession and its strong desire to establish and justify a unique and recognized role for itself in the health-care field. Chiropractic is one of the few professions that devotes specific courses in each of its academic years to discussion of its history, philosophy, ethics, and principles of practice.

Chiropractic is approaching the centennial of the first adjustment in 1885. The profession has been referred to as "one of the most remarkable social phenomena in American history" by Inglis [1963] and as a "medical and social protest movement" [Gibbons, 1980]. It cannot, however, be taken out of context from the very old practice of spinal manipulation, which forms the cornerstone of chiropractic practice. Robert Anderson, in Chapter 1, elegantly describes the widespread use of manipulation as a healing method in multiple cultures throughout history and around the world. He describes the setting in the 19th century and the evolution of this practice that allowed for the development of a profession dedicated to manipulation. His observation that orthodox medical practitioners in the 19th century expressed ambivalence toward and disdain for the practice of manipulation is probably the reason why chiropractic was forced to develop outside of the mainstream of medical specialties.

The difficulties of starting a new profession are almost insurmountable, especially when it starts with the teaching of a clinical skill to persons who, for the most part, were not university trained, where facilities were makeshift, and where both theory and practice had yet to evolve beyond ideas and techniques learned by apprenticeship. Russ Gibbons, in Chapter 2, reviews positions taken by many of the early leaders of the profession. The conflict between associations, colleges, and personalities is a major part of chiropractic history and folklore. It is only by studying the works and ideas of D. D. Palmer, B. J.

Palmer, Aleck Gregory, Arthur Forrester, Willard Carver, Hugh and Vinton Logan, James Firth, and others that an understanding of the basis for the internal dissension and debate that have persisted to some extent into modern times can be found.

The conflicting opinions, the multiple theories and philosophies, as well as adjusting techniques of each of the major schools and dominant personalities in the early chiropractic years, are reviewed in depth by Gerry Waagen and Virgil Strang in Chapter 3. The interaction between vitalism and science in the various theories used to explain chiropractic practice and the conflict between these two approaches by different chiropractic educators have been a prominent part of chiropractic search for an identity separate from medicine. Reed Phillips and Robert Mootz, in Chapter 4, demonstrate that this conflict has not yet been resolved. They use the terms materialism and holism to explain the two prominent forces that dominate chiropractic theory. They then attempt to form a contemporary paradigm for chiropractic and stress the importance of a rational chiropractic theory. It is clear from these chapters, however, that the debate over the philosophy of chiropractic will continue into the foreseeable future.

The evolution of chiropractic from an ostracized group of practitioners to an accepted health-care profession has been the subject of intense study by sociologists. Ian Coulter, in Chapter 5, reviews the role sociology has played in labeling and defining the position of chiropractors in American society. The writings of social scientists on the evolution of chiropractic are reviewed in depth and demonstrate that the perception of chiropractic has been impacted as much or more by outside influences as by changes within the profession. The tremendous growth and acceptance of chiropractic around the world are illustrated in Appendix A by an international team of coauthors. Chiropractic, initially considered a uniquely American phenomenon, is growing rapidly in Australia, Europe, Japan, and South Africa, and gaining a foothold in a growing number of Third World, Middle Eastern, and Eastern countries. Already, government commissions in New Zealand, research from

England, and clinical practice methods from Switzerland and Australia are having a major impact on the American chiropractic scene.

Despite the input of the most educated and experienced of chiropractic authorities, four of whom have doctorate degrees in fields ranging from history, anthropology, and sociology to biological science and epidemiology, the five chapters in this section still seem to explain inadequately the success of chiropractic. Recent studies by Kane et al. (1974) and Cherkin and MacCormack (1989) have shown that chiropractic care is accepted by patients to a much greater extent than comparable medical care. Recently published controlled comparative trials (Meade et al., 1990; Waagen et al., 1990) also suggest that chiropractic care is significantly more effective than family practice medicine to a point that seems to exceed the results of clinical trials purely on the effectiveness of manipulation as a treatment modality. The essence of chiropractic philosophy and its appeal to the public remain enigmatic. It is clear that further research, discussion, and debate are necessary. Study of the historical roots, sociology, and philosophical basis of chiropractic is likely to remain an intricate part of every chiropractic student's education.

Scott Haldeman

References

Cherkin DC, and MacCormack FA. Patient evaluations of low back pain care from family physicians and chiropractors. *West J Med* 1989;150:351–355.

Gibbons RW. The evolution of chiropractic: Medical and social protest in America. In Haldeman S, ed. *Modern developments in the principles and practice of chiropractic.* New York: Appleton-Century-Croft;1980:3–24.

Inglis B. *The case for unorthodox medicine.* New York: G.P. Putnam; 1963.

Kane RL, Oslen D, and Lymaster C, et al. Manipulating the patient—A comparison of physician and chiropractor care. *Lancet* 1974;1:1333–1336.

Meade TW, Dyer S, and Browne W, et al. Low back pain of mechanical origin: Randomised comparison of chiropractic and hospital outpatient treatment. *Br Med J* 1990;300:1431–1437.

Waagen GN, DeBoer K, and Hansen BA, et al. A prospective comparative trial of general practice medical care, chiropractic manipulative therapy and sham manipulation in the management of patients with chronic or repetitive low back pain. Abstract, International Society for the Study of the Lumbar Spine, Annual Meeting, Boston, June 13–17, 1990.

chapter 1

Spinal Manipulation Before Chiropractic

Robert Anderson

- **MANUAL THERAPY IN SMALL-SCALE COMMUNITIES**
- **MANIPULATION IN ASIAN CIVILIZATIONS**
- **MANIPULATION IN ANCIENT WESTERN CIVILIZATION**

- **EUROPE FROM ANTIQUITY TO THE 19TH CENTURY**
- **TRADITIONAL AND MEDICAL INFLUENCES ON PALMER**
- **CONCLUSION**
- **REFERENCES**

Back and neck pain afflict humanity in communities everywhere (Kelsey, 1982; Anderson, 1987a). Throughout the world, people also attempt to treat pain of spinal origin, but not all methods work successfully. One method of treatment is administering spinal manipulation. For certain kinds of back pain, spinal manipulation can be demonstrably beneficial (Cassidy and Kirkaldy-Willis, 1988). Historically, spinal manipulation has been practiced in many, although not in all, parts of the world. Wherever spinal manipulation has been practiced, it has been used to treat musculoskeletal disorders and, much less frequently, visceral disease.

Reaching at least two and a half millennia into the past, Western physicians and surgeons also practiced spinal manipulation. In the century or two before chiropractic was born, however, orthodox medical practitioners abandoned this form of manual therapy, leaving spinal manipulation to persist as a folk specialty of uneducated bonesetters. For a time, only books and papers gathering dust on library shelves survived to document manipulative techniques considered quite orthodox from antiquity until the 17th century. Almost unnoticed, an occasional medical iconoclast continued even into the 19th century to practice or advocate spinal manipulation in Great Britain, but not in the United States.

In the 19th century, many hardworking Americans in rural and industrial communities suffered from back and neck pain, but almost nobody in the United States at that time was practicing spinal manipulation to give them relief. One family of English bonesetters migrated to New England (Joy, 1954), and at least one individual bonesetter apparently ventured into the vast wilderness of frontier America (Terrett, 1986). Bonesetters were rare in the United States, however, and quite unavailable to most farmers and workers who needed spinal care. Daniel David Palmer helped to fill this vacuum when he created the chiropractic profession. Much of what Palmer achieved was already put in place by another healer located in the American Midwest, Andrew Taylor Still, the founder of osteopathy. But although Still and Palmer made spinal manipulative therapy available in North America, and eventually around the world, they did not originate these American practices out of thin air.

Utilizing a worldwide ethnographic and historical perspective, ways in which spinal manipulation was practiced in various parts of the world before the end of the 19th century will be examined. Like Venus, chiropractic materialized fully formed as a new profession on the American frontier, but spinal manipulation has roots that spread both deep and wide.

Manual Therapy in Small-Scale Communities

In many parts of the world, people reside in small communities remote from the sophistication of cities

Acknowledgment

I am grateful to Dr. Allan Terrett for helpful comments on an early draft of this chapter. Of course, I assume sole responsibility for it in its final form.

and professions. They live out their lives in relative isolation as peasants in rural agricultural villages, as tribal peoples practicing horticulture deep in rain forest environments, or as nomadic herders moving over vast landscapes infrequently traveled by physicians and surgeons. Because back pain is pandemic, it occurs in these folk and tribal communities. What resources do such peoples have for coping with the problem?

Many people know of no methods of treatment that work. In a village in Central Asia, where nearly half of the adult population was found to be experiencing at least mild spinal pain at the time of examination by Western physicians, no effective treatment was available (Anderson, 1984). Bonesetters are well known in that part of the world; several are located in the capital city of Kathmandu (Durkin-Longley, 1982). None was found in the village under investigation, however.

Several shamans did practice their occult craft in the community, and although there are areas of the world where shamans are known to treat back pain with success (Murphy, 1981; Anderson, 1989), no such skills were known by these practitioners. A local tavern keeper, reflecting the influence of contemporary medicine, kept a syringe for injecting penicillin. His treatment was dangerous as well as useless. In short, the need alone did not create a successful healing art for back pain in this community. Villagers suffered silently, accepting back pain as an inevitable concomitant of aging.

Other isolated communities are more fortunate. For example, bonesetters (*hueseros, componedores*) and massagers (*sobadores*) are found throughout Hispanic America. *Sobadores,* who are usually women, practice their healing art as a sideline, and are described as practicing massage. Massage, although not curative, can provide transient palliative benefits.

Anthropologists have not looked closely at what massage actually involves in societies of small scale. A single investigation into the work of one *sobador* revealed that a primitive form of nonspecific spinal adjusting was offered (Fig. 1–1). The practitioner who was studied provided at least temporary relief to most of those who sought him out (Anderson, 1987b). It is possible that folk massagers throughout Latin America practice indigenous forms of spinal manipulation, but field research is needed to explore that possibility.

Elsewhere in the world, other forms of spinal adjusting have been described. The *lomilomi* of Hawaii provides an example of a practice known throughout Oceania as well as parts of Asia such as China, Japan, and, more distantly, India. The *lomilomi,* usually a woman, practices massage, but,

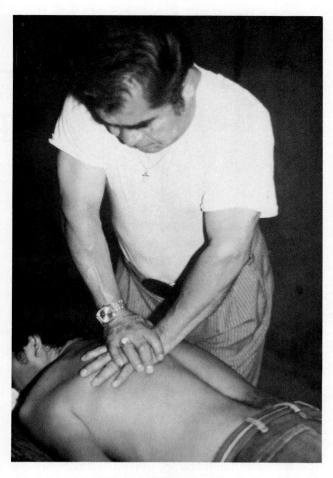

Figure 1–1. Manipulation of the thoracic spine by a contemporary folk practitioner (*sobador*) in Mexico.

in addition to soft tissue work, may manipulate spinal vertebrae by the imprecise technique of walking on the back. On an anecdotal basis, back tramping has been described as effective for the treatment of lumbago and sciatica (Handy, 1934; Anderson, 1982a).

The ethnomedicine of early Europe and Great Britain also included spinal manipulation. Bonesetters practiced hands-on treatment of the spine in peasant and early industrial communities before these traditional part-time practitioners fell almost to extinction under the pressures of modernization. Some walked on backs (Fig. 1–2). Others applied traction by lifting the sufferer off the ground and giving a hearty shake (Schiotz and Cyriax, 1974). Once numerous and widely located, bonesetters persisted until the recent past in a few places, for example, Finland (Hernesniemi, 1983), Russia (Tropkin, 1988), and Norway and Wales (Simon Leyson, personal communication).

A few English bonesetters migrated to New England where some communities benefited from

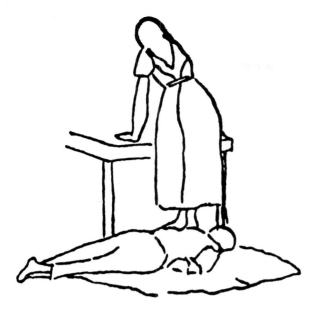

Figure 1-2. The tramping cure performed by a German peasant, probably in the 19th century. (*From Schiotz and Cyriax, 1974, p. 19, with permission.*)

their treatment (Joy, 1954). It is possible that bonesetters exerted an influence when chiropractic was founded. Daniel David Palmer may have been instructed by a bonesetter trained in the English tradition (Terrett, 1986). It is also possible that he was influenced by Bohemian folk practitioners who migrated to the United States from what is now Czechoslovakia. An early chiropractic text shows a photo of an old Bohemian immigrant giving a spinal

adjustment as he learned it not far from Prague in the mid-19th century (Fig. 1–3). The technique looks superficially like the technique of D.D. Palmer, because the old immigrant is shown leaning over his prone patient in the process of applying a thrust with his two hands joined together (Smith et al., 1906).

Just as not much is known about spinal manipulation in small communities throughout the world for the treatment of musculoskeletal problems (type M disorders), neither is it clear the extent to which spinal manipulation was used as a way to treat organic disease (type O disorders). Far away, in a part of the world quite distant from the Midwest, ethnographic evidence does document a rare example of the treatment of visceral disorders by means of spinal manipulation. In Indonesia the *balian*, a kind of community healer found on the island of Bali, functions as a general practitioner who treats both type M and type O problems. The *balian* relies on ritual, indigenous medications and massage. ''Massage is a popular therapy for a wide range of complaints,'' according to one research team, ''from aches and pains in the joints, lethargy, and fatigue to impotence, dysentery, headaches, influenza, sprains and strains, and . . . seizures and childlessness.'' Further, the *balian* carries out a form of massage that includes ''chiropractic-like manipulations'' (Connor et al., 1986, pp. 177, 179).

In most parts of the world, however, spinal manipulation in small-scale communities seems to have been used solely for painful joint and muscle problems (Schiotz and Cyriax, 1974). Mexican *sobadores*, for example, do not treat visceral disease by spinal

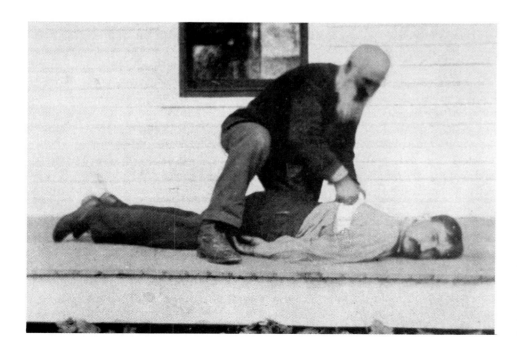

Figure 1-3. A 19th century migrant from Bohemia (Czechoslovakia) administering a spinal adjustment. (*From Smith et al., 1906, p.11, courtesy of David D. Palmer Health Sciences Library, Palmer College of Chiropractic.*)

manipulation, even though, in addition to massage and manipulation for stiffness and soreness, *sobadores* massage the stomach for "blockage" (*empacho*) and apply pressure to the roof of the mouth for "fallen fontanelle" (*mollera caida*) (Kay, 1977; Anderson, 1983a).

Although it appears that type O disorders were not widely treated by spinal manipulation in small-scale societies, it may be that we are misled by the failure of ethnographers to explore this subject adequately. The old Bohemain bonesetter referred to earlier acknowledged that he himself was cured of blood poisoning as a young person by spinal manipulation. If blood poisoning was treated by spinal adjusting, what other nonmusculoskeletal diseases were also treated in this manner by Czechoslovakian folk healers? To the extent that these practices accurately portray peasant methods of curing, was Palmer aware of them when he treated the deafness of his first chiropractic patient? Historians still have work to do on these questions.

Manipulation in Asian Civilizations

Anthropologists find it useful to distinguish healers who are trained in the oral traditions of small-scale communities from book-educated professional physicians found only in large, complex civilizations (Anderson, 1972). With the emergence of the world's first cities and states in the Far East (particularly China) and the Middle East (including adjacent North Africa and Southeastern Europe), professional physicians increasingly distinguished themselves from folk practitioners as they moved beyond prehistoric oral traditions to develop complex medical systems based in part on the elaboration of written texts. In both of these regions, physicians practiced spinal manipulation.

Medical attitudes toward the spine during the earliest dynasties in China are not known, despite claims to the contrary (Wardwell, 1987), but a medical text written about 2000 years ago during the Han Dynasty, *The Yellow Emperor's Classic of Internal Medicine* [*Huang Ti Nei Ching Su Wen*], describes massage and exercises. Massage may well have included mobilization and manipulation, but the *Yellow Emperor's Classic* is too vague on this point to allow us to be sure (Veith, 1966).

Many centuries later, in 1749, we find excellent evidence that spinal manipulation was practiced (Fig. 1–4). One drawing in *The Golden Mirror of Medicine* [*I Tzung Chin Chien*] illustrates a form of gravity traction used for treatment of the lumbar spine (Mindich, 1987). The drawing depicts a patient standing on a small stack of bricks or tiles while

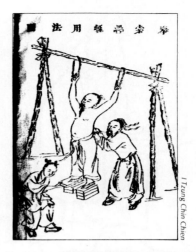

I Tzung Chin Chien

Figure 1–4. An 18th century method for traction and alignment of the spine. (*Courtesy of Dr. Huang Min-der and the Free China Review, vol 37, No. 2, p. 21.*)

hanging from two ropes, one held in each hand, while the practitioner appears to be applying force by hand on a lumbar vertebra. Simultaneously, an assistant is pulling one tile after the other out from under the patient to increase the force of gravity (von Rottauscher and von Rottauscher, 1972, pp. 143–144).

In the Peoples' Republic of China today, as well as in the Republic of China on Taiwan and in other centers of Chinese culture, spinal manipulation is still practiced for type M disorders. The treatment of chronic lumbar pain continues to be carried out using gravity traction, which requires the patient to hang from a bar. Back tramping, described earlier, is also practiced, but so too are lumbar and cervical adjusting techniques using both long and short lever arms for mobilization and manipulation (Anhui Medical School Hospital, 1983, pp. 48, 51, 117; Kuo, 1988; Wong, 1979, pp. 53, 56, 115).

In the Far East, type O disorders are also treated in part with manual therapy applied to the spine. The theory behind Chinese massage, as with acupuncture, includes the principle that the specific effect may take place at some distance from the area directly under the massager's hands (Huard and Wong, 1972, pp. 52–53). Chinese medical theory acknowledges the spine "as a canal linking the cerebral cavities with the genitalia" (Huard and Wong, 1972, p. 54; Anderson 1983b), and Chinese practitioners apply manual therapy to the spine to cure type O problems. Through deep massage at the occiput, for example, massagers find that they can bring down high blood pressure. Peptic ulcer is treated by thumb pressure applied along both sides of the vertebral column along with pressure applied on acupuncture points and abdominal massage, all of which may be supplemented by herbal remedies, rest, relaxation, and a dietary regimen (Anhui Medical School Hospital, 1983, pp. 191–194). Although the theory and practice of traditional Chinese medicine include manual spinal therapy, this therapeutic method is, for the most part, subordinate to acupuncture and herbalism in the treatment of both type M and type O disorders.

Manipulation in Ancient Western Civilization

Around the eastern Mediterranean as early as 5000 years ago, rich agricultural civilizations grew out of Neolithic village roots in Egypt, Mesopotamia, Greece, and Rome. Within this fertile crescent, the origins of Western medicine were forged by an emergent class of physicians. Did ancient medicine include manipulation?

The earliest of these civilizations appeared almost simultaneously in Mesopotamia and Egypt. In both, medical theory was suffused with belief in the efficacy of magic. Babylonian and Assyrian physicians treated rheumatism, arthritis, and sciatica primarily with incantations. There is no evidence that these disorders were treated with spinal manipulation (Sigerist, 1951, p. 483).

More is known of the history of medicine in ancient Egypt. What was it like? Authorities agree: "Egyptian medical documents contain a hodge-podge of home remedies based on a lore of herbs and of sympathetic magic, outright witch-doctoring in the forms of charms and incantations, and shrewd observation on the functions of the body" (Wilson, 1951, p. 56; see also Breasted, 1967, pp. 85–86).

It may well be that Egyptian medicine began to move toward a more empirically based practice in the field of orthopedic surgery. Evidence indicates that Egyptians diagnosed musculoskeletal disorders, especially broken bones, as having a natural causation and cure (Wilson, 1951, p. 57; Mertz, 1964, p. 70). From the evidence of mummies as well as of skeletal remains, it is clear that osteoarthritis was very common, particularly in the spinal column (Osler, 1988). This painful disorder, however, was treated on the same principles as other diseases with incantations and drugs (Dawson, 1953, p. 50). No papyrus, temple inscription, or other evidence provides any factual basis for describing spinal manipulation in ancient Egypt. One can see small indications of the promise of scientific medicine in some of the practices and principles of Egyptian physicians, particularly in their growing knowledge of anatomy as stimulated by the custom of mummification. It

was Greece, however, that became committed to a philosophy of scientific objectivity.

It is in Greece that we find the first unimpeachable historical evidence of the practice of spinal manipulation anywhere in the world, even though the practice there must have been much older, as it is already well elaborated and complex in the earliest historical evidence. Despite claims to the contrary (Lowe, 1979; Wardwell, 1987), however, we have no sure knowledge of the practice of spinal manipulation before the fifth century BC.

The first physician clearly to describe techniques of spinal manipulation was none other than Hippocrates in his book *On Joints*. In this work, he identifies two contrasting techniques of spinal manipulation for two kinds of spinal disorder. The first disorder described is a scoliotic curvature of the spine. The spinal manipulation, known as succussion, consisted of gravity traction carried out in a more forceful manner than the Chinese procedure described earlier.

> If then one desires to do succussion, the following is the proper arrangement. One should cover the ladder with transverse leather or linen pillows, well tied on, to a rather greater length and breadth than the patient's body will occupy. Next, the patient should be laid on his back upon the ladder; and then his feet should be tied at the ankles to the ladder, without being separated, with a strong but soft band. Fasten besides a band above and below each of the knees, and also at the hips; but the flanks and chest should have bandages passed loosely round them, so as not to interfere with the succussion. Tie also the hands, extended along the sides, to the body itself, and not to the ladder. When you have arranged things thus, lift the ladder against some high tower or house-gable. The ground where you do the succussion should be solid, and the assistants who lift well trained, that they may let it down smoothly, neatly, vertically, and at once, so that neither the ladder shall come to the ground unevenly, nor they themselves be pulled forwards. (Withington, 1928, pp. 285–286)

The second disorder described is a pronounced subluxation in which "one of the vertebrae necessarily appears to stand out more prominently, and those on either side less so" (Withington, 1928, pp. 297–298). The treatment for this disorder required spinal adjustment using a specialized adjusting table. Chiropractors who apply heat before adjusting will be interested to note that Hippocrates did the same. "Give the patient a vapour bath if possible," he advised, "or one with plenty of hot water" (Withington, 1928, p. 297). The patient was then placed prone on a board covered with cloaks or other material to make it soft but not yielding. Hippocrates adjusted his patients under traction, although he does indicate that one can use either traction alone or manipulation alone. His adjusting table was equipped with poles at each end, to which straps were attached for the leverage that was needed to apply tractive force. One strap wrapped around the chest and under the arms was pulled to apply a force toward the head; a second one around the hips was pulled toward the feet. An assistant at each end tugged at the straps to distract the spine. Wheels and axles could be set up if more force was needed. While the patient was under traction, the physician or a trained assistant administered a spinal thrust.

In refractory cases, practitioners could even use a leverage feature of this adjusting table (Fig. 1–5). The table could be equipped with a wooden bar attached by a hinge at one side either to a vertical post in the ground or into a hole in the wall. Passing transversely across the back of the patient from its fulcrum, the arm could be pulled down on a small leather pillow or thickness of cloth located on the subluxation by the adjuster who, with an assistant or two if more weight was needed, pressed the bar downward across the malpositioned vertebra (Withington, 1928, pp. 297–301; Schiotz and Cyriax, 1974, pp. 5–9).

Hippocrates considered spinal manipulation safe even when it was done with less specificity. He indicated that the adjustment could be done on a patient under traction by sitting on the subluxation, by sitting and hopping up and down, or by mobilizing

the lesion with one's foot. From two Roman authors who wrote much later, we learn that mobilizing with one's foot could include standing on the subluxation (Appollonius, AD. 60–80, cited in Schiotz and Cyriax, 1974) or walking on it (Galen, AD 131–202, cited in Schiotz and Cyriax, 1974).

Hippocrates clearly recommended spinal manipulation for two kinds of type M disorder: curvature of the spine and subluxation of a vertebra. It has been said that he also practiced spinal manipulation in the treatment of type O disorders, but not one shred of evidence available at this time supports that belief (Lomax, 1975, 1977; Wardwell, 1987). The ultimate origin in Europe of the concept of treating organic disease by spinal adjusting still eludes us.

Europe From Antiquity to the 19th Century

The influence of Hippocrates was immense. Although his method of succussion was not widely emulated, his method of adjusting vertebral subluxations using an adjusting table persisted for more than 2000 years. To the east this method became a part of Islamic medical practice. During the Middle Ages, Avicenna of Baghdad included this technique in his influential medical book, which helped diffuse it throughout the Middle East. At the end of the Middle Ages, a Latin translation of Avicenna's work was published in Europe, contributing to the renaissance of Western medicine. During the 16th century, the method of Hippocrates also appeared in the writings

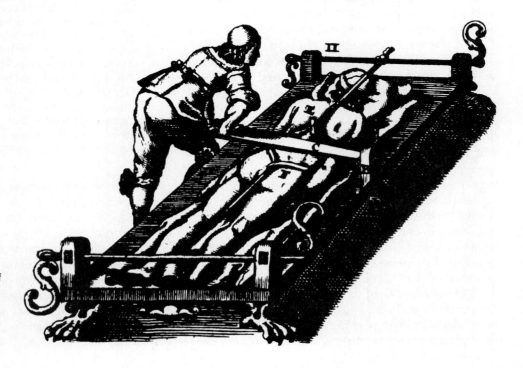

Figure 1–5. Treatment table and manipulative technique of Hippocrates as still practiced in the 17th century. (*From Scultetus*, The Surgeon's Store-House, *1674. Courtesy of Yale Medical Library*.)

of influential Western European medical authorities including Guido Guidi and Ambroise Paré.

In the 17th century, in addition to the work of Avicenna, a physician might encounter a brief reference to methods of manipulation of the extremities in *The Compleat Bone-Setter* by Friar Thomas Moulton (1656, pp. 20–21) or a description of the Hippocratic method of spinal manipulation and the table of Hippocrates in *The Surgeons Store-House* by Johannis Scultetus (see Fig. 1–5), which was published in English in 1674 and in Latin in 1693 (Anderson, 1983c; Schiotz and Cyriax, 1974, pp. 9–14, 188).

Despite the venerable age of Hippocrates's method spinal adjusting soon after went into decline. By the 19th century, surgeons had largely abandoned it for the treatment of subluxations. In 1837, a French surgeon wrote of the ''almost immediate cure'' of cases of lumbago treated with spinal manipulation (cited in Schiotz and Cyriax, 1974, pp. 59–60), but such references were unusual, and the tenor of the medical literature had become openly critical. A London publication in 1833, describing the Hippocratic table as it had been transmitted by Paré, recommended that it be used with great caution in the treatment of scoliosis (Fig. 1–6): ''Although the principle on which such extensions and manipulations were applied was erroneous, they might be beneficial in some cases, and the reputation acquired for them, by these instances of success, covered the mischief which must have resulted from their indiscriminate employment in all cases of spinal distortion'' (Beale, 1833, pp. 306–311). As late as 1841, a British doctor, describing the method of Hippocrates, observed that ''great objections'' were raised to this method, which was being used in a potentially harmful way for the treatment of scoliosis, ''without the probability of gaining any ultimate good.'' Referring to a recently deceased physician who advocated this method, the same doctor wrote:

I had many opportunities of observing that he kept the patient constantly in the recumbent position, producing extension of the spine by fixing the upper part of it, placing around the pelvis a firm belt, which was attached to a windlass at the lower part of the couch, the patient being in the facial recumbent position; and when sufficient extension had been made the Doctor would employ pressure against the spinous and other processes of the vertebrae, keeping up such application of pressure for nearly an hour. The patient's back was rubbed for some time by a nurse before he used the extension and pressure alluded to. (Tuson, 1841)

It is not entirely clear why nearly all physicians and surgeons abandoned spinal manipulation. They may have given it up in the treatment of adult scoliosis in part because they judged that it was ineffective. Whether for scoliosis or for subluxations, however, spinal manipulation probably was given up because it could be dangerous.

Doctors grew increasingly wary of applying pressure to joints, which not infrequently were invaded and weakened by tuberculosis, a scourge of endemic proportions at that time. As early as the 18th century, Sir Percival Pott wrote that spinal caries had become quite common and that manipulating a tubercular joint could have disastrous consequences. Nineteenth century surgeons worried greatly about manipulating tubercular vertebrae that could disintegrate or, because of a manipulation, fail to undergo a gradual autofusion, as it is ''to this alone, that we are to look for the patient's recovery'' (Lomax, 1975; Tuson, 1841; Brodie, 1850).

Syphilis might also weaken bone, but it seems likely that doctors worried more about danger to themselves. Syphilis was as feared as AIDS is in our time because no effective cure was known. Better to medicate than to manipulate and thus avoid expo-

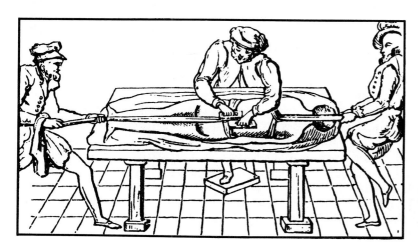

Figure 1–6. Version of the treatment table and manipulative technique of Hippocrates as modified for the treatment of scoliosis by Ambroise Paré in the 16th century. (*From Beale, 1833, p. 307.*)

sure to a fearful disease that frequently resulted in disfigurement, sickness, and death (Fossgreen, cited in Anderson, 1983c).

Although physicians backed away from spinal manipulation, patients did not. People suffering from rheumatism, lumbago, or sciatica continued to seek out practitioners who could provide relief by means of manual therapy. They found their way to folk practitioners known as bonesetters. Where did bonesetters learn to manipulate spines? In part they may have learned by imitating physicians. As long ago as in the time of ancient Greece, doctors employed assistants. One can well imagine unlettered helpers setting up for themselves time and again when fellow villagers or early industrial working people approached them for treatment.

The more massive force of imitation was probably in the other direction, however. It must not be forgotten that bonesetting was a widespread technique of village healers in various parts of Europe, and that it occurred in other parts of the world. On the principle that widespread cultural traits are likely to be old, the age-area hypothesis, it seems probable that spinal manipulation was originally practiced by folk practitioners long before the rise of medicine as a profession. This possibility is also suggested by the fact that folk practitioners did not use the treatment table of Hippocrates, but relied on more generic techniques.

Anthropological research into the history of Europe identifies two highly differentiated cultural traditions that coexisted for centuries—those of unlettered villagers with their so-called ''Little Traditions,'' and those of literate urban elites with their ''Great Tradition.'' Clearly these cultures interacted in a dialectic of acculturation and differentiation. Over time, the Little Traditions' unschooled healers and the Great Tradition's learned physicians each practiced their own versions of spinal manipulation. In a complex and fluctuating give-and-take of imitation and differentiation, one curative tradition undoubtedly borrowed and modified what existed in the other in a process of mutual influence (Redfield, 1956; Anderson, 1971).

As a part of the Great Tradition, the medical literature until the first half of the 19th century described both spinal manipulation and a relationship between a painful vertebra and more remote manifestations of type M and type O disorders. This was a literature unfamiliar to most doctors. As one writer put it, speaking of the relationship between pressure on a vertebral segment and pain in a diseased part at some distance away, ''This symptom has been carefully noticed by a few, superficially by several, but totally neglected by the great majority of Practitioners'' (Monell, 1845, p. 20).

In addition to descriptions of spinal manipulation, and for the most part separate from them, some books from early in the 19th century included occasional references to a relationship between the spine and type O disorders (Fig. 1–7). For example, Monell observed that ''when acute Rheumatism attacks any part, the pain of that part is increased by pressure on the spine at that point from whence the nerves distributed to the diseased part arise'' (Monell, 1845, p. 21). In addition Stanley noted that ''the internal organs, especially of the abdomen and pelvis, variously participate in the nervous derangements ensuing from disease in the spine'' (Stanley, 1849, p. 318).

Perhaps the most influential publication to elaborate the concept of a spinal origin of organic disease was a book published in 1843 by J. Evans Riadore, Fellow of the Royal College of Surgeons. Riadore took the position that, because spinal nerves reach out to every organ and muscle in the body, ''we cannot be otherwise than prepared to hear of a lengthened catalogue of maladies that are either engendered, continued or the consequence of spinal irritation.'' He illustrated this point by noting that disorders of the digestive organs result from irritation of the spinal nerves exiting the intervertebral foramena at T6 through T8. He noted that what we would today call disk and facet degeneration might be involved at those levels. The treatment was to perform a spinal adjustment (cited in Schiotz and Cyriax, 1974, pp. 71–72)!

By the end of the 19th century, one detects a curious ambivalence toward spinal manipulation on the part of physicians for type M disorders. On the one hand, it was a well-established part of medical culture to express utter disdain for bonesetters and their folk practices. British physicians who, before the Medical Act of 1858, ''cheerfully sent patients to bonesetters for manipulation,'' subsequently did their best to put bonesetter out of business (Schiotz and Cyriax, 1974, p. 72). On the other hand, physicians had to recognize how popular bonesetters were with people who sought them out.

This ambivalence on the part of the medical establishment was apparent when James Paget, one of the most famous surgeons of his time, recommended in *The Lancet* that doctors would do well to observe bonesetters and learn from them (Paget, 1867). Paget could hardly be called a supporter of unorthodox practitioners, because he referred to them as ''enemies'' and ascribed their success more to luck than to wit. Nevertheless, his message was: ''Learn to imitate what is good and avoid what is bad in the practice of bonesetters.'' His article must have raised eyebrows, but it failed in its avowed purpose. Doctors as a whole continued to deprecate joint manipulation (Anderson, 1983d).

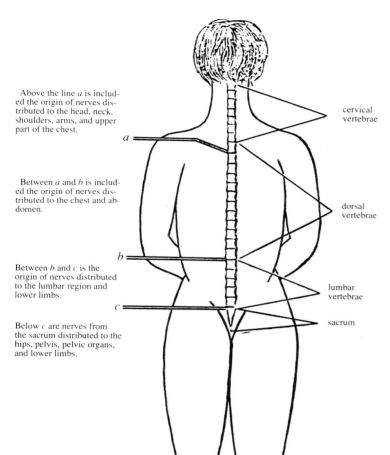

Above the line *a* is included the origin of nerves distributed to the head, neck, shoulders, arms, and upper part of the chest.

Between *a* and *b* is included the origin of nerves distributed to the chest and abdomen.

Between *b* and *c* is the origin of nerves distributed to the lumbar region and lower limbs.

Below *c* are nerves from the sacrum distributed to the hips, pelvis, pelvic organs, and lower limbs.

a

b

c

cervical vertebrae

dorsal vertebrae

lumbar vertebrae

sacrum

Figure 1–7. Prechiropractic medical drawing illustrating the existence of relationships between spinal nerve roots and more distant parts of the body. (*From Monell, 1845, p. 20.*)

The ambivalence of physicians found further expression in one practitioner who was unusually open-minded. Wharton Hood, defying current medical ethics, apprenticed himself to a bonesetter. He eventually became skilled enough to treat the patient overload of his busy teacher. On the basis of his training, he concluded that manipulation was beneficial and safe. Publishing in *The Lancet* 4 years after James Paget, Hood offered the medical profession a technical manual on extremity adjusting techniques (Fig. 1–8). Hood did not, however, describe techniques of spinal manipulation (Hood, 1871; Anderson, 1981).

A quarter of a century after Paget and Hood, Daniel David Palmer performed the first chiropractic adjustment. Nevertheless, the medical literature on spinal manipulation immediately before 1895 was sparse in comparison with early in the century (Schiotz and Cyriax, 1974; Sollman, 1987). It was also sparse for some years after, which suggests that doctors were not talking much about it at that time. Occasional medical endorsements of manipulation did appear, however, including one in 1910 that stated, ''It is very remarkable that the medical pro-

fession should so long have neglected such a wide field of therapeutics'' (cited in Schiotz and Cyriax, 1974, p. 61). In 1915 Frank Romer released *Modern Bonesetting for the Medical Profession,* but this was long after Palmer's work began (Anderson, 1981). Not until the 1920s and 1930s did books by physicians on spinal manipulation become more available.

Traditional and Medical Influences on Palmer

Palmer was eclectic. He was probably influenced by a bonesetter who spent some time in Davenport, Iowa, even though bonesetters were not found in most American communities. The itinerant healer may have had family connections to bonesetters in England, but we know very little about that episode in the evolution of chiropractic (Terrett, 1986). The bonesetting tradition appears to have influenced Andrew Still, who founded osteopathy in Kirksville, Missouri, sometime during the 1880s. Dr. Still referred to himself for a time as ''The Lightning Bonesetter'' (Gevitz, 1982).

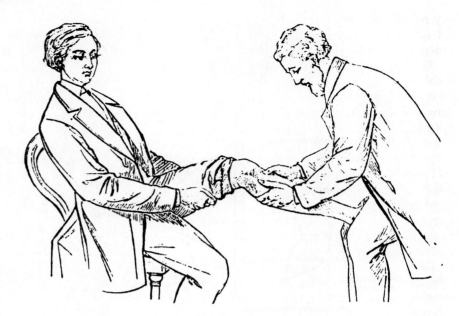

Figure 1–8. Manipulation of the knee by a 19th century bonesetter. (*From Hood*, 1871, p. 346.)

Palmer appears also to have been directly influenced by osteopaths. In 1892, Still established the American College of Osteopathy within a day's travel from Davenport, Iowa, where Palmer founded chiropractic 3 years later. Palmer probably spent a few days visiting Dr. Still, who vigorously advocated osteopathic manipulation for the treatment of type M and type O disorders. It is reasonable to think that Palmer was influenced by osteopathy, even though his method of adjusting was different and he did not accept the major explanatory concept of early osteopathy that attributed disease to vascular rather than neuronal mechanisms (Gevitz, 1982).

Palmer was also influenced by physicians and surgeons through his extensive reading of medical publications, especially books and articles written before 1850. The first physician known to use the term *subluxation* was Johannes Hieronymi in his published dissertation of 1746 (cited in Terrett, 1987). It is improbable that Palmer was directly familiar with the work of Hieronymi, but he apparently had read the work of two physicians, William and Daniel Griffin, who described "spinal irritation" as causes of visceral diseases in 1834. Palmer may also have been influenced by the publications of Edward Harrison dating from 1820 and 1821. Allen Terrett notes that Harrison used the word *subluxation*, that he recognized both type M and type O disorders as caused by subluxations, and that he used the spinous and transverse processes as levers for adjusting subluxations. "The fundamental hypotheses of chiropractic had been repeatedly stated in the medical literature well before the birth of D.D. Palmer" (Terrett, 1987, p. 32).

Conclusion

Although back pain is found everywhere, not every society is equipped to treat it with spinal manipulation. From ethnographic studies in remote communities we know that people may simply live with their pain and dysfunction without receiving effective treatment. Spinal manipulation does occur widely throughout the world, however. On a regional level, it occurs throughout Hispanic America, Eurasia, and Oceania. It is particularly notable that back tramping has been documented in various parts of Asia, Oceania, and Europe, including historic China and ancient Greece. Finally, there is reason to suspect that as more refined ethnochiropractic research on the exact nature of native techniques of massage is carried out, manipulation will be found to exist even more widely throughout the world.

At the two extremes of the Old World, Asia and Europe, civilizations emerged in the Bronze and Iron Ages in which the occupation of physician and surgeon took health care out of the oral tradition of folk healing and transformed it into a written tradition of professional practitioners. In these cultures, spinal adjusting and spinal traction were elaborated as treatment modalities within professional medicine.

In the West, the oldest known description of spinal adjusting is that of Hippocrates who wrote in the fifth century BC. He described a positioning of the hands and a concern with the angle of the adjustment that anticipates the technique of Palmer by nearly two and a half thousand years. The technique of Hippocrates included the application of spinal manipulation under traction, a method that became very nonspecific when it included the use of levers and sitting or standing on the patient. It also included a treatment table of unique design.

For centuries during which we have no direct archival records of how people in the small communities of peasant Europe were treating back pain, we know that the techniques of ancient Greece endured as a part of professional medical and surgical care. That ceased to be true during the 18th and early 19th centuries, with the rare exception of a few British and French physicians who prescribed spinal manipulation in spite of the chorus of disdain that was directed against bonesetters. Bonesetters had replaced surgeons in the practice of spinal manipulation during the half century before Palmer and for a quarter of a century after.

Palmer was well read in the medicosurgical literature that described spinal manipulation. He knew of the methods of bonesetters and was acquainted with osteopathic techniques. It is a truism for those who investigate the process of creativity that nothing under the sun is truly new. Every discovery builds on previous ones. It is unlikely that Palmer developed chiropractic theory and method whole cloth out of his own intellect. Rather, he drew deeply from the manipulation traditions of medicine, bonesetting, and osteopathy. The significance of his achievement is in no way lessened by these historical findings.

Palmer filled a vacuum in American culture by advocating spinal adjusting as a health-care option for a population of hardworking people who otherwise were inadequately served (Anderson, 1982b). Because he trained relatively uneducated aspirants to become chiropractors, he resurrected from history the role of the folk practitioner who was skilled in providing needed health services on the margins of the established medical profession. In pronouncing each graduate a Doctor of Chiropractic (DC), he simultaneously resuscitated an ancient health-care role, that of the professional physician or surgeon who functioned as an esteemed practitioner of spinal manipulation.

People in our time suffer from spinal disorders that are as old as the species itself. Chiropractors offer effective methods of treatment for type M spinal disorders. Many also continue to treat type O disorders by spinal adjusting (Anderson, 1990). In providing these services, they draw sustenance from deep roots and widely distant branches that were consolidated, transformed, and energized by D.D. Palmer, the founder of chiropractic.

References

Anderson R. *Traditional Europe: A study in anthropology and history.* Belmont, Calif: Wadsworth; 1971.

_____ . *Anthropology: A perspective on man.* Belmont, Calif: Wadsworth; 1972.

_____ . Wharton Hood, M.D., The Rejected Father of Manual Medicine. *Arch Calif Chiropractic Assoc* 1981;5(2):59–63.

_____ . Hawaiian therapeutic massage. *World-Wide Rep* 1982a; 24(5):4A.

_____ . An historical perspective on the founder of chiropractic. *Arch Calif Chiropractic Assoc* 1982b;6(1):61–66.

_____ . The Bagelmacher in Israel. *Calif Chiropractic Assoc J* 1983a;8(8):12.

_____ . An American contribution to Third World medicine: Spinal manipulative therapy. In John H. Morgan, ed. *Third World medicine and social change.* Lanham, NY: University Press of America; 1983b:17–27.

_____ . On doctors and bonesetters in the 16th and 17th centuries. *Chiropractic Hist* 1983c;3(I):11–15.

_____ . Medical prejudice: the case of bonesetting. *Eur J Chiropractic* 1983d;31:5–12.

_____ An orthopedic ethnography in rural Nepal. *Med Anthropol* 1984; 8(1):45–59.

_____ . Investigating back pain: The implications of two village studies in South Asia. In Paul Hockings, ed. *Dimensions of social life: Essays in honor of David G. Mandelbaum.* Berlin: Mouton de Gruyter; 1987a:385–396.

_____ . The treatment of musculoskeletal disorders by a Mexican bonesetter (*sobador*). *Soc Sci Med* 1987b;24(1):43–46.

_____ . The shaman as healer: What happened? *Am Back Society Newslett* 1989;6(2):9.

_____ . Chiropractors for and against vaccines. *Med Anthropol* 1990; 12:169–186.

Anhui Medical School Hospital. *Chinese massage therapy: A handbook of therapeutic massage.* Hor Ming Lee and Gregory Whincup, trans. Boulder, Colo: Shambala Press; 1983.

Beale LJ. *A treatise on the distortions and deformities of the human body. Exhibiting a concise view of the nature and treatment to the principal malformations and distortions of the chest, spine, and limbs.* London: John Churchill; 1833.

Breasted JH. *A history of Egypt.* New York: Bantam Books; 1967 (First published, 1905.)

Brodie, Sir Benjamin C. *Pathological and surgical observations on the diseases of the joints.* 5th ed. London: Longman, Brown, Green, and Longmans; 1850.

Cassidy JD and Kirkaldy-Willis WH. Manipulation. In Kirkaldy-Willis WH, ed. *Managing low back pain.* 2nd ed. New York: Churchill-Livingstone; 1988.

Connor L, Asch P, and Asch T. *Jero Tapakan: Balinese healer.* Cambridge: Cambridge University Press; 1986.

Dawson WR. Egypt's place in medical history. In E. Ashworth Underwood, ed. *Science, medicine and history: Essays on the evolution of scientific thought and medical practice. Written in honour of Charles Singer.* London: Oxford University Press; 1953:47–60.

Durkin-Longley, S. *Ayurveda in Nepal: A medical belief system in action.* Department of Anthropology, University of Wisconsin, Madison; 1982. PhD dissertation.

Gevitz N. *The D.O.'s: Osteopathic medicine in America.* Baltimore: Johns Hopkins University Press; 1982.

Handy ESC, Pukui MK, and Livermore K. Outline of Hawaiian physical therapeutics. *Bernice P. Bishop Mus Bull* 1934;126.

Hernesniemi A. Nikamankasittelijat Laakarin Nakokulmasta. *Suomen Laakarilehti* 1983;4:286–287.

Hood WH. On the so-called bone-setting, its nature and results. *Lancet* 1871; No. 6, pp. 304–310; No.7, pp. 344–349.

Huard P and Wong M. *Chinese medicine.* New York: McGraw-Hill; 1972.

Joy RJT. The natural bonesetters with special reference to the Sweet family of Rhode Island: A study of an early phase of orthopedics. *Bull Hist Med* 1954;28:416–441.

Kay MA. Health and illness in a Mexican-American barrio. In Spicer EH, ed. *Ethnic medicine in the Southwest.* Tucson, Ariz: University of Arizona Press; 1977:96–168.

Kelsey JL. *Epidemiology of musculoskeletal disorders.* Monographs in Epidemiology and Biostatistics, vol 3. New York: Oxford University Press; 1982.

Kuo PF. Manual medicine as practiced in China. *Manual Med* 1988; 3:95–99.

Lomax E. Manipulative therapy: A historical perspective from ancient times to the modern era. In Goldstein M, ed. *The research status of spinal manipulative therapy.* DHEW publication (NIH) 76–998. Bethesda, Md: U.S. Department of Health, Education and Welfare; 1975:11–A.

Lomax E. Manipulative therapy: An historical perspective. In Buerger AA, and Tobis JS, eds. *Approaches to the validation of manipulation therapy.* Springfield, ILL: Charles C Thomas; 1977.

Lowe JC. The original contingencies hypothesis. *Digest Chiropractic Econ* 1979;21:4.

Mertz B. *Temples, tombs and hieroglyphs: The story of the Egyptians.* New York: Dell; 1964.

Mindich JH. Five millennia of medical practice. *Free China Rev* 1987;37(2):10–27.

Monell GC. *Rheumatism, acute and chronic: A prize essay.* New York: H.G. Langley; 1845.

Moulton T. The *compleat bone-setter.* Revised and enlarged by Robert Turner. (Archives, Royal College of Surgeons, London; 1656.)

Murphy R. Review of *The Way of the Shaman: A Guide to Power and Healing* by Michael Harner. *Am Anthropol* 1981;83:714–715.

Osler, Sir William. Early Egyptian medical practices. *JAMA* 1988; 259(II):1725. (From a lecture given at Yale University, 1913.)

Paget J. Cases that bone-setters cure. *Br Med J* 1867;1:1–4.

Redfield R. *Peasant society and culture: An anthropological approach to civilization.* Chicago: University of Chicago Press; 1956.

von Rottauscher W. and von Rottauscher A. *Chinese folk medicine.* Marion Palmedo, trans. New York: New American Library; 1972.

Schiotz EH and Cyriax J. *Manipulation past and present.* London: William Heinemann Medical Books; 1974.

Sigerist HE. *A history of medicine.* vol I: *Primitive and archaic medicine.* New York: Oxford University Press; 1951.

Smith OG, Langworthy SM, Paxon MC. *A textbook of modernized chiropractic.* Cedar Rapids, Iowa: Langworthy; 1906:vol 1.

Sollmann AH. Manipulative therapy of the spine. *Dynam Chiropractic* February 1, 1987, pp. 28–31. (Abstracted by Eleonore Blaurock-Busch from *5000 Years of Manual Medicine,* Munich, 1974.)

Stanley E. *Treatise on diseases of the bones.* London: Longman, Brown, Green, and Longmans; 1849.

Terrett AGJ. The genius of D.D. Palmer. *J Aust Chiropractors' Assoc* 1986;16(4):150–158.

Terrett AG. The search for the subluxation: An investigation of medical literature to 1895. *Chiropractic Hist* 1987;7 (I):29–33.

Tropkin A. The miracle worker from Kobelyaki. *Soviet Life* 1988; 6(381):32–34.

Tuson, EW. *The cause and treatment of curvature of the spine, and diseases of the vertebral column.* London: John Churchill; 1841.

Veith I. *Huang Ti Nei Ching Su Wen [The Yellow Emperor's classic of internal medicine].* Berkeley: University of California Press; 1966.

Wardwell WI. Before the Palmers: An overview of chiropractic's antecedents. *Chiropractic Hist* 1987;7:27–33.

Wilson JH. *The culture of ancient Egypt.* Chicago: University of Chicago Press; 1951.

Withington ET. *Hippocrates, with an English translation.* Cambridge, Mass: Harvard University Press; 1928.

Wong PP. *Modern Chinese massotherapy.* Hong Kong: Medicine and Health Publishing Co; 1979.

chapter 2

Medical and Social Protest as Part of Hidden American History

Russell W. Gibbons

- **THE POPULAR HEALTH MOVEMENT: REBELLION TO HEROIC MEDICINE**
- **THE EMERGENCE OF MANIPULATION THERAPY**
- **B. J. PALMER: BARNUM WITH SCIENCE**
- **THE OLD SCHOOL CONVERTS: MEDICAL ALLIES AND CRITICS**
- **THE SURVIVAL YEARS AND EDUCATIONAL REFORM**
- **CONCLUSION: GOING TO JAIL FOR CHIROPRACTIC**
- **REFERENCES**

For much of the century, the inevitable demise of chiropractic has been predicted by various leaders of American medicine and by social scientists who have studied dissenting groups. These physicians and scientists opined that chiropractors, as they began to share the fundamentals of basic science, would discard their allegedly unproven therapeutic baggage and embrace orthodox medicine. So too, it was reasoned, would a more educated populace shun the services of chiropractors.

On both points, however, chiropractic's doomsayers were proven wrong. Chiropractors enter the final decade of this century, in which they mark their centennial, as a growing and respected alternative to orthodox medicine. Government and private sector investigations, moreover, reveal a high degree of patient satisfaction with chiropractic services (USDHEW, 1969; Quebec Royal Commission, 1975; New Zealand Commission, 1979; Meade, et al, 1990). Those who predicted chiropractic's demise could well look to the toil and turmoil of its troubled evolution to find the reasons for its survival.

Chiropractic history parallels other great American social transformations that occurred during its near century of existence. Not surprisingly, much if not all of chiropractic's history is a chronicle of struggle and strife, of conflict and schism, and of massive internal reform and professional maturation. Indeed, the early history of chiropractic displays the characteristics and dynamics of other grass roots social protest movements. For, like the abolitionists, chiropractors were systematically persecuted and driven from town to town. Like the feminists and suffragettes, chiropractors were made objects of ridicule. And like the civil rights workers of more recent times, chiropractors were intimidated and subverted by agents and provocateurs. In the finest traditions of reform movements, they were imprisoned for their beliefs, as this account from California testifies:

> In just one year (1921), 450 of approximately 600 chiropractors were hauled into court and convicted of practicing without a license. They were given jail sentences or the alternative of a fine. They chose to go to jail. (Inglis, 1963)

If this record is disquieting to those who believe that the merits of any healing art should be decided through the dispassionate process of scientific inquiry and not in the uninformed court of public opinion, then let us recall that the ascendancy of "scientific medicine" in the early part of this century came not through the rational evidence of the laboratory but through the political process. It was the landmark indictment of orthodox medical education by the Rockefellers, through Abraham Flexner, that resulted in the emergence of the regular school of medicine as a political presence (Flexner, 1910/1967). Let us turn first, then, to consider the state of the medical arts just prior to the advent of Daniel David Palmer, the founder of chiropractic (Fig. 2–1).

The Popular Health Movement: Rebellion to Heroic Medicine

The healing business was undergoing a difficult transition to a professional and scientific basis in the second half of the 19th century, the same period that would see the emergence of the Still and Palmer schools.

"Heroic" medicine was the rule of the day. Physicians of the regular school employed therapies that were drastic and often debilitating. Their therapeutic regimen included bloodletting and purges, often administered until the patient fainted. The primitive state of medicine in that period produced a swelling chorus of public outrage that crystallized into a medical protest movement.

The feminist writers Ehrenreich and English (1978) have called this protest against the ravages of heroic medicine the Popular Health Movement and have linked it to the early women's movement of the 1830s and the Workingmen's party of the same period. Swapping medical horror stories, members of various women's circles began to swap home remedies and then systematically sought out ways to extend their knowledge and skills. Today's "know your body" courses had their distant roots in the "Ladies Physiological Societies" of the pre–Civil

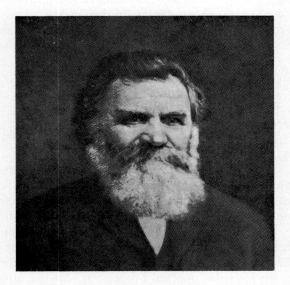

Figure 2–1. Daniel David Palmer, 1845–1913. Founder of the last dissenting school of American medicine, he announced chiropractic in 1895. (*From the B. J. Palmer Special Collection, David D. Palmer Health Sciences Library, Davenport, Iowa.*)

War period, in which the universal ideology was a distrust of the regular school of medicine. During this period, Fanny Wright, an intellectual leader and rouser of workers' rights and women's suffrage, established a People's Hall of Science in New York's Bowery, where public instruction in physiology was one of the most popular offerings.

At the same time, a poor New Hampshire farmer was piecing together a healing system that would become the basis of the first real alternative to the regular school. Samuel Thomson had watched his wife suffer and his mother die at the hands of the regulars' heroic therapy. He reacted by reconstructing the system of folk medicine he had learned as a farm boy from a female lay healer and midwife. His practice was accepted by the people he visited, because most of them also had experienced disaster at the hands of the regular school physicians.

Thomson's medical philosophy was as important as his set of techniques. His goal was to remove healing from the marketplace and utterly democratize it: every person should be his or her own healer. To this end Thomson set out to spread his healing system as widely as possible among the American people. He set up hundreds of Friendly Botanical Societies, in which people met to share information and study the Thomsonian system. Five Thomsonian journals were published, and at its height the Thomsonian movement claimed 4 million adherents out of a total U.S. population of 17 million (Ehrenreich and English, 1978).

Other healing systems followed the Thomsonians. The first true drugless alternative, the Hygienic Movement of Sylvester Graham, called for the eating of raw fruits and vegetables and whole-grain breads and cereals. Although recalled today only through the cracker named after him, his forces combined with the Thomsonians to triumph over orthodoxy. Ehrenreich and English (1976) summarize this period by observing that

> Every state that had a restrictive physician-licensing law softened it or repealed it in the 1830s. Some, like Alabama and Delaware, simply changed their laws to exempt Thomsonian and other popular kinds of irregular healers from prosecution. This was an enormous victory for "people's medicine." At least one of the movement's principles, anti-monopolism, had been driven home. (p. 4)

The decline of the Thomsonian and the Hygienic movements occurred about the same time, but for different reasons. Hydropathy had flourished "because it championed the most comforting and efficacious elements of hygienic and hands-on medical care'' (Cayleff, 1988). Like many of the alternative political and religious movements that flourished and then as quickly disappeared in mid-19th century America, their followers soon lost faith in the monocausal philosophies that had originally attracted them. Organizationally, they could not attain the leadership and public posture that would have been necessary to confront their allopathic adversaries, who had begun the long process of standardization and exclusion of all ''nonscientific'' healers from the ranks of recognized healers (Starr, 1982).

These dissenters were followed by a distinctive American-born sect, eclectic medicine, and a European import, homeopathy. Both would gather thousands of unorthodox physicians and millions of adherents through the last quarter of the 19th century, yet both would eventually lose out in the competition with the ''successful sect,'' allopathy. The eclectics, disorganized to the point that they engaged in combat between factions for the possession of a Cincinnati medical school (''wielding knives, pistols, chisels, bludgeons and blunderbusses''), all but disappeared. A temporary revival, however, gave the eclectics life into the 20th century (Numbers, 1972; Rothstein, 1972).

Eclectic and homeopathic medicine differed in their philosophical approaches to healing, but each demonstrated how American medicine was to be constantly changing, rejecting and then accepting some of the more attractive tenets of their sectarian branches. Eclectism, as its name suggests, was a broad-scope outgrowth of the botanical movements of the early and mid-19th century. It achieved popularity in many rural environments, but the post-Flexner reform period reduced its practitioners from 4752 in 1900 to a few hundred 50 years later. Its last school closed in 1939 (Rothstein, 1972).

Homeopathy was the largest and most significant challenge to regular medicine in the last century. A German physician, Samuel Christian Hahnemann, had quit his practice in disillusionment of traditional forms. He developed a theory that disease could be cured by drugs that produced in a healthy person the symptoms found in those who were sick. The movement found quick acceptance in America and presented a serious alternative to the regular school. Its decline began in the decade after the Flexner report, although the 1980s have produced a revival of sorts in North America (Kaufman, 1971).

Their larger and better-organized rivals, the homeopaths, would parallel the eclectic's survival. With a strong European tradition that centered around its founder, Samuel Hahnemann, homeopathy prospered in the United States for much of the 19th century. Wealthy patrons endowed many homeopathic hospitals and schools, enabling homeo-

paths to attain respectability within the medical profession while holding unorthodox views. Yet following the Flexner report in 1910, all but their better institutions succumbed to rising standards, and the frontal allopathic assault on their very ideology caused the last homeopathic school to close within two decades. Homeopathic hospitals were forced to accept allopathic orthodoxy, and only the hospital in Philadelphia bearing the founder's name recalls their once influential role in medicine (Kaufman, 1971).

It was not just the public, however, but many of those in the academic world and those who were exploring the biological and physical sciences in a university setting who were skeptical of the role of medicine and the process of educating physicians. As America charged into the post–Civil War period, Harvard University felt that its informal alliance of colleges should elevate their standards to earn affiliation. Thus in 1870, President Samuel Elliot of Harvard wrote to the Dean of the Faculty of Medicine, suggesting that he adopt written examinations for the medical degree rather than the customary 5-minute oral examinations. ''Written examinations are impossible in the medical school,'' the dean replied, ''for the majority of the students cannot write well enough'' (Hall, 1974). The dean's response epitomized the state of medical education at that time, this in an institution that was generally regarded as second only to Johns Hopkins as a hallmark of medical schooling in the United States.

The leader of the reform movement in medical education, Abraham Flexner, would write just four decades later of the two goals intertwined with the founding of the American Medical Association (AMA)—adequate preliminary schooling and uniform standards—''that neither of these propositions has even yet been realized'' (Flexner, 1910/1967).

The reform movement in medicine seemed to be following the model of the big fish eating the little fish. The health dissidents were swallowed up, their palatable heretical doctrine was digested or discarded, and the allopathic shark came to dominate the health-care sea. While this process occurred, as the last quarter of the 19th century began, the seedbed for new schools of medical protest were being laid in the prairie states of Iowa, Kansas, and Missouri.

The Emergence of Manipulation Therapy

Andrew Taylor Still (Fig. 2–2) was a country doctor with only a few months' training at a Kansas City school that would be long closed by the time that Flexner denounced virtually all of medical educa-

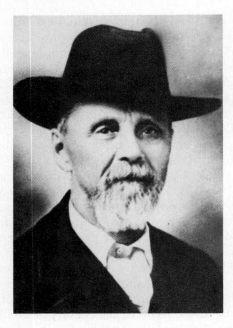

Figure 2-2. Andrew Taylor Still, 1826–1916. He launched his osteopathic school 5 years before Palmer in his Missouri "mecca" of Kirksville. *(From the American Osteopathic Association.)*

tion. An epidemic of spinal meningitis took the lives of three of Still's children, and like Thomson and Hahnemann, he sought an alternative system. In June 1874, in the small northeast Missouri town of Kirksville, Still "flung to the breeze the banner of osteopathy" (Booth, 1924). It took 18 years for Still, who by then was 66, to open his American School of Osteopathy.

It is inevitable that osteopathy and chiropractic are lumped together in both public perception and the abbreviated literature that treats both in medical history. Although different in cultural and social background, both Still and Palmer had many similarities and both advertised themselves as magnetics in the 1880s in Missouri and Iowa communities within 3 hours' traveling time from the other.

While both were categorized as "back doctors" or "rubbing doctors" after the turn of the century, there was a distinctive separation in osteopathic and chiropractic principles. Original osteopathic treatment as taught by Still emphasized indirect manipulation (Gevitz, 1982). Still advanced his "lesion osteopath" concept just as Palmer would embrace the "subluxation chiropractor."

Closer to the Mississippi River, another healer was making his reputation. Daniel David Palmer, born in the Canadian backwoods in 1845, had been an itinerant tradesman, had taught school, and was involved in making and losing several small mercantile fortunes in Illinois and Iowa before establishing

himself as a magnetic healer in Burlington, Iowa, in 1886. Within the next decade, he attracted patients from throughout the Midwest, and he began his own study of the anatomy and physiology of the human body (Gielow, 1982). Palmer was 50 that hot September day in 1895 when Harvey Lillard came into his office in the Putnam building on the east end of Brady Street in Davenport's tenderloin district. That day the creative act was laid for chiropractic, named by the Reverend Samuel H. Weed, a Palmer patient.

Chiropractic's growth years began in 1896 when Palmer began instruction on the fourth floor of the Putnam building as Dr. Palmer's School and Cure, and later as the Palmer Institute and Chiropractic Infirmary (Fig. 2-3). Through 1902 only 15 graduates sat under "Old Dad Chiro." Among those obtaining a degree that year was Bartlett Joshua Palmer, who had just turned 21.

D.D. began to collect the notes and papers that he would publish in 1910 in Portland, Oregon, as *The Chiropractor's Adjuster* (Palmer, 1910). One friendly historian found it

> Mosaic in its dicta and Platonic in its thoroughness . . . flaying allopathy in particular, he denounced the use of drugs and discussed the cure of almost every disease from abasia to zymosis. . . . (it) teemed with maxims, controversy, satire, poetry and irrelevancies, but withal, revealed a genius that must have impressed his offended colleagues. (*Dictionary of American Biography,* 1934)

And offended colleagues there would be for all of the three decades in the public life of D. D. Palmer as healer.

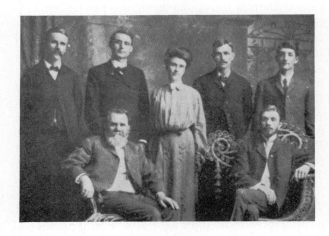

Figure 2-3. Early Palmer School faculty, circa 1906. *(From the B. J. Palmer Special Collection, David D. Palmer Health Sciences Library, Davenport, Iowa.)*

Like the doctrines that he published about his new school, Palmer's movements were erratic. After divesting his interest in the school, infirmary, and osteological collection to his son, the founder left Davenport as an itinerant chiropractic proselytizer, practitioner, and teacher. He traveled to the Indian Territory, to Oregon, and finally to California, returning to Davenport in 1913 as a discoverer denied. He died in Los Angeles 3 months later, after being struck by an automobile in the school lyceum parade. The car was driven by B.J., and unsubstantiated charges of patricide would linger for years (*Dictionary of American Biography*, 1934; Gibbons, 1977).

The egocentric character of chiropractic leadership, as manifested in its early training institutions and in its volatile technique debates, may have evolved from the charismatic nature of the Palmers. Daniel David Palmer and his son Bartlett Joshua were cut from the tough postfrontier stock of rugged individualists (Fig. 2–4). Both would bridge the last days of folk medicine with a popular suspicion of orthodox healing and of the sciences that were seeking out and obtaining the support of the massive philanthropies that were being established on the wealth of industrial and banking fortunes. Their family, including B.J.'s wife Mabel, an anatomist with medical school training, and their son David Daniel,

would constitute the "first family of chiropractic" (Fig. 2–5).

In retrospect, the senior Palmer is gaining increased stature within the profession that he founded as it approaches its centennial. French historian–chiropractor Pierre Louis Gaucher-Perslherbe, in a classic work published in France in 1985, establishes D. D. Palmer as a self-educated scholar with an excellent working knowledge of the medical and scientific theories of the period (Gaucher, 1985). He writes: "we may well ask, how many American or even European doctors of the day would have been able to quote in the same breath Cabriolus, Morgagni, Cheselden and Fallopius?" as did the elder Palmer in his 1910 book.

B. J. Palmer: Barnum with Science

It is difficult to discuss chiropractic history without relating the life, the eccentricities, and the exceptional charisma of Bartlett Joshua Palmer (Fig. 2–6). Though he was a font of endless words, writing at least 30 volumes of varying lengths, editing two of chiropractic's earliest publications for over half a century, and speaking thousands of hours over radio and television, B.J. in many ways remains an enigma.

B.J.'s accomplishments, as well as his tyrannical leadership, are well known to those who have explored chiropractic history. He was a self-described genius of chiropractic, and on reflection, there may be some truth in that assertion that withstands scrutiny. His brilliant organizational mind left little room for dissenters, and he ruthlessly cast out those who opposed him on issues he saw as critically affecting the profession. From the inception of the Palmer properties on Brady Street Hill, there was an injunction to write only to Dr. B. J. Palmer, or to "address all correspondence to firm and not individuals" (*Palmer College Archives*, 1960). He maintained control to a suffocating degree, yet at the same time retained the passionate loyalty of most of those who were on his staff and faculty (Gibbons, 1987).

Those who met B.J. at a Palmer School lyceum or encountered him in the early years of chiropractic reported a religious-like experience. Almost from the first days of his presidency of the Palmer School of Chiropractic B.J. wore his hair long, flowing over his shoulders. He was usually attired in a white linen suit, with his long, black, silk bow tie coming halfway to the waist. A fellow iconolast of the early 20th century was Elbert Hubbard, a lecturer, writer, essayist (*A Message to Garcia*), and editor who wore similar attire and became a friend of B.J. "He was a

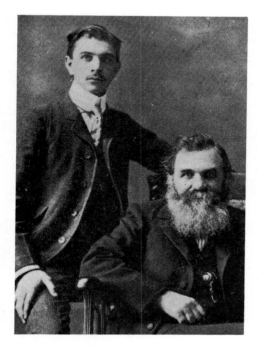

Figure 2–4. A young B. J. Palmer, circa 1904, who would be the self-styled "developer" of chiropractic, with his father, the unchallenged founder. (*From the B. J. Palmer Special Collection, David D. Palmer Health Sciences Library, Davenport, Iowa.*)

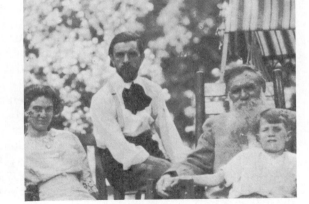

Figure 2–5. The "first family" of chiropractic, circa 1913: Mabel and B. J. Palmer with son David Daniel, who in time would head the Palmer school. *(From the B. J. Palmer Special Collection, David D. Palmer Health Sciences Library, Davenport, Iowa.)*

striking figure," wrote Hubbard, and it was B.J.'s figure that would dominate the chiropractic landscape for two thirds of its existence. He emulated Hubbard and played P. T. Barnum in popularizing the chiropractic story. To his school came other leading political and social dissenters, including William Jennings Bryan (Fig. 2–7) and Eugene Debs.

B.J. jealously watched over the ideological flame of chiropractic, which, he maintained, was his alone to keep. His financial judgments and decisions were absolute. For a good part of two decades he was the undisputed leader of the profession. Yet, from 1924 to his death in 1961 he was a titular leader only, keeping the flame for a fundamentalist minority and doing battle with most of the profession, which he saw as following the osteopathic moth into the seductive allopathic flame.

Yet B.J. the entrepreneur, and ideologue, provided the environment that advanced both the physical and the biological sciences in the Davenport mecca of chiropractic (Fig. 2–8). The osteological laboratory and museum, which were started by the founder, were expanded to the point that an investi-

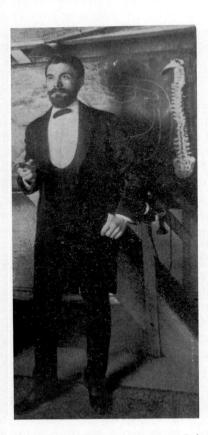

Figure 2–6. Taking over the presidency of the Palmer School in 1906, B.J. would preside at the "Fountainhead" for more than half a century. *(From the B. J. Palmer Special Collection, David D. Palmer Health Sciences Library, Davenport, Iowa.)*

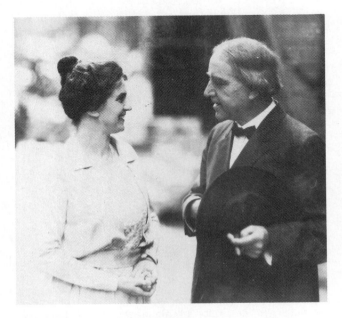

Figure 2–7. Mabel Palmer with William Jennings Bryan on campus, 1912. *(From the B. J. Palmer Special Collection, David D. Palmer Health Sciences Library, Davenport, Iowa.)*

THE PALMER SCHOOL OF CHIROPRACTIC

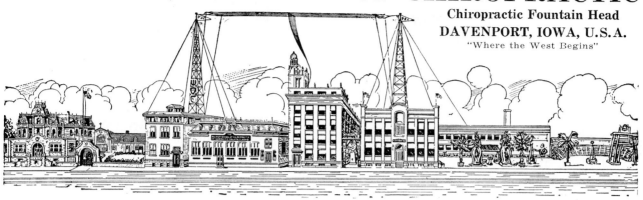

**Chiropractic Fountain Head
DAVENPORT, IOWA, U.S.A.**
"Where the West Begins"

Figure 2–8. The Palmer School, circa 1925, had become the "Chiropractic Fountainhead," complete with the nation's second commercial radio station. *(From the B. J. Palmer Special Collection, David D. Palmer Health Sciences Library, Davenport, Iowa.)*

gating team from the Council on Medical Education and Hospitals of the AMA declared in 1928 that it "was without doubt, the best collection of human spines in existence" (AMA, 1928). The x-ray laboratories, which B.J. established only 13 years after Roentgen, were among the first and the finest in healing institutions. In 1934, in cooperation with physiologists and a medical team in Dresden, Germany, he secured the first wet specimen transparency of the spinal canal in the upper cervical region. And the next year, he established a research clinic in the school's classroom building, where he received the most difficult of medically diagnosed diseases.

The equipment and facilities of the clinic made it one of the finest in the Midwest, with a full medical and nursing staff, a complete diagnostic laboratory, and a physical medicine section. B.J. also secured ownership of Clear View Sanatorium and operated it as a chiropractic facility for mental patients, offering clinical experience for senior Palmer students for some 20 years (Quigley, 1983). His 1935 instrument for reading brain waves and their conduction through the spinal cord was a prototype of today's electroencephalogram.

Science was always in conflict with hucksterism, however, during B.J.'s tenure as chiropractic's neodeveloper. "I will sell chiropractic, serve chiropractic, and save chiropractic if it will take me twenty lifetimes to do it," he would write (Palmer, 1933). And B.J. set forth to sell, serve, and save in the best of the Barnum tradition. In August 1924, under a tent set up on the east end of the campus, B.J. announced the neurocalometer, a pioneer heat-sensing device used to determine the existence of a subluxation. B.J.'s lyceum address was given an advance

billing as "The Hour Has Struck," and chiropractors who came by the thousands were led to believe that the very future of the profession would be decided at this historic occasion. A critical consensus agreed that it was historic, but only in that it marked the decline of B.J.'s unquestioned leadership. Recalled a participant:

> Who shall forget that torrid night under the tent when B. J. spoke . . . in that philippic he maligned chiropractic . . . said many ugly things to the field. It was the hour that nearly rimracked and slaughtered and destroyed chiropractic. (Bealle, 1947)

A massive wave of defections followed after the 1924 lyceum, although a hard core of believers would hold to B.J.'s assertion that "no chiropractor can practice chiropractic without an NCM (neurocalometer) . . . no chiropractor can render an efficient, competent or honest service without the NCM" (Palmer, 1933).

For the next generation, the spokesmen of broad-scope chiropractic maintained that B.J. had forfeited any right to responsible professional leadership and that to them had passed the difficult task to elevate their marginal calling to a level that would receive serious consideration in academic and health-care circles. The public perception of osteopaths and chiropractors as but different types of "back doctors" belied the reality that chiropractic was lagging far behind its osteopathic "cousins" in educational standards, school equipment, faculty, and clinical opportunities (Gevitz, 1982, 1988).

The Old School Converts: Medical Allies and Critics

Other chiropractic heads included those who had made the transition from previous schools of medical dissent or from mainline "allopathy" itself. They would find themselves on opposite sides of the emerging internal debate within chiropractic, in which those who maintained that they represented the original "purist" philosophy of the senior Palmer were in conflict with those who advocated a more broad-scope approach.

Within chiropractic literature, the conflict has survived to this day, despite the disdain of a new generation of practitioners educated in the basic medical sciences. "Straight" versus "mixer" was an ideological confrontation that divided the first pioneers of the profession, who sought a following among their own graduates and those of the competing factions.

Indeed, D. D. Palmer spent fully 185 pages in his book in critical commentary of his son B. J. Palmer, of his osteopathic counterpart A. T. Still, and of Willard Carver (Fig. 2–9), who would challenge B.J. for the leadership mantle after the founder's death. In that same context he derided the views of five of his own graduates who launched

competing schools and journals and authored their own volumes on chiropractic—A. P. Davis, Solon Massey Langworthy, Oakley Smith (Fig. 2–10), Joy Loban, and J. Allen Howard (Donahue, 1990).

Prominent on this landscape of itinerant healing dissenters was A. P. Davis, a graduate of both the regular and the homeopathic schools in the 1880s, who was one of Still's first osteopathic graduates, joining him on the faculty at his Kirksville school before taking up chiropractic under D.D. In 1903 Davis made a sworn statement that the two schools were distinct and separate in theory and application, which was widely used in early Palmer tracts (Palmer, 1904; *Palmer College Archives*).

An early Palmer medical associate, Alva A. Gregory, conducted a school with the founder in Oklahoma City while it was still the Indian Territory. He later broke with Palmer in a dispute over the nature of the spinal subluxation, arguing that instead of displaced vertebrae, there was a "relaxation of spinal ligaments."

Another physician, Arthur L. Forster, president of the National School, which had begun after a curriculum dispute with B.J. in 1906, expressed qualifications as to Palmer's monocausal theories:

> Palmer, however, fell into one serious error. He did as so many before him have done. He became

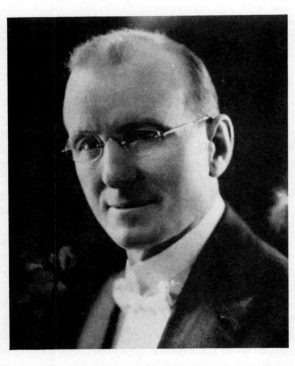

Figure 2–9. Willard Carver, an Iowa attorney who represented D. D. Palmer, took up chiropractic and became a rival to both Palmers as author, writer, school president, and philosopher. *(From the Logan College Archives.)*

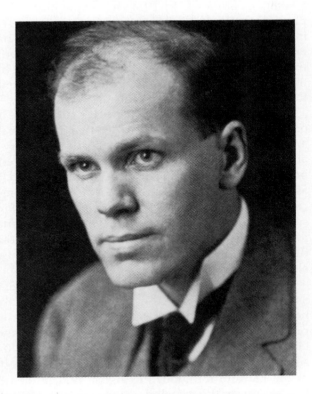

Figure 2–10. Oakley Smith, a medical student who studied under D. D. Palmer, helped organize the first competing school in 1904. *(From the B. J. Palmer Special Collection, David D. Palmer Health Sciences Library, Davenport, Iowa.)*

overzealous. He claimed that all disease is due to subluxations of the vertebrae and that all diseases could be eradicated by adjustment of the vertebrae. He derided all other forms of therapy, and persistent in his original views to the end. (Forster, 1915)

Gregory and Forster continued in association with chiropractic throughout their professional lives, unlike others who viewed it as a money-making opportunity in the era of declining fringe medicine. Four physicians in LaFayette, Indiana, for instance, ran a "college" in which they said "our short way teaches you how to do the reductions on patients in a few weeks' time." The self-styled president listed himself as a graduate of Bellevue Hospital and a Chicago medical school (United College of Chiropractic, 1915).

Philosophical divisions within early chiropractic can be traced to the early students of D. D. Palmer, including Gregory and S. M. Langworthy. Willard Carver, Palmer's attorney, took up chiropractic and moved to Oklahoma where he was in ideological conflict with the Palmers for almost four decades. The senior Palmer's emphasis on "tone" later became known as the segmental theory of chiropractic.

Carver evolved what came to be known as the structural theory, based on the principles of body mechanics. B. J. Palmer did not depart from his father's concepts of the adjustment until 1935, when he advanced emphasis on the atlas in his book *The Subluxation Specific—The Adjustment Specific*, which led to the "above down, inside out" theory.

Earlier James Firth, a leading chiropractic diagnostician, left the Palmer School with three faculty colleagues to form the Lincoln College. Foster's associates at the National College in Chicago, William Schultze and J. Allen Howard, provided an opposite polar point for broad-scope theory and practice. All of these chiropractic theorists published books and journals and established schools (Gibbons, 1981a).

Some, starting with B.J. and Langworthy, launched organizations, where political and legislative tactics became the issue. Personal style and philosophical direction led to other splits, such as that of Joy M. Loban in 1910. Technique and ideology would later gain followers for the Logans (Hugh and Vinton), Joseph Janse at National, and W. A. Budden at Western States (Gibbons, 1977, 1981b).

Unity in chiropractic has been an elusive goal since the 1905–1906 organization of the original and rival American (ACA) and Universal (UCA) chiropractic associations. Later, a 1930 merger would form the National Chiropractic Association (NCA), which in 1963 reverted to the ACA. B.J.'s International Chiropractors association (ICA) and the NCA–

ACA would continue to reflect the purist broad-scope split through midcentury.

D. D. Palmer's itinerant school history was repeated by many of the early "school men." Gregory was associated with an Indianapolis school as well as his Oklahoma City ventures. Two of the four 19th century Palmer graduates were pioneer school heads: A. P. Davis was president of a neuropathic school in Washington and a short-lived osteopathic school in Pittsburgh as well as Texas and Michigan institutions, and Oakley Smith was dean of the American School in Cedar Rapids before he launched his naprapathic school in Chicago in 1906. Other pioneer M.D. chiropractors like G. H. Patchin and J. Shelby Riley presided over schools in New York, Boston, Washington, Detroit, and Fort Wayne.

Carver, Palmer's early nemesis, branched out from Oklahoma to Washington, Denver, and New York City (Carver, 1923). B.J.'s philosophy protege, Joy Loban, launched the rival Universal College three blocks down Brady Hill, then went to a Washington school, joined the Pittsburgh College, and merged it with the troubled Universal in 1919 (Dye, 1939). T. F. Ratledge began institutions in Arkansas and Oklahoma before starting the Los Angeles school. Although some of these may not have been within the brush of B.J.'s charge that many schools owners were "the curse of chiropractic, the army of scholastic pretenders who, leech-like, have fastened themselves to the pedagogical phase of the vocation," there was little doubt that less than altrustic motives predominated (International Association of Chiropractic Schools and Colleges, 1917).

The Survival Years and Educational Reform

Educational reform took about a generation to accomplish after the 1910 Flexner report on medical education. Osteopaths were able to limit their "lesionist-full practice rights" debate within their one organization, and gradually raised entrance standards to 2 years of college and 4 professional years of study. They eliminated marginal schools and reduced their number to eight, building new facilities and maintaining osteopathic hospital opportunities (Givitz, 1988).

Chiropractic, fearful of losing matriculants because of course length and also unable to upgrade their institutions as long as the 18-month course was accepted as "standard," was to wait fully to midcentury before reform became a serious undertaking. By the time of the watershed 1924 lyceum event, more than half of the states had legalized chiropractic (Fig. 2–11), with only a handful requiring more than 18 months. The state of chiropractic education just 4 years after the death of D. D. Palmer is revealed in this assertion by one "school man" at an organization meeting of an early, abortive group called the International Association of Chiropractic Schools and Colleges (1917): "We should not be wasting the time of our students with such medical subjects (as) chemistry, bacteriology and microscopy . . . our time should be on palpation and adjustment."

These remarks were not challenged by some 12 other school presidents in attendance, at least 4 of whom claimed MD degrees and some medical standing. B. J. Palmer's insistence that 18 months was sufficient delayed reform for much of four decades. The consequences would be reflected in the various states that adopted so-called basic science laws, ostensively to examine medical, osteopathic, and chiropractic candidates before they took their own licensing board. The 1930 pass rate for seven of these boards was MDs, 88%; DOs, 55%; and DCs, 22% (Gevitz, 1988). For several states, the basic science tactic effectively dried up new chiropractors for a full generation.

A 1922 survey by an inspector retained by the UCA resulted in a report of 25 institutional visits, about half of which were negative, with the suggestion that "commercial possibilities" may have been the prime motivation of many of their proprietary owners and managers. Ten years later a scathing denunciation came from the Committee on the Costs of Medical Care, which sought to compile data on chiropractic education. The survey's author, Louis Reed of the University of Chicago, said flatly that chiropractic schools could not "be taken seriously as educational institutions" (Wiese and Ferguson, 1988; Reed, 1932).

Yet before the Reed survey, the Council on Medical Education of the AMA had damned with faint praise the physical plant and equipment of the Los Angeles college while at the same time dismissing the medical faculty of Chicago's National College as "having no standing whatsoever in the medical profession in America" (AMA, 1928).

In truth, chiropractic education reflected the demographic highs and lows of this "troublesome sect," as Fishbein described it. Growth years followed World War I and continued through the 1924 neurocalometer debacle. Coupled with the economic depression that came 5 years later, the student population rapidly descended, as did the number of schools (Reed found 79 schools in 1921 and 21 in 1932, with attendance declining "from more than 5,000 to less than 2,000" in that 6-year span). The fortunes of the Palmer school constituted a barometer for chiropractic itself, experiencing a rollercoaster descent from 2100 to 300 students in 1923–1930 (Reed, 1932; Gibbons, 1980).

The 1930s became a survival mode for the profession, with broad-scope schools turning out naturopaths and forging alliances with occasional remnants of the eclectics, homeopaths, and ill-defined "drugless physicians." The purists continued their feuding, but succumbed to the domination of B. J.

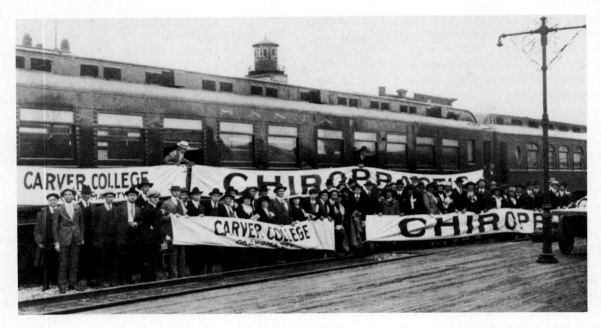

Figure 2-11. Concerted lobbying by chiropractors and their patients resulted in legislation in most of the states by the end of the 1920s. *(From the Logan College Archives.)*

Palmer. School heads such as Hugh Logan, T. J. Ratledge, Carl S. Cleveland, James Drain, and Craig Kightlinger were not "mixers" but they were not all within B.J.'s solar system (Gibbons, 1980). Cleveland's Kansas City College (Fig. 2–12) stressed "hands only" as did these other institutions.

The demographics of chiropractic practitioners and students plummeted to dangerous levels during World War II, the War Manpower Board denying them exemption from the draft as needed health professionals. Yet by 1946 the cycle repeated the 1918 upswing of returning veterans, this time thousands of chiropractic students being supported by the government under the G.I. Bill. The schools, rejuvenated, began the long, agonizing process of self-reform, prodded by the new Director of Education of the National Chiropractic Association, John J. Nugent.

The hard times of the Great Depression brought chiropractic schools to a critical state. The NCA met in Hollywood, California, and formed a Commission on Educational Standards, which in time would become the Committee on Accreditation. It was viewed with suspicion by the majority of the proprietary institutions, even those designated as "mixer," and the rival Palmer group, the ICA, countered with its own Chiropractic Educational Commission which required little more than an affirmation of "straight" philosophy to gain listing on its "approved" list (Gibbons, 1980; Wardwell, 1988).

Into this fray came a unique individual, a former West Pointer turned chiropractor who combined an inspiration for chiropractic politics and an art of persuasion to begin a 25-year career in the reformation of chiropractic education. John J. Nugent had graduated from the National University of Dublin before coming to Davenport to study chiropractic.

In June 1922, only a year after he had matriculated at the Palmer School, Nugent came into conflict with the developer of chiropractic and was expelled for "disloyalty, disrespect and insult to the President" (*Fountain Head News* 1959;55:14), yet 3 weeks later was reinstated by faculty action. The personal enmity between the two men would continue for four decades.

John Nugent was named the Director of Education of the NCA and proceeded to visit every institution purporting to offer the DC degree in his lifetime, perhaps traveling with Flexner's report as his subliminal guide. Some of these visits were covert in nature, for Nugent, as he would later relate, had "become a name hated in much of chiropractic" and a self-described "symbol of revolt against Palmer" leadership (Gibbons, 1985; Wardwell, 1988).

By 1950, with enrollment in chiropractic schools again swelling because of returning veterans, much of Nugent's reforms had been in place: the 4-year course had become standard, most states had enacted amendments to their chiropractic acts requiring the minimum, and all but a few schools had become nonprofit institutions.

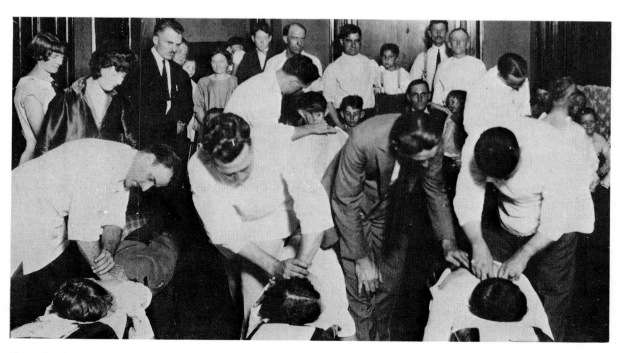

Figure 2–12. Palpation class at Cleveland college, Kansas city, circa 1922. The "hands-only" approach kept chiropractic distinctive. *(From Cleveland College.)*

Critics of chiropractic educational progress tend to make the comparative arguments of post-Flexner medical reform and that of the osteopaths in the 1910–1940 period. There are, however, several qualifications to understand the delay in standardization for the 4-year course and the 2-year preprofessional requirement in chiropractic. Osteopathic historian Norman Gevitz says that the DOs, "biting the bullet," adopted the 2-year requirement in 1940, fully expecting that their enrollments would decline (Gevitz, 1988).

World War II drastically affected the student pool in all professional schools, but for chiropractic the numbers became critical. With the 1945–1946 upturn, all schools looked toward expansion. Medical education had been the first to tap the federal font during the New Deal, and with the Hill–Burton Act in 1946, both medical and osteopathic teaching hospitals realized millions for new hospital construction. The U.S. Public Health Service in 1951 also included osteopathic schools in its teaching grants.

For chiropractic, however, there was no funding from the public sector. Proposals for professional endowment, such as that of the Chiropractic Research Foundation in 1944, did not realize any substantial amounts. NCA's Nugent continued on a virtual one-man campaign of reforming chiropractic education, negotiating the merger of smaller schools, overseeing the transfer of proprietary to professionally owned institutions, and writing standards for revised curriculums, strengthened faculties, and greater clinical opportunities.

With the death of B. J. Palmer in 1961, the slow process of unified educational standards would enter its last stage. The 4-year course became universal, some 40 years after the DOs. Nugent, whom B. J. Palmer had once called "the anti-christ of chiropractic," was largely unrecognized for his work and died virtually unnoticed in 1979. His place as "the Abraham Flexner of chiropractic" seems ensured, his memorial being the acceptance of its schools by the higher education community (Gibbons, 1985).

Conclusion: Going to Jail for Chiropractic

If chiropractic's survival is to be credited to an ideology as much as to the social factors that developed to its advantage, then this should be attributed not to the broad-scope advocates so much as to the purists. To B. J. Palmer and the fundamentalist school must be accorded the motivation that did stamp it with a distinctive label within the therapeutic marketplace, something recognized by public identification as well as by allopathic condemnation. For although broad-scope advocates may have elevated the practice closer to the threshold of respectability and subsequent acceptability by the scientific mainline, the purist concept provided the separate identity during a period when chiropractic's continued existence was doubted by many.

Morris Fishbein, (1889–1976) the long-time editor of the *Journal of the American Medical Association* and onetime AMA secretary, liked to predict "an early relapse and a not far-distant end" for chiropractic when lecturing on what he called the "medical cults" (Fishbein, 1925). Yet in 1969, seven years before he died, the chiropractors that he held in such abject contempt were to rub professional elbows with orthopedists, neurophysiologists, and manipulative specialists at an international conference sponsored by the National Institutes of Health.

That day, however, was not to come until the doors of countless jailhouses, county lockups, and prison farms were to close on the practitioners of the last surviving reform school of healing. The first arrests began before chiropractic completed its first decade, when B. J. Palmer was conducting an itinerant practice in West Virginia. In January 1904 a warrant was issued for his "unlawfully treating persons as a physician" in Barbour County. Two years later the trial of D. D. Palmer in Davenport (Fig. 2–13) and the Morikubo case in Wisconsin resulted in a conviction and acquittal for the same charge of "practicing medicine without a license." The Morikubo defense involved former Wisconsin Lieutenant Governor Tom Morris representing a Japanese-American chiropractor in a LaCrosse, Wisconsin, trial, and was successful and set the precedent for thousands of other cases in the decades to follow.

The prosecutions continued well past mid-century, with investigators from the medical boards in New York and Massachusetts, the last bastions of orthodoxy, seeking arrests whenever the legislative initiative of the medical lobby called for them. A mass arrest of 100 chiropractors in New York City in 1922 followed the abortive California prosecutions and helped to launch the laymen's movement, called the American Bureau of Chiropractic (ABC). Led by William Werner, this group marshalled enough support to fill Madison Square Garden in 1935, cheering such chiropractic boosters as Happy Chandler, the populist lieutenant governor of Tennessee (and later baseball commissioner), and Edward Lodge Curran, a priest–attorney who was a prominent follower of Father Charles Coughlin.

Yet as late as 1949, a well-known Manhattan husband-and-wife team, whose patients included the late Ambassador Joseph Kennedy, was sent to jail after their refusal to tell the court that they would "desist in the practice of medicine without a li-

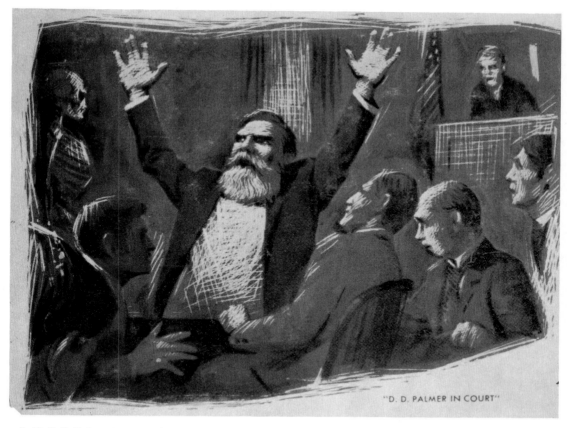

"D. D. PALMER IN COURT"

Figure 2–13. D. D. Palmer in court, 1913. The founder was the first chiropractor to go to jail for the practice of medicine, and hundreds would follow him. *(From Jonorm Publishing Company.)*

cense." From the Women's House of Detention, Katherine (Kitty) Scallon would write a friend of her concern for her husband, Mack Scallon, who was serving his time on Hart's Island:

> Being here is sometimes like a bad dream, when you think of it being for nothing but doing good . . . I felt down-hearted when the news came that Mabel (Palmer) died, but I would always perk up when I thought of chiropractic and the many people it had helped . . . and then I'd throw my shoulders back and be ready and willing to make any sacrifice to help free our beloved science. (K. Scallon, 1949 to M. Garfunkle, 1949, Sherman College Library Collection, Spartanburg, SC)

Thus did the evangelical character of early chiropractic transcend to midcentury, when more complicated times would confront those who challenged the supremacy of the marketplace of healing. The zeal of the early pioneers, reflected in Palmer associate Howard Nutting, an uncle of Willard Carver, was that its practitioners "keep bravely on until the flag

of chiropractic is unfurled in every town and hamlet" (Nutting, 1915).

The systematic persecution and prosecution that have been visited on chiropractors and their institutions for most of this century, "in a virulence unequaled in the annals even of the medical profession" (Inglis, 1963), provides insight into the nature of chiropractic as true social protest.

Facing continued opposition from medicine, excluded from any dialogue or intercourse with the scientific and biological communities, dismissed by the agencies of higher education in both public and private sectors, chiropractic achieved political protection through legislative enactments while on a holding action in the other areas. Patient belief translated to public support. Chiropractors shared the passion and action of their times, earning the right to full maturation in the second half of the century.

References

American Medical Association (AMA). Report of investigations, Council on Medical Education and Hospitals. *JAMA* 1928;99:20.

Bealle M. *Medical Mussolini*. Washington, DC: Columbia Press; 1947.

Booth ER. *History of osteopathy.* Kirksville, Mo: American School of Osteopathy; 1924.

Carver W. *Chiropractic Red Book.* Oklahoma City; 1923.

Cayleff SE. The water cure movement. In Gevitz N, ed. *Other healers.* Baltimore, Md: Johns Hopkins University Press.

Dictionary of American Biography (DAB). vol 14. New York: Charles Scribner; 1934.

Donahue J. Revised index. *Chiropractic Hist* 1990;10:2.

Dye A. *The evolution of chiropractic.* Philadelphia: 1939.

Ehrenreich B and English D. *Witches, midwives and nurses.* Old Westbury, NY: Feminist Press; 1976.

Ehrenreich B and English D. *For her own good.* New York: Anchor/Doubleday; 1978.

Fishbein. *The medical follies.* New York: Boni & Liveright; 1925.

Flexner A. *Medical education in the United States.* New York: Times-Arno Press: 1910; 1967 reprint.

Forster AL. *Principles and practice of spinal adjustment.* Chicago: National School of Chiropractic; 1915.

Gaucher PL. *A mended statue: Chiropractic's early concepts.* E. Weeks, trans. LeMans: Jupiles; 1985.

Gevitz N. *The D.O.s: Osteopathic medicine in America.* Baltimore, Md: Johns Hopkins University Press; 1982.

Gevitz N (ed). *Other healers.* Baltimore, Md: Johns Hopkins University Press; 1988.

Gibbons RW. Chiropractic in America: The historical conflicts of cultism and science. *J Popular Culture* 1977;11(3):720–731.

Gibbons RW. The rise of the chiropractic educational establishment, 1897–1980. In *Who's Who in Chiropractic.* Littleton, Colo: Who's Who Publishing Co; 1980.

Gibbons RW. 1981a. ''Physician-chiropractors: Medical presence in the evolution of chiropractic. *Bull Hist Med* 1981a;55:233–245.

Gibbons RW. Solon Massey Langworthy: Keeper of the flame during the ''lost years'' of chiropractic. *Chiropractic Hist* 1981b;1:14–21.

Gibbons RW. Chiropractic's Abraham Flexner: The lonely journey of John J. Nugent, 1935–1963. *Chiropractic Hist* 1985;5:44–51.

Gibbons RW. Assessing the oracle at the fountainhead: B. J. Palmer and his times, 1902–1961. *Chiropractic Hist* 1987;7:1.

Gielow V. 1982. *Old Dad Chiro: A biography of D. D. Palmer.* Davenport, Iowa: Badwin.

Hall TE. *The contributions of John Martin Littlejohn to osteopathy.* London: Maidstone Osteopathic Clinic; 1974.

Inglis B. *The case for unorthodox medicine.* New York: G. P. Putnam; 1963.

International Association of Chiropractic Schools and Colleges. Minutes of organization meeting, August 1917. Palmer College Archives.

Kaufman M. *Homeopathy in America: The rise and fall of an American medical heresy.* Baltimore, Md: Johns Hopkins University Press; 1971.

Meade TW, et al. Low back pain: Random comparison of chiropractic and outpatient treatment. *Brit Med J.* 1990;300:6737.

New Zealand Commission. *Status of chiropractic.* Auckland: New Zealand Commission on Inquiry on Chiropractic; 1979.

Numbers R. The making of an eclectic physician. *Bull Hist Med* 1972;47:2.

Nutting H. A glorious future. *Chiropractor* 1915;11:1.

Palmer BJ. *The Chiropractor.* Davenport, Iowa: Palmer School of Chiropractic Press; 1918:vol 14, p. 20.

Palmer BJ. Comments by B.J. *Fountainhead News* 1933;29:12.

Palmer DD. *Chiropractor* 1904;1:4.

Palmer DD. *The chiropractor's adjuster.* Portland, Oreg: Portland Publishing Co; 1910.

Palmer DD. Letter. *Natl Chiropractic J* 1936;6:3.

Palmer College archives. Davenport, Iowa: David D. Palmer Health Sciences Library; 1960.

Quebec Royal Commission. *Study of chiropractic, osteopathy and naturopathy.* Montreal: Province of Quebec; 1975.

Quigley WL. Pioneering mental health: Institutional psychiatric care in chiropractic. *Chiropractic Hist* 1983;3:69–73.

Reed L. *The healing cults.* Chicago, Ill: University of Chicago Press; 1932.

Rothstein WG. *American physicians in the nineteenth century.* Baltimore, Md: Johns Hopkins University Press; 1972.

Starr P. *The social transformation of American medicine.* New York: Basic Books; 1982.

United College of Chiropractic. Announcements. Lafayette, Ind; 1915.

U.S. Department of Health, Education & Welfare (USDHEW). *Independent practitioners under medicare.* Washington, DC: U.S. Government Printing Press; 1969.

Wardwell WI. Limited, marginal, and quasi-practitioners. In Freeman HE, ed. *Handbook of medical sociology.* 2nd ed. Englewood Cliffs, NH: Prentice-Hall; 1972.

Wardwell WI. Chiropractors: Evolution to acceptance. In Gevitz, N, ed. *Other healers.* Baltimore, Md: Johns Hopkins Press; 1988.

Wiese G and Ferguson A. How many chiropractic schools? *Chiropractic Hist* 1988;8:1.

chapter 3

Origin and Development of Traditional Chiropractic Philosophy

Gerald Waagen
Virgil Strang

- **CHIROPRACTIC'S ORIGINS**
  Daniel David Palmer
- **VITALISM**
  Bartlett Joshua Palmer
  Ralph W. Stephenson
  William David Harper
- **SCIENCE**
  Willard Carver
  A. Earl Homewood
  C. O. Watkins
  Joseph Janse

  Fred W. Illi
  Henry J. Gillet
- **SKEPTICAL INQUIRY AS THE DISTINGUISHING FEATURE OF SCIENCE**
- **ROLE OF PHILOSOPHY IN CHIROPRACTIC'S SURVIVAL**
- **CONCLUSION**
- **REFERENCES**

The origin of chiropractic can be dated to a specific time and place, September 18, 1895, in Davenport, Iowa, when a magnetic healer named Daniel David Palmer gave a patient a chiropractic adjustment. In retrospect, the founding and subsequent development of a structural, spinal-based system of health care such as chiropractic seems almost inevitable. It is probably true, however, that without a strong philosophical basis, chiropractic would never have become a viable form of health care. That philosophical foundation was provided initially by D. D. Palmer. He drew from diverse sources to create a comprehensive philosophical system that was internally consistent. A dualism can be recognized in Palmer's philosophy that consists of elements derived either from metaphysical, spiritual, mystical, or vitalist sources, and elements derived from the science of the time. Although present, the duality is not obvious in Palmer's writings. That duality became apparent in the works of his philosophical successors.

The metaphysical components of Palmer's philosophy were developed by individuals here referred to as proponents of vitalism. Those who concentrated instead on a mechanistic study of chiropractic

developed chiropractic science. Differences between proponents of either philosophic focus were differences of emphasis, not kind, and the divergence of opinion has never been very substantial. Vitalists advocated scientific research, and those in the science pathway accepted in general the metaphysical concepts elucidated by Palmer.

The approach taken in this chapter is historical. Ten philosophers have been chosen to represent important aspects of the development of traditional chi-

Acknowledgments

We gratefully acknowledge the generous assistance of Robert Mootz, DC, Gale Lewellen, MS, J. Keating, PhD, K. F. DeBoer, PhD, and Victor Strang, DC, for helpful discussion and corrections of fact and concept. Figure 3–1 was prepared by Peter Fysh, DC, Palmer College of Chiropractic West, Sunnyvale, California.

G.W. thanks the Anatomy Department of Palmer College of Chiropractic in Davenport, Iowa, for providing him with time, encouragement, and tolerance while he was working on the chapter; and he appreciates the graciousness and dedication of the staff of the David D. Palmer Health Sciences Library, who have, over in the years, conscientiously acquired important historical documents in the Archives, and help scholars use those sources.

Glenda Wiese provided the photographs of the philosophers from the Archives, David D. Palmer Health Sciences Library, in Davenport, Iowa.

ropractic philosophy. They include chiropractic's founder, D. D. Palmer; three vitalists, B. J. Palmer, R. W. Stephenson, and W. D. Harper; and six scientists, W. Carver, C. O. Watkins, A. E. Homewood, J. Janse, F. W. Illi, and H. J. Gillette. For each, a brief biography is given, their contributions to chiropractic philosophy are described, and relations to predecessors and followers are discussed.

Chiropractic's Origins

When D. D. Palmer gave the first chiropractic adjustment, the social climate was conducive to the development of such an unorthodox form of health care. The most important factor that contributed to the origin of chiropractic was the medical protest or medical reform movement of the 1800s. The medical concept of a vertebral subluxation and the tradition of bonesetting as a nonmedical form of treatment for many ailments were factors that had indirect influence on the development of D. D. Palmer's philosophy and method of health care.

A popular medical protest movement had arisen in the earlier part of the 19th century in response to heroic medical treatments, which often did more harm than good to patients. Medical treatment had little rational basis and consisted largely of bloodletting and surgery (which was both septic and unnecessary), along with the administration of various poisons and heavy metals, which were used as medications to purge the patient of unknown or poorly understood maladies.

The medical reform movement consisted of lifestyle recommendations and professional alternatives to orthodox medicine. The primary lifestyle changes were recommendations for improving personal hygiene (e.g., bathing frequently), eating fresh or uncooked fruits and vegetables, and regular exercise in the fresh air, all of which were scoffed at or opposed by orthodox medical practice. Those reasonable lifestyle changes of the medical reform movement were eventually incorporated into orthodox medical practice. Important professional alternatives to orthodox medicine that arose during the latter 1800s were homeopathy, osteopathy, naturopathy, and magnetic healing. All of these schools of theory and therapy were characterized by their relative harmlessness. Even if they did not directly benefit the patient, they did not result in substantial harm.

Chiropractic also traces its philosophical roots in part to that zeitgeist of the times, which was responsive to drugless, noninvasive forms of health care. Because they had an economic stake in health care, practitioners of orthodox medicine did not enthusiastically support other alternative health-care pro-

viders. Three outcomes were possible in the competition between orthodox medicine and the alternative providers: (1) elimination of one or the other; (2) incorporation of the alternative providers into orthodox medicine; (3) coexistence, either friendly or adversarial. To some degree, it is likely that combinations of all of these relationships and interactions occurred to virtually all of the forms of nonorthodox health care. In the United States chiropractic has coexisted with orthodox medicine since its inception.

Although Daniel David Palmer claimed to have been the first to use the term *subluxation* (1910), the first recorded use of the term was by a medical practitioner. In 1746 the physician Hieronymi used *subluxation* to refer to a vertebral segment that exhibited decreased mobility and slight malposition (Lomax, 1975). In 1820, an English physician, Edward Harrison, noted that the spinal cord is compressed by the subluxation and that organs innervated by related nerves will be disturbed as a result (Lomax, 1975). Palmer emphasized that modification of nerve impulse transmission caused by subluxation of spinal joints resulted in physiologic dysfunction or disease. That concept of the relation between nerves and organs was similar to the medical concept of "tone" and was invoked by Palmer to explain the nature of the relationship between the subluxation and disease. Deficient or excessive tone resulted from the effect of a subluxation on a nerve. Nerve vibration to and from an organ would result in disease when it caused either deficient or excessive tone. It is reasonable to assume that D. D. Palmer borrowed the term and concept of tone and vertebral subluxation from medical writings (Terrett, 1987).

Although D. D. Palmer acknowledged Dr. Jim Atkinson as a mentor (Palmer, 1910), there is no evidence that Atkinson taught any specific form of manual therapy. There is not doubt, however, that in practice chiropractic was similar to an ancient art known as bonesetting. In certain families (i.e., the Sweets of Rhode Island, the Ortmans of South Dakota), the art of hands-on therapy was passed from one generation to the next, or to a person with manual dexterity who was interested and capable of learning the art (Gibbons, 1980). It has also been described in the writings of Hippocrates and others throughout the world (Lomax, 1975).

Periodically, a medical physician would become interested in bonesetting and refer patients to bonesetters, but there was never a formal relationship between bonesetting and orthodox medicine. A few physicians learned the art themselves and tried to convince others of the importance of manual therapy (Lomax 1975). In 1871, for example, referring to the treatment methods of the eminent bonesetter Richard Hutton, Wharton Hood wrote that "bone setting

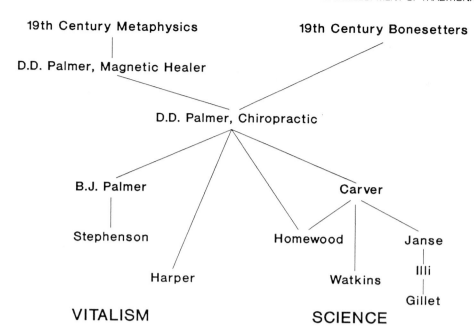

Figure 3–1. Origin and development of traditional chiropractic philosophy.

may be defined as the art of overcoming by sudden flexion and extension, any impediments to the free motion of joints'' (Lomax, 1975).

Bonesetting preceded Andrew Taylor Still's foundation of osteopathy in 1874, which, in turn, preceded Palmer's 1895 origination of chiropractic (Still, 1910; Palmer, 1910). Although osteopathy emerged about two decades before chiropractic, no clear evidence has been put forth that bonesetting made a direct contribution to osteopathy or chiropractic. Further, it has not been proved that Still taught D. D. Palmer the rudiments of manual therapy. Knowingly or unknowingly, however, chiropractic furthered the tradition of bonesetting. Bonesetting and certain components of osteopathy may be considered the practical precursors of chiropractic (Wardwell, 1987) (Fig. 3–1).

Unlike the lay bonesetters, chiropractors developed a legitimate health-care profession by offering graduate degrees and seeking licensure, as did the allopathic physicians and surgeons. Perhaps a lack of clearly articulated philosophy contributed to the gradual attrition of the bonesetters. Conversely, the combination of chiropractic's efforts to obtain social legitimacy and its emphasis on strong philosophic premises may explain, in part, its successful defense against organized medical persecution (Keating and Mootz, 1989).

Daniel David Palmer

The ''founder'' of chiropractic, Daniel David Palmer (Fig. 3–2), was born in 1845 in Canada. Although

Palmer's formal education did not continue past the age of 11, he read voraciously and, in his later years, carried a ''traveling library'' (Donahue, 1987). Palmer was a self-taught man whose knowledge of philosophy and the science of his day was consider-

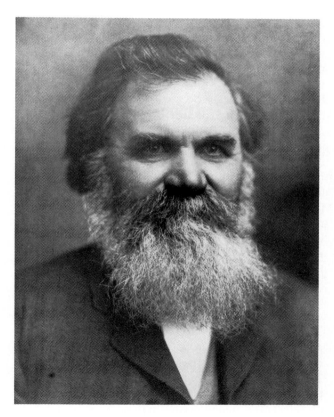

Figure 3–2. Daniel David Palmer.

able (Gaucher, 1986). He emigrated to Iowa in 1865, where he found work as a schoolmaster. In 1886, his interests in 19th-century philosophical concepts led him to become a magnetic healer. As a magnetic healer Palmer influenced the temperature, energy, or electrical flow in a patient by directional rubbing, stroking, kneading, or manipulation of specific regions of the patient's body (Gielow, 1983).

The first chiropractic adjustment was performed on September 18, 1895, and the Palmer School of Magnetic Cure was incorporated in 1896. Palmer enlisted the help of a friend to coin the term *chiropractic* from Greek roots meaning "done by hand" (Lomax, 1975). Palmer was jailed for 23 days for practicing medicine without a license in 1906. His conviction, along with legal action against other chiropractors, may have provided impetus to the vitalist elements in chiropractic philosophy (Mootz and Keating, 1989). After his release from jail, Palmer sold the school (renamed the Palmer School and Infirmary of Chiropractic) to his son Bartlett Joshua Palmer. He established numerous schools of chiropractic throughout the United States prior to his death in 1913 in Los Angeles.

The initial question about health care that perplexed Palmer was, "Why does one man get sick when others who work at the same bench or live in the same house, do not? If they eat the same food and breathe the same air, why does one person contract a disease and another remain healthy?" (Palmer, 1910). He reasoned that vertebral dysarthria was the primary cause of disease. His further deduction of a correlation between vertebral dysarthria, for which he used the term *subluxation*, and neurologic manifestations was the most significant of Palmer's concepts (Gaucher, 1986).

Palmer described the subluxation as a vertebral segment that is not frankly dislocated, but is out of normal anatomic relationship to the adjacent segments. He considered a decrease of motion to be one of the key features of a subluxation. The mediating factor between the subluxation and disease was the nervous system. All subluxations were thought to involve nerves and nerve transmission changes. The pathogenic result of a subluxation was, according to Palmer, loss of normal functioning of the nerves.

Because it is known what books he carried in his traveling library (Donahue, 1987), it is reasonable to assume that D. D. Palmer was familiar with certain 19th-century concepts. Sources for his philosophy probably included metaphysics (a movement arising from the transcendentalism of Emerson during the 1830s), theosophy (a mystical system involving matter and life), spiritualism (the concept that the spirit of a deceased healer could be used to heal), vitalism (the belief that the principles that govern life are different from the principles of inanimate matter), and the biologic sciences, especially neurology (Donahue, 1987).

The vitalistic and spiritualistic elements in Palmer's philosophy of chiropractic included concepts that Palmer called innate intelligence, universal intelligence, mind, life, and soul.

Universal intelligence is defined as the life force, power, or source of creation, which is expressed in the individual as innate intelligence. Palmer argued that universal intelligence strives to express itself and improve itself individually as innate intelligence. This guiding innate intelligence allows the individual to make himself better physically, mentally, and spiritually (Donahue, 1986). Palmer reasoned that the innate intelligence controls and coordinates bodily activity by receiving and sending information via the nerves.

He described the mind as a dual entity: the innate, or individual part of universal intelligence; and the educated, or acquired part of the mind, which is developed throughout life. Each mental attribute contributed to the existence of the other, according to D. D. Palmer. Although the concept of innate became the cornerstone of the vitalist philosophy of B. J. Palmer, it is impossible to describe the philosophy of D. D. Palmer as favoring either vitalism or science. He clearly thought that both were important.

D. D. Palmer described the ability of the body to heal itself without entering the classic dispute between vitalists and naturalists, wherein the former claim that the principles that explain how life functions are different from the laws that govern nonliving matter. Perhaps he considered the controversy to be irrelevant, because he wrote as though all matter were imbued with life.

D. D. Palmer clearly delineated major philosophical differences between orthodox medicine and chiropractic. One primary distinction is that, although allopathic medicine perceives the cause of disease to be a result of the environment overwhelming an individual, chiropractic follows a more holistic perspective, which argues that the problem lies within the organism. Specifically, a structural problem within the spine contributes to diminished neurologic ability to cope with the environment, and the ability of the body to heal itself is decreased. Palmer believed the cause of most disease is displaced vertebrae; the disease is an effect of that displacement. Diseases are not cured, and the patient is not treated. Palmer wrote, "I don't cure diseases, I adjust displaced vertebrae." In place of a method of treatment, the chiropractor brings abnormal parts to a proper relative position. Illness is essentially a functional problem and becomes structural or organic only as an end process (Terrett, 1986).

Vitalism

The philosophy of D. D. Palmer included the two related elements of vitalism and science. Three chiropractic philosophers were major proponents of this vitalist tradition: B. J. Palmer, Ralph W. Stevenson, and William D. Harper. Stephenson was a disciple of B. J. Palmer. Harper was a vitalist in the sense that he apparently considered the concept of life force to be more important than mechanical explanations of chiropractic practice. Vitalists did not depart from chiropractic philosophy: they continued essentially unchanged the basic doctrine of the vitalism/science blend established by D. D. Palmer. B. J. Palmer and Harper both established research institutes and called for scientific research.

Bartlett Joshua Palmer

Bartlett Joshua Palmer was born in What Cheer, Iowa, in 1882 (Fig. 3–3). He became known as the ''developer'' of chiropractic. Palmer was described as charismatic and brilliant in an organizational sense. He had a flair for the flamboyant as well as the scientific, and was a leader who, with his written and spoken words, motivated thousands of people. Although he did not graduate from high school, B. J. Palmer became the president of five corporations.

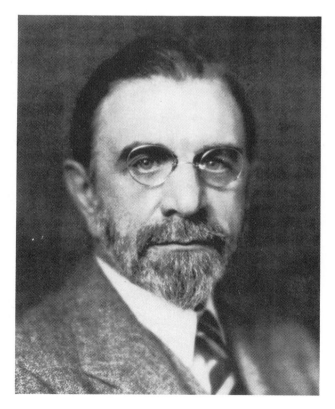

Figure 3–3. Bartlett Joshua Palmer.

He was a world traveler, and was considered an important collector of art. He wrote more than 37 books, and for more than 50 years he edited two of chiropractic's earliest periodicals. He was a television and radio lecturer, and a dominant force in three chiropractic professional organizations.

B. J. Palmer was president of the Palmer School of Chiropractic from 1904 to 1961. He developed an osteologic laboratory and museum that were highly acclaimed, and established roentgenology facilities that were among the finest in healing institutions of the times. The B. J. Palmer Research Clinic was established in 1935, and the Clearview Sanitarium in Davenport was owned by the college for about 10 years (1951–1961). Palmer also developed an instrument for recording brain waves that might be considered the forerunner of the electroencephalograph (Gibbons, 1980). It is believed by some that, for most of the first half of the 20th century, B. J. Palmer was the primary force that prevented chiropractic from being consumed by the medical profession (Gibbons, 1980). Palmer died at his winter home in Sarasota, Florida, in May 1961.

The philosophy of B. J. Palmer was primarily a development of the vitalistic, life-force aspects of the philosophy of D. D. Palmer. Three distinct ideas can be discerned in the philosophy of B. J. Palmer: (1) the ''principle of chiropractic''; (2) the ''big idea,'' a mystical concept; and (3) a comprehensive and unique life view that included detailed descriptions of health, disease, chiropractic care, and related matters.

The ''principle of chiropractic'' was a succinct description of chiropractic practice. The principle can be summarized as follows: a chiropractic adjustment reduces a vertebral subluxation, which normalizes function of the nervous system, thereby allowing the body to heal itself unimpeded. For a number of years, B. J. Palmer emphasized the importance (based on his empirical clinical perceptions) of subluxations of the occipitoatlantoaxial region of the cervical spine. He promoted the distinctiveness of the chiropractic approach as adjustments given by hand only for the removal of subluxation, which he considered to be the major impediment to restoration and maintenance of health. It logically followed that chiropractors should not concern themselves with ''treatment of disease''(B. J. Palmer, 1958).

B. J. Palmer's second construct, the ''big idea,'' is derived from D. D. Palmer's vitalistic concept of innate intelligence. When innate is in control, the person is healthy and perfectly functional. It is only necessary to let innate express itself and everything the person does will be functionally ideal (Smallie, 1988; Strang, 1987).

A corollary to the ''big idea'' as expressed by

B. J. Palmer was a peculiar belief in the perfection of the incoming (afferent) sensory system. B. J. Palmer's use of the concept "above-down, inside-out" to describe the relationship of universal and innate intelligence with a body implied that he believed that the incoming nervous impulses were not affected by subluxations. Innate always has adequate information to function perfectly; if there are dysfunctions, they are always in the efferent or outgoing system.

Ralph W. Stephenson

Ralph W. Stephenson (Fig. 3–4) summarized B. J. Palmer's ideas in his textbook on chiropractic philosophy (Stephenson, 1927). Stephenson was born in Lincoln, Illinois, in 1879, and graduated from Iowa State University in Ames before entering chiropractic school. After completing his chiropractic degree at the Palmer School of Chiropractic in 1921, he joined the faculty as an instructor of philosophy, later becoming the chairman of the technique department. He published many articles on chiropractic philosophy and technique, and three books: *The Art of Chiropractic* (1927), *Chiropractic Textbook* (1927), and *System of Adjusting the Spine* (1954).

In the *Chiropractic Textbook*, Stephenson identified 33 principles of chiropractic science, including such concepts as innate, cycles, and the meric system. Stephenson wrote that the forces of innate intelligence operate via the nerves. Interference with nerve transmission contributed to subluxations in the spinal column.

Stephenson illustrated the functioning of the body using cyclic diagrams. The simple "safety-pin" cycle is an abstraction that includes only afferent and efferent transmission between tissue and brain cells (Fig. 3–5) (Stephenson, 1927, p. 9). The "normal complete" cycle (Fig. 3–6) (Stephenson, 1927, p. 10) consists of 31 steps, 15 afferent and 16 efferent, and is "the outline of the story of the normal functioning of Innate in the body" (Stephenson, 1927, p.8). The "vertemere" cycle (Fig. 3–7) (Stephenson, 1927, p. 77) adds the cycle from brain to a vertebral segment to the normal complete cycle. "The Vertemere Cycle is the cycle from Innate Brain to the tissues, holding in situ the vertebra in question. A subluxation impinging a nerve from brain to organ also impinges the nerves supplying its own tissues, and that is why it exists as a subluxation" (Stephenson, 1927, p. 76). Stephenson further asserted that the vertemere cycle was the basis for the art or technique of chiropractic (Stephenson, 1927, p. 76).

The concepts of "ease" and "disease" are related to the functioning cycles. "Ease" is present when the cycles are functioning properly; however, when there is a disturbance of the afferent–efferent cycle there is a lack of ease, or "dis-ease," which is caused by a subluxation. It is reasoned that the structural intervention of chiropractic spinal adjustment restores normal function (Stephenson, 1927, pp. 80–90).

Stephenson often used the term *incoordination* instead of disease for sickness. He used the term *insanity* to refer to pathologic tissue function. Body tissue pathology was therefore physical insanity, and brain tissue pathology was mental insanity (Stephenson, 1927, p. 97).

Stephenson also emphasized the role of the circulatory or "serous" systems. He pointed out, in his own way, that the potential for systemic toxicity was facilitated by this system. Any substance retained in the serous circulation that could not be used by the body was considered a poison (Stephenson, 1927, pp. 105–108). This concept helped to develop and perpetuate chiropractic as a drugless health-care discipline.

Another concept described by Stephenson (1927, pp. 342–343) was the "meric" system. This was one of the first attempts by chiropractors to map out nerve distributions and relate them to vertebral segments and physiologic function. Although unrefined, it served as a model to explain empirical observations of chiropractic adjustments on patients. It at-

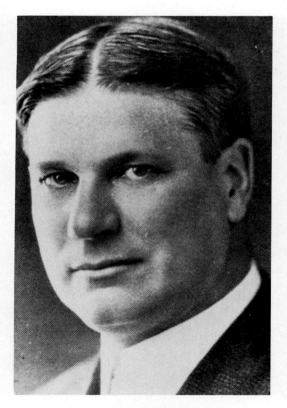

Figure 3-4. Ralph W. Stephenson.

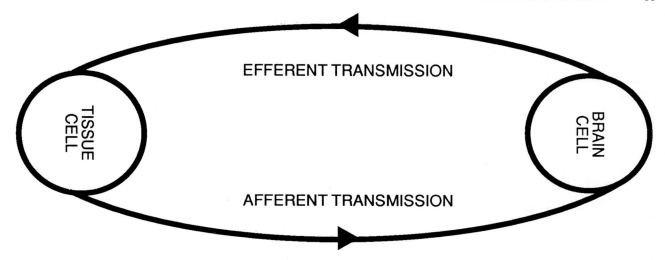

Figure 3-5. The simple "safety pin" cycle.

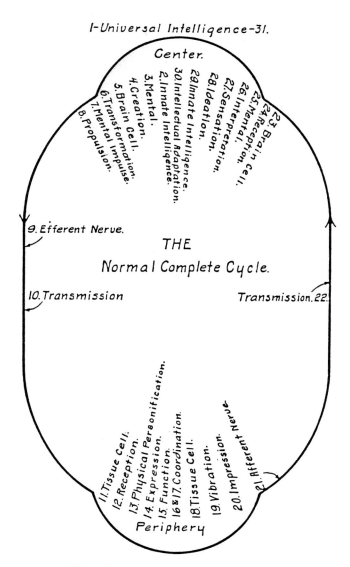

Figure 3-6. The "normal complete" cycle.

tempted to correlate segmental dysfunction with systemic and visceral disorders, and preceded the modern osteopathic and chiropractic dysfunction models of hypersympathicotonia and somatovisceral reflexes (Korr, 1978).

William David Harper

The third major vitalist, William David Harper (Fig. 3-8), was born in 1908 in Big Spring, Texas. He attended the Massachusetts Institute of Technology, receiving an engineering degree (1933), and then graduated from Texas Chiropractic College (TCC) in Pasadena, Texas (1942). He practiced chiropractic in Massachusetts from 1942 to 1949. In 1949, he moved back to Texas, where he held various faculty and administrative positions at TCC for the next 30 years. He was the president of TCC from 1966 to 1976. Harper lectured throughout the United States for 37 years. During the 1970s, he served as a research consultant to TCC, where the W. D. Harper Clinic and Research Center was built. His written works include a pamphlet for TCC, *What Is Chiropractic?*; the text, *Anything Can Cause Anything* (1974); and numerous articles for chiropractic journals.

Harper's philosophical position could most accurately be described as "scientific mysticism," through which he sought the ultimate cause of health. According to Harper, the philosophy of D. D. Palmer can be summarized by six principles. The first two principles are that consciousness, or irritability, occurs at a cellular level (principle 1) and an organism level (principle 2). The third principle is the simple cycle or the simple reflex arc. The first part of the reflex is initiated by an environmental perturbation, which results in sensory nerve transmission to the brain. The arc is completed when innate responds via a motor nerve. The fourth principle is

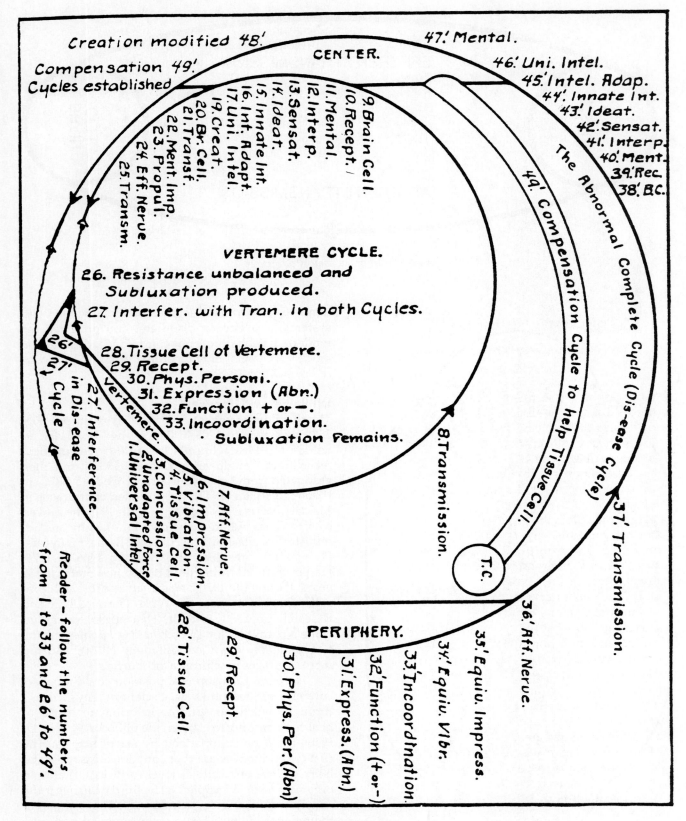

Figure 3-7. The "vertemere" cycle.

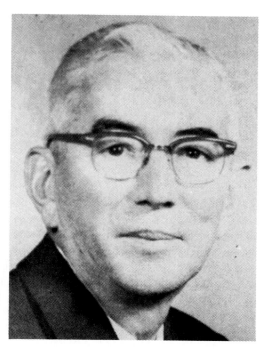

Figure 3-8. William David Harper.

that the response is normal in a healthy person, but if there is disease, the response is abnormal. The abnormal function is caused by mechanical, chemical, or psychologic environmental factors. Innate always functions perfectly, the correct impulse is always initiated by innate; the abnormal results, either too much or too little nerve impulse, occurs because of the condition of the transmitting nervous system. The fifth principle is that there are no new functions; abnormal functions are normal functions at the wrong time. The sixth principle is that dysfunction may be caused environmentally by physical (i.e., trauma), chemical (i.e., poisons), or psychologic irritation of the motor nerves.

The contributions of B. J. Palmer, Stephenson, and Harper represent the mystical–vitalist tradition of chiropractic philosophy. It is clear that their perspectives were derived in part from observations of clinical events and from their understanding of the biologic, physiologic, and anatomic sciences of the time. The philosophical systems erected by B. J. Palmer, Stephenson, and Harper are isolated systems, which diverged greatly from the philosophy of D. D. Palmer. There was one principle, however, that was common to these three and to anyone who worked in the vitalist tradition.

Permeating the chiropractic philosophical tradition beginning with D. D. Palmer and continuing through B. J. Palmer, Stephenson, and Harper, is the principle of innate healing. That principle also remains central to the philosophical positions of those whose writings emphasize scientific or pragmatic explanations. Confusion and polarization have resulted from attempts to superimpose vitalistic concepts on known, tangible phenomena. D. D. Palmer's dualism consisted of (1) the intangible chiropractic metaphor that acknowledged and described the body's ability to self-heal and (2) the chiropractic principle that describes a relationship between body structure and physiologic function. The metaphor describes the intangible constructs of a belief system; i.e., universal intelligence, which permeates all things, is expressed in the individual as innate intelligence. The chiropractic principle describes a tangible, measurable phenomenon; i.e., a chiropractic adjustment reduces a structural vertebral lesion (the subluxation), which alters the functioning of a body.

The metaphor can only be supported by logic, faith, and consensus. The principle is more amenable to evaluation via scientific inquiry. B. J. Palmer, Stephenson, and Harper consciously or unconsciously attempted to integrate these concepts into a single chiropractic philosophy. To the uninitiated, this seemed like cultism, but to the ostracized chiropractor trying to stay out of jail for practicing medicine without a license, this did provide a legally defensible distinction between medicine and chiropractic (Mootz and Keating, 1989). This philosophy also served to galvanize and organize chiropractors around a central, intuitively appealing model to explain what they saw in their practices every day.

Science

The term *science* has been chosen to represent the contribution to traditional chiropractic philosophy of six leaders who fostered the gradual development of chiropractic science. Their contributions, however, were more those of enthusiasm than accuracy, but their efforts must not be belittled. The modern science of chiropractic has evolved from the accomplishments of these men, their colleagues, and successors.

Willard Carver

Willard Carver (Fig. 3-9) was born in Maysville, Iowa, on July 14, 1866. Carver received his law degree from Drake University in Iowa, and practiced law for 15 years. Carver and D. D. Palmer were friends before the discovery of chiropractic. His mother is reputed to have been one of Palmer's first patients. Because of this friendship, Carver defended him in 1903, in Scott County, Iowa, when Palmer had been arrested for practicing medicine without a license.

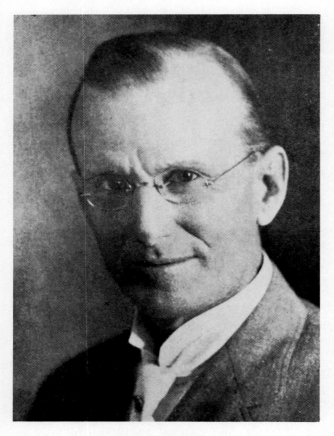

Figure 3-9. Willard Carver.

Carver initially saw himself as an observer of the embryonic chiropractic profession, and later as the counselor and lawyer-advocate for the profession. When D. D. Palmer sold the chiropractic school to his son B. J. Palmer in 1906, Carver's feelings, changed. Carver did not feel the same kinship to B. J. Palmer that he had with D. D. Palmer.

Deciding to take up the study of chiropractic himself, Carver graduated from the Charles Ray Parker School of Chiropractic in 1906 and opened the Carver Chiropractic College in Oklahoma City that same year. Carver also founded chiropractic schools in New York City (1919), Washington, D.C. (1922), and Denver (1923). All of these schools eventually merged with other institutions. Carver wrote and published 18 books, but is best known for *Carver's Chiropractic Analysis* (1921). Carver had a naturalistic view of chiropractic; e.g., instead of Innate he referred to the physiologic processes that reconstruct the body.

Carver disagreed with D. D. Palmer about the nature of the subluxation. Palmer thought of a subluxation as a single dysfunctional segment of the spine, but Carver considered subluxations to be the result of abnormal curves of the spine caused by muscular imbalance. If there is excessive innervation to a set of muscles, Carver maintained, the muscles on the opposite side will, by way of compensation, react with more contraction and so create an imbalance and a subluxation. This condition he named the complex opposed rotational scoliosis (Carver, 1921).

Like D. D. Palmer, Carver believed that doctors do not and cannot heal. Doctors only may aid in restoring relationship so that physiologic processes may reconstruct the body back to its original condition. In addition to restoring relationship, the doctor must, in Carver's opinion, also use suggestion as a means of healing. He defined *suggestion* as any information obtained in any manner. Carver argued that suggestion is the basis of all systems of healing. "We find the same percent of cures among the 'medicine men' of the savages and we find no higher percent of restorations among the 'practitioners of medicine,' faith has produced substantially all of the efficacious results that have occurred" (Carver, 1924, p. 40). Carver considered healing to be accomplished by suggestion first transmitted to the brain, then to the soul, and finally to every part of the body via the nervous system. He believed that the function of the adjustment was to remove occlusion so that the influence of suggestion could effect normal function of the body.

A. Earl Homewood

A. Earl Homewood (Fig. 3–10) was influenced by both D. D. Palmer and Carver (see Fig. 3–1). Homewood was born in Toronto, Ontario, Canada, in 1916. He graduated as a doctor of physical therapy from the University of Natural Healing Arts, in Denver, Colorado (1941); he received the doctor of chiropractic degree from Western States Chiropractic College in Portland, Oregon (1942), and from that same college he received the bachelor of therapeutic arts (1948). He also received degrees in naturopathy

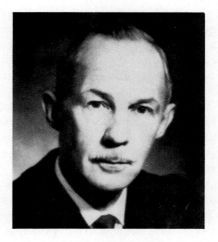

Figure 3-10. A. Earl Homewood.

(Philadelphia College of Naturopathy, 1953) and law (Blackstone School of Law, Chicago, 1960).

From 1945 to 1980, Homewood held various faculty and administrative positions, including president, at Canadian Memorial Chiropractic College, Los Angeles College of Chiropractic, and the Western States Chiropractic College. His writings include *Neurodynamics of the Vertebral Subluxation,* (1962) *Chiropractic and Care, Chiropractic and the Law,* and numerous articles in chiropractic journals.

Homewood continued to use D. D. Palmer's terms, innate and universal intelligence, when referring to the body's ability to heal itself. He explicitly agreed, however, with Carver's abnormal curves of the spine, rather than Palmer's single-segment concept of subluxation. In Homewood's opinion, Palmer's primary concept was that subluxations cause an excess of efferent nerve impulses. A subluxation is not a partial dislocation that impinges on a nerve; the problem is that excessive motor nerve impulses cause contraction of muscles, resulting in tenderness and pain. The mechanism of that excessive nerve function is irritation caused by imbalanced muscular contraction.

Homewood wrote that a disturbed neural supply via the reflexes is the cause of disease, reminiscent of the 19th-century theory of spinal irritation as a cause of disease. According to that concept, a disease in the liver, for example, could be caused by abnormal innervation of the organ. Homewood noted that all organ-systems are connected via the nervous system, and therefore all organs are functionally interrelated. Those relations were described by Homewood as reflexes, which include viscerosensory, viscerovisceral, somatovisceral, and psychovisceral reflexes. Like Carver, Homewood attempted to integrate observation and reproducibility into his models in a scientific fashion.

C.O. Watkins

C. O. Watkins (Fig. 3–11) was born in Eagle Grove, Iowa, in 1909. He was the founder of one of the first accrediting associations for chiropractic education, held numerous political positions in chiropractic, and was the editor and publisher of an early periodical, *The Chirolite,* from 1929 until 1941. C. O. Watkins' role in the development of chiropractic science was primarily political. Although he did not actively participate in scientific inquiry himself, he wrote (Watkins, 1944) and lectured extensively on the need to critically investigate chiropractic as a science. He was one of the first chiropractic spokespersons to challenge the need for vitalism of any kind in chiropractic (Keating, 1987). In both a temporal and philosophical sense, Watkins followed Carver (see Fig. 3–1).

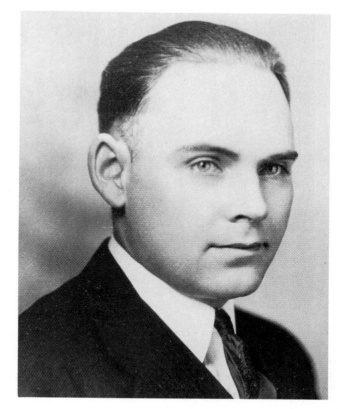

Figure 3–11. C. O. Watkins.

Joseph Janse

Almost from the time of the inception of chiropractic, there were two large schools—the Palmer College of Chiropractic in Davenport, Iowa, and the National School of Chiropractic in Chicago, Illinois. Joseph Janse (Fig. 3–12) was the president of National College from 1945 to 1980. In that influential position, Janse combined the metaphysical concept of innate (Janse, 1975) as expressed by D. D. Palmer and the naturalism of Carver into a mechanistic philosophy of chiropractic.

Joseph Janse was born August 1909 in Middleburg, Holland. After receiving higher education in Utah (1930–1933), he graduated from the National College of Chiropractic in Chicago and joined the faculty that same year (1938). A few years later, he was appointed president of National College. Janse lectured and presented papers extensively at conferences, symposia, and meetings. He was a coauthor of the text *Chiropractic Principles and Technic* (1947). Janse enthusiastically encouraged and assisted scientific understanding of chiropractic. In addition to his own efforts, he provided facilities and support for Fred Illi's anatomic investigations.

Janse's conception of the subluxation did not differ substantially from that of D. D. Palmer. In practical terms, according to Janse, a subluxation oc-

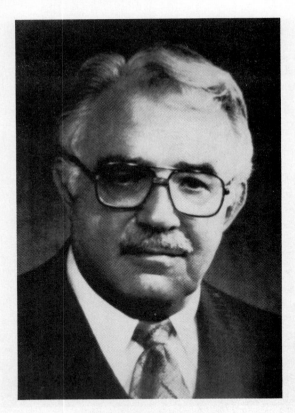

Figure 3–12. Joseph Janse.

curs when normal motion is exceeded and osseous movement causes pressure on a nerve. The essential feature of a subluxation is that the vertebra is relatively fixed in its abnormal position and no longer takes part in the normal movements of the spine. If a vertebra possesses normal mobility, it is not considered to be subluxated. The cure of disease by adjustment of subluxated vertebrae is therefore accomplished by the conversion of rigid segments into movable units.

Janse's European origins may have influenced his mechanistic view of chiropractic philosophy. At any rate, it can be noted that after Janse, further development of this branch of chiropractic occurred primarily in Europe. Discussion of the development of traditional chiropractic philosophy will be completed by describing the contributions of the Europeans Illi and Gillet.

Fred W. Illi

Fred W. Illi (Fig. 3–13) was born in Switzerland in 1901. Illi received his chiropractic degree from the Universal Chiropractic College in Pittsburg, Pennsylvania (1927). Among other accomplishments, Dr. Illi was founder–director of an institute for the study of clinical biomechanics in Geneva, Switzerland, and published findings of himself and co-workers (Illi, 1951) pertaining to spine and pelvic mechanics.

According to Illi, chiropractors are the practitioners who are most competent at locating and correcting common disturbances of the human spine to reestablish normalcy of function. Like Janse, Illi thought that humans are prone to structural disturbances of the spine caused by erect posture and the change of the spine from a horizontal to a vertical weight-bearing position.

Illi asserted that one of the primary results of the change in posture was freely moveable sacroiliac joints, which are subject to immense stresses. Subluxation of the sacroiliac joint is present when the articulating surfaces of the joint are misaligned. When that happens, there is a unilateral shifting of the pelvis. If that functional change continues it becomes structural and may result in herniation of the intervertebral disks at spinal segments above the pelvis. Symptoms of the herniation include backache and unilateral sciatic neuralgia. An additional predisposing condition to suffering from vertebral subluxations is the reduction in general physical activity by humans in the modern world, with a consequent reduction in spinal health and decreased ability to withstand the forces of gravity.

Illi also directly addressed the relationship between the allopathic medical community and chiropractic. In a letter to the Swiss government, he wrote that the diagnostic terms *rheumatism* and *neuralgia* are used as catchall terms by the medical profession with no substantial knowledge of the basic etiology.

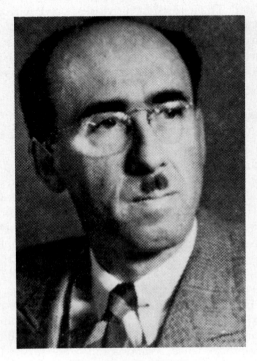

Figure 3–13. Fred W. Illi.

He asserted that most frequently the conditions described by those terms are caused by distortions resulting from spinal and pelvic mechanical dysfunctions. The primary task of the doctor of chiropractic consists in reducing those distortions of the pelvis, spine, and occiput. Illi recommended that chiropractic be considered the proper form of therapy for those conditions.

Henry J. Gillet

The European mechanistic approach to chiropractic research was also diligently pursued by Gillet and his co-workers in Belgium. Henry J. Gillet (Fig. 3–14) was born in Winnipeg, Canada, May 23, 1907. He graduated from the Palmer School of Chiropractic (1928), and opened a private office in Brussels, Belgium, where he practiced chiropractic for the next 48 years. He was a writer, researcher, private practitioner, and lecturer who contributed many anatomic and biomechanical theories to the science of chiropractic.

Gillet (1952) analyzed the subluxation into its component features, and concluded that the term *fixation* is more accurate than subluxation as descriptive of the clinical phenomenon with which the chiropractor deals. He did not consider fixation to be completely accurate as a term, however, because vertebrae are not normally fixed or ankylosed to each other; there is, instead, a reduction of mobility caused by varying degrees of dysfunction of the articular soft tissues, muscles, ligaments, or synovial

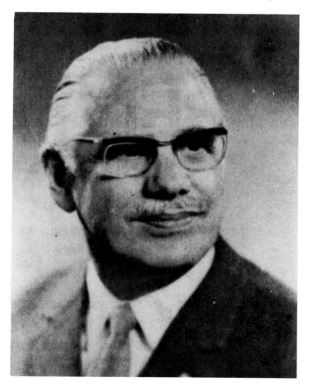

Figure 3–14. Henry J. Gillet.

bursae. Gillet studied both the contributions of the various soft tissues to dysfunction and the amount of dysfunction present by means of motion studies and laid the groundwork for many current investigations.

Skeptical Inquiry as the Distinguishing Feature of Science

As the founder of chiropractic, D. D. Palmer contributed chiropractic's two key components or principles: (1) an untestable metaphor for self-healing and (2) a testable principle that describes a relationship between anatomic structure and nervous system activity. Although D. D. Palmer apparently ignored the differences between these components, his vitalistic successors did not.

B. J. Palmer, R. W. Stephenson, and W. D. Harper made use of biologic principles of their times to support their vitalistic premises. But even though careful observations and documentation were abundant in much of the work of those individuals, there was never a hint of skeptical inquiry in their studies or writings. The wisdom of ''innate intelligence'' was never questioned and publications and investigations began with a dogmatic, vitalistic premise.

The six philosophers beginning with Carver demonstrated the rudiments of critical thinking about chiropractic science, philosophy, and art. They all supported unbiased inquiry into their models and supported and encouraged a certain amount of critical investigation into the chiropractic principle. All but Watkins, however, accepted and perpetuated D. D. Palmer's metaphor of self-healing. Although the others were somewhat critical, they were not uncomfortable with this vitalistic premise. Watkins, on the other hand, consistently called for mainstream science and scholarly activity within the profession. For their part, these original chiropractic scientists contributed to the model-building movement within the rest of the academic and health-care fields that is evident in chiropractic today.

Role of Philosophy in Chiropractic's Survival

Two fundamental principles run as threads through the vitalist and science paths of chiropractic philosophy, one primary and the other secondary. The primary principle is that healing is done by the patient. The secondary principle is that chiropractic care consists of adjusting subluxations of the spine by hand only. Chiropractic is a specific type of health care characterized not by ailment treated but by method of treatment. A corollary to the second principle, described D. D. Palmer, is that the chiropractor adjusts all dysfunctional joints of the body, not just those of the spine (Palmer, 1910). An alternative to the restriction of adjusting by hand only is the proposition that the chiropractor will use all methods to adjust subluxations except drugs and major surgery. This alternative has traditionally been associated with Janse and the National School in Chicago.

The first principle, patients heal themselves, is a vitalist concept; the life force, which is called *innate* in chiropractic, is considered to effect healing of a body with an intact nervous system. Subluxations interfere with normal function, and when they are removed the body heals itself. This is a vitalist concept because the belief in the innate power of healing implies that the living body has intrinsic recuperative powers and is, in that sense, different from other forms of matter. Philosophers of the vitalist trend vigorously elaborated the metaphysical concepts involved in the first principle. They paid little attention to mechanical explanations of chiropractic.

Traditional chiropractic philosophy is considered to consist of the philosophy of health care described by D. D. Palmer and his successors up to modern times. That philosophy has allowed chiropractic to remain distinct from other healing arts. Chiropractic was one of many types of health care that arose during the 19th century as part of a protest movement against orthodox medicine. The decrease in alternate forms of health care such as homeopathy and naturopathy can probably be attributed to their relative ineffectiveness compared with orthodox medicine as the latter advanced during the 1900s. Osteopathy began, like chiropractic, as a specific form of therapy. Possibly because it lacked a separatist philosophy, osteopathy eventually became allied with orthodox medicine.

A distinctive philosophy has proved to be the virtue of chiropractic, and it is probably the primary reason chiropractic has survived into modern times. If chiropractic is to continue it will probably do so only if it retains a distinct philosophical identity. Historically, chiropractic's identity has been shaped by both the vitalist and science paths of philosophical development. The essential chiropractic philosophy established by D. D. Palmer is present in both of these philosophical currents. The differences between the two are those of emphasis and are not irreconcilable.

Conclusion

The question must be raised of how a chiropractic separatist philosophy might fare in the modern sci-

entific world and, more specifically, in the rational academic, scientific world of modern health care as exemplified by orthodox medicine. If continued scientific investigation of chiropractic were to elucidate the underlying principles, would such an undertaking undermine chiropractic's philosophical tenets and destroy the identity of the discipline and so the discipline itself? Must chiropractic be prepared to abandon its philosophy, and its identity, to adapt to scientific discoveries? These questions, of course, cannot be answered with certainty. It is reasonable, however, to expect that if chiropractic is to survive in any form, its distinctive philosophy must be maintained, and there need not be any conflict between such a philosophy and the findings of science (Smallie, 1988).

References

Carver W. *Carver's chiropractic analysis.* Oklahoma City; Warden-Ebright; Published privately by the author. 1921.

Carver W. *Scientific catechism;* Oklahoma City, OK: Carver Chiropractic College 1924.

Donahue JH. DD Palmer and innate intelligence. Development, division and derision. *Chiropractic Hist* 1986;6:31–38.

Donahue JH. DD Palmer and the metaphysical movement in the 19th century. *Chiropractic Hist* 1987 7(1):23–28

Gaucher-Perslherbe PL. *La chiropractique: Contribution a l'historie d'une discipline marginalise.* Le Mans: France; 1986. (English translation by Elizabeth Weeks) unpublished ms.

Gibbons RW. The evolution of chiropractic: Medical and social protest in America, In Haldeman S, ed. *Modern developments in the principles and practice of chiropractic. New York: Appleton-Century-Crofts; 1980.

Gielow V. *Old dad chiro: A biography of D. D. Palmer, founder of chiropractic.* Davenport, Iowa: Bawden Bros.; 1981.

Gillett H. *Belgian chiropractic research.* Brussels, Belgium: Published privately by the author; 1952.

Harper WD. *Anything can cause anything, a correlation of Dr. Daniel David Palmer's Principles of Chiropractic.* 3rd ed. Pasadena, Texas: Published privately by the author. 1974.

Homewood AE, *The neurodynamics of vertebral subluxation.* Willowdale, Ontario, Canada: Chiropractic publishers; 1962.

Illi FW. *The vertebral column, life-line of the body.* Lombard, Illinois: National College of Chiropractic; 1951.

Janse J et al. *Chiropractic principles and technic;* 2nd ed. Chicago, Illinois: National College of Chiropractic 1947.

Janse J. History of the development of chiropractic concepts; chiropractic terminology, pp 25–42. In Goldstein M, ed. NINCDS Monograph No. 15, The research status of spinal manipulative therapy, U.S. Department of Health, Education, and Welfare; Washington, DC. 1975.

Keating JC Jr. and Claude O. Watkins: Pioneer advocate for clinical scientific chiropractic. *Chiropractic Hist* 1987; 7(2):11–15.

Keating JC and Mootz RD. The influence of political medicine on chiropractic dogma: implications for scientific development. JMPT. 1989; 12(5):393–397.

Korr IM, ed. *The neurobiologic mechanisms of manipulative therapy.* NY: Plenum Press; 1978.

Lomax E. Manipulative therapy: A historical perspective from ancient times to the modern era. In Goldstein M, ed. *The research status of spinal manipulative therapy.* NINCDS Monograph No. 15, U.S. Department of Health, Education, and Welfare Washington, DC, 1975.

Mootz RD and Keating JC. The chiropractic tradition, what was medicine's role? *ICA Int Rev Chiropractic* 1989; July/August: 53–57.

Palmer BJ. *The Subluxation Adjustment Specific.* Davenport, Iowa: Palmer School of Chiropractic; 1934.

Palmer BJ. *Palmer's law of life,* Davenport, Iowa: Palmer School of Chiropractic: 1958.

Palmer DD. *The Chiropractor,* Davenport, Iowa: Palmer School of Chiropractic: 1904–1906

Palmer DD. *The chiropractor's adjuster, the science, art and philosophy of chiropractic.* Portland Ore.: Portland Printing House; 1910.

Smallie P. *The opening of the chiropractic mind.* Stockton, CA: World-wide books; 1988.

Stephenson RW. *Chiropractic textbook.* Davenport, Iowa: Palmer School of Chiropractic; 1927.

Still AT. *Osteopathic research and practice.* Kirksville, Mo: Published by the author: 1895.

Strang, VV, *Essential principles of chiropractic.* Davenport, Iowa: Palmer College of Chiropractic: 1984.

Terrett AGJ. *The genius of D. D. Palmer. J Austral Chiropractic Assoc* 1986; 16:150–158.

Terrett AGJ. The search for the subluxation: An investigation of medical literature to 1985. *Chiropractic Hist* 1987; 7(1):29–33.

Wardwell WI. Before the Palmers: an overview of chiropractic's antecendents. *Chiropractic Hist* 1987;7(2):27–34.

Watkins CO. *The basic principles of chiropractic government.* Sidney, Australia: Published by the author; 1944.

Contemporary Chiropractic Philosophy

Reed B. Phillips
Robert D. Mootz

- **CHIROPRACTIC PHILOSOPHY OR PHILOSOPHY?**
- **MATERIALISM: THE ORIGIN OF CHIROPRACTIC'S TESTABLE PRINCIPLE**
- **HOLISM: THE ORIGIN OF CHIROPRACTIC'S UNTESTABLE METAPHOR**
- **THE CHIROPRACTIC DISTINCTION**
- **TRADITIONAL VERSUS CONTEMPORARY CHIROPRACTIC PHILOSOPHY**

- **AN APPLIED CHIROPRACTIC PARADIGM**
- **BENEFITS OF A RATIONAL CONSENSUS-BASED PARADIGM**
- **THEORY AND COHERENCE OF PURPOSE**
- **THE RATIONAL MODEL OF CONTEMPORARY CHIROPRACTIC**
- **CONCLUSION**
- **REFERENCES**

Truth is the object of philosophy,
But not always the object of philosophers.
—John Churton Collins

Contemporary chiropractic philosophy finds its roots in the dynamics of the mind–body struggle. It recognizes and respects the power of the unknown, accepts the limits of science, but also recognizes the role that critical scientific inquiry plays in the acquisition of new knowledge. This philosophy provides a clear identity for chiropractic art and science. Chiropractic philosophy has no fear of acceptance by or absorption into the mainstream; rather, it seeks integration into the greater world of philosophy and science, encouraging social acceptance and duly deserved benefits.

Chiropractic Philosophy or Philosophy?

The origins of traditional chiropractic philosophy can be found in the dualistic ontology of vitalism versus materialism. Despite claims of uniqueness from some chiropractic traditionalists (Stephenson, 1927; Barge, 1988), a perusal of philosophic writings re-veals antecedents to concepts such as universal and innate intelligence, adaptation, harmony, and the state of ''dis-ease'' resulting from imbalance or interference in these forces. In Hall's (1969) writings on the *Ideas of Life and Matter,* he discusses the formulations of life–matter that began with the early Greek philosophers. The very roots of vitalism stem from Plato's view that life is a nonmaterial entity imposed on matter, causing it to display life-as-action. The opposing mechanistic perspective suggests that the increasingly complex organization of higher life forms permits the appearance (or emergence) in them of new modes of life with new functions and behavior.

The imposition of force on matter as described by Stephenson (1927) in his list of *Thirty-three Principles* is akin to the formulations discussed by Hall. The concept of a universal intelligence (an all-pervading energy) is a common assumption of materialism according to Collingwood (1924, p. 167). If one ponders the ''intelligence'' of universal intelligence, then the concept of a teleologic principle found in the philosophy of holism becomes prominent. The relationship between life and matter is a philosophical entanglement founded in antiquity, formulated in metaphysical constructs, and expressed in philosophical materialism and holism.

When D. D. Palmer drew upon 19th-century metaphysics, philosophy, and science in the articulation of his perspective of health, disease, mind, and body, he laid his foundations on the deterministic constructs of holism and materialism (Donahue, 1987).

Weiant's (1981) description of five classic disciplines of philosophy helps put Palmer's chiropractic philosophy in perspective. *Ontology* attempts to evaluate the nature of reality. Idealism (vitalism) suggests that thought is an entity that creates and sustains matter. On the other hand, the materialist (mechanist) believes that thought is a by-product of physical events (i.e., consciousness is the result of neurochemistry of the brain). Either view by itself can be termed monistic. The dualist would argue that both realities can occur. Holism can be applied as either a vitalistic or a dualistic concept.

The remaining disciplines include *epistemology*, which examines the nature of human knowledge; *ethics*, which is concerned with the nature of right and wrong; *aesthetics*, which examines beauty; and *logic*. Establishing truth in ontology, epistemology, ethics, and aesthetics can only be accomplished by consensus. Agreement can be reached through common belief, experience, culture, or disposition. But the absoluteness of any construct within these domains cannot be "proved" or "disproved."

The final discipline, logic, attempts to explore the nature of "correct inference." By the use of deductive and/or inductive reasoning, any given consistent premise can lead to the same conclusion with application of an identical reasoning algorithm. The Renaissance saw development and refinement of logic with the inclusion of organized skepticism as a means to test the soundness of a logical conclusion. The addition of testing (or experimentation) gave birth to a new algorithm, the scientific method. Contemporary chiropractic philosophy is best understood within the context of those components that are testable (materialism) and those that are not (vitalism or holism).

Materialism: The Origin of Chiropractic's Testable Principle

The essence of materialism is the assertion that an indifferent substrate is behind the various facts that are observed. Materialism seeks to understand the nature of the universe and the mechanisms that account for changes. Materialism can be based on the assumption of an all-pervading energy, as opposed to the presence of some "universal essence" (Ledermann, 1970, p. 3). Ledermann illustrates the energy principle in the medical model by noting that

illness is explained as "an energy block preventing an exchange of energy between molecules; treatment would consist of removing such a block." In chiropractic, the block would be "subluxation" and the energy, "innate intelligence." The difference is that energy ought to be identifiable and measurable, whereas "intelligence" implies being and consciousness and can never be quantified mechanistically. The role of innate intelligence in healing therefore can be neither supported nor refuted.

Materialism is mechanistic. All explanations of life–matter relationships are based on natural laws. The secrets of life are carried in the chemical substances of DNA; the function of thinking is a neurochemical process. In chiropractic, the mechanistic (or testable) principle is that a spinal adjustment removes a subluxation and thereby affects physiologic function. This mechanistic principle is inherently quantifiable and can, therefore, be operationally defined and measured. This aspect of the chiropractic philosophy lends itself to the critical inquiry of the scientific process. The adjustment serves as the independent variable, subluxation is a mediating variable, and a change in physiologic function is therefore the dependent variable. All the while it is acknowledged that there is some as yet unmeasurable commodity of energy that drives the machine. This formulation creates a tangible, testable hypothesis. In this process, new knowledge is gained, but absolute truth is never attained. Materialism and its mechanistic procedures fail to explain the purpose behind the life–matter or mind–body relationship, nor does it try to. Chiropractic's mechanistic principle is merely the way in which the clinician and scientist can describe and investigate that which is observed on his or her patients (Keating and Mootz, 1987).

Holism: The Origin of Chiropractic's Untestable Metaphor

Holism is a philosophical approach to the integration of body, mind, and spirit. Within it there is recognition that health depends on obedience to natural laws and that deviation from these laws can result in illness. Holism is based on the philosophy of teleology, which asserts that there is a design or purpose in nature. An idealistic or vitalistic component can be seen in teleology. Based on the vitalism and metaphysics of his time, D. D. Palmer provided chiropractic a teleologic metaphor when he expounded the concept that there is a "universal intelligence" that is manifest in living things as an "innate intelligence," which provides purpose, balance, and direction to all biologic function (Palmer, 1910).

The classic medical concept of homeostasis also has its roots in the teleology of holism. Ledermann (1970) describes the application of holistic philosophy to medicine:

> Psychotherapists and physicians as well as surgeons who treat patients for physical ailments rely on the holistic response from the mind or the body. The stimulation whether by word or by drug or by any other physical agent is intended to call forth a whole-making result, which is the same sort of result which is present when mind or body answer to the ''normal'' stimuli which arise from within it or which arrive from without. The centers of regulations within the central nervous system and the effectors which are connected with these centers in the different organs all point to the existence of a holistic principle which is manifest throughout the body and mind. (p. 24)

The great advances in 20th-century medicine, however, have usually come from the mechanistic application of the scientific method (i.e., antibiotics for infectious disease). This in turn has reinforced the mechanistic philosophy in typical medical practice, thereby suffocating any significant widespread emphasis on holism. Unfortunately, this reductionist approach has failed to provide the answers to the chronic degenerative diseases. An increased emphasis on holistic philosophy by the chiropractor may be part of the reason why patients with degenerative disease seek out chiropractic care.

The concept of a holistic agent is difficult to approach with scientific methodology. Like ontology, it cannot be measured, tested, or operationally defined. Holism defies current methods of mechanistic determinism and reductionism because it is not finite. Yet in practice, physicians implicitly rely on the presence of a holistic power in their patients:

> They cannot measure this power in units, but they attempt to gauge its strength. A surgeon for instance who envisages a major operation on a patient must assess this person's capacity to stand up to the strain of the operation, and he must therefore estimate his vitality, his holistic power. Any doctor is concerned with the holistic recuperative power of his patients. (Ledermann, 1970, pp. 34–35)

Yet, holism can be taken to a dogmatic extreme. If trusted implicitly, the holistic application of any method of natural healing may fail to prevent illness or restore health. In the presence of a viable non-holistic alternative, contemporary society dictates the application of such an approach when natural methods are insufficient. As Ledermann (1970, pp. 32–33) states, ''the unspecific approach is thus limited, and it is the duty of the therapist to assess each patient's condition and to apply specific measures, based on the mechanistic–materialistic approach, if necessary.'' A *complete* reliance on a holistic universal intelligence entails dogma and is not acceptable in current chiropractic philosophy or practice. Figure 4–1 illustrates both the testable materialistic component and the untestable metaphor that make up chiropractic philosophy.

The Testable Principle

Chiropractic Adjustment
↓
Restoration of Structure Integrity
↓
Improvement in Health Status

Materialistic:

- operational definitions possible

- lends itself to scientific inquiry

The Untestable Metaphor

Universal Intelligence
↓
Innate Intelligence
↓
Body Physiology

Vitalistic:

- origin of holism within chiropractic

- cannot be proven or disproven

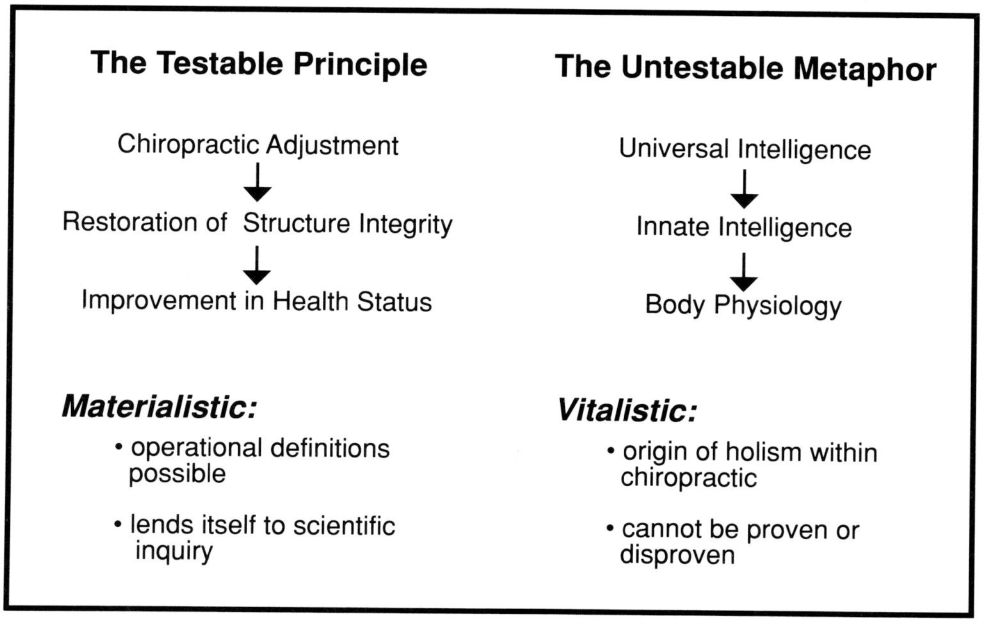

Figure 4–1. Chiropractic's dualistic philosophy.

The Chiropractic Distinction

Philosophy has been an integral part of chiropractic from its inception. Although chiropractic shares much with other health-care professions, its emphasis on and application of philosophy have been in intense contrast to modern medicine. In addition, chiropractic philosophy gravitates toward the naturopathic approach to health care (Black, 1988). By comparison, the allopathic model suggests that disease is the result of an environmental agent's virulence overwhelming the host organism. The appropriate solution is to counter the environment agent, as in the example of countering a bacterial infection with an antibiotic. Because the cause is environmental in nature, the solution is to counter the perceived environmental factor. The naturopathic approach provides a differing perception as to the nature of disease causation. As Palmer (1910) originally queried, why would one individual working in the identical environment become sick when the other remained healthy? The naturopath's answer is decreased host resistance. The appropriate solution would be to direct treatment at the host to strengthen it, regardless of the nature of any environmental agents.

The homeopathic model shares the concept of disease causation with the allopathic tradition, in which disease is viewed as the result of environmental virulence. The homeopath's solution, however, leans toward the naturopathic approach. The homeopath attempts to trigger a latent host response to the environment by providing a mild stimulus that parallels the disease from the environment.

Chiropractic philosophy and practice exhibit characteristics of holism and naturopathy. But what makes it distinct from these? Strang's (1984) biologic spectrum emphasizes a key difference with traditional perspectives. An organism is in a constant state of flux between the extremes of ideal functional wellness and death. In traditional medicine, an organism must cross an arbitrary threshold toward death on the spectrum (the clinically identifiable disease state) to merit therapeutic intervention. The chiropractor is more concerned with assessing the direction in which the organism is headed on the spectrum. So long as the movement is toward wellness, no intervention is required. If movement appears to be in the opposite direction, intervention is indicated even in the absence of clinically manifest indications of a recognized disease state.

Chiropractic's uniqueness when contrasted with naturopathy and osteopathy is less obvious. Although chiropractic shares with naturopathy a concern for proper diet, lifestyle, and a healthy environment, chiropractic emphasizes the importance of musculoskeletal integrity for the promotion of un-hindered neurophysiology. Further, chiropractic constantly observes the stricture *do no harm*, stimulating advancement of the most conservative approaches over other options. This therapeutic conservatism continues to foster mainstream chiropractic as a completely drugless (as well as nonsurgical) healing art. Although osteopathy shares an interest in the manual care of body structures with chiropractic, osteopathy as a whole has always embraced pharmacologic and surgical interventions as well. And if not by design, there is a major effort among chiropractic practitioners to communicate and explain in the most easily understood way what the chiropractor does to his or her patients.

Black (1988) asserts that society at large is displaying a return to vitalism and turning away from the mechanistic approach found in double-blind scientific trials as the sole source for new knowledge in health care. Bryner (1987) questions the value of vitalism in chiropractic philosophy, and Keating (1988) deplores the inability of the profession to deal with scientific and philosophical criticism. Total reliance on either philosophical basis represents extremism and impedes the understanding and balance that can accrue from the useful influences of each.

Traditional Versus Contemporary Chiropractic Philosophy

Both traditional and contemporary chiropractic philosophy display the dualism of testable principle (materialism) and untestable metaphor (holism) (Fig. 4–1); however, contemporary chiropractic philosophy displays a new perspective that escaped the early traditionalists. There is recognition that the untestable constructs of holism cannot be used to rationalize explanations for clinically observed phenomena. There is new appreciation for and understanding of the nature of scientific inquiry. Contemporary chiropractic philosophers understand that the scientific method is one of the valuable tools in the artillery of philosophy.

Modern-day chiropractic also recognizes that confidence in chiropractic methods is not a substitute for substantive description, observation, evaluation, and communication of chiropractic concepts to society at large. It is philosophy that will formulate the future of health care and chiropractic's role in it, and not the dogma and rhetoric that have characterized uncritical doctrines in medicine and chiropractic alike. Many of the self-proclaimed chiropractic philosophers of today continue to confuse medical bashing and chiropractic enthusiasm for philosophy. Even B. J. Palmer made the distinction between being excited and proud about what chiropractors do and philosophy (Palmer, 1924).

Contemporary chiropractic philosophy provides direction for the theoretical development and model building of the future. It retains the value of holism and its teleologic underpinnings and, at the same time, incorporates new knowledge formulated in a mechanistic, scientific approach. It is a dynamic philosophy that is responsive to historical contexts and cognizant of cultural influences. It is a philosophy that provides meaning and purpose for day-to-day practice and scholarly investigation, as well as rational input to social opinion and decision making.

An Applied Chiropractic Paradigm

The defining characteristics of any profession are the perspectives its members bring to the problems they face. This is what Kuhn (1970) termed *paradigm consensus*. Such consensus is evident when knowledge is applied to scholarly and practical problem solving in a systematic manner. To attain paradigm consensus, it is requisite that the majority of the professionals defined by the paradigm accept the process. A paradigm shift occurs when conflicting observations and experiences disrupt the familiar and the conventional. New insights arise to explain apparent contradictions. Finally, a more comprehensive perspective comes to the forefront and transforms traditional knowledge and resolves the conflicts. This new paradigm becomes the organizing framework for explorations in both research and practice.

Diversity within chiropractic stems largely from philosophical origins rather than from contradictions within the body of knowledge produced by legitimate scientific inquiry. In part, contradictory scientific findings are lacking because of the sparsity of research activity within chiropractic. Are philosophical contradictions equatable to scientific ones as an indicator of a fomenting paradigm shift in a Kuhnian sense? Or, is the establishment of a beachhead of science within chiropractic initiating a paradigm shift?

Coulter asserts that chiropractic may actually consist of several distinct paradigms (1990). A Kuhnian construct paradigm can be seen in Palmer's initial discovery of the therapeutic effect of a spinal adjustment. The initial development of a construct paradigm leads to the formulation of subsequent ones. Importance is ascribed to metaphysical paradigms in the beginning of any new science. Chiropractic's a priori assumption of the existence of universal and innate intelligence constitutes a metaphysical paradigm that provides a particular way of looking at the world. Coulter argues that although such presuppositions may be ontologic, as even D. D. Palmer recognized, they can also be the foundations for theoretical commitments. Over time, the value and usefulness of this paradigm diminish, and in

chiropractic, this has spawned abundant controversy. Next, Palmer's holistic conceptions make up a philosophical paradigm regarding the nature of health.

Chiropractic's philosophic paradigm differentiates between predisposing causes of disease and aggravating factors. This forms the basis of the chiropractic emphasis on "natural" remedies. Coulter also describes chiropractic as having separate sociologic and research paradigms based on the political and scientific behaviors the chiropractic profession had demonstrated. More interestingly, he characterizes chiropractic as an "alternative" paradigm, which along with allopathy has outlived the three other competing health-care paradigms of naturopathy, osteopathy, and homeopathy. Although chiropractic displays the characteristics of having a distinct paradigm(s), Coulter (1990) notes that this "has not lead to the research tradition generally associated with scientific paradigms."

Contemplation of contemporary chiropractic philosophy requires new consideration of the chiropractic paradigm. It is in an evolutionary flux. Philosophical disputes are likely to prevent professional consensus until scientific inquiry produces an adequate knowledge base for harmony. As the knowledge base expands, the paradigm will become more clearly defined and its articulation will be more precise. The evolving paradigm of contemporary chiropractic philosophy embraces the structure–function relationship, accepts the unmeasurableness nestled within holism, and seeks knowledge founded on application of the scientific method and grounded in rationalism. The new paradigm is a dynamic one, responsive to and interactive with its environment, much like the subject of the paradigm itself, the human body in health and disease.

The degree to which there is agreement on basic terminology and concepts reveals the extent of development of the paradigm. In chiropractic, the emergence of an accruing body of scholarly work is fostering consensus. Such principles as homeostasis, the capacity for self-healing, the centrality and vulnerability of the nervous system, the musculoskeletal expression of pathophysiology, and the impact of lifestyle on health remain the cornerstones on which the paradigm rests.

Benefits of a Rational Consensus-Based Paradigm

A paradigm represents patterns that become the cohering glue of a theoretical model. Theory is a belief that is used as the basis for action. But it is a belief based on documented observation of predictable phenomena. Theory is fundamentally interdependent with practice. It serves to harness communication between doctor and patient and lay the groundwork for confidence (by both) in the therapy administered. Theory is an abstract of experience and as such represents a systematized accounting for observed phenomena. The more developed the theory, the more useful it is clinically as it begets predictability in the nature of the relationship between different phenomena. The resultant control that is provided is of particular interest to the chiropractor, for theory will dictate the method of practice. The theory of a pinched nerve as a cause for back pain or a heart ailment will most likely provoke a different therapy than the theory of a torn muscle for back pain or vascular ischemia as a cause for heart pain. Theory invokes control.

Although chiropractic theory still longs for development and refinement, its philosophical and political evolution is stimulating the attainment of knowledge and a maturity that may very well help to resolve the remnants of disunity and professional conflict. Theory affects the way people comprehend and process information. The application of theory in practice creates a challenge to thinking, yielding new clinical skills and the purposeful application of the art.

Paradigm and theory guide education, research, and practice. As expertise accumulates within the profession, recognition follows that pries open the doors of competition with other disciplines for access to resources for continued theory development. Chiropractic's ability as a profession to remain autonomous and competitive for resource allocation is directly related to the power derived from its theoretical development. In the absence of a well-developed and *well-documented* theoretical basis, the future of chiropractic as a profession will be in the hands of anecdotal evidence alone.

The social justification for chiropractic services rests in part on the evidence that such services make a visible and valued difference. When practice characteristics are theoretically grounded, external challenges to chiropractic's efficacy can be countered through the explanatory and predictive power of theory. Well-developed theory becomes a normative pattern for justifying practice procedures and thereby serves as a source of internal control for the profession as well.

Theory and Coherence of Purpose

Coherence of professional purpose is closely linked with professional autonomy and internal control. The absence of coherence is evident when chiropractic doctors have difficulty agreeing on what it is they are about and how they plan to arrive at a stated purpose. In the absence of well-developed theory, arguments over purpose become meaningless and the danger of absorption into a more theoretically founded health-care system becomes very real. As Coulter (1990) argues, "the rhetoric of chiropractic should not be used to determine (its paradigm), a full analysis of all the competing claims should."

Theory development contributes to professional autonomy by allowing chiropractic doctors to better control and produce a valued societal goal. Theory directs the efforts toward fulfillment of that goal through communication and agreement both within the profession and with society at large. Accepting individual and professional responsibility for the development of purposeful chiropractic theory contributes to coherency of purpose. That purpose should be to provide a model for a rational approach to the practice of chiropractic.

The Rational Model of Contemporary Chiropractic

"Perspective" and "balance" are perhaps the two words that best characterize chiropractic's rational model. While maintaining conceptual intimacy with the holistic perspective, contemporary chiropractic embraces critical investigation and development in all aspects of its approach to health care. Despite insurmountable odds resulting from medical and social ostracism, chiropractic has become the second largest healing art in North America. It has attained governmental recognition for its practice, and, in the absence of virtually any external funding, it has developed and achieved governmentally accredited doctoral programs at chiropractic schools worldwide. The soundness of its philosophical foundations has, in part, contributed to its success.

Chiropractic's social and philosophic evolution has produced a model that incorporates diagnostic and therapeutic procedures that are safe, practical, reliable, and effective. This new rational model is sensitive to, and interactive with, the needs and expectations of patients, providers, scholars, and society at large. The model is a reflection of a scientifically based curriculum that continues to emphasize the importance of solutions over palliation.

The rational chiropractic model of health care is wellness oriented as opposed to sickness oriented. It is concerned with the person who is ill rather than with the illness that is attached to a person. This holistic mindset mandates personalized cooperative care. The approach is conservative, trusting in the inherent recuperative ability of the body, cognizant of the dynamics between lifestyle, environment, and health. Although the focus is on the person, chiropractic seeks to understand the cause of the person's illness in an effort to eradicate it, rather than palliate associated symptoms. There is recognition of the centrality of the nervous system and its intimate relationship with both the structural and the regulatory capacities of the body. The multifactorial nature of influences (structural, chemical, and psychologic), on the nervous system is appreciated. The chiropractic model is vigilant in balancing benefit and risk, and it recognizes as imperative the need to monitor progress and effectiveness through appropriate diagnostic procedures.

Of recognized importance is the need to prevent unnecessary barriers in the doctor–patient encounter. The chiropractic model is a patient-centered, hands-on approach intent on influencing function through structure. The chiropractic doctor is an early interventionist emphasizing timely diagnosis and treatment of functional, reversible conditions. Figure 4–2 illustrates the general components of the contemporary model of chiropractic.

Conclusion

Contemporary chiropractic philosophy embraces the best of old and new. It is a blend of experience, conviction, critical thinking, openmindedness, and appreciation of the natural order of things. It is composed of the tangible, testable principle that structure affects function, and the untestable, metaphorical recognition that life is self-sustaining and the doctor's aim is to foster the establishment and maintenance of an organism–environment dynamic that is the most conducive to functional well-being.

Contemporary chiropractic philosophy recognizes that it is a part of the greater body of philoso-

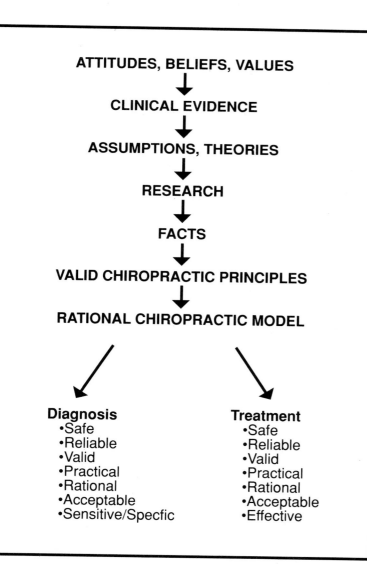

Figure 4–2. The rational model of chiropractic is founded on a belief system connected to clinical evidence and validated by the methods of science.

phy and science in general. It distinguishes between what is known and what is believed. It embraces the holistic paradigm of wellness while insisting on deterministic materialism for the establishment of valid chiropractic principles. It understands that the role of a philosophical foundation is to be the beacon for theoretical development. And it holds the patient's best interest as primary. Chiropractic will make its contributions to the further elucidation of the mind–body conflict and the holism–materialism debate as will the other fields within the sciences and arts. Yet it recognizes that this is primarily the domain of philosophy at large. Chiropractic philosophy teaches that failure to fill the void of knowledge within its own discipline carries the greatest risk that this void will be filled by scientists outside the profession who would then have a legitimate claim to chiropractic theory and practice.

Any health-care system works to serve the individual patient. As Strang (1980) pointed out in a lecture at Palmer College of Chiropractic in May 1980, the original franchise of any profession, by definition, is to put itself out of business. As dentistry succeeds in its purpose, we will have a world without cavities and gum disease, and a world with little use for the dentist. Chiropractic must not lose sight of its original franchise. Disease prevention and health promotion through structural integrity and harmony with the environment are chiropractic's purpose. We have a long way to go.

References

Barge F. Dr. Barge speaks for the record. In Peterson D, ed. *MPI's Dynamic. Chiropractic* 1988;6(25):3.

Black D. *Health at the Crossroads.* Springville, Utah: Tapestry Press; 1988.

Bryner P. Isn't it time to abandon anachronistic terminology? *J Aust Chiropractor's Assoc* 1987;17(2):53–59.

Collingwood RC. *Speculum Mentis on the Map of Knowledge.* Oxford: Clarendon Press; 1924.

Coulter ID. The chiropractic paradigm. *J Manipulative Physiol Ther* 1990;13(5):279–287.

Donahue J. D.D. Palmer and the metaphysical movement in the 19th century. *Chiropractic Hist* 1987;7(1):23–28.

Hall TS. *Ideas of Life and Matter,* vol 1. Chicago/London: University of Chicago Press; 1969:18–20.

Keating JC. Science, politics, and the subluxation. *AM J Chiropractic Med* 1988;1(3):107–110.

Keating JC, and Mootz RD. Five contributions to a philosophy of the science of chiropractic. *J Manipulative Physiol Ther* 1987;10(1):25–29.

Kuhn T. *The Structure of Scientific Revolutions.* Chicago: University of Chicago Press; 1970.

Ledermann EK. *Philosophy and Medicine.* Philadelphia: JB Lippincott; 1970.

Palmer DD. *The Science, Art, and Philosophy of Chiropractic.* Portland, Oreg.: Portland Printing House; 1910.

Palmer BJ. *Lyceum Address.* Davenport, Iowa: Palmer School of Chiropractic; 1924.

Stephenson RW. *Chiropractic Textbook.* Davenport, Iowa: Palmer School of Chiropractic; 1927.

Strang VV. *The Essential Principles of Chiropractic.* Davenport, Iowa: Palmer College of Chiropractic; 1984:20–22.

Weiant CW. Chiropractic philosophy: The misnomer that plagues the profession. *Arch Calif Chiropractic Assoc* 1981;5(1):15–22.

chapter 5

The Sociology of Chiropractic: Future Options and Directions

Ian Douglas Coulter

- **THE EARLY YEARS**
- **THE LATER WRITINGS**
- **THE CHANGING PERSPECTIVE**
- **THE LESSONS**
- **FUTURE OPTIONS AND DIRECTIONS**

The Chiropractor as a Specialist
The Chiropractor as an Alternate Healer
Evaluating the Options
- **CONCLUSION**
- **REFERENCES**

The sociological writings on chiropractic are interesting as much for what they illustrate about sociology as for what they teach about chiropractic. From the early 1950s until around the mid-1970s, these writings frequently reflected the same cultural bias against chiropractic as found in society at large. Furthermore, their portrayal of chiropractic had a tremendous influence on how chiropractic was perceived by other professions. This point is crucial in understanding the history of chiropractic, particularly in understanding its struggle for legitimacy. The writings of social scientists are extremely influential in this process of legitimation, and pejorative descriptions such as marginal profession, alternative profession, and psuedoprofession can adversely influence the legitimacy of professional groups. Few groups were as negatively labeled as chiropractic.

Sociological writings have a unique ability to act back on the very reality they set out to describe, and because of that, they have an ideologic immediacy that is lacking in most of the sciences. The purpose in this chapter is therefore not only to present the information provided by sociologists about the various aspects of chiropractic, but to present a critical context within which to view these writings.

The Early Years

The early sociological writings on chiropractic were characterized by an interest in the esoteric features of the profession rather than on giving a descriptive account (Coulter, 1983a). The focus was on the assumed marginality of chiropractic, its cultism, its professionalism or lack of it, and its deviant theory of disease.

The writings of Wardwell were the first to introduce chiropractic as a serious subject for sociologic study. His original article (Wardwell, 1952) introduced the concept of marginality to describe the status of chiropractic. By using this concept, he conveyed the fact that the chiropractor's role was not as well institutionalized as that of the medical physician. Chiropractors were judged to be marginal in five areas: (1) the amount of technical competence they possessed, (2) the breadth of their scope of practice, (3) their legal status, (4) their income, and (5) their prestige. In a later article, Wardwell (1955) examined the psychologic reactions of chiropractors to tension and frustration that result from a marginal role.

Wardwell's early writings (1952, 1955) had several major effects on the sociology of chiropractic. First, for some 30 years Wardwell's work was accepted as definitive, and few, if any, writers failed to acknowledge his work as their starting point. Even as late as 1970, writers such as Naegele (1970) would still state, ''My justification for concentrating on chiropractors is that Walter Wardwell's excellent study of this group is available.'' Second, the conceptualization of chiropractic as a marginal profession was adopted virtually without exception by sociologists (and other social scientists), and no substantive critique was offered of the premises underlying its use. Marginality became one of the accepted and self-evident "facts" about chiropractic. Subsequent investigations were therefore not aimed at examining marginality as a hypothesis but at illustrating some of its consequences. Finally, whether intended or not, the label reinforced negative connotations about the role of chiropractic. This consequence can be illustrated by examining some of the literature that followed Wardwell's.

The Later Writings

Offering an anthropologic account of the popularity and growth of chiropractic in Iowa, McCorkle (1961) conceded that chiropractic was the most "influential" of the alternative health-care systems but, nevertheless, titled his paper "Chiropractic: A *Deviant* Theory of Disease and Treatment in Contemporary Western Culture." Leis (1971) and Lin (1972), although focusing on professionalization, both chose chiropractic as an interesting case study because of its so-called deviancy. In the case of Sternberg (1969), chiropractic was studied explicitly for the purpose of examining how students of chiropractic cope with the problem of stigma. All of the studies mentioned portray chiropractors either as a group struggling toward professionalism or as a group that has acquired some but not all of the characteristics of a profession. Evans (1973a,b) continued this focus on what chiropractic needed to do to achieve professional status. Rootman and Mills (1974) provided an interesting analysis of the differences between American and Canadian chiropractors with regard to professional behavior. White and Skipper (1971) also took as their premise that chiropractic was a marginal profession and attempted to examine the factors influencing an individual's decision to engage in a chiropractic career.

The negative labeling of chiropractic reached a new level in two publications written by sociologists: Roebuck and Hunter (1972), who focused on health-care quackery, and Cowie and Roebuck (1975), who presented chiropractic as deviant. Both studies purported to establish that important labeling groups in the United States saw chiropractic as deviant or marginal; both therefore concluded that chiropractic had a deviant or marginal role in health care. Cowie and Roebuck went on to state, "It is ironic that even Roebuck and Hunter, who have delineated the labeling bodies in this section, have contributed to the deviant image of chiropractic by publishing an article which designates it as such to a scientific reading public" (p. 4).

Other terms used to describe (and label) chiropractic include *heterodox*, as opposed to orthodox (Hewitt and Wood, 1975; Baer 1984); *caste* (Anderson, 1981); and *outcaste* (Weisner, 1983). Cobb (1977), also viewing chiropractic within the perspective of anthropology, continued the same tradition of negative characterization by asserting "writers of every persuasion are unanimous in their contention that the chiropractic theory of disease causation has no scientific validity," and "Chiropractic has, over the years, taken on a variety of apparent professional trappings." Cobb undertook to explain how such a group could obtain legitimacy, and argued that a new era of pluralism has been the coattail on which chiropractic was riding.

During this period, Wardwell continued to publish on chiropractic (1962, 1976, 1979, 1980a–c, 1981), but his later writings explored, for the most part, changes in the status of the profession (from a marginal to a limited medical profession, as opposed to a parallel profession) and postulated possible directions in which chiropractic might go.

What was the impact of this body of studies on chiropractic? For the student of chiropractic, the results can be confusing and depressing. On the one hand, the body of literature in the social sciences gives very little factual information about chiropractic. As stated at the outset, the social sciences have not systematically investigated chiropractic on the basis of empirical data but have, instead, focused on the conceptualization of the role of the profession in society and in theorizing either about the causes or the effects of that role. Whatever the term actually used, the interest of social scientists has been in investigating chiropractic as a hybrid and an oddity within the health-care system. Those focusing on chiropractic have begun with the explicit (or implicit) assumption that this is indeed the case. The overall effect is to reinforce the impression that chiropractic is not a profession, or that it is a quasi-profession or a group on the way to becoming a profession, and that chiropractic is somehow unorthodox, deviant, or a caste. An investigation of the reasons why this happened is a fitting subject for the field of the sociology of sociology, but those reasons have been explored by Rosenthal (1981) and Coulter (1983a,b).

The Changing Perspective

The publication of a Sociological Symposium (1978, vol. 22) on chiropractic marked the beginning of a new era in the sociology of chiropractic. Although most of the writers still begin by acknowledging Wardwell, they also recognize that the earlier conceptualizations were not based on empirical data. Schmitt (1978), for example, examines theories about chiropractic in relation to utilization data. Moreover, writers such as Wild (1978) acknowledge that the focus on marginality is no longer appropriate and that it is in all likelihood a politically created marginality. In the same publication, Notz (1978) introduces the idea of chiropractic as a distinct paradigm.

In their work, Kelner and colleagues (1980) dispensed entirely with the earlier conceptualization and, in the most extensive study on chiropractic to that time, focused on an empirical description of chiropractic education, practice, and patients. A major departure was their use of random samples and extensive participation surveys. Their study also looked at the evidence for considering chiropractic as an alternative paradigm of health care by focusing on the doctor–patient health encounter and on the model of education. A series of articles resulting from this study explored in greater depth subjects such as the chiropractic curriculum (Coulter, 1981), the chiropractic model of education (Coulter, 1983b), the chiropractic patient (Coulter, 1985), and the chiropractor's role (Coulter, 1986b). Caplan (1984) advanced the alternative paradigm argument further by maintaining that if chiropractors become the musculoskeletal experts that medicine is increasingly willing to accept, they will in fact lose their distinctive health paradigm.

This perspective was further modified by Willis' work (1983) on medical dominance, the first to examine chiropractic within a Marxian framework. This work again avoids labeling chiropractic and focuses on the political attempts by medicine (including its use of labels) to exclude chiropractic. In focus and method, Willis' study represents a complete break with earlier sociologic writings. This work has been expanded in the work by Coulter (1991a) which focuses specifically on ideology and hegemony.

At the same time, a new perspective also was emerging in medical writing about chiropractic. This change was heralded by an editorial in the *American Journal of Public Health* by Silver (1980) supporting the first publication by that journal of an article on chiropractic (Yesalis et al., 1980). As Silver noted, it was becoming increasingly necessary for health planners and administrators to become familiar with chiropractic. Coulehan, in three articles (1985a–c), concluded that chiropractic could help physicians to understand the clinical art of medicine. In Canada, Kirkaldy-Willis and Cassidy (1985) published a series of articles reporting on the joint work of a chiropractor and an orthopedic surgeon over a 10-year period, and Imrie and Barbutto (1988) also published a book combining chiropractic and medical approaches to back care.

The Lessons

There are lessons to be drawn from a critical assessment of the way articles on chiropractic were written as well as from the information they provide about the nature of chiropractic itself. The first lesson is that extreme caution must be exercised in using these studies. In many instances, the conceptualizations of chiropractic are not based on empirical data and are little more than exercises in labeling. Furthermore, the labels themselves seriously distort the data that were assembled.

Second, the amount of good, reliable data on chiropractic, despite more than 30 years of writings, is extremely modest; however, the literature does provide startling evidence of one major change. From the late 1940s, when some chiropractors were being prosecuted and jailed for practicing medicine without a license, to the late 1980s, a radical transformation occurred in the way chiropractic was perceived. Social scientists were increasingly willing to look at chiropractic as an alternative form of health care, or as a speciality within the health-care system. In addition, chiropractic achieved widespread social acceptance. Increasingly, chiropractic is covered by various legislative statutes applicable to other health professions. Chiropractic services are now often covered by health insurance plans, and, in some instances, chiropractors have access to facilities from which they were once excluded (e.g., hospitals). It is therefore increasingly difficult to portray chiropractic as a marginal profession or as playing a marginal role in health care.

Whatever the status of chiropractic in the past, by the late 1980s it became clear that chiropractic had established for itself a secure niche within the health-care system. This does not mean it lacks opponents or that some fairly powerful groups, such as medicine, remain unwilling to accept chiropractic. But it does mean that, despite such powerful opponents, chiropractic has flourished. Its educational institutions are secure, they continue to attract large numbers of increasingly qualified students, the number of practitioners is growing, and significant achievements have been made on the political front. Whereas the survival of chiropractic was once problematic, the question now is simply what future role it will develop within the health-care system.

Future Options and Directions

Perhaps the liveliest debates within the sociology of chiropractic concern the question of where chiropractic is headed in the future. At the risk of oversimplifying this discussion, there are two answers to this question. Some maintain that, in the future, chiropractors will assume a role as health-care specialists. Others see chiropractors as providing broad-based alternative health care.

The Chiropractor as a Specialist

The position of chiropractors as specialists has been forcefully advanced by De Boer and Waagen (1986), who unequivocally state that "chiropractors are musculoskeletal specialists who primarily treat patients with back pain or other musculoskeletal problems." This is also the position of Wardwell (1980a–c), who has written more extensively on this topic than perhaps any other social scientist.

Wardwell maintains that chiropractic could, in fact, take one of five separate directions in the future. The first would be to fuse with medicine, either by joining it voluntarily, as did homeopathy and osteopathy, or by being taken over by medicine. A second possibility would be to practice under medical supervision, as do physical therapists. Third, chiropractic could simply disappear. Fourth, chiropractic could retain its present status as marginal or parallel to medicine. The fifth possibility is to become a limited medical profession such as dentistry, podiatry, and optometry.

For Wardwell, the fifth possibility reflects the reality of the way many chiropractors now practice. Furthermore, he sees this option as an attractive alternative with advantages to the health-care system:

> The reality is that chiropractors frequently refer patients to M.D.'s or other providers for conditions beyond their scope of practice, and that more and more M.D.'s are referring patients to chiropractors, though usually for a narrow range of neuromusculoskeletal conditions and especially if the patients do not respond well to medical treatments. Hence, many chiropractors already practice as limited medical practitioners in that they restrict their scope to practice a fairly narrow range of conditions that they believe they can help.
>
> Were chiropractors to adopt the "limited practitioner" model, they would continue to practice independent of physicians but give up their former cultist claims that they use a completely different theory of health and illness and can treat nearly all illnesses better than physicians.

Finally, Wardwell (1980b, p.436) states that "the most appropriate solution is for chiropractic to compromise its original principles and to become a limited medical profession."

Wardwell (1981) has also isolated specific social pressures that are encouraging chiropractic to go in this direction. These include the financial reimbursement practices of third-party payers, who typically pay for only a narrow range of chiropractic services and nothing else. Licensure requirements and public opinion reinforce this limited practice option. The presumed benefits of becoming a limited practitioner would include diminished medical opposition, increased recognition, more medical referrals, more generous third-party reimbursements, and perhaps greater public utilization.

Within chiropractic itself, there is considerable support for Wardwell's conception of the future of chiropractic. Writers such as Ford (1980), Keating (1988), Donahue (1986, 1987, 1988), and Nykoliation and colleagues (1986) have all, in one form or another, challenged the traditional philosophy underpinning chiropractic's claim as an alternative paradigm and have postulated more constrained roles.

The Chiropractor as an Alternate Healer

At the same time that many chiropractors and social scientists are recommending a retrenchment of chiropractic, a new group of observers is advancing the status of chiropractic as an alternative health-care paradigm and exhorting the profession to protect and preserve that status. Evans (1975), for example, focused on the chiropractor at the level of primary care, asserting that a unique patient–practitioner relationship positioned chiropractic in the future as a primary-contact healing profession. Coulehan (1985c) has more recently made the same argument by concentrating on the clinical art of chiropractic.

In their study, Kelner and colleagues (1980) paid particular attention to the healing encounter in chiropractic practice. This study was unique in that it involved participant observation and interviews of more than 600 randomly chosen patients. The study was able to document that, although musculoskeletal conditions formed the overwhelming majority of the conditions presented to the chiropractor, the care was greatly expanded into such areas as nutrition, exercise, weight, stress, and posture. Coulter (1986b), using empirical data from this study, argued that the more correct conceptualization of the chiropractic role was that of a limited alternative. This study also clearly established the importance, and place, or diagnosis within the practice of chiropractic. Further work by Kelner and colleagues (1981) also placed chiropractic among the other health practitioners.

Morinis (1980) argued that it was the philosophy of chiropractic, not the technique, that made it distinct. His concern, as an observer, was that chiropractors attempting to follow the specialist route would end up destroying the very basis of chiropractic. There is an increasing interest being shown in the philosophical basis of chiropractic (Donahue 1987, Keating 1988, Coulter 1989, 1990a, 1991b).

Perhaps the fullest discussion of this issue, however, is given by Caplan (1984). His position is distinct in that his discussion begins with the premise that chiropractic is a unique and potentially valuable paradigm of health care. What Wardwell sees as cultist, Caplan (1984) sees as a genuine alternative, intellectual paradigm: ''It seems that the chiropractic paradigm is not so much unscientific as it is a *different* science.'' Like Morinis, Caplan is worried that chiropractors are assisting in their own subjugation by giving up their unique paradigm; unlike Wardwell, he sees strong social trends that will make this paradigm socially attractive. Caplan sees the self-care and holistic health-care movements as two trends that are contributing to the demand for alternative health care and that embrace the ideas of chiropractic. Allied with this is the ongoing critique of allopathic medicine. With widespread popular support, chiropractic has the opportunity to establish itself as equal to, but distinct from, traditional medicine.

One might also argue that the model of education for chiropractic is distinct from that of medicine and introduces the student to a distinct paradigm (Coulter, 1983b). Indeed, it is incumbent that chiropractic education preserve and develop the chiropractor as a holistic practitioner (Coulter, 1986a). Chiropractors have traditionally operated as wellness practitioners, using a broad-based paradigm, and have been extensively involved in lifestyle counseling (Coulter, 1988). The recent consumer movements have now made the chiropractic paradigm very attractive, and chiropractic is well situated to take advantage of this social movement. The extent, therefore, to which chiropractic represents a distinct paradigm, perhaps an alternative one, has now become a topic for serious investigation (Coulter, 1990).

Evaluating the Options

In evaluating the two opposing predictions of the future of chiropractic, it is necessary to distinguish the context of the discussion. The likely outcome depends on whether or not the discussion is centered on the internal dynamics of chiropractic itself (its schisms, debates, disagreements, etc.), on the health-care system and the histories of the various health professions to date, or on the whole society and the broad social and cultural movements that are occurring.

For the present author, the latter context is the more useful. The health-care system does not work independently within society, and it is being drastically affected by economic and sociocultural factors such as the feminist, consumer, and holistic health/wellness movements. These factors are, in turn, in-terrelated. For its part, chiropractic is not immune from such social events. An internalist account of chiropractic, therefore, will give a very limited understanding of its future. Chiropractic's internal dynamics, however, will greatly affect the profession's ability to respond to social changes. If, for example, internal forces drive chiropractic in the direction of becoming a neuromusculoskeletal specialty at the same time the general public is seeking generalist, holistic practitioners, chiropractic could find itself left out of a movement embracing those ideas it has historically championed.

Chiropractors have traditionally treated neuromusculoskeletal problems but have expanded their interests into what is now termed wellness care. They have been involved at various times and in various places with a variety of health problems; however, these health problems have seldom been the life-threatening, pathologic conditions focused on by medicine. Even in the area of gastrointestinal problems, and the viscerosomatic area, chiropractors have focused on lifestyle-related problems (arising from stress, inappropriate diet, etc.). It may be argued then that chiropractors have been involved in wellness care as opposed to sick care. Few chiropractic patients die from the conditions presented to the chiropractor for treatment. From this perspective, the conflict between medicine and chiropractic, which at one level has been seen as an economic conflict (i.e., the result of economic competition), has been a case of false interpretation. Chiropractic has not competed successfully with medicine for illness care. The serious pathologies, traumas, and so on have always been treated predominantly by medicine and will, in all likelihood, continue to be so. Chiropractic has competed successfully in the area of lifestyle-related conditions (sprain and strain, posture, diet, stress, etc.). Because this area is also an area of increased interest to health-care planners and the public, and because its focus is inherently preventive, chiropractors are well situated for the future. As Coulehan (1985a) has noted, chiropractic philosophy, with its concept of holistic care (mind, body, and spirit), gives its clinical practice a decided edge over allopathic medicine in this regard.

The ultimate outcome will depend, in part, on chiropractic education. For much of its history, chiropractic has been more progressive in its educational program. For example, it has been much more involved in nutrition education than has allopathic medicine. Moreover, many aspects of chiropractic practice, some of which chiropractors performed almost intuitively (e.g., health promotion) are now disciplines in their own right. For chiropractors to keep a competitive edge in the very components of their alternative paradigm that makes them attractive, they will need a more systematic presentation of these subject matters in their education. Whereas in the past, chiropractic education has been driven in the direction of the basic biologic sciences for legitimacy, in the future it will have to turn increasingly to the social sciences, humanities, and other health sciences.

Conclusion

In modern society, professional groups and others are greatly influenced by the pronouncements made by social scientists. One has only to consider the tremendous impact Freudian psychology has had on how we experience and interpret psychologic phenomena to appreciate this influence. Over the past 30 years, chiropractic has been similarly affected by sociologists' writings about it.

First, it has been affected by the small number of social scientists who have shown any interest. Although this is changing, given the status of chiropractic as the second or third largest primary-contact health profession in North America, this neglect is worthy of comment.

Second, chiropractic has been affected by the conceptualizations of chiropractic proposed by the social scientists. Until very recently, even where the social scientists could be considered sympathetic (in the sense of accepting chiropractic as a worthy topic of investigation), their writings have been characterized by unacknowledged biases. Parts of the chiropractic paradigm have been labeled apriori as cultist and unorthodox, and not as the result of empirical investigation. (The extent to which chiropractic has been, or is, a cult would be an interesting research topic.)

Looked at within the history of ideas, the original concepts of Palmer form a consistent part of positivistic philosophy of the 19th century. Social scientists, therefore, have not been averse to advising chiropractic to give up its cultist elements, its unscientific premises, its unorthodox metaphysical beliefs, for positions more acceptable to groups such as medicine. Much work is still needed before a coherent, and more objective, sociologic account of chiropractic will be available. When it is available, it will document one of the more interesting stories in the survival and development of an alternative health profession and will contribute significantly to our understanding of the social processes that influence such survival.

References

Anderson RT. Medicine, chiropractic and caste. *Anthropol Quart* 1981;54:157.

Baer HA. A comparative view of a heterodox health system: Chiropractic in America and Britain. *Med Anthropol* 1984;8:151.

Caplan RL. Chiropractic. In Salmon JW, ed. *Alternative Medicines: Popular and Policy Perspectives.* New York: Tavistock; 1984.

Cobb AK. Pluralistic legitimation of an alternative therapy system: The case of chiropractic. *Med Anthropol* 1977;1:1.

Coulehan JL. A Chiropractic and the clinical art. *Soc Sci Med* 1985a;21:383.

Coulehan JL. Adjustment, the hands and healing. *Culture, Med Psychiatry* 1985b;9:353.

Coulehan JL. Hands on practice: An examination of the evaluation of clinical chiropractic. *Chiropractic Hist* 1985c;5:53.

Coulter ID. The chiropractic curriculum: A problem of integration. *J Manipulative Physiol Ther* 1981;4:147.

Coulter ID. Chiropractic observed: Thirty years of changing sociological perspectives. *Chiropractic Hist* 1983a;3:43.

Coulter ID. Chiropractic and medical education. A contrast in models of health and illness. *J Canad Chiropractic Assoc* 1983b;27:151.

Coulter ID. The chiropractic patient: A social profile. *J Canad Chiropractic Assoc* 1985;29:25.

Coulter ID. Chiropractic physicians for the twenty-first century. *J Canad Chiropractic Assoc* 1986a;30:127.

Coulter ID. The chiropractic role: Marginal, supplemental or alternative health care? An empirical reconsideration. In Coburn D and Torrance D, eds. *Health in Canada.* Toronto: Fitzhenry & Whiteside; 1986b.

Coulter ID. The patient, the practitioner, and wellness—Paradigm lost, paradigm gained. *J Manipulative Physiol Ther* 1990a;13:107.

Coulter ID. The chiropractic paradigm. *J Manipulative Physiol Ther* 1990b;13:5.

Coulter ID. The chiropractic wars on the energy within. *Am J Chiro Med* 1989;2:64.

Coulter ID. Of clouds and clocks and chiropractors: Toward a theory of irrationality *Am J Chiro Med* 1990c;3:84.

Coulter ID. Philosophy of science and chiropractic research. *J Manipulative Physiol Ther* 1991b;14:130.

Coulter ID. Sociological studies of the role of the chiropractor: An exercise in ideological hegemony? *J Manipulative Physiol Ther* 1991a;14:51.

Cowie JB and Roebuck JB. *An Ethnography of a Chiropractic Clinic: Definitions of a Deviant Situation.* New York: Free Press; 1975.

De Boer K and Waagen G. The future role of the chiropractor in the health care system. *J Manipulative Physiol Ther* 1986;9:225.

Donahue J. D. D. Palmer and innate intelligence: Development, division and derision. *Chiropractic Hist* 1986;6:31.

Donahue J. D. D. Palmer and the metaphysical movement in the 19th century. *Chiropractic Hist* 1987;7:23.

Donahue J. Dis-ease in our principles. The case against innate intelligence. *Am J Chiropractic Med* 1988;1:86.

Evans GD. Treatment technologies and publics. Their relevance to achieving professional status. *J Canad Chiropractic Assoc* 1973a;21:11.

Evans GD. A sociology of chiropractic. *J Canad Chiropractic Assoc* 1973b;21:6.

Evans GD. The role of the chiropractor at the primary care level. *J Canad Chiropractic Assoc* 1975;12:14.

Ford CW. As a man thinketh: Toward a new paradigm of chiropractic healing. *J Manipulative Physiol Ther* 1980;254:3.

Hewitt D and Wood PHN. Heterodox practitioners and the availability of specialist advice. *Rheumatol Rehab* 1975;14:191.

Imrie D and Barbutto L. *The Back Power Program.* Toronto: Stoddart; 1988.

Keating JC. Science and politics and the subluxation. *Am J Chiropractic Med* 1988;1:107.

Kelner M, Hall O, and Coulter I. *Chiropractors Do They Help.* Toronto: Fitzhenry & Whiteside; 1980.

Kelner M, Hall O, and Coulter I. Chiropractors and their competitors. In K. Lundy, B. Warme (Eds), *Work in the Canadian Context. Continuity Despite Change.* Toronto: Butterworths;1981:125.

Kirkaldy-Willis WH and Cassidy JD. Spinal manipulation in the treatment of low back pain. *Canad Fam Physician* 1985;31:535.

Leis GL. *The Professionalization of Chiropractic.* Ph.D. thesis, State University of New York; 1971.

Lin PL. *The Chiropractor, Chiropractic and Process: A Study of the Sociology of an Occupation.* Ph.D. thesis, University of Missouri;1972.

McCorkle T. Chiropractic: A deviant theory of disease and treatment in contemporary Western culture. *Hum Organization* 1961;20:20.

Morinis FA. Theory and practice in chiropractic. An anthropological perspective. *J Canad Chiropractic Assoc* 1980;24:114.

Naegele KO. *Health and Healing.* San Francisco: Jossey-Bass; 1970:105.

Notz M. Paradigm identification and organizational structure: An overview of the chiropractic health care profession. *Sociol Symp* 1978;22:18.

Nykoliation JW, Cassidy JD, Arthur BE, and Wedge JH. An algorithm for the management of scoliosis. *J Manipulative Physiol Ther* 1986;9:1.

Roebuck JB and Hunter B. The awareness of health care quackery as deviant behaviour. *J Health Hum Behav* 1972;15:3.

Rootman I and Mills DL. Professional behavior of American and Canadian chiropractors. *J Health Soc Behav* 1974;15(March):3.

Rosenthal SF. Marginal or mainstream: Two studies of contemporary chiropractic. *Sociol Focus* 1981;14:271.

Schmitt M. The utilization of chiropractors. *Sociol Symp* 1978;22:55.

Silver GA. Chiropractic—Professional controversy and public policy. *Am J Public Health* 1980;70:348.

Sternberg D. *Boys in Plight. A Case Study of Chiropractic Students Confronting a Medically Oriented Society.* Ph.D. thesis, New York University; 1969.

Wardwell W. A marginal professional role: the chiropractor. *Soc Forces* 1952;30:339.

Wardwell W. The reductions of strain in a marginal role. *Am J Sociol* 1955;61:16.

Wardwell W. *Limited, marginal, and quasi-practitioners.* In Freedman HE, Levine G, and Reeder LS, eds. *Handbook of Medical Sociology.* Englewood Cliffs, NJ: Prentice-Hall; 1962.

Wardwell W. Whither Chiropractic. *Digest Chiropractic Econ* 1976;18.

Wardwell W. Social factors in the survival of chiropractic. *Sociol Symp* 1978;22:6.

Wardwell W. Limited and marginal practitioners. In Freedman HE, Levine G, and Reeder LS, eds. *Handbook of Medical Sociology,* 3rd ed. Englewood Cliffs, NJ: Prentice-Hall; 1979.

Wardwell W. The present and future role of the chiropractor. In Haldeman S, ed. *Modern Developments in the Principles and Practice of Chiropractic.* New York: Appleton-Century-Croft; 1980a.

Wardwell W. The triumph of chiropractic—And then what? *J Sociol Soc Welfare* 1980b; 7(3):425–429, 436.

Wardwell W. A sounding board—Future of chiropractic. *N Engl J Med* 1980c;302:688.

Wardwell W. Chiropractors—Challengers of medical domination. *Res Sociol Health Care* 1981;2:207.

Weisner D. A caste and outcaste system in medicine. *Soc Sci Med* 1983;17:475.

White M and Skipper JK. The chiropractic physician: A study of career contingencies. *J Health Soc Behav* 1971;12:300.

Wild PB. Social origins and ideology of chiropractors: An empirical study of the socialization of the chiropractic student. *Sociol Symp* 1978;22:33.

Willis E. *Medical Domination.* Sydney: George Allen & Unwin; 1983.

Yesalis CE et al. Does chiropractic utilization substitute for less available medical services. *Am J Public Health* 1980;70:415.

II

Physiological and Biomechanical Principles

Chiropractic theory over the past 95 years has been a major focus of criticism and a slowly evolving process within the chiropractic profession. One of the major problems has been the difficulty of medical and chiropractic scientists, despite extensive research, to document the cause of back pain and dysfunction. Dr. Nachemson, Chief of Orthopedic Surgery in Goteborg, Sweden, as recently as 1985 stated that only 20% of patients with acute back pain can be given a precise pathoanatomic diagnosis. The breakdown between symptomatology and pathology is even more evident in patients with chronic back pain [Haldeman et al., 1988]. It is therefore not unexpected that many original theories explaining chiropractic results have not stood up to intensive research.

Research on the spine within both chiropractic and medical institutions has, however, become progressively more sophisticated, and current chiropractic theories are constantly being modified to reflect this research. The primary focus of these theories has been in three distinct but interacting fields: neurophysiology, spinal biomechanics, and pathophysiology.

Neurophysiologic concepts of importance to chiropractic theories are discussed in Chapters 6 through 11. Rauschning sets the stage by reviewing the anatomic relationships between neural elements and the vertebrae. His outstanding sectional anatomic photographs allow one to visualize the structures referred to in the remaining chapters. Classical chiropractic theory proposed by D. D. Palmer and B. J. Palmer related to nerve root compression. The understanding of the physiology of nerve root compression has, however, undergone extensive changes since the Palmers first discussed this process. Dahlin and his colleagues have been conducting research into the effects of nerve root compression for a number of years and present, in Chapter 7, a detailed discussion of current theory on the effects of compression on nerve roots and surrounding vascular and membranous structures. The majority of patients who present to chiropractors do so for pain. Recent changes in pain physiology and concepts presented in

Chapter 10 are therefore of major importance in understanding treatment offered these patients. Interaction between the somatic and visceral nervous systems has held particular interest to chiropractors and formed the basis for the theories of Homewood [1963]. Chiropractors in the past relied on certain osteopathic researchers such as Korr [1976] to justify these concepts. Modern research, by Sato and co-workers, has described many of the details of these reflexes and this is reviewed in depth in Chapter 8. Swenson in Chapter 9 describes how these reflexes have been investigated in the clinical setting and discusses some of the limitations of the clinical research done to date. The intense interest by chiropractors in these reflex studies is driven by a body of anecdotal observation and opinion that spinal abnormalities are capable of causing disturbances in visceral organ function and the general health of a patient. The research in support of this idea and the theories on which these opinions are based are described in Chapter 11 by Dhami and De Boer.

An understanding of spinal biomechanics has played an integral part in the development of chiropractic theory. The adjustment has always been considered the direct application of a force resulting in a specific mechanical response in the spine. It is therefore essential that biomechanical concepts be understood before chiropractic diagnostic and adjusting procedures can be applied. Moroney in Chapter 12, reviews the biomechanics of the cervical spine while Farfan, in Chapter 13, describes the biomechanical principles in the lumbar spine which are important in the genesis of spinal symptoms. Triano in Chapter 18 reviews the intricate relationship between these biomechanical principles and the physiology of both the normal and abnormal spine.

Research on the pathophysiology of specific spinal structures has advanced significantly over the past decade and has been incorporated into chiropractic theory. The three structures which have been most intimately discussed in the chiropractic literature are described in Chapters 15, 16 and 17. Bishop discusses in detail the structure and chemistry of the intervertebral disc and how it changes with aging and injury. Giles reviews the zygapophyseal joints as a source of pain and pathology, Cassidy and Mierau review the controversial area of sacroiliac joint structure, function and pathology.

After reading this section it should become evident that current chiropractic theory is dependent on an integral knowledge of the anatomy and physiology of the spine and its neural elements, the biomechanical relationship between vertebrae, and the pathophysiology of various spinal structures. As these chapters show, there remain significant gaps in both research and understanding in these fields that, it is hoped, will be satisfied in the future. Nonetheless, there is currently sufficient research to establish well-formulated theories on the mechanism of action of chiropractic care.

Scott Haldeman

References

Haldeman S, Shouka M, Robboy S. Computed tomography, electrodiagnostic and clinical findings in chronic Workers' Compensation patients with back and leg pain. *Spine* 1988;13:345–350.

Homewood AE. *The Neurodynamics of the Vertebral Subluxation.* Willowdale, Ontario: Chiropractic Publishers; 1963.

Korr IM. The spinal cord as organizer of disease processes. Some preliminary perspectives. *J Am Osteopath Assoc* 1976;76:89–99.

Nachemson AL. Advances in low back pain. *Clin Orthop* 1985;200:266–278.

chapter 6

Spinal Anatomy: The Relationship of Structures

Wolfgang Rauschning

- **METHODOLOGY**
- **VERTEBRAL COLUMN VERSUS SPINE**
- **EFFECT OF MOTION ON STRUCTURAL RELATIONS**

- **CERVICAL SPINE**
- **THORACIC SPINE**
- **LUMBAR SPINE**

The human spine is extremely complex, both with respect to its supporting structures and its neural elements and blood vessels. In addition, the various portions of the spine such as the craniovertebral junction, cervical spine, thoracic spine, lumbar spine, and sacrum are highly dissimilar. A systematic description of the plethora of the spine's morphologic features would clearly exceed the scope of an anatomic chapter geared toward the understanding of basic anatomic facts, which the author considers potentially significant for the practice of the readers whom this book addresses.

Several contributors to this textbook elaborate on aspects of spinal anatomy, pathophysiology, and biomechanics. The anatomy of the intervertebral discs and of the facet joints is here described only as far as the topographic relationships of the neurovascular structures are concerned. The systematic and descriptive anatomy of the spine is taught in excellent classical textbooks and scientific articles dealing with specialized morphologic topics.

Methodology

Modern computerized sectional imaging modalities such as x-ray computed tomography (CT), ultrasonography (US), and magnetic resonance imaging (MRI) have in the past decade prompted a great number of sectional anatomic investigations in which diagnostic scans are correlated with sectional anatomic images. The illustrations in this chapter have been selected from an image database of more than 18,000 images of the spine, all of which show undistorted relationships of the soft tissues to the bony structures. In addition to the normal anatomy in different planes in the neutral posture, the functional anatomic relationships are exemplified in physiologic postures and movements.

Conventional dissection, by definition, entails the destruction of layers of tissues, which inevitably leads to distortion of topographic relationships. Conventional histologic examinations necessitate fixation and decalcification, which leads to shrinkage and deformation of essential neurovascular relationships. The images in this chapter are cryosectional surface images from frozen cadaveric spines. As the whole torso or portions of the spine were frozen in situ, the relationships of the spinal soft tissues to the vertebrae were "frozen" in neutral postures or in typical and clinically significant functional positions. The spinal segments were also x-rayed and examined with a CT scanner in the axial, sagittal, coronal, or oblique planes. Specimens were then sectioned on a heavy-duty sledge cryomicrotome, using a surface cryoplaning technique developed by the author in 1977. Photographs of the leading surface of the block taken at submillimeter cutting height intervals render undistorted images in which structures can be recognized by their natural colors and texture. More importantly, the spatial relationships are preserved in every specimen.

Vertebral Column Versus Spine

For didactic reasons it may be advisable to distinguish between the vertebral column and the spine. *Vertebral column* designates the multisegmentally mobile osseoligamentous construct that has multiple physiologic curvatures in the sagittal plane. It renders stability and support to the trunk, head, and upper extremities and enables active mobility through a highly complex array of inter- and paraspinal muscles.

Spine as a term encompasses more than the musculoskeletal elements of the vertebral column. It houses osseoligamentous spaces that accommodate, protect, and transmit vital and delicate neurovascular structures. These spaces are the vertebral canal and the two foramina or *root canals* at each intervertebral spinal level. Root canal morphology significantly varies from one vertebral level to the next. These mobile conduits also display a wide and significant range of individual variations with respect to canal size and configuration.

Mobility and the pattern of motion vary greatly between various regions of the spine. Every spinal motion segment has a typical range and pattern of motion that is determined by the shape and three-dimensional arrangement of bony and articular surfaces, intervening discs, ligaments, and joint capsules. Motion is also determined and controlled by the insertion and origin of the muscles attaching to the spine and their mass, fiber composition, and orientation in space. Most mobile are the cervical spine and the mid- and lower lumbar spine.

Effect of Motion on Structural Relations

Movement of the vertebral column affects the size and volume of the vertebral canal and foramina (root canals). These canals contain the spinal cord and the lumbosacral roots of the cauda equina. Both the spinal cord and cauda equina are contained and ensheathed by the thecal sac, a tubular structure that is continuous at the foramen magnum level with the thecae of the skull. The dura mater spinalis continues into the dura mater of the skull (pachymeninx). The former is completely lined internally by the arachnoid membrane (leptomeninx) and contains the cerebrospinal fluid (CSF) in which the spinal cord and the cauda equina roots and some subarachnoid blood vessels float freely. The neural thecal envelopes are affixed to the vertebral column at the level of the neuroforamina, where a variable number of cauda equina roots converge toward strut-shaped infundibular expansions of the thecal sac, the root sleeves, or the root sheaths. Free intrathecal roots become ensheathed by the meninges in the foramen. Whereas the arachnoid membrane terminates at the medial border of the ganglion, the dura is contiguous with the capsule of the ganglion and then becomes the perineurium of the segmental spinal nerves.

This important point at which the CSF compartment terminates is best visualized by myelography; functional myelography displays the movement of the roots and the spinal cord inside the thecal sac. The spinal cord as well as the cauda equina roots moves anteriorly in the prone position and in flexion. They move posteriorly in the supine position and in extension. Lateral movement occurs in lateral bending and in the lateral decubitus position. Especially in the upper cervical spine, rotatory movement is induced to the spinal cord by the pulling effect exerted by the segmental nerve roots.

Although the intrathecal neural elements are mobile, the thecal sac is segmentally attached to the vertebral column by several important ligaments and membranes. Some of these are commonly known as the Hoffman ligaments. The thecal sac does not expand appreciably when intrathecal pressure rises because the dura is not very elastic, but the thecal sac and the root sleeves cannot resist compression. The size of the vertebral canal and its volume increase slightly in flexion and decrease in extension. Size and volume of the intervertebral root canals increase and decrease more dramatically in flexion versus extension. These volume changes are most pronounced in the cervical spine.

Epidural fat and epidural veins surround the thecal sac. A plexus of veins behind the vertebral bodies is somewhat arbitrarily called the anterior internal venous plexus; thinner and less voluminous veins underneath each lamina constitute the posterior internal spinal veins. The contents of the vertebral canal and the root canals can be conceived of as a hydraulic system in which the filling and emptying of the epidural veins and sinuses facilitate large and almost instantaneous variations in the volume of the canals.

Cervical Spine

In the upper cervical spine and craniocervical junction, the assimilation of the body of C-1 onto the body of C-2 forms the unique atlantoaxial motion segment in which roughly half of the rotatory movement of the entire cervical spine occurs. The atlantoaxial articulation, similar to the shoulder joint, lacks bony congruity and stability. Ligaments and joint capsules resist excessive motion. A true synovial joint is found between the lateral masses of the atlas and axis, between the anterior arch of the atlas and the odontoid process, and also between the transverse ligament (or, rather, the transverse portion of the cruciate ligament) and the dens. Far stronger than the transverse ligament and probably more important are the alar ligaments and the tectorial membrane which anchor the odontoid process directly to the skull base.

The tip of the odontoid process abuts the lowermost portion of the pons and most of the medulla oblongata with its vital nuclei (Fig. 6–1). Posteriorly, the commonly wide cisterna magna provides some spatial reserve for a translatory movement of the dens posteriorly. The posterior elements of the cervical spine are comparatively thin, elastic, and resilient. These elements include the ligamentum flavum between the laminae, sparse strands of interspinous process ligament, and the flaccid joint capsules.

The spinous processes of the cervical spine are short and usually have bifid tips. Contrary to many textbook descriptions and biomechanical concepts, there is no supraspinous ligament (Fig. 6–2). A midsagittal (median) septum of fibrous strands extends posteriorly in the midline and attaches to the strong, thick, yellow ligamentum nuchae. This ligament is

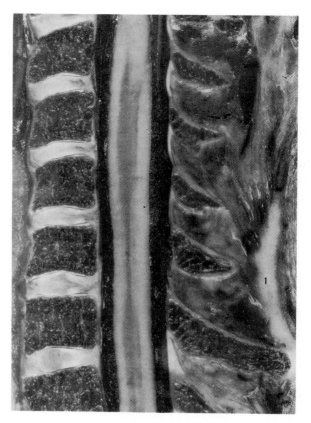

Figure 6–2. Midsagittal section through the mid- and lower cervical spine of a young female. The intervertebral discs display normal configuration and intrinsic architecture. Note the thick layers of the anterior anulus fibrosus, which is slightly bulging, and the thinner, straight posterior anular margins. The cerebrospinal fluid displays dark. Posteriorly, the short spinous processes are linked by the thin interlaminar ligamenta flava from which strands of connective tissue run to the thick, elastic ligamentum nuchae (*1*), which expands from C-7 (*2*) to the occipital tubercle. Note the absence of a supraspinous ligament in the cervical spine.

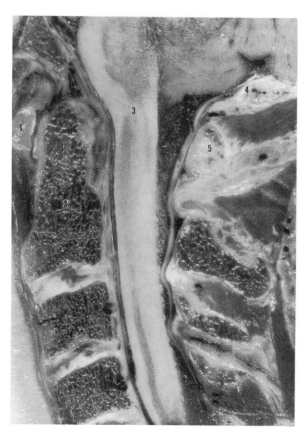

Figure 6–1. Midsagittal section through the upper cervical spine and foramen magnum of a 44-year-old male. There is moderate arthrosis of the joint between the anterior arch of the atlas (*1*) and the dens (*2*) and slight degeneration of the intervertebral discs. Note also the medulla oblongata (*3*), the atlantooccipital membrane (*4*), the posterior arch of atlas (*5*),

continuous with the superficial layers of the thoracic aponeurosis and runs from the spinous process of C-7 to the tubercle of the occiput. In the neutral position, the ligamentum flavum bulges slightly anteriorly. This bulge is more pronounced in extension and it decreases or disappears in flexion. The anterior wall of the cervical vertebral canal is perfectly straight in normal specimens. In extension, this wall displays no bulge from the discs, but a segmental ''shingling'' during retrolisthesis of the upper vertebra in relation to the lower vertebra caused by the obliquity of the facet joints, which induces translatory displacement by coupled motion.

In the cervical spine, the discs allow a sagittal sliding movement, but the uncinate processes effectively resist lateral translation. This might have deleterious effects on the vertebral artery, which is tightly held in the costotransverse foramina of C-3 to C-6. The vertebral artery runs through a knee-shaped bony tunnel in the lateral mass of the axis and curves around the lateral aspect of the highly mobile atlantoaxial joint. Hypermobility or instability at this level and/or osteoarthrotic lipping of the joint surfaces may erode the artery or cause arterial thrombosis.

Figure 6–3 displays meniscoid synovial folds in the facet joints of the midcervical spine. Although the morphology, innervation, and radiographic appearance of these folds or tags have been studied extensively, little is known about their function and their potential role in posttraumatic, degenerative

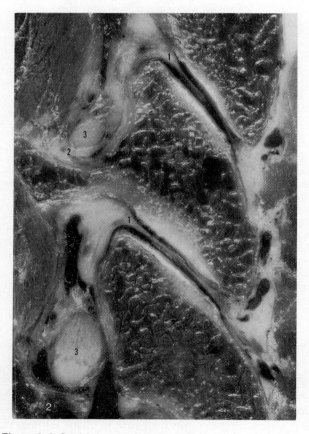

Figure 6–3. Sagittal section through the lateral portion of normal facet joints in the lower cervical spine. The articular processes are oriented at an angle of 70° to the horizontal plane. This obliquity accounts for the fact that, in extension, the vertebra above is forced to slide posteriorly (retrolisthesis) on the vertebra below. Typical for the middle and lower cervical spine are the meniscoid synovial folds (1), which emanate from the entire circumference of the joint capsules and project 2 to 3 mm toward the center of the joints. Anteriorly, the articular process is connected with the furrow-shaped transverse process (2). The nerve root and ganglion (3) lie immediately superior to this furrow.

and inflammatory neck pain. The author has observed significant posttraumatic changes such as fresh ruptures, entrapment, and late fibrosis of these meniscoids.

In the cervical spine below C-2, the segmental nerves have to pass a distance of about 2 cm from the piercing of the thecal sac to the tubercles of the transverse process. Whereas the lumbar nerves invariably curve around the inner and inferior border of the pedicle of the upper vertebra of each motion segment, the cervical nerves run over the upper or cranial aspect of the pedicle and continue laterally in an anteroinferiorly sloping direction on top of the transverse process. This process is a composite of the transverse process proper posteriorly and an assimilated rib equivalent (anlage) anteriorly. Both processes are connected lateral to the costotransverse foramen by the distally convex intertransverse bar. The cervical nerve passes in a slit between the scalenus muscles, which attach to the tubercles of the transverse process and the rib anlage process.

Figure 6–4 shows the relationships between the nerve root of C-6 and the vertebral artery in a specimen that had been frozen in marked flexion. Note the filling of the epidural veins which, rather than being a rete of veins, constitute venous sinuses that can fill and empty rapidly. Extension decreases the sagittal diameter of the cervical vertebral canal for two reasons. First, retrolisthesis of the upper vertebra of the motion segment pushes its lower endplate toward the unyielding spinal cord, which is "bound" anterolaterally by the roots that are affixed to the walls of the root canals by the ligaments. Second, in the neutral position the ligamentum flavum is in a state of tension similar to a stretched rubber band. In extension it retracts and thickens by volume redistribution, which occurs underneath the lamina. These dynamic effects of extension movement are even more dramatic in the root canals because the posterior translation of the lower endplate of the upper vertebra pushes and sometimes compresses the neural bundle against the anterior surface of the superior articular process.

The so-called "root" is a complex structure, composed of highly dissimilar structural and neurophysiologic elements: the root sleeve, housing intrathecal motor and sensory roots; the highly vascularized and pressure-sensitive dorsal root ganglion; and the postganglionic composite spinal nerve. At the ganglion level, the motor root is clearly discernible as a structure separate from the ganglion. Thus, pressure exerted on the "root" may trigger different neurodysfunctional phenomena, depending on which component of the root is compressed. Terms such as *root complex* and *root bundle* could be used to designate this complex composition of the root.

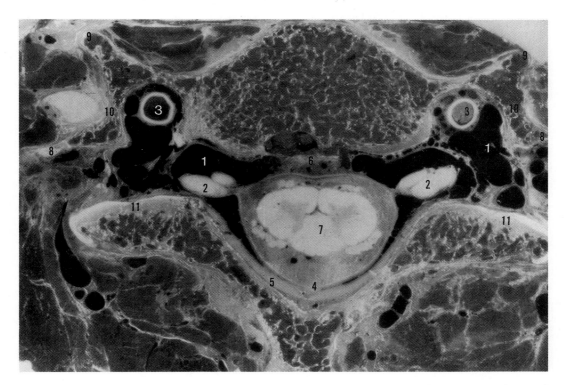

Figure 6–4. Axial (horizontal) section through C-6 of a specimen that had been positioned and frozen in flexion. The wedge shape of the articular processes (cf. Fig. 6–3) causes enlargement of the root canals and marked widening of the epidural and perineural venous plexus (*1*), which is filled with black cadaveric blood. The root sleeves (*2*) are suspended in these sinusoids, and each carries a thin motor and thicker sensory root. The vertebral arteries (*3*) are also surrounded by venous expansions. The thecal sac (*4*) is closely attached to the sublaminar ligamentum flavum (*5*) posteriorly and to the posterior longitudinal ligament (*6*) anteriorly. The spinal cord (*7*) floats freely in the CSF compartment (subarachnoid space); its gray and white matter are clearly distinguished. The complex transverse process is composed of the transverse process proper (terminating in the posterior tubercle) (*8*) and an anterior portion derived from the rib anlage, which carries the anterior tubercle (*9*). Both are connected by the distally convex intertransverse bar (*10*). Note that, owing to the position of flexion, the inferior articular process of C-6 (*11*) lacks its articulating counterpart, the superior articular process of C-7, causing the appearance of a "naked facet."

In its long canal, the root sleeve, ganglion, and nerve cannot yield superiorly because the cervical roots lie in a deep oblique groove at the anterior aspect of the process. Not infrequently, the uncinate process curves posteriorly, further immobilizing the root. In spondylotic specimens it may be completely encased by bone anteriorly because of the uncinate spurring. Compromise of the vertebral canal size and compression of the spinal cord have been observed when the lower endplate carries spondylotic spurs, ridges, or flanges, especially when the spine is extended (Figs. 6–5 and 6–6) and when the posterior longitudinal ligament is ossified.

Thoracic Spine

In the thoracic spine, the spinal cord occupies a relatively small proportion of the vertebral canal. The cord is quite mobile in the subarachnoid compartment. Small segmental intrathecal nerve roots run obliquely in the inferior and lateral direction. Contrary to the spinal cord intumescence at the cervicothoracic junction and the conus medullaris region, the thoracic nerve roots and nerves are thin (Fig. 6–7 and 6–8). In the upper thoracic spine, the nerves lie midway between the pedicles. Toward the lower thoracic spine the root complex with its small, spherical ganglion increasingly comes in closer contact with the pedicle of the vertebra under which it exits. In the thoracic foramina, sparse lobuli of fat and large venous plexuses surround the nerve root and ganglion.

Thoracic facet joint capsules are thin toward the vertebral canal and foramina. Their articular surfaces are oriented in a slightly oblique coronal plane. The ligamentum flavum in the thoracic and lumbar spine inserts into a relatively small surface at the upper margin of the lower lamina and into a significantly larger osseous area of the upper lamina. It covers

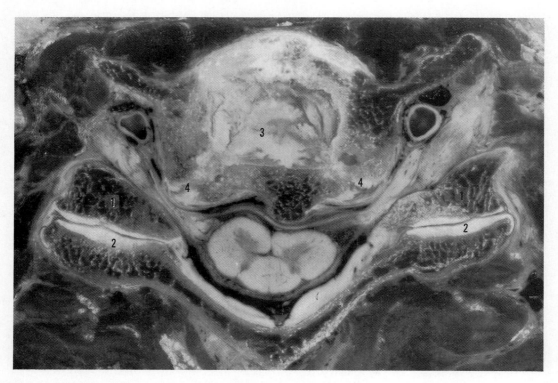

Figure 6–5. Axial section through the C5–C6 motion segment of a specimen that had been frozen *in situ* in extension. The wedge shape of the articular processes (cf. Fig. 6–3) causes retrolisthesis of the suprajacent vertebra, which in turn markedly decreases the sagittal dimensions of the vertebral canal (spinal canal) and root canals (intervertebral foramina). This decrease in volume causes complete emptying of the epidural and periradicular venous sinusoids. Posteriorly, the superior articular process of C-5 (*1*) is driven like a wedge underneath the inferior process of C-6 (*2*). Anteriorly, the lower endplate of C-5 (see also Fig. 6–6) is translating posteriorly. The thickening of the sublaminar ligamenta flava further accentuates this stenosis. The intervertebral disc (*3*) is degenerated. There also is marked uncovertebral arthrosis (*4*). Note the compression of the motor roots by the uncovertebral osteophytes (*5*).

and occupies the portion of the lamina that slopes posteriorly. Thus, the posterior wall of the vertebral canal consists predominantly of ligamentum flavum, interrupted only by narrow bands of laminar bone. Typical of the thoracic spine are its limited mobility and the segmental anchorage of the ribs, which articulate with their heads at each disc level with two adjacent vertebrae in true synovial articulations. In addition, the ribs articulate with the club-shaped costotransverse processes. These junctures are reinforced by an array of particularly strong ligaments.

Lumbar Spine

At the thoracolumbar junction, the intervertebral discs rapidly increase in height (Fig. 6–9). The anterior wall of the vertebral canal is straight, and the intervertebral discs show no tendency of bulging into the canal. Normally, the thecal sac is wide and occupies the whole vertebral canal. The thickest portion of the conus medullaris usually lies at the T-11 and T-12 levels. Anterior and posterior bundles of cauda equina roots emerge from the anterolateral and posterolateral sulci of the spinal cord and of the conus on each side. Contrary to the cervical and upper thoracic roots, which form by stepwise fusion of small filaments or rootlets, the lumbosacral roots emerge directly from the cord without intermittent rootlets. In axial cross section, the conus area with the dorsal and ventral root bundles takes the shape of a butterfly. In the lumbar spine, the intervertebral discs further increase in thickness relative to the height of the vertebrae. Whereas the discs of L-1 and L-2 have a straight posterior margin, the discs of L-3, L-4, and L-5 have a distinctly posteriorly convex, bulging configuration (Fig. 6–10).

In contrast to the discs in the thoracic spine, where the peripheral layers of the anulus fibrosus insert into the apophyseal ring, the lower lumbar discs feature insertion of the outer anular lamellae beyond

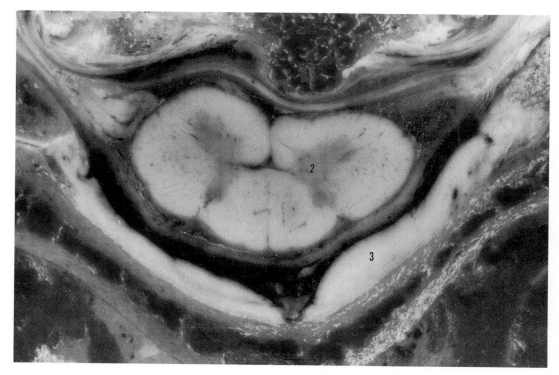

Figure 6–6. Closeup image of Figure 6–5, showing the vertebral canal and the entrance of the root canals. The lower endplate of C5 carries a pointed spondylophyte (*1*) close to the midline which not only indents the dura mater but also compresses the spinal cord. The butterfly shape of the gray matter (*2*) is clearly seen, as are the numerous blood vessels inside the spinal cord. The thickening caused by retraction (volume redistribution) of the ligamentum flavum is

the assimilated ring apophysis into the periosteum and Sharpey's fibers of the vertebral body. This normal architecture of the discs can be seen in sagittal CT and MRI scans and should not be confused with pathologic bulging of the discs as a result of degeneration or instability.

In horizontal cross sections, the vertebral bodies of the cervical, thoracic, and upper lumbar spine as well as their intervening discs have a more or less distinctly concave posterior margin. The only exception is the L-5 body and the lumbosacral disc, which always have a posteriorly convex or at least straight posterior border. In the lumbar spine, the thecal sac is normally round (Fig. 6–11). The location of the roots in the thecal sac varies with posture and movement as described for the cervical spinal cord.

Normal movement in the lumbar spine entails less anterior and posterior translatory movement than in the cervical spine because the facet joints have a less pronounced slope. Considerable interindividual variations exist. In spines with developmentally short pedicles and borderline dimensions of the vertebral canal diameter, even slight hypermobility or compromise by functional or structural degenerative lesions, fracture fragments, or translation movement may compromise the intraspinal blood vessels and neural elements.

The thick lumbar roots with their voluminous ganglia and the postganglionic lumbar spinal nerves snugly follow the medial and inferior aspect of the pedicles. Owing to their size, they normally occupy a large proportion of the lumbar root canals. Hypermobility and/or reduction of the intervertebral disc height (e.g., following chemonucleolysis) may cause a relatively sudden decrease in foramen dimensions and compression of the root. This may be further accentuated by the concomitant destabilization of the disc, especially in extension and/or rotation movements. Figure 6–12 shows the undistorted relationships between the nerve roots and the vertebral column in a specimen that had been frozen in moderate extension.

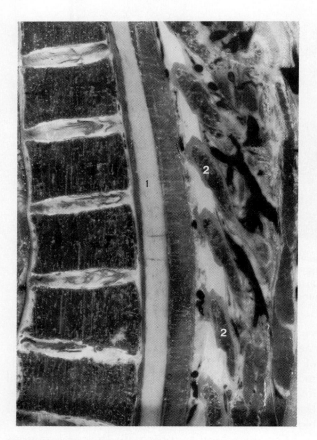

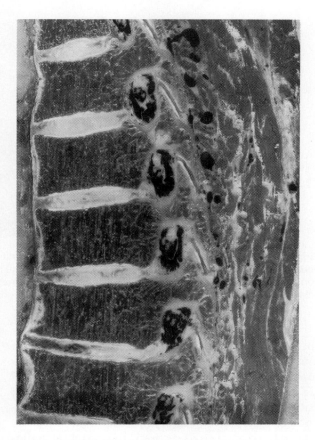

Figure 6–7. Midsagittal section through the midthoracic spine of an elderly male adult. Note the moderate to severe multilevel disc degeneration, producing slight kyphosis, which causes the spinal cord (*1*) to lie anteriorly in the vertebral canal. Posteriorly, the broad laminae (*2*) overlie each other like shingles, "hiding" the interlaminar ligamentum flavum from a posterior view. Adjacent to the laminae engorged veins of the posterior external venous plexus are seen. The ligamentum flavum at each level attaches to a wide area at the inferior and anterior surfaces of the suprajacent lamina and on a much smaller surface of the upper rim and posterior margin of the infrajacent lamina.

Figure 6–8. Sagittal section through the foramina and facet joints of the specimen in Figure 6–7. The thoracic vertebrae are square. In the mid- and lower thoracic spine the upper margin of the pedicles is flush with or slightly elevated above the upper vertebral endplate. The thoracic foramina are located behind the lower portion of each vertebra and not at the level of the motion segment. They contain veins and some areolar fat tissue. The nerve roots are very small in relation to the foramen. There is marked degeneration of the lowest intervertebral disc and also anterior endplate ridging.

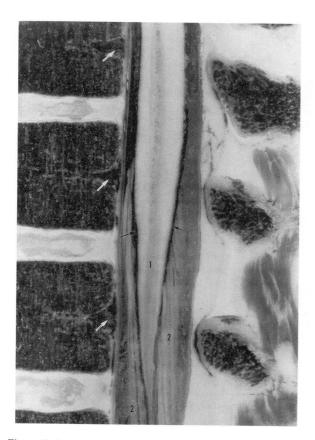

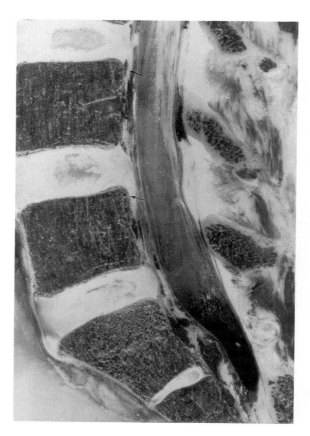

Figure 6–9. Midsagittal section through the vertebral canal at the thoracolumbar junction housing the conus medullaris (*1*) and the heavy bundles of the cauda equina (*2*). The cauda equina roots emerge directly from the conus. Some carry wider medullary feeder arteries. The tip of the conus is composed of gray matter. On the anterior and posterior surfaces of the conus, the anterior and posterior spinal arteries are seen (*closed arrow*). Note that the posterior margin of the intervertebral discs is perfectly straight, and the endplates are roughly parallel. Posteriorly in the midportion of the vertebral bodies, osseous foramina allow the veins of the vertebral body to communicate with the ventral internal vertebral venous plexus (*open arrows*).

Figure 6–10. Sagittal section through the lower lumbar spine (L3–L4 disc) to the upper sacrum slightly to the right of the midline of a young male adult. The intervertebral discs are thick in relation to the vertebral body height. Their posterior anular margin markedly bulges into the vertebral canal. The peripheral anular layers attach to the apophyseal rings of the vertebrae and also blend with the periosteum beyond the ring apophysis (*arrow*). The cul de sac terminates at the level of the second sacral segment slightly inferior to the fused S1–S2 junction.

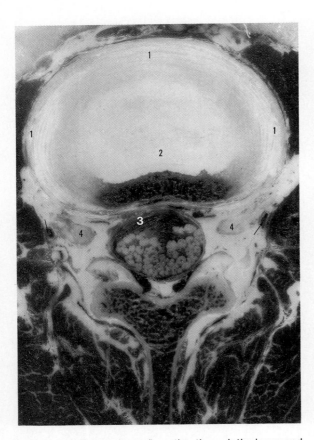

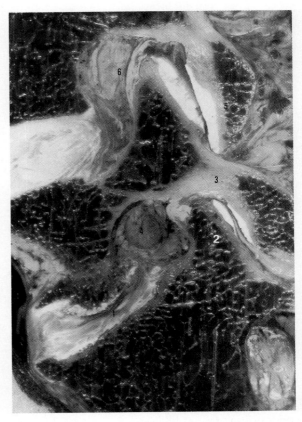

Figure 6–11. Axial (horizontal) section through the lower end-plate of L-3. In this slightly oblique tangential cut through the upper disc compartment, the strong anterior and lateral anular layers are clearly outlined (*1*); in the center the cartilaginous endplate is displayed (*2*). The thecal sac is round and firmly affixed to the lower endplate of L-3 (*3*). Lateral and slightly anteriorly, the dorsal root ganglia (*4*) lie embedded in foraminal fat tissue. Immediately lateral to the ganglia are located the segmental radicular arteries (*arrows*). Posterolaterally, the thecal sac abuts the uppermost portion of the interlaminar ligamentum flavum, which also constitutes the elastic capsule of the facet joints. Posteriorly, the constituents of the erector spinae muscle are demarcated by fascicular planes and fat.

Figure 6–12. Sagittal section through the foramina and facet joints of the lower lumbar spine of a middle-aged female. The spine was positioned in extension and then frozen *in situ*. At L5–S1 the disc is degenerated (*1*). The collapse of the disc and the loss of disc height cause the superior articular process of the sacrum (*2*) to impact on the pars interarticularis of L-5 (*3*). Little movement occurs at L5–S1. This stable situation is also reflected by ample areolar fat tissue and veins surrounding the L-5 dorsal root ganglion (*4*). By contrast, marked mobility occurs at the L4–L5 segment. L-4 is rotated posteriorly on L-5, causing its inferior articular process (*5*) to slide inferiorly and slightly posteriorly until its lower tip hugs the pars interarticularis of L-5. In extension, the superior articular process of L-5 moves superiorly and markedly anteriorly into the upper portion of the foramen, compressing and flattening the L-4 dorsal root ganglion (*6*) from posteriorly in the subpedicular notch.

chapter 7

Physiology of Nerve Compression

Lars B. Dahlin
Sten H. Holm
Björn L. Rydevik
Göran Lundborg

The pathophysiology of nerve compression and spinal nerve root compression is complex. To gain an understanding of these lesions it is important to have basic knowledge about the normal structure and function of the peripheral nerve trunk as well as of the spinal nerve root (Fig. 7–1). A nerve trunk and a spinal nerve root consist of several different tissue components that all react in different ways to trauma. The present chapter reviews the basic microanatomy of the peripheral nerve and the spinal nerve root as well as the way they respond to compression. Important pathophysiological findings are related to clinical symptoms.

Microanatomy of the Peripheral Nerve Trunk

Connective Tissue

The peripheral nerve trunk is a composite structure consisting of connective tissue elements and a rich network of microvessels, all of which serve the purpose of supporting the axons. The connective tissue elements are arranged in three layers: the epineurium, the perineurium, and the endoneurium (Fig. 7–2) (Sunderland, 1978; Thomas and Olsson, 1984). The axons are closely packed within the endoneurium. Bundles of axons are surrounded by the perineurium, which is a lamellated sheath consisting of flattened perineurial cells that together act as a diffusion barrier (Olsson, 1966; Olsson and Reese, 1969, 1971). A bundle of axons together with the perineurium is called a fascicle, and a peripheral nerve consists of several fascicles. The amount of endoneurium as well as perineurium varies between different nerves, as well as along the same nerve trunk. This variation probably reflects the need for extra mechanical protection at some locations in the extremities. Several fascicles are embedded in the loose connective tissue called the epineurium.

Endoneurial Fluid Pressure

The interstitial fluid pressure inside the fascicle (endoneurial fluid pressure, EFP) is slightly greater than

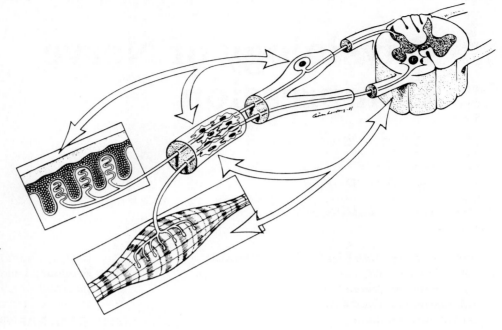

Figure 7-1. Anatomical arrangement of motor and sensory neurons and their target organs. Arrows indicate the interaction between nerve cell bodies, Schwann cells, and their target tissue. *(From Lundborg, 1988, p.2, with permission.)*

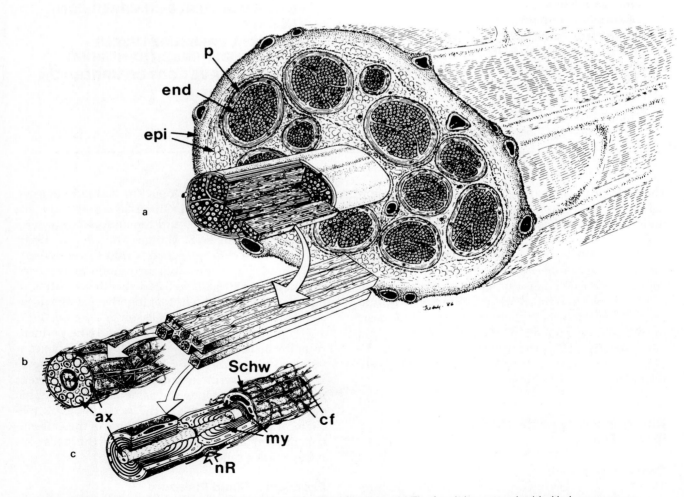

Figure 7-2. Microanatomy of a peripheral nerve with several fascicles. (*a*) The fascicles are embedded in loose connective tissue, and each fascicle is surrounded by a perineurium (p). The intrafascicular tissue elements are located around the nerve fibers. (*b*) Nonmyelinated and (*c*) myelinated epi = epineurium, end = endoneurium, Schw = Schwann

that of the surrounding tissues (Low et al., 1977; Myers et al., 1978; Hargens et al., 1978; Chen et al., 1976). Different neuropathies or trauma can further increase the EFP which may affect nerve function (Myers and Powell, 1981).

Microcirculation

The peripheral nerve trunk is very well vascularized and receives its blood supply from vessels originating in nearby arteries and veins (Lundborg, 1970, 1975, 1988). When these vessels reach the epineurium (Fig. 7–3), they divide into ascending and descending branches which run longitudinally along the epineurium, anastomosing with plexuses located in the epineurium, perineurium, and endoneurium. The intrafascicular vascular bed extends along the whole length of the nerve and consists mainly of capillaries that communicate with the extrafascicular vessels, through numerous anastomoses that often pierce obliquely through the perineural layer (Lundborg, 1975, 1988; Myers et al., 1982). The endoneurial capillaries are normally not permeable to proteins, and thus play a crucial role in the regulation of the *milieu interieur* of the endoneurial space by acting as diffusion barriers (Olsson et al., 1971).

Nerve Fibers

The nerve fibers are myelinated or nonmyelinated, and both types are surrounded by Schwann cells. In myelinated nerve fibers, one axon is associated with only one Schwann cell, and the membrane of the cytoplasm of the Schwann cell is wrapped around the axon, thereby forming the myelin sheath. However, the Schwann cells of the nonmyelinated fibers are arranged in a different way; i.e., a great number of axons are located in troughs in the Schwann cell (Berthold, 1978). In the myelinated fibers the different Schwann cells meet each other at the nodes of Ranvier, where the exchange of different ions takes place, thereby allowing the so-called saltatory propagation of impulses from node to node. In nonmyelinated fibers the propagation of impulses is more continuous. The nerve conduction velocity is dependent on the type of nerve fibers as well as the diameter of the fiber. In general, Myelinated nerve fibers have a higher nerve conduction velocity than do nonmyelinated fibers, and large-diameter myelinated fibers have greater conduction velocities than thinner myelinated fibers (Gasser and Erlanger, 1929; Dahlin et al., 1989).

Axonal Transport

The bidirectional transport that occurs in a neuron consists of transport from the cell body out to the periphery (anterograde axonal transport) and from the periphery up to the cell body (retrograde axonal transport). Anterograde transport can roughly be divided into two groups. Fast transport (20–410 mm/day), involves mainly small vesicular organelles

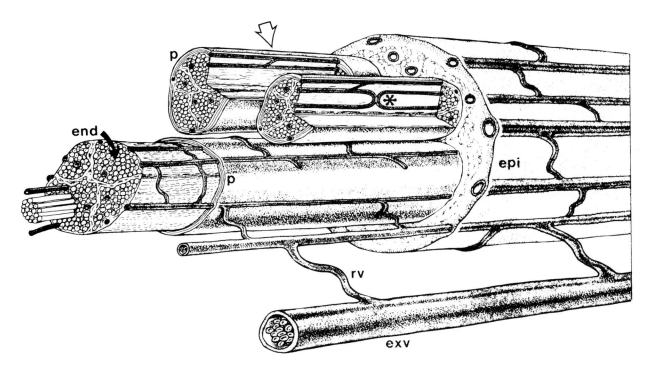

Figure 7–3. Intraneural microvascular network of a peripheral nerve. Vessels present in all nerve layers are fed by extrinsic vessels (exv) via regional feeding vessels (rv). The asterisk indicates a capillary loop, and the arrowhead indicates vessels piercing the perineurium (p) obliquely. Epi = epineurium, end = endoneurium. (*From Lundborg, 1988, p 43, with permission.*)

and both membranous and soluble materials. Fast transport is critically dependent on an adequate supply of energy (Ochs, 1974). Slow transport (0.1–30 mm/day) involves proteins, but the composition and amount is different from that of fast transport. Examples of proteins transported by slow transport are actin and the subunit proteins of microtubules and neurofilaments (Black and Lasek, 1980; Brady and Lasek, 1982; McLean et al., 1983; Dahlin, 1986).

The velocity of retrograde transport is roughly half of that reported for anterograde transport. The functions of retrograde transport are recycling of materials originally transported from the cell body to the axon terminal and transfer of information about the status of the axon, its terminals, its target cells, and its general environment (Varon and Adler, 1980; Bisby, 1982). One of the best known examples of the so-called neuronotrophic factors (proteins presumably supplied by the neuron's target territory, incorporated by the axon terminals, and retrogradely transported to operate on the nerve cell body) (Varon and Adler, 1980) is nerve growth factor (NGF), which affects sensory and sympathetic neurons (Levi-Montalcini, 1976; Thoenen and Barde, 1980). Neuronotrophic factors may not only be of importance normally, but may be of even more importance after nerve trauma and during subsequent cellular repair. Furthermore, retrograde transport may not only be of "positive" importance for the body but may also have a "negative influence" on the organism. Different viruses, such as the herpes simplex virus, are incorporated at axon terminals and transferred up the axon by retrograde transport to the nerve cell body where the viruses exert their effects (Kristensson, 1982).

Anatomy and Physiology of Spinal Nerve Roots

The spinal nerve roots are the anatomic nerve structures connecting the peripheral nervous system and the central nervous system. Within the lumbar subarachnoid space, the dorsal and ventral lumbosacral nerve roots from the cauda equina. The nerve roots pass through confined spaces in the spine, where pathological changes of various kinds may cause nerve root deformation or dysfunction. The spinal nerve roots structurally differ from the peripheral nerves. Consequently, the nerve roots may not react to compression in the same way as peripheral nerves (Rydevik et al., 1984; Rydevik and Garfin, 1989). Furthermore, spinal nerve roots are not as homogeneous in structure as peripheral nerves. Spinal nerve roots in the cauda equina, for example, differ structurally from the nerve roots located at the level of the

intervertebral foramina. At this latter location, the nerve root complex comprises both motor and sensory roots, as well as a dorsal root ganglion. The nerve roots in the cauda equina have a very sparse connective tissue network and are enclosed by a very thin sheath. Because of the sparse connective tissue network in the nerve roots of the cauda equina, these roots may be more susceptible to mechanical compression than the spinal nerve roots located in the intervertebral foramina.

Peripheral Nerve Compression

Nerve compression injuries may be acute, in association with trauma, or chronic as in nerve entrapments. The clinical symptoms that patients may notice vary from slight paresthesias and motor weakness to complete loss of sensory and motor function. Sometimes pain may occur after trauma and, surprisingly, chronic pain conditions may occur after minor nerve injuries. To understand the nature of nerve compression injuries, it is important to differentiate between effects on various tissue components and effects produced by various compression levels.

Low Pressure Levels (20–150 mm Hg)

Effect on Microcirculation. Impairment of intraneural blood flow is probably of major importance in the pathophysiology of carpal tunnel syndrome (CTS), i.e., compression of the median nerve in the carpal tunnel at the wrist (Sunderland, 1976). Compression of a peripheral nerve at pressures around 20 to 30 mm Hg will impair venular blood flow in the tibial nerve of rabbits (Rydevik et al., 1981; Ogata and Naito, 1986). When the applied pressure is increased to 60 to 80 mm Hg or higher there is a complete stop in the circulation in the compressed segment (Bentley and Schlapp, 1943; Rydevik et al., 1981; Matsumoto, 1983; Ogata and Naito, 1986). Sunderland originally suggested that this initial lesion in carpal tunnel syndrome, i.e., intrafascicular anoxia resulting from obstruction of the venular flow and ischemia, leads to intrafascicular edema and an increase in intrafascicular pressure with subsequent impairment of intraneural blood flow. It has been shown experimentally that in trafascicular edema may occur after compression and that this edema may increase the endoneurial fluid pressure (Rydevik and Lundborg, 1977; Lundborg et al., 1983; Powell and Myers, 1986). The edema that occurs in the fascicles is most pronounced subperineurially but may also occur perivascularly and endoneurially (Powell and Myers, 1986). In examination of the nerve fiber injuries that occur, it is obvious that subperineurial fibers are more often damaged than those at the core of the fascicle.

The anatomic arrangement that exists in the fascicles, i.e., the vessels in the endoneurial space communicate with the extrafascicular vessels by anastomoses piercing obliquely through the perineurial layer, is important because, with increased EFP, this arrangement may constitute a possible obstruction that will impair intrafascicular blood flow (Lundborg, 1975; Lundborg et al., 1983). Computer modeling demonstrates that elevation of EFP can deform cylindric vessels in the perineurium into eliptic shapes, thereby reducing the cross-sectional area of the lumen (Myers et al., 1986). The epineurial fibrosis that may occur after chronic compression may also create further mechanical problems for the transperineurial vessels, inducing venous stasis. This mechanism may also explain the reduced nerve blood flow observed in diabetic neuropathy (Powell, 1983; Tuck et al., 1984) and the increased susceptibility to nerve compression in that condition (Brown et al., 1980; Dahlin et al., 1986b, 1987a).

Impairment of the microcirculation in the compressed segment of a peripheral nerve may be of great pathophysiological importance at low pressure levels. This assumption is supported by the clinical observation that patients with carpal tunnel syndrome may recover immediately after decompression of the median nerve. Furthermore, studies in volunteers without signs of nerve compression indicate that there is a critical pressure level threshold at about 40 to 50 mm Hg at which peripheral nerve viability is acutely jeopardized (Lundborg et al., 1982; Gelberman et al., 1983). Hypertensive subjects show an increased resistance to peripheral nerve compression, as demonstrated by the fact that corresponding functional changes are induced first at 60 to 70 mm Hg compression if the patient has high blood pressure (Szabo et al., 1983).

Effect on Axonal Transport. Axonal transport is an energy-requiring process, and impairment of intraneural microcirculation may inhibit this process. Compression of a peripheral nerve in an experimental model at pressures as low as 20 to 30 mm Hg for 2 to 8 hours inhibited anterograde as well as retrograde axonal transport (Fig. 7–4) (Dahlin, 1986). The inhibition of axonal transport at increasing pressure levels or compression at longer periods will induce a *graded effect* on the transport (Rydevik et al., 1980; Dahlin et al., 1984, 1986c; Dahlin and McLean, 1986).

The blockage of axonal transport may have a serious effect on the functional state of the neuron. Inhibition of fast and slow anterograde transport may adversely affect the transmitter function at the axon terminals and can impair the transport of different cytoskeletal elements down the axon to the peripheral parts of the axon. This may, if the pressure is high enough or if the compression is applied for a sufficient period, induce degeneration of the axon distal to the compression site.

Impairment of retrograde transport may induce a regenerative response in the nerve cell body by disturbing the transport of neuronotrophic factors (Dahlin et al., 1987b; Archer, 1987). These changes consist of morphologic as well as biochemical alterations in the nerve cell body. The morphologic changes (Fig. 7–5) consist of changes in the size of the cell and nuclear volume, an eccentric position of the nucleus, as well as dispersion of the Nissl substance in the cytoplasm of the cell (chromatolysis) (Nissl, 1892; Barron, 1983; Dahlin et al., 1987b). The metabolic changes in the nerve cell bodies include an increase in RNA synthesis and a subsequent increase in protein synthesis (Grafstein and McQuarrie, 1978). It should be noted that there is not an increase in the synthesis of *all* proteins in the cell but, generally, there is a shift away from the production of materials required for transmitter function toward the production of structural components required for restitution of the axon (Skene, 1984; Archer, 1987). There are variations in these classical reactions that are related to the type of axonal lesion, as well as the age and species of the animal (Torvik, 1976).

Diabetes as a Contributory Factor. Many diabetic patients suffer from different types of neurologic disorders (Brown and Asbury, 1984). One such disorder is entrapment neuropathy, which can affect nerves in the upper as well as the lower extremities. Clinical observations (Mulder et al., 1961) as well as a number of morphologic and ultrastructural studies (Brown et al., 1980; Sharma et al., 1981) indicate that diabetes may make the axons of the peripheral nerve more vulnerable to injury. Compression of a peripheral nerve at 30mm Hg for 3 hours in an animal with experimentally induced diabetes produced a more pronounced inhibition of fast axonal transport at the site of compression than produced in controls (Dahlin et al., 1986b). The mechanism underlying this increased susceptibility to damage is probably related to the accumulation of a metabolite of glucose (sorbitol) and subsequent edema, which may in turn affect intraneural microcirculation (Powell, 1983; Tuck et al., 1984; Low et al., 1985; Dahlin et al., 1986b; 1987a; McLean, 1988).

Structural and Functional Changes Compression of a peripheral nerve may also induce injuries to an axon and its Schwann cells. At very low pressures (30–50 mm Hg) a segmental demyelination associated with Schwann cell necrosis may occur, and at a pressure that induces ischemia and endoneurial

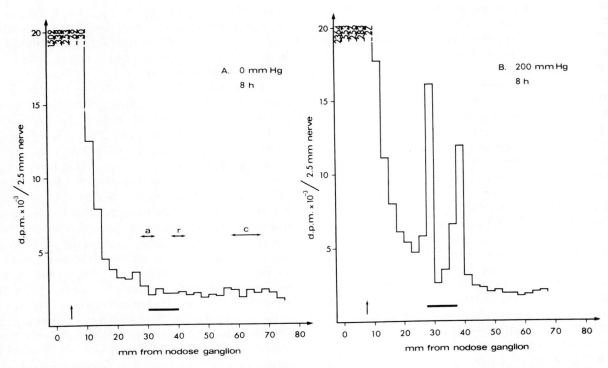

Figure 7-4. Effects of compression on anterograde and retrograde axonal transport. Profiles of radiolabeled proteins in rabbit vagus nerves 24 hours after radiolabeling in the nodose ganglia. Nerves were compressed at 0 mm Hg (sham compression) and 200 mm Hg for 8 hours. Black horizontal bars indicate the site of compression, and vertical arrows indicate ligatures to exclude slow transport. Sham compression induced no inhibition of axonal transport. Compression at 200 mm Hg induced marked inhibition of axonal transport at distal (retrograde transport) and proximal (anterograde transport) edges of the compressed segment. (*From Dahlin et al., 1986c, p. 224, with permission.*)

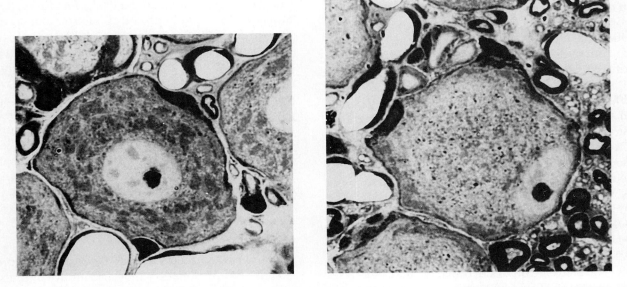

Figure 7-5. Nerve cell bodies from ganglia in which the vagus nerves had been compressed at (*A*) 0 mm Hg and (*B*) 30 mm of Hg for 2 hours, 7 days before evaluation of morphology. The nerve cell body in (B) exhibits dispersed Nissl substances and peripheral displacement of the nucleus. Methylene blue and Azur II, x 1,200. (*From Dahlin et al., 1987b, p. 613, with permission.*)

edema (80 mm Hg), injuries to the axons have been observed (Rydevik and Nordborg, 1980; Powell and Myers, 1986). The injuries are more pronounced subperineurially as compared with the observed changes in the core of the fascicles (Spinner and Spencer, 1974; Powell and Myers, 1986). It should be noted that the endoneurial edema has been observed to be most pronounced subperineurially but occurs also perivascularly and endoneurially (Powell and Myers, 1986). The intraneural topography of individual fascicles in a peripheral nerve is also important with respect to the loss of function that may be seen, because a superficially located fascicle may suffer more from compression than a deeply located, more protected fascicle (Lundborg, personal communication).

Nerve function can also be affected by compression. This has been studied by several researchers using different pressure levels as well as different modes of pressure application. It is difficult to compare results of all these studies accurately, but generally at least 130 to 150 mm Hg has to be applied to the nerve to block conduction within a few hours in experimental models (see, for example, Bentley and Schlapp, 1943; Matsumoto, 1983). A human model has also been developed to study the effects of nerve function during experimental application of external compression to the carpal tunnel. A low pressure (30 mm of Hg) can induce neurophysiological changes and paresthesias in the median nerve–innervated fingers; higher pressure (60 and 90 mm Hg) can induce rapid and complete block of conduction in sensory fibers. This loss of function preceded the block in motor fibers (Lundborg et al., 1982).

High Pressure Levels (200–1000 Hg)

Structural and Functional Changes. When a peripheral nerve is compressed at a high pressure level, there are pronounced and characteristic changes in the structure of the nerve fibers. These changes have been extensively studied by Ochoa et al. (1972). Their electron microscopic study of single teased fibers showed that there was a characteristic displacement of the node of Ranvier in large myelinated nerve fibers following compression (Fig. 7–6). The paranodal myelin was stretched at one side of the node and invaginated into the paranodal myelin on the other side. These changes were maximal beneath the edges of the cuff. The nodes were always displaced away from the cuff toward the uncompressed tissue. This phenomenon seems to be caused by the pressure gradient within the nerve between its compressed and uncompressed parts. The lesion is followed by demyelination (Ochoa et al., 1972; Rydevik

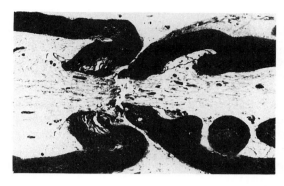

Figure 7–6. Low-power ultrastructural appearance of a single fiber from a compressed nerve showing the typical invagination of one paranode by the adjacent one. The displacement is from right to left. (*From Ochoa et al., 1972, p. 435,*

and Nordborg, 1980) and, usually, subsequent remyelination within weeks or months.

The reason the large-diameter myelinated nerve fibers are affected may be that these fibers normally have a narrowing of the axon at the node (Berthold, 1978). This would make movement of the axoplasm difficult, resulting in the observed displacement of the nodal axolemma. Large fibers may also be subjected to greater deformation than thinner fibers at a given pressure (MacGregor et al., 1975). Thin nonmyelinated nerve fibers are therefore more resistant to compression injuries than are myelinated fibers (Fowler and Ochoa, 1975; Dahlin et al., 1989).

The pressure gradient between the compressed and uncompressed parts of the nerve is important in understanding the ultrastructural changes observed when comparing experiments in which whole oxygenated nerves are subjected to high pressures within a pressure chamber (Grundfest, 1936) with experiments in which nerves are subjected to local compression. In the former experiments, the nerves withstand very high pressure without impairment of conduction, but when local compression is applied to the nerve, the conduction properties are affected at comparatively low pressures (Bentley and Schlapp, 1943; Denny-Brown and Brenner, 1944; Rydevik and Nordborg, 1980; Dahlin et al. 1986c). The location of the lesion in the nerve fibers during compression, i.e., injury to the nerve fibers at the edges with sparing at the center of the compressed segment, is termed the *edge effect*.

There is a marked deterioration of conduction properties of the myelinated nerve fibers during compression at high pressures (Rydevik and Nordborg 1980; Dahlin et al., 1986a, 1989); however, the effects on nonmyelinated nerve fibers are not so pronounced (Dahlin et al., 1989). A very high pressure (600 mm Hg) is needed to block the conduction in these thin fibers. Thinner myelinated fibers are more susceptible to deprivation of oxygen than thicker ones, whereas nonmyelinated fibers differ in response according to the method used to induce ischemia (Dahlin et al. 1989).

Mechanical Deformation Versus Ischemia

There has for many years been a debate concerning the importance of mechanical deformation versus ischemia as source of the impaired nerve function (Bentley and Schlapp, 1943; Denny-Brown and Brenner, 1944; Ochoa et al., 1972; Fowler et al., 1972; Gilliatt, 1975, 1980; Rydevik and Nordborg, 1980). At these high pressures, the more important factor is probably the mechanical deformation of the nerve fibers and not the induced ischemia, although intraneural vessels are also injured. Compression at high pressure can induce a "no-reflow phenomenon" in the intraneural blood vessels in a previously compressed nerve segment, indicating that there may be a persistent impairment of intraneural microcirculation caused by mechanical injury to the blood vessels (Rydevik et al., 1981). The mechanical injury is, in a similar way as for nerve fibers, concentrated mainly at the edges of the compressed segment. There is also leakage from the intraneural microvessels with formation of an endoneurial edema (Rydevik and Lundborg, 1977).

Nerve Entrapments

Chronic compression lesions represent the combined effect of a persistent inflammatory reaction in the nerve and a direct mechanical injury to the nerve fibers. This impingement on the nerve will increase vascular permeability, produce a chronic edema, and form an intraneural scar. Impairment of intraneural microvascular flow as well as repeated mechanical trauma to the fibers may result in myelin damage and axonal degeneration. Several experimental models are used to study the pathoanatomy and pathophysiology of chronic nerve entrapment (Fullerton and Gilliatt 1967a, b; Ochoa and Marotte, 1973; Horiuchi, 1983; Nemoto, 1983; MacKinnon et al., 1984). A consistent finding in the model in guinea pigs, with a naturally developing entrapment lesion, is an asymmetry of the myelin sheath on either side of the entrapment. Moreover, the sheath appears to be thinned at the end of the internodal segment close to the center of the lesion, and thickened and swollen at the opposite side—a picture giving the impression of tadpoles or sperm swimming from the center of the lesion. Ultrastructural analysis has revealed that the terminal lobes of the inner myelin lamellae are detached from the axolemma at the

node, with retraction of the myelin along the internode and the corresponding aspect of myelin at the other end of the internode (Fullerton and Gilliatt, 1967a, b; Ochoa and Marotte, 1973). In more advanced stages, a prominent paranodal demyelination with partial exposure of the axon and even Wallerian degeneration may be seen. This picture has also been seen in median and ulnar nerves in humans (Neary and Eames, 1975).

Stages of Nerve Compression Injury

Even if a nerve compression injury represents a mixed lesion with varying extents of damage in various fiber populations, it may still be possible to define various stages of nerve compression injuries (Seddon, 1943, 1972; Sunderland, 1978; Lundborg, 1988). Deprivation of oxygen, based on a circulatory arrest induced by slight local compression, may inhibit impulse transmission in structurally intact nerve fibers. This may be termed *physiological conduction block*. An example of this block occurs when one leg is crossed over the opposite knee, producing pressure on the peroneal nerve that the person notices as the foot "goes to sleep." This condition is, however, immediately reversible when the pressure is released.

The term *neurapraxia* (Seddon, 1943, 1972) is used to describe a local conduction block in which axonal continuity is preserved and conduction within the compressed segment is recovered within weeks or months. The pathophysiologic basis for this block is supposed to be local myelin damage at the nodes of Ranvier (Ochoa et al., 1982), together with endoneurial edema formation (Rydevik and Lundborg, 1977; Lundborg, 1988). The condition will diminish when the local myelin damage has been repaired. In this condition there is usually a complete paralysis, although the function of the sensory sympathetic fibers is often spared (Seddon, 1943). An example of this condition is "Saturday night palsy," produced when the radial nerve is compressed against the humerus. In the more detailed classification of nerve injuries by Sunderland (1978) neurapraxia is called a "type I lesion," implying local myelin damage in a preserved nerve fiber without Wallerian degeneration.

When there is a loss of continuity in the axon but the endoneurial tubes remain intact, the term *axonotmesis* is used. Wallerian degeneration will hereby be induced and axons will have to regenerate in preserved endoneurial tubes for functional recovery. Because the endoneurial tubes are preserved, the prognosis is good. Sunderland called this lesion type II.

Seddon used the term *neurotmesis* to describe a lesion in which the nerve either has been completely severed or has been so disorganized by scar tissue that spontaneous recovery will not occur (Seddon, 1972). Sunderland has, however, divided this lesion in three subgroups, in which type III implies a loss of continuity of the axon and endoneurial tubes, with the perineurium still intact. In those cases, the continuity and orientation of endoneurial pathways are lost and there usually will be an intrafascicular fibrosis. If the continuity of the perineurium is lost but the epineurium is preserved, the lesion is called type IV. Finally, if the continuity of the entire nerve trunk is lost the lesion is called type V. Sunderland's type III to V lesions (neurotmesis) require surgery if functional recovery is to be expected.

Clinical Pressure Levels and Double Crush Syndrome

Using newly developed technologies, the pressure on the median nerve in the carpal canal has been measured at levels of 30 to 110 mm Hg (depending on the position of the hand) in patients with symptoms of carpal tunnel syndrome (Gelberman et al., 1981). The range for a control group was 2.5 to 31 mm Hg. On the basis of these experimental findings, it can be assumed that the intracellular transport of proteins and the microcirculation in compressed neurons will be disturbed, and that edema will ensue.

Interestingly, there is an overrepresentation of carpal tunnel syndrome in patients suffering from cervical radiculopathy (''double crush syndrome'') (Upton and McComas, 1973; Hurst et al., 1985). It has been suggested that the proximal compression of a nerve may render the distal parts of the axon more susceptible to compression. The observed effects of compression on axonal transport make such a theory highly plausible. Aproximal compression may decrease anterograde axonal transport, which would inhibit delivery of necessary materials to the axon and its terminals, making the distal parts of the axon more vulnerable to compression. However, the opposite event may also occur: a distal lesion affecting retrograde axonal transport may induce a lack of neuronotrophic factors in the cell body and thereby affect the cell body's production of substances transported by anterograde axonal transport. Such mechanisms may make the *proximal* part of the axon more susceptible to compression (Dahlin et al., 1986c, 1987b; Archer, 1987). This theory, ''reversed double crush syndrome,'' may explain why a simple carpal tunnel release sometimes can produce symptoms of a proximal lesion (Carrol and Hurst, 1982).

In conclusion, acute and chronic compression of

a peripheral nerve may affect the function of the nerve fibers by different mechanisms, all contributing to the symptoms seen in patients with nerve compression syndroms (Fig. 7–7).

Spinal Nerve Root Compression

Spinal nerve roots are frequently subjected to mechanical deformation produced by trauma and degenerative conditions of the spine. In some cases, such deformation is associated with symptoms like paresthesias, motor weakness, and pain. Mechanical deformation of spinal nerve roots affects all tissue components of these structures, i.e., nerve fibers, blood vessels, and connective tissue elements. As mentioned earlier, nerve roots are less homogeneous structures than peripheral nerves, and the structure of nerve roots is different at the level of the cauda equina and the level of the intervertebral foramina. Thus, experimental data obtained at one specific anatomic site may not be applicable to other locations. Previous research has been very limited on the problems related to spinal nerve root compression, but there are a large amount of data regarding the pathophysiology of peripheral nerve compression.

Gelfan and Tarlov (1956) studied the effects of compression on the spinal cord, nerve roots, and peripheral nerves. The results from this study indicate that the spinal cord and nerve roots seem to be less resistant to compression than peripheral nerves. Similar conclusions were drawn by Sharpless (1975), who compared the effects of compression on conduction properties of peripheral nerves and spinal nerve roots.

The physiological effects of nerve root compression have been analyzed by Olmarker and co-workers in a porcine model, in which the nerve roots of the cauda equina were subjected to graded, acute compression in vivo. (Olmarker et al., 1987, 1988; Pedowitz et al., 1988). The effects of various pressure levels on nerve root blood flow, solute transport to the nerve root tissue, and impulse conduction across the compressed cauda equina segment were analyzed. Data obtained indicate that even low-pressure compression of the nerve roots (in the range 5–10 mm Hg) may induce venous congestion in the intraneural microcirculation (Olmarker et al., 1989b). Complete ischemia in the compressed nerve root segments occurs at approximately 130 mm Hg compression in this model, a pressure level that correlates with the mean arterial blood pressure of the experimental animal. Analyses of the transport ^{3}H-labeled methyl glucose to the nerve root tissue during graded compression indicate that there is approximately 45% reduction of the solute transport to

ACUTE EFFECTS   CHRONIC EFFECTS

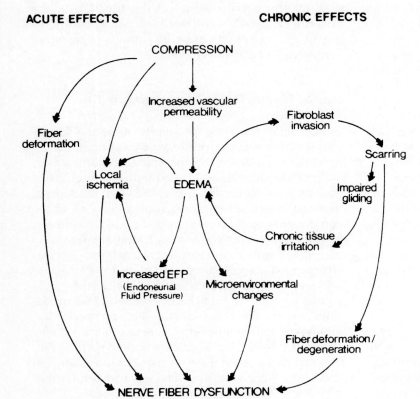

Figure 7-7. Acute and chronic effects of compression on intraneural tissues. (*From Lundborg, 1988, p. 64, with permission.*)

the compressed nerve root segments during compression at 10 mm Hg (Olmarker et al., 1990). Intraneural edema, as seen with fluorescence microscopy by extravasation of serum albumin labeled with Evans blue, was induced after compression at 50 mm Hg for 2 minutes or longer (Olmarker et al., 1989a). Electrophysiologic analysis using this model has shown that compression at 100 mm Hg for 2 hours leads to a pronounced impairment of both afferent nerve root conduction (75% reduction of the recorded compound nerve action potential amplitude) and efferent nerve root conduction (45% reduction of the recorded electromyogram amplitude) (Pedowitz et al., 1988). Impulse conduction in motor nerve roots seemed to recover faster and to a more complete degree than in the sensory nerve roots following decompression in this acute nerve root compression model. Sham application of the compression device for 2 hours as well as compression at 50 mm Hg for the same period did not induce any significant changes in efferent or afferent nerve root conduction.

Mechanical compression of the nerve roots may produce acute and chronic impairment of the blood supply and transport of nutrients to the nerve tissue in the cauda equina. Furthermore, the clearance of waste products from the nerve root tissue may be impaired as a result of such mechanical compression. These kinds of alterations in metabolic balance may

be further potentiated by chronic tissue changes such as fibrosis in and around the nerve root tissue. Chronic nerve root impingement may lead to demyelination of the nerve fibers at the level of compression. Such demyelinated nerve fibers are likely to be pain sensitive (Weinstein et al., 1989); however, detailed mechanisms regarding the morphologic and physiologic changes associated with various kinds of nerve root deformation are still incompletely understood.

Conclusion

Compression of the peripheral nerve trunk and the spinal nerve root will induce marked changes in microcirculation and nutrition of the nerve trunk and nerve root. The vascular permeability is increased, which produces an endoneurial edema, thereby increasing the endoneurial fluid pressure. This may contribute, along with the direct mechanical effects, to the observed structural changes in the nerve. Electrophysiologic changes are observed during and after compression with impairment of impulse conduction. Intraneural transport—axonal transport—is blocked by compression, and this event may be involved in the establishment of a double crush syndrome; that is, compression of a peripheral nerve trunk at one level will make other parts of the same nerve trunk more susceptible to another trauma. The experimental findings correlate well to the pressure levels found clinically in patients with, for example, carpal tunnel syndrome. Diabetes mellitus may confer on the peripheral nerve an increased vulnerability to trauma. Increased knowledge about the pathophysiology of nerve compression is important to an understanding of different clinical compression syndromes and improvement of their treatment.

References

Archer DR. *Axonal Transport and Related Responses to Nerve Injury.* Thesis. University of Liverpool; 1987.

Barron KD. Comparative observations on the cytologic reactions of central and peripheral nerve cells to axotomy. In Kao CC, Bunge RP, Reier PJ, eds. *Spinal Cord Reconstruction.* New York: Raven Press; 1983:7–40.

Bentley FH and Schlapp W. The effects of pressure on conduction in peripheral nerve. *J Physiol* 1943;102:72–82.

Berthold CH. Morphology of normal peripheral axons. In Waxman SG, ed. *Physiology and Pathobiology of Axons.* New York: Raven Press; 1978:3–63.

Bisby MA. Functions of retrograde axonal transport. *Fed Proc* 1982;41:2307–2311.

Black MM and Lasek RJ. Slow components of axonal transport: Two cytoskeletal networks. *J Cell Biol* 1980;86:616–623.

Brady ST and Lasek RJ. The slow components of axonal transport: Movements, compositions and organization. In Weiss DG, ed. *Axoplasmic Transport.* Berlin/Heidelberg: Springer-Verlag; 1982:206–217.

Brown MJ and Asbury AK: Diabetic neuropathy. *Ann Neurol* 1984;15:2–12.

Brown MJ, Sumner AJ, and Greene DA, et al. Distal neuropathy in experimental diabetes mellitus. *Ann Neurol* 1980;8:168–178.

Carrol RE and Hurst LC. The relationship of thoracic outlet syndrome and carpal tunnel syndrome. *Clin Orthop* 1982;164:149–153.

Chen HI, Granger HJ, and Taylor AE. Interaction of capillary, interstitial, and lymphatic forces in the canine hindpaw. *Circ Res* 1976;39:245–254.

Dahlin LB. *Nerve compression and axonal transport. Experimental studies on anterograde and retrograde anoxal transport and nerve cell body changes in peripheral nerve subjected to graded compression.* Thesis, Gothenburg University; 1986.

Dahlin LB, Archer DR, and McLean WG. Treatment with an aldose reductase inhibitor can reduce the inhibition of fast axonal transport following nerve compression in the streptozotocin-diabetic rat. *Diabetologia* 1987a;30:414–418.

Dahlin LB, Danielsen N, and Ehira T, et al. Mechanical effects of compression of peripheral nerves. *J Biomech Eng* 1986a;108:120–122.

Dahlin LB and McLean WG. Effects of graded experimental compression on slow and fast axonal transport in rabbit vagus nerve. *J Neurol Sci* 1986;72:10–30.

Dahlin LB, Meiri KF, and McLean WG, et al. Effects of nerve compression on fast axonal transport in streptozotocin-induced diabetes mellitus. An experimental study in the sciatic nerve of rats. *Diabetologia* 1986b;29:180–185.

Dahlin LB, Nordborg C, and Lundborg G. Morphological changes in nerve cell bodies induced by experimental graded nerve compression. *Exp Neurol* 1987b;95:611–621.

Dahlin LB, Rydevik B, and McLean WG, et al. Changes in fast axonal transport during experimental nerve compression at low pressures. *Exp Neurol* 1984;84:29–36.

Dahlin LB, Shyu BC, and Danielsen N, et al. Effects of nerve com-

pression or ischemia on conduction properties of myelinated and unmyelinated nerve fibres. *Acta Physiol Scand* 1989;136:97–105.

Dahlin LB, Sjöstrand J, and McLean WG. Graded inhibition of retrograde axonal transport by compression of rabbit vagus nerve. *J Neurol Sci* 1986c;76:221–230.

Denny-Brown D and Brenner C. Paralysis of nerve induced by direct pressure and by tourniquet. *Arch Neurol Psychiatry* 1944;51:1–26.

Fowler TJ, Danta G, and Gilliat RW. Recovery of nerve conduction after a pneumatic tourniquet: Observations on the hind limb of the baboon. *J Neurol Neurosurg Psychiatry* 1972;5:638–647.

Fowler TJ and Ochoa J. Unmyelinated fibres in normal and compressed peripheral nerves of the baboon: A quantitative electron microscopic study. *Neuropathol Appl Neurobiol* 1975;1:247–265.

Fullerton PM and Gilliatt RW. Pressure neuropathy in the hindfoot of the guinea-pig. *J Neurol Neurosurg Psychiatry* 1967a;30:18–25.

Fullerton PM and Gilliatt RW. Median and ulnar neuropathy in the guinea-pig. *J Neurol Neurosurg Psychiatry* 1967b;30:393–403.

Gasser HS and Erlanger J. The role of fiber size in the establishment of a nerve block by pressure or cocaine. *Am J Physiol* 1929;88:581–591.

Gelberman RH, Hergenroeder PT, and Hargens AR, et al. The carpal tunnel syndrome. A study of carpal canal pressures. *J Bone Joint Surg [Am]* 1981;63:380–383.

Gelberman RH, Szabo RM, and Williamson RV, et al. Tissue pressure threshold for peripheral nerve viability. *Clin Orthop Relat Res* 1983;178:285–291.

Gelfan S and Tarlov IM. Physiology of spinal cord, nerve root and peripheral nerve compression. *Am J Physiol* 1956;185:217–229.

Gilliatt RW. Peripheral nerve compression and entrapment. In AF Lant, ed. *The Oliver Sharpey Lecture. 11th Symposium on Advanced Medicine. Proceedings of the Royal College of Physicians.* London Pitman; 1975:144–163.

Gilliatt RW. Acute compression block. In AJ Sumner, ed. *The Physiology of Peripheral Nerve Disease.* Company, Philadelphia/London/Toronto, WB Saunders; 1980;287–315.

Grafstein B and McQuarrie IG. Role of the nerve cell body in axonal regeneration. In CW Cotman, ed. *Neuronal Plasticity.* New York: Raven Press; 1978:155–195.

Grundfest H. Effects of hydrostatic pressures upon the excitability, the recovery, and the potential sequence of frog nerve. *Cold Spring Harbor Symp Quant Biol* 1936;4:179–187.

Hargens AR, Akeson WH, and Mubarak SJ, et al. Fluid balance within the canine anterolateral compartment and its relationship to compartment syndromes. *J Bone Joint Surg [Am]* 1978;60:499–505.

Horiuchi Y. An experimental study on peripheral nerve lesions—Compression neuropathy. *J Jn Orthop Assoc* 1983;57:789–803.

Hurst LC, Weissberg D, and Carroll RE. The relationship of the double crush to carpal tunnel syndrome (an analysis of 1,000 cases of carpal tunnel syndrome). *J Hand Surg* 1985;10B:202–204.

Kristensson K. Implications of axoplasmic transport for the spread of virus infections in the nervous system. In Weiss DG and Gorio A, eds. *Axoplasmic Transport in Physiology and Pathology.* Berlin/Heidelberg: Springer-Verlag; 1982:153–158.

Levi-Montalcini R. The nerve growth factor: Its role in growth, differentiation and function of the sympathetic axon. *Prog Brain Res* 1976;45:235–258.

Low P, Marchand G, Knox F, and Dyck PJ. Measurement of endoneurial fluid pressure with polyethylene matrix capsules. *Brain Res* 1977;122:373–377.

Low PA, Nukada H, and Schmelzer JD, et al. Endoneurial oxygen tension and radial topography in nerve edema. *Brain Res* 1985;341:147–154.

Lundborg G. Ischemic nerve injury. Experimental studies on intraneural microvascular pathophysiology and nerve function in a limb subjected to temporary circulatory arrest. *Scand J Plast Reconstruct Surg Suppl* 1970;6.

Lundborg G. Structure and function of the intraneural microvessels as related to trauma, edema formation, and nerve function. *J Bone Joint Surg [Am]* 1975;57:938–948.

Lundborg G. *Nerve Injury and Repair.* London/Edinburgh: Churchill/Livingstone; 1988.

Lundborg G, Gelberman RH, and Minteer-Convery M, et al. Median nerve compression in the carpal tunnel—Functional response to experimentally induced controlled pressure. *J Hand Surg* 1982;7:252–259.

Lundborg G, Myers R, and Powell H. Nerve compression injury and increased endoneurial fluid pressure: A ''miniature compartment syndrome.'' *J Neurol Neurosurg Psychiatry* 1983; 46:1119–1124.

MacGregor RJ, Sharpless SK, and Luttges MW. A pressure vessel model for nerve compression. *J Neurol Sci* 1975;24:299–304.

MacKinnon SE, Dellon AL, and Hudson A, et al. Chronic nerve compression: An experimental model in the rat. *Ann Plast Surg* 1984;13:112–120.

Matsumoto N. An experimental study on compression neuropathy—Measurement of blood flow with the hydrogen washout technique. *J Jpn Orthop Assoc* 1983;7:805–816.

McLean WG. Pressure-induced inhibition of fast axonal transport of proteins in the rabbit vagus nerve in galactose neuropathy: Prevention by an aldose reductase inhibitor. *Diabetologia* 1988;31:443–448.

McLean WG, McKay AL, and Sjöstrand J. Electrophoretic analysis of axonally transported proteins in rabbit vagus nerve. *J Neurobiol* 1983;14:227–236.

Mulder DW, Lambert EH, Bastrom JA, and Sprague RG. The neuropathies associated with diabetes mellitus. A clinical and electromyography study of 103 unselected diabetic patients. *Neurology* 1961;11:275–284.

Myers RR, Mizisin AP, and Powell HC, et al. Reduced nerve blood flow in hexachlorophene neuropathy. Relationship to elevated endoneurial fluid pressure. *J Neuropathol Exp Neurol* 1982; 41:391–399.

Myers RR, Murakami H, and Powell HC. Reduced nerve blood flow in edematous neuropathies—A biochemical mechanism. *Microvasc Res* 1986;32:145–151.

Myers RR and Powell HC. Endoneurial fluid pressure in peripheral neuropathies. In Hargens AR, ed. *Tissue Fluid Pressure and Composition.* Baltimore/London: Williams & Wilkins; 1981:193–207.

Myers RR, Powell HC, and Costello ML, et al. Endoneurial fluid pressure: Direct measurement with micropipettes. *Brain Res* 1978;148:510–515.

Neary D and Eames RA. The pathology of ulnar nerve compression in man. *Neuropathol Appl Neurobiol* 1975;1:69–88.

Nemoto K. An experimental study on the vulnerability of the peripheral nerve. *J Jpn Orthop Assoc* 1983;57:1773–1786.

Nissl F. Uber die Veranderungen der Ganglienzellen am Facialiskern des Kaninchens nach Ausreissung der Nerven. *Allg Z Psychiat* 1892;48:197.

Ochoa J, Fowler TJ, and Gilliatt RW. Anatomical changes in peripheral nerves compressed by a pneumatic tourniquet. *Anat* 1972;113:433–455.

Ochoa J and Marotte L. The nature of the nerve lesion caused by chronic entrapment in the guinea-pig. *J Neurol Sci* 1973;19:491–499.

Ochoa J, Torebjörk HE, Culp WJ, and Schady W. Abnormal spontaneous activity in single sensory nerve fibers in humans. *Muscle Nerve* 1982;5:S74–S77.

Ochs S. Energy metabolism and supply of P to the fast axoplasmic transport mechanism in nerve. *Fed Proc* 1974;33:1049–1058.

Ogata K and Naito M. Blood flow of peripheral nerve. Effects of dissection, stretching and compression. *J Hand Surg* 1986; 118: 10–14.

Olmarker K, Rydevik B, Hansson T, and Holm S. Compression-induced changes of the nutritional supply to the porcine cauda equina. *J Spinal Disord* 1990;3:25–29.

Olmarker K, Rydevik B, and Holm S. *Intraneural Edema Formation in Spinal Nerve Roots of the Porcine Cauda Equina Induced by Experimental, Graded Compression.* Transactions, Orthopaedic Research Society, annual meeting, Atlanta, Ga., February 1988.

Olmarker K, Rydevik B, and Holm S. Edema formation in spinal nerve roots induced by graded, experimental compression. An experimental study on the pig cauda equina with special reference to differences in effects between rapid and slow onset of compression. *Spine* 1989a;14:569–573.

Olmarker K, Rydevik B, Holm S, and Bagge U. Effects of experimental graded compression on blood flow in spinal nerve roots. A vital microscopic study on the porcine cauda equina. *J Orthop Res,* 1989b;7:817–823.

Olmarker K, Rydevik B, and Holm S, et al. *Graded Compression of the Porcine Cauda Equina Modifies Nerve Root Nutrition, Blood Flow and Impulse Conduction.* Abstract, Orthopaedic Research Society, 33rd annual meeting, San Francisco, January 1987.

Olsson Y. Studies on vascular permeability in peripheral nerves. I. Distribution of circulating fluorescent serum albumin in normal, crushed and sectioned rat sciatic nerve. *Acta Neuropathol* 1966;7:1–15.

Olsson Y, Kristensson K, and Klatzo I. Permeability of blood vessels and connective tissue sheaths in the peripheral nervous system to exogenous proteins. *Acta Neuropathol Suppl V* 1971:61–69.

Olsson Y and Reese TS. Inaccessibility of the endoneurium of mouse sciatic nerve to exogenous proteins. *Anat Rec* 1969; 163:318.

Olsson Y and Reese TS. Permeability of vasa nervorum and perineurium in mouse sciatic nerve studied by fluorescence and electron microscopy. *J Neuropathol Exp Neurol* 1971;30:105.

Pedowitz RA, Rydevik B, and Hargens AR, et al. *Motor and Sensory Nerve Root Conduction Deficit Induced by Acute Graded Compression of the Pig Cauda Equina.* Transactions, Orthopaedic Research Society, 34th annual meeting, Atlanta, Ga. February 1988.

Powell HC. Pathology of diabetic neuropathy: New observations, new hypotheses. *Lab Invest* 1983;49:515–518.

Powell HC and Myers RR. Pathology of experimental nerve compression. *Lab Invest* 1986;55:91–100.

Rydevik B, Brown M, and Lundborg G. Pathoanatomy and pathophysiology of nerve root compression. *Spine* 1984;9:7–15.

Rydevik B and Garfin S. Spinal nerve root compression. In Szabo RM ed. *Nerve Compression Syndromes—Diagnosis and Treatment.* Thorofare, NJ: Slack; 1989.

Rydevik B and Lundborg G. Permeability of intraneural microvessels and perineurium following acute graded experimental nerve compression. *Scand J Plast Reconstruct Surg* 1977;11:179–187.

Rydevik B, Lundborg G, and Bagge U. Effects of graded compression on intraneural blood flow. An in vivo study on rabbit tibial nerve. *J Hand Surg* 1981;6:3–12.

Rydevik BL, McLean WG, and Sjöstrand J, et al. Blockage of axonal transport induced by acute, graded compression of the rabbit vagus nerve. *J Neurol Neurosurg Psychiatry* 1980;43:690–698.

Rydevik B and Nordborg C. Changes in nerve function and nerve fibre structure induced by acute, graded compression. *J Neurol Neurosurg Psychiatry* 1980;43:1070–1082.

Seddon H. Three types of nerve injury. *Brain* 1943;66:237–288.

Seddon H. *Surgical Disorders of the Peripheral Nerves.* Edinburgh: Churchill Livingstone; 1972.

Sharma AK, Bajada S, and Thomas PK. Influence of streptozotocin-induced diabetes on myelinated nerve fibre maturation and on body growth in the rat. *Acta Neuropathol* 1981;53:257–265.

Sharpless SK. Susceptibility of spinal roots to compression block: The research status of spinal manipulative therapy. In Goldstein M, ed. *NINCDS Monograph No.15.* Washington, DC: U.S. Government Printing Office; 1975:155–161.

Skene JHP. Growth-associated proteins and the curious dichotomies of nerve regeneration. *Cell* 1984;37:697–700.

Spinner M and Spencer PS. Nerve compression lesions of the upper extremity. A clinical and experimental review. *Clin Orthop Relat Res* 1974;104:46–67.

Sunderland S. The nerve lesion in the carpal tunnel syndrome. *J Neurol Neurosurg Psychiatry* 1976;39:615–626.

Sunderland S. *Nerves and Nerve Injuries,* 2nd ed. Edinburgh/London/New York: Churchill Livingstone; 1978.

Szabo RM, Gelberman RH, and Williamson RV, et al. Effects of increased systemic blood pressure on the tissue fluid pressure threshold of peripheral nerve. *J Orthop Res* 1983;1:172–178.

Thoenen H and Barde Y-A. Physiology of nerve growth factor. *Physiol Rev* 1980;60:1284–1335.

Thomas PK and Olsson Y. Microscopic anatomy and function of the connective tissue components of peripheral nerve. In Dyck PJ, Thomas PK, Lambert EH, and Bunge R, eds. *Peripheral Neuropathy,* vol. 1. Philadelphia: WB Saunders; 1984:97–120.

Torvik A. Central chromotolysis and the axon reaction: A reappraisal. *Neuropatol Appl Neurobiol* 1976;2:423–432.

Tuck RR, Schmelzer, and Low PA. Endoneurial blood flow and oxygen tension in the sciatic nerves of rats with experimental diabetic neuropathy. *Brain* 1984;107:935–950.

Upton ARM and McComas AJ. The double crush in nerve-entrapment syndromes. *Lancet* 1973;2:359–362.

Varon S and Adler R. Nerve growth factors and control of nerve growth. *Curr Top Dev Bio* 1980;16:207–252.

Weinstein JN, La Motte R, and Rydevik B, et al. Nerve. In Frymoyer JW, Gordon SL, eds. *New Perspectives on Low Back Pain.* Parke Ridge, Ill: American Academy of Orthopaedic Surgeons; 1989:35–130.

Spinal Reflex Physiology

Akio Sato

Manipulation performed by chiropractors excites somatic afferent fibers in the musculoskeletal structures of the spine. These afferent excitations may, in turn, provoke reflex responses affecting skeletal muscle, autonomic, hormonal, and immunologic functions. An understanding of spinal reflex physiology is, therefore, fundamental to comprehending the effects of manipulation. Spinal reflexes are essentially propriospinal, but are modulated by supraspinal factors. In this chapter, the basic principles of three major spinal reflexes are described: (1) somatosomatic reflexes, (2) viscerosomatic reflexes, and (3) somatovisceral reflexes.

Basic Principles
of Reflex Physiology

The term *reflex* was first used to describe somatic motor spinal reflexes in the late 18th century. Re-

flexes generally are accepted as being characterized by the following:

1. They are involuntary responses.
2. They are not related to learning; i.e., they have a hereditary basis.
3. They show stereotypical, predictable response patterns.
4. They are not conditioned by consciousness.
5. They require relatively short latent periods from the time of stimulus to the beginning of the response.
6. They are purposeful, i.e., involved in the regulation of physiologic functions or behaviors.
7. They consist of a receptor, afferent pathway, integrative center, efferent pathway, and effector.
8. They do not include the cerebral cortex as an integrative center.

The fundamental components of a reflex pathway are shown in Figure 8–1. These consist of a stim-

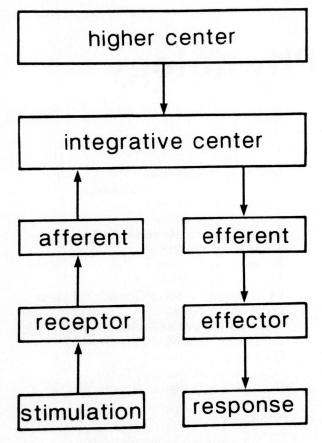

Figure 8-1. Diagram of a reflex.

ulus-activated receptor, transmission via an afferent nerve fiber to an integrative center, efferent transmission of the information to the effector, and induction of a reflex response. This pathway is called a reflex arc. Additionally, the magnitude of the reflex response is often detected by the receptor, which frequently contributes negative feedback control of the reflex system. These common characteristics are well illustrated by the somatic motor reflexes, the responses of which are usually visible to the naked eye. Many reflexes, such as autonomic responses, are not as obvious. For example, blood pressure is maintained at a steady level by the baroreflex mechanism (Heymans and Neil, 1958). Information from the baroreceptor is transmitted by baroreceptor afferent fibers to the integrative center in the brain stem and spinal cord. The efferent pathway is composed of autonomic sympathetic and parasympathetic nerves. The effectors for the baroreflex include tissues in the heart, blood vessels, and adrenal medullary glands. From the adrenal medullary glands, catecholamine hormones including adrenaline, noradrenaline, and dopamine are secreted. These hormones constitute a portion of the reflex response.

The concept of the reflex has undergone a gradual expansion. Sometimes a hormone can be the major part of the efferent path of the reflex. In the well-known milk-ejection reflex, for example, the efferent path is secretion of oxytocin from the posterior lobe of the pituitary gland (Cross and Green, 1959; Harris, 1955). In the case of reflex regulation of parathyroid hormone secretion by low serum calcium levels, the low Ca^{2+} concentration in blood itself acts as an afferent path. The parathyroid gland functions as an integrative center, and parathyroid hormone as an efferent path. There are other examples of reflexes having an organization somewhat different from the classic pattern described above. For example, an axon reflex has no integrative center. A ganglionic reflex has an integrative center located in a peripheral autonomic ganglion. And a conditioned reflex has partial involvement of the cerebral cortex.

The general concept of reflexes has changed in another important way. Although most reflexes have been regarded as immutable responses to a particular stimulus under certain physiologic parameters, it is clear that there are a variety of physiologic and pathologic situations that can alter long-term reflex function. A common example is the facilitation of the monosynaptic muscle stretch reflex that occurs after damage to corticospinal pathways. This facilitation has been attributed to anatomic reorganization (sprouting) of afferent fibers in the spinal cord (Goldberger and Murray, 1985). On a more physiologic level, the flexor reflex (a withdrawal response to painful stimuli) has been shown to be altered for days after an intense period of stimulation (Steinmetz et al., 1985). Additionally, the flexor reflex is known to be altered at the spinal cord level by classical conditioning paradigms (Beggs et al., 1983; Durkovic, 1975), indicating that there is a degree of simple "learning" that can affect reflex function. Additionally, physiologic processes such as habituation can decrease reflex responses (Groves and Thompson, 1970). In the case of autonomic reflexes, the endogenous opioid system has been proposed to be one mechanism whereby responses may be modulated. Indeed, opiates have been shown to selectively suppress certain components of somatoautonomic reflexes (Sato et al., 1986). Despite advancements in the understanding of physiologic modulation of reflex function, this remains a poorly understood topic.

Reflexes are important for maintaining somatic, autonomic, and endocrinologic processes at functional levels. Alternatively, these various functions are regulated mainly by two systems: one is by reflexes and the other is by descending order from the higher centers. Such orders include a programming system of motor control and emotional influence on the autonomic and hormonal responses. Some components of central pathways of reflex arcs and some components of descending command information from the higher centers overlap or occupy the same neuronal structures.

Reflexes can be divided into four types based on the contributions of somatic and autonomic nerves to the efferent and afferent paths of the reflexes.

1. Somatosomatic reflexes: reflexes whose afferents and efferents are somatic nerve fibers.
2. Viscerovisceral reflexes: reflexes whose afferents and efferents are visceral sensory fibers and autonomic nerve fibers.
3. Somatovisceral reflexes (= somatoautonomic reflexes): reflexes whose afferents are somatic sensory fibers and whose efferents are autonomic efferent nerve fibers.
4. Viscerosomatic reflexes (= visceromotor reflexes): reflexes whose afferents are visceral sensory fibers and whose efferents are somatic motor nerve fibers.

In this chapter, mainly spinal reflexes are introduced, with attention focused on somatosomatic, viscerosomatic, and somatovisceral reflexes.

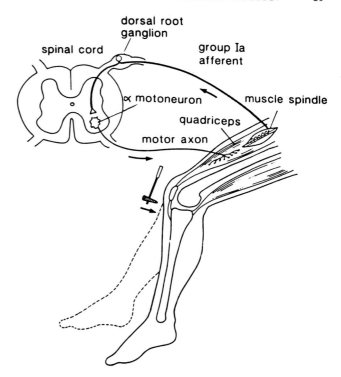

Figure 8-2. Diagram of the stretch reflex. The information from muscle spindles is conducted to the spinal cord through group Ia afferent fibers, exciting the alpha motoneuron.

Somatosomatic Reflex

Stretch Reflex

The knee-jerk and ankle-jerk reflexes are typical muscle stretch reflexes. Although they are sometimes called "tendon reflexes," receptors located in tendons are not responsible for these reflexes. The slight and instantaneous stretching of muscles connected to the tendon induced by striking the tendon (such as the patellar or Achilles tendon) excites muscle spindle stretch receptors within the muscle belly. Afferent information from the muscle stretch receptors produces the reflex contraction of the corresponding muscles through connections within the spinal cord (Fig. 8-2). The efferent limb of the stretch reflex characteristically results in contraction of muscle fibers of the same muscles (homonymous muscles) from which the afferents arise. For this reason, muscle stretch reflexes are proprioceptive reflexes.

Functionally, the stretch reflex has a negative feedback on motion of the body part. For example, if a muscle under resting conditions happens to be stretched for any reason, there is an increase in afferent discharges originating in its muscle spindles. This will reflexively contract the muscle, causing it to attempt to return to its resting length. This feedback mechanism helps to maintain the length of a muscle

or degree of contraction at a constant level. This is important for the maintenance of muscle tone, posture, and the position of joints.

The afferent limb of the stretch reflex comprises thick myelinated group Ia fibers, which conduct the afferent information of the muscle spindle to the central nervous system. In the spinal cord, this information is transmitted to alpha motoneurons located in the ventral horn, exciting the alpha motoneurons that connect to the homonymous muscle (see Fig. 8-2). As there is only one synapse in this reflex arc (within the spinal cord), the stretch reflex is a typical example of a monosynaptic reflex.

Role of the Gamma Motoneuron. The muscle spindle consists of groups of intrafusal muscle fibers. These fibers are arranged in parallel with the extrafusal muscle fibers, which constitute the bulk of the muscle and which are controlled by alpha motoneurons (Fig. 8-3). Intrafusal muscle fibers, which are responsible for activation of Ia afferent fibers, receive motor innervation by gamma efferent motoneurons. Nerve impulses conducted by axons of the gamma motoneurons to the intrafusal muscle fibers are capable of increasing group Ia afferent discharges from the muscle spindle, thereby augmenting stretch reflex sensitivity.

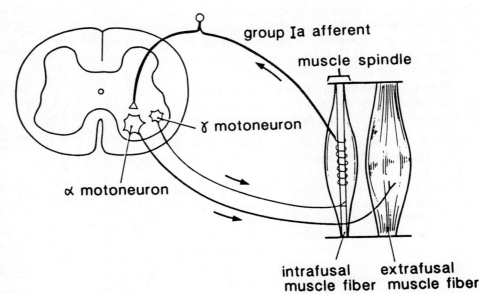

Figure 8-3. Role of the gamma motoneuron. Excitation of a gamma motoneuron increases group Ia afferent discharges from the muscle spindle, augmenting the sensitivity of the stretch reflex.

Recurrent Inhibition of Renshaw. An axon of the alpha motoneuron may branch inside the spinal cord, sending a collateral fiber to stimulate an interneuron called a Renshaw cell (Fig. 8-4). The Renshaw cell, in turn, sends an inhibitory axon to the alpha motoneuron. Excessive excitation of the alpha motoneuron can be prevented by this recurrent inhibitory circuit.

Presynaptic Inhibition of Group Ia Pathways. There is an axoaxonic synapse on the spinal terminal of group Ia afferent fibers originating from the muscle spindle. When this axoaxonic synapse is excited, synaptic transmission from the afferent group Ia

fiber to the alpha motoneuron is inhibited. This inhibition is called presynaptic inhibition. Presynaptic inhibitory mechanisms thereby modulate the input of group Ia fibers.

Role of Golgi Tendon Organs. The musculotendinous connections located at either end of the muscle fibers contain receptors called Golgi tendon organs (Fig. 8-5). These receptors are sensitive to muscle tension, whereas the muscle spindles are sensitive to muscle length. When a muscle contracts and increases its tension (e.g., from activation of the stretch reflex), muscle tendons are stretched, and their tendon organs are excited. The excitation is

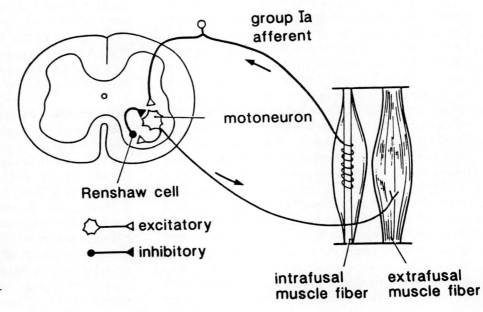

Figure 8-4. Diagram of the recurrent inhibition of Renshaw. An alpha motoneuron may branch a collateral axon to the Renshaw cell, which inhibits the alpha motoneuron.

conducted into the spinal cord through group Ib afferent fibers, exciting inhibitory interneurons in the spinal cord. These interneurons in turn inhibit the alpha motoneurons innervating the homonymous and synergist muscles. Excessive stretch reflexes of the muscle and excessive development of tension of the muscle can thus be prevented by inhibitory modulation.

Reciprocal Inhibition. Many joints have at least two different functional groups of muscles that act in an antagonistic manner. The muscle groups directly contributing to the motion of the joint under consideration are called agonists; those opposing the action are termed antagonists.

During the knee-jerk reflex, the agonist muscle group includes the quadriceps muscles, which extend the knee. A tap on the patellar tendon stretches these muscles, thereby exciting the muscle spindle. In addition to exciting monosynaptic alpha motoneurons of agonist (extensor) muscles, the afferent discharges of the group Ia fibers from these spindles excite inhibitory interneurons that connect to the alpha motoneurons innervating antagonist (flexor) muscles (Fig. 8–6). The antagonist alpha motoneuron is therefore reciprocally inhibited, and the tone of the antagonist muscles is decreased. This inhibition of antagonist muscle is called reciprocal inhibition, group Ia inhibition, or reciprocal antagonist inhibition. In this case, there is one inhibitory interneuron in the spinal cord between the group Ia fiber terminal and the antagonistic alpha motoneuron, making the pathway disynaptic. When there are more than two synapses within a central reflex arc, the reflex is called a polysynaptic reflex.

Flexor Reflex

Afferent information from other receptors can also produce motor reflexes. For example, when the foot of an animal touches a hot surface, or a mechanical nociceptive stimulus is applied to the foot, the lower extremity undergoes a coordinated withdrawal, characterized by flexion at many joints, so as to escape from the stimulus. This reflex response is termed the flexor reflex, flexion reflex, or withdrawal reflex (Fig. 8–7). During this reflex, as flexor muscles contract, the extensor muscles relax, facilitating the flexion of the joints. This coordinated reflex is regulated using polysynaptic reflex pathways.

Afferent fibers that elicit flexor reflexes are called flexor reflex afferents. As opposed to the thick myelinated group Ia or group Ib fibers responsible for stretch or tendon reflexes, afferent fibers mediating the flexor reflex are much thinner, ranging in group II, III, and IV fibers of skin, muscle, and joints.

This flexor reflex is physiologically significant in producing rapid reflex escape from nociceptive stimulation. In addition to a protective function, this reflex seems to play a role in regulating the movement of joints during walking, as group II afferent fibers, which are excited by innocuous stimulation of skin and muscle, are also able to evoke flexor reflexes.

Crossed Extensor Reflex

When a strong stimulus such as nociceptive stimulation is applied to the skin of one foot, not only is flexion of the ipsilateral leg produced, but there is also extension of the contralateral leg (see Fig. 8–7). This extension of the contralateral leg is called the crossed extensor reflex or crossed extension reflex. This reflex may have a physiologic role in causing the contralateral leg to bear the body's weight while the ipsilateral flexor reflex occurs. This inhibition of the contralateral flexor motoneuron occurs also polysynaptically.

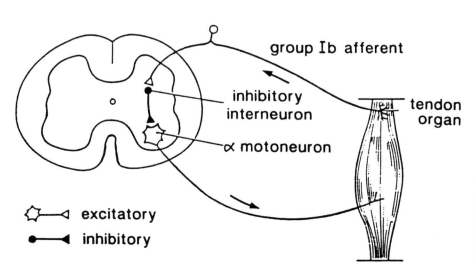

Figure 8-5. Reflex pathway from Golgi tendon organ to alpha motoneuron. The information from the tendon organ is conducted through group Ib afferent fibers to the spinal cord, exciting the inhibitory interneuron, which inhibits the alpha motoneuron.

group Ib afferent

inhibitory interneuron

tendon organ

α motoneuron

excitatory

inhibitory

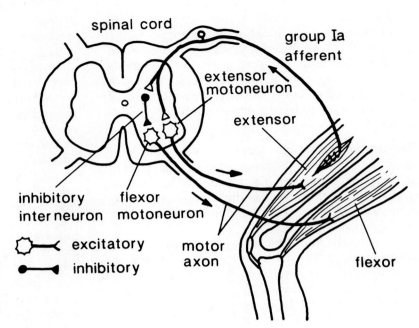

Figure 8–6. Diagram of reciprocal inhibition on the stretch reflex. When an extensor muscle is stretched, the extensor muscle (agonist) contracts (the stretch reflex) and the flexor muscle (antagonist) is reciprocally relaxed through the excitation of the inhibitory interneuron.

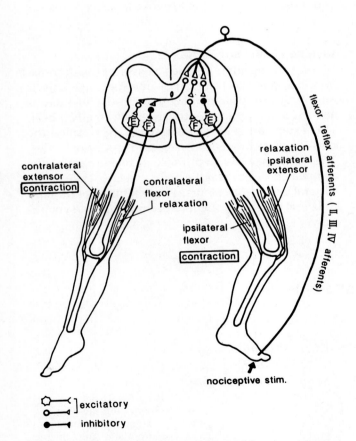

Figure 8–7. Diagram of the flexor reflex and the crossed extensor reflex. E = extensor motoneuron, F = flexor motoneuron. When nociceptive stimulation is applied to the foot, the ipsilateral flexors contract and extensors relax, while the contralateral flexors relax and extensors contract.

Cutaneous Reflexes

The motor reflexes that are activated following cutaneous stimulation are termed cutaneous reflexes. These reflexes are mediated through interneurons at the spinal level and are thus polysynaptic. Pressure stimulation on a foot pad causes an extension of joints of the lower limb through the excitation of extensor muscles. This extension is called the extensor thrust (Sherrington, 1906). Cutaneous tactile stimulation of a foot results in extension of the same foot digit (Engberg, 1964). These reflexes appear to be important during walking and may help to stabilize the extension of the foot during stance.

The monosynaptic muscle stretch reflex in the quadriceps muscles can be facilitated by tactile stimulation of the skin covering the quadriceps muscle and inhibited by stimulation of skin areas located distant from the muscle (Hagbarth, 1952). As tactile stimulation of different skin areas has varying results, cutaneous stimulation is considered to play an important role in control of motor functions.

As mentioned previously, weak mechanical stimulation of certain skin areas occasionally produces contraction of extensor muscles, resulting in an extensor thrust. Intense stimulation of the same skin area often produces the opposite effect, i.e., a flexor reflex. Thus, the particular cutaneous reflex response elicited depends not only on the particular skin area stimulated, but also on the quality of the stimulus.

Cutaneous reflexes are observed not only in extremity muscles, but also in trunk muscles. For example, scratching the abdominal skin causes reflex contraction of the abdominal muscles (the abdominal reflex). Stroking the medial thigh causes reflex contraction of the cremaster muscle (cremasteric reflex).

Long Spinal Reflex

The reflexes mentioned so far, including the stretch reflex, flexor reflex, and cutaneous reflex, have reflex arcs within the same segment or, at the most, within a few segments of the spinal cord. Thus, they are called segmental reflexes. There are long spinal reflexes, too. They are characterized by reflex arcs that include multiple spinal segments. Two examples of long spinal reflexes, the interlimb reflex and the scratch reflex, are described here.

Interlimb Reflex. Nociceptive stimulation to the forepaw of a decerebrated animal produces flexion of the same forelimb (flexor reflex), extension of the contralateral forelimb (crossed extensor reflex), extension of the ipsilateral hind limb, and flexion of the contralateral hind limb (Sherrington, 1906). Similarly, stimulation of the hind limb produces flexion of the same hind limb, extension of the contralateral hind limb, extension of the ipsilateral forelimb, and flexion of the contralateral forelimb. These reflexes are called the forelimb–hind limb and hind limb–forelimb reflexes, respectively. As it is possible to produce them in spinal-sectioned animals, these reflexes are patterned in the spinal cord. Obviously, reflex pathways within the cervical cord and lumbosacral spinal cord interconnect by descending and ascending propriospinal neurons. These interlimb reflexes apparently contribute to coordinated movements of the forelimb and hind limb during walking.

Scratch Reflex. In chronic spinal-sectioned dogs, either rubbing of the skin of the back or slight movement of the hair of the back causes the ipsilateral hind limb to scratch the stimulated skin area. This reflex is called the scratch reflex (Sherrington, 1906). This reflex includes an orienting component, in which the hind limb finds the stimulated area, and a component of rhythmic extension and flexion of the hind limb. Cutaneous afferent information from the back skin enters the spinal cord, where it produces the rhythmic excitations of motoneurons innervating hind limb flexor and extensor muscles with a frequency of about 4 Hz. The frequency of these rhythmic movements is rather constant, regardless of the particular frequency of cutaneous stimulation. Rhythmic movements of the hind limb can be seen even after the lumbosacral dorsal roots are severed, indicating that these movements are not due to hind limb afferent feedback control. These movements may be produced by a spinal rhythmic generator that organizes the flexion and extension movements of the hind limb.

Viscerosomatic Reflex

The reflex contraction of somatic muscle produced by the stimulation of visceral afferent nerves is called the viscerosomatic reflex or visceromotor reflex. Viscerosomatic reflexes commonly operate during the control of respiration and micturition and under several other physiologic conditions.

During respiration, the rhythm of the diaphragm and intercostal muscles is controlled, through the motor nerves, primarily by the respiratory regulatory centers in the brain stem. This rhythmic respiratory movement is also controlled by reflex action. Visceral sensory information is transmitted from pulmonary stretch receptors and chemoreceptors in the blood vessels to the respiratory regulatory centers in the brain stem through visceral afferent nerves (vagus and glossopharyngeal nerves). This information then influences motoneurons innervating respiratory muscles, thereby controlling respiration via a medullary reflex.

During regulation of micturition, afferent information from the stretch receptors of the bladder controls the contractility of the external sphincter muscle of the urethra, which is composed of striated muscle fibers. When the bladder is distended by urine, afferent information is transmitted into the spinal cord through the visceral afferents (pelvic nerve) and integrated within the central nervous system. This afferent activity triggers an increase in efferent nerve activity of the somatic pudendal nerve, thus contracting the external sphincter muscles of the urethra. This prevents incontinence. During micturition, the bladder contracts strongly, and as intravesical pressure increases, the sphincter muscles of the urethra relax, allowing passage of urine through the urethra. There are centers for these bladder–urethral external sphincter muscle reflexes in both the brain stem and the spinal cord.

If the gastrointestinal tract is severely distended, visceral afferent activation may cause reflex contraction of the abdominal muscles and the muscles of the extremities (Miller, 1924). In spinal-sectioned cats, a single electrical shock to the splanchnic afferent nerve produces evoked reflex discharges in spinal motor nerves at various segmental levels (Downman, 1955). This reflex is strongest in the segments of the abdominal muscles, which are innervated by T10 to T12, the region where the splanchnic afferent nerve fibers enter mainly the spinal cord. It has therefore, been suggested that these viscerosomatic reflexes are segmentally organized.

Pathologic viscerosomatic reflexes can be recognized in some visceral diseases. When visceral organs are abnormally distended or inflamed, visceral pain input frequently results in contractions of abdominal muscles. This is especially true when the inflammation spreads to the parietal peritoneum. Such a reflex contraction of abdominal muscles is useful both for the protection of the abdominal organs and for the diagnosis of diseases. This reflex is called muscular defense or involuntary guarding.

Somatovisceral Reflex

It has long been known that stimulation of skin or muscle produces changes in visceral function (see reviews by Sato and Schmidt, 1973, 1987; Sato et al., 1979a,b; Aihara et al., 1979). For example, in cases of abdominal pain caused by spasmodic intestinal contractions, warming the area of skin innervated by the same segment of spinal cord that innervates the diseased portion of intestinal tract will inhibit intestinal movements and relieve the pain. This somatointestinal reflex occurs because afferent stimulation from temperature receptors in the skin heightens the activity of sympathetic efferents innervating the intestine at the same spinal segment level. Other well-known examples of somatoautonomic reflexes include the somatocardiac reflex, in which stimulation of the skin causes changes in heart rate, and the somatovesical reflex, in which stimulation of the skin of the perineum initiates micturition in patients with chronic spinal cord injury.

The neural mechanisms involved in somatovisceral reflexes in humans are very difficult to investigate, because these reflexes are greatly influenced by emotional factors following somatic sensory stimulations.

The physiologic mechanisms underlying somatovisceral reflexes are gradually being elucidated by experiments using anesthetized animals, thereby eliminating emotional factors. Somatovisceral reflexes may be broadly classified, on the basis of their reflex pathways, as spinal reflexes (the reflex center is the spinal cord) and supraspinal reflexes (the reflex center is a part of the central nervous system higher than the spinal cord) (Sato and Schmidt, 1971, 1973). The manifestations of spinal or supraspinal reflexes vary according to the type of stimulation or effector involved.

Some examples of somatosympathetic reflex discharges are shown in Fig. 8–8. In the case depicted in this figure, sympathetic reflex discharges are recorded from the lumber white rami (L1 WR)

and electrical stimuli are delivered to the spinal nerves L1 to L4, to the dorsal roots L7 to S1, and also to cutaneous and muscle hind limb nerves (SU, GS). As is evident in the figure, one characteristic of spinal reflexes (early spinal reflex component) is that the size of the reflex response varies according to the particular spinal segment stimulated. That is, when the afferents transmitting somatic sensory input and the efferents innervating effectors are at the same or nearby spinal segmental level, the spinal reflex is large; if the spinal segments of afferent and efferent pathways are far from each other, the spinal reflex is small. Conversely, somatosympathetic reflex responses that are mediated supraspinally (late supraspinal reflex component) are relatively constant in size, regardless of the segmental level of somatic afferent input.

The neural mechanisms of the principal somatovisceral reflexes elucidated by Sato and co-workers over the past two decades are introduced here.

Somatocardiac Reflex

It has long been known from clinical studies that the heart rate can be changed by somatic afferent stimulation. Systematic electrophysiologic studies of this subject were started in 1958 by Schaefer's group, who were the first to recognize that the central reflex pathway for somatocardiac sympathetic reflex discharges is supraspinal (Sell et al., 1958). Their studies were continued by Coote and Downman (1966) who identified a spinal sympathetic reflex component in the somatocardiac reflex. Sato and colleagues extended this work by analyzing correlations between autonomic nerve activity and cardiac response following somatic sensory stimulations (Kaufman et al., 1977; Sato and Schmidt, 1987; Sato et al., 1979a, 1981).

Cutaneocardiac Reflex. In a majority of anesthetized cats and rats with normal body temperature, a reflex increase in heart rate is elicited after natural stimulation, such as pinching (noxious mechanical stimulation, Fig. 8–9A–D) or rubbing (innocuous mechanical stimulation) anywhere on the surface of the body. Innocuous stimulation produces a weak and inconsistent increase in heart rate; noxious stimulation causes a consistent marked reflex increase in heart rate. This cutaneocardiac acceleration reflex is produced mainly by an augmentation of cardiac sympathetic efferent nerve activity. In spinal-sectioned animals, only stimulation of the chest skin produces a reflex increase in heart rate, and this increase is small (Fig. 8–9, N–Q). Thus, in an animal with an intact central nervous system, the supraspinal reflex component, which is large and diffuse, dominates the small, segmentally organized sympa-

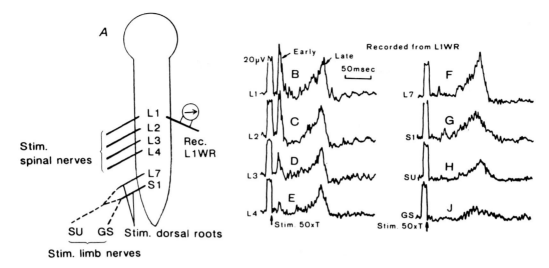

Figure 8–8. Somatosympathetic reflex discharges. (*A*) Schematic diagram of the arrangement of the stimulation and recording electrodes in a cat. WR = white ramus. (*B–J*) Tracings of sympathetic reflexes recorded from the L1 WR. Single stimuli (indicated by arrows) were given at the end of the calibration pulses to the spinal nerves (L1–L4), the dorsal roots (L7–S1), and the limb cutaneous nerve (sural nerve, SU) and muscle nerve (gastrocnemius and soleus nerve, GS) with 50 times threshold (50xT) intensity. Note early spinal reflex and late supraspinal reflex components. *(Modified*

thetic reflex component of the cutaneocardiac acceleration reflex.

A reflex increase in heart rate occurs in anesthetized cats after thermal stimulation of the skin. The threshold temperature for evoking cardiac acceleration is between 13 and 19°C for cold stimulation and about 40°C for warm stimulation. Either innocuous warming (below 40°C) or innocuous cooling (above 13°C) causes a small reflex increase in heart rate. Stimulation by heat (above 45°C) and cold (below

10°C) in the noxious ranges produces a larger increase in heart rate.

Musculocardiac Reflex. When injected into a muscle artery of the hind limb, algesic substances such as potassium chloride and bradykinin, which are known to excite the thin myelinated group III and unmyelinated group IV muscle afferents, can change heart rate. Injection of potassium chloride regularly induces an acceleration of heart rate and an

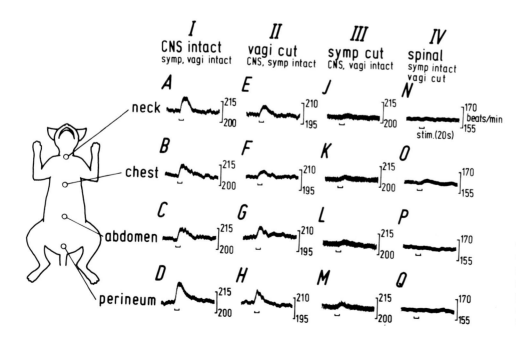

Figure 8–9. Effect on heart rate of pinching various skin areas under different conditions. The skin of the neck, chest, abdomen, and perineum was pinched for 20 seconds. *(From Kaufman et al., 1977, p. 105, with permission.)*

increase in blood pressure. With bradykinin, both accelerations and decelerations can be observed.

Electrical Stimulation of Cutaneous and Muscle Afferents.

In anesthetized cats, the heart rate changes when cutaneous and muscle afferents of the hind limb nerve are stimulated electrically. Repetitive stimulation of cutaneous group II afferents of the hind limb does not change the heart rate. Activation of cutaneous group III afferent fibers usually leads to an increase in heart rate. Increases in heart rate are invariably seen when repetitive stimulation is delivered to the smallest cutaneous afferents, the group IV afferents (Fig. 8–10). This reflex increase in heart rate is produced by an increase in cardiac sympathetic efferent nerve activity (Fig. 8–10). Activation of large-diameter group I and II muscle afferents does not affect heart rate, whereas group III muscle afferent volleys provoke bradycardia or tachycardia. The nature of the response depends on the precise characteristics of the experimental situation but is difficult to predict or to modify. Stimulation of group IV muscle afferents invariably induces definite increases in heart rate.

Articulocardiac Reflex.

Activation of small-diameter knee-joint afferents influences such cardiovascular functions as heart rate, blood pressure, and cardiac sympathetic efferent nerve activity in anesthetized cats. These effects are particularly pronounced when the joint receptors are sensitized by inflammation. Although movements of a normal knee joint through the normal range do not have any significant influence on heart rate in a cat with an intact central nervous system, movements of normal joints beyond this range induce heart rate changes of the same order of magnitude as those elicited by pinching a paw. In inflamed joints, movements in the normal working range of the joint are just as powerful in their cardiovascular effects as noxious stimuli in normal joints. Forceful movements of inflamed joints produce even more potent increases in heart rate than intense noxious stimulation of normal tissue.

Somatogastrointestinal Reflex

Somatogastrointestinal reflexes are well known clinically, and the influence of somatic afferent stimulation on gastrointestinal motility has been reported for dogs, cats, monkeys, and humans. The neural mechanisms of cutaneogastric reflexes have been investigated in anesthetized rats by recording gastric motility and autonomic efferent nerve activity (Sato et al., 1975; Aihara et al., 1979; Sato and Schmidt, 1987). Expansion of the pyloric antrum causes rhythmic contractile waves corresponding to gastric peristaltic movements. Pinching of the abdominal skin

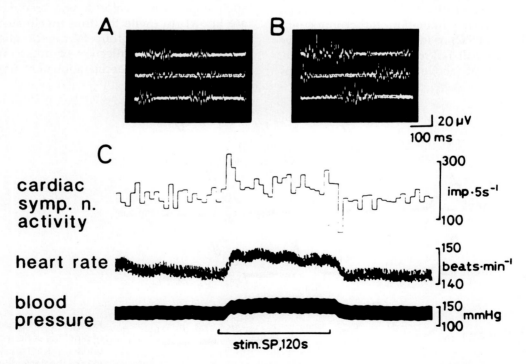

Figure 8–10. Effect of group IV cutaneous afferent volleys on cardiovascular function. Cardiac sympathetic efferent discharges (A) in control condition, and (B) during electrical stimulation of the hind limb cutaneous nerve (superficial peroneal nerve, SP) with 200 times threshold intensity at 10 Hz. (C) Simultaneous recording of cardiac sympathetic

usually inhibits gastric motility (Fig. 8–11A), whereas pinching the hind paw sometimes facilitates gastric motility in anesthetized rats. In anesthetized cats, however, these reflex responses are less marked and the facilitatory response cannot be observed.

The neural mechanisms involved in both reflex inhibition and facilitation of rat gastric motility by stimulation of the abdominal skin and hind paw have been determined. Abdominal skin stimulation markedly and consistently increases gastric sympathetic efferent (splanchnic) nerve activity without significantly altering gastric vagal efferent nerve activity (Fig. 8–11B). The increase in gastric sympathetic efferent nerve activity causes reflex inhibition of gastric motility produced by pinching the abdominal skin. Hind paw stimulation increases gastric vagal efferent nerve activity, whereas gastric sympathetic efferent nerve activity is only slightly increased. The increase in gastric vagal efferent nerve activity apparently is responsible for the reflex facilitation of gastric motility produced by hind paw pinching.

The inhibition of gastric motility caused by pinching the abdominal skin is essentially un-changed after spinal transection at the C1 level, indicating that the spinal cord plays a predominant role in this somatogastric inhibitory reflex (Fig. 8–11D). Additionally, the strongly segmental organization for this reflex response in animals with intact central nervous systems further suggests that the inhibitory reflex is integrated in the spinal cord. A similar organization has been described for both the inhibitory cutaneoduodenal reflex (Sato and Terui, 1976) and the inhibitory cutaneointestinal reflex to noxious stimulation of abdominal skin.

Single electrical stimuli delivered to lower intercostal afferent nerves produce reflex discharges in the splanchnic nerve. These reflex discharges are integrated at the spinal level, and consist of an early spinal reflex discharge from excitation of group II and III afferent fibers and a late spinal reflex discharge from activation of group IV afferent fibers. Similar reflexes are seen in both intact and spinal-sectioned rats, further reinforcing the spinal nature of the reflexes. Both early and late spinal splanchnic efferent reflex discharges apparently contribute to the inhibition of gastrointestinal motility by increas-

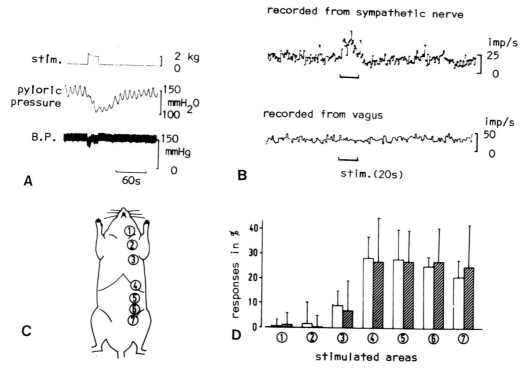

Figure 8–11. Effect of skin pinching on intraluminal pyloric pressure of rat. (*A*) Sample recording of pyloric pressure when the abdominal skin was pinched. (*B*) Recordings of efferent mass discharge activity of gastric sympathetic nerve branches and vagal branches. (*C*) Various skin areas used for stimulation. (*D*) Magnitude of reflex responses elicited by stimulation of skin areas shown in (*C*). White columns indicate responses of rats with central neuraxis intact; hatched columns indicate responses of spinal-sectioned rats. (*Modified from Sato et al., 1975, pp. 153, 155, and 156, with permission.*)

ing splanchnic sympathetic nerve activity after stimulation of abdominal skin.

Somatovesical Reflex

Cutaneous stimulation of the perineal area evokes micturition in chronic spinal-sectioned patients and animals (Sato et al., 1977, 1979b; Sato and Schmidt, 1987). This cutaneous stimulation evokes contraction of the quiescent bladder, while inhibiting the large rhythmic micturition contractions.

Cutaneovesical Reflex. When the urinary bladder is slightly expanded, it has a quiescent, or small, rapidly fluctuating tonus. Innocuous or noxious mechanical stimulation of the perineal skin produces a transient increase in intravesical pressure as a result of a reflex increase in efferent discharges of the vesical branch of the pelvic nerve, a parasympathetic nerve (Fig. 8–12: I,D). Hypogastric (sympathetic) nerves are not essential for this vesical reflex re-

sponse. Perineal stimulation produces reflex bladder contractions whether the spinal cord is intact or transected above the sacral level. This suggests that the excitatory cutaneovesical reflex is a propriospinal and segmental dominated reflex.

When the urinary bladder is expanded further, large, slow rhythmic micturition contractions synchronized with burst discharges of the parasympathetic pelvic efferent nerve are initiated. These micturition contractions are completely abolished either by bilateral destruction of the pelvic nerve branches or by spinal transection at the cervical or middle thoracic level. These rhythmic micturition contractions must therefore be initiated by pelvic efferent nerve activity resulting from a reflex integrated in supraspinal structures. Noxious stimulation of perineal, abdominal, or chest skin produces in this order of inhibiting effectiveness a reflex inhibition of micturition contractions (Fig. 8–12: II, III, F–H). The inhibition results from the depression of burst discharges

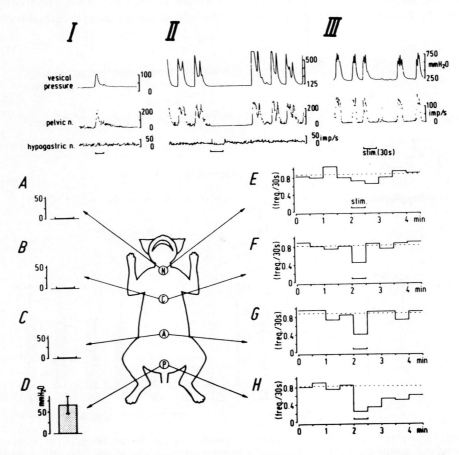

Figure 8-12. Effect of pinching the skin for 30 seconds on vesical pressure and vesical autonomic efferent nerve activity. I, II, and III are simultaneous recordings of vesical pressure, pelvic efferent nerve activity, and hypogastric efferent nerve activity. (*A–D*) Reflex changes in the peak amplitude of vesical pressure after pinching the skin when the bladder is quiescent. (*E–H*) Peristimulus–time histograms of the large, rhythmic micturition contractions. The ordinates represent frequency of the large micturition contractions per 30 seconds. (*Modified from Sato et al. 1977, pp. 112 and 114, with permission.*)

in the pelvic efferent nerve. The wide area of skin over which noxious stimulation produces effective inhibition indicates that there is an intermediate degree of segmental organization of somatopelvic reflexes when compared with the other responses mentioned earlier. Sympathetic hypogastric nerves do not appear to be essential in producing this cutaneovesical inhibitory reflex response.

Application of thermal stimulation of various temperatures to the perineal skin produces responses similar to those evoked by mechanical stimulation. Thermal stimulation in the nonnoxious range causes a small and inconsistent response, whereas thermal stimulation in the noxious range generates a consistent excitatory (when the bladder is quiescent) or inhibitory (when the bladder is expanded) response.

Musculovesical Reflex. Micturition contractions are also inhibited when muscle afferent activity in hind limb nerves is evoked by close intraarterial injection of algesic substances, such as potassium chloride and bradykinin. This inhibition is brought about by depression of the rhythmic burst discharges of the parasympathetic pelvic efferent nerves. On the other hand, when the bladder is quiescent, the effect on the bladder of algesic chemical stimulation of the hind limb muscle afferents is excitatory, because of a reflex increase in pelvic efferent nerve activity.

Electrical Stimulation of Somatic Afferents. Repetitive electrical stimulation of group III and IV cutaneous and muscle afferents has an excitatory effect on the quiescent bladder and an inhibitory effect on the bladder during large, rhythmic micturition contractions. On the other hand, stimulation of group I (muscle afferent) and II (cutaneous and muscle) afferents is ineffective.

Chronic Spinal-Sectioned Cats. Somatovesical reflexes were studied in cats whose spinal cords were transected at the midthoracic level many months earlier (Sato et al., 1983). When the bladder is empty and quiescent, brief repetitive electrical stimulation of a hind limb somatic nerve increases the pelvic efferent nerve activity, which in turn results in reflex vesical contractions (Fig. 8–13A). When the bladder is expanded, there are spontaneous, large, rhythmic micturition contractions. These observations contradict the view held since Barrington (1925) that the center for generating the rhythmic micturition contractions is in the brain stem. Micturition contractions in chronic spinal-sectioned cats, as in normal cats, are induced by rhythmic burst discharges in pelvic efferent nerves from the lower spinal cord. Electrical stimulation of hind limb nerves produces an initial, transient vesical contraction, followed by long-lasting inhibition of the rhythmic micturition contractions of the expanded bladder as a result of depression of pelvic rhythmic burst discharges (Fig. 8–13B).

Somatosudomotor Reflex

Activation of sweat glands produces changes in both the voltage and the impedance of the skin. A reflex change in skin potential or impedance produced by various stimuli, including emotional stimuli, is called the ''galvanic skin reflex'' (GSR) or the ''electrodermal reflex'' (EDR) (see a review by Wang, 1964). Cat paws have sweat glands and are often used to study the GSR.

In spinal-sectioned cats the GSR can be either excited or inhibited by pinching the skin or stimulating cutaneous afferent nerves originating from various spinal segments (Sato and Schmidt, 1987). Generally speaking, there is a tendency for the GSR to be inhibited when the afferent input enters spinal seg-

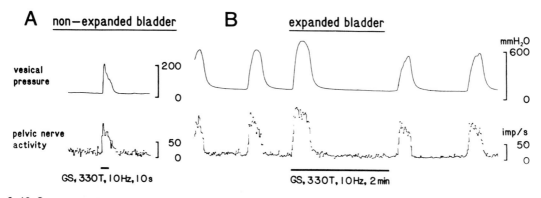

Figure 8–13. Cutaneovesical reflex in chronic spinal cats. Changes in bladder contractility and pelvic efferent nerve activity in response to repeated electrical stimulation of the hind limb muscle nerve (gastrocnemius and soleus nerve, GS) in a cat 12 months after spinal transection. *(From Sato et al., 1983, p. 353, with permission.)*

ments near the outflow of the sudomotor sympathetic nerve fibers to the corresponding paw, whereas excitation occurs when the input is to distant segments. Interestingly, an inhibitory GSR is produced more frequently by ipsilateral than by contralateral cutaneous stimulation. It seems reasonable to assume that this phenomenon results from a mechanism similar to the one that produces hemihidrosis in human beings (Takagi and Sakurai, 1950). Hemihidrosis in humans is a condition in which excessive perspiration occurs contralateral to the side of the body to which pressure is applied and reduced perspiration occurs ipsilateral to the side to which pressure is applied.

Somatoadrenal Medullary Reflex

Visceral function is influenced by circulating hormones in addition to autonomic nerve activity. Although many recent studies have dealt with the effects of somatic afferent stimulation on autonomic nerve activity, the possibility of similar somatohormonal secretion reflexes has received little attention. Recently, Sato's laboratory has demonstrated

that adrenal sympathetic nerve activity and catecholamine secretion from the adrenal gland are modulated reflexively by somatic afferent activity (Araki et al., 1984; Sato, 1987; Sato and Schmidt, 1987).

Cutaneoadrenal Reflex. Noxious pinching of the lower chest or hind paw produces reflex increases in both adrenal sympathetic efferent nerve activity and catecholamine secretion from the adrenal medulla (Fig. 8–14A and B) in anesthetized rats and cats. Pinching the lower chest for 3 minutes elicits a longer-lasting response than does similar hind paw stimulation, i.e., 7 to 17 minutes (for lower chest pinching) and 1 minute (for hind paw pinching) after cessation of the stimulation. After spinal transection at the C1–C2 level, only stimulation in the lower chest region is capable of producing a reflex response (Fig. 8–15A and B).

As opposed to the increased adrenal secretion and nerve activity elicited by pinching, innocuous brushing of the lower chest or hind limb skin in anesthetized but otherwise intact rats produces reflex inhibition of both adrenal sympathetic nerve activity and catecholamine secretion. This inhibition is re-

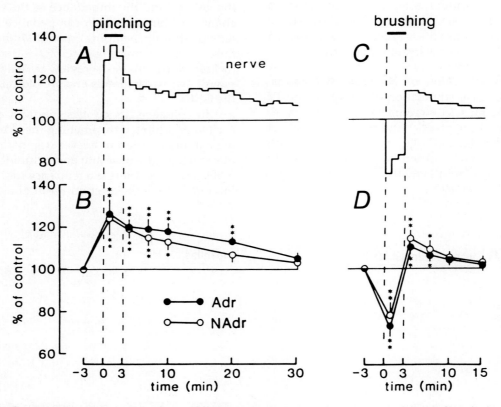

Figure 8–14. Cutaneoadrenal medullary reflexes. Effects on adrenal sympathetic nerve activity (*A, C*) and adrenal catecholamine secretion (*B, D*) during stimulation of lower chest skin by pinching (*A, B*) or by gentle brushing (*C, D*). In (A) and (C), values indicate means of the mean response of each animal. In (B) and (D), values indicate means ± SE of the mean response of each animal. *(Modified from Araki et al., 1984, pp. 293 and 294, with permission.)*

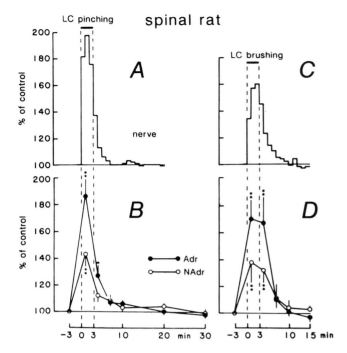

Figure 8–15. Cutaneoadrenal medullary reflexes in spinal rats. Effects on adrenal sympathetic nerve activity (*A, C*) and adrenal catecholamine secretion (*B, D*) during stimulation of lower chest skin by pinching (*A, B*) or by gentle brushing (*C, D*) in spinal rats. *(Modified from Araki et al., 1984, pp. 295 and 296, with permission.)*

stricted to the stimulation period (Fig. 8–14C and D). Some slight increases in both nerve activity and secretion rates occur after cessation of the brushing stimulation as a rebound response. There is some species variability in inhibitory adrenal reflexes as these reflexes cannot be produced in anesthetized cats. After the spinal cord is severed in rats, brushing the lower chest or hind limb skin does not produce inhibition but, rather, has the opposite effect: a reflex increase in both nerve activity and catecholamine secretion (Fig. 8–15C and D). Therefore, noxious or innocuous cutaneous stimulation can reflexively modulate the secretion of adrenal medullary hormones via the central nervous system by augmenting or depressing activity in the adrenal sympathetic efferent nerve.

Both cold and warm stimulation of portions of the abdominal skin in the noxious range (below 10°C or above 45°C) causes reflex increases in both adrenal nerve activity and adrenal catecholamine secretion. Conversely, stimulation in the innocuous range (between 13 and 40°C) does not produce significant changes in these variables. In contrast to the response to mechanical stimuli, there is no inhibitory adrenal medullary reflex response to innocuous thermal stimulation. This suggests some degree of mo-

dality specificity in the type of somatic afferent fibers capable of producing inhibitory adrenal medullary reflex responses.

Articuloadrenal Medullary Reflex. Articular stimulation such as rhythmic flexion and extension, as well as rhythmic inward and outward rotation of a knee joint, within the physiologic range of motion, changes neither nerve activity nor adrenal catecholamine secretion. Static outward rotation in the normal working range also has no effect; however, as soon as this static rotation is extended into the noxious range (i.e., beyond the normal range of motion), significant increases in both of these variables are elicited. Additionally, these articuloadrenal medullary reflexes are greatly augmented in animals whose knee joints are artificially inflamed. In these animals, reflex responses are elicited by knee-joint movements that are within normal ranges. Apparently a supraspinal contribution to the reflex response of the sympathoadrenal medullary function is evoked by knee-joint stimulation, as spinal transection at the C2 level completely abolishes the response.

Mechanical stimulation of the thoracic or lumbar vertebral joint in anesthetized rats causes an initial decline in adrenal nerve activity followed by a subsequent increase, which is attributed to baroreceptor effects secondary to a reflex depressor response of blood pressure.

Electrical Stimulation of Somatic Afferent Nerves. Electrical stimulation of somatic afferent nerves at high intensity, activating both myelinated (A β and Aδ, or groups II and III) and unmyelinated (C, or group IV) afferent fibers, produces increases in adrenal nerve activity nearly identical to those induced by noxious mechanical or thermal stimulation of the skin innervated by the nerves tested. On the other hand, low-intensity electrical stimulation, activating myelinated afferent fibers alone, produces inhibitory responses similar in character and duration to the responses evoked by innocuous mechanical stimulation of the skin in rats.

Single-shock stimulation of the 13th thoracic nerve (rats have 13 thoracic nerves) evokes various reflex components in the adrenal nerve in rats. These components, in the temporal order in which they appear, are (1) initial depression of spontaneous activity (the early depression), (2) reflex discharge resulting from activation of A afferent fibers (the A-reflex), (3) subsequent reflex discharge resulting from activation of C afferent fibers (the C-reflex), and (4) postexcitatory depression. It has been suggested that the decrease in sympathetic nerve activity that occurs during repetitive electrical stimulation of myelinated afferent fibers is due to summation of both the early and postexcitatory depression components evoked by a single-shock stimulation. On the other hand, the increase in activity during repetitive stimulation of both myelinated and unmyelinated afferent fibers is due to summation of the C-reflex components elicited by a single-shock stimulation. In cats, A-reflex, C-reflex, and postexcitatory depression appear on a single electrical stimulation; however, no early depression is observed. The lack of early depression may relate to the fact that neither brushing of the skin nor innocuous movements of the normal knee joint produce any significant inhibitory response in cats.

Conclusion

The basic sciences have demonstrated a variety of reflex responses that can be investigated in animals. In general, these responses arise from stimuli that may be classified as somatic or visceral and, in turn, produce responses in somatic or visceral (autonomic) motor systems. Most of the well-characterized somatic reflexes are patterned primarily at the spinal cord level. Visceral reflex responses may have an integrative center in the spinal cord or in the brain stem, depending on the particular response under consideration. Although reflexes are, by definition, largely outside the realm of direct voluntary control, there are many factors that may influence overall reflex response. Generally, these factors are poorly understood and have only recently come under intense scrutiny. Although many aspects of reflex function are more readily investigated in animals, most studies of reflex function in pathologic states are better performed in the ultimate clinical model, humans.

References

Aihara Y, Nakamura H, Sato A, and Simpson A. Neural control of gastric motility with special reference to cutaneo-gastric reflexes. In Brooks C McC, Koizumi K, and Sato A, eds. *Integrative Functions of the Autonomic Nervous System.* Tokyo: University of Tokyo Press/Amsterdam: Elsevier/North-Holland; 1979:38–49.

Araki T, Ito K, Kurosawa M, and Sato A. Responses of adrenal sympathetic nerve activity and catecholamine secretion to cutaneous stimulation in anesthetized rats. *Neuroscience* 1984; 12:289–299.

Barrington FJF. The effect of lesions of the hind- and mid-brain on micturition. *Q J Exp Physiol* 1925;15:81–102.

Beggs AL, Steinmetz JE, Romano AG, and Patterson MM. Extinction and retention of a classically conditioned flexor nerve response in acute spinal cats. *Behav Neurosci* 1983;97:530–540.

Coote JH, and Downman CBB. Central pathways of some autonomic reflex discharges. *J Physiol (Lond)* 1966;183:714–729.

Cross BA, and Green JD. Activity of single neurons in the hypo-thalamus: Effect of osmotic and other stimuli. *J Physiol (Lond)* 1959;148:554–569.

Downman CBB. Skeletal muscle reflexes or splanchnic and intercostal nerve origin in acute spinal and decerebrate cats. *J Neurophysiol* 1955;18:217–235.

Durkovic RG. Classical conditioning, sensitization and habituation of the flexion reflex of the spinal cat. *Physiol Behav* 1975; 14:297–304.

Engberg I. Reflexes to foot muscles in the cat. *Acta Physiol Scand* 1964;62 (suppl. 235):1–64.

Goldberger ME and Murray M. Recovery of function and anatomical plasticity after damage to the adult and neonatal spinal cord. In Cotman CW, ed. *Synaptic Plasticity.* New York: Guilford Press; 1985:77–110.

Groves PM and Thompson RF. Habituation: A dual process theory. *Psychol Rev* 1970;77:419–450.

Hagbarth K-E. Excitatory and inhibitory skin areas for flexor and extensor motoneurons. *Acta Physiol Scand* 1952;26(suppl. 94): 1–58.

Harris GM. *Neural Control of the Pituitary Gland.* Monogragh of the Physiology Society. London: Arnold; 1955.

Heymans C, and Neil E. *Reflexogenic Areas of the Cardiovascular System.* London: Churchill; 1958.

Kaufman A, Sato A, Sato Y, and Sugimoto H. Reflex changes in heart rate after mechanical and thermal stimulation of the skin at various segmental levels in cats. *Neuroscience* 1977;2:103–109.

Miller FR. Viscero-motor reflexes, II. *Am J Physiol* 1924;71:84–89.

Sato A. Neural mechanisms of somatic sensory regulation of catecholamine secretion from the adrenal gland. *Adv Biophys* 1987;23:39–80.

Sato A, Sato Y, and Schmidt RF. The effects of somatic afferent activity on the heart rate. In Brooks C McC, Koizumi K, and Sato A, eds. *Integrative Functions of the Autonomic Nervous System.* Tokyo: University of Tokyo Press/Amsterdam: Elsevier/North - Holland; 1979a:275–282.

Sato A, Sato Y, and Schmidt RF. Somatic afferents and their effects on bladder function. In Brooks C McC, Koizumi K, and Sato A, eds. *Integrative Functions of the Autonomic Nervous System.* Tokyo: University of Tokyo Press/Amsterdam: Elsevier/North - Holland; 1979b:309–318.

Sato A, Sato Y, and Schmidt RF. Heart rate changes reflecting modifications of efferent cardiac sympathetic outflow by cutaneous and muscle afferent volleys. *J Auton Nerv Syst* 1981;4:231–247.

Sato A, Sato Y, Schmidt RF, and Torigata Y. Somato-vesical reflexes in chronic spinal cats. *J Auton Nerv Syst* 1983;7:351–362.

Sato A, Sato Y, Shimada F, and Torigata Y. Changes in gastric motility produced by nociceptive stimulation of the skin in rats. *Brain Res* 1975;87:151–159.

Sato A, Sato Y, Sugimoto H, and Terui N. Reflex changes in the urinary bladder after mechanical and thermal stimulation of the skin at various segmental levels in cats. *Neuroscience* 1977; 2:111–117.

Sato A, Sato Y, Suzuki A, and Swenson RS. The effects of morphine administered intrathecally on somatosympathetic reflex discharges in anesthetized cats. *Neurosci Lett* 1986;71:345–350.

Sato A, and Schmidt RF. Spinal and supraspinal components of the reflex discharges into lumbar and thoracic white rami. *J Physiol (Lond)* 1971;212:839–850.

Sato A, and Schmidt RF. Somatosympathetic reflexes: Afferent fibers, central pathways, discharge characteristics. *Physiol Rev* 1973;53:916–947.

Sato A, and Schmidt RF. The modulation of visceral functions by somatic afferent activity. *Jpn J Physiol* 1987;37:1–17.

Sato Y, and Terui N. Changes in duodenal motility produced by noxious mechanical stimulation of the skin in rats. *Neurosci Lett* 1976;2:189–193.

Sell R, Erdelyi A, and Schaefer H. Untersuchungen uber den Einflu peripherer Nervenreizung auf die sympatheische Aktivitat. *Arch Ges Physiol* 1958;267:566–581.

Sherrington CS. *The Integrative Action of the Nervous System.* New Haven, Conn: Yale University Press; 1906.

Steinmetz JE, Beggs AL, Molea D, and Patterson MM. Long-term relation of a peripherally induced flexor reflex alteration in rats. *Brain Res* 1985;327:312–315.

Takagi K, and Sakurai R. A sweet reflex due to pressure on the body surface. *Jpn J Physiol* 1950;1:22–28.

Wang GH. *The Neural Control of Sweating.* Madison: University of Wisconsin Press, 1964:1–130.

chapter 9

Clinical Investigations of Reflex Function

Rand S. Swenson

Reflex mechanisms have been invoked to explain a wide array of clinical observations. While many of these mechanisms have substantial foundation in animal research (see Chapter 8), human research into reflex function has lagged. This is due largely to the necessary technical limitations placed on experimental protocols involving human subjects. Despite these significant obstacles, much work has been accomplished in the area of human reflex physiology and pathophysiology. This chapter represents an attempt to summarize some of this research, especially as it relates to chiropractic. Nonetheless, wide gaps exist in our ability to extrapolate from reflex functions in animals to clinical observation of end-organ effects. Therefore, we will attempt to define some promising areas for further research.

For the purposes of the present discussion we consider all studies or observations made on humans as being "clinical." Of course, some of these observations have a much greater impact on clinical practice than do others; however, they are all potentially of clinical importance. Additionally, some spheres of reflex function are much better understood than others. This does not necessarily reflect the relative importance of the particular reflex function to clinical practice, but rather often reflects the presence or absence of appropriate tools for study of that function in human subjects. Despite the improvement in technological capacity to investigate reflex function in humans, we trust that the reader will come away with renewed appreciation for the awesome task confronting investigators attempting to study reflex function in human health and disease.

Reflexes Defined

Reflexes may be defined as involuntary responses to stimuli. The minimum criteria for a reflex are the presence of a receptor, a conductive/integrative pathway (simple though it may be), and an effector, by which the response may be observed. All classes of sensory stimuli may provide the receptive component of reflexes. Additionally, emotional stimuli may evoke reflex responses that are rather complex in nature. Generally, in clinical research on reflex function, such emotional responses are regarded as a factor to be controlled rather than investigated. This is especially true considering the tremendous difficulty encountered in attempting to standardize emotional stimuli as well as the extreme diversity of responses between subjects (Heller et al., 1984; Hodes et al., 1985). The potent influences of emotional state on "tone" in the autonomic nervous system make this a very important concern in studies of autonomic nervous system reflex function in humans.

From the above definition of *reflex* it should be apparent that to investigate true reflex phenomena it is necessary to be certain that the observed responses are not voluntary. This is especially true whenever investigating somatic reflex function because the voluntary control system of the somatic nervous system is very well developed. Additionally, it is becoming increasingly clear that voluntary control of autonomic functions cannot be ruled out. Not all responses to a stimulus, then, can be properly classified as reflex in nature. This is a point to bear in mind when considering the results of any study of human reflex physiology or pathophysiology.

The following discussion concentrates on the two major categories of reflex response: somatic and visceral reflexes. Certain reflex responses that are not readily categorized are discussed in a subsequent section.

Clinical Studies of Somatic Reflexes

Somatosomatic reflexes constitute that class of reflexes that have both their receptor and effector in somatic tissue. The discussion focuses on the axial musculoskeletal system, however, the majority of work has been done on the extremities. Although it may be safe to assume that axial and appendicular structures show a great deal of similarity in response to somatic stimuli, it is equally clear that there are likely to be areas of difference. Because appendicular neuromuscular structures are much more accessible, the majority of clinical research has been done on the extremities. Therefore, care must be taken in extrapolation from data derived from studies on limb muscles to spinal muscular physiology.

H-Reflex

Undoubtedly, the best-known and most widely applied clinical reflex is the "monosynaptic" myotatic reflex. This reflex, which can be tested clinically by use of a reflex hammer, can be elicited and measured electrically (Magladery et al., 1951, Burke et al., 1983). This electrical response is known as the Hoffmann's reflex (H-reflex). Although the reflex is most commonly elicited in the triceps surae muscle (an electrical measure of the Achilles reflex) it can be evoked in other appendicular muscles (Deschuytere et al., 1976, 1983). The H-reflex can be quantitated and followed longitudinally. This quantification and standardization are aided by expressing the response as a ratio of the reflex muscular response elicited by electrical stimulation of the muscle afferent nerve fibers to the response elicited by direct maximal stimulation of the motor nerve (H/M$_{max}$ ratio). Alternatively, it may be expressed as the ratio of the threshold stimulation intensity necessary to evoke

the reflex necessary for direct muscle response (Davies and Lader, 1985). Clinically, the H-reflex has been used to demonstrate damage to the innervation of the triceps surae muscle, i.e., damage to the sciatic nerve or to the first sacral nerve root. In the case of nerve lesions, as one might imagine, the reflex diminishes both when expressed in absolute numbers and when expressed in terms the of H/M$_{max}$ ratio; however, the H-reflex is of interest beyond this relatively simple, straightforward application.

The H-reflex is now known to be more complex than previously thought, consisting of both mono- and polysynaptic reflex pathways (Burke et al., 1984). The magnitude of the reflex response is dependent on the level of excitability of alpha motor neurons (Davies, 1984; Verrier, 1985). Therefore, the response may provide an index of ongoing input from voluntary and other reflex neuronal pathways impinging on the motor neuron pool.

The convergence of inputs on alpha motor neurons is illustrated by the influence of the voluntary "set" of muscles on the reflex. It has been shown that the H-reflex increases preparatory to volitional activation of a muscle (Frank, 1986). The convergence of voluntary and reflex pathways on the motor neuron "sets" the neuron for activating the muscle (Etnyr and Abraham, 1986). Additionally, the H-reflex has been shown to be decreased by passive muscle stretch (Robinson et al., 1982) and increased by voluntary muscle contraction (Deschuytere et al., 1983; Magladery et al., 1951; Tanaka, 1974; Upton et al., 1971).

It is noteworthy that some afferent inputs that are incapable of evoking responses by themselves do have the ability to change the excitability of motor neurons. A prime example is the augmentation and inhibition that may be observed in triceps surae H-reflexes as a result of tonic neck input (Rossi et al., 1985, 1987; Traccis et al., 1987). In the normal adult, afferent inputs from cervical spinal joints and muscles are not capable of eliciting tonic neck reflexes, i.e., overt contractions of skeletal muscle (these reflexes may be visible in newborns and in individuals with nervous system damage). Despite this inability to elicit overt movements in normal adults, cervical receptors can be shown to make significant input to lower-extremity motor neurons by their ability to alter H-reflex responses (Rossi et al., 1985, 1987; Traccis et al., 1987). From these data it is clear that it is not necessary for reflex inputs from cervical spinal joints and muscles to have observable effects on motor activity to demonstrate that they have an effect on postural reflex function. Furthermore, these studies serve to extend the concept of reflexes, as they show that there can be reflex modulation of the strength and threshold of another reflex response.

Humphries and Triano (1989) have recently applied H-reflex electrophysiology to the study of nonradicular low back pain. H/M$_{max}$ was found to be significantly greater in a population of low-back-pain sufferers than in a group of normal subjects. This augmentation of somatic reflex function in nonradicular back pain is quite the opposite of the pattern that would be expected had these patients been manifesting signs of nerve injury. The most obvious, and probably the best explanation for the increase in the H-reflex, is an increase in reflex excitability in motor neuron pools secondary to converging pain input evoked by spinal or paraspinal pathology. These investigators also have shown that the augmented H-reflexes generally diminish toward normal with time and therapy, paralleling a decline in symptomatology. These findings provide a fertile ground for clinical investigation of therapy for low back pain that is not solely dependent on symptomatology as an outcome measure.

Joint and muscle afferents are not the only sensory systems capable of modulating muscle activity. It has been demonstrated that cutaneous stimulation can affect electrical activity of thigh muscles during normal stride (Kanda and Sato, 1983). This has been explained functionally on the basis of inputs from the sole of the foot influencing stance and gait. Despite the finding that stimulation of lower-extremity skin can influence lower limb muscles, it is not clear whether cutaneous receptors from other parts of the body can affect tone and reflex function. It is probable that more sensitive measures will be necessary for complete elucidation of the motor effects of cutaneous sensory input.

Flexor Reflex

The flexor reflex is another response that may be evoked and recorded in humans (Willer, 1977, 1983). It is not nearly as well studied as the H-reflex, probably because it is not as closely tied to a clinically observable phenomenon as the H-reflex is tied to myotatic reflexes. The flexor reflex has, however, proved to be of increasing utility in the study of pain and analgesia in humans, as it represents an electrical measure of reflex withdrawal from painful stimuli (Huzon, 1973; Meinck et al., 1985; Willer, 1977). It has a shorter latency than voluntary withdrawal and therefore represents an initial, involuntary response to pain (Huzon, 1973; Meinck et al., 1985). Unlike the H-reflex, the effects of posture, ongoing voluntary activity, and other stimuli (cutaneous, muscle afferent, etc.) on flexor reflex threshold and strength are not well understood. Ironically, in the midst of this general lack of understanding of afferent interaction, it is from studies of flexor reflexes that some of the more convincing clinical data have been gathered in

support of transcutaneous electrical nerve stimulation (TENS) and acupuncture. Studies have shown diminished flexor responses in the face of electroacupuncture (Boureau et al., 1979) and TENS (Chan and Tsang, 1987). These data, in conjunction with similar reports from laboratory animal research, present a formidable framework against which hypotheses concerning the antinociceptive properties of these therapeutic modalities may be tested. It is probable that the coming decade will find evidence of interaction between other afferent systems (including spinal afferents) and flexor reflexes. For example, it would be interesting to test the diminished pain perception observed following manipulation (Terrett and Vernon, 1984) against an objective measure of nociceptive function such as the flexor reflex. It is likely that the flexor reflex will assume an expanding role in the clinical investigation of the physiology of pain.

Paraspinal Musculature

By comparison with the aforementioned reflexes in the extremities, less is known about reflex function of axial musculature. Paraspinal musculature is electromyographically silent in normal subjects at rest (Floyd and Silver, 1955). Therefore, any observed activity in these muscles under resting conditions must result from voluntary and reflex input. It would be reasonable to assume that sustained patterns of activity in these muscle groups at rest would be reflex in origin. From the clinical observation that lumbar paraspinal musculature appears to be ''in spasm'' in many low-back-pain patients has evolved the hypothesis that reflexes triggered by pain afferents are probably active in these patients to produce the ''spasm'' (see Flor and Turk, 1984; Nouwen and Bush, 1984); however, this hypothesis has been challenged by a variety of studies that fail to show increased electromyographic activity in paraspinal muscles of patients with back pain (Collins et al., 1982; Kravitz et al., 1981; Miller, 1985; Wolf and Basmajian, 1978). Although there are a few reports to the contrary (Grabel, 1973; Hoyt et al., 1981), if one accepts that the bulk of data indicate that the clinically observed ''spasm'' is not due to increased tonic activity or contraction of muscle, an alternative explanation must be sought. Although it is beyond the scope of this chapter to further explore this question, help may be forthcoming from literature concerning trigger points, where changes in muscle consistency without change in tonic activity have been recognized for many years (see Travel and Simons, 1983).

Although there is little evidence to suggest change in back muscle tone in low back pain, there is evidence for alteration in muscle function, possibly of a reflex nature. Denslow and co-workers (Denslow, 1942; Denslow and Hassett, 1942; Denslow et al., 1947) have reported that electrical responses (contractions) are frequently evoked in paraspinal muscles following pressure stimulation over the spinus process of vertebral segments with "osteopathic lesions." Such responses are not seen when normal segments are similarly stimulated. The inference is that these responses are pathophysiologic reflexes, although an alternative explanation considers that the responses may be partially explained by voluntary "guarding" in response to noxious stimuli.

Further evidence of abnormal reflex physiology in back pain patients derives from study of "flexion relaxation" in lumbar paraspinal muscles. During normal flexion excursion of the lumbar spine, paraspinal muscles that initially contract to lower the spine to the flexed position subsequently relax and achieve electrical silence in the flexed posture (Floyd and Silver, 1955). In many patients with low back pain, paraspinal muscles fail to achieve this relaxed state at the limits of motion, and instead continue their pattern of high electrical activity initiated at the onset of flexion (Floyd and Silver, 1955; Triano and Schultz, 1987). Although this may be interpreted as a "voluntary guarding" in response to painful movement, the reproducibility of the response suggests a reflex origin, i.e., "involuntary guarding."

As can be seen from the preceding discussion, advancement in clinical understanding of somatosomatic reflexes has been largely dependent on electromyographic technology. Although these techniques have proven to be extremely useful in some spheres of somatic reflex physiology, much remains to be explored. The capacity of therapeutic interventions to alter reflex responses in patients with spinal pathology needs to be assessed.

Further advances in clinical study of somatosomatic reflexes may come from development of new technologies for measuring motor neuronal activity. More likely, however, it will be dependent on improving our ability to quantify electromyographic signals (Davies, 1984) and to obtain stable, reproducible reflex responses from a variety of muscle groups over a prolonged period.

Clinical Studies of Visceral Reflexes

The autonomic nervous system (ANS) is known to participate in the control of more aspects of physiology than was ever previously appreciated; however, clinical understanding of ANS function has not kept pace with the explosion of basic science knowledge. This has largely resulted from the relatively crude measures that are available to the clinician for quantifying ANS function (Hilsted, 1984). Additionally, because it has not been convincingly demonstrated that direct measurement of ANS activity is of appreciable clinical value, it would be difficult to justify direct invasive monitoring of the system. Therefore, clinicians have generally been content to record end-organ effects of ANS activity. The role of the ANS in pathophysiology has generally been inferred from these end-organ effects and from the response of the system to pharmacologic agents known to influence autonomics. An additional problem exists in the quantification of tonic activity, as this requires procedures for measurement that are stable over time and reasonably consistent between individuals. At present, there is no ideal measure for sympathetic tone; however, experiments examining adrenergic receptors on blood elements may afford some hope for the future (Bannister et al., 1981; Davies et al., 1982). The relatively crude and indirect methods that have generally been employed in clinical studies of ANS function are largely responsible for our limited knowledge of autonomic function in disease states. Clinically significant autonomic reflexes may be classified a psychovisceral, viscerovisceral, and somatovisceral.

Psychovisceral Reflexes

Psychovisceral refers to the potent effect of emotions, especially those relating to stress, on autonomic (Goldstein, 1987; Vingerhoets, 1985) and neuroendocrine (Molitch and Hou, 1983; Syvalahti, 1987) function. Short-term psychovisceral reflexes have been employed as one means of assessing autonomic function (Heard, 1964; Hodes et al., 1985; Sleight et al., 1978). These methods generally use some mental stressor, such as arithmetic or unpleasant noise, while monitoring blood pressure or heart rate. It has been shown, for example, that hypertensive individuals manifest an increased sympathetic response to such stress (Dustan, 1987; Herd et al., 1987). A well-recognized example of longer-duration stress in clinical medicine is the development of gastric ulcers in heavily stressed patients, such as those in an intensive care unit (Hillman, 1985; Marrone and Silen, 1984; Silen, 1987). Recently, data have been accumulating relative to possible involvement of stress-related neural and neuroendocrine responses in such diverse processes as hypertension (Cinciripini, 1986a; Herd et al., 1987), cardiac arrhythmia (Cinciripini, 1986b; Dimsdale et al., 1987), atherosclerosis (Cinciripini, 1986b; Clarkson et al., 1987; Manuck et al., 1987; Schneiderman, 1987) diabetes mellitus (Surivit and Feinglos, 1988), certain autoimmune conditions (Kochler, 1985; Wallace, 1987), and alterations in adrenal medullary function (McCarty et al., 1988). Furthermore, increased adrenal medullary function may be a factor in the development of hypertension (Majewski and Rand, 1986; Snider, 1983). Although relationships have been described between stress and certain clinical syndromes as well as between stress and immune response (Tecoma and Huey, 1985; Palmblad, 1987), much remains to be investigated regarding the physiologic mechanisms involved. Deeper understanding of autonomic involvement in stress responses in humans will depend on development of methods to accurately measure sympathetic and parasympathetic tone, as well as methods for assessing organ-system effects.

Viscerovisceral Reflexes

Clinical evaluation of the ANS heavily depends on measurement of viscerovisceral reflexes (Bannister, 1983b; Hillsted, 1984; O'Brien et al., 1986; Vita et al., 1986). Orthostatic measurements are commonly performed on patients and depend on an intact ANS for cardiovascular responses to upright posture. Normal responses result mainly from vasoconstriction in the lower limbs to maintain blood pressure or, failing this, from increases in cardiac output (heart rate and stroke volume). If the sympathetic innervation to both the legs and the heart has failed (or if blood volume is depleted beyond the capacity of the ANS to respond), then profound orthostatic hypotension results. Other useful measures of autonomic function that depend on intact viscerovisceral reflexes include beat-to-beat variability in heart rate, which is lost with destruction of the autonomic innervation of the heart; Valsalva's maneuver, which produces slowing of the heart with intact autonomics; gastric emptying (measured with a nuclear medicine scan), which is delayed with autonomic (particularly parasympathetic) neuropathy; and cystometry, which depends on intact parasympathetic innervation to evoke normal contraction to bladder distention. It is noteworthy that migraine sufferers manifest diminished sympathetic responses to a variety of visceral as well as somatic stimuli (Gotoh et al., 1984; Rubin et al., 1985).

Despite the well-known participation of visceral reflexes such as the baroreceptor response in homeostatic regulation of body functions, there is little evidence to suggest that alteration of visceral reflex function may cause pathology. In this regard, there is some support (though not conclusive) that altered baroreceptor sensitivity may contribute to the development of systemic hypertension (Bristow et al., 1969; Shimada et al., 1986; Sleight, 1984).

Somatovisceral Reflexes

There are a few somatoautonomic reflexes with proven clinical utility. Among the best described is the ciliospinal reflex by which pupillary dilation may be observed following a noxious stimulation of the neck (Reeves and Posner, 1969). This response is mediated predominantly by sympathetic activation at the spinal cord level; however, it is not routinely quantitated. The cold pressor test is another somatoautonomic reflex that has been used in clinical evaluation of the autonomic nervous system. Normally, immersion of a hand in ice water results in a reflex increase in heart rate and blood pressure that is dependent on intact sympathetics (Ewing, 1983).

Clinical Measurement of Autonomic Reflex Function

The clinical measures used to assess the ANS are well suited to the detection of failure of autonomic function, but are crude, at best, for assessing the absolute level of autonomic reflex functioning. Additionally, there is no clinical method for determination of autonomic tone except in few organ-systems where minute-to-minute variability in function may be recorded. The cardiovascular system, which is under tonic control of the ANS, is certainly the most amenable to such evaluation, and even here the interpretation of autonomic tone from physiologic variables is indirect (Hilsted, 1984; O'Brien et al., 1986; Vita et al., 1986).

Activity in identifiable autonomic nerve fibers in human peripheral nerves has been successfully recorded (see Vallbo et al., 1979). This technique is capable not only of demonstrating responses to stimuli but also of assessing the degree of ongoing autonomic activity. Unfortunately, such methods are clinically impractical and, even from a scientific perspective, such studies require sampling of many units before any conclusions may be drawn. Additionally, only selected autonomic fibers, i.e., sympathetic nerve fibers that are distributed to appendicular structures (blood vessels, skin, sweat glands, etc.); may be sampled, the autonomics to visceral organs are inaccessible with this technique. Probably the most useful thing to come out of these studies to this point is the finding that sympathetic nerve fibers in human peripheral nerve are functionally similar to those of other vertebrates. This may provide some confidence when attempting to extrapolate data from laboratory experiments to human beings.

As the major clinical tests of autonomic function are best suited to determination of loss of autonomic innervation, it is not surprising that numerous disorders have been found that do just that (see Bannister, 1983a; McLeod and Tuck, 1987). Examples include diabetes mellitus, uremia, multiple sclerosis, Parkinson's, amyloidosis, Guillian–Barré, and alcoholism. Most hypotheses regarding ANS participation in pathology, however, have focused on the possibility of increased sympathetic nervous system activity (Korr, 1978). This remains an unproven hypothesis, although there is a significant body of literature suggesting that increased sympathetic function may be etiologic in "essential" hypertension (Dustan, 1987; Sleight, 1984; Tuck, 1986). Even here, it is not clear whether the increase in sympathetic activity is present only at the inception of the disorder or whether it persists throughout its course. Despite the finding that autonomic reflexes are altered in hypertensives (Bristow et al., 1969; Shimada et al., 1986), it remains to be proved whether this alteration in neural function is the primary cause of the hypertension.

Some of the most convincing data supporting the hypothesis of sympathetic hyperactivity in humans comes from studies of galvanic skin resistance (GSR). GSR is predominantly an index of sudomotor activity and, as such, reflects the level of sympathetic tone in the region (Thomas and Kawahata, 1962). The GSR that is measured under basal conditions is a reflection of tonic activity in the sympathetic nervous system, along with whatever reflex activity may be ongoing at the time of recording. It has been shown, for example, that pain produces local decreases in GSR (i.e., local sympathetic activation) presumably by a reflex mechanism (Riley and Richter, 1975; Yamagata et al., 1976); however, demonstration of generalized increases in sympathetic activity has proven somewhat problematic. Collins and colleagues (1982) found that patients with chronic low back pain had generally increased skin conductance (i.e., decreased GSR and increased sympathetic activity). On the other hand, Naifeh and co-workers (1983) failed to show any significant increases in resting GSR in patients with postoperative pain. Additionally, these postoperative pain patients showed blunted reflex changes in GSR to a variety of maneuvers designed to increase sympathetic activity (Naifeh et al., 1983). This correlated with decreased heart rate responses in postsurgical patients to mental arithmetic, Valsalva's maneuver, and dive reflex (Heller et al., 1984). It is not clear how these findings relate to the previously discussed regional sympathetic hyperactivity in painful areas; however, the findings of regional differences in sympathetic activity suggest the presence of ongoing local reflex activity. Furthermore, it is likely that the results of cardiovascular reflex testing would be different if evaluated in areas of sympathetic hyperactivity. This possibility awaits exploration.

Korr and colleagues (1958, 1962, 1964; Wright et al., 1960), who mapped GSR in paraspinal regions, concluded that stable patterns of variability in GSR can be identified in human subjects. Additionally, they found that these patterns could be associated with "osteopathic lesions" of the spinal column and that the patterns were altered by manipulative therapy.

Thermography also provides some supportive evidence for the hypothesis that spinal pathophysiology can influence autonomic function. Thermography is a measure of heat loss from the most superficial aspects of the skin and, therefore, largely represents blood flow through small vessels of the skin. The predominant control of this circulation is sympathetic, although other local factors such as axon reflexes and neurohumoral factors are known to play a part (Uematsu and Long, 1976). Two recent reviews have concluded that recognizable thermographic patterns are established in a population of back pain patients (Gillstrom, 1985, Newman et al., 1984). These patterns, which are particularly evident in patients with sciatic root involvement (Wexler, 1978), include localized regions of increased temperature, suggesting active vasodilation, probably mediated through axon reflexes from involvement of nocioceptive afferent fibers. Additionally, a much wider region of decreased temperature can be identified, suggesting increased sympathetic activity. The finding that cool regions are not randomly distributed suggests local reflex mediation rather than generalized stress reaction to pain.

Effects of Spinal Manipulation on Autonomic Function

Clinical studies that have attempted to examine effects of spinal manipulation on autonomic function have been founded on one of two hypotheses: (1) the manipulation is capable of evoking autonomic reflex responses, or (2) the manipulation is capable of interrupting reflexes that have been established by spinal pathology.

The majority of reports implicating spinal manipulation in autonomic reflex changes have considered effects on cardiovascular function. Although rarely have these reports speculated on the physiologic mechanism of response, it can be hypothesized that more immediate effects would be of reflex origin, whereas more sustained changes may represent correction of spinal dysfunction, thereby eliminating ongoing pathologic reflexes. Studies examining cardiovascular changes in normal subjects have suggested some activation of sympathetics by manipulation in cervical, upper thoracic, or lower thoracic regions (Clymer et al., 1972; Tran and Kirby, 1977a,b; Wickes, 1980). These studies have employed measures of heart rate and blood pressure as well as doppler pulse signal to assess ANS tone. Only short-term responses were observed by these authors, and potential longer-term responses were not evaluated. One confounding variable that was not controlled in the aforementioned reports is the direct mechanical effects of manipulation on intra-abdominal and intrathoracic pressures, and thereby on venous return. Therefore, the possibility exists that these experiments were recording changes evoked by visceroviseral reflexes or mechanical effects rather than spinovisceral responses. Reexploration of this topic, searching for regional differences in autonomic response, would appear to be a reasonable subject for future investigation, as this would diminish the likelihood of responses being attributable to visceroviseral responses or to generalized "defense" or "orienting" responses (Hodes et al., 1985).

Many clinical reports have evaluated effects of a course of manipulative treatment on blood pressure (see Crawford et al., 1986). By and large these studies suggest a diminution in blood pressure of hypertensive patients (Fischera and Celander, 1969; Hood, 1974; Norris, 1964); however, these studies have been uncontrolled or poorly controlled, and have failed to recognize the statistical principle or "regression to the mean." This principle states that any group that is selected for its divergence from the average value in a population will have subsequent measurements closer to the average value regardless of treatment (or lack of it). The only way to address this issue in clinical research is through appropriately matched controls. Such controlled investigation of this topic is clearly necessary.

Reflex Sympathetic Dystrophy

It would be remiss to ignore the recent interest in so-called "reflex sympathetic dystrophy" (RSD) in this discussion of autonomic reflex function. This syndrome, which goes by a number of synonyms, apparently represents a spectrum of chronic pain disorders following tissue injury (Christensen and Henriksen, 1983; Headley, 1987; Schwartzman and McLellan, 1987). This trauma may involve extensive damage to nerve fibers, i.e., classic causalgia, or may represent response to relatively trivial injury. The fundamental pattern observed consists of prolongation and exacerbation of pain (causalgia-like, burning), along with some degree of dystrophic and vascular change. These dystrophic changes go through a series of stages, often beginning with swelling and cyanosis either in the area of injury or occasionally remote (usually distal) to the site of trauma. There may be progression to atrophy of affected tissues

(skin, bone, muscle) and loss of joint mobility with fibrosis. This phenomenon has been easiest to observe in the distal portion of the limbs; however, it may occur, albeit with fewer apparent changes in overlying skin, in more proximal portions of the musculoskeletal system. The marked early vascular changes in microcirculation suggest autonomic effects (Christensen and Henriksen, 1983; Sylvest et al., 1977), although the role of local factors and of axon reflexes in this response is poorly understood.

Most theories concerning the etiology of the regional sympathotonia in RSD focus on the possibility of sustained reflex activation of sympathetic nerve fibers. Presumably, it is the pain afferents that result in this abnormal reflex. According to this hypothesis, the increase in sympathetic activity not only results in the vascular changes, but further sensitizes and/or activates pain fibers (Blumberg and Janig, 1984; Devor, 1983). Although this attractive hypothesis cannot be regarded as conclusively proved, there is substantial clinical support for it. Blockade of sympathetics to the affected region, either surgically or with local anesthetic, frequently eliminates the pain. Furthermore, temporary blockade with local anesthetic often produces permanent relief in these patients. This supports the contention that the pathophysiologic process is reflex in nature, and that the reflex is self-sustaining. Of course, much work remains to be done on this topic and the underlying mechanisms that have been proposed are still largely speculative.

"Special" Reflexes

There are a few reflexes of possible clinical significance that are not as well known as those described earlier. First, there has been a growing appreciation for the possible role of axon reflexes in certain clinical situations. An axon reflex, as opposed to the reflexes we discussed earlier, is defined as a reflex that requires only one neuron. This neuron, generally a pain afferent neuron, not only conveys the pain sensation to the central nervous system, but also releases neurohumoral substances from its peripheral terminals. This produces local and regional vascular changes and may be capable of affecting local smooth muscle. Although this mechanism has long been known to be responsible for the flare reaction in "wheal and flare" from local trauma, it has recently become a topic of some interest as a possible mechanism in asthma (Barnes, 1986).

Viscerosomatic reflexes do not command as much attention as they once did. Earlier in this century physicians relied to a much greater extent on physical signs such as body habitus and posture for the diagnosis of internal disorders. Therefore, many of the early physical diagnosis texts discussed the patterns of muscle "spasm" attendant with internal pathology. The classic work of Pottenger (1953) reflects the interest that this subject once enjoyed. Recent deemphasis of many elements of physical diagnosis has occurred coincident with an increase in the use of more direct (and invasive) tests of internal disease.

Conclusion

Although reflexes have long been a part of clinical practice there are many aspects that are poorly understood. The clinical understandings of reflexes has generally lagged behind basic sciences, especially in the area of visceral reflex physiology. This is probably due to the relatively crude clinical measures applied to the investigation of these reflexes in humans; however, basic science research suffers from problems in identifying good animal models of clinical disease and in ethical restraints governing the use of animals in experiments studying chronic pathology. The coming years will see an improvement in our ability to monitor reflex functions in humans. This should permit expansion of understanding of reflex involvement in many clinical situations.

One of the large remaining questions in reflex physiology that await appropriate investigative tools is the issue of facilitation of neuronal reflex pathways. Although basic science research suggests that neuronal pathways may be facilitated through repeated use, this often hypothesized mechanism requires further delineation prior to acceptance as significant in human disease.

References

Bannister R. *Autonomic Failure.* Oxford: Oxford University Press; 1983a.

Bannister R. Clinical studies of autonomic function and dysfunction. *J Auton Nerv Syst* 1983b;7:233–237.

Bannister R, Boylston AW, Davies B, et al. Beta receptor numbers and thermodynamics in denervation supersensitivity. *J Physiol (Lond)* 1981; 319:369–377.

Barnes PJ. Asthma as an axon reflex. *Lancet* (Feb. 1986): 242–245.

Blumberg H and Janig W. Discharge pattern of afferent fibers from a neuroma. *Pain* 1984;20:335–354.

Boureau F, Willer JC, and Yamaguchi Y. Effets d'une stimulation electrique hetero-segmentaire percutanee (electro-acupuncture) sur le reflexe nociceptif de flexion chez l'homme. *Ann Anesthes Fr* 1979;5:422–426.

Bristow JD, Honour AJ, Pickering GW, et al. Diminished baroreceptor sensitivity in high blood pressure. *Circulation* 1969;39:48–54.

Burke D, Gandevia SC, and McKeon B. The afferent volleys responsible for spinal proprioceptive reflexes in man. *J Physiol (Lond)* 1983;339:535–552.

Burke D, Gandevia SC, and McKeon B. Monosynaptic and oligosynaptic contributions to human ankle jerk and H-reflex. *J Neurophys* 1984;52:435–448.

Chan CWY, and Tsang H. Inhibition of the human flexion reflex by low intensity, high frequency transcutaneous electrical nerve stimulation (TENS) has a gradual onset and offset. *Pain* 1987;28:239–253.

Christensen K, and Henriksen O. The reflex sympathetic dystrophy syndrome. *Scand J Rheumatol* 1983;12:263–267.

Cinciripini PM. Cognitive stress and cardiovascular reactivity. I. Relationship to hypertension. *Am Heart J* 1986a;112:1044–1050.

Cinciripini PM. Cognitive stress and cardiovascular reactivity. II. Relationship to atherosclerosis, arrhythmia and cognitive control. *Am Heart J* 1986b;112:1051–1065.

Clarkson TB, Kaplan JR, Adams MR, and Manuck SB. Psychosocial influences on the pathogenesis of atherosclerosis among nonhuman primates. *Circulation* 1987;76(suppl. I):29–40.

Clymer D, Levin F, and Sculthorpe R. Effects of osteopathic manipulation on several different physiologic functions. *J Am Osteopath Assoc* 1972;72:204–207.

Collins GA, Cohen MJ, Naliboff BD, and Schandler SL. Comparative analysis of paraspinal and frontal EMG, heart rate and skin conductance in chronic low back pain patients and normals to various postures and stress. *Scand J Rehab Med* 1982;14:39–46.

Crawford JP, Hickson GS, and Wiles MR. The management of hypertensive diseases: A review of spinal manipulation and the efficacy of conservative therapeusis. *J Manip Physiol Ther* 1986;9:27–32.

Davies B, Sudera D, Sagnella G, et al. Increased numbers of alpha-receptors in sympathetic denervation supersensitivity in man. *J Clin Invest* 1982;69:779–784.

Davies TW. Definition of human reflex excitability by statistical analysis of quantal EMG responses. *Brain Res* 1984;293:386–389.

Davies TW, and Lader MH. Determination of excitability in human proprioceptive reflexes: Analysis and characteristics of EMG thresholds of postural muscle. *Brain Res* 1985;339:19–26.

Denslow JS. An analysis of the variability of spinal reflex thresholds. *J Neurophysiol* 1944;7:207–215.

Denslow JS, and Hassett CC. The central excitatory state associated with postural abnormalities. *J Neurophysiol* 1942;5:393–402.

Denslow JS, Korr IM, and Krems AD. Quantitative studies of chronic facilitation in human motor neuron pools. *Am J Physiol* 1947;150:229–238.

Deschuytere J, DeKeyser C, Deschuytere M, and Rosselle N. H reflexes in muscles of the lower and upper limbs in man: Identification and clinical significance. *Adv Neurol* 1983;39:951–960.

Deschuytere J, Rosselle N, and DeKeyser C. Monosynaptic reflexes in the superficial forearm flexors in man and their clinical significance. *J Neurol Neurosurg Psychiatry* 1976;39:555–565.

Devor MJ. Nerve pathophysiology and mechanisms of pain in causalgia. *J Auton Nerve Syst.* 1983;7:371–384.

Dimsdale JE, Ruberman W, Carleton RA, et al. Sudden cardiac death. Stress and cardiac arrhythmia. *Circulation* 1987;76(suppl. I):198–201.

Dustan HP. Essential hypertension: Neural considerations. *Med Clin North Am* 1987;71:897–905.

Etnyr BR and Abraham LD. H-reflex changes during static stretching and two variations of proprioceptive neuromuscular facilitation techniques. *Electroencephalogr Clin Neurophysiol* 1986; 63:174–182.

Ewing DJ. Practical bedside investigations of diabetic autonomic Failure. In Bannister R, ed. *Autonomic Failure.* Oxford: Oxford University Press; 1983.

Fischera AP and Celander DR. Effect of osteopathic manipulative therapy on autonomic tone as evidenced by blood pressure change and activity of the fibrinolytic system. *J Am Osteopath Assoc* 1969;68:1036–1038.

Flor H and Turk DC. Etiological theories and treatments for chronic back pain. I. Somatic models and interventions. *Pain* 1984;19:105–121.

Floyd WF and Silver PHS. The function of the erectores spinae muscles in certain movements and postures in man. *J Physiol (Lond)* 1955;129:184–203.

Frank A. Spinal motor preparation in humans. *Electroencephalogr Clin Neurophysiol* 1986;63:361–370.

Gillstrom P. Thermography in low back pain and sciatica. *Arch Orthop Trauma Surg* 1985;104:31–36.

Goldstein DS. Stress induced activation of the sympathetic nervous system. *Bailliere's Clin Endocrinol Metab* 1987;1:253–278.

Gotoh F, Komatsumoto S, Araki N, and Gomi S. Noradrenergic nervous activity in migraine. *Arch Neurol* 1984;41:951–955.

Grabel JA. Electromyographic study of low back muscle tension in subjects with and without chronic low back pain. *Dis Abstr Int* 1973;34(B):2929–2930.

Headley B. Historical perspective of causalgia. *Phys Ther.* 1987;67:1370–1374.

Heard GE. The psychogalvanic response in the study of sympathetic activity. *Br J Surg* 1964;51:629–631.

Heller PH, Perry F, Naifeh K, et al. Cardiovascular autonomic response during preoperative stress and postoperative pain. *Pain* 1984;18:33–40.

Herd JA, Falkner B, Anderson DE, et al. Psychopathologic factors in hypertension. *Circulation* 1987;76(suppl. I):89–94.

Hillman K. Acute stress ulceration. *Anaesth Intensive Care* 1985;13:230–240.

Hilsted J. Testing for autonomic neuropathy. *Ann Clin Res.* 1984;16:128–135.

Hodes RL, Cook EW, and Lang PJ. Individual differences in autonomic response: Conditioned association or conditioned fear? *Psychophysiology* 1985;22:545–556.

Hood RP. Blood pressure results in 75 abnormal cases. *Digest Chiropractic Econ* 1974;16:36–38.

Hoyt WH, Hunt HH, and DePauw MA. Electromyographic assessment of chronic low back pain syndrome. *J Am Osteopath Assoc* 1981;80:728–730.

Humphreys CR, Triano JJ, and Brandl MJ. Sensitivity study of H-reflex alterations in idiopathic low back pain patients vs. a healthy population. *J Manip Physiol Ther* 1989;12:71–78.

Huzon M. Exteroceptive reflexes to stimulation of the sural nerve in man. In Desmedt JE, ed. *New Developments in Electromyography and Clinical Neurophysiology*, vol. 3. Basel: Karger.

Kanda K and Sato H. Reflex responses of human thigh muscles to non-noxious sural stimulation during stepping. *Brain Res* 1983;288:378–380.

Kochler T. Stress and rheumatoid arthritis. *J Psychosom Res* 1985;29:655–663.

Korr IM. Sustained sympathotonia as a factor in disease. In Korr IM, ed. *The Neurobiologic Mechanisms in Manipulative Therapy.* New York: Plenum Press. 1978:229–268.

Korr IM, Thomas PE, and Wright HM. Patterns of electrical skin resistance in man. *Acta Neuroveg* 1958;17:77–96.

Korr IM, Wright HM, and Chace JA. Cutaneous patterns of sympathetic activity in clinical abnormalities of the musculoskeletal system. *Acta Neuroveg* 1964;25:589–606.

Korr IM, Wright HM, and Thomas PE. Effect of experimental myofascial insult on cutaneous patterns of sympathetic activity in man. *Acta Neuroveg* 1962;23:329–355.

Kravitz E, Moore ME, and Glaros A. Paralumbar muscle activity in chronic low back pain. *Arch Phys Med Rehab* 1981;62:172–176.

Magladery JW, Porter WE, Park AM, and Teasdall RD. Electrophysiological studies of nerve and reflex activity in normal man. 4. The two neurone reflex and identification of certain action potentials from spinal roots and cord. *Bull Johns Hopkins Hosp* 1951;88:449–519.

Majewski H and Rand MJ. A possible role of epinephrine in the development of hypertension. *Med Res Rev* 1986;6:467–486.

Manuck SB, Henry JP, Anderson DE, et al., Biobehavioral mechanisms in coronary artery disease: Chronic stress. *Circulation* 1987;76 (suppl. I):158–163.

Marrone GC and Silen W. Pathogenesis, diagnosis and treatment of acute gastric mucosal lesions. *Clin Gastroenterol* 1984;13:635–650.

McCarty R, Horwatt K, and Konarska M. Chronic stress and sympathetic-adrenal medullary responsiveness. *Soc Sci Med* 1988;26:333–341.

McLeod JG and Tuck RR. Disorders of the autonomic nervous system: Part 1. Pathophysiology and clinical features. *Ann Neurol* 1987;21:419–430.

Meinck H-M, Kuster S, Bencke R, and Conrad B. The flexor reflex—Influence of stimulus parameters on the reflex response. *Electroencephalogr Clin Neurophysiol* 1985;61:287–298.

Miller DJ. Comparison of electromyographic activity in the lumbar paraspinal muscles of subjects with and without chronic low back pain. *Phys Ther* 1985;65:1347–1354.

Molitch ME and Hou SH. Neuroendocrine alterations in systemic disease. *Clin Endocrinol Metab* 1983;12:825–851.

Naifeh K, Heller P, Perry F, et al. Basal skin resistance as a measure of autonomic function during clinical pain. *Pain* 1983;16:277–283.

Newman RI, Seres JL, and Miller EB. Liquid crystal thermography in the evaluation of chronic back pain: A comparative study. *Pain* 1984;20:293–305.

Norris T. A study of the effect of manipulation on blood pressure. *Year Book Acad Appl Osteopathy* 1964:184–188.

Nouwen A and Bush C. The relationship between paraspinal EMG and chronic low back pain. *Pain* 1984;20:109–123.

O'Brien IAD, O'Hare P, and Corrall RJM. Heart rate variability in healthy subjects: Effect of age and the derivation of normal ranges for tests of autonomic function. *Br Heart J* 1986;55:348–354.

Palmbald JE. Stress-related modulation of immunity: A review of human studies. *Cancer Detect Prev Suppl* 1987;1:57–64.

Pottenger FM. *Symptoms of Visceral Disease.* St Louis, Mo.: Mosby; 1953.

Reeves AG and Posner JB. The ciliospinal response in man. *Neurology, Minneap.* 1969;19:1145–1152.

Riley LH and Richter CP. Uses of the electrical skin resistance method in the study of patients with neck and upper extremity pain. *Johns Hopkins Med J* 1975;137:69–74.

Robinson KL, McComas AJ, and Belanger AY. Control of soleus motoneuron excitability during muscle stretch in man. *J Neurol Neurosurg Psychiatry* 1982;45:699–704.

Rossi A, Mazzocchio R, Mondelli M, and Scarpini C. Postural neck reflexes involving the lower limb extensor motoneurons in man. *Electromyogr Clin Neurophysiol* 1987;27:195–201.

Rossi A, Rossi B, and Santarcangello E. Influences of neck vibration on lower limb extensor muscles in man. *Arch Ital Biol* 1985;123:241–253.

Rubin LS, Graham D, Pasker R, and Calhoun W. Autonomic nervous system dysfunction in common migraine. *Headache* 1985;25:40–48.

Schneiderman N. Psychophysiologic factors in atherogenesis and coronary artery disease. *Circulation* 1987;76 (Suppl. I):41–47.

Schwartzman RJ and McLellan TL. Reflex sympathetic dystrophy. *Arch Neurol* 1987;44:555–561.

Shimada K, Kitazumi T, Ogura H, et al., Differences in age-independent effects on blood pressure on baroreflex sensitivity between normal and hypertensive subjects. *Clin Sci* 1986;70:489–494.

Silen W. The clinical problem of stress ulcers. *Clin Invest Med* 1987;10:270–274.

Sleight P. Hemodynamics in hypertension and heart failure. *Am J Med* 1984;76:3–13.

Sleight P, Fox P, Lopez R, and Brooks DE. The effect of mental arithmetic on blood pressure variability and baroreflex sensitivity in man. *Clin Sci Mol Med* 1978;55:381s–382s.

Snider SR. Dopamine: An important neurohormone of the sympathoadrenal system. *Endocrine Rev* 1983;4:291–309.

Surivit RS and Feinglos MN. Stress and the autonomic nervous system in type II diabetes. A hypothesis. *Diabetes Care* 1988;11:83–85.

Sylvest J Jensen EM, Siggard-Anderson J, and Pedersen L. Reflex sympathetic dystrophy, resting blood flow and muscle temperature as diagnostic criteria. *Scand J Rehab Med* 1977;9:25–29.

Syvalahti E. Endocrine and immune adaptation in stress. *Ann Clin Res* 1987;19:70–77.

Tanaka R. Reciprocal Ia inhibition during voluntary movements in man. *Exp Brain Res* 1974;21:529–540.

Tecoma ES and Huey LY. Psychic distress and the immune response. *Life Sci* 1985;36:1799–1812.

Terrett ACJ and Vernon H. Manipulation and pain tolerance. *Am J Phys Med* 1984;63:217–225.

Thomas PE and Kawahata A. Neural factors underlying variations in electrical resistance of apparently nonsweating skin. *J Appl Physiol* 1962;17:999–1002.

Traccis S, Rosati G, Patraskakis S, et al. Influence of neck receptors on soleus motoneuron excitability in man. *Exp Neurol* 1987;95:76–84.

Tran T and Kirby J. The effects of upper cervical adjustment upon the normal physiology of the heart. *ACA J Chiropractic* 1977a;11:S58–S62.

Tran T and Kirby J. The effects of upper thoracic adjustment upon the normal physiology of the heart. *ACA J Chiropractic* 1977b;11:S25–S28.

Travel JG and Simons DG. *Myofascial Pain and Dysfunction*. Baltimore/London: William Wilkins; 1983.

Triano JJ and Schultz AB. Correlation of objective measure of trunk motions and muscle function with low-back disability rating. *Spine* 1987;12:561–565.

Tuck ML. The sympathetic nervous system in essential hypertension. *Am Heart J* 1986;112:877–886.

Uematsu S and Long DM. Thermography in chronic pain. In Uematsu S, ed. *Medical Thermography. Theory and Clinical Applications.* Los Angeles: Brentwood; 1976:52–68.

Upton ARM, McComas AJ, and Sica REP. Potentiation of "late" responses evoked in muscles during effort. *J Neurol Neurosurg Psychiatry* 1971; 34:699–711.

Vallbo AB, Hagbarth K-E, Torebjork HE, and Wallin BG. Somatosensory, proprioceptive and sympathetic activity in human peripheral nerve. *Physiol Rev* 1979;59:919–957.

Verrier MC. Alterations in H reflex magnitude by variations in baseline EMG excitability. *Electroencephalogr Clin Neurophysiol* 1985;60:492–499.

Vingerhoets AJ. The role of the parasympathetic division of the autonomic nervous system in stress and the emotions. *Int J Psychosom* 1985;32:28–34.

Vita G, Princi P, Calabro R, et al. Cardiovascular reflex tests. *J Neurol Sci* 1986;75:263–274.

Wallace DJ. The role of stress and trauma in rheumatoid arthritis and systemic lupus erythematosus. *Semin Arthritis Rheum* 1987;16:153–157.

Wexler EC. Peripheral thermographic manifestations of lumbar disk disease. *Appl Radiol* 1978;7:53–58.

Wickes D. Effects of thoracolumbar spinal manipulation on arterial flow in the lower extremity. *J Manip Physiol Ther* 1980;3:3–6.

Willer JC. Comparative study of perceived pain and nociceptive flexion reflex in man. *Pain* 1977;3:69–80.

Willer JC. Nociceptive flexion reflexes as a tool for pain research in man. *Adv Neurol* 1983;39:809–827.

Wolf SL and Basmajian JV. Assessment of paraspinal electromyographic activity in normal subjects and chronic back pain patients using a muscle biofeedback device. In Asmussen A, ed. *Biomechanics VIB* Baltimore, Md.: University Park Press; 1978.

Wright HM, Korr IM, and Thomas PE. Local and regional variations in cutaneous vasomotor tone of the human trunk. *Acta Neuroveg* 1960;22:33–52.

Yamagata S, Ishikawa M, Saijo M, et al. A diagnostic reevaluation of electrical skin resistance, skin temperature and deeper tenderness in patients with abdominal pain. *Tohoku J Exp Med* 1976;118(suppl.): 183–189.

chapter 10

Systemic Effects of Spinal Lesions

Muhammed Shahid Ilyas Dhami
Kenneth F. DeBoer

The question of whether chiropractors or other practitioners can alleviate or cure certain diseases of internal organs by somatic manipulation is fraught with controversy. Even though it is a central tenet of chiropractic philosophy that treatment is not given per se for *any* disorder directly, many if not most chiropractors report anecdotally that patients with many types of visceral disorders often improve under their care. In this chapter our purpose is to evaluate current understanding of the relationships between spinal lesions or associated somatic dysfunction and systemic (internal organ) functions (or dysfunction). We approach this task from the standpoint that what one would most like to know is what can, and does, go wrong with a particular organ or system when a particular vertebral or musculoskeletal dysfunction, or particular somatic stimulus, is present. Our survey of existing information is rather wide ranging but concentrates on the central area of documenting somatovisceral phenomena. Unfortunately, little direct experimental work yet exists on the exact title topic but whatever exists, in our opinion, is at least consistent with current chiropractic principles and practices and, at best, signals encouragement for further clinical and experimental research.

Spinovisceral Relationships

When internal physiologic systems are affected or altered as a result of changes in some spinal or paraspinal structure, the phenomenon generally falls under the rubric of somatovisceral reflex, even though the true relationship is usually unknown, indirect, and possibly "nonreflex." For the manipulatory disciplines, there are two opposite sides (pathogenic and therapeutic) to these somatovisceral phenomena. A central tenet of both osteopathy and chiropractic is that certain lesions in the spinal column, variously called subluxations (vertebral subluxation complex) (Haldeman, 1975, 1980), osteopathic lesions (Hoag et al., 1969), somatic dysfunctions (Patterson and Steinmetz, 1986), spinal dysarthrias (Hildebrandt, 1977), and a variety of other terms (Haldeman, 1977), can cause changes in internal organ function that may proceed to the disease state. Equally significant is the corollary that through the use of artful manipulation, these foci of spinal irritation can be alleviated and thereby beneficially affect internal organ functioning.

Clinical observations of patients who report "improvement" of internal, visceral disorders after chiropractic or osteopathic therapy prompted the postulated spinovisceral relationship. Clinical improvement of a variety of visceral disorders was claimed by Palmer (1910) and Still (1910) soon after the births of both chiropractic and osteopathy, and a steady flow of similar reports has continued to the present. The claims are based on case reports, anecdotes, and clinical lore, most of which are scientifically unsound. Although this large body of literature cannot be exhaustively reviewed here, the evidence therein is interesting and provocative at the very least. The range of viscera and organ systems claimed to be affected is also impressive, as indicated in Tables 10-1 and 10-2.

In addition, several symposia and other forums have produced additional discussions, and occasionally data, on the possible relationships of visceral disorders to spinal lesions or spinal manipulations (Lewit, 1978; Korr, 1978; Buerger and Tobis, 1975; Goldstein, 1975; Mazzarelli, 1982). A book by Hartmann and Schwartz (1973) summarized claims in which chiropractic spinal adjustments resulted in improvement in various mental and learning disabilities.

Similar reports relating spinal lesions to internal dysfunction also abound in the early biomedical literature (e.g., Ussher, 1940; Wills and Atsatt, 1934). Carnett (1927) thought that spinal lesions at T6–10 were related to gallbladder disease as well as ''pseudoappendicitis attacks.'' Davis (1950) related dorsal spinal ''radiculitis'' with ''cardiac arrhythmia.'' Urinary retention was reported in a case of an asymptomatic protruded lumbar disc by Love and Emmett (1967) from the Mayo Clinic. Kellgren (1939) presented quite convincing case histories showing that trigger points or other abnormalities of specific spinal or paraspinal structures either caused or simulated epigastric pain, angina, nausea, appendicitis, cholecystitis, and renal or ureteral pain. Lewis and Kellgren (1939) and Maigne (1972) found that paraspinal stimulation along the spinous process of T1 produced chest pain that simulated angina. ''Spinal joint lesions'' brought on by ''ruptured discs'' were reported to produce angina symptoms in patients by Josey and Murphy (1946). MacDonald and Hargrave-Wilson (1935) similarly found causes of gallbladder disease ''cured'' by manipulation of T7 and T8 joint lesions, in which the spinal joints apparently caused referred pain that mimicked gallbladder disease. The gallbladder was later found to be healthy.

More recently, somewhat more rigorous clinical case reports on spinovisceral relationships have been related by Kunert (1965), Lewit (1978), Rychlikova (1975), and others. Kunert (1965) concluded, on the basis of careful clinical case histories, that mild spinal lesions often appeared to be a contributing factor to various heart and other visceral disorders. Even more frequently, spinal lesions have appeared to

TABLE 10-1. PARTIAL LIST OF ORGANIC DISORDERS REPORTED TO BE RELATED TO SPINAL LESIONS OR AFFECTED BY CHIROPRACTIC MANIPULATION.

Organic Disorder	References
Barre-Lieou syndrome	Luisetto et al., 1982
Vertebral autonomic dysfunction	Johnson, 1981
Migraine	Watkins, 1951; Wight, 1978
Asthma	Wiles and Diakow, 1982; Darabiloff, 1969
High blood pressure	Wiles and Diakow, 1982; Hood, 1974
Cardiac arrythmia	Egli, 1965; Tran and Kirby, 1977
Dysmenorrhea	Thomason et al., 1979
Ulcers	Paprocki, 1969; Hildebrandt, 1976
Colic and constipation	Reiss, 1960; Martin, 1977
Pulmonary diseases	Triano, 1976
Endocrine function	Chapman, 1963
Low blood sugar and hyperinsulinism	Goodheart, 1965
Abdominal discomfort, bloating or fullness; ileocecal valve	Brunarski, 1980; Goodheart, 1967
Miscellaneous organ disorders, e.g., stomach, colon, rectum, small intestine, bladder, spleen, pancreas, gallbladder, livers, kidney, uterus, ureters	Paprocki, 1969; Mears, 1972

TABLE 10-2. PARTIAL LIST OF DISORDERS REPORTED TO BE RELIEVED BY OSTEOPATHIC SPINAL MANIPULATION.

Organic Disorder	Reference
High blood pressure	Miller, 1966; Norris, 1964; Northup, 1960
Asthma	Wilson, 1946
Fibrinolysis and autonomic tone	Celander et al., 1968
Emphysema	Foelliner et al., 1968
Chronic obstructive pulmonary disease	Howell et al. 1975; Miller, 1977
Pulmonary infection	Purse, 1966
Resistance to stress in rats	Greenspan and Melchilor, 1966
Peptic ulcers	Hay, 1939
Other nonspecific gastro intestinal disease	Robuck, 1947; Tweed, 1931
Irritable bowel syndrome	Masterson, 1985
Coronary arterial disease	Richmond, 1942
Renal disease	Hix, 1960

simulate heart disease, angina, dyspepsia, and the like. From this latter perspective, if spinal lesions are able to cause misdiagnosis of organic visceral disease, then the possibility of using manual manipulation to relieve the spinal lesion becomes a very attractive differential diagnostic procedure.

Lewit (1978) may be the most active current allopathic physician attempting to clarify and document the long postulated spinovisceral pathological pathway. He has published numerous case history reports in which various types of vertebral manipulation have apparently led directly to clinical cure or improvement in asthma (Lewit, 1978), peptic ulcer (Rychlikova, 1975), Meniere's disease (Lewit, 1961), and many other diagnosed conditions (Lewit, 1963, 1971, 1978). Barre-Lieou syndrome (Maigne, 1972) has also been reported to be helped by manipulation.

Most of the studies and reports from the three major groups of medical professionals are rather poor from a strictly scientific point of view. In most cases the studies are significantly flawed, lacking control patients, large numbers of carefully accumulated homogeneous groups of subjects, rigidly specified diagnostic criteria, statistical analysis, as well as many of the other elementary ingredients of a well-designed clinical study. Nevertheless, the honest and often pioneering clinical observations made by a large number of able clinicians over many decades, in many lands, and from differing outlooks are in many ways impressive. At the very least, the hypothesis that relatively mild somatic spinal lesions can cause, contribute to, or simulate visceral disease merits more than out-of-hand rejection. Fiske (1987) states categorically that various abdominal pains referred from spinal joint dysfunctions are often mistaken for colic, appendicitis, or gallbladder or other visceral pain by both chiropractors and medical doctors. If these visceral illnesses can be alleviated by spinal manipulation, as often seems the case, patients would be saved from enormous medical costs, unnecessary surgery, drugs, and so on. It is regrettable that neither the manipulative professions nor the allopathic community has performed the relevant experimental and epidemologic studies to determine the true incidence and mechanics of such "simulated" visceral disorders vis-à-vis true reflexively caused spinovisceral disorders.

Studies in animals and recent data from humans provide more convincing evidence of the spinovisceral connection (Fiske, 1987). Beal (1983) and Beal and Dvorak (1984) found that osteopathic spinal lesions (somatic dysfunctions), as detected by palpation of the spine by multiple osteopathic examiners, were well correlated by segmental level with visceral disease such as peptic ulcer, esophagitis, pancreatitis,

gastric outlet obstruction, and, particularly, hypertension. DeBoer and McKnight (1988a) found that blood pressure decreased after a single cervical spinal manipulation in a group of 53 chiropractic students. Of interest in that study is that the studied population was presumed to comprise healthy, normotensive students, and no effect on blood pressure was expected. Nevertheless, the actual effect of relieving a putative cervical subluxation by a single manipulation was striking in those students who happened to have an initial blood pressure reading in the borderline hypertensive range. In *those* particular students the blood pressure decrease was clinically significant, and the magnitude of the effect caused the group mean also to be statistically significant.

Mannino (1979) measured serum aldosterone levels in 10 normotensive and 35 hypertensive patients. There was a significant drop in aldosterone following osteopathic spinal manipulative therapy, but not after sham manipulations. This effect was seen in hypertensive patients, but not in normotensive patients. Blood pressure, however, did not decrease significantly following osteopathic manipulative therapy in either group. Thus, Mannino may have been the first to demonstrate a direct or indirect effect of somatic stimulation on endocrine function.

It is common clinical experience to observe a variety of visceral disturbances following spinal cord injuries, even after comparatively mild lesions. Sexual dysfunction (Perese et al., 1976), gastric (Fealey et al., 1984) and colonic (Aaronson et al., 1985) motility disturbances (Berlly and Wilmot, 1984), and other organ malfunctions (Pedersen, 1983) have been amply documented. Many gastrointestinal disturbances such as gastric stasis, altered upper gastrointestinal propulsive and myoelectric activity, and food transit and intraluminal pressure abnormalities have been repeatedly reported in response to a large number of noxious or mild somatic stimuli applied to vertebral or extremity somatic structures (Camillieri et al., 1984; Matsumoto et al., 1972; Perret and Hesser, 1960; Halter and Pflug, 1980; Porreca and Burks, 1983; Bueno et al., 1978).

Recently Glick and colleagues (1982, 1984) and others (Aaronson et al., 1985) have carefully described both colonic and bladder myoelectric dysfunction in both multiple sclerosis patients and low-spinal-cord–injured patients. These workers showed the central importance of spinal connections below the level of the injury in causing or maintaining altered visceral function. Moreover, they found evidence of altered spinal cord reflexes even in the presence of normal peripheral nerves and the corresponding segmental interneurons in the spinal cord.

Korr (1947) reported evidence of heightened reflex reactivity in spinal cord areas associated with palpable osteopathic lesions. He found reliable increases in galvanic skin response (GSR) readings at specific cord levels and named them *facilitated segments*. It has long been a key hypothesis of osteopaths and chiropractors that locally altered somatovisceral reflexes arising from a traumatized spinal joint constitute a vicious cycle of altered afferent and efferent traffic, which leads to a facilitated or hyperactive spinal segment (Korr, 1947, 1979a,b; Patterson and Steinmetz, 1986; Haldeman, 1980; Perl, 1975). This hyperactivity leads to further altered neural activity, both locally and within the cord, which in turn causes further alteration of local somatic tissue, e.g., muscle splinting. This facilitated segment is putatively located at a definite spinal level, leading to altered sympathetic and parasympathetic outflow, which in turn has a profound effect on local blood flow as well as ongoing neural and visceral activity (Sato and Terui, 1976). The local signs of the facilitated segment are regarded as constituting the features of the classical putative osteopathic lesion or chiropractic subluxation, e.g., altered joint function, tenderness, tissue texture, and temperature changes (Haldeman, 1977, 1980, 1981). Figure 10–1 illustrates a common conception of how biomechanical or other spinal lesions influence visceral activity via somato-sympathetic or somatovisceral reflexes.

Somatovisceral Reflexes in Animals

Beginning in the mid-1970s, Sato and colleagues (1975a,b) elegantly showed a direct connection between skin and/or somatic afferent nerve stimulation on heart rate, gastric and duodenal motility, and bladder activity in cats and rats. Changes in gastrointestinal activity were monitored by pressure changes

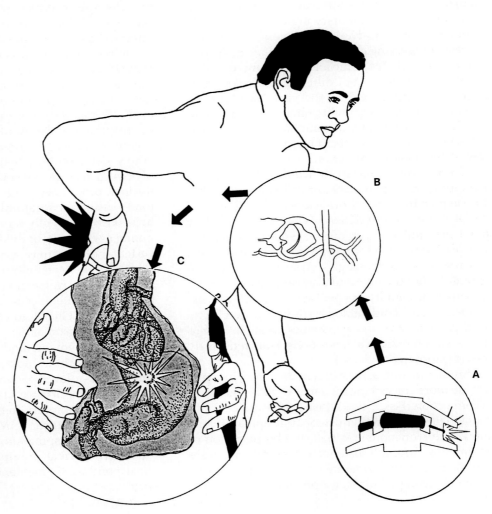

Figure 10–1. Common conceptualization of biomechanical or spinal lesions relating to visceral activity via somato-sympathetic reflexes. Spinal lesions (*A*) lead to altered neural activity (*B*), which may relate to altered visceral activity (*C*).

in balloons inserted in anesthetized animals. Using changes in phasic pressure amplitude and frequency as outcome variables, they stimulated numerous somatic sites by pinching with a mosquito forceps. In both cats (Ito et al., 1979) and rats (Sato et al., 1975a,b) the studies demonstrated that gastric motility was either inhibited or facilitated according to the somatic site stimulated. Paraspinal stimulation inhibited gastric motility, which was later convincingly shown to result from increased somatosympathetic reflex activity (Kametani et al., 1978, 1979). Lateral skin stimulation usually, but not always, facilitated gastric activity. Pinching was carried out at virtually every vertebral level and was inhibitory from approximately T1 to T10 (Kametani et al., 1978). Cutaneous abdominal stimuli were even more inhibitory (Sato et al., 1980).

Abdominal skin stimuli produced similar effects on spontaneous duodenal and jejunal motility in rats (Sato and Terui, 1976; Koizumi et al., 1980). Heart rates were also significantly affected during the period of stimulation (Kaufman et al., 1977). Cardiac reflex responses, however, were not segmentally related, whereas somatogastric inhibition in response to noxious skin stimulation was (Sato, 1980; Kametani et al., 1979). These effects were immediate neural reflexes, not hormonally mediated phenomena (Sato et al., 1981). Sectioning the spinal cord did not abolish the segmentally induced gastrointestinal inhibition, which indicates a segmental, spinal somatosympathetic inhibitory reflex. Cord sectioning did, however, abolish the increased gastric motility, which therefore appears to be primarily supraspinally mediated (Kametani et al., 1979).

Sato and colleagues (1975a, 1980) in similar work using cats documented the existence, as well as the segmental relationships, of somatovisceral responses. They noted altered bladder activity in response to somatic (skin) afferent nerve stimuli, although not from dorsally located paraspinal superficial afferents. Similarly, specific somatosympathic reflex activity of the adrenal medulla was observed after stimulation of dorsal spinal afferent nerves (Araki et al., 1981; Ito et al., 1979; Sato et al., 1981). Reflex increases of adrenal epinephrine that lasted longer than the neural excitation were observed following cutaneous pinching of ventral abdominal skin.

In another study on anesthetized cats, Sato and colleagues (Sato et al., 1984) showed that T3 and T4 dorsal nerve stimulation was highly effective in activating somatosympathetic reflexes to the heart, which implies that there is a rather direct segmental connection between a peripheral afferent nerve and ongoing visceral function. Of perhaps even greater interest was the finding (Schaible et al., 1987) that passive move-

ment of an inflamed knee joint increased inferior cardiac nerve impulses and also blood pressure in anesthetized cats. In this study, carageenin was injected into the knee joint capsule to produce an experimental joint lesion. This type of lesion is possibly reminiscent of the putative spinal joint inflammation postulated to cause a vertebral lesion, i.e., chiropractic subluxation or osteopathic lesion.

If Sato's finding could be replicated in an experimentally induced subluxation in which inflamed spinal joints were produced, perhaps a more direct model of chiropractically relevant somatovisceral reflex connections could be established. Yochum and Rowe (1985) found that osteoarthrities, either of natural occurrence in the cervical spine of humans or carageenin-induced in rabbit and sheep knee joints, produced "subluxation" (actually "luxation" from the chiropractic standpoint) (Fiske, 1979) of these joints. In a recent study, He et al. (1988) found that knee joints injected with carageenin caused joint receptor nerve traffic alteration, both at rest and at different positions of the limb. After nonnoxious pressure over the affected muscle, altered nerve traffic occurred in the spinal cord as well as in both alpha and gamma motor neurons. This may explain the positive feedback (vicious cycle), whereby inflammation produces abnormal muscle intrafusal and extrafusal activity that, in turn, alters the normal position of the joint slightly, which then by abnormal activity in the joint receptors causes still greater alpha and gamma motor neuron activity and thereby more muscle abnormality, and so on.

A significant barrier to further understanding these relationships is the lack of a relevant experimental animal model. DeBoer (1981) reported a statistically successful method of inducing vertebral lesions (VLs) in rabbit cervical and thoracic spines. He was able to mechanically rotate and displace a single thoracic vertebral segment by using an activator-type gun device. VLs were reliably produced and detected by independent, blinded palpators for several weeks following placement of the lesions. In this work, however, no attempt was made to monitor any physiologic changes following placement of the lesion, even though the problem of verifying the actual presence of the VL was solved.

Surgical means of inducing subluxations are currently being actively explored in the author's laboratory. In one approach, a thin stainless-steel bar 2.5 cm long × 5 mm wide is wedged between adjacent thoracic spinous processes in the midthoracic spine (DeBoer and McKnight, 1988b). Figure 10–2 depicts how this bar produces a definite VL, specifically a rotatory misalignment of adjacent motor units. In this recently completed study, six of six rabbits implanted with this device showed clear evidence of

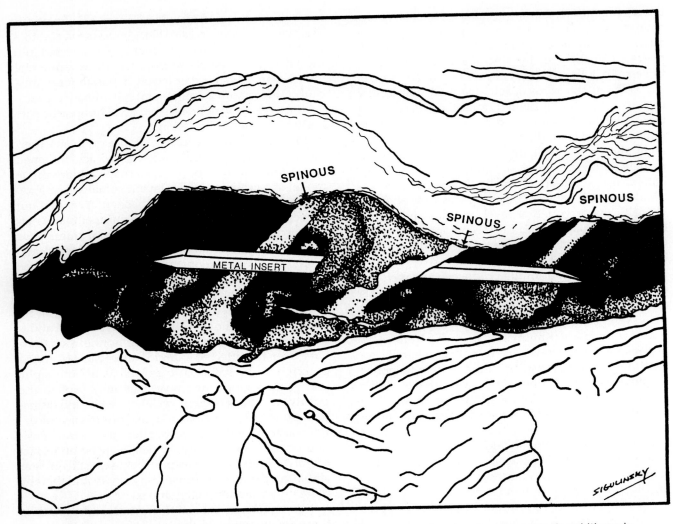

Figure 10–2. Surgical induction of "subluxation" between adjacent thoracic spinous processes in the midthoracic spine by implantation of a thin stainless-steel bar (2.5 mm long x 5.0 mm wide).

the induced VL several days to several months after the operation. In an earlier preliminary experiment DeBoer (1984) used similar devices to produce a mechanical misalignment lesion in rabbits. Gastric electromyographic activity was evaluated as a physiologic response measure. Chronically implanted silver–silver chloride electrodes at various sites on the serosa of the upper gastrointestinal tract were used to obtain high-quality electromyographic (EMG) tracings of slow-wave activity (SW) and spike-burst activity (SB). Both SW and SB are related to neuromuscular activity in general and to the ongoing contractile activity of the gut in particular. Changes in SW and SB from long-term recordings of EMG before and again after induction of experimental VLs in these rabbits were tabulated and analyzed. Although some differences were noted (e.g., power spectral density changes in SW), the large variability,

the small number of animals, and the extreme difficulties of visually analyzing large amounts of continually recorded data made conclusive generalizations unwarranted.

Further evidence for an effect of spinal lesions on gastrointestinal electromyographic activity was obtained in a recent experiment by DeBoer et al. (1988). In this experiment the acute effects of an acute vertebral lesion on gut myoelectric activity were determined using a method reminiscent of Sato's approach. Again, normal rabbits displaying normal gastric and duodenal EMG tracings from chronic implanted electrodes were used. Figure 10–3 illustrates a typical chart recorder trace from an undisturbed rabbit before manually applying a lesioning force designed to rotate and anteriorly displace a vertebra and thus simulate a somatic dysfunction, or subluxation. Figure 10–4 illustrates the type of force

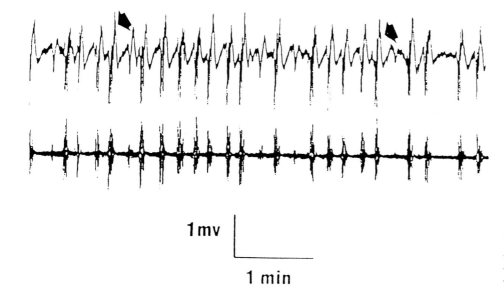

1mv

1 min

Figure 10–3. Chart recording from the stomach of an undisturbed rabbit before manual application of lesioning force designed to rotate and anteriorly displace vertebrae to stimulate somatic dysfunction or subluxation. Top trace is raw unfiltered electromyogram showing slow-wave activity. Bottom trace is same signal filtered (1–1000 Hz) to remove slow-wave activity and show spike activity.

applied and the putative spinal lesion produced. Gastrointestinal EMG activity was recorded during the entire period of the lesioning. Results clearly showed (Fig. 10–5) that this stimulus profoundly altered ongoing gut activity. Vertebral lesions were applied at T1, T6, T12, and L3 and, as Table 10–3 shows, inhibition of gastric motility as measured by EMG activity was most clear at T6.

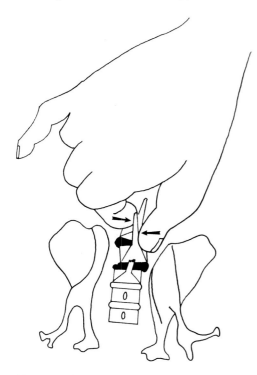

Figure 10–4. Illustration of the type of manual force applied and the putative acute spinal lesion produced.

Neurobiologic and Biochemical Effects of Spinal Manipulation

Recently, biochemical and neurobiological investigations have begun to add significant understanding to the field. Spinal manipulation is hypothesized to produce significant short-term bursts of proprioceptive transmission in the large-caliber myelinated alpha afferent fibers arising from the spinal joint capsules and ligaments and in the muscle spindles of the local paraspinal musculature. These large-fiber signals are believed to modulate the interneuronal pool via the dorsal spinal root ganglion and the substantia gelatinosa and to act to close the gate on pain transmission (Wyke, 1987). Evidence exists that sensorimotor reflex connections are also influenced by manipulation via stimulation of the segmental motor pools (Vernon et al., 1986). Together, these effects may result in a reduction of both pain and muscle hypertonicity, the two most evident clinical effects of manipulation.

Less attention has been paid to the role of neurotransmitters, especially serotonin, noradrenaline, and substance P (Gitelman, 1975; Badalamenti et al., 1987). A review by Pressman and Nickles (1984) considered the broad range of potential neurotransmitter effects. By placing spinal manipulation within the generic group of ''stimulus-producing analgesic'' (SPA) modalities, Pressman and Nickles (1984) implicate the same neuroendocrine model involved in transcutaneous electrical nerve stimulation (TENS) and acupuncture.

The model of spinal antinociception proposed for TENS and acupuncture would seem equally fitting for spinal manipulation. Thus, short-term

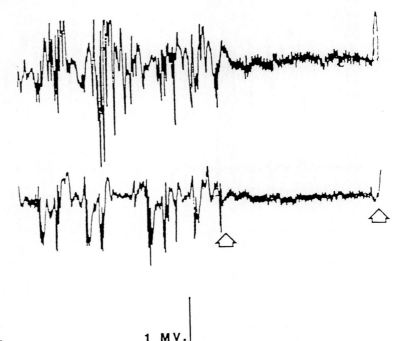

1 M V.

1 MIN.

Figure 10-5. Gastrointestinal electromyographic activity (unfiltered, 0.03–1000 Hz) during the entire period of manual lesion (between arrows), which caused cessation of gut activity. Top trace from stomach, bottom trace from proximal duodenum.

bursts, presumably of high-intensity alpha afferent transmission, may activate a "spinal gate" and block pain. The neurons of the substantia gelatinosa are enkephalinergic; thus, a local spinal or segmental release of enkephalin might be expected with spinal manipulation. However, ascending tracts are also implicated in antinociception. Spinal manipulation may indeed be involved in the feedback loop that involves hindbrain nuclei and their descending inhibitory pathways (Cervero and Wolstencroft, 1984). The most cephalad projections reported for acupuncture and TENS involve activation of the hypothalamic-pituitary axis, presumably through somesthetic projections in the thalamus and sensory cortex. Plasma β-endorphins arise almost exclusively from the pituitary gland. Plasma β-endorphin is purported to act more like a hormone than a neurotransmitter and, indeed, a precise correlation of endorphin increases

TABLE 10-3. MEAN GASTRIC ELECTROMYOGRAPHIC MYOELECTRIC ACTIVITY.[a]

Site of VL	Mean Interval		Mean Difference	t, n, p
	Experimental	Control		
T1	47.56	21.60	25.96	$t = 1.94$ $n = 6$ $p > 0.05$
T6	78.60	25.35	53.25	$t = 6.46$ $n = 10$ $p < 0.001$
T12	32.29	23.49	8.80	$t = 2.20$ $n = 6$ $p > 0.05$
L3	25.16	20.12	5.04	$t = 1.05$ $n = 8$ $p > 0.05$

[a]*Expressed as seconds between consecutive spikes in conscious rabbits during a 2-minute application of a vertebral lesion. Vertebral lesions were applied at four different locations. Related-sample t tests were used with two-tailed tests of significance [n = 15]. The EMG inhibition after VL at T6 is striking.*

in the cerebrospinal fluid and plasma compartments has been disputed (Clement-Jones et al., 1980). The two compartments may function differently with regard to increases in β-endorphins produced by various therapeutic agencies (manipulation). In other words, plasma β-endorphin is only a selective outcome of a more complex set of responses (as yet poorly understood).

Mechanism of Pain Modulation and Analgesia by Endorphins

Endorphins are neurotransmitters at most of the synaptic relay points of the major pain pathways, ranging from sites in the dorsal horn of the spinal cord, periaqueductal gray, to the thalamus and cortex. Because endorphins are located in regions critical to the relay or integration of somatosensory information, they may influence transmission at multiple levels of the nervous system. Pituitary pools of endorphins that may interact with peripheral nerves via the systemic circulation or gain access to the brain are important for the chiropractic care of chronic pain sufferers. Both physical and psychic stressors provoke a secretion of β-endorphins into systemic plasma in humans (Millan, 1981).

After the discovery of endogenous opiate-like peptides, a number of studies showed that enkaphlin-like and β-endorphin-like substances are elevated in the cerebrospinal fluid (CSF) of patients after local stimulation of brain regions, producing analgesia (Akil et al., 1978; Almay et al., 1978; Hosobuchi et al., 1979). A schematic illustration of the major components of a descending system that contributes to the analgesic action of opiates and of electrical brain stimulation is depicted in Figure 10–6. The model is based on the original structure proposed by Basbaum and Fields (1978, 1984). Highlighted in stippling are the connections between the projection neurons of the periaqueductal gray (PAG) and various subregions of the rostral ventral medulla (the nucleus raphe magnus, NRM; the nucleus reticularis magnocellularis, Rmc; and the nucleus reticularis paragigantocellularis lateralis, Rpgl. The latter project via the dorsolateral funiculus to the spinal dorsal horn, where they inhibit nociceptive neurons. The inhibitory action of the spinal cord may be via direct postsynaptic inhibition or via opioid peptide-containing endorphin interneurons (indicated by stripes and ''E''). There are other endorphin links illustrated at the level of PAG and rostral medulla; however, their connections are not indicated. Inputs to the PAG (one of which is a hypothalamic β-endorphin pathway) are also illustrated, as is the noradrenergic (NE) contribution to bulbospinal con-

trol. The ascending components of this system are indicated by the unfilled symbols. These include afferent inputs, projection neurons of the dorsal horn, and their collaterals into the medulla and PAG. The ascending input to the PAG and raphe nucleus is presumed to derive, in part, from collaterals of neurons of the nucleus reticularis gigantocellularis (Rgc).

This model implicates three opioid peptide (E) links. These may involve enkephalin or dynorphin neurons. Basbaum and Fields (1984) indicated that cortical and diencephalic sites may provide inputs to the PAG. An important component in this system is the β-endorphin from the hypothalamus; however, it is not known as yet how opiates activate output neurons or how noradrenergic neurons fit into the activation process. What is the functional consequence of coexistence of neurotransmitters/neuromodulators in a single neuron? Do 5-hydroxytryptophan and N terminals interact at the level of the spinal cord? How do various endogenous opioid peptides interact? Is there an opiate receptor specific for analgesia? Despite these questions, it seems clear that pain modulation is a behaviorally significant physiologic process, using a discrete central nervous system involving the release of opioid peptides, biogenic amines, and other neurotransmitters in its function.

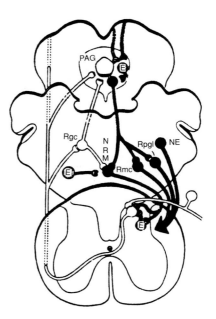

Figure 10–6. Schematic illustration of the major components of a descending system that contributes to the analgesic action of opiates and of electrical brain stimulation. See text for explanation. PAG = periaqueductal gray, NRM = nucleus raphe magnus, Rmc = nucleus reticularis magnocellularis, Rpgl = nucleus reticularis paragigantocellularis lateralis, E = endorphin interneuron. (*From Basbaum and Fields, 1984, p. 330, with permission.*)

Relation of Endorphin to Pain Conditions

Chronic Pain

The pain threshold and tolerance level in patients suffering from chronic pain may be related to endorphinergic pathways. Endorphinergic mechanisms appear to modulate both the perception and stimulus of pain (Davis, 1983). Patients with chronic pain syndrome and high CSF levels of endorphins had greater pain tolerance and a higher pain threshold than those with lower levels (Von Knorring et al., 1978). Another study showed that the CSF endorphins were low in patients with pain of organic etiology in comparison with patients with psychogenic pain (Almay et al., 1978). The level of CSF endorphins in patients appears to correlate with their need for narcotics in the postoperative state (Tamsen et al., 1982). Basal endorphin levels can be used to predict how much narcotic a patient will need to control pain in the postoperative period (Tamsen et al., 1980). Akil and co-workers (1976) suggested that chronic pain may deplete neurons of endorphins, thus impairing their function. This was further supported by another study in which experimental pain thresholds were measured in patients with chronic pain; naloxone and placebo did not alter pain thresholds (Lindblom and Tegner, 1979).

Jogging

Plasma β-endorphin levels have been shown to increase after a marathon (Colt et al., 1981). Analgesia produced by long-distance running is blocked by naloxone (Haier et al., 1981). Running and bicycling have been shown to increase other hormones, e.g., plasma prolactin and growth hormone (Noel et al., 1972). Similarly, strenuous exercise and running have been reported to increase plasma cortisol, presumably through stimulation of release of adrenocorticotropin (ACTH) (Noel et al., 1972; Davies and Few, 1973), although the effect of exercise on plasma ACTH levels in humans has not been well established.

In rats, both ACTH and β-endorphin are secreted into the peripheral blood in response to swimming (Fraioli et al., 1980). Shyu et al., (1982) reported that long-lasting muscle exercise (jogging), acupuncture, and low-frequency electrical stimulation of afferent nerve fibers produce discharges in muscle afferent nerve fibers (Group III) that modulate central endorphin mechanisms and result in analgesic effects. Recent reports by Hatfield and associates (1987) demonstrated that older men respond to graded exercise with serum β-endorphin levels similar to those of younger men and that the effective results imply an association between circulating β-endorphin and specified psychologic variables. In some cases, clinical syndromes of insensitivity to pain are related to endorphin excess (Dehen et al., 1978).

Low Back Pain

Johansson and co-workers (1980) demonstrated a significantly lower level of β-endorphins in CSF of ten patients with chronic back pain; this finding was recently corroborated by Puig et al. (1982). Several studies have shown that spinal manipulative therapy (SMT) reduces back pain, at least in the short term (Waagen et al., 1986). Long-term parallel studies of β-endorphin levels are needed.

Placebo Mechanisms

Levine et al. (1978) suggested that placebo-induced analgesia might be mediated through endorphinergic neuronal tracts. Naloxone increased pain in patients who had molar extractions. A group of patients who had previously experienced an analgesic response to a placebo injection of physiologic sodium chloride were more vigorous in their pain increase in response to naloxone. Placebo analgesic response may be considered the result of recruitment by environmental influences (such as reassurance) of brain pain-suppressing mechanisms.

Somatic Stimulation and Endorphins

Acupuncture analgesia appears dependent on opiate-like hormones: hypophysectomy reduces the analgesic effect of acupuncture in animals (Pomerantz et al., 1977) and humans (Szczudlik and Andrezej, 1983). Naloxone blocks acupuncture analgesia (Mayer et al., 1977). Whether naloxone would block the β-endorphin rise seen after spinal manipulation (Vernon et al., 1986) remains to be investigated. Electroacupuncture seems dependent on β-endorphins (Abbate et al., 1980; Cheng, 1980), although some aspects of electroacupuncture appear to have non-adrenergic contributions as well (Chapman et al., 1973). Figure 10–7 depicts the modulation of the endorphin system at low- and high-frequency electroacupuncture via the spinal cord. An increase in CSF endorphins after electroacupuncture (Sjolund et al., 1977) also supports the idea of endorphin-mediated analgesia; however, hypnotically induced reduction in pain appreciation does not appear to be affected by naloxone in humans (Barber and Mayer, 1977).

Cervical Spinal Manipulation and β-Endorphins

To investigate whether or not spinal manipulation might exert its pain-relieving effect through activa-

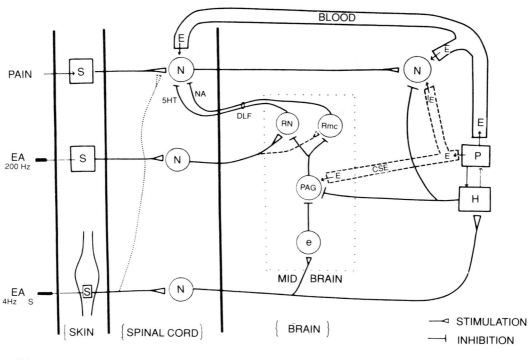

Figure 10–7. At low frequency (4 Hz), electroacupuncture (EA) may stimulate the midbrain (PAG) to release enkephalins, which will indirectly stimulate the raphe nucleus (RN) and/or reticular magnocellular nucleus (Rmc) to send a descending inhibition on the spinal cord pain cells. Serotonin (5-hydroxytryptamine [5-HT] and noradrenaline (NA) are probably the neurotransmitters involved in the RN and Rmc systems, respectively. In parallel, EA may also stimulate the hypothalamus (H) and pituitary (P) to rlease β-endorphine or dynorphin. The pituitary endorphins may either penetrate the blood–brain barrier or backflow to the hypothalamus or cerebrospinal fluid (CSF) and bind to the opiate receptors in the spinal cord and the brain. In addition, low-frequency (4-Hz) EA may cause the segmental release of endorphins from the spinal cord interneurons and their binding to the opiate receptors in the pain transmission cells. High-frequency (200-Hz) EA appears to stimulate directly the RN and Rmc descending inhibitory systems, bypassing the endorphin system. S = sensory receptor, N = interneuron, e = enkephalinergic neuron, E = endorphin (b-endorphin or dynorphin), PAG = periaqueductal gray, DLF = dorsolateral funiculus. (*From Vernon et al., 1986, p. 119, with permission.*)

tion of the endogenous opiate system, Vernon and colleagues (1986) examined the effect of cervical spinal manipulation on plasma β-endorphin levels in 27 healthy male subjects. Figure 10–8 shows the plasma β-endorphin levels both before and after spinal adjustment. To control for any differences in baseline levels among subjects, each subject's postintervention levels were expressed as percentages of the mean of the subject's two baseline levels. These percentage data were analyzed using repeated analyses of variance (ANOVAs), which showed significant differences among groups ($p < 0.005$) and among times ($p < 0.002$). After the initial increase, β-endorphin levels tended to decrease as the time after intervention increased. A one-way ANOVA

showed very highly significant differences among the three groups at 5 minutes ($p < 0.0001$).

Because this study was confined to plasma β-endorphin, it was concluded that the minimal stimulus generated by this experimental maneuver was sufficient to induce a mild elevation in the hypothalamic–pituitary axis, resulting in a slight response of plasma β-endorphin (Fig. 10–9).

It is possible that this release phenomenon may be dose dependent. It has been shown that high-intensity, low-frequency TENS can selectively produce increases in plasma β-endorphin (Hughes et al., 1984). The quality and quantity of peripheral stimulation may be an important determinant of the pituitary endorphin response. A response more substan-

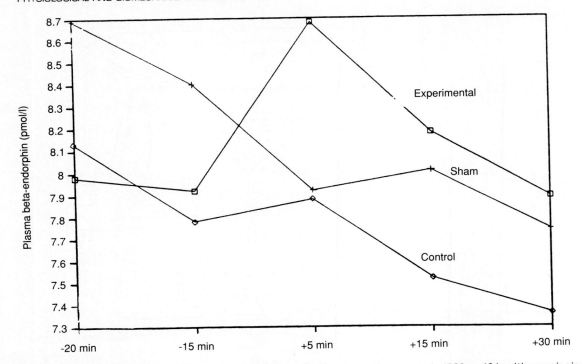

Figure 10–8. Plot of mean β-endorphin levels before and after SMT. (*From Vernon et al., 1986, p. 121, with permission.*)

tial than that found in this study might therefore be induced by a higher dosage of spinal manipulation (either at one time or in series).

The authors consider, however, that their study approaches this phenomenon from a ''minimalist'' point of view. Only one manipulation was performed, and this constitutes the minimum act sufficient to distinguish sham from active treatment. The amount of somatic stimulation from a single manipulation is therefore minimum and expectations of outcome were correspondingly low. A recent report by Christian and colleagues (1988) suggested that ma-

nipulative therapy does not activate the hypothamic–pituitary–adrenal axis; hence, no change in β-endorphin and cortisol was found. The extent to which this elevation in plasma β-endorphin manifests itself clinically has not been determined as yet.

Spinal Cord and Melatonin

In view of the chiropractic emphasis on the spine, it is interesting that many types of dysfunctions of the spinal column may disrupt the endogenous clock

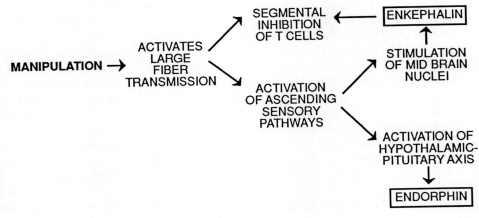

Figure 10–9. Conceptual model of the neurohormonal effects of spinal manipulation. (*From Vernon et al., 1986, p. 122, with permission.*)

Cervical Spinal Cord Lesions Disrupt the Rhythm

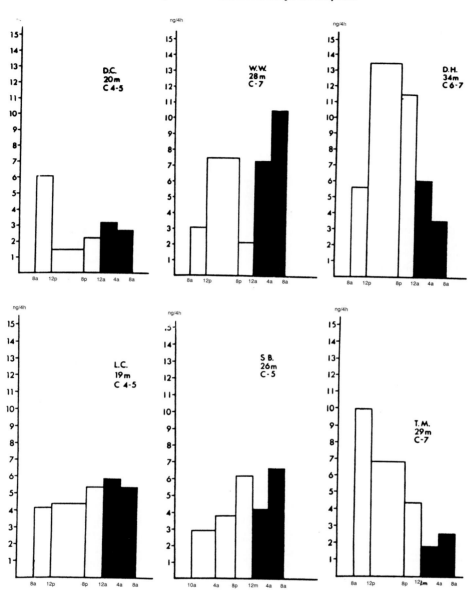

Figure 10-10. Urinary melatonin levels per 4- or 8-hour collection periods for each of six quadriplegic subjects. Data are expressed as nanograms per 4- or 8-hour interval. Age, sex, and level of transection are indicated for each subject. (*From Kneisley et al., 1978a, p. 313, with permission.*)

that controls melatonin rhythmicity (Reppert et al., 1981; Tattersall et al., 1986). Other studies have shown that there is a deficiency of melatonin in humans with cluster headaches (Chazot et al., 1984) and cervical spinal cord lesions and autonomic failure (Claus-Walker and Halstead, 1982). Lesions of the periventricular nucleus area of the hypothalmus have been shown to disrupt the suprachiasmic spinal cord circuit in the melatonin rhythm-generating system. Figures 10–10 and 10–11 show that quadraplegic subjects do not exhibit normal day–night variation in melatonin excretion (Kneisley et al., 1978a, b). Further, spinal injury disrupts other endocrine

rhythms like serum cortisol, aldosterone, and growth hormone (Fig. 10–12).

Additional factors such as inactivity and position may also modify the melatonin rhythm in humans. Lynch and colleagues (1975) reported that urinary melatonin rhythm was disrupted in three young patients who were kept immobilized in bed with healing leg fractures. A deficiency in melatonin may exacerbate depression, peptic ulcer, sexual dysfunction, and stress (Naurizi, 1984). Recently, melatonin has also been implicated as causing analgesia in mice in a dose-related response (Lakin et al., 1981). The decrease in susceptibility to pain

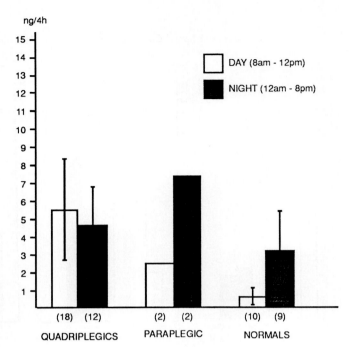

Figure 10–11. Melatonin content of urine during sleep (12 AM–8 AM; shaded bar) and while awake (8 AM–12 PM) among normal persons, quadriplegic subjects, and one paraplegic subject. Content is expressed as nanograms of melatonin per time period (mean + SD). Numbers in parentheses represent the number of urine collections for each time period. (*From Kneisley et al., 1978a, p. 318, with permission.*)

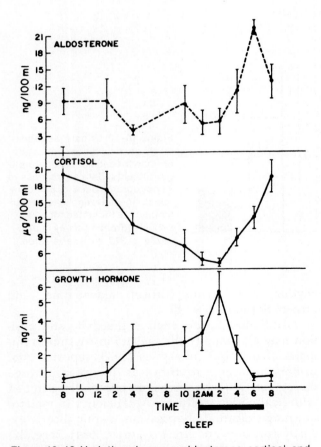

Figure 10–12. Variations in serum aldosterone, cortisol, and growth hormone over a 24-hour period in six quadriplegic subjects. Blood was sampled via an indwelling catheter at the times indicated. Data are expressed as means ± SE. (*From Kneisley et al., 1978a, p. 319, with permission.*)

was not observed in animals in which melatonin administration was followed by the opiate antagonist naloxone.

Manipulation and Melatonin

As noted earlier, the pineal hormone melatonin has been implicated in a variety of spine-related physiologic mechanisms as well as disorders. Melatonin secretion (Cardinali, 1983; Klein et al., 1981) seems to be controlled by sympathetic neurons, as evidenced by the fact that propranolol blocks the nighttime secretion of melatonin. Moreover, the 24-hour rhythm of secretion is absent in patients with transection of the cervical spinal cord (Kneisley et al., 1978a,b) and patients with chronic autonomic failure (Vaughan et al., 1979). These studies suggest a role of sympathetic neurons in secretion of melatonin through the pathways shown in Figure 10–13.

As melatonin is found in both CSF and peripheral blood, it may exert its effect on the central nervous system, the peripheral (nonneural) system, or both. However, the release or synthesis of melatonin is under the direct control of sympathetic neurons. Consequently, any change in sympathetic activity may directly affect melatonin secretion or synthesis. Melatonin also has several strong effects on the hypothalamus. Some mechanisms of action of melatonin on the hypothalamus are listed in Table 10–4.

An increasing body of evidence now proposes that the sympathetic superior cervical ganglion (SCG) may be a peripheral center of integration of

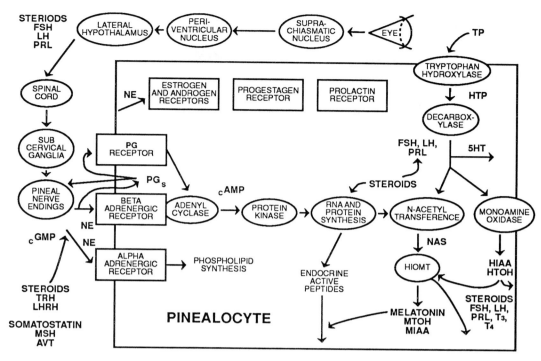

Figure 10-13. Schematic summary of the mechanisms for neuronal and hormonal control of pineal secretory activity. The major driving force for the circadian variation in melatonin synthesis is given by neural signals originating in the retina and reaching the pineal via its sympathetic nerves. The released norepinephrine (NE) interacts with alpha- and beta-adrenoreceptors, which are coupled to phospholipid synthesis and adenylcyclase, respectively. Prostaglandins (PGs) are involved in this metabolic sequence, affecting cyclic AMP (cAMP) synthesis. The increase in cAMP induced by NE leads to the activation of protein kinase and results, via RNA and protein synthesis, in an increase in the number of N-acetyltransferase (NAS) and hydroxyindole-O-methyltransferase (HIOMT) molecules. Both enzymes play a central role in melatonin biosynthesis, which starts with the uptake of the amino acid tryptophan (TP) from the bloodstream. TP is readily converted into 5-hydroxytryptophan (HTP) by the enzyme tryptophan hydroxylase, and is decarboxylated to serotonin (5-HT) by relatively nonspecific decarboxylase. There is a precipitous drop in pineal 5-HT concentration at night, because of oxidative deamination, which yields 5-hydoxyindoleacetic acid (HIAA) and 5-hydroxytryptophol (HTOH) and increased melatonin biosynthesis. Final products of HIOMT include melatonin, 5-methoxytryptophol (MTOH), and 5-methylindoleacetic acid (MIAA). The control mechanism for the synthesis of endocrine-active peptides is unknown; some data suggest that melatonin may be involved in their regulation. Sites for hormone regulation include pineal cells, through different hormone receptors; pineal nerve endings; sympathetic ganglia; and descending sympathetic pathways. LH = luteinizing hormone, LHRH = luteinizing hormone-releasing hormone, MSH = melanocyte-stimulating hormone, FSH = follicle-stimulating hormone, PRL = prolactin, T_3 = triiodothyronine, T_4 = thyroxine, TRH = thyrotropin-releasing hormone.(*From Cardinali, 1983, p. 5, with permission.*)

neural and endocrine signals. In addition to innervating significant neuroendocrine structures, SCGs are active points of summation for hormone signals (Cardinali, 1981; Cardinali et al., 1982; Klein et al., 1983).

TABLE 10-4. MECHANISMS OF ACTION OF MELATONIN ON THE HYPOTHALAMUS

1. Action on serotonin receptors
2. Binding to specific receptors in medial basal hypothalamus
3. Inhibition of protein synthesis throughout hypothalamus
4. Inhibition of hypothalamic microtubule protein content
5. Impairment of fast axonal transport and induction of ultrastructural changes in nerve endings of the median eminence
6. Inhibition of hypothalamic monoamine oxidase
7. Inhibition of prostaglandin E_2 and cyclic AMP synthesis

Source. *Cardinali and Ritta, 1983; Vacas et al., 1981.*

There is evidence that melatonin secretion may be disrupted by a lesion of the cervical spinal cord (Kneisley et al., 1978b). These alterations may occur in the pineal organ as a result of a lesion within the cervical spinal cord interrupting descending sympathetic neurons to the superior cervical ganglia.

Is there any effect on melatonin excretion in patients with a subluxated cervical spinal cord? Although there is no conclusive evidence at this time, we hypothesize that cervical spinal subluxations may modify melatonin rhythmicity in patients with neck pain, specifically, that we would observe an increase in melatonin secretion after SMT. Preliminary investigations in healthy males and females showed an increase in melatonin after a single cervical spinal manipulation (Dhami and Coyle, 1986). These find-

TABLE 10–5. EFFECT OF SPINAL MANIPULATION ON PLASMA MELATONIN AND SERUM PITUITARY HORMONES DURING FOLLICULAR PHASE IN FEMALE SUBJECTS [a]

Hormone (units)	Time Period			
	0800 h	0900 h	1000 h	1200 h
Melatonin (pg/mL				
Control (N=5)	39 ± 7.2	32 ± 5.5	25 ± 4.2	19 ± 3.4
Manipulated (N=8)	37 ± 10.3	30 ± 7.4	31 ± 5.3*	26 ± 4.2
LH (IU/L)				
Control (N=5)	8 ± 1.1	7 ± 2.8	8 ± 2.3	8 ± 1.6
Manipulated (N=6)	7 ± 2.4	8 ± 1.9	10 ± 1.8*	8 ± 2.4
FSH (IU/L)				
Control (N=5)	5 ± 1.3	6 ± 2.5	7 ± 1.4	7 ± 1.8
Manipulated (N=6)	7 ± 2.7	7 ± 1.8	11 ± 2.6*	8 ± 1.2
Prolactin (ng/mL)				
Control (N=5)	8 ± 2.0	9 ± 1.7	8 ± 1.9	8 ± 2.1
Manipulated (N=6)	10 ± 3.3	9 ± 2.6	12 ± 2.2*	11 ± 2.7

[a]Subjects manipulated at 0900 H.
* Values differ significantly from control group, $p < 0.05$.
From Dhami and Coyle (1986), with permission.

ings (Tables 10–5 through 10–8) suggest that the human pineal is regulated by the central nervous system and that neurons arising in or coursing through the spinal cord are important for the generation of a normal pineal rhythm in humans.

Conclusion

The most compelling reason for continuing to believe that there is a relationship between spinal lesions and internal functioning (malfunctioning) remains the clinical and anecdotal reports of adventitious improvements in various disorders concomitant with therapy designed to remove spinal lesions. This evidence is not and cannot be conclusive but only encouraging and tantalizing. Rigorous answers must be sought experimentally. Swenson's chapter in this book is particularly interesting and relevant to some of the concepts with which we have dealt.

Along with some clinical supportive data, a plethora of neurophysiologic and psychophysiologic

TABLE 10–6. EFFECT OF SPINAL MANIPULATION ON PLASMA MELATONIN AND SERUM PITUITARY HORMONES DURING MENSTRUAL MIDCYCLE IN FEMALE SUBJECTS [a]

Hormone (units)	Time Period			
	0800 h	0900 h	1000 h	200 h
Melatonin (pg/mL)				
Control (N = 4)	70 ± 21.7	62 ± 8.8	41 ± 9.3	58 ± 6.2
Manipulated (N = 5)	59 ± 9.9	58 ± 7.7	47 ± 7.4	27 ± 5.6
LH (IU.L)				
Control (N = 4)	16 ± 3.3	17 ± 2.6	16 ± 2.8	17 ± 2.6
Manipulated (N = 5)	18 ± 2.5	19 ± 3.4	21 ± 3.1*	18 ± 2.8
FSH (IU/L)				
Control (N = 4)	12 ± 2.1	11 ± 1.4	12 ± 1.8	12 ± 2.3
Manipulated (N = 5)	11 ± 1.7	12 ± 2.2	14 ± 2.0	13 ± 1.8
Prolactin (mg/mL)				
Control (N = 4)	14 ± 1.0	15 ± 2.4	15 ± 1.5	14 ± 1.9
Manipulated (N = 5)	15 ± 2.1	16 ± 2.7	17 ± 1.8	16 ± 1.3

* Value differs significantly from group, $p < 0.05$
[a]Subjects manipulated at 0900 h).
From Dhami and Coyle (1986), with permission.

TABLE 10–7. EFFECT OF SPINAL MANIPULATION ON PLASMA MELATONIN AND SERUM PITUITARY HORMONES DURING LUTEAL PHASE IN FEMALE SUBJECTS [a]

Hormone (Units)	Time Period			
	0800 h	**0900 h**	**1000 h**	**1200 h**
Melatonin [pg/mL]				
Control [N = 5]	49 ± 4.6	25 ± 3.5	22 ± 2.9	16 ± 2.4
Manipulated [N = 5]	35 ± 7.3	29 ± 4.4	20 ± 3.7	18 ± 2.7
LH [IU/L]				
Control [N = 5]	5 ± 2.0	4 ± 1.5	4 ± 1.7	5 ± 1
Manipulated [N = 5]	4 ± 1.5	5 ± 2.1	6 ± 1.4[*]	5 ± 1
FSH [IU/L]				
Control [N = 5]	3 ± 0.8	4 ± 1.1	4 ± 0.8	4 ± 1.4
Manipulated [N = 5]	4 ± 1.2	5 ± 1.8	6 ± 1.2[*]	5 ± 1.9
Prolactin [ng/mL]				
Control [N = 5]	19 ± 2.5	20 ± 2.2	21 ± 2.7	19 ± 1.8
Manipulated [N = 5]	20 ± 1.7	21 ± 3.4	24 ± 2.1[*]	22 ± 3.1

[a]Subjects manipulated at 0900 h.
[*] Values differ significantly from group, $p < 0.05$.
From Dhami and Coyle (1986), with permission.

data are in line with the concept. Although admittedly weak, the tactic of trying to establish a relationship between a nidus in the spine and internal visceral change by establishing general concordance between known neuroanatomic and neurophysiologic facts provides some additional measure of support. Other chapters in this book, especially Spinal Reflex Physiology by Sato (Chapter 8) and Physiology of Spinal Pain by Haldeman (Chapter 13), reinforce the connection. In the most intensively studied cases, both experimental and clinical, a substantial direct or indirect change in organ function has been found in association with somatospinal stimuli. We conclude that the studies of neurophysiologic reflex relations are uniformly supportive, as illustrated in a wide variety of situations from gastric motility to endocrine changes. It is painfully obvious from a survey of the literature, however, that the reality of

vertebrogenic visceral lesions (and manipulative correction) remains an open question that can be resolved only with experimental and clinical research on a large scale in the future. We urge that future research focus on which spinal lesion produces what disorder (dysfunction) through which mechanism(s). The impetus for such work is strong.

The strongest conclusion we make is that the use of manipulation in differentiating "true" viscerogenic from somatogenic or vertebrogenic disease or pain may increasingly be an attractive role.

References

Aaronson MJ, Freed MM, and Burakoff R. Colonic myoelectric activity in persons with spinal cord injury. *Dig Dis Sci* 1985;30: 295–300.
Abbate D, Santamaria A, Brambilla A, et al. Beta-endorphin and electroacupuncture. *Lancet* 1980;2:1309–1315.
Akil H, Mayer DJ, and Liebeskind JC. Antagonism of stimulation

TABLE 10–8. EFFECT OF SPINAL MANIPULATION ON URINARY 6-HYDROXYMELATONIN[a] DURING FOLLICULAR, MIDCYCLE, AND LUTEAL PHASES IN FEMALE SUBJECTS

Phase	Time Period	
	0800–0900 h[b]	**1000–1200 h[b]**
Follicular		
Control [N = 5]	1.7 ± 0.3	3.0 ± 0.4
Manipulated [N = 6]	1.4 ± 0.4	4.3 ± 2.3[**]
Midcycle		
Control [N = 4]	2.2 ± 0.6	4.2 ± 1.7
Manipulated [N = 5]	1.8 ± 0.7	3.9 ± 1.1
Luteal		
Control [N = 5]	1.4 ± 0.4	3.5 ± 1.3
Manipulated [N = 5]	1.9 ± 0.6	3.8 ± 0.9

[a]Expressed as ng/mL urine.
[b]Correlation coefficient with plasma melatonin (r = 0.78–0.91)
[**] Value differs significantly from control group, $p < 0.05$ (df) = 18).
From Dhami and Coyle (1986), with permission.

produces analgesia by naloxone, a narcotic antagonist. *Science* 1976;191:961–969.

Akil H, Richardson DE, and Hughes J. Enkephalin-like material elevated in ventricular cerebro-spinal fluid of pain patients after analgetic focal stimulation. *Science* 1978;201:463–470.

Almay BGL, Johansson F, Von Knorring L, et al. Endorphins in chronic pain. I. Differences in CSF endorphin levels between organic and psychogenic pain syndromes. *Pain* 1978;5:153–157.

Arabiloff B. Bronchial asthma—A case report. *J Clin Chiropractic* 1969;24:40–42.

Araki T, Ito K, Kurosawa M, and Sato A. The somato-adrenal medullary reflexes in rats. *J Auton Nerv Syst* 1981;3:161–170.

Badalamenti MA, Dee R, and Ghillani R, et al. Mechanical stimulation of dorsal root ganglia induces increased production of substance P: A mechanism for pain following nerve root compression? *Spine* 1987;12:552–555.

Barber J and Mayer DJ. Evaluation of the efficacy and neural mechanisms of hypnotic analgesia procedure in experimental and clinical dental pain. *Pain* 1977;4:441–446.

Basbaum AI and Fields HL. Endogenous pain control mechanism: Review and hypothesis. *Ann Neurol* 1978;4:451–462.

Basbaum AI and Fields HL. Endogenous pain control systems: Brain stem spinal pathways and endorphin circuitry. *Annu Rev Neurosci* 1984;7:309–338.

Beal MC. Palpatory testing for somatic dysfunction in patients with cardiovascular disease. *J Am Osteopath Assoc* 1983;82:822:831.

Beal MC and Dvorak J. Palpatory examination of the spine: A comparison of the results of two methods and their relationships to visceral disease. *Manual Med* 1984;1:25–32.

Berlly MH and Wilmot CB. Acute abdominal emergencies during the first four weeks after spinal cord injury. *Arch Phys Med Rehab* 1984;65:687–690.

Brunarski DJ. Functional considerations of spinal manipulative therapy. *J Am Chiropractic Assoc* 1980;14:S63–S68.

Bueno L, Ferre JP, and Ruckebusch Y. Effects of anesthesia and surgical procedures on intestinal myoelectric activity in rats. *Dig Dis Sci* 1978;23:690–695.

Buerger AA and Tobis JS. *Approaches to the Validation of Manipulative Therapy.* Springfield, Ill; Charles C Thomas; 1975.

Camillieri M, Malagelada JR, Kao PC, and Zinsmeister AR. Effect of somatovisceral reflexes and selective dermatomal stimulation on postcibal antral pressure activity. *Am J Physiol* 1984; 247: G703–G708.

Cardinali DP. Molecular mechanisms of neuroendocrine integration in the central nervous system: An approach through the study of the pineal gland and its innervating sympathetic pathway. *Psychoneuroendocrinology* 1983;8:3–30.

Cardinali DP. Melatonin. A mammalian pineal hormone. *Endocrinology* 1981;2:327–346.

Cardinali DP, Pisariv MA, and Barontini M, et al. Efferent neuroendocrine pathways or sympathetic superior cervical ganglia. *Neuroendocrinology* 1982;35:248–254.

Cardinali DP and Ritta NM. The role of prostaglandins in neuroendocrine junction. Studies in the pineal gland and the hypothalamus. 1983:2–6.

Carnett JB. The simulation of gall bladder disease by intercostal neuralgia of the abdominal wall. *Ann Surg* 1927;86:747–757.

Celander E, Koenig AJ, and Celander DR. Effects of osteopathic manipulative therapy on autonomic tone as evidenced by blood pressure changes and activity of the fibrinolytic system. *J Am Osteopath Assoc* 1968;67:1037–1038.

Cervero F and Wolstencroft JH. A positive feedback loop between spinal cord nociceptive pathways and antinociceptive areas in the cat's brain stem. *Pain* 1984;20:125–131.

Chapman CR, Murphy TM, and Butler SH. Analgesic strengths of 33 percent nitrous oxide: A signal detection theory evaluation. *Science* 1973;179:1246–1253.

Chapman F. *An Endocrine Interpretation of Chapman's Reflexes.* Davenport, Iowa: Palmer College of Chiropractic; 1963.

Chazot G, Claustrat B, and Brun J, et al. A chronobiological study of melatonin, cortisol, growth hormone and prolactin secretion in cluster headache. *Cephalalgia* 1984;4:213–220.

Cheng RSS. *Mechanisms of Electroacupuncture Analgesia as Related to Endorphins and Monoamines: An Intricate System Is Proposed.* Thesis. Toronto: University of Toronto: 1980.

Christian GF, Stan GJ, Sissons D, et al. Immunoreactive ACTH, β-endorphin, and cortisol levels in plasma following spinal manipulative therapy. *Spine* 1988;13:1411–1417.

Claus-Walker J and Halstead LS. Metabolic and endocrine changes in spinal cord injury. 1. Consequences of partial decentralization of the autonomic nervous system. *Arch Phys Med Rehab* 1982;63:569–575.

Clement-Jones V, Lowry PJ, and Rees LH, et al. Development of a specific extracted radioimmunoassay for methionine enkephalin in human plasma and CSF. *J Endocrinol* 1980;86:231–237

Colt EWD, Wardlaw, and Frantz AG. The effect of running on plasma beta endorphins. *Life Sci* 1981;28:1637–1641.

Davies CTM and Few JD. Effects of exercise on adrenocorticol function. *J Appl Physiol* 1973;35:887–891.

Davis D. Respiration manifestations of dorsal spine radiculitis simulating cardiac asthma. *Ann Intern Med* 1950;32:954–959.

Davis GC. Endorphins and pain. *Psychiatr Clin North Am* 1983; 6:473–487.

DeBoer RF. An attempt to induce vertebral lesions in rabbits by mechanical irritation. *J Manipulative Physiol Ther* 1981;4:119–128.

DeBoer KF. Gastrointestinal myoelectric activity in rabbits with vertebral lesions: Preliminary report. *Eur J Chiropractic* 1984; 32:131–142.

DeBoer KF and McKnight ME. Effects of cervical spine adjustments on blood pressure. *J Manipulative Physiol Ther* 1988a; 11:261–266.

DeBoer KF and McKnight ME. Surgical model of a chronic subluxation in rabbits. *J Manipulative Physiol Ther* 1988b;11:366–372.

DeBoer KF, Schultz M, and McKnight ME. Acute effects of spinal manipulation on gastrointestinal myoelectric activity in conscious rabbits. *Manual Med* 1988;3:85–94.

Dehen H, Willer JC, and Prier S, et al. Congenital insensitivity to pain and the morphine-like analgesic system. *Pain* 1978;5:351–356.

Dhami MSI and Coyle BA. *Evidence for Sympathetic Neuron Stimulation by Cervical Spinal Manipulation.* Proceedings Conf. Res. Educ., CCA, San Diego, Calif, June 28, 1986.

Egli AB. Spine and heart. Vertebrogenous cardiac syndromes. *Ann Swiss Chiropractic Assoc* 1965;4:95–105.

Fealey RD, Szurszewski JH, Merritt JL, and DiMagno EP. Effect of traumatic spinal cord transection on human upper gastrointestinal motility and gastric emptying. *Gastroenterology* 1984;87:69–75.

Fiske F. Specific adjustment to control blood pressure. *J Am Osteopath Assoc* 1979;25:435–437.

Fiske JW. *Medical Text of Neck and Back Pain.* Springfield, Ill: Charles C Thomas; 1987.

Foellner RP, Taylor RM, Marjan G, and Kelso AF. Proposed study to evaluate the effects of osteopathic manipulative therapy in the treatment of the emphysema patient. *J Am Osteopath Assoc* 1968;67:131–132.

Fraioli F, Morreti C, and Paolucci D, et al. Physical exercise stimulates marked concomitant release of beta-endorphin and adrenocorticotropic hormone (ACTH) in peripheral blood in man. *Experientia* 1980;36:987–989.

Gitelman R. Spinal manipulation in the relief of pain. In Goldstein M, *The Research Status of SMT.* (Monograph) Washington, DC:

NINCDS; 1975. DHEW Publication (NIH) 76–998, pp. 277–285.

Glick ME, Meshkinpour H, and Haldeman S, et al. Colonic dysfunction in multiple sclerosis. *Gastroenterology* 1982;83:1002–1007.

Glick ME, Meshkinpour H, and Haldeman S, et al. Colonic dysfunction in patients with thoracic spinal cord injury. *Gastroenterology* 1984;86:287–294.

Goldstein M, ed. *The Research Status of Spinal Manipulative Therapy.* Bethesda, Md: DHEW; 1975: NINCDS Monograph 15.

Goodheart G. The ileo-cecal valve syndrome. *Digest Chiropractic Econ* 1967;9:32–35.

Goodheart GJ. Low blood sugar and hyperinsulinism. *Digest Chiropractic Econ* 1965;7:12–15.

Greenspan J and Melchior J. The effect of osteopathic manipulative treatment on the resistance of rats to stressful situations. *J Am Osteopath Assoc* 1966;65:1205–1209.

Haier RJ, Quid K, and Mills JSC Naloxone alters pain perception after jogging. *Psychiatry Res* 1981;5:231–235.

Haldeman SC. The pathophysiology of the spinal subluxation. In Goldstein M, ed. *The Research Status of Spinal Manipulative Therapy.* Bethesda, Md: DHEW; 1975: NINCDS Monograph 15, pp. 217–226.

Haldeman SC. The clinical basis for discussion of mechanisms of manipulative therapy. In Korr IM, ed. *The Neurobiologic Mechanisms in Manipulative Therapy.* New York: Plenum Press; 1977:53–75.

Haldeman SC, ed. *Modern Developments in the Principles and Practice of Chiropractic.* New York: Appleton-Century-Crofts; 1980.

Haldeman SC. Pain physiology as a neurological model for manipulation. *Manual Med* 1981;19:5–11.

Halter JB and Pflug AE. Effects of sympathetic blockage by spinal anesthesia on pancreatic islet function in man. *Am J Physiol* 1980;239:E150–E155.

Hartmann GW and Schwartz HS, eds. *Mental Health and Chiropractic, a Multiple Disciplinary Approach.* New York: Sessions; 1973.

Hatfield BD, Goldfarb AH, Sforzo GA, et al. Serum beta-endorphin and effective responses to graded exercise in young and elderly men. *J Gerontol* 1987;42:429–431.

Hay J. The importance of faulty structural relations in etiology and treatment of peptic ulcer. *J Am Osteopath Assoc* 1939;39:162–165.

He X, Proske U, Schaible H-G, and Schmidt RF. Acute inflammation of the knee joint in the cat: Altered responses of flexor motoneurons to ligament movements. *J Neurophysiol* 1988;59:326–340.

Hildebrandt RW, ed. *Principles and Practice of Chiropractic.* Lombard, Ill: National College of Chiropractic; 1976.

Hildebrandt RW. *Chiropractic Spinography.* Des Plaines, Ill: Hilmark; 1977.

Hix EL. Influence of the autonomic innervation on renal function. *Acad Appl Osteopath Year Book* 1960:137–142.

Hoag JM, Cole WV, and Bradford SG, eds. *Osteopathic Medicine.* New York: McGraw-Hill; 1969.

Hood RP. Blood pressure results in 75 abnormal cases. *Digest Chiropractic Econ* 1974;16:36–38.

Hosobuchi Y, Rossier J, and Bloom FE, et al. Stimulation of human periaqueductal gray for pain relief increases immunoreactive beta-endorphin in ventricular fluid. *Science* 1979;203:279–284.

Howell RK, Allen TW, and Kappler RE. The influence of osteopathic manipulative therapy in the management of patients with chronic obstructive lung disease. *J Am Osteopath Assoc* 1975;74:149–159.

Hughes GS, Lichstein PR, Whitelock D, and Harker C. Response of plasma beta-endorphins to transcutaneous electrical nerve stimulation in healthy subjects. *Phys Ther* 1984;64:1062–1066.

Ito K, Kim P, Sato A, and Torigata Y. Reflex changes in gastric motility produced by nociceptive stimulation of the skin in anesthetized cats. In Ito M, ed. *Integrative Control Functions of the Brain*, vol. II. Amsterdam: Elsevier/North-Holland; 1979.

Johansson F, Almay BGL, Von Knorring L, et al. Predictors for the outcome of treatment with high frequency transcutaneous electric nerve stimulation with chronic pain. *Pain* 1980;9:55–62.

Johnston RJ. Vertebrogenic autonomic dysfunction—Subjective symptoms: A prospective study. *J Can Chiropractic Assoc* 1981;25:51–57.

Josey AI and Murphy F. Ruptured intravertebral disc simulating angina pectoralis. *JAMA* 1946;131:581–587.

Kametani H, Sato A, Sato Y, and Simpson A. Neural mechanisms of reflex facilitation and inhibition of gastric motility to stimulation of various skin areas in rats. *J Physiol* 1979;294:407–418.

Kametani H, Sato A, Sato Y, and Ueki K. Reflex facilitation and inhibition of gastric motility from various skin areas in rats. In Ito M, ed. *Integrative Control Functions of the Brain*, vol. 1. Tokyo: Kondansha Scientific; 1978.

Kaufman A, Sato A, Sato Y, and Sugimoto H. Reflex changes in heart rate after mechanical and thermal stimulation of the skin at various sigmental levels in cats. *Neuroscience* 1977;2:103–109.

Kellgren JH. Somatic simulating visceral pain. *Clin Sci Mol Med* 1939;4:303–309.

Klein DC, Namboodiri MAA, and Auerbach DA. The melatonin rhythm generating system: Developmental aspects. *Life Sci* 1981;28:1975–1986.

Klein DC, Smoot R, and Weller JL, et al. Lesions of the paralenticular nucleus area suprachismatic–spinal cord circuit in the melatonin rhythm generating system. *Brain Res Bull* 1983;10:647–659.

Kneisley LW, Moskowitz MA, and Lynch HJ. Cervical spinal cord lesions disrupt the rhythm in human melatonin excretion. *J Neural Transm* 1978a;13:311–323.

Kneisley LW, Moskowitz MA, and Lynch HJ, et al. The 24-hour rhythm of secretion of melatonin is absent with transection of cervical spinal cord. *J Neural Transm* 1978b;11:11–19.

Koizumi K, Sato A, and Terui N. Role of somatic afferents in the autonomic system control of intestinal motility. *Brain Res* 1980;182:85–97.

Korr IM. Neural basis of osteopathic lesions. *J Am Osteopath Assoc* 1947;47:191.

Korr IM, ed. *The Neurologic Mechanisms in Manipulative Therapy.* New York: Plenum Press, 1978:119–168.

Korr IM. The spinal cord as organizer of disease process: Part II—The peripheral autonomic nervous system. *J Am Osteopath Assoc* 1979a;79:82–90.

Korr IM. The spinal cord as organizer of disease processes: Part III—Hyperactivity of sympathetic innervation as a common factor in disease. *J Am Osteopath Assoc* 1979b;79:232–237.

Kunert W. Functional disorders of internal organs due to vertebral lesions. *Ciba Symp* 1965;13:85–96.

Lakin ML, Miller CH, and Stott ML, et al. Involvement of the pineal gland and melatonin in murine analgesia. *Life Sci* 1981;29:2543–2551.

Levine JD, Gordon NE, and Fields HL. The mechanism of placebo analgesia. *Lancet* 1978;2:654–659.

Lewis T and Kellgren JH. Observations relating to referred pain. *Clin Sci* 1939;4:47–71.

Lewit K. Menieres disease and the cervical spine. *Rev Czech Med* 1961;7:129–139.

Lewit K. Results of manipulative treatment on childhood migraines. *Hippocrates* 1963;34:308–316.

Lewit K. Ligament pain and anteflexion headache. *Eur Neurol* 1971;5:365–378.

Lewit K. The contribution of clinical observation to neurobiological mechanisms in manipulative therapy. In Korr IM, ed. *The*

Neurobiologic Mechanisms in Manipulative Therapy. New York; Plenum Press; 1978:3–25.

Lindbolm U and Tegner R. Are the endorphins active in clinical pain state? Narcotic antagonism in chronic pain patients. *Pain* 1979;7:65–71.

Love JG and Emmett JL. 'Asymptomatic' protruded lumbar disc as a cause of urinary retention—Preliminary report. *Mayo Clin Proc* 1967;42:249–257.

Luisetto G, Spano D, and Steiner W. et al. Plasma levels of β-endorphin and calcitonin before and after manipulative treatment of patients with cervical arthrosis and Barri's syndrome. In Mazzarelli JP, ed. *Chiropractic Intraprofessional Research.* Toronto: Edizioni Minerva Medica; 1982:47–52.

Lynch HJ, Wurtman RJ, and Moskowitz MA. Daily rhythm in human urinary melatonin. *Science* 1975;187:69–71.

MacDonald G and Hargrave-Wilson W. *The Osteopathic Lesion.* London: Heinemann; 1935.

Maigne R. Post cervical syndrome of Barre-Lieou and subjective syndrome of head trauma. In Liberson WT, ed. *Orthopedic Medicine: A New Approach to Vertebral Manipulations.* Springfield, Ill: Charles C Thomas; 1972:192–206.

Mannino JR. The application of neurologic reflexes to the treatment of hypertension. *J Am Osteopath Assoc* 1979;79:225–231.

Martin RJ, ed. *Dynamics of Correction of Abnormal Function.* Sierra Madre, Calif: R.J. Martin; 1977:163–165.

Masterson EV. Irritable bowel syndrome: An osteopathic approach. *Osteopath Ann* 1985;12:12–18.

Matsumoto T, Hayes MF, DeLaurentis D, and Miyata M. Evaluation of acupuncture in management of gastrointestinal atony following vagotomy. *Surg Forum* 1972;23:401–402.

Mayer DJ, Price DD, and Rafil. Antagonism of acupuncture analgesia in man by the narcotic antagonist naloxone. *Brain Res* 1977;121:368–373.

Mazzarelli J, ed. *Chiropractic Intraprofessional Research.* Toronto: Edizioni Minerva Medica; 1982.

Mears DB. Analysis and adjustment of the occiput and cervical spine. *Digest Chiropractic Econ* 1972;15:80–82.

Millan MJ. Stress and endogenous opioid peptides, a review. In Emrich HE, ed. *The Role of Endorphins in Psychopharmacology.* Basel: Karger; 1981:49–67.

Miller AD. A review of hypertension and its management by osteopathic manipulative therapy. *Year Book Acad Appl Osteopathy* 1966:30–36.

Miller WD. Treatment of visceral disorders by manipulative therapy. In Korr IM, ed. *The Neurobiologic Mechanisms in Manipulative Therapy.* New York: Plenum Press; 1977: NINCDS Monograph 2, pp. 53–75.

Naurizi CP. Disorders of the pineal gland associated with depression, peptic ulcer and sexual dysfunction. *South Med J* 1984;77:1516–1518.

Noel GL, Suh HK, Stone G, and Frantz AG. Human prolactin and growth hormone release during surgery and other conditions of stress. *J Clin Endocrinol Metab* 1972;35:840–851.

Norris T. A study of the effect of manipulation on blood pressure. *Year Book Acad Appl Osteopathy* 1964:184–188.

Northup TL. Manipulative management of hypertension. *J Am Osteopath Assoc* 1960;60:973–978.

Palmer DD. *Textbook of the Science, Art and Philosophy of Chiropractic.* Portland, Oreg: Portland Printing House; 1910.

Paprocki CC. Gastrointestinal disorders. *ACA J Chiropractic* 1969(Suppl. III):s49–s55.

Patterson MM and Steinmetz JE. Long-lasting alterations of spinal reflexes: A basis for somatic dysfunction. *Manual Med* 1986; 2:38–42.

Pedersen E. Regulation of bladder and colon–rectum in patients with spinal lesions. *J Auton Nerv Syst* 1983;7:329–338.

Perese DM, Prezio JA, and Perese EF. Sexual dysfunction caused by injuries of the cervical spinal cord without paralysis. *Spine* 1976;1:149–154.

Perl ER. Pain: spinal and peripheral nerve factors. In Goldstein M, ed. *The Research Status of Spinal Manipulative Therapy.* Bethesda, Md: DHEW; 1975:NINCDS Monograph 15.

Perret G and Hesser FH. Studies on gastric motility in the cat. *Gastroenterology* 1960;38:219–230.

Pomerantz B, Cheng R, and Law R. Acupuncture reduces electrophysiological and behavioral responses to noxious stimuli: Pituitary is implicated. *Exp Neurol* 1977;54:172–177.

Porreca F and Burks TF. The spinal cord as a site of opioid effects on gastrointestinal transit in the mouse. *J Pharmacol Exp Ther* 1983;227:22–27.

Pressman AH and Nickles SL. Neurophysiological and nutritional considerations of pain control. *J Manipulative Physiol Ther* 1984;7:219–229.

Puig MM, Laorden ML, and Miralles FS, et al. Endorphin levels in cerebrospinal fluid of patients with postoperative and chronic pain. *Anesthesiology* 1982;57:1–4.

Purse FM. Manipulative therapy of upper respiratory infection in children. *J Am Osteopath Assoc* 1966;65:964–971.

Reiss EH. Visceral disorders and their relationship to backache. *J Natl Chiropractic Assoc* 1960:17–19,60–62.

Reppert SM, Perlow MJ, and Ungerleider LG, et al. Effects of damage to the suprachiasmatic area of the anterior hypothalamus on the daily melatonin and cortisol rhythms in the rhesus monkey. *J Neurosci* 1981;1:1414–1425.

Richmond WG. Influence of somatic manipulation in coronary artery disease evaluated by a controlled method. *J Am Osteopath Assoc* 1942;41:217–225.

Robuck SV. Osteopathic management of gastric and duodenal ulcers. *J Am Osteopath Assoc* 1947;46:465–468.

Rychlikova E. Vertebrogenic disorders in internal affections, their importance in therapy. pp. 94–95. In Lewit K and Gutzmann G, eds. *Rehabilitacia, Proceedings of the 10th Congress, International Federation of Manipulative Medicine, Prague;* 1975:suppl. 10–11 pp. 94–95.

Sato A. Physiological studies of the somatoautonomic reflexes. In Haldeman SC, ed. *Modern Developments in the Principles and Practices of Chiropractic.* New York: Appleton-Century-Croft; 1980:93–105.

Sato A, Sato Y, and Schmidt RF. Reflex bladder activity induced by electrical stimulation of hind limb somatic afferents in the cat. *J Auton Nerv Syst* 1980;1:229–241.

Sato A, Sato Y, and Schmidt RF. Heart rate changes reflecting modifications of efferent cardiac sympathetic outflow by cutaneous and muscular afferent volleys. *J Auton Nerv Syst* 1981;4:231–247.

Sato A, Sato Y, Shimada F, and Torigata Y. Changes in gastric motility produced by nociceptive stimulation of the skin in rats. *Brain Res* 1975a;87:151–159.

Sato A, Sato Y, Shimada F, and Torigata Y. Changes in vescical function produced by cutaneous stimulation in rats. *Brain Res* 1975b;94:465–474.

Sato A, Sato Y, and Swenson RS. Effects of morphine on somatocardiac sympathetic reflexes in spinalized cats. *J Auton Nerv Syst* 1985;12:175–184.

Sato A and Swenson RS. Sympathetic nervous system response to mechanical stress of the spinal column in rats. *J Manipulative Physiol Ther* 1984;7:141–148.

Sato Y and Terui N. Changes in duodenal motility produced by noxious mechanical stimulation of the skin in rats. *Neurosci Lett* 1976;2:189–193.

Schaible H-G, Schmidt RF, and Willis WD. Enhancement of the responses or ascending tract cells in the cat spinal cord by acute inflammation of the knee joint. *Exp Brain Res* 1987;66:489–499.

Shyu B-C, Andersson SA, and Thoren P. Endorphin mediated increase in pain threshold induced by long-lasting exercise in rats. *Life Sci* 1982;30:833–840.

Sjolund B, Terrenius L, and Ericksson M. Increase in cerebrospinal fluid levels of endorphins after electropuncture. *Acta Physiol Scand* 1977;100:382–390.

Still AT. *Osteopathy: Research and Practice.* Kirksville, Mo; 1910.

Szczudlik A and Andrezej L. Plasma immunoreactive beta-endorphin and enkephalin concentration in healthy subjects before and after electropuncture. *Acupunct Electrother Res* 1983;8:127–137.

Tamsen A, Hartvig P, and Dahlstrom B, et al. Endorphins and on-demand pain relief. *Lancet* 1980;1:769–773.

Tamsen A, Sakurada T, and Wahlstrom A, et al. Postoperative demand for analgesics in relation to individual levels of endorphins and substance P in cerebrospinal fluid. *Pain* 1982;13:171–177.

Tattersall JEH, Cerrero F, and Lumb BM. Viscerosomatic neurons in the lower thoracic spinal cord of the cat: Excitation and inhibition evoked by splanchnic and somatic nerve volleys and by stimulation of brain stem nuclei. *J Neurophysiol* 1986;56:1411–1423.

Thomason PR, Fisher BL, Carpenter PA, and Fike GL. Effectiveness of spinal manipulative therapy in treatment of primary dysmenorrhea: A pilot study. *J Manipulative Physiol Ther* 1979;2:104–145.

Tran TA and Kirby JD. The effects of upper cervical adjustment on the normal physiology of the heart. *J Am Chiropractic Assoc* 1977;14:s59–s62.

Triano JJ. Case study: Chronic obstruction and restrictive pulmonary disease complicated by congestive heart failure. *Digest Chiropractic Econ* 1976;18:52–53.

Tweed L. Change in the digestive juices due to vertebral lesions. *J Am Osteopath Assoc* 1931;31:83–85.

Ussher NT. The viscerospinal syndrome—A new concept of visceromotor and sensory changes in relation to deranged spinal structures. *Ann Intern Med* 1940;13:2057–2090.

Vacas MI, Sarmiento MIK, and Cardinali DP. Melatonin increases cGMP and decreases cAMP levels in rat medial basal hypothalamus *in vitro. Brain Res* 1981;225:207–211.

Vaughan GM, McDonald SD, and Jordan LM, et al. The 24-hour rhythm of secretion of melatonin in patients with chronic autonomic failure. *Psychoneuroendocrinology* 1979;4:351–356.

Vernon HT, Dhami MSI, Howley TP, and Annett R. Spinal manipulation and beta-endorphin: A controlled study of the effect of a spinal manipulation on plasma beta-endorphin levels in normal males. *J Manipulative Physiol Ther* 1986;9:115–123.

Von Knorring L, Almay BGL, and Johansson F, et al. Pain perception and endorphin levels in cerebrospinal fluid. *Pain* 1978;4:359–362.

Waagen GN, SC Haldeman, and G Cook, et al. Short term trial of spinal adjustments for the relief of low back pain. *Manual Med* 1986;2:63–67.

Watkins RJ. A chiropractic explanation of migraine and how it can be corrected. *J Natl Chiropractic Assoc* 1951;22:50–55.

Wight JS. Migraine: A statistical analysis of chiropractic treatment. *ACA J Chiropractic* 1978;12:S63–S67.

Wiles MR and Diakow P. Chiropractic and visceral disease: A brief survey. *J Can Chiropractic Assoc* 1982;26:65–68.

Wills I and Atsatt RF. The viscerospinal syndrome: A confusing factor in surgical diagnosis. *Arch Surg* 1934;29:661–668.

Wilson PT. The osteopathic treatment of asthma. *J Am Osteopath Assoc* 1946;46:491–492.

Wyke BD. The neurology of low back pain. In Jason MIV, ed. *The Lumbar Spine and Back Pain,* 3rd ed. New York: Churchill Livingstone; 1987.

Yochum TR and Rowe LF. Arthritides of the upper cervical complex. In Glasgow EF, Twomey FT, Scull ER, et al., eds. *Aspects of Manipulative Therapy.* New York: Churchill Livingstone; 1985: 23–33.

Biomechanics of the Cervical Spine

Sean P. Moroney

- **BIOMECHANICALLY RELEVANT CERVICAL ANATOMY**
  The Lower Cervical Cervical Spine
  The Upper Cervical Spine
  The Cervical Ligaments
- **KINEMATICS OF THE LOWER CERVICAL SPINE**

- **KINEMATICS OF THE UPPER CERVICAL SPINE**
- **THE KINETICS OF THE CERVICAL SPINE**
- **THE SPINAL CORD AND NERVE ROOTS**
- **THE VERTEBRAL ARTERY**
- **CONCLUSION**
- **REFERENCES**

The human neck is a remarkable structure, possessing a wide range of mobility in nearly every direction. Situated in a highly vulnerable area between the relatively massive skull and the relatively immobile trunk, the neck has the potential of incurring potentially fatal or disabling injuries that, in other regions of the body, would have milder sequelae.

The neck functions as a conduit for the major vessels and nerves passing to and from the cranium, for the tubes of the digestive and respiratory systems, and for the spinal cord passing from the cranium to the trunk. This latter passage occurs along the slender, but highly flexible, cervical spinal column.

In most vertebrates (with such exceptions as the whales, in which the cervical spine is largely vestigial), the movement of the cervical spine facilitates contact of the end organs of all of the special senses (with the exception of touch) with the environment. An organism's ability to direct its vision, olfaction, has obvious consequences for its survival. The movements of the cervical spine are those of flexion and extension, lateral bending, rotation, and circumduction of the head and neck. In addition, cervical muscle groups suspend and move the shoulder girdle and act to elevate the thoracic inlet. A pronounced coupling of movements is evident, particularly between lateral bending and rotation.

Biomechanically Relevant Cervical Anatomy

The cervical spine is composed of two functionally distinct but interacting components: the upper cervical spine, consisting of the articulations between the occiput, the atlas, and the axis; and the lower cervical spine, consisting of the articulations from C2–C3 through C7–T1.

The Lower Cervical Spine

The vertebrae of the lower cervical spine, from C-3 to T1, are characterized by an architecture that basically resembles (but with significant differences) that found within the thoracic and lumbar regions. The vertebrae comprising these lower cervical motion segments are small, having broad bodies with laterally raised uncinate processes on the upper surfaces, and having sloping posterior arches, which enclose a relatively large triangular vertebral foramen. The vertebral bodies gradually increase in size down to C-7. As in other regions of the spine, this is associated with an increase in weight-bearing load at more inferior levels. The upper surfaces of the transverse processes are grooved to contain and restrain the spinal nerve roots as they exit the spinal canal. Perforating each transverse process is a transverse foramen, through which pass (and are thereby anchored) the vertebral artery (except at C-7), the vertebral veins, and the sympathetic nerves.

The articular processes are stacked laterally to the bodies in the form of pillars. The posterior joints on the superior and inferior aspects of these pillars (also known as zygapophyses or apophyseal joints) are true synovial joints. Their almost flat, but not entirely congruent, surfaces lie approximately in the same plane, which is oriented at about 45 degrees to the horizontal and at 90 degrees to the midsagittal plane. The angle of inclination to the horizontal plane increases from the lower to the upper cervical spine. The area of the facets is approximately two-thirds the area of the intervertebral disc; despite this, cervical joints are not primarily weight bearing. A fibrocartilaginous meniscus is commonly found in these joints in normal and abnormal spines. The cervical joint capsules, which are lax, are richly innervated, particularly with nociceptive fibers, more so than in the lumbar or thoracic area. This heightened innervation may be associated with a greater degree of kinesthetic sense for the cervical region.

The intervertebral discs of the cervical spine resemble the discs of the lower regions of the spine. As in the lumbar and thoracic regions, the discs constitute approximately one quarter of the length of the cervical spine. The discs are sellar in shape on both the upper and lower surfaces and are thicker anteriorly, giving the cervical spine its typical lordotic appearance. Relative to the height of the cervical bodies, the cervical discs are larger than discs in lower regions of the spine; the ratio of disc height to body height ranges from 0.33 to 0.5. This relatively greater vertical dimension facilitates the greater flexibility of the neck. The disc is thickest at C6-7, freely permitting motion yet stopping excessive movement. Bland (1987) notes that the occurrence of the vacuum phenomenon (gas pockets within the disc) in the cervical spine is a relatively frequent event; it is probably due to local subatmospheric pressures.

Each cervical disc has a typical annulus fibrosus with the characteristic laminar fibrocartilaginous composition. The annulus is attached to the circumference of the upper and lower surfaces of the vertebral bodies. The nucleus pulposus, placed slightly to the anterior of the disc, has a volume of approximately 0.2 mL. Within its salt- and water-rich interior is found a meshwork of proteoglycan and collagen fibers. Through their hydrophilic properties, the proteoglycans are largely responsible for the ability of the nucleus to hold and retain water in the presence of physical and osmotic pressures, and to thereby exhibit resilience to applied loads. The nucleus pulposus redirects axial forces radially to the annulus, the fibers of which are then subjected to tension. The annulus as well as the cartilaginous end plates of the vertebrae may thereby play a role in ab-

sorbing and dissipating energy. During waking hours, weight bearing leads to disc dehydration and a consequent loss of height of the cervical column; rehydration due to unloading during nightly rest tends to restore its original height. With age, however, the nucleus pulposus progressively dehydrates and loses its intrinsic height. Because of consequent changes in the ability to resist such forces as shearing, fissuring may develop as the disc is gradually transformed into fibrocartilage.

The uncovertebral joints, also known as the joints of Luschka, are not present until the early part of the second decade of life. In the first decade, a child's cervical discs are highly elastic. As they gradually lose some of their elasticity, however, clefts due to shearing stresses occur in the posterolateral area of the annulus in the vicinity of the developing uncinate processes on the lateral margins of C-3 to C-7. These joints later develop articular cartilage, joint capsules, synovial membranes, joint spaces, and subchondral bone. By virtue of their position, the uncovertebral joints form a barrier to posterolateral protrusion of the disc, but still allow the potential for direct posterior protrusion into the cord. Sherk and Parke (1989) and Bland (1987) note that past consideration of the development by fissuring within the posterolateral region of the annulus of the uncovertebral joints led earlier anatomists to view these joints as products of degeneration, rather than as true joints. The thesis that these are normal structures appears now to be well established. Bland (1987), however, notes that the earlier point of view is given support by the fact that, from the fourth to the sixth decades, some of the fissures that develop within the disc (primarily in a transverse direction) may be associated with synovial lining.

The Upper Cervical Spine

The upper cervical spine, also termed the occipitoatlantoaxial complex, is comprised of the occiput, the atlas (C-1), and the axis (C-2). The upper cervical vertebrae have a unique architecture that is directly related to their important biomechanical function. The eye of the novice would be most struck by the absence of a body in the atlas and by the presence of the vertically oriented peg-like projection, the dens or odontoid process, from the body of the axis. This unique anatomic structure gives the second cervical vertebra its name and is responsible for the exceptionally large range of axial motion available to the cervical spine. The upper cervical region is also unique in that no intervertebral discs are present.

The atlas is mounted on the dens of the axis like a ring or wheel on an eccentrically placed axle. Bony masses on the lateral aspects of the ring form the articulations with the occiput and the axis. The atlas is the only vertebra in which the superior facets directly overlie the inferior facets. A midline synovial articulation is also present between the anterior arch and the dens.

The superior facets of the atlas are ellipsoidal in shape and are cupped to the correspondingly congruent occipital condyles. Ellipsoidal joints display different radii of curvature depending on the plane in which they are sectioned; unlike a ball-and-socket, or spheroidal joint, they tend to be predominantly biaxial, with two primary modes of movement. The inferior facets tend to be nearly flat or mildly convex in the anteroposterior direction and mildly concave in the mediolateral direction. The facets face inferiorly and medially to the corresponding surfaces of C-2. The atlas is the widest vertebra, from the tip of one transverse process to the other, above C-7. This lateral extent gives a substantial mechanical advantage and leverage to its attached muscles for the rotation of the head; however, because the transverse foramina are situated more laterally, the vertebral arteries are at comparatively greater risk of inquiry.

The articular facets of the axis are slightly convex in both directions and face superiorly and laterally for articulation with the atlas. Two synovial cavities are present on the dens in the midline; one articulates with the anterior arch of the atlas and the other provides a spacing between the dens and the transverse ligament of the atlas. The dens has a narrow waist where it is crossed by this ligament. The dens tapers superiorly—sometimes sharply—to its tip, providing extended sagittal motion in translation and rotation. The inferior aspect of C-2 resembles a typical cervical vertebra in appearance and articulation.

The Cervical Ligaments

The ligaments, particularly in the lower cervical spine, resemble those of the thoracic and lumbar regions. The anterior longitudinal ligament is strong but narrow and is more firmly attached to the anterior surfaces of the intervertebral discs than to the vertebral bodies. The posterior longitudinal ligament, a uniformly broader structure here than in the lumbar region, is firmly attached to the discs but minimally to the bodies. This tends to make the anterior surface of the vertebral canal smooth. The ligamenta flava, consisting primarily of the protein elastin, have the important property of stretching under tension and of retracting without any bulging or folding; this absence of bulging is particularly important in the position of full extension. The ligamentum nuchae, however, unlike the supraspinous ligaments that are its analogues in the lower spinal segments is vestigial and resembles the ligamentum flavum in its composition and elastic properties.

In the upper cervical spine, the anterior longitudinal ligament and the posterior longitudinal liga-

ment are continued as the anterior atlanto-occipital membrane and the tectorial membrane, respectively. The posterior atlanto-occipital membrane links the posterior margin of the foramen magnum with the posterior arch of the atlas. Calcification of this membrane, along its margin at the arcuate foramen, gives rise to the ponticulus posticus, a structure that may contribute to compression of the vertebral artery; this condition may become clinically significant when the artery is pathologically altered. Direct ligamentous connections between the occiput and the odontoid process are made by the vestigial apical ligament and the strong round alar ligaments. The transverse ligament of the atlas, on the posterior aspect of the dens, links the lateral masses of the atlas across the interior of its ring and forms the posterior part of the pivot joint.

Most of the cervical musculature, as measured by cross-sectional area, is found posteriorly and laterally. Besides having extensions of the larger extensor muscles of the lower spine, the cervical spine is similarly equipped with analogues of the smaller intersegmental muscles. In addition, a unique array of bending and rotational muscles, the recti and the obliqui, is found in the upper cervical region.

Kinematics of the Lower Cervical Spine

The motion segments of the lower cervical spine produce movement by acting as a unit, without selectivity or preferential mobility of any specific motion segment. In general, movements are coupled. That is, rotations about separate axes may occur simultaneously when a segment moves in response to a given force. Similarly, translations along an axis may accompany certain rotations. Representative values of the ranges of intersegmental motion are presented in Table 11–1.

To better appreciate the nature of cervical movements, it is worth reconsidering the accepted anatomic reference system. Anatomic textbooks com-

TABLE 11–1. REPRESENTATIVE RANGES OF MOTION OF THE LOWER CERVICAL SPINE

	Flexion Extension (degrees)	Lateral Bending (degrees)	Axial Rotation (degrees)
C-2–C-3	8	10	9
C-3–C-4	13	11	11
C-4–C-5	12	11	12
C-5–C-6	17	8	10
C-6–C-7	16	7	9
C-7–T-1	9	4	8

After Jofe et al. (1989), p. 65 with permission.

monly present three body planes: the sagittal, the coronal, and the transverse. The intersections of these planes correspond to the X–, Y–, and Z– axes of the three-dimensional coordinate system. Translations along and rotations about any of these three axes are defined as primary, or pure, movements. The combination of the three possible modes of translation and the three possible modes of rotation gives rise to the six possible degrees of freedom in an unconstrained system (Fig. 11–1); constraints such as the presence of ligaments and/or joint geometry, tend, in general, to reduce the number of degrees of freedom available. When movement occurs at some specific joint that cannot be characterized as a pure movement, the movement is described as being coupled, or linked, about separate axes. Clearly, al-

though when an object moves in simple rotation, it is reasonable to think that it is moving about some single axis at any instant of time. If it is recognized that this axis may not be oriented parallel to any one of the three primary axes, then it can be seen that the observation of two rotations about two axes, or coupling of primary movements, reduces to the expression of a single degree of freedom.

Rotations are usually characterized as occurring about some center of motion. For very simple devices, such as a potter's wheel, the axis of rotation is fixed in space and all the points of the object describe circular arcs about it. Seldom, though, does this kinematic situation prevail in the human body. Movements at the joints of the body are primarily rotational in nature. But because of geometric irreg-

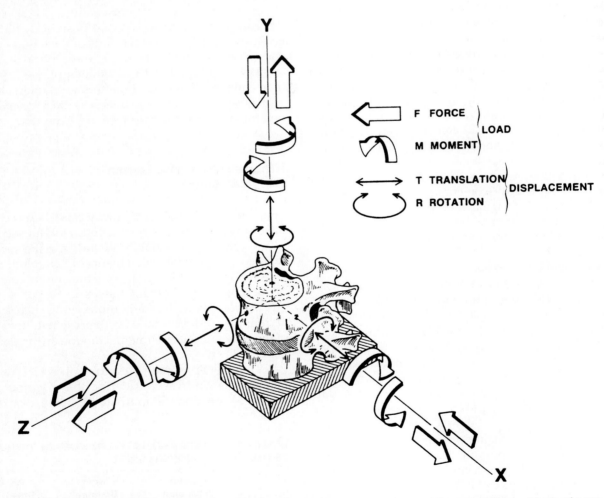

Figure 11–1. A three-dimensional coordinate system has been placed at the center of the upper vertebral body of a motion segment. The coordinate system is fixed in space. To document the complete mechanical behavior of the spine motion segment, six forces along and six moments or torques about the three axes of the coordinate system are applied. These 12 load components are depicted. The application of any one of the load components produces displacement of the upper vertebra with respect to the lower vertebra. The displacement consists of translation and rotation. These two motions can be further divided with respect to the coordinate axes. Thus, the three-dimensional displacement has six components, three translations along and three rotations about the three axes of the coordinate system. These are also shown. (*From White and Panjabi [1978], p. 38, with permission.*)

ularities in articular surfaces and changes in the material properties of tissues undergoing gradual deformations, the center of motion is rarely, if ever, fixed at any one point. This situation is amplified when pathological changes are present in the region under consideration. It has become customary in the analysis of joint motion to calculate the location of the center of rotation from one instant to another. Nordin and Frankel (1989) have provided a concise description of this method (based on last century's work by Reuleaux) as applied to the knee. The method may be applied in exactly the same manner to the cervical spine. The primary clinical utility of the method may be the characterization of abnormal patterns of movement based on the spatial path outlined by the moving instant centers. Further work remains to be done in this area, especially for the cervical spine.

Flexion and extension of the cervical column generally involves little out-of-plane movement on the part of the vertebrae. Penning (1960) analyzed a series of normal cervical radiographs and calculated the centers of flexion–extension motion for the lower cervical spine (Fig. 11–2). The movement of a superior vertebra was found to describe an approximately circular movement about a point in the vertebra below. In general, as successively lower motion segments were examined, the center of motion was found at successively higher locations within the inferior vertebra. The center of motion for C2 was

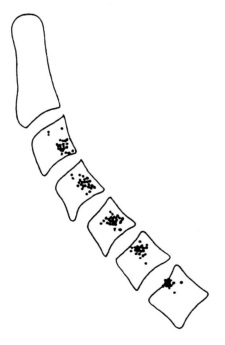

Figure 11–2. Centers of flexion–extension motion for C2-7 in the absence of radiographic evidence of disc degeneration. Note the regional differences in the mean location of the centers of motion. (*From Penning [1989], p. 35, with permission.*)

found to be situated typically near the posterior inferior margin of the body of C-3. For C-6, the instant center was found to be situated at approximately the midpoint of the superior surface of the inferior vertebra.

These findings imply that, because the distance from the object in motion to the center of motion is decreasing (because the radius of curvature is smaller at lower levels of the lower cervical spine), the path traced by C-2 flexing on C-3 will be flat relative to the more arcuate path of C-6 flexing on C-7. The movement at the top of the spine then may be described as gliding, whereas the movement at the base may be characterized as tilting in nature. This is consistent with the findings of Lysell (1969). The greater degree of gliding possible in the upper reaches of the lower cervical spine might indicate potentially greater instability under transverse loading at that level.

The cervical intervertebral disc, representing an anterior symphysis joint of the motion segment, contributes to the identity of the motion patterns in the cervical spine. Rolander (1966) demonstrated that excision of the posterior facets in lumbar vertebrae had a surprisingly negligible influence on the movement pattern of the motion segment. Although caution should be exercised in extrapolating data from one region of the spine to another, the basic similarities in the anatomic structures suggest that the cervical disc may play a significant role in determining movement patterns. Raynor and colleagues (1986) found that removal of cervical facets caused little change in anteroposterior motion under applied forces; however, the coupled movements of lateral bending appeared to be reduced under the action of similar forces.

Intervertebral discs generally tend to be more freely movable in bending (either flexion–extension or lateral bending) than in twisting or shearing. This is evident in sagittal movements. In full flexion, the spinal curvature changes from the neutral mild lordosis to a curvature concave to the anterior. The anterior margin of the disc is compressed, whereas the posterior fibers are stretched. The anterior longitudinal ligament is slackened, whereas the posterior longitudinal ligament is stretched. The nucleus pulposus is displaced slightly to the posterior as the superior body of each motion segment translates anteriorly by a minute amount. The articular facets of the superior vertebrae glide upward on those beneath, whereas the intervertebral foramina enlarge in cross-sectional area. In full extension, all of these configurational changes are reversed. In lateral bending and rotation, the disc is similarly wedged on the side of lateral bending; the intervertebral foramina are reduced in size on the ipsilateral side and enlarged on the contralateral side.

Lateral bending and rotation of the lower cervical spine are generally discussed together, because there is a significant amount of coupling between these movements. To understand their simultaneous occurrence, it is necessary to consider the facet geometry at work. As discussed above, the articular facets are parallel and inclined at an angle of 45 degrees to the horizontal. When, for example, leftward rotation of the head on the neck takes place, the articular facets on the left side of the lower cervical column glide in an anterior and superior direction, whereas those on the right side of the column glide in a posterior and inferior direction. This has the effect of rotating the spinous processes to the left and of elevating the left side of each vertebra with respect to the right side. It is this latter movement, a tilting of the vertebra to the right, that constitutes lateral bending. A similar analysis, for the case of lateral bending of the head and neck, will be left to the reader.

A different analysis, presented by Penning (1989), that integrates all components of the motion segment might be more illustrative. As stated, the facet surfaces lie approximately in a plane; it is then reasonable to consider that movement may occur about an axis perpendicular to this plane. The facets would then glide on each other along an arc about this axis. The plane in question was visualized using the imaging capabilities of a computed tomography (CT) scanner. Because the uncinate processes were present in the image, in this plane and in planes parallel to this plane (Fig. 11–3), it was reasonable to consider that their presence might induce a circular rotational motion about some point within the vertebral body. The analysis of a series of similar parallel planes in the same segment permitted the construction of an axis for this movement. The axis plainly has an oblique orientation with respect to the conventional anatomic planes, as discussed earlier. The combined movement of lateral bending–rotation thus would be resolved in the standard system of conventional planes into two distinct, but coupled, movements. Lysell (1969) made a similar determination of a center of rotation, but not of an axis, within the anterior part of the vertebral body. He found that during rotation of the head, the spinal rotational movements were larger than the coupled lateral bending. Conversely, during lateral bending of the head and neck, the spinal lateral bending movements were larger than the coupled rotations. This latter finding suggests that the spatial orientation of the axis of rotation–lateral bending may not have a constant orientation with the anatomic planes.

During lateral bending of a lumbar vertebra, the disc tends to deform and move in the direction of bending. This tendency can exist in the cervical spine as well, where the anterior part of the cervical disc is

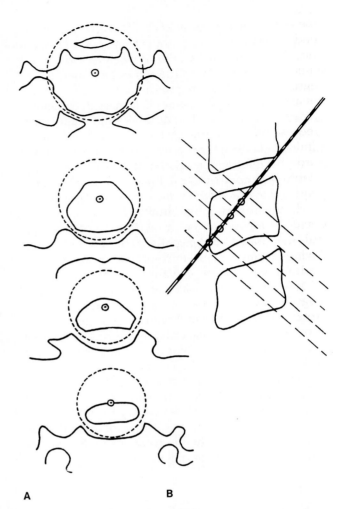

A   **B**

Figure 11–3. (A) Schematic drawings of CT sections of the cervical vertebrae taken parallel to the plane of the intervertebral joints. The centers of the circles drawn through the uncovertebral joints correspond to centers of joint motion. **(B)** The centers are transferred to a drawing of a lateral radiograph showing the corresponding CT levels and are connected by a line representing the instantaneous axis of rotational motion, in this case between C-2 and C-3. (*From Penning [1989], p. 44, with permission.*)

similar to the lumbar disc. The posterior part of the disc, however, is supported by the uncinate processes, the presence of which may suffice to cause translation of the posterior part of the disc in the direction opposite bending. These opposite translations of different parts of the disc are, in essence, a torsion of the disc that generates, in turn, a rotation of the upper vertebra on the lower. The direction of this rotation is consistent with that observed, suggesting that, for lateral bending, the instant center may be found in the upper vertebral body. Jofe and colleagues (1989) state that the location is entirely speculative.

The axes of rotation of the lower cervical vertebrae, for flexion–extension and rotation–lateral bending, are generically illustrated in Figure 11–4. This illustration suggests that the lower cervical motion segment may be regarded as a system with 2 degrees of rotational freedom. The amount of rotational coupling with lateral bending varies throughout the lower cervical column. At C-2, there are 2 degrees of rotation for every 3 degrees of lateral bending; this may be expressed as a ratio of two-thirds, or 0.67. In contrast, at C-7 there is 1 degree of rotation for every 7.5 degrees of lateral bending; this may be expressed as a ratio of 1/7.5, or 0.13.

In the lower cervical spine, a horizontal translation of 2.7 mm is considered the upper limit of normal movement of one vertebra on another in flexion–extension. If these measurements are made from radiographs, the value is increased to 3.5 mm to account for the effects of radiographic magnification. Values in excess of these are interpreted as indications of instability owing to trauma or other factors.

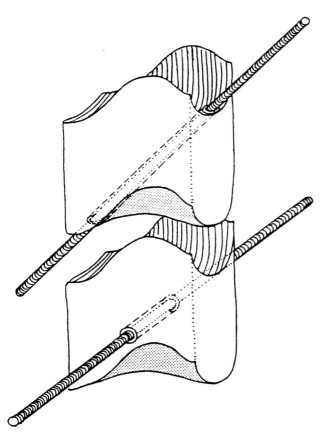

Figure 11–4. The axes of motion in the typical human cervical motion segment. The upper axis is for rotation–lateral flexion; the lower axis is for flexion–extension (left lateral and slightly dorsal view). (*From Penning [1989], p. 46, with permission.*)

Kinematics of the Upper Cervical Spine

The unique capabilities of the upper region of the cervical spine are especially manifest in axial rotation, where the special ring-and-peg mechanism of C-1 to C-2 accounts for nearly half of the total rotation at this level. Because of lower resistance to motion at this level, it is possible for movement to occur without involvement of the lower cervical spine. Representative values of ranges of motion of the motion segments of this level are presented in Table 11–2. Because of the shorter radius of curvature of the occipital condyles and superior surface of the lateral masses of the atlas in the sagittal plane, as compared with the radius of curvature in the coronal plane, the instant center of rotation for flexion–extension is located more inferiorly than the center of rotation for lateral bending (Fig. 11–5).

As viewed on a radiograph, the posterior arch of the atlas remains approximately midway between the basiocciput and the spinous process of C-2 as the neck is positioned in flexion and extension. A paradoxical motion may, however, occur in the upper cervical spine during flexion–extension of the neck as a whole. A result of this motion is that the occiput will begin to extend on the atlas toward the end of the motion. At the end of the range of motion, less flexion will be evident at this level than in the midrange. This can be due to the translation of the skull relative to the atlas, as may occur at the end of neck flexion when the chin strikes the chest. An attempt to continue the motion can only continue with translation of the chin inferiorly on the sternum, causing a pull on the posterior arch toward the skull. This effect can be more dramatically illustrated in radiographs of the chin-in and chin-out configurations. When standing upright, an individual may be asked to project his or her head anteriorly while keeping the eyes level. This anterior movement of the head induces forward flexion of the neck, but, because the head is held level, the atlanto-occipital joint is forced into extension. In essence, the cervical spine is

TABLE 11-2. REPRESENTATIVE RANGES OF MOTION OF THE UPPER CERVICAL SPINE

Motion Segment	Motion	Range of Motion (degrees)
Occiput–C-1	Flexion–extension	13
	Lateral bending	8
	Axial rotation	10
C-1–C-2	Flexion–extension	10
	Lateral bending	0
	Axial rotation	65

After from Jofe et al. [1989], p. 62 with permission.

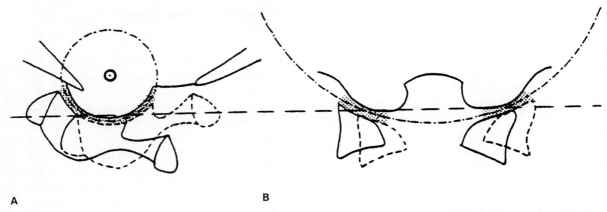

Figure 11–5. Atlanto-occipital movement diagrams. **(A)** Diagram of flexion–extension (in sagittal view) (*solid line* indicates flexion; *broken line* indicates extension). The center of motion forms a circle passing through the atlanto-occipital joints (*shaded area*). **(B)** Diagram of lateral flexion (in coronal view) diagram with the center of motion forming a circle passing through the atlanto-occipital joints (*solid line* indicates left lateral flexion; *broken line* indicates right lateral flexion). (*From Penning [1989], p. 48, with permission.*)

forced into an S configuration with a kyphotic curve below C-2 and a lordotic curve above C-2. In the chin-out configuration, the skull is translated posteriorly and the S configuration is established in a reverse manner. The greatest range of motion between the upper cervical segments in flexion and extension are induced by these maneuvers.

Axial rotation of the upper cervical complex occurs predominantly at the atlantoaxial articulation. Until recently, it was considered that the geometry of the atlanto-occipital joints precluded any axial rotation. Clark and colleagues (1986) measured a mean axial rotation of 4.8 degrees at the atlanto-occipital articulation. This would seem to imply that, based on the geometry of the joints, some separation of the apposing surfaces must be occurring. As rotation takes place through approximately 45 degrees in each direction about the eccentrically placed odontoid process (approximately 50% of the rotation of the entire cervical spine), the vertebral canal is reduced in cross-sectional area by about one-third. This occurrence, however, poses a minimal problem for the spinal cord, because the canal is especially capacious here.

Rotation of the atlas about the axis takes place with an axis of rotation through the dens. The transverse ligament of the atlas plays a crucial role in providing stability of the complex during this movement. Tension in the contralateral alar ligament is the primary restraint on rotation. When the contralateral alar ligament severed, rotation may be increased by as much as 30%. Jofe and co-workers (1989) identified fibers of the alar ligaments that attach to the occiput and to the lateral masses of the atlas. They stated that lateral bending was checked by the contralateral upper (occipital) and by the ipsilateral lower (atlanteal) alar ligaments. It may be pos-

sible that damage to this ligament and a subsequent inability to restrain movement of the atlas on the axis may irritate the vertebral artery and joint capsules, giving rise to an array of clinical symptoms.

During pure lateral flexion of the upper cervical spine, the approximation of the occipital condyle to the axis on the side of bending acts to force the wedge-shaped ipsilateral lateral mass of the atlas into the side of bending. Rotation of the cervical spine is coupled with lateral flexion. Consequently, turning the head to one side causes the vertebrae to laterally flex to that side; this movement is seen as high as the level of the axis. However, because the eyes are generally kept level during pure rotation, a compensating lateral flexion in the upper cervical spine must occur. Consequently, the atlas is forced to glide toward the contralateral side of the neck during axial twisting.

There appears to be minimal translation between the occiput and the atlas during normal movements. The atlantoaxial articulation, however, presents a different picture. The lateral articulations involve convex surfaces in contact over a relatively small area. As rotation occurs to one side from the neutral midposition, the atlas may be seen (especially on radiographs) to descend vertically to a lower position. This is simply due to the fact that the highest elevation of the atlas on the axis is in the midposition. This motion has been characterized by Henke (1863) as that of a ''double-threaded screw.''

The Kinetics of the Cervical Spine

Besides being a mechanism with kinematic properties, the cervical spine is a structure that must, in its various configurations, be subject to a variety of forces and moments and that, under these loads, must perform in a totally life-supporting way for the optimum benefit of the individual. The behavior of a system as structurally complex as this depends on the interplay of its material properties, the geometry of its components, the types of external forces (e.g., gravity, impact) to which it is subjected. Additional factors that must be taken into account include the internal forces within the spine (e.g., muscle forces), the points of application and directions of application of external forces, the loading modes used, the rate of loading, the initial configuration of the cervical spine, and the relative position of the head, neck, and thorax. There is considerable variability in the tissue properties and geometries from one individual to another. In addition, these factors may vary with the age of the individual. Physiological conditions, such as pregnancy, are known to affect properties such as the extensibility of ligaments. A totally encyclopedic catalog of spinal responses to all conceivable mechanical scenarios has not yet been assembled.

Among the material properties to be considered are the failure levels of the components of the spine. When loading is applied at or in excess of these levels, the typical response of the component is an irreversible change in function under any subsequently applied loads. Values such as those presented in Table 11–3 represent averages determined through experimentation on a large number of specimens; the range of variation between individual specimens is often quite wide.

Often the behavior of a specimen under a specific type of mechanical load is given in terms of the stiffness of the material. Larger values of stiffness imply a small degree of flexibility. Put another way, the larger the degree of stiffness, the smaller the deformation induced by a given load. The data in Table 11–4 are the results of a series of separate studies on different levels of the cervical spine. Liu (1981), and Coffee and colleagues (1987) differentiated between the middle and lower cervical spine. Coffee et al. in-

TABLE 11-3. FAILURE LEVELS OF CERVICAL COMPONENTS

Structure	Failure Load
Cervical vertebral body	2800–4200 N
Transverse ligament of C-1	1000 N
Anterior longitudinal ligament	340 N
Posterior longitudinal ligament	180 N
Cervical disc (compression)	3200 N
Cervical disc (tension)	1000 N
Cervical disc (torsion)	6 N-m

From Crowell et al. (1989), p. 83 with permission.

TABLE 11-4. CERVICAL MOTION SEGMENT STIFFNESS

	Translational Stiffness (x 10^5 N/m)				
Region	**Compr**	**Tension**	**+Shear**	**−Shear**	**Lateral Shear**
Middle	36.9	5.9	—	—	—
Lower	41.2	5.8	—	—	—
Middle	51.8	9.0	5.80	2.2	—
Lower	13.6	2.0	1.04	1.3	—
All	10.8	3.9	1.40	0.50	1.2
All	1.4	0.52	0.34	0.52	0.52

	Rotational Stiffness ($\times$ 10 N-m/radian)			
Region	**Flexion**	**Extension**	**Lateral Bend**	**Axial Rotation**
Middle	2.9	7.1	15.8	17.6
Lower	16.9	14.8	21.9	22.5
Middle	8.6	—	—	—
Lower	16.6	19.1	—	—
All	15.2	18.6	17.2	14.9
All	—	—	—	—

From Crowell et al. (1989) p. 84 with permission.

dicated that the midcervical region, from C-2 to C-4, had greater axial and shear stiffnesses than the lower cervical region, from C-5 to C-7; bending stiffness in flexion was greater in the lower region than in the midregion. The data of Moroney (1988a) and of Panjabi and colleagues (1986) in Crowell et al. (1989) did not make this distinction. In the former study, a large number of degenerated specimens were tested, possibly obscuring regional differences in stiffness. The stiffness values listed in Table 11–4 are not constants for a given tissue but, in fact, vary with the loading level applied. Figure 11–6 shows that stiffness (defined here as the slope of the load–displacement curve) is small for low applied load levels. This would imply that the motion segment, under small loads, has a ''neutral zone'' in which it exhibits a high degree of flexibility and may have an indeterminate equilibrium position.

Spinal loading may come from external sources. These forces and moments, if of sufficient magnitude, may be responsible for a variety of injuries, including fractures, dislocations, and ligament disruptions. Orthopedic texts, such as Turek (1984), deal with the several consequences of these mechanical events.

An important mode of loading of spinal motion segments is due to muscular contraction forces. Of particular interest are the forces associated with maximum voluntary exertions. Muscles act along different lines of action and contract with different levels of intensity. Their force contributions can be many and varied. Because these individual forces cannot

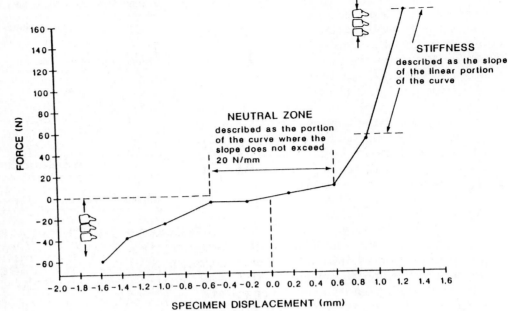

Figure 11-6. Load–displacement curve for a cervical spinal motion segment. If the stiffness is measured below the steep portion of the curve, reported values will be substantially lower than other estimates. *(From Crowell [1989], p. 85, with permission.)*

be measured directly, a computer simulation model is necessary to estimate the forces acting on a spinal motion segment. A model typically incorporates a number of assumptions, which may have a limited level of realism but should give the investigator an estimate of the quantities under analysis. Typically, a multimuscle array such as that of the midcervical spine is assumed to have all muscles contracting at the same intensity.

Moroney and co-workers (1988B) reported the results of a study in which maximal voluntary strengths in bending and torsion were measured. The muscle forces were calculated, and the reaction forces of shear and compression at the C4-5 disc were calculated. The mean voluntary neck strengths ranged as high as 29.7 Nm (for maximal attempted extension). The calculations of the muscle forces were correlated with the electromyographic signals recorded from the skin surface in the region overlying the muscles in question. The mean predicted joint reaction forces are tabulated in Table 11–5. The maximum calculated compression force is lower than the mean failure strength for cervical discs and vertebral bodies reported in Table 11-3. This suggests that the structures within the neck are at least strong enough to withstand the effects of internal forces.

The Spinal Cord and Nerve Roots

The spinal cord is cushioned and suspended within the subarachnoid space by the surrounding cerebro-

spinal fluid. In addition, the fibrofatty tissues and venous plexuses of the epidural space isolate the cord from the movements of the laminae. The cervical enlargement, the largest region of the cord, is found between C-3 and T-2. Interestingly, the canal is widest in the region of C-1 to C-3 where, as mentioned earlier, the movements of C-1 in full rotation have the potential of markedly reducing the space available to the cord.

Geometric changes of the spinal cord take place during spinal movements. In extension, the cord thickens due to the development of transverse folding and slackening of the dentate ligaments. In addition, the posteroinferior margin of the vertebral bodies protrude into the canal during extension, reducing its sagittal diameter by 1 to 2 mm. Space within the canal becomes minimal in this configuration of the spine. In flexion, the cord increases its length by approximately 3 cm (about 25% of its length at rest). The lengths of the anterior and poste-

TABLE 11-5. MEAN PREDICTED MOTION SEGMENT REACTIONS FORCES DURING MAXIMAL EXERTIONS

Exercise	Lateral Shear [N]	Anteroposterior Shear [N]	Compression [N]
Relaxed	0	−2	122
Left twist	33	70	778
Extension	0	135	1164
Flexion	0	31	558
Left bending	125	93	758

From Moroney et al. [1988b] p. 719, with permission.

rior walls of the canal are increased by approximately 1.5 and 5 cm, respectively. As the cord is pulled superiorly, the dura is also pulled upward, increasing the level of tension in the nerve roots. Any foldings of the cord or dura are smoothed, and the dentate ligaments are tensed.

The nerve root occupies approximately one-fourth to one-third of the space of the intervertebral foramen, with the remainder of the space being taken up by the blood and lymphatic vessels of the spinal column and by connective tissues. The least mobile nerves in the cervical column, and those potentially most subject to axial deformations, are the fourth, fifth, sixth, and seventh cervical nerves. These are anchored within the gutter of the transverse process by connective tissue attachments, preventing the possibility of traction and avulsion from the cord by forces originating from the shoulder girdle and the upper extremity. As with the spinal cord, flexion tends to straighten the root sleeves, bringing them in close contact with the inferior and medial margins of the pedicles. In extension, the sleeves slacken and develop transverse folds. In lateral flexion, the nerve roots on the convex side become taut, whereas those on the concave side became slack.

The Vertebral Artery

Along each side of the cervical column from C-6 to C-1, the vertebral artery passes through the transverse foramina as it courses toward the skull and its intersection with the intracranial vessels (Fig. 11–7). At the level of C-2, the transverse foramen is directed superiorly and laterally toward the next foramen in C-1. As the vessel makes this crossing, it forms a loop of approximately 1.5 to 2 cm outside the canal. Another loop is formed as it leaves C-1 and passes behind the lateral mass for entry into the vertebral canal. The slack in the C-1 to C-2 loop at the transverse foramen is taken out during rotation. The vertebral artery then follows a tortuous path as it makes a pair of U-turns inward toward the cord.

Circulation through the vertebral artery can be compromised by changes in its caliber as it is stretched and by kinking. Selecki (1969) demonstrated that when the head and neck are rotated to one side, kinking sufficient to alter blood flow to the cranium can develop in the contralateral artery at about 30 degrees of rotation. After about 45 degrees of rotation, the ipsilateral artery also begins to exhibit similar changes. Under normal conditions, if one vertebral artery is occluded by rotation, there is generally sufficient vascular supply to the brain from other sources, such as the contralateral vertebral artery, that the person is usually unaware of any changes. Pathological changes in one artery, for example, a decrease in functional caliber due to atherosclerotic plaquing, may render the circulatory supply asymmetric. When the head and neck are then rotated to the affected side, the pathological artery is unable to supply sufficient blood to the brain. Symptoms such as visual disturbances, vomiting, nausea, and vertigo may develop.

Conclusion

The cervical spine is designed to accommodate a wide range of motion with minimal effect on the

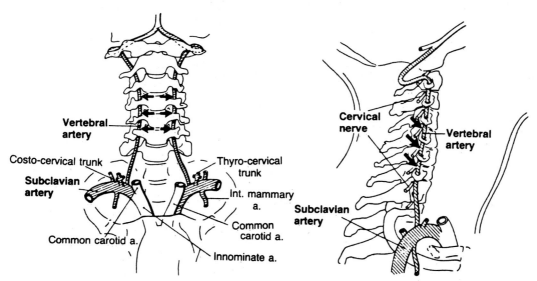

Figure 11–7. Anteroposterior and lateral views of the vertebral artery to show anatomic divisions and sites of compression. *Arrows* indicate the most common sites of compression of the vertebral artery by osteophytes. (*From Turek [1984], with permission.*)

structures of the central nervous system. In addition, the nerve roots in the lower part of the cervical spine are anchored within their intervertebral foramina. The extreme rotations sustainable in the neck can have profound effects on the vascular supply to the brain through the pairs of vertebral arteries, especially when one of these is compromised.

Trauma to or pathological processes within the cervical spine can have clinical ramifications in the cranium above (e.g., headache) or in the extremities and body below (e.g., the cervical nerves to the diaphragm and the upper extremities). The neck is extremely vulnerable to injuries induced by mechanisms of acceleration and deceleration, to which our modern way of life predisposes us and for which no totally adequate protective device has as yet been designed. Due to its location, structure, and function, it is not altogether surprising that chiropractic care was focused on the cervical spine (especially on its upper region) for so long and with such intensity.

References

Bland JH. *Disorders of the Cervical Spine: Diagnosis and Medical Management.* Philadelphia: W. B. Saunders Co.; 1987:54.

Clark CR, Goel VK, Galles K, and Liu YK. *Kinematics of the Occipito-atlanto-axial Complex.* Transaction, Cervical Spine Research Society, 1986.

Coffee MS, Edwards WT, Hayes WC, and White AA III. *Mechanical Responses and Strength of the Human Cervical Spine.* Exhibit, Am. Spinal Injury Assoc. meeting, Boston, March 1987.

Crowell RR, Edwards WT, and White AA III. Mechanisms of injury in the cervical spine: experimental evidence and biomechanical modelling. In *The Cervical Spine,* 2nd ed., The Cervical Spine Research Society Editorial Committee. Philadelphia: Lippincott; 1989:70–90.

Henke, W. *Handbuch der Anatomie und Mechanik der Gelenke.* Leipzig and Heideberg, 1863.

Jofe MH, White AA, and Panjabi MM. Clinically relevant kinematics of the cervical spine. In *The Cervical Spine,* 2nd ed., The Cervical Spine Research Society Editorial Committee. Philadelphia: Lippincott; 1989:57–69.

Liu YK, Krieger KW, and Njus G, et al. *Investigation of Cervical Spine Dynamics.* Aerospace Medical Research laboratory (AMRL-TR-138), WPAFB, Ohio, 1981.

Lysell E. Motion in the cervical spine. An experimental study on autopsy specimens. *Acta Ortop Scand* (Suppl) 1969;123:54.

Moroney SP, Schultz AB, Miller JAA, and Andersson GBJ. Load-displacement properties of lower cervical spine motion segments. *J Biomechanics* 1988a;21:769–779.

Moroney SP, Schultz AB, and Miller JAA. Analysis and measurement of neck loads. *J Orthop Res* 1988b;6:713–720.

Nordin M, and Frankel VH. *Basic Biomechanics of the Musculoskeletal System,* 2nd ed. Philadelphia: Lea & Febiger; 1989:118.

Panjabi MM, Summers DJ, and Pelker RR, et al. Three-dimensional load-displacement curves due to forces on the cervical spine. *J Orthop Res* 1986;4:152.

Penning L. Functioneel rontgenonderzoek bij degeneratieve en traumatische aandoeningen der laag-cervicale bewegingssegmenten. Thesis, Groningen, 1960:3–13.

Penning L. Functional anatomy of joints and discs. In *The Cervical Spine,* 2nd ed., The Cervical Spine Research Society Editorial Committee. Philadelphia: Lippincott; 1989:33–56.

Raynor R, Moskouich R, Zidel P, and Pugh J. Alterations in primary and coupled neck motions following facetectomies. Presentation Cervical Spine Research Society, December 1986.

Rolander SD. Motion of the lumbar spine with special reference to the stabilizing effect of posterior fusion. An experimental study on autopsy specimens. *Acta Ortop Scand* (Suppl) 1966;90:86.

Selecki BR. The effects of rotation of the atlas on the axis: Experimental work. *Med J Aust* 1969;1:1012.

Sherk HH, and Parke WW. Developmental anatomy. In *The Cervical Spine,* 2nd ed., The Cervical Spine Research Society Editorial Committee. Philadelphia: Lippincott, 1989:9–10.

Turek S. *Orthopaedics: Principles and Their Application.* Vol 1 & 2, 4th ed. Philadelphia: J.B. Lippincott Company; 1984.

White AA, and Panjabi MM. *Clinical Biomechanics of the Spine.* Philadelphia: Lippincott; 1979.

chapter 12

Biomechanics of the Lumbar Spine

H. F. Farfan

- **THE EVOLUTION OF HUMAN SPINAL MOTION**
- **THE BASIC PRINCIPLE OF BIOMECHANICS**
- **THE USE OF MUSCLE TO CONTROL STRESS**
- **FLEXION–EXTENSION AND COMPRESSION LOAD**
- **THE ABDOMINAL MECHANISM**
- **MECHANISMS OF INJURY**

- **DEGENERATION OR TRAUMA**
- **PATHOLOGICAL SEQUENCE OF FRACTURED END PLATE**
- **PATHOLOGICAL SEQUENCE OF TORSIONAL OVERLOAD**
- **THE AREAS OF MAXIMUM STRESS**
- **COMBINED POSTERIOR FACET AND DISC DAMAGE**
- **CONCLUSION**
- **REFERENCES**

An understanding of how the normal spine functions is essential to understand its various malfunctions. The study of the mechanics of the spine shows that it functions according to the laws of conservation of energy, that is, it functions at minimum stress, and the stress is equal in all its joints. Malfunctions are due to an overload of the mechanical elements, principally the intervertebral joints. This may take one of two forms: (1) compression overload, or (2) torsional overload. They have different symptomatology and different pathology, and require different forms of treatment.

The Evolution of Human Spinal Motion

Fishes swim with side-to-side motions of the spine, which seems to call for equal muscular development of back and front of the spine. The spine bends laterally about its long axis, and the fins are used mainly as stabilizers. The same musculature is used in animals that emerged onto land. The two sets of paired limbs are used as stabilizers, but with a difference. The animal uses these appendages as pivots that stick into the ground, and about which it can rotate its body. The ordinary tetrapod motion is advancement of a forefoot on one side and a hind foot on the other. The animal now lifts and advances its other two feet, imparting a sinuous motion to the spine.

This gives to the animal an asymmetry of muscular development. To the lateral bend, there is added a small degree of axial rotation. The lateral bend is the force behind the motion. It appears that the muscular power of the legs is not required to accomplish this motion. In snakes, the requirement for a pivot is served by the presence of motile scales. There is no call for powerful extensor–flexor muscles. This tetrapod motion is also part of the human heritage, as evidenced by the crawling of an infant. It has sunk down into our subconscious and appears in sleep and in the decerebrate animal (Fig. 12–1).

Improvements in the tetrapod motion can take a different form such as the gallop. This is a fully developed ancient method of progression. In this mode of motion, there is simultaneous advancement of the forelimbs and extension of the hindlimbs, alternating with simultaneous retraction of the forelimbs and advancement of the hindlimbs. An important feature of this method of progression is the alternate flexion and extension of the spine. This development marks a great departure from the dinosaurs, and is seen to predominate in all species, except birds. In humans, this motion also predominates, and is the basic motion of the spine.

In the gallop, the main musculature must be

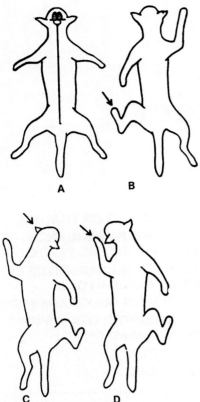

Figure 12–1. The tetrapod motion noted in the decerebrate animals. The advancement of the forefoot on one side is accompanied by advancement of the hind foot on the other side and pivoting motion of the spine.

from flexion and extension. There must also be lateral bend for regular tetrapod motion, and there must be a slight axial rotation.

Birds and humans habitually stand on two feet. In this position, they can walk. In birds, however, there is an almost rigid connection between the forelimbs and hindlimbs, which makes the animal rotate from side to side with each step. Compensating movements must be made with the neck and tail to balance the angular momentum. Because of the rigidity of the spine between forelimbs and hindlimbs, there is little call for lateral bend, or extension-flexion.

In humans, the mobility of the spine has been retained, and walking is accomplished by another mechanism, that is, by axial pelvic rotation. The movement of lateral bend, inherited from earlier animal forms, cannot produce axial rotation in a straight spine. In the presence of a curved spine (lordosis), however, axial rotation is produced by a lateral bend of the spine. Thus, with alternate right and left lateral bend, the pelvis is forced to rotate to the left, then to the right. At the same time, the shoulders are forced to rotate in the opposite direction to the pel-

vis. This mechanism still requires the pegs (lower extremities) to permit progression. Thus, lateral flexion of the spine drives the axial rotation of the spine. The axial skeleton must transmit the torque. The higher the speed of forward progression, the more torque required. This is the reason why experimentally the torque strength of the axial skeleton is increased by flexion of the spine or by compression.

The habitual motions of the spine are flexion-extension and lateral bend–axial rotation. Flexion-extension is the older of these two basic motions. Axial rotation is a later evolutionary adjustment. Flexion–extension motion (sagittal plane) is, therefore, better protected by evolutionary adaptation.

The Basic Principle of Biomechanics

In the performance of any given task, the musculoskeletal system seems to function in a fashion that minimizes energy expenditure. Where ligaments are available for a task, the task will tend to be shifted as much as possible to the ligaments as ligaments are passive structures and low-energy users compared with muscle.

As an energy saver, the alternating rotation of the shoulders and pelvis forms a mechanism similar to the vertical pendulum of a clock. Apart from saving energy, there is stability to this motion. In any motion, however, muscles are required to work to control and coordinate the movement. For example, flexing the elbow is a task in which gravity can be used as the motor force, no muscle performing the movement. With the arm abducted, no muscle action is necessary to produce flexion at the elbow. However, the triceps is involved in braking the fall of the forearm and hand. The muscle, innervation, guides and controls the movement.

Imagine having two elbow joints in series. The motion could be accomplished by motion at one or other joints, or else motion at both. This would require a higher degree of coordination between the muscles and ligaments that control the two joints. The problem of control of movement in the spine is more complex because of its several joints.

The Use of Muscle to Control Stress

Flexing forward to touch the hands to the ground bears a superficial resemblance to the motion at the elbow. Under the force of gravity, the body is allowed to flex forward. The motion stops, however, because the ligaments provide a brake, just at the

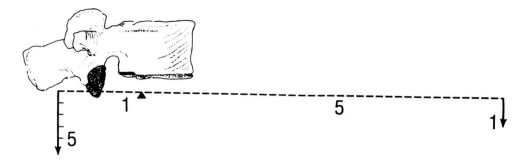

Figure 12–2. The turning movements of the abdominal and posterior spinal muscles on the posterior facets. The rotational force exerted on the joints is equal to the force multiplied by the distance from the center of rotation.

limit of spinal motion permitted by the spinal ligaments, at about 45 degrees of forward rotation. The lower arc of motion is arrested by the hamstring muscles, which stop the forward rotation of the pelvis, after a forward rotation of about 40 degrees. In this motion, more than one spinal joint is involved in the first arc of motion, and two joints, the sacroiliac joints and the hips, are involved in the second arc of motion.

The degree of coordination between muscle joint and ligament requires a high degree of sophistication. Add to this the requirement that stress be equal at all joints, and it is possible to get an idea of the complexity of the controlling system and the possibilities for failure.

If the abdominal muscles are used to flex the spine forward, all joints move in a sequence that is the exact opposite of the straightening-up movement. It can be shown that, by actively flexing forward with the abdominal muscles, the stress at the intervertebral joints is reduced. If an additional load is being manipulated, it is mandatory to use the abdominal muscles, both to flex forward and to straighten up. Clinically the active use of the abdominal muscles relieves the pain associated with lifting an object.

Flexion–Extension and Compression Load

The horizontal body experiences the least axial compression load. This is especially true when the muscles are paralyzed by sleep. The moment the body is vertical, sitting or standing, there is axial compression. It does not help to stand on the hands, because the body weight is distributed equally between the upper body and the hips with the lower extremities. The center of gravity of the body is approximately at the level of the second sacral segment.

The spine, without its musculature, can support only 5 pounds without collapsing. This means that

the musculature, by active contraction, maintains the upright posture.

When a muscle contracts across a joint, it exerts a compression force at the joint, between its point of origin and its point of insertion. It also exerts a turning movement, that is, force multiplied by distance from center of rotation (Fig. 12–2). It may also exert a shear force, depending on the angle of the muscle to the joint (Fig. 12–3). By changing the local geometry, the stress at the joint can be changed.

A ligament, however, cannot contract. It can be stretched and, when stretched, it develops a tension that also exerts a turning movement, a shear, and a compression. These combined muscular and ligamentous forces have effects on the intervertebral

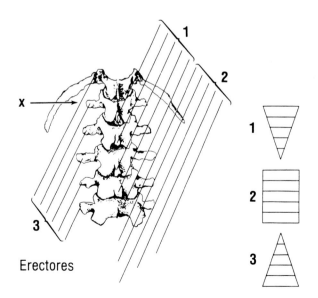

Figure 12–3. The shear force is exerted on a joint when there is an angle between the muscle and a joint. The horizontal force exerted by the components of erectores muscle (1, 2, 3) on different vertebrae is dependent on the length of the muscle (X) and the angle of the muscle and the joint.

joint, which is constructed to support all shear with the facet joints and posterior ligaments, and to support all compression with the disc.

The mechanism of the disc joint is analogous to standing on a plank placed across an inflated innertube of a car tire. When standing in the middle, there is compression on both sides, and the plank moves down in proportion to the load. To flex forward or backward, the position of the load must be changed. The load cannot be applied past the midpoint of the tire. Thus, to change the angle of the disc, the center of pressure of the disc, also called the instantaneous center of motion, is changed. To change the center of pressure, a muscle must develop tension in a ligament. The disc itself may be regarded as being frictionless, because the force incident to it is always at right angles through full range of motion.

Should an individual not use the full range of motion at the joint, abnormal forces will develop, mostly of a shear nature, affecting both facet joints and disc. For example, after abdominal surgery or pregnancy, there is loss of the natural rhythm of flexion at the lumbosacral joint, and early deterioration of disc and facets occurs, being most obvious in the facet joints and loss of posterior disc thickness.

The process takes 15 to 20 years to develop and accounts for the considerable number of persons over age 40 with low back pain that radiates to the hips and lateral thighs.

The Abdominal Mechanism

There are two types of ligaments in the spine. There are those, such as the interspinous ligaments, that are attached directly to bone, and develop tension as the vertebrae move, stretching them. There are others that are attached to muscle, and the muscle can raise the tension in the ligament.

The internal oblique and transversus abdominal muscles are both attached to the middle sheet of the lumbodorsal fascia. By their contraction, they can raise the tension in this sheet of fascia. Normally, as tension is applied to this fascia, the fascia tends to narrow like a nylon stocking. If this narrowing is blocked by a muscle attached to its side, the tension in the fascia may rise to a value higher than the muscle force alone (biaxial stress). To produce a maximum effect, the abdominal cavity must be pressurized slightly to give it a rounded shape.

Mechanisms of Injury

Movement in the sagittal plane induces a rise in compression loads, and may produce compressional failures. Lateral bend and axial torsion are movements in off-sagittal plane and occur with asymmetrical lifts and asymmetrical motions. They may result in a different type of injury called the torsional injury. These injuries are not due to pure tension, as there is always a certain compressional component as well as an element of lateral bend.

The basic requirement of normal function is minimized stress, equalized in all joints. To achieve this, the muscles, the ligaments, and the joints have to be coordinated across the full range of motion. Any deviation from this could cause an injury to the joint (disc). The ligaments and muscles are virtually impossible to injure, except by direct trauma. Although muscle fatigue can be postulated as the cause of injury, muscle fatigue should upset the coordination at the joint, with resulting injury to the joint, and not to the muscle itself.

Under normal circumstances, the body does not use its full reserves. Even the weightlifter does not use his or her full capacity to lift. There seems to be about 40% of capacity left untapped at maximum lift. This reserve is the safety factor and may be tapped under serious mental stress, or under the influence of drugs.

In sedentary activity, individuals seldom exert themselves more than 10 to 15% of their capacity. A heavy manual laborer may exert 30 to 40% of capacity on rare occasions. However, considering the incoordination in a system whose very existence depends on coordination of its components, it is not difficult to decide that this is the dominant cause of spinal failure.

Coordination involves the motion of the spinal joints through full range. If part of this range has been lost, there inevitably will be a loss of lifting capacity. The key to rehabilitation is the use of the fullest range of motion possible.

The best method of lifting is the method that produces the lowest stress in the intervertebral joints. Therefore, the posterior ligaments must be brought into play. The spine must be flexed, and the abdominal muscles tightened, to bring the posterior midline ligaments and the lumbodorsal fascia into play. At the same time, the spine must be as close as possible to the object lifted, to reduce to a minimum the leverage of the load (load multiplied by distance from the spine). The fully flexed spine seems incompatible with requirements for reduced leverage of the load, until it is remembered that full flexion of the spine can be obtained while the spine is maintained in the vertical position.

To carry loads safely, the faster the speed of walking, the more torque strength is required. As mentioned, during flexion both the lifting strength and the torque strength are increased. Thus, just as the weight of the object to be carried determines the degree of lordosis, the degree of lordosis controls the speed of walking.

Degeneration or Trauma

There is abundant evidence to suggest that degeneration is healing in the presence of repeated trauma. Consider a sprained interphalangeal joint of a finger. The injury is to the ligament that holds the joint surfaces together. When the ligament is ripped, the articular surfaces just slide off. They receive no injury. When the dislocation is reduced, the ligament heals by scar formation outside of the articular surfaces. The scar, like all scars, contracts, thus returning the injured ligament to its original state.

On the other hand, when a disc is sprained, it is the ligament that holds the end plates together that is torn. This ligament is the annulus, and differs from the finger joint. It is located between the end plates. Scarring of this ligament will cause the end plates to come closer together. Hence the radiographic finding of a narrowed disc.

Pathological Sequence of Fractured End Plate

The fractured end plate is the most common pathological finding in the lumbar spine. Original descriptions of this lesion are to be found in the pathological studies reported by Andrae (1929) and Schmorl (1926). In studying these lesions at a later date, Key (1949) came to the conclusion that the Schmorl's nodes, as they came to be called, represented healing fractures of the end plates.

Four types—not necessarily four grades—of this injury exist in the laboratory (Fig. 12–4): (1) Subend plate compression fractures of cancellous bone. The overlying end plate and cartilage are intact and, therefore, still maintain the normal fluid barriers between the disc and vertebral body. (2) Fractures of the end plate and cartilage, which open a communication between disc and vertebral body. These fractures are of three types: (a) fissure fractures of the end plate; (b) depressed fractures of the end plate; and (c) fissures or depressed fractures with disc material forced into the vertebral body.

These fractures can all be created in the laboratory by compression of the vertebra–disc–vertebra unit. The application of axial load through the annulus causes bending stresses in the end plate. A linear fracture of the end plate can be produced in this matter even when the nucleus has been removed (Lamy, 1978). Larger bending stresses can be induced in the end plate when the nucleus is present. This is not to

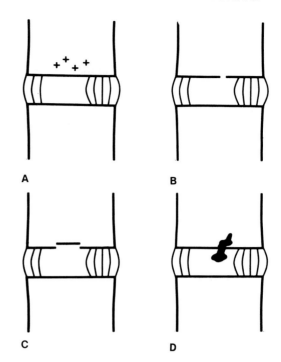

Figure 12–4. Various types of fractured end plate: **(A)** subchondral; **(B)** fissure fracture; **(C)** depressed fracture; **(D)** fracture with trapped disc material.

say that the fracture occurs because the pressure in the disc is increased. Any firm material in the center of the disc, such as degenerated disc material, will act like a punch and produce a punched-out fracture of the end plate.

A rise of pressure in the disc itself will not cause a fractured end plate. By stretching the disc apart, however, the increased pressure ruptures the annulus. A fracture of the end plate can result if the end plates are restrained by a compressive force. This is the normal state of affairs when intradiscal pressure is increased. The fractured end plate, although it heals, remains weak. Under normal conditions, the end plate can withstand high injection pressures in the disc. When Schmorl's nodes are present, however, very little injection pressure is required to reopen the communication between disc and vertebral body (Farfan, 1973). The disc with a fractured end plate loses some of its stiffness. However, it does retain, in great measure, its capacity to support axial compression, because the main resistance to axial compression is provided by the vertebral body cortex, the peripheral ring of the end plate, and the annulus.

The loss of the fluid seal between disc and vertebral body can greatly affect the disc–vertebra unit as a whole when accelerated loadings are applied, as in heavy lifting, rapid flexion–extension, or repeated motions. This is because of the hydraulic augmentation of the vertebral body's resistance to compression. As the vertebral body is compressed, its fluid content is expelled through the resistance of its cancellous bone. The more rapidly the fluid has to be expelled, the greater will be the resistance offered by the porous cancellous bone. Therefore, this mechanism ensures that, with rapid loading, the vertebral body becomes strengthened by this mechanism. With fractures of the end plate, as with fractures of the peripheral cortex, this mechanism is impaired (Fig. 12–5).

After a fractured end plate, the spine cannot be expected to handle loads that can only be manipulated at high speed. For people of great strength, this limit would be in the neighborhood of 57 kg/m but, for people of average strength, this limit would be much less, probably half of this.

A fractured end plate allows fluid to leak from the disc space at a much faster rate than normal. Thus, as the day goes by, disc thickness is reduced with its loss of fluid and the facet joints gradually sublux, producing pain. If the fluid is restored to the disc its thickness is regained, and the symptoms disappear. This occurs with repeated hyperextensions, the most ancient exercise for low back problems (Goldthwaite, 1911). Thus, hyperextension exercises will help most patients with a fractured end plate, and they work well in the older age group, where fractured end plates are common.

Schmorl's nodes tend to propagate from one end plate to the next, in a sequence consistent with the hydraulic compartmentalization of the spine. Discs and vertebral bodies are initially separate compartments. Fractures of one end plate extend the compartment to include one disc and one vertebra; the second fracture will extend the compartment to include either the neighboring disc or the adjacent vertebral body. The most common location of the Schmorl's node in the lumbar spine is in the upper two lumbar vertebrae, where they seem to be of little clinical significance. They may occur, however, in the lower lumbar spine, caused by the sudden impact of a fall on the buttocks or, possibly, by heavy lifting. There seems to be no reason to expect these injuries to be painless. However, because they are undisplaced fractures in cancellous bone, one may expect rapid healing, accompanied by rapid resolution of symptoms.

In those instances in which disc material is trapped in the fracture, it is not known whether the healing is delayed. In the laboratory, such displaced fragments may sometimes be extracted from the vertebral body by distracting the disc. Although this in vitro situation does not compare with that in life, it is possible that this phenomenon might well account for the success of a sudden manipulative elongation of the spine.

The axial compression overload does its principal damage to the disc, and not to the facet joints. The facet joints of L1-2, L2-3, and L3-4 in all positions of the spine are in line with the axial overload. Those of the last two lumbar vertebrae come close to this alignment when the spine is in flexion, the position assumed for a heavy lift. This leaves them safe from the compressive overload.

The late sequelae of end plate fractures have not been studied in any experimental model. It must be extrapolated from what is known of the healing pro-

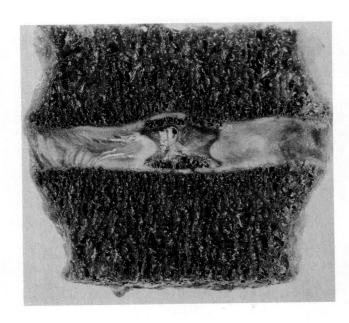

Figure 12–5. Natural fractured end plate. (*From Farfan HF: Mechanical Disorders of the Low Back. Philadelphia, Lea & Febiger, 1973. Modified from Farfan HF: J Bone Joint Surg 54A:492, 1972.*)

cess to arrive at the probable sequence of events. At the onset, the disc loses its content, and there is bleeding into the disc from the vertebral body. This is rapidly followed by invasion of the disc cavity by granulation tissue, which accounts for the digestion or gradual resolution of the avascular end plate cartilage and inner annulus. With the loss of disc material, the disc loses its thickness and the adjacent vertebrae come closer and closer together. The remaining viable outer annulus is pushed gradually over the end plate rim, causing osteophyte formation.

Accompanying the loss of disc thickness, the facet joints subluxate, becoming arthritic and painful, especially when subjected to weight bearing, i.e., prolonged standing or sitting, particularly if the spine is forced in extension or flexion (Figs. 12–6 and 12–7). Furthermore, the subluxation of the facets may result in lateral entrapment of the nerve root, the superior facet coming quite close to the nerve as it passes outward around the pedicle of the vertebra above (Fig. 12–8). Such a joint does not have any increased mobility, and it gets stiffer and stiffer with passing years. Its progression often leads to a natural ankylosis or fusion. It seems unlikely that mobilization of such a joint could do anything except produce

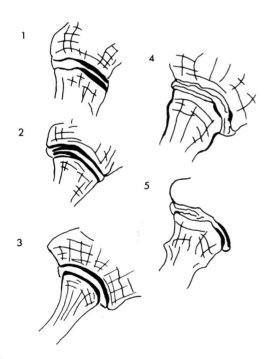

Figure 12–6. Degeneration of facet joints. **(1)** normal; **(2)** fragmentation cartilage; **(3)** loss of cartilage, early osteoporosis; **(4)** crush fracture of base articular process, synovial invasion of widened joint and advancing osteoporosis; **(5)** almost total loss of cartilage, further synovial invasion of joint space, osteoporosis. *(From Farfan HF: Mechanical Disorders of the Low Back. Philadelphia, Lea & Febiger, 1973. Modified from Farfan HF: J Bone Joint Surg 54A:492, 1972.)*

an inflammatory response that, in turn, would only increase the stiffness or, at worse, initiate the lateral entrapment syndrome.

In the entire sequence outlined above, there is no mention of disc protrusion. This is because, with compression axial overload, the disc may bulge, but never sufficiently enough to interfere with the neural canal content. The high axial loads in life are generated in the flexed position and with forward flexion when the posterior disc annulus does not bulge backward into the canal. In fact, it becomes flattened or even slightly concave.

In a very special set of circumstances, high compression loads may result in disc protrusion into the neural canal. This particular situation may arise with a sudden fall on the buttocks, which finds the intervertebral joint unconstrained by tight ligaments (spine not fully flexed) and the muscles inactive.

In the laboratory, the intervertebral joint is found to be very resistant to compression axial load, withstanding nearly 1 ton of compression before failure. It requires a lift of over 180 kg to produce compression loads of this order in young, healthy individuals. By comparison, the intervertebral joint is very susceptible to torsion, requiring a one-handed lift of less than 45 kg to generate the 9.4-kg/m of torque required to damage the joint (Farfan et al., 1970).

Pathological Sequence of Torsional Overload

Lumbar joints are not all equally sensitive to torsion. The joint with a more rounded disc shape tends to be less sensitive to torsion than that with a more oval shape. The lower lumbar joints should, therefore, be expected to be the first to fail (Farfan et al., 1972). Furthermore, the L-5 vertebra in 60 to 70% of individuals is either deeply seated in the pelvis or articulated closely with the pelvis by means of short iliotransverse ligaments. In either case, the L-5 vertebra and, therefore, the joint between it and the sacrum, are protected from torsional stresses (MacGibbon and Farfan, 1979). The L5-S1 joint is also protected from torsional stress by reason of the lumbar curve. Generally speaking, L-5 joints with large lumbosacral angles would tend to feel less torsional strain than those with small lumbosacral angles (Kraus, 1976). These combinations of antitorsional devices make the L4-5 disc, two to one, the most common lumbar joint affected by torsion.

This may be viewed in another way. For walking or running, it is necessary to have a fixed lumbar curve and distal lumbar joints able to withstand greater torsional stress. The natural evolution is to-

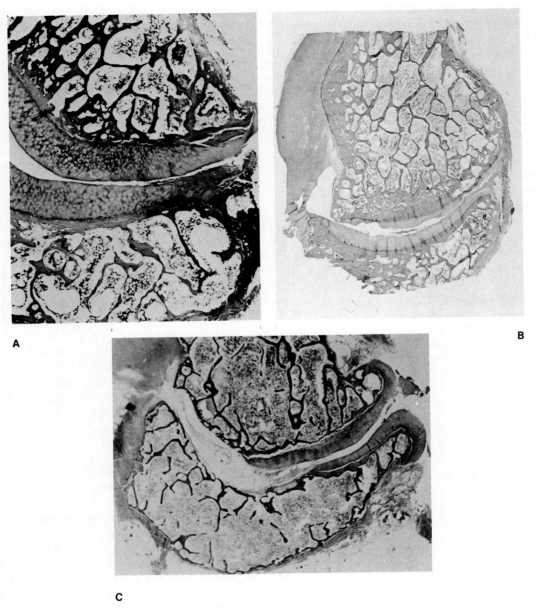

Figure 12–7. (A) Normal facet. **(B)** Early degeneration of articular cartilage. Note mass of new bone formation at the inferior margin of the lamina closer to the facet. **(C)** Ulcerations are more advanced. Note tongue of synovial tissue growing into the joint from its ventral aspect.

ward fixation of the two joints above the sacral promontory, giving them much greater torque capacity. Flexion will be maintained by increasing the flexibility at L3-4.

In the presence of such antitorsional devices, the L-5 to S-1 disc can still be injured by axial compression loads. It is exactly in such "protected" joints that one can look for the probable sequences of "pure" axial compression overload.

When torsion is applied to an intervertebral joint, the center of motion is found to be within the disc (Fig. 12–9). Resistance to torsion is offered

mainly by the facet joints and discs in almost equal proportion. When injuries occur, they occur simultaneously in the posterior elements and in the disc (Farfan et al., 1971).

Injuries in the facet joints are basically those of compression subchondral fractures on either side of the articulation. The tissue response is effusion, synovitis, and limitation of motion, all of which are probably pain-producing responses. One can expect fibrillation of cartilage, loss of articular cartilage, possibly the presence of loose bodies in the joint, and chronic synovitis (see Fig. 12–7). In more than 500

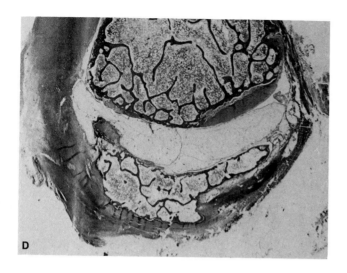

Figure 12-7 *(cont'd).* **(D)** Marked erosion of articular cartilage on both sides of joint with loss of subchondral bone and thinning of the bony trabeculae on both sides of the joint. Large fatty synovial mass separating the articular surfaces. (*From Farfan HF: Mechanical Disorders of the Low Back. Philadelphia, Lea & Febiger, 1973. Modified from Farfan HF: J Bone Joint Surg 54A:492, 1972.*)

operations on facet joints, these cadaveric pathologies have been confirmed. Of these, loose body formation is quite a rare finding and, in no case has a nipped synovial fringe been recognized. In addition, isolated injuries to supraspinous or interspinous ligaments, ligamentum flavum, and facet capsules have not been recognized during surgery. This is supported by laboratory studies that, while indicating that facet capsules and supraspinous and interspinous ligaments contribute to torque strength, have shown no gross injury at the point of failure of the whole joint.

The tissue reaction to intra-articular damage and chronic synovitis affects the juxta-articular bone of the articular processes. Bone in this region becomes osteoporotic and subject to compression fracture. These compression fractures have been found in cadaver specimens and also at surgery. Facet joint arthritis and fractures of the articular process, both in the same spinal segment, can be expected to give rise

to referred pain. Putti (1927) was of the opinion that facet joint arthritis alone could explain most of the symptomatology in mechanical disorders of the back.

One comment should be made relative to the classic loss of lumbar lordosis accompanying intervertebral joint disease. The loss of lordosis cannot be ascribed to "muscle spasm." Without exception, the paravertebral muscles are behind the axis of flexion–extension motion in the disc. Contraction of these muscles, therefore, would produce extension or increased lordosis. On the other hand, axial rotation at the intervertebral joint is accompanied by flexion at the joint. This would explain both the loss of lordosis and the rotoscoliosis. However, this cannot be the whole story, because it does not offer an explanation for alternating scoliosis, a problem that will be referred to later.

The effects of torsion on the disc under laboratory conditions are spectacular. At the point of maxi-

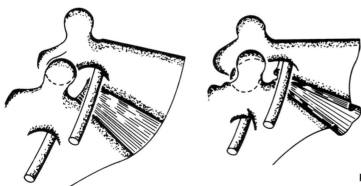

Figure 12-8. Collapse of lumbosacral joint brings superior facet of L-5 close to the pedicle of the vertebra above.

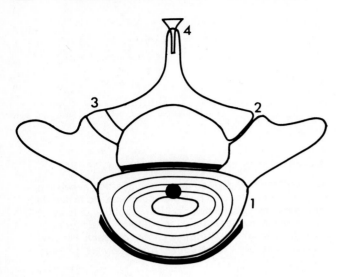

Figure 12-9. Parts of the intervertebral joint that resist torsion. These include: (1) disc and its anterior and posterior longitudinal ligaments which may be considered as integral components of the disc; (2) bony facet articulations; (3) capsules of the facet articulations; (4) the supraspinous and other intervertebral ligaments; as well as the musculature. *(From Farfan HF: Mechanical Disorders of the Low Back. Philadelphia, Lea & Febiger, 1973. Modified from Farfan HF: J Bone Joint Surg 54A:492, 1972.)*

mal torsion, the disc "gives" suddenly with loud snapping sounds. In fact, it can be said to "slip" in almost exactly the same sense that a car clutch slips. The annulus becomes distorted all around its periphery, but in greater degree at the posterolateral angles. Here, the outer annulus fibers subjacent to the longitudinal ligaments are ripped off the end plate on one side over a considerable distance. The inner annular layers and nucleus remain undistributed and there is no injury to the end plate.

The distortion of the outer annulus may be large enough to interfere with neural canal content, and it may stretch the posterior longitudinal ligament. In the rabbit, this annular ligament injury elicits a polymorphonuclear response, followed by granulation tissue accompanied by an invasion of the outer annulus with new small vascular channels. There is some reason to believe that the same reaction occurs in humans (Sullivan et al., 1971).

Such soft tissue distortion of the annulus and the posterior longitudinal ligament, both well supplied with nerve endings, is undoubtedly a source of pain, whether or not the distortion interferes with the nerve roots. Theoretically, at this stage, the distorted annulus may be reduced, possibly by derotation in flexion. At this stage, the circular cicatrization of the damaged annulus may return the annulus to its original shape and location.

When torsion is repeatedly applied to the disc, in the laboratory over a given angle of arc, its resistance to torsion to this arc of motion is almost completely lost. Left to recover, much of its torque strength will return. If the test is performed after removing a small window of annulus for purposes of observation, it is seen that the inner annular layers begin to separate and gradually work themselves free, bulging up and out through the window. This separation of inner annular fibers is not uncommonly seen in degenerated discs, where almost entire whorls of loose tissue can be found.

It is not evident that loose annular tissue, found in degenerated discs, is caused by repeated torsion. It is only important that it occurs. Furthermore, there is some evidence that, under certain conditions, these loose bits of material can be induced to move within the disc cavity. It is clear that disc protrusions could not occur unless disc material could be induced to move. When a disc cavity is injected with silastic glue, and the glue is allowed to set, the glue sets with a firm rubbery consistency, not unlike that of disc material removed at surgery. (The normal disc accepts only a small amount of material, somewhat less than 1 ml.) To accept more, the disc already must be degenerated to some degree. When a disc prepared in this manner is subjected to repeated torsion, the little pellet of silastic glue is found to track through the disc material toward the posterolateral angle. When larger volumes of silastic glue have been used, the material has, on occasion, been forced out through the annulus.

Thus, there occurs the phenomenon of loose material in the disc that can be induced to move under certain circumstances, even in the presence of discs with a still intact outer annulus. It is possible that such loose material may be forced up under the sensitive posterior outer annulus by a compressional or torsional force, much like a melon seed from between the finger and thumb. A manipulation might possibly dislodge this fragment from its pain-producing position to a more medial one, nearer the center of the disc. Also, this material might be moved from one side to the other, resulting in a sudden switch of clinical signs and symptoms. It can be imagined readily that manipulation might also force loose material irretrievably through the annulus.\

The Areas of Maximum Stress

As previously mentioned, torsion affects the disc, causing distortion and eventual avulsion of the annulus from one end plate. The site of maximum distortion and avulsion is at the location of maximum stress. This point of maximal stress is dictated by the shape of the disc in the following areas: (1) midpoint posteriorly in discs with rounded posterior outlines; (2) the posterolateral angle at the medial pedicular margins in discs with flat posterior outlines; and (3) laterally in discs with lozenge-shaped outlines (Fig. 12–10).

Where the disc shapes are absolutely symmetrical, then the highest stress concentrations would be bilaterally placed and similar. When the disc is asymmetrically formed, however, stress concentrations

occur on only one side, usually on the more hypoplastic side. The hypoplastic side is indicated by axial tomography, or sometimes in simple radiographs when it is marked by a more oblique or smaller facet joint (Fig. 12–11). The hypoplastic side is, therefore, the weak side, the side on which disc problems arise, and to which the rotoscoliosis occurs in the majority of instances. Repeated torsion will, therefore, repeatedly affect the weakest side, rupturing annular fibers in deeper and deeper layers, until finally a communication between the outer annulus and the disc nucleus is created. This radial fissure, as it is known, indicates that the joint has reached the point of instability and abnormal motion that can often be demonstrated (Fig. 12–12).

Beside indicating the stage of instability attained, the radial fissure provides a channel through the outer annulus, through which disc material can be extruded. Although relatively late in the process, the radial fissure may form early, with a rapidly progressing clinical course. It remains, nevertheless, relatively uncommon to find a true extrusion of disc material.

In the vast majority of disc injuries, ingrowth of granulation tissue occurs, with its concomitant vascularization from the end plate or from the outer layers of annulus. This tissue response digests or hydrolizes the disc content. Although not commonly thought of as scar formation, this reaction, in the

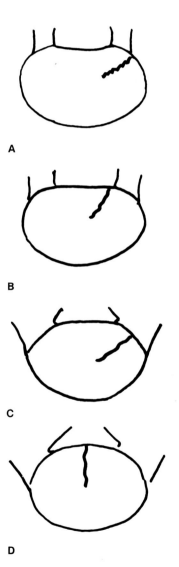

A

B

C

D

Figure 12–10. Radial fissures seem to occur at locations of torsional stress concentrations that in turn depend on the shape of the disc. The various lumbar disc outlines are shown. **(A)** Upper lumbar, fissures from lateral to the pedicle. **(B)** Most common, L-4. **(C)** Common, L-5 (more commonly the L-5 has a shape as in **D**). **(D)** Not uncommon at L-4. (*From Farfan HF: Orthop Clin N Am 8:13, 1977.*)

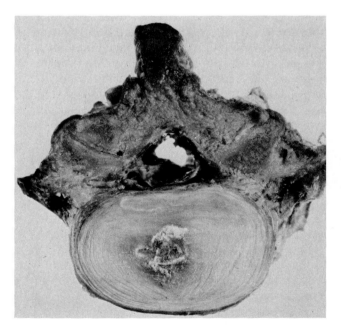

Figure 12–11. Grossly asymmetric intervertebral joint, obvious in both facet joint and disc. (*From Farfan HF: Mechanical Disorders of the Low Back. Philadelphia, Lea & Febiger, 1973. Modified from Farfan HF: J Bone Joint Surg 54A:492, 1972*)

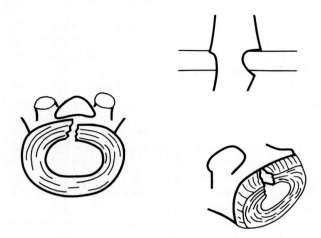

Figure 12–12. The nature of disc protrusion. Note separation of annulus only on one side. The lesion in life is covered partly by a posterior longitudinal ligament and by inflammatory exudate. (*From Farfan HF: Clin Neurosurg 25:284, 1979.*)

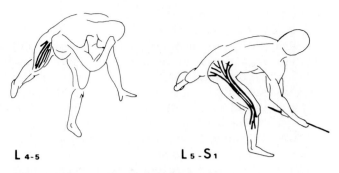

Figure 12–13. Facet syndromes. (See text.)

normally avascular disc, removes loose fragments of tissue and tends to stabilize the remainder. The usual outcome is a loss of loose material for extrusion, a good reason for temporizing and allowing nature to do its bit.

The healing process in this instance is also imperfect, as it was in the case of the fractured end plate. In cadaveric material, the disc, with even the earliest signs of degeneration, always shows less resistance to torsion than a normal disc. This ensures that, when torsional overload is applied a second time, it will be the same joint that is injured, the other joints in the column being protected, as it were, by the presence of the one that is strained. The progression is always at the same joint, in contrast to the compressional overload that strikes successively neighboring discs.

Combined Posterior Facet and Disc Damage

It remains now to consider the combined effects of arthritic facets and damaged discs on the patient. Because of the arthritic facets, positions of extension or of flexion, if prolonged, will give backache and, with further aggravation, will cause referred pain in the buttocks and lateral thigh (Fig. 12–13).

Because of loss of annular tissue, resistance to both compression and torsional loads is impaired. Heavy lifting of any kind, especially when the load is carried asymmetrically, as in one-hand lifting, may cause the patient to experience difficulty. Such a condition is, of course, a serious threat to normal lifestyles.

Healing cannot be expected to progress any faster than that of a healing ligament, which is the major component of the annulus. It takes at least 6 weeks for a damaged ligament to regain 80% of its tensile strength. The acute inflammatory response of the facet joints may recover rapidly, but the induced synovitis also takes a long time to settle.

Certain other conditions occur in a joint that has been damaged by torsion, and these conditions are best understood if one keeps in mind that the disc and posterior elements are injured simultaneously.

The deformation of the neural arch on one side may be so severe that it may never regain its original shape. When rotation is forced, the long, superior articular process of the rotated vertebra is jammed against the short, sturdy, unyielding, superior facet of the vertebra below. The result is that the superior articular process is bent backward and medially (Fig. 12–14).

In the meantime, the inferior process on the opposite side is not greatly distorted, because the only resistance to its motion is the capsular ligament of the distracted facet. The pedicle on this side, however, is displaced medially, taking its nerve root with it. In this way, with a rotation of 9 degrees, the displacing pedicle may stretch the nerve root by 1 cm, which is probably enough to result in compromise of its function, leading to a neuropathic syndrome, without the necessity of having a disc protrusion or extrusion (Fig. 12–15).

This type of nerve root impairment may be of extreme clinical importance, both for the practitioner of spinal manipulation as well as for the surgeon. Relief of symptoms could be expected with restoration of normal alignment by rotation. For the surgeon, it explains a large group of patients explored without disc protrusion being found (the "hidden" disc of Dandy, 1942). It could also explain certain false-positive myelograms, in which the defect in the column of dye results from inability to fill the nerve sheath because the nerve root was tightly drawn against the pedicle.

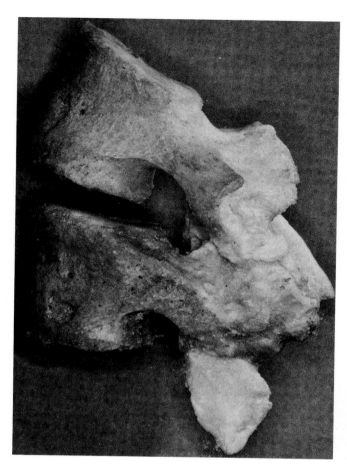

Figure 12–14. The wide angle between the inferior articular process and the pedicle is well demonstrated. This deformation allows the vertebra above to slip forward. (*From Farfan HF: Mechanical Disorders of the Low Back. Philadelphia, Lea & Febiger, 1973. Modified from Farfan HF: J Bone Joint Surg 54A:492, 1972.*)

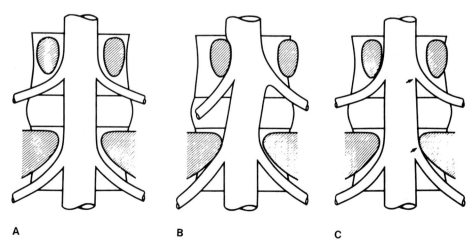

A   B   C

Figure 12–15. The rotation effect on nerve roots. **(A)** Neutral. **(B)** L-4 has been rotated to the patient's left stretching L-4 and L-5 roots on patient's left side. A temporary situation. **(C)** The spine has been derotated but because the vertebral body is now forward on the right side, it is the L-5 nerve root which is stretched over the back of the body of L-5, and its pedicle.

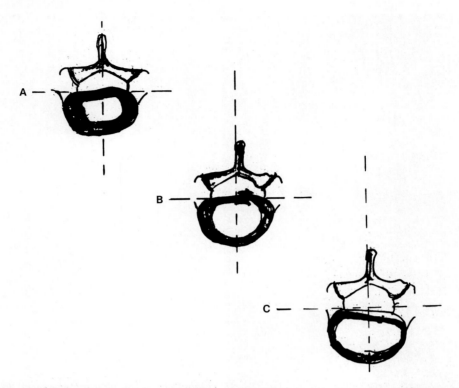

Figure 12–16. Degenerative spondylolisthesis: the progression from original rotation injury. **(A)** Left facet joint is cracked and there is distortion of the annulus with subsequent degeneration. **(B)** The degeneration has progressed in both facet joints, making the arch weaker so that it is subject to the crush fracture and deformation. **(C)** Deformation of arch allows listhesis to develop. (*From Farfan HF: Orthop Clin N Am 8:15, 1977.*)

When torsion is removed, the deformed arch may not recover and may remain with a skewed look. The disc, because it is damaged at the same time, permits the deformed neural arch to settle once more, so that the gross relationship of lamina and facet joints is restored. The vertebral body, however, has now rotated forward on the deformed side. This has the effect of causing an abrupt change of direction of the neural canal, causing the neural content to be drawn tight to the undisplaced side. This may cause a restriction of the cauda equina. If, in addition, one considers that the facet joints may be swollen and arthritic, and the disc distorted, it can be seen that the cauda equina as well as its circulation may be impeded, thereby giving rise to the syndrome of spinal stenosis. When the displacement of the vertebral body becomes obvious, the condition is known as degenerative spondylolisthesis (Fig. 12–16).

In these late gross disturbances of the intervertebral joint, there seems little to gain by mobilization of the joint. As with the lateral entrapment syndrome due to collapse of disc thickness, the condition has passed beyond the scope of the practitioner of spinal manipulation.

Conclusion

It is important to recognize the two major types of injury to the low back: compression overload and torsional overload. Distinction between these two entities will make the treatment simple and more effective.

It is also important to recognize the progression of changes as the initial injury heals or fails to heal. The resulting multiplicity of disease stages still should be recognized by the original diagnosis.

References

Andrae R: Uber knorpelnoschiten am Hinter endeder wirbelandechelin berech des spinalkanals. *Beitr Pathol* 1929; 82:464.

Dandy WE. Recent advances in the diagnosis and treatment of ruptured intervertebral discs. *Ann Surg* 1942;115:514.

Farfan HF. *Mechanical Disorders of the Low Back.* Philadelphia: Lea & Febiger; 1973.

Farfan HF, Cossette JW, and Robertson GH, et al. The effects of torsion on the lumbar intervertebral joints: The role of torsion in the production of disc degeneration. *J Bone Joint Surg* 1970; 52A:468.

Farfan HF, Huberdeau RM, and Dubow HI. Lumbar intervertebral disc degeneration; The influence of geometrical features on the pattern of disc degeneration. *J Bone Joint Surg* 1972;54A:492.

Farfan HF, Cossette JW, Robertson GH, and Wells RV. The instantaneous center of rotation of the third lumbar intervertebral joint. *J Biomech* 1971;4:149.

Goldthwaite JE. The lumbosacral articulation. An explanation of many cases of ''lumbago,'' ''sciatica'' and ''paraplegia.'' *Boston Med Surg* 1911;164:365.

Key JA. The intervertebral disc: Anatomy, physiology and pathology. *Am Acad Orthop Surg* 1949;6:27.

Kraus H. Effect of lordosis on the stress in the lumbar spine. *Clin Orthop* 1976;117:56.

Lamy C. Mechanism of failure of the vertebral body end plate. Unpublished, 1978.

MacGibbon B, and Farfan HF. Are all lumbar spines the same—radiological survey. *Spine* 1979;4:258.

Putti V. New conceptions in the pathogenesis of sciatic pain. *Lancet* 1927;2:53.

Schmorl G. Die pathologische anatomie der wirbelsaule. *Verh Dtsch, Ges Orthop* 1926;21:3.

Sullivan JD, Farfan HF, and Kahn DS. Pathological changes with intervertebral joint rotational instability in the rabbit. *Can J Surg* 1971;14:71.

chapter 13

The Neurophysiology of Spinal Pain

Scott Haldeman

Musculoskeletal and spinal pain are the most common symptoms treated by chiropractors. Both Vear (1972) and Breen (1977) report that over 90% of patients seeking chiropractic care do so for musculoskeletal pain. Over 50% of these patients are looking for relief of low back pain. In addition, most research into the effectiveness of manipulation and chiropractic care has looked at pain relief as a primary indicator of successful care.

It has been estimated that up to 90% of the population will suffer from back pain in their lifetime. Nagi et al. (1973) noted that 18% of the population between the ages of 18 and 64 have persistent back pain. These facts illustrate why it is so important for the practicing chiropractor to comprehend the phys-

iological mechanisms that are involved in the genesis and treatment of spinal pain.

Conceptual Models and Definitions of Pain

During the past decade, major changes have taken place in the conceptualization of spinal pain. The changes in pain research and theory have been so drastic that chiropractors who studied the neurophysiology of pain as recently as 5 years ago will find their knowledge out of date regarding current thinking on the generation and treatment of spinal pain.

The most obvious change is the realization that

there is no such thing as an independent, well-defined, and isolated stimulus-dependent pain system. Pain had been described in the past as a process initiated by tissue damage, where impulses follow along specific fibers to the spinal cord and then along designated spinal pathways to the central nervous system where they stimulate specific centers. Wall (1989a), however, cited convincing reasons why this fixed stimulus-response relationship cannot be used as a model for pain. He notes that not all pain stimuli are known or presently detectable. Furthermore, no stimulus can exist in isolation. Its central effect depends on the presence of other peripheral stimuli and on the activity of the central nervous system. In addition, there are plastic changes in neural connections, particularly after injury. These changes influence the way in which the nervous system responds to pain. These observations have changed the conceptualization of the mechanism of pain from a tight, well-understood, electrical-type diagrammatic system to a flexible system that interacts with all other stimuli and involves virtually all aspects of the nervous system.

The second reason for the deviation from the traditional stimulus–response theory is the realization that there is an intimate relationship between emotional factors and pain response. Signs of emotional distress are the most clearly recognizable evidence that a person suffers from pain. Early models of pain inferred that the emotional changes were simply a reaction to a primary sensory stimulus. Craig (1989), on reviewing past theories, suggests that the psychophysiological cognitive and affective processes were treated as if they were sources of experimental errors that had to be controlled. These theories suggested that if the course of pain was eliminated by surgical or medical methods the emotional component would go away. The observation that surgical and medical approaches were often not able to eliminate pain in all situations and that the emotional response did not always correlate with the amount of sensory input has led to modification of these early concepts.

Melzack and Wall (1965) were the first to modify this theory by suggesting that pain stimuli simultaneously activated affect–motivational and sensory–discriminative components of pain. This model gave equal emphasis to these two components of pain. Evidence supporting this theory came from the observation that psychological and physical interventions may influence one component of pain but not another (Johnson and Rice, 1974; Martelli et al., 1987). Gracely et al. (1978), for example, demonstrated that anxiolytics, such as diazepam, reduce the affective discomfort rather than the sensory–intensity components of pain. On the other hand, the

narcotic fentanyl reduces the sensory intensity of pain without changing the unpleasantness of pain (Gracely et al., 1982).

This model, however, does not fully describe all observed pain phenomena. It is becoming increasingly evident that there is a close interaction between the discriminative and affective components of pain. Pain symptoms are very prevalent in psychiatric patients, particularly among those suffering anxiety-based and exogenous depression disorders (Merskey, 1986). Romano and Turner (1985) found that 50% of patients with pain and depression develop the two disorders simultaneously. Patients with emotional distress, on the other hand, often develop pain complaints to provide a legitimate access to care (Craig 1989). This allows these patients to express psychological distress in a socially acceptable manner. The search for a primary organic source of pain and pain stimulus reduction-oriented care is often unsuccessful in these patients.

These factors have led the taxonomy committee of the International Association for the Study of Pain, chaired by Merskey (1979), to define pain as ''an unpleasant sensory and emotional experience associated with actual or potential tissue damage, or described in terms of such damage.'' They offer a number of comments that are equally important:

> Pain is always subjective.
>
> It is unquestionably a sensation in a part of the body but it is also always unpleasant and therefore an emotional experience.
>
> May people report pain in the absence of tissue damage or any likely pathophysiologic cause.
>
> Activity induced in a nociceptor and nociceptive pathways by a noxious stimulus is not pain, which is always a psychological state, even though we may well appreciate that pain most often has a proximate physical cause.
>
> If they regard their experience (pain reported for psychological reasons) as pain and if they report it in the same ways as pain caused by tissue damage, it should be accepted as pain.

Principles of Nociception

One of the vital functions of the nervous system is to protect the body against injury or threat of injury. This requires that injury be detected by the receptor system and that this information be transferred to the central nervous system. The receptor system must be able to detect and transfer details concerning the location and intensity of the injury or noxious stimuli irrespective of the type of energy that is causing the injury.

Much nociception research has been carried out on skin receptors in animals, because of their easy access. Unfortunately, research results on animals may not be transferred readily to humans, although such research often has clinical correlations. Of greater importance is the fact that research on cutaneous receptors cannot always be extrapolated to deeper tissues, which are most commonly associated with spinal pain. Despite these shortcomings, animal-based research has established some basic principles of nociception.

The idea that there is only one class of nociceptor has probably never been widely acknowledged. There are multiple nociceptors in tissues. In the skin, for example, nociception has been demonstrated to occur on stimulation of (1) C-fiber mechano-heat receptors, which respond to thermal stimuli between 38 and 50°C in a graded manner; (2) A-delta fiber mechano-heat nociceptors, which respond to higher temperatures and conduct at a higher velocity; (3) C-fiber mechanoreceptors, which do not respond to heat and have a low threshold for mechanical stimuli; and (4) receptors responsive to cold stimuli. In addition nonnociceptors may signal pain under certain circumstances. Campbell et al. (1988), for example, noted that low threshold mechanoreceptors may signal pain under causalgic conditions.

Pain should not be considered an all-or-none phenomenon. Nociception is a graduated response. C fibers reactive to mechanical and heat stimuli show a graduated response curve; the greater the stimulus, the greater the response. This not only occurs because of the recruitment of more fibers by the larger stimulus, but also through a graduated response by individual fibers to increasing stimulus intensity (La Motte and Campbell, 1978). Individual receptors also respond differently to different intensities of stimuli. For example, C-fiber nociceptors respond at temperatures up to 50°C, whereas A-delta nociceptors have thresholds of above 50°C. These fibers also respond to different levels of mechanical stimuli and have been divided into so-called high-threshold and low-threshold nociceptors.

Furthermore, the idea that each receptor responds to only a single stimulus type is not valid. Nociceptors respond to different classes of stimuli. Although certain receptors respond to fairly specific temperature ranges, virtually all nociceptors studied to date respond to mechanical stimuli (Campbell et al., 1989). The response to mechanical stimuli, however, may not be painful when applied to fibers that produce painful responses to heat. This has been explained by the possibility that heat tends to stimulate larger skin areas than local pressure.

An additional principal of nociception is that nociceptors become sensitized after injury. Injured tissue is well known to be hyperalgesic. This means that the application of a stimulus that is not normally painful can cause pain when applied to an injured area. This is one of the reasons why pain often accompanies inflammation. Moreover, hyperalgesia not only occurs at the site of injury but also in surrounding uninjured areas, so-called secondary hyperalgesia (Lewis, 1935). The mechanism of hyperalgesia is thought to be the result of sensitization of receptors, thereby reducing their threshold. Tissues injured by one stimulus, e.g., heat, also become sensitive to other stimuli, e.g., mechanical. This has led to the speculation that both peripheral and central mechanisms for hyperalgesia may occur (Campbell et al., 1989). The central mechanism may involve enhanced synaptic efficacy between central pain-signaling neurons or changing central inhibitory input.

Finally, nociceptors may become chemically sensitized. Injury to tissues causes the local release of numerous chemicals as part of the inflammatory process and result in the sensitization of nociceptors. These chemical agents include bradykinin, prostaglandins, leukotrienes, serotonin, histamine, substance P, thromboxanes, platelet activating factor, and free radicals. These agents have been shown to cause pain when applied to free nerve endings (Keele and Armstrong, 1964, 1968; Lim, 1970). Some of these agents appear to be released from mast cells, possibly in a sequential manner, because these cells show degranulation during inflammatory responses (Nennesmo and Kristensson, 1981). Campbell et al., (1989) feel that sensitization of nociceptors is the primary mechanism of hyperalgesia owing to inflammation. Sensitization probably relates to changes in sodium conductance in the receptor region brought about by the action of these chemicals on multiple interacting intracellular messenger systems. Substance P is of particular interest because it is felt to be released from unmyelinated afferent fibers upon antidromic axon reflex activation, resulting in the flare response that characterizes inflammation.

Spinal Pain Syndromes

A wide variety of pain syndromes relating to spinal or paraspinal tissue have been defined. The nature of spinal pain varies with such factors as age of the individual at onset, nature and location of injury to the spine, intensity, duration, aggravating and relieving factors, areas of the body to which the pain radiates, and response to treatment.

The literature on spinal pain syndromes is so confusing that systematic classification is impossible. There are, however, a large number of named pain syndromes or diagnoses that have been considered to originate from the irritation of spinal or paraspinal tissues. These diagnoses can be divided into syndromes in which the pain is primarily felt close to the spine and those in which the pain radiates some distance from the spine (Table 13–1). Certain syndromes, such as suboccipital headaches, brachial neuralgia, and lumbago, simply describe the area where pain is felt. Anteflexion headache and lumbar hyperextension syndrome describe syndromes that are aggravated by a particular movement. Sacroiliac pain, postural low back pain, and muscle contraction headaches refer to the supposed etiology of the syndromes, whereas myofascial pain and disc syndrome suggest that the pathogenesis of the pain is understood. This type of terminology reflects the confusion that continues to exist in the understanding of spinal pain and the difficulty clinicians are having in communicating their impression of the disorder from which a particular patient is suffering.

The problem, in part, is due to a general lack of understanding of the pathogenesis of spinal pain. A review of the literature in search of a single etiologic factor that could explain all spinal pain can be very frustrating. There are clinicians and scientists of considerable repute who have implicated each of the various spinal and paraspinal tissues in the etiology of spinal pain, and for most of the tissues there are at least two or three pathological processes that are considered possible causes of the noxious stimulus. Table 13–2 lists the more commonly quoted etiologic factors that are thought to be responsible for spinal pain.

Clinicians need a working model of spinal pain to make sense of the growing scientific and clinical literature on spinal pain and to use the available knowledge on the subject in the practical management of patients. A logical place to start is with the neurophysiological processes that are involved in the genesis of pain in spinal and paraspinal tissues.

Pain-Sensitive Structures in Spinal Tissues

Nerve terminals that might act as pain receptors have been sought in virtually all spinal tissues. Free nerve endings, which appear as complex arborizations of fine, unmyelinated axons under the light microscope (Weddell et al., 1954; Wyke, 1970), have been found most commonly. These endings, which are thought to undergo continuous fragmentation and regeneration, are separated from the intercellular matrix by a basement membrane (Cauna, 1968). Lim (1970) suggests that the anionic receptor sites in pain terminals may be located in the basement membrane surrounding each Schwann cell and its associated axon.

Nerve endings having the potential to react to noxious stimuli are found in a number of spinal and paraspinal tissues. These tissues and their nerve supply make up a spinal nociceptor system and include the following:

1. The skin and subcutaneous tissues of the back contain a dense subepithelial meshwork of thin unmyelinated fibers with fine nerve terminals ramifying between epithelial cells of the skin surface.
2. The paraspinal ligaments—including longitudinal, flaval, interspinous, and sacroiliac ligaments—contain fine nerve endings that have been shown to weave between bundles of ligamentous fibers (Jackson et al., 1966; Wyke, 1970). These fibers are most dense in the posterior longitudinal ligament and least dense in the flaval and interspinous ligaments.
3. The fibrous capsules of the posterior zygapophyseal and sacroiliac joints are innervated through a plexus of fine unmyelinated fibers (Pederson et al., 1956; Wyke, 1970; and see Giles, Chapter 5.)
4. The periosteal covering of the vertebral bodies and arches has a dense plexus of unmy-

TABLE 13–1. PAIN SYNDROMES ORIGINATING FROM IRRITATION OF SPINAL OR PARASPINAL TISSUES

Spinal Pain Syndromes	Referred Pain Syndromes
Suboccipital headache	Occipitofrontal headache
Anteflexion headache	Referred paresthesias
Cervical syndrome	Muscle contraction headache
Acute neck strain	Brachial neuralgia
Chronic neck pain	Cervical or pseudoangina
Quadratus lumborum syndrome	Intercostal neuralgia
Myofascial pain syndrome	Pseudoappendicitis
Fibrositis	Pseudocholecystitis
Psoas syndrome	Sciatalgia
Disc syndrome	Neurogenic claudication
Lumbago	Notalgia paresthetica
Lumbosacral strain	Reflex sympathetic dystrophy
Lumbar hyperextension syndrome	

**TABLE 13-2. FACTORS IMPLICATED
IN THE PATHOGENESIS OF SPINAL PAIN**

Factor	Pathological Process
Intervertebral disc	Degeneration
	Herniation
	Discitis
	Internal disc derangement
Posterior joints	Congenital assymetry
	Subluxation
	Fixation or locking
	Sacrolization or lumbarization
	Rheumatoid or osteoarthritis
Vertebral body	Spondylosis
	Osteoporosis
	Intraosseous hypertension
Ligaments	Acute strain
	Chronic strain
	Laxity or instability
Muscles	Poor muscle tone
	Muscle spasm
	Myofascial pain
Nerve root	Compression
	Stretch
	Inflammation
Sacroiliac joint	Subluxation
	Trauma
	Fixation
	Inflammation
Psychological status	Depression
	Anxiety

elinated nerve fibers that is continuous with the plexus innervating the articular capsule, fasciae, aponeuroses, and tendons (Hirsch et al., 1963; Jackson et al., 1966; Wyke, 1970).

5. The dura mater and epidural adipose tissue contain a plexus of unmyelinated fibers that is more dense in the anterior dural fibers than in the posterior fibers and more dense in the dura itself than in the epidural adipose tissue (Edgar and Nundy, 1966; Wyke, 1970).

6. The walls of arteries and arterioles supplying spinal and paraspinal tissues contain nerves that are carried into the cancellous bone of the vertebral bodies, sacrum, and ilium by blood vessels that supply the bone and can, therefore, be irritated by pathological changes occurring within the bone (Hirsch et al., 1963; Jackson et al., 1966).

7. The adventitial sheaths of the epidural and paravertebral veins have a nerve supply that extends the nociceptor system throughout the epidural and extravertebral connective tissue (Pederson et al., 1956; Wyke, 1970).

8. The paraspinal muscles obtain their nociceptive innervation primarily through the perivascular plexus of nerves lying within the adventitial sheaths of arteries, arterioles, and veins (Iggo, 1961; Lim et al., 1961).

9. The annulus fibrosis contains a fine plexus of nerve fibers in the outer loose connective tissue fibers that is continuous with the periosteum of the vertebral bodies (Stilwell, 1956; Hirsch et al., 1963).

Nachemson (1969) has shown that degenerated intervertebral discs released acidic substances, which may diffuse through the annulus fibrosis and activate nerve endings in the posterior longitudinal ligament, dura mater, and epidural tissues. It has also been demonstrated that degenerating articular cartilage can release inflammatory agents, which may irritate nerve endings in the joint capsule (Melmon et al., 1967; Zvaifler, 1973). The close approximation of the posterior facets, nerve root, and disc and the possibility that inflammatory agents released by irritation of any of these structures could stimulate the same plexus of nerve fibers might be one reason why it is so difficult to differentiate clinically the pain originating from these structures (Fig. 13-1).

Spinal pain may, in certain patients, be due to the subthreshold stimulation of more than one spinal structure through the previously discussed mechanism of hyperalgesia. This could explain the observation by Smith and Wright (1944) that pressure on a nerve root was more likely to cause sciatica if the nerve root was sensitized by disc herniation. The fact that disc herniation by itself need not be painful (Friberg and Hirsch, 1949) also suggests that

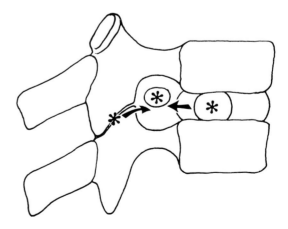

Figure 13-1. The posterior joints, nerve root, and intervertebral disc are in close proximity to each other. Inflammatory agents released from trauma to these structures may stimulate the same nociceptive receptors. (*From Haldeman S. 1978. In AA Buerger and JS Tobis, eds. Approaches to the*

more than one factor is often responsible for spinal pain. This is further supported by the work of Perl (1971) and Sicuteri (1967) who have demonstrated that the threshold for pain in skin and muscle may be lowered by previous tissue damage, repeated nerve stimulation, or muscle ischemia. In the spine, the lowering of the pain threshold by one stimulus may be so great that previously innocuous stimuli could become painful.

Afferent Pathways from Spinal and Paraspinal Tissues

The plexus of nerve fibers that make up the spinal nociceptor system sends impulses to the spinal cord by unmyelinated C (less than 2 μm in diameter) or group IV nerve fibers and, to a lesser extent, by small myelinated A-delta (2 to 5 μm in diameter) or group III nerve fibers. These slow-conducting nerve fibers reach the spinal cord through a number of peripheral pathways (Wyke, 1970, 1976; Brodal, 1969). These pathways are illustrated in Figures 13–2 through 13–5.

The posterior primary ramus of the spinal nerves is commonly made up of three branches (Fig. 13–2). The afferent nerve fibers, which segmentally innervate the skin of the back in a dermatomal fashion, join with muscular branches from the dorsal paraspinal muscles to form the lateral and intermediate branches of the posterior primary rami of the spinal nerves. The medial branch of the posterior primary rami of the spinal nerves is made up of afferent fibers from sensory receptors in the posterior apophyseal joints, the sacroiliac joints, the interspinous ligaments, the walls of blood vessels supplying the paraspinal muscles, the vertebral bodies and their arches, as well as the periosteum, fascia, tendons, and aponeurosis of the spine and paraspinal tissues. The apophyseal joints and posterior structures commonly receive an overlapping innervation from the nerve root above and below the structure, explaining why exact segmental localization of pain is very difficult (Fig. 13–3). In addition, cervical and lumbosacral nerve roots commonly have intersegmental connections (Pederson et al., 1956; Mulligan 1957; Pallie, 1959). The fact that these connections do not exist in the dorsal spine might explain the apparent ability of patients to localize dorsal spine pain more accurately than lumbar pain.

Recurrent meningeal (sinuvertebral) nerves arise from each spinal nerve distal to the dorsal root ganglion and turn back through the intervertebral foramen to supply the posterior longitudinal ligament, the ligamentum flavum, the anterior dura mater, the epidural fat tissue and veins, and the walls of blood vessels supplying the vertebral bodies (Fig. 13–4). Wiberg (1949) describes three patterns of distribution of the sinuvertebral nerve in the lumbar spine and notes that in certain people an afferent branch may

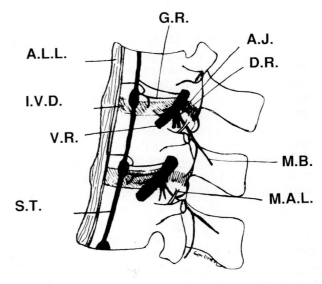

Figure 13–3. Lateral view of the nerves innervating the spinal structure. The medial branch (M.B.) of the dorsal primary ramus (D.R.) travels under the mammilloaccessory ligament (M.A.L.) to innervate the apophyseal joints (A.J.) and other posterior structures. The gray rami communicantes (G.R.), as well as direct branches to the intervertebral disc (I.V.D.), originate from the ventral ramus (V.R.) and travel by the sympathetic trunk (S.T.) to the anterior longitudinal ligaments (A.L.L.) and other anterior structures. (*Drawing by Emile Goubran, MD.*)

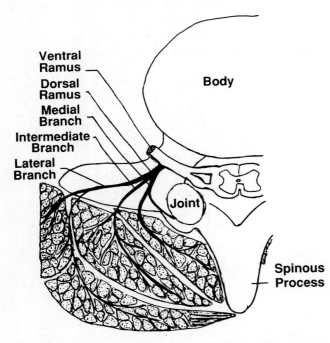

Figure 13–2. The innervation of the posterior elements of the spine by the posterior rami of the spinal nerves. (*Drawing by Emile Goubran, MD.*)

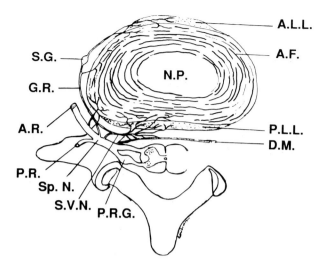

Figure 13–4. The sinuvertebral nerve (S.V.N.) and gray rami communicantes (G.R.), as well as small direct branches to the disc originate from the anterior primary ramus (A.R.) of the spinal nerve (Sp.N.) at the level of its division from the posterior primary ramus (P.R.) and distal to the posterior root ganglion (P.R.G.). The sinuvertebral nerve innervates the posterior aspects of the disc, posterior longitudinal ligament (P.L.L.) and dura mater (D.M.). The gray ramus carries fibers in the sympathetic plexus through the sympathetic ganglion (S.G.) to innervate the anterior and lateral aspects of the superficial annulus fibrosis (A.F.) and anterior longitudinal ligament (A.L.L.). The nucleus pulposus (N.P.) is without direct nerve supply. (*Drawing by Emile Goubran, MD.*)

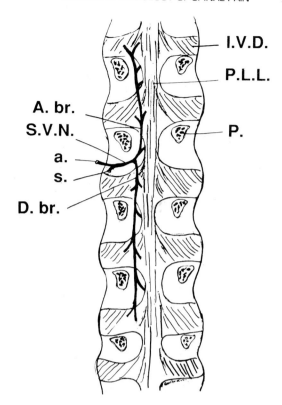

Figure 13–5. The sinuvertebral nerve (S.V.N.) originating from the autonomic branch (a) and the somatic branch (s) divides into an ascending branch (A.br.) and descending branch (D.br.) to pass medial to the pedicles (P.) and innervate the posterior longitudinal ligament (P.L.L.) and intervertebral disc (I.V.D.). (*Drawing by Emile Goubran, MD.*)

ascend or descend up to two vertebral segments to innervate the posterior longitudinal ligament at that level (Fig. 13–5). This anatomic observation may account for poor localization of lumbar pain and why it may be felt to arise one or two segments removed from the irritable lesion (Wyke, 1970).

Three other groups of slow-conducting nerve fibers innervate the spinal cord. Centripedal branches of the paravertebral plexus of nerve fibers extend the length of the vertebral column and innervate the paravertebral venous plexus, longitudinal ligaments, dura mater, epidural fat, vertebral periosteum, and related connective tissue structures (Wyke, 1970). In addition, each primary spinal ventral ramus receives one or more rami communicantes from the sympathetic trunk around the concavity of the vertebral body (Figs. 13–3 and 4). These rami communicantes provide branches to the anterior longitudinal ligament and the anterior and lateral surfaces of the intervertebral discs (Bogduk et al., 1981). Finally, Bogduk et al. (1981) dissected direct branches from the primary ventral rami (Figs. 13–3 and 4) to the posterior lateral aspect of the adjacent intervertebral discs, which he clearly separated from the sinovertebral nerves.

The Termination of Primary Afferent Fibers

The primary nociceptive afferent fibers have their cell bodies in the dorsal root ganglion. The axon of these ganglion cells often follows a highly convoluted glomerular path and then divides into central and peripheral branches (Lee et al., 1986). The central processes enter the spinal cord through the dorsal roots, where the A and C fibers separate into bundles (Fig. 13–6). Primary afferents, particularly unmyelinated ones, are also found in ventral roots, but it is still not clear to what extent they penetrate the spinal cord and participate in nociceptive function. In the dorsal root, the small diameter fibers assume a lateral or anterior position, whereas the larger diameter nerve fibers tend to separate from them more medially (Ranson, 1914; Brodal, 1969).

The dorsal root fibers penetrate the spinal cord, where many of them bifurcate, one branch ascending and one descending. C fibers tend to travel in the most lateral part of the white matter including the Lissauers' tract, and A fibers more medially (Rethelyi and Szentagothai, 1973). The fibers can spread rostrocaudally up to 14 segments in the cervical region in certain animals, although this appears to be less for C fibers and may only be one to three segments above and below the entry level in the thoracic and lumbar regions (Szentagothai, 1964; Imai and Kusama, 1969).

The termination of collateral nerve endings from primary afferent fibers has been determined from numerous staining and electrophysiological methods. Each afferent modality appears to have a fairly unique dorsal horn distribution. The large myelinated fibers from low threshold afferent receptors have been studied by Brown (1981) and Woolf (1987). The hair follicle afferents end in flame-shaped arbors, primarily in the lateral aspects of lamina II and III, whereas mechanoreceptors from the skin spread their endings more diffusely and medially in lamina II through V. Rapidly adapting mechanoreceptors appear to end more medially than the slowly adapting mechanoreceptors (Fig. 13–6).

Small myelinated (A-delta) fibers end at two levels. The first is a fine arborization, mostly in lamina I and dorsal lamina II. The second is in the deeper layers of lamina IV and V. C fiber collaterals, on the other hand, tend to penetrate the dorsal gray matter and terminate in the superficial (lamina I) layers of the dorsal horn. Substance P, which is known to be localized in these afferents, is concentrated in Lissauers' tract as well as the superficial lamina I and II of the dorsal horn (Hokfelt et al., 1975).

Muscle afferent fibers differ from their cutaneous counterparts by terminating in lamina I and in laminae V to VI. There does not appear to be any significant endings in laminae II to IV. The lamina VI endings are in the sites that contain the cells of origin of the spinocerebellar tracts (Molander and Grant, 1987).

Chronic Peripheral Nerve Pain

The injury of peripheral nerves is commonly associated with ongoing chronic pain after the source of injury, such as inflammation, trauma or compression, has been removed. Although some of the mechanisms by which this may occur are due to changes in the central nervous system, there are a number of processes at the site of nerve injury and healing that can explain part of the phenomenon of chronic pain.

When a nerve is originally injured there is a very brief injury potential that can be felt as acute pain. This may be followed by localized inflammation and the process of nociception discussed earlier in this chapter. The elimination of the inflammatory process and the healing of the injured nerves, however, results in a number of changes that make the nerve capable of generating pain in a chronic fashion in the absence of specific nociceptive stimuli.

The regeneration of nerves that have been cut or severely injured starts through the formation of an end-bulb at the proximal stump of the nerve (Devor, 1989). Fine axon sprouts appear from the end-bulb and elongate in an attempt to reach the peripheral target tissue. If progress of the sprout is blocked, then a tangled mass or neuroma is formed. The end-bulb, sprouts, and the neuroma, unlike peripheral nerve axons, are able to generate impulses spontaneously or produce prolonged responses to a broad range of stimuli (Calvin, 1980). Thus, these neuromas become sensitive to very minor mechanical stimuli as well as to changes in temperature and ischemia. Similarly, these endings become sensitive to sympathetic stimulation. They are specifically sensitive to noradrenaline, which may be released from sympathetic fibers caught in the neuroma (Nunn et al., 1982). This process has been used to explain, at

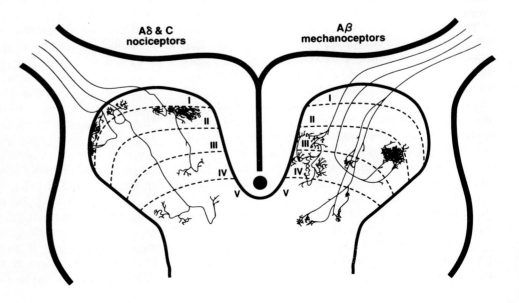

Figure 13–6. The termination of the primary sensory nerve endings in the dorsal horn. The smaller C fibers separate laterally and terminate in lamina I. The Aδ fibers, also more lateral, end in a fine arborization in lamina I and II and have a second ending in lamina IV and V. The larger mechanoreceptor myelinated Aβ fibers separate medially to end in lamina II through V depending on their origin.

least in part, the pain associated with causalgia and reflex sympathetic dystrophy (Devor, 1983).

Another property of injured nerve fibers and neuromas is that of "cross-talk." This is the situation where activity in one nerve is not isolated, as is the case in normal nerve fibers. Instead, activity in one nerve can spread to adjacent fibers. This occurs in neuromas due to the intimate contact of unmyelinated sprouting. Numerous mechanisms for this action has been described (Devor, 1989), among them ephaptic transmission of electrical potentials, release of neuroactive peptides from the peripheral endings of cells, and crossed after-discharge amplification of stimuli. These processes can lead to prolonged generation of barrages of impulses in large numbers of nerves from minor stimulation of only a few fibers.

The Spinal Cord

The Dorsal Horn

The dorsal horn of the spinal cord is the primary location for the interaction and integration of nociceptive stimuli, nonnociceptive stimuli and central pain controlling mechanisms. It is at this level where the intimate interaction between these systems determine which spinal reflexes may be generated and the nature and degree of information that will be transmitted to higher centers. Although the exact mechanisms through which this occurs have yet to be fully worked out, there is a growing amount of research that allows some insight into this integration process.

The cell bodies of neurons in the dorsal horn have been classified according to size, shape, and orientation within six laminae (Rexed, 1952). As noted before, small myelinated A-delta afferents terminate mainly in laminae I, II and V, whereas the unmyelinated C afferents terminate in laminae I and II. The dendritic distribution of cells in each of these laminae have been defined by anatomic and physiological means and allow for integration of activity between laminae in fairly specific patterns. There is, however, some discrepancy between the morphological distribution of cells in specific layers and their physiological patterns of activity, which has yet to be explained (Wall, 1989b).

Primary Sensory Afferents

The primary sensory afferents interact with dorsal horn cells through a number of neurotransmitters. These have been divided by Jessel and Dodd (1989) into specific subgroups. The first includes those transmitters with fast excitatory postsynaptic actions on spinal neurons. These appear to be either L-glutamate or a closely related compound (Haldeman and

McLennan, 1972) that probably is associated with cutaneous and 1A afferent synapses. Adenosine triphosphate (ATP) may be a fast transmitter in low threshold mechanosensitive C fibers. The second subgroup includes several peptides including substance P and various kinins that produce slow excitatory postsynaptic potentials in dorsal horn cells. These peptides are localized primarily in the superficial dorsal horn layers and are felt to modify the responses to the rapidly acting sensory transmitters (Jessel and Dodd, 1989).

The receptive fields of the primary sensory afferents have been studied extensively by electrophysiological methods. The receptive fields for each of the primary stimuli have been determined but are considerably less well defined than initially anticipated. Wall (1989b) describes five classes of dorsal horn cells: (1) low threshold (A-beta) mechanoreceptors, which are found in all laminae but concentrate in lamina IV; (2) thermoreceptor cells concentrating in lamina I and to a lesser extent in laminae III, IV, and V; (3) movement detection cells, which are found in lamina VI; (4) nociceptive-specific neurons; (A-delta and C fibers), which are found primarily in lamina I and to a lesser extent in laminae IV and V; and (5) wide dynamic range neurons, which respond to multiple stimuli from A-beta and C fibers and exist in all laminae.

The Integration of Responses

In the dorsal horn there is no fixed relationship between the input and output of specific cells. The way in which the afferent barrage of new information is processed is mediated by inputs from other parts of the periphery and from the brain. This process results in the highly variable relationship between the nature of an injury and the pain response to the injury. These integrative processes can be divided according to their time sequence into three processes (Wall, 1989b).

Rapid Gate Control. Rapid gate control is the process whereby coincidental activation of large-diameter mechanical stimuli inhibits the response of dorsal horn cells to nociceptive input. This is the most rapid integrative process, lasting milliseconds to seconds, and was first demonstrated by Wall and Cronley-Dillon in 1960 and incorporated into the now famous "gate control" theory of pain proposed by Melzack and Wall (1965). The basic premise that nociceptive input can be inhibited by sensory input from nonnociceptors and from higher brain centers has been repeatedly confirmed (Pomeranz et al., 1968; Price and Wagman, 1973; Burgess, 1978).

This theory has been used to explain a number of treatment modalities. Counterirritation and acupuncture are traditional methods of relieving pain in which a large number of sensory receptors are stimulated, often in the vicinity of the primary painful lesion (Kerr, 1975). There are a number of reports in the literature demonstrating that these procedures can relieve pain (Gammon and Starr, 1941; Stewart et al., 1977). The utilization of trigger point manipulation for the relief of spinal problems may well work through this neural mechanism. The fact that the trigger and acupuncture points have a very similar distribution (Melzack et al., 1977) further suggests a similar mode of action.

Another demonstration of this theory is the observation that partial nerve injury causes or potentiates pain. A number of disorders selectively destroy large-diameter nerve fibers. These disorders include postherpetic neuralgia (Noordenbos, 1959), tabes dorsalis (Brodal, 1969), rheumatoid vasculitis (Weller et al., 1970), and diabetes (Greenbaum et al., 1964). These disorders are often associated with a severe, painful peripheral neuropathy, which at times can mimic radicular pain (Child and Yates, 1978). Nerve compression similarly affects large nerve fibers before small nerve fibers (Haldeman and Meyer, 1970). The question arises whether chronic neuropathies of this type might potentiate the pain that results from minor spinal injuries. Wyke (1976) quotes the observation by Ochoa and Mair (1969) that there is a selective degeneration of large-diameter nerve fibers with increasing age in adult life to explain the diminishing pain tolerance that characterizes older patients. There is, however, some disagreement with this point of view. Dyck et al. (1976) was unable to find any correlation between the amount of pain in peripheral neuropathies and the ratio of small to large nerve fiber degeneration. They also pointed out that certain diseases, such as Friedrich's ataxia, which are characterized by a highly selective large-diameter nerve fiber loss, are not inevitably accompanied by pain. It is likely that many other factors play an important role in the modification of pain in peripheral nerve diseases.

Slow Sensitivity Control. When C fibers from muscles and joints are stimulated for about 20 sec, Wall and Woolf (1984) recorded a rise in excitability in the spinal cord. The excitability dropped after 5 min, followed by a second rise that lasted over 1 hr. The long latency, long duration response produces a large expansion of the receptor fields and can cause nociceptive-specific cells to respond to light stimuli as well as to intense stimuli (Cook et al., 1987). The response is triggered by the arrival of impulses but is sustained by an intrinsic spinal cord process.

This integrative process appears to be due to a different transmitter system that is responsible for rapid excitation of second order neurons. Wall and Woolf (1986) demonstrated that cutting peripheral C fibers causes a change in the peptide content in these cells. When chronically cut to the point where the peptide has changed, only the rapid excitation of dorsal horns remain. The ability to produce prolonged facilitation is no longer present. Wall (1989b) feels that the process of prolonged facilitation or slow sensitivity may be one factor responsible for wide-spreading, slow-onset tenderness that occurs after an injury to deep muscles or joints.

Prolonged Connectivity Control. There is increasing research demonstrating plasticity in the dorsal horn receptor fields based on the input from the periphery and higher centers. The majority of this research has been on the effects of peripheral nerve injury. When a peripheral nerve is cut, the immediate effect is the abolition of the receptor fields of cells that are normally excited by the cut afferents (Devor and Wall, 1981). This is followed over a period of days by a collapse of the presynaptic and postsynaptic inhibitory mechanisms that normally regulate the cells which have been deafferented. These cells become much more excitable, often to the point where they begin to respond to afferents that were previously ineffective. These cells then adopt a larger and different receptor field (Wall, 1989a). These processes are felt to be mediated by the transport of neurochemical substances, such as nerve growth factor (Fitzgerald et al., 1985), rather than by either the fast or slow neurotransmitters.

This process is currently being proposed to explain the often severe pain processes associated with nerve injury including central pain, deafferentation syndromes, causalgia, and reflex sympathetic dystrophy. Wall (1989b) feels that many of the chronic or prolonged painful diseases result from pathological changes occurring within the dorsal horn. These changes produce a state of increased excitability where pain can be triggered by normally non-nociceptive inputs.

Referred Pain from Spinal Structures

The convergence of afferent fibers from skin, viscera, and muscles onto the same cells of the spinal cord (Selzer and Spencer, 1967; Pomeranz et al., 1968) has provided an explanation for the clinical phenomenon of referred pain. The classic experiments of Kellgren and Lewis (1939), recently confirmed by Feinstein (1978), that irritation of spinal and paraspinal tissues by the injection of hypertonic saline can mimic a variety of visceral pain syndromes is one example of referred pain from the spine. The ability of a spinal lesion to mimic the pain of such disorders as angina pectoris, appendicitis, cholecystitis (Kellgren and Lewis, 1939) may, in part, explain the anecdotal reporting of successful treatment of such disorders by practitioners of spinal manipulative therapy.

Central Pain Transmission

As in other areas of pain physiology, there has been a shift in the conceptualization of the central pain pathways. Prior descriptions of independent pathways with well-defined functions have not held up under close scrutiny. The nociceptive somatosensory pathways are now perceived as a series of parallel ascending systems with overlapping functions. Nociceptive information ascends in the brain through the various pathways listed below. However, the distinction between these pathways tends to blur when one realizes that a given neuron in the spinal cord may send collateral projections to several different nuclei in the brainstem.

The basic function of these pathways is to carry sensory discriminative as well as motivation-affective components of pain sensation. In addition, impulses in these pathways trigger both reflex motor and autonomic responses through their connections with specific nuclei. Furthermore, impulses in these pathways appear capable of activating the descending pain control or analgesic system.

The description of the specific pathways is based on the primary termination of its fibers and is not to be interpreted as the exclusive connection that one might infer from the pathway's name. Many authors find that a functional division is of greater value (Wyke, 1976; Dennis and Melzack, 1977). The so-called discriminative system is responsible for determining the location and quality of the painful stimulus, whereas the motivational–affective system is responsible for the emotional responses to pain.

The Discriminative Ascending Pain Pathways

Neospinothalamic Tract. The neospinothalamic tract has been known to be involved in the transmission of pain impulses since Spiller (1905) discovered that pain sensation in humans was diminished after lesions of the ventrolateral quadrant of the spinal cord. Mehler et al. (1960) states that this tract contains the phylogenetically more recent of the anterolateral tracts involved in pain transmission. This tract is considered to be the most direct pathway through which pain impulses from the spinal cord can reach the thalamus (Dennis and Melzack, 1977). It is made up of large diameter fibers having the ability to conduct impulses rapidly (Wyke, 1976). This pathway is not exclusively for the passage of pain impulses,

however. Pomeranz et al. (1968) found that 30% of the nerve units in this tract responded exclusively to noxious stimulation, whereas the other 70% showed polymodal responses to a wide variety of tactile, temperature, and noxious stimuli. The nerve fibers in this tract cross the midline in the spinal cord and ascend in the ventrolateral spinal funiculus. They pass through the lower brainstem in close association with the medial lemniscus and end in the ventral posterolateral nucleus of the thalamus (Getz, 1952; Lund and Webster, 1967). These tracts have also been found to terminate on other thalamic nuclei and certain subthalamic nuclei.

Dorsal Column Postsynaptic Tract. This system is traditionally viewed as carrying only innocuous tactile and proprioceptive impulses. Uddenberg (1968), however, found that over 25% of axons in the dorsal columns of the cat exhibited sustained, high frequency discharges to noxious stimuli. These observations have been confirmed by Angaut-Petit (1975). The nociceptive relays in the dorsal columns differ from the relays of other sensations carried in this funiculus. The proprioceptive relay is by the primary afferent neuron with its cell body in the dorsal root ganglia. The nociceptive relay, on the other hand, is by second-order neurons or postsynaptic dorsal column fibers whose cell bodies are in the dorsal horn of the spinal cord (Angaut-Petit, 1972, 1975). The final destination of these neurons is as yet undetermined. Dennis and Melzack (1977), however, feel that these neurons very likely follow the same course as the other dorsal column fibers to the thalamus, especially the ventroposterolateral nucleus.

Spinocervicothalamic Tract. This pathway ascends in the dorsolateral funiculus to the lateral cervical nucleus. The efferents from the lateral cervical nucleus cross the midline to ascend in the medial lemniscus to the ventroposterolateral nucleus of the thalamus (Dennis and Melzack, 1977). Originally thought to be present only in lower animals, this tract has now been demonstrated in humans (Kircher and Ha, 1968). The fact, however, that the lateral cervical nucleus can only be demonstrated in 50 to 60% of human cadavers (Truex et al., 1970) has led to the suggestion that it may be vestigial in humans. This pathway is intimately involved with the transmission of pain impulses in cats, and Dennis and Melzack (1977) feel that it probably serves a similar function in humans.

Comparison of Discriminative System Pathways. In reviewing the literature and comparing the properties of these three pathways, Dennis and Melzack (1977) feel that the modalities they represent are qualitatively similar and include touch, pain, and temperature. However, there do appear to be minor differences in the type of sensation carried by each pathway; the neospinothalamic tract having a greater pain representation than the other pathways. These tracts all originate from the dorsal horn of the spinal gray matter, conduct at similar velocities, and project predominantly to the nuclei of the lateral thalamus as illustrated (Fig. 13–7). The tracts differ somewhat in the anatomic pathways they follow and the specific thalamic nuclei to which they project. There are also, apparently, some differences in the type of central inhibitory control that can be exerted on these three systems.

Dennis and Melzack have used these data to speculate on the rationale of having three systems for discriminative pain transmission. They feel that this arrangement may allow the response to pain to vary depending on what the person is doing at the time. Conceivably this could occur through inhibition or facilitation of these three nociceptive systems depending on the behavioral state of the body. This may be one explanation why patients with spinal pain show such tremendous variation in their response to pain at different times of the day and under differing circumstances.

The Motivational-affective Pain Pathways

The three pathways of the nonspecific motivational–affective system are illustrated in Figure 13–8. They make up a system rather than individual tracts with specific functions. This system appears to be less important in the perception and localization of pain. Instead, it is responsible for the less conscious spinal, brainstem, and affective responses to pain. It is through this system that an individual automatically withdraws from pain, changes blood pressure, respiratory and heart rate, and passes information to the hypothalamus and limbic system to bring about emotional responses to noxious stimuli.

Paleospinothalamic Tract. The paleospinothalamic tract projects to the midline and intralaminar thalamic nuclei rather than to the ventroposterolateral thalamus, which is the terminal nucleus of the discriminative system. The cells of this tract are located primarily in the deeper lamina (VI to IX) of the dorsal horn of the spinal cord (Albe-Fessard et al., 1974). The fibers for the most part cross the midline in the spinal cord; however, some fibers may ascend ipsilaterally. They ascend in the ventrolateral fasciculus together with the neospinothalamic nuclei, separating medially from the latter tract in the diencephalon to terminate in the medial thalamic nuclei (Dennis and Melzack, 1977).

Spinoreticular Tract. The spinoreticular tract originates from spinal cord cells similar to those of

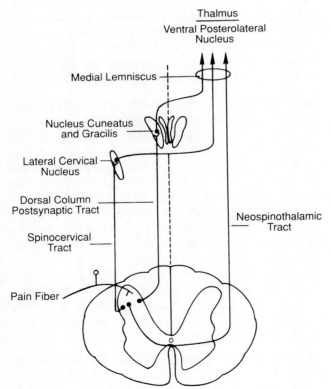

Figure 13–7. The three major pathways of the discriminative pain system between the dorsal horn and the thalamus.

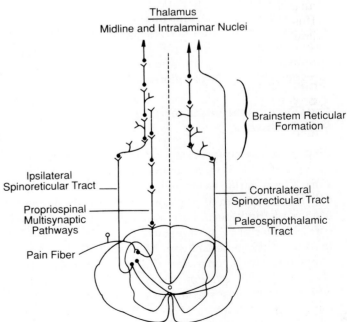

Figure 13–8. The major pathways of the motivational–affective pain system between the dorsal horn and the various

the paleospinothalamic tract and ascends in close approximation to this tract. It differs from the paleospinothalamic tract in that a high percentage of these fibers ascend ipsilaterally (Kerr and Lippman, 1973). The fibers separate from the spinothalamic tracts in the brainstem at various levels to terminate in a number of reticular formation nuclei (Pompeiano, 1973). Reticular formation neurons in turn project to the periaqueductal gray matter where they interact with the descending inhibitory system. There are projections to the mesencephalic nuclei, the dorsal and posterior hypothalamus, and the midline and intralaminar nuclei of the thalamus (Casey and Jones, 1978). The nociceptive input to the reticular formation has been found to be diffuse, poorly somatotopic, and highly convergent with other sensory modalities (Dennis and Melzack, 1977). The paleospinothalamic and spinoreticular fibers have also been shown to conduct at a slower rate than either the dorsal column or neospinothalamic fibers (Feltz et al., 1967).

Multisynaptic Ascending and Descending Propriospinal System.

This system exists in the spinal cord and connects different levels of the cord. The various components of the fasciculi proprii have been reviewed by Nathan and Smith (1959) who include the ground bundles and Lissauer's tract, as well as the cornicommissural, coma, and septomarginal tracts under this heading. These fibers mediate all those functions that continue after the spinal cord has been transected. Hannington-Kiff (1974) feels that these fibers also ascend to the brainstem reticular formation and are partly responsible for the diffuse, nonspecific, persistent responses to painful stimuli.

Endogenous Pain Control Mechanisms

Clinical pain management is difficult because patients with apparently similar injuries show great variation in their pain response. The observation that severely wounded soldiers could block out pain completely was responsible, in part, for the proposal by Melzack and Wall (1965) of the existence of a central mechanism for inhibiting pain sensation. Since then, a number of researchers (Reynolds, 1969; Mayer and Liebeskind, 1974; Adams, 1976) have found that direct stimulation of the medial brainstem and other brain structures in animals and humans can produce almost complete analgesia.

The most consistent results occur on electrical stimulation of the central periaqueductal gray matter of the brainstem reticular formation. The effects are not considered causally related to the reward properties of certain brain centers because it often occurs at electrode sites that do not support self-stimulation (Mayer and Liebeskind, 1974). The inhibition of spinal cord neurons on stimulation of the central gray matter can persist for up to 5 min beyond the actual period of brain stimulation (Liebeskind et al., 1973) and may develop gradually, achieving maximum effect after about 5 min of stimulation (Melzack and Melinkoff, 1974). This latter observation has been considered to be due to recruitment of additional inhibitory neurons and has led to the suggestion that acupuncture analgesia, which shows a similar buildup of inhibition, may be due to activation of the reticular formation. Direct stimulation of dorsal column tracts can similarly cause significant inhibition of pain (Brown and Martin, 1973) presumably by activating inhibitory descending pathways originating in the reticular formation.

The neurons in the periaqueductal gray matter that are responsible for the descending inhibition of spinal neurons have been shown to be the site of action of the opiate analgesics (Kuhar et al., 1973; Adams, 1976; Fields and Anderson, 1978). These sites have been found to be rich in peptides with morphine-like analgesic properties known as endorphins (Hughes et al., 1975; Simantov et al., 1976). The importance of these endorphins in the modulation of pain is becoming better understood as research progresses. A relationship between pain tolerance and cerebrospinal fluid (CSF) levels of endorphins has been noted (Knorring et al., 1978), which led to the suggestion that endorphins are one of the physiological factors that contribute to pain threshold and pain tolerance levels. Patients with severe psychological depressive disorders have been found to be relatively insensitive to pain (Knorring et al., 1974) and to possess increased CSF endorphin levels (Almay et al., 1978). Of similar interest is the observation that acupuncture analgesia can be blocked by naloxone, an antagonist of the opiate analgesics (Sjolund and Eriksson, 1976), and that in certain patients increased endorphin levels in the CSF can be found after electroacupuncture (Sjolund et al., 1977). This suggests that in addition to a spinal gate-control inhibitory mechanism, acupuncture may have a central analgesic action mediated through a release of endorphins.

Another neurochemical agent that appears to be intimately involved in the central inhibitory mechanism is serotonin, or 5-hydroxy-tryptamine. This agent is thought to be one of the primary neurotransmitters in both ascending and descending spinal pathways involved with the modulation of pain sensation. The evidence in favor of this role for serotonin has been reviewed by Messing and Lytle (1977).

Brain serotonin, which is synthesized from the amino acid precursor tryptophan, has been found to decrease when animals have been fed tryptophan-free diets (Fernstrom and Wurtman, 1971). These animals have, in turn, been found to be hyperalgesic to electroshock (Lytle et al., 1975), thus suggesting the potential clinical significance of the neurotransmitter. Moldofsky and Warsh (1978) have further suggested that there may be a measurable changes in free levels of plasma tryptophan in patients with chronic pain such as "fibrobrositis." Attempts to treat these patients by modifying dietary tryptophan, however, proved to be unsuccessful.

The primary pathways that are thought to be important in the descending inhibitory mechanism are shown in Figure 13–9. The periaqueductal gray matter (PAG) can be activated through both ascending dorsal column system pathways (Brown and Martin, 1973) or by descending pathways from higher centers in the frontal cortex or hypothalamus. The PAG,

in turn, appears to inhibit the spinal cord nociceptor neurons directly through tryptaminergic inhibitory pathways and indirectly through pathways using substance P as a transmitter, causing the release of endorphins in the spinal cord (Hughes, 1978). The transmitter released at primary sensory terminals appears to be either glutamate (Haldeman and Mc-Lennan, 1972) or substance P (Krnjevic and Morris, 1974; Hokfelt et al., 1975). This complex interaction of neural pathways and chemical transmitters determines whether pain impulses will be permitted to pass from primary to second-order neurons in the spinal cord.

The pathways in Figure 13–9 illustrate the extent of the central pain control system. It extends from the frontal cortex and hypothalamus through the thalamus, the periaqueductal gray matter, the medullary reticular nuclei, to the spinal cord. It also receives both excitatory and inhibitory inputs from peripheral nerves, both high threshold and low threshold. It is further affected by the various connections between these centers and other parts of the nervous system.

Central Responses to Pain

The response of the brain to painful stimuli is extremely complex. There are very few higher functions that are not influenced to a greater or lesser extent by this extremely powerful sensory stimulus. Figure 13–10 illustrates those central functions that have been demonstrated to be influenced specifically by painful stimuli.

Perception and Localization

The rapid oligosynaptic ascending pathway from the ventral posterolateral thalamus projects to the postcentral region of the parietal cerebral cortex. This primary somatosensory cortex has a strict somatotopic spatial distribution of neurons, which have been named the homunculus (Penfield and Rasmussen, 1950). The back and neck have a relatively small homuncular area of representation in the lateral parasagittal region of the postcentral gyrus. This may account, in part, for the poor ability to localize accurately spinal pain from these regions. Stimulation of the nociceptive pathways to the primary sensory cortex results in the specific anatomic localization of the stimulus and the recognition of the nature of the stimulus; i.e., whether it is throbbing, pricking, pressing, bursting, or burning (Wyke, 1968; Nashold et al., 1972).

Much of the localization and perception of pain is felt to be secondary to concomitant stimulation of mechanoreceptors. This conclusion comes from the

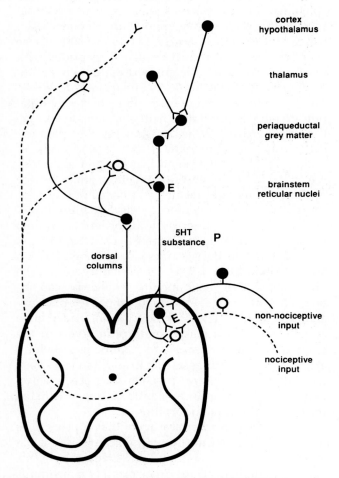

Figure 13–9. The primary pathways associated with the central pain control mechanism. This mechanism can be influenced by incoming afferent impulses or by central mechanisms in the cerebral cortex, hypothalamus, and brainstem.

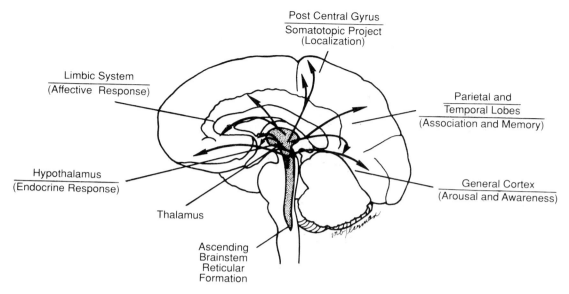

Figure 13-10. The major areas of the brain affected by nociceptive input and that, in turn, influence the response of the person to pain stimuli.

observation that exclusive stimulation of nociceptors results in little or no activation of postcentral cortical neurons (Mountcastle and Powell, 1959). At the same time, direct stimulation of the primary and secondary cortex in unanesthetized patients does not result in the sensation of pain although it does evoke a variety of nonpainful somatic sensations (Penfield and Rasmussen, 1950).

Motivational-affective Response

The distinctly unpleasant emotional sensation that is the hallmark of pain appears to arise from the phylogenetically older part of the brain known as the limbic system. This complex system of centers and pathways provides the mechanism whereby a pain stimulus is perceived as uncomfortable, aching, or hurting. Activation of the limbic system by painful stimuli occurs primarily by neural connections between the intralaminar and medial thalamic nuclei to the cingulate gyrus and orbitofrontal cortex (Purpura and Yahr, 1966; Brodal, 1969).

Destruction of pathways or nuclei within the limbic circuit, such as the orbitofrontothalamic projection system, the medial thalamus, or the cingulate gyrus, results in a loss of this affective component to pain (Wyke, 1968; Cassinari and Pagni, 1969; White and Sweet, 1969). When these pathways or nuclei have been surgically destroyed in humans through procedures such as orbitofrontal leukotomies or stereotactic surgery in attempts to reduce pain, patients have noted that they are still aware of the fact that something is wrong with the body and can local-

ize the sensation (through an intact somatosensory cortex). These patients, however, no longer complain of discomfort or pain (Nemiah, 1962; White and Sweet, 1969).

General Arousal and Sensory Focusing

For the cerebral cortex to receive and interpret a sensory stimulus and bring this sensation into consciousness, it is necessary that the individual be awake and alert. The mechanism to achieve the state of general awareness or wakefulness and to focus attention on a particular stimulus appears to lie in the brainstem reticular formation.

The reticular activating system extends from the medulla to the thalamus and has both ascending and descending components (Bowsher, 1976). Activation of the ascending reticulothalamic pathways by stimulating specific reticular formation nuclei causes generalized cerebral arousal, which can be determined both clinically and through electroencephalography (Pompeiano, 1973). Similar arousal responses can be obtained by stimulating peripheral sensory receptors that connect directly with neurons in the reticular formation. Destruction of the medial reticular formation while sparing the long sensory tracts to the cortex results in permanent coma despite the fact that sensory input can still reach the cortex (French, 1960).

The reticular formation is also, in part, responsible for the focusing of attention on specific sensations. The exact manner in which this takes place is still unknown. One possible mechanism is by modulating the input by the descending inhibitory pathways from the periaqueductal nuclei involved in the endorphin system. This mechanism could, conceivably, close the ''gate'' to all sensations other than that on which attention was being focused (Melzack and Wall, 1965; Mayer and Liebeskind, 1974).

Establishment of Memory Engrams

The exact electrochemical process through which memory engrams are established in the brain is unknown. The storage and retrieval of memory, however, is of major importance in the interpretation of sensory input and allows an individual to correlate the nature, intensity, and associated sensations of the immediate stimulus with previous sensory experiences. This, in turn, allows for an appropriate response to the sensation.

The major storage site for memory engrams appears to be in the temporal lobes, which receive thalamocortical projections from the medial thalamic nuclei (Purpura and Yahr, 1966; Brodal, 1969). The establishment of memory engrams for painful experiences has been noted to be a function of the intensity of the stimulus, the length of time the stimulus lasts, and the frequency with which it is repeated (Wyke, 1976).

Visceral–hormonal Response

The hypothalamus is considered to be one of the major centers for the control of sympathetic and parasympathetic activity as well as hormonal function (Haymaker et al., 1969). Input to the hypothalamus is by medial thalamic nuclei, the reticular formation, and the limbic system (Martini et al., 1971). It is by these inputs that the viscerohormonal responses to pain are mediated. These responses include cardiovascular, gastrointestinal, and hormonal changes (Engel, 1959; Black, 1970). Many of the cardiovascular and gastrointestinal responses are mediated through spinal or lower brainstem reflexes. These responses are modified and coordinated, in turn, by higher centers in the cortex and the hypothalamus. The discovery of a direct effect of enkephalins and opiate antagonists on the secretion of pituitary hormones (Rivier et al., 1977; Graffenried et al., 1978; Stubbs et al., 1978) together with the growing number of metabolic and neuronal functions that are being found to be influenced by these natural peptides, has led to the suggestion that there may be an enkephalinergic system that has a physiologic role in providing a link between perception, behavior, neuroendocrine regulation, endocrine secretion, and metabolism (Stubbs et al., 1978).

Evaluating Spinal Pain

When reviewing the neurophysiology of pain it is very easy to dissociate physiology from a specific clinical situation. However, an understanding of the physiologic mechanisms of pain and the specific anatomic, physiologic, and psychological characteristics of the spinal pain syndromes is essential if one is to approach patients with these problems in a logical manner.

Figure 13–11 presents a conceptual model that provides one method of evaluating a patient with spinal pain. In this model, spinal pain is not equated with any one pathological disturbance, such as disc disease or myofascial pain. Instead, it is viewed as the sum of all the anatomic, physiologic, pathological, psychological, and environmental processes that are known to influence pain. These processes may be present to a greater or lesser extent in any one patient. It is unlikely that any patient with pain can be considered to have only a single localized pathological lesion uninfluenced by psychological factors, sensory input from other receptors, or the general status of the nervous system.

Figure 13–11 has been simplified to include only a few components of pain, ignoring for simplicity's sake environmental, metabolic, and other factors that may be of importance. Similarly, the origin of each of the major components of spinal pain has been reduced to a few examples rather than an extensive list of all possibilities. The component marked ''nociceptor input'' could include any one or combination of the pathological processes that were listed in Table 13–2. These processes can result in tissue destruction and are potential causes of primary back pain (Wyke, 1976). The nonnociceptor input comes from rubbing, heating, or cooling the skin, and from muscle activity, joint movement, or any therapeutic (mustard plaster, electrocutaneous stimulators, etc.) means of stimulating peripheral receptors. This input may have the effect of closing the ''gating mechanism'' in the central nervous system, thereby inhibiting pain. Selective nerve injury caused by systemic diseases such as diabetes and rheumatoid arthritis, or by nerve compression, may also influence the manner in which the painful and nonpainful sensations interact. The possibility that the pain is being felt some distance from a pathological process must be taken into account. Thus, referred pain may be from visceral or somatic structures and may be the primary cause of pain or simply contribute to the discomfort a patient is experiencing. The psychological factors for anxiety, depression, or secondary gain are important components in the central modification of the pain signal and play a

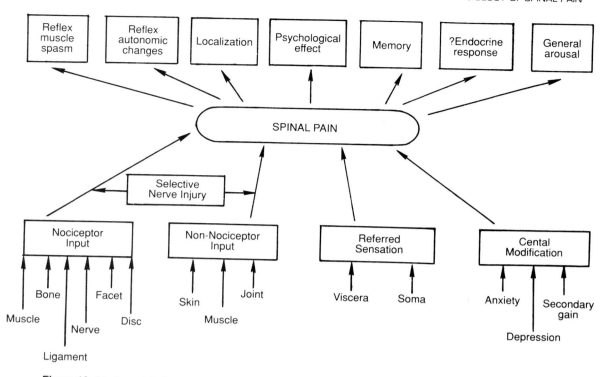

Figure 13–11. A model of some of the factors that make up and influence the sensation of spinal pain.

large part in determining just how the patient will respond to his or her pain.

The impact of spinal pain, in turn, is on virtually all aspects of central nervous system function, and the response to pain is dependent on the overall status of the nervous system. If a complaint of acute spinal pain is viewed as a composite of all these factors, then it should be possible to determine, with thorough examination procedures, the relative importance of these factors in any particular patient.

One of the most crucial points that must be made when reviewing a patient in pain is that there may be an apparent dissociation between observed pathology and patient symptoms (Haldeman et al., 1988). This is especially true in patients with chronic pain. Such patients often appear to act in totally different ways than do those with acute pain. This can no longer be viewed as some vague or inherent psychological status of a patient. Very specific physiological changes occur in chronic pain situations. These changes are listed in Table 13–3. They can occur in the periphery as hyperalgesia or sensitization of peripheral nociceptors. The healing process after nerve injury can result in neuroma formation, which may cause increased sensitivity of nerve endings to sympathetic activity or mechanical stimuli and can cause cross-talk between different nerves. Changes in the input into the spinal cord, in turn,

can cause plastic changes in neuronal connections with loss of presynaptic and postsynaptic inhibition and expansion of receptor fields. The brainstem can modify pain input by changing the degree of activity in the endogenous pain control mechanisms. The entire response of the patient is, in addition, influenced by the patient's coping skills, degree of depression, and general psychological status.

The final analysis of a particular patient's pain status, therefore, must take into account the chronicity of the pain with particular emphasis on the over-

TABLE 13–3. PHYSIOLOGIC CHANGES OCCURRING IN CHRONIC PAIN SITUATIONS

Component	Physiologic Manifestation
Brainstem	Endogenous pain Control mechanisms
Cortex	Depression Coping mechanisms
Periphery	Sensitization Hyperalgesia
Nerve injury	Hypersensitivity Sympathetic sensitivity Cross-talk
Spinal cord	Expansion of receptor fields Loss of inhibition Neuroplasticity

all status of the nervous system and the existence of all past and present painful stimuli, traumatic events, and psychological responses.

References

Adams JE. Naloxone reversal of analgesia produced by brain stimulation in the human. *Pain* 1976;2:161.

Albe-Fessard D, Levante A, and Lamour Y. Origin of spinothalamic and spinoreticular pathways in cats and monkeys. In Bonica JJ, ed. *Pain. Advances in Neurology*, vol. 4. New York: Raven Press; 1974.

Almay BGL, Johansson F, and von Knorring L, et al. Endorphins in chronic pain. Differences in CSF endorphin levels between organic and psychogenic pain syndromes. *Pain* 1978;5:153.

Anguat-Petit D. Post-synaptic fibers in the dorsal columns and their relay in the nucleus gracilis. *Brain Res* 1972;48:380.

Angaut-Petit D. The dorsal column system. I. Existence of long ascending post-synaptic fibers in the cat's fasciculus gracilis. *Exp Brain Res* 1975;22:457.

Black P. *The Physiological Correlates of Emotion*. New York: Academic Press; 1970.

Bogduk N, Tynan W, and Wilson AE. The nerve supply to the human lumbar intervertebral discs. *J Anat* 1981;132:39–56.

Bowsher D. Role of the reticular formation in responses to noxious stimulation. *Pain* 1976;2:361.

Breen AC. Chiropractors and the treatment of back pain. *Rheumatol Rehabil* 1977;16:46.

Brodal A. *Neurological Anatomy in Relation to Clinical Medicine*, 2d ed. London: Oxford University Press; 1969.

Brown AG. The termination of cutaneous nerve fibers in the spinal cord. *Trends in Neuroscience*, 1981;4:64–67.

Brown AG, and Martin HF. Activation of descending control of the spinocervical tract by impulses ascending the dorsal columns and relaying through the dorsal column nuclei. *J Physiol* 1973;235:535.

Burgess PR. Peripheral modulation: Neurophysiological observations. *Neurosci Res Program Bull* 1978;16:160.

Calvin W. Some design features of axons and how neuralgias may defeat them. In Bonica JJ, Albe-Fassard D, Lieboskind JC, eds. *Advances in Pain Research and Therapy*, vol 3. New York: Raven Press; 1980:297–309.

Campbell JN, Raja SN, and Cohen RH et al. Peripheral neural mechanisms of nociception. In Wall PD and Melzack R, eds. *Textbook of Pain*. New York: Churchill-Livingston; 1989.

Campbell JN, Raja SN, Meyer RA, and MacKinnon SE. Myelinated afferents signal the hyperalgesia associated with nerve injury. *Pain* 1988;32:89–94.

Casey KL, and Jones EG. VI Suprasegmental mechanisms. An overview of ascending pathways: Brainstem and thalamus. *Neurosci Res Program Bull* 1978;16:103.

Cassinari V, and Pagni CA. *Central Pain. A Neurosurgical Survey*. Cambridge, MA: Harvard University Press; 1969.

Cauna N. Light and electron-microscopical structure of sensory end organs in human skin. In Kenshalo DR, ed. *The Skin Senses*. Springfield, IL: Thomas; 1968.

Child DL, and Yates DAH. Radicular pain in diabetes. *Rheumatol Rehabil* 1978;17:195.

Cook AJ, Woolf CJ, Wall PD, and McMohan SB. Dynamic receptive field plasticity in rat spinal cord dorsal horn following C-primary afferent input. *Nature* 1987;325:151–153.

Craig DK. Emotional aspects of pain. In Wall PD and Melzack R, eds. *Textbook of Pain*. New York: Churchill-Livingston; 1989.

Dennis SG and Melzack R. Pain-signalling systems in the dorsal and ventral spinal cord. *Pain* 1977;4:97.

Devor M. Nerve pathophysiology and mechanisms of pain in causalgia. *J Anatomic Nervous System*, 1983;7:371–384.

Devor M. The pathophysiology of damaged peripheral nerves. In Wall PD and Melzack R eds. *Textbook of Pain*, 2nd edition. New York: Churchill-Livingston; 1989, Chapter 3.

Devor M, and Wall PD. The effect of peripheral nerve injury on receptor fields of cells in the cat spinal cord. *J Comp Neurol*, 1981;199:277–291.

Dyck PJ, Lambert EH, and O'Brien PL. Pain in peripheral neuropathy related to rate and kind of fiber degeneration. *Neurology* 1976;26:466.

Edgar MA, and Nundy S. Innervation of the spinal dura mater. *J Neurol Nerosurg Psychiatr* 1966;29:530.

Engel BT. Some physiological correlates of hunger and pain. *J Exp Psychol* 1959;57:389.

Feinstein B. Referred pain from paravertebral structures. In Buerger AA, and Tobis JS, eds. *Approaches to the Validation of Manipulation Therapy*. Springfield, IL: Thomas; 1978.

Feltz P, Krauthamer G, and Albe-Fessard D. Neurons of the medial diencephalon. I. Somatosensory responses and caudate inhibition. *J Neurophysiol* 1967;30:55.

Fernstrom JC, and Wurtman RJ. Effect of chronic corn consumption on serotonin content of rat brain. *Nature (New Biol)* 1971;234–62.

Fields LH, and Anderson SD. Evidence that raphespinal neurons mediate opiate and midbrain stimulation produced analgesias. *Pain* 1978;5:333.

Fitzgerald M, Wall PD, Coedert M, and Emson PC. Nerve growth factor counteracts the neurophysiological and neurochemical effects of chronic sciatic nerve injury. *Brain Res* 1985;232:131–141.

French JD. The reticular formation. In Field J, Magoun HW, and Hall VE, eds. *Handbook of Physiology*. Washington: American Physiological Society; 1960.

Friberg S, and Hirsch C. Anatomical and clinical studies on lumbar disc degeneration. *Acta Orthop Scand* 1949;19:222.

Gammon GD, and Starr J. Studies on the relief of pain by counterirritation. *J Clin Invest* 1941;20:13.

Getz G. The termination of spinothalamic fibers in the cat as studied by the method of terminal degeneration. *Acta Anat* (Basel) 1952;16:271.

Gracely RH, Dabner R, and McGrath P. Fentanyl reduces the intensity of painful tooth pulp sensation: Controlling for detection of active drugs. *Anesth Analg* 1982;61:751–755.

Gracely RH, McGrath P, and Dubner R. Validity and sensitivity scales of sensory and affective verbal pain descriptors. *Pain* 1978;5:19–29.

Graffenried B von, del Pozo E, and Roubiech J, et al. Effects of the synthetic enkephalin analogue. FK 33–824 in man. *Nature* 1978;272:729.

Greenbaum D, Richardson PC, Salmon MV, and Urich H. Pathological observations on six cases of diabetic neuropathy. *Brain* 1964;87:201.

Haldeman S, and Meyer BJ. The effect of constriction on the conduction of the action potential in the sciatic nerve. *South African Med J* 1970;44:903.

Haldeman S, and McLennan H. The antagonistic action of glutamic acid diethylester towards amino acid-induced and synaptic excitations of central neurons. *Brain Res* 1972;45:393.

Haldeman S. Why one cause of back pain? In Buerger AA and Tobis JS, eds. *Approaches to the Validation of Manipulative Therapy*.

Haldeman S, Shouka M, and Robboy S. Computed tomography, electrodiagnostic and clinical findings in chronic Workers' Compensation patients with back and leg pain. *Spine 13* 1988;3:345–350.

Hannington-Kiff JG. *Pain Relief*. London: Heinemann; 1974.

Haymaker W, Anderson E, and Nauta WJH, eds. *The Hypothalamus*. Springfield, IL: Thomas; 1969.

Hirsch C, Inglemark BE, and Miller M. The anatomical basis for low back pain: Studies on the presence of sensory nerve endings in ligamentous, capsular, and intervertebral disc structures in the human lumbar spine. *Acta Orthoped Scand* 1963;33:1.

Hokfelt T, Kellerth JO, Nilsson G, and Pernow B. Experimental immunohistochemical studies on the localization and distribution of substance P in cat primary sensory neurons. *Brain Res* 1975;100:235–252.

Hughes J. Intrinsic factors and the opiate receptor system. *Neurosci Res Program Bull* 1978;16:141.

Hughes J, Smith TW, and Kosterlitz HW, et al. Identification of two related pentapeptides from the brain with potent opiate antagonist activity. *Nature* 1975;258:577.

Iggo A. Non-myelinated afferent fibers from mammalian skeletal muscle. *J Physiol* 1961;155:52P.

Imai Y, and Kusama T. Distribution of the dorsal root fibers in the cat. An experimental study with the Nanta method. *Brain Res* 1969;13:338–359.

Jackson HC, Windelmann RK, and Bickel WH. Nerve endings in the human lumbar spinal column and related structures. *J Bone Joint Surg* 1966;48A:1272.

Jessel TM, and Dodd J. Functional chemistry of primary afferent neurons. In Wall PD and Melzack R, eds. *Textbook of Pain,* 2nd edition. New York: Churchill-Livingston; 1989.

Johnson JE, and Rice VH. Sensory and distress components of pain. *Nursing Res* 1974;23:203–209.

Keele CA, and Armstrong D. *Substances Producing Pain and Itch.* London: Arnold; 1964.

Keele CA, and Armstrong D. Mediators of pain. In Lim RKS, ed. *Pharmacology of Pain.* Oxford: Pergamon Press; 1968.

Kellgren JH, and Lewis T. Observations related to referred pain, visceromotor reflexes and other associated phenomena. *Clin Sci* 1939;4:47.

Kerr, FWL. Pain, a central inhibitory balance theory. *Mayo Clin Proc* 1975;50:685.

Kerr FWL, and Lippman HH. Ascending degeneration following anterolateral cordotomy and midline myelotomy in the primate. *Anat Rec* 1973;175:356.

Kircher C, and Ha H. The nucleus cervicalis lateralis in primates including man. *Anat Rec* 1968;160:376.

Knorring L von, Almay BGL, Johansson F, and Terenius L. Pain perception and endorphin levels in cerebrospinal fluid. *Pain* 1978;5:359.

Knorring L von, Espvall M, and Pettis C. Averaged evoked responses, pain measures and personality variables in patients with depressive disorders. *Acta Psychol Scand* (Suppl) 1974;255:99.

Krnjevic K, and Morris ME. An excitatory action of substance P on cuneate neurons. *Can J Physiol Pharmacol* 1974;52:736.

Kuhar MJ, Pert CB, and Snyder SM. Regional distribution of opiate receptor binding in monkey and human brain. *Nature* 1973;245:447.

LaMotte RH, and Campbell JN. Comparison of responses of warm and nociceptive C-fiber afferents in monkeys with human judgements of thermal pain. *J Neurophysiology* 1978;41:509–528.

Lee KH, Chung K, Chung JHC, and Coggeshall RE. Correlation of cell body size, axon size, and signal conduction velocity for individually labeled dorsal root ganglion cells in the cat. *J Comparative Neurology* 1986;243:335–346.

Lewis T. Experiments relating to cutaneous hyperalgesia and its spread through somatic fibers. *Clin Sci* 1935;2:373–423.

Liebeskind JC, Guilbaud G, Besson JM, and Oliveras JL: Analgesia from electrical stimulation of the periaqueductal gray matter in the cat: Behavioral observations and inhibitory effects on spinal cord interneurons. *Brain Res* 1973;50:441.

Lim RKS. Pain. *Ann Rev Physiol* 1970;32:269.

Lim RKS, Guzman F, and Rodgers DW. Note on the muscle receptors concerned with pain. In Barker D, ed. *Symposium on Muscle Receptors.* Hong Kong: Hong Kong University Press; 1961.

Lund RD, and Webster KW. Thalamic afferents from the spinal cord and trigeminal nuclei: An experimental anatomical study in the rat. *J Comp Neurol* 1967;130:313.

Lytle LD, Messing RB, Fisher L, and Phebus L. Effects of chronic corn consumption on brain serotonin and the response to electric shock. *Science* 1975;190:692.

Martelli MF, Auerbach SM, Alexander J, and Mercuri LG. Stress management in the health care setting: Matching interventions with patient coping styles. *J Consulting and Clinical Psychology* 1987;55:201–207.

Martini L, Molla M, Fraschini F, eds. *The Hypothalamus.* New York: Academic Press; 1971.

Mayer DJ, and Liebeskind JC: Pain reduction by focal electrical stimulation of the brain: An anatomical and behavioral analysis. *Brain Res* 1974;68:73.

Mehler WR, Feferman ME, and Nauta WJH. Ascending axon degeneration following anterolateral cordotomy. An experimental study in the monkey. *Brain* 1960;83:718.

Melmon KL, Webster ME, Goldfinger SE, and Seegmiller JE. The presence of a kinin in inflammatory synovial effusion from arthritides of varying etiologies. *Arthritis Rheumat* 1967;10:13.

Melzack R, and Melinkoff DF. Analgesia produced by brain stimulation: Evidence of a prolonged onset period. *Expt Neurol* 1974;43:369.

Melzack R, Stillwell DM, and Fox EJ. Trigger points and acupuncture points for pain: Correlations and implications. *Pain* 1977;3:3.

Melzack R, and Wall PD. Pain mechanisms: A new theory. *Science* 1965;150:971.

Merskey H. Pain terms: A list with definitions and notes on usage. Recommended by the IASP subcommittee on taxonomy. *Pain* 1979;6:249–252.

Merskey H. Psychiatry and pain. In Sternbach RA, ed. *The Psychology of Pain.* New York: Raven Press; 1986:97–120.

Messing RB, and Lytle LD. Serotonin-containing neurons: Their possible role in pain and analgesia. *Pain* 1977;4:1.

Molander C, and Grant G: Spinal cord projections from hindlimb muscle nerves in the rat studied by transganglionic transport of HRP or WGA-HRP or DSMO-HRP. *J Comparative Neurol* 1987;260:246–256.

Moldofsky H, and Warsh JJ. Plasma tryptophan and musculoskeletal pain in non-articular rheumatism ("fibrositis syndrome"). *Pain* 1978;5:65.

Mountcastle VB, and Powell TPS. Central nervous mechanisms subserving position sense and kinesthesis. *Bull Johns Hopkins Hosp* 1959;105:173.

Mulligan JH. The innervation of the ligaments attached to the bodies of the vertebrae. *J Anat* 1957;91:455.

Nachemson A. Interdiscal measurements of pH in patients with rhizopathies. *Acta Orthop Scand* 1969;40:23.

Nashold BS, Somjen G, and Friedman H. Paresthesias and EEG potentials evoked by stimulation of dorsal funiculi in man. *Esp Neurol* 1972;36:273.

Nagi SZ, Riley LE, and Newby LG. A social epidemiology of back-pain in a general population. *J Chron Dis* 1973;26:769.

Nathan PW, and Smith MC. Fasciculi proprii of the spinal cord in man. *Brain* 1959;82:610.

Nemiah JC. The effect of leukotomy on pain. *Psychosomat Med* 1962;24:75.

Nennesmo I, and Kristensson C. Somatopetal axonal transport of fluorescent lectins, distribution patterns and cytophotometric quantification in mouse peripheral neurons. *Neuroscience Letters* 1981;27:243–248.

Noordenbos W. *Pain. Problems Pertaining to the Transmission of Nerve Impulses Which Give Rise to Pain.* Amsterdam: Elsevier; 1959.

Nunn D, Gregy J, Ambrose W, and Hanker J. Histochemical study of autonomic fiber sprouting in traumatic neuroma. *J Dental Research* 1982;61:258.

Ochoa J, and Mair WGP. The normal sural nerve in man. II. Changes in the axons and Schwann cells due to aging. *Acta Neuropathol* 1969;13:217.

Pallie, W. The intersegmental anastomoses of posterior spinal rootlets and their significance. *J Neurosurg* 1959;16:188.

Pederson HS, Blanch CFJ, and Gardner ED. The anatomy of the lumbosacral posterior rami and meningeal branches of spinal nerves (sinuvertebral nerves) with an experimental study of their function. *J Bone Joint Surg* 1956;38A:337.

Penfield W, and Rasmussen T. *The Cerebral Cortex on Man: A Clinical Study of Localization of Function.* New York: Macmillan; 1950.

Perl EP. Is pain a specific sensation? *J Psychiatr Res* 1971;8:273.

Pomeranz B, Wall PD, and Weber WV. Cord cells responding to fine myelinated afferents from viscera, muscle and skin. *J Physiol* 1968;99:511.

Pompeiano O. Reticular formation. In Iggo A, ed. *Handbook of Sensory Physiology. Vol 2. Somatosensory System.* Berlin: Springer-Verlag; 1973.

Price DD, and Wagman IH. Relationships between pre and postsynaptic effects of A and C fiber inputs to dorsal horn of M Mulatta. *Exp Neurol* 1973;40:90.

Purpura DP, and Yahr MD, eds. *The Thalamus.* New York: Columbia University Press; 1966.

Ranson SW. The tract of Lissauer and the substantia gelatinosa Rolandi. *Am J Anat* 1914;16:97.

Rethelyi M, and Szentagothi J. Distribution and connections of afferent fibers in the spinal cord. In Iggo A, ed. *Handbook of Sensory Physiology,* vol. 2. Berlin: Springer-Verlag; 1973:207–250.

Rexed B. The cytoarchitectonic organization of the spinal cord in the cat. *J Comparative Neurology* 1952;96:415–495.

Reynolds DV. Surgery in the rat during electrical analgesia induced by focal brain stimulation. *Science* 1969;164:444–445.

Rivier C, Vale W, Ling N, and Brown M, et al. Stimulation in vivo of the secretion of prolactin and growth hormone by B-endorphin. *Endocrinol* 1977;100:238.

Romano JM, and Turner JA. Chronic pain and depression: Does the evidence support a relationship? *Psychological Bull,* 1985;97:18–34.

Selzer ME, and Spencer WA. Convergence and reciprocal inhibition of visceral and cutaneous afferents in the spinal cord. *Fed Proc,* 1967;26:433.

Sicuteri F. *Vaso-neuroactive Substances and Their Implication in Vascular Pain.* Research and Clinical Studies in Headache. Basel: Karger, 1967.

Simantov R, Keehar MJ, Pasternak GW, and Snyder SH. The regional distribution of a morphine-like factor enkephalin in monkey brain. *Brain Res* 1976;106:189.

Sjolund R, and Eriksson M. Electro-acupuncture and endogenous morphines. *Lancet* 1976;2:1085.

Sjolund R, Terenius L, and Eriksson M. Increased cerebrospinal fluid levels of endorphins after electroacupuncture. *Acta Physiol Scand* 1977;100:382.

Smith M, and Wright V. Sciatica and the intervertebral disc, *J Bone Joint Surg* 1944;40A:1401.

Spiller WG. The occasional clinical resemblance between caries of the vertebrae and lumbothoracic syringomyelia, and the location within the spinal cord of the fibers for the sensation of pain and temperature. *Univ P Med Bull* 1905;18:147.

Stewart D, Thomson J, and Oswal I. Acupuncture analgesia: An experimental investigation. *Brit Med J* 1977;1:67.

Stilwell DL. The nerve supply of the vertebral column and its associated structures in the monkey. *Anat Rec* 1956;125:139.

Stubbs WA, Jones A, Edwards CRW, Delitala G, et al. Hormonal and metabolic responses to an enkephalin analogue in normal man. *Lancet* 1978;2:1225.

Szentagothai J. Neuronal and synaptic arrangement in the substantia gelatinosa. *J Comp Neurol* 1964;122:219.

Truex RC, Taylor MS, Smythe MQ, and Gildenberg PL. The lateral cervical nucleus of cat, dog and man. *J Comp Neurol* 1970;139:93.

Uddenberg N. Differential localization in dorsal funiculus of fibers originating from different receptors. *Exp Brain Res* 1968;4:367.

Vear HJ. A study into the complaints of patients seeking chiropractic care. *J Can Chiropr Assn* 1972;16:9.

Wall PD. Introduction. In Wall PD and Melzack R, eds. *Textbook of Pain.* New York: Churchill-Livingston; 1989a.

Wall PD. The dorsal horn. In Wall PD and Melzack R eds. *Textbook of Pain,* 2nd edition. New York: Churchill-Livingston; 1989b.

Wall PD, and Cronly-Dillon JR. Pain, itch and vibration. *Arch Neurol* 1960;2:365–375.

Wall PD, and Woolf CJ. Muscle but not cutaneous C-afferent input produces prolonged increases in the excitability of the flexion reflex in the rat. *Physiol* 1984;356:443–458.

Wall PD, and Woolf CJ. The brief and the prolonged facilitatory effects of unmyelinated afferent input on the rat spinal cord are independently influenced by peripheral nerve injury. *Neurosciences* 1986;17:1199–1206.

Weddell G, Pallie W, and Palmer E. The morphology of peripheral nerve terminations in the skin. *Quart J Microscop Sci* 1954;95:483.

Weller RO, Bruchner FE, and Chamberlain MA. Rheumatoid neuropathy: A histological and electrophysiological study. *J Neurol Neurosurg Psychiatr* 1970;33:592.

White JC, and Sweet WH. *Pain and the Neurosurgeon: A Forty Years' Experience.* Springfield, IL: Thomas; 1969.

Wiberg G. Back pain in relation to the nerve supply of the intervertebral disc. *Acta Orthopaed Scand* 1949;19:211.

Woolf CJ. Central termination of cutaneous mechanoreceptor afferents in the rat lumbar cord. *J Comparative Neurol* 1987;261:105–119.

Wyke BD. The neurology of facial pain. *Br J Hosp Med* 1968;1:46.

Wyke B. Neurological basis of thoracic spinal pain. *Rheumatology and Physical Medicine* 1970;10:356.

Wyke B. Neurological aspects of low back pain. In Jayson M ed. *The Lumbar Spine and Back Pain.* New York: Grune & Stratton; 1976.

Zvaifler NJ. The immunopathology of joint inflammation in rheumatoid arthritis. *Adv Immunol* 1973;16:265.

chapter 14

Pathophysiology of the Intervertebral Disc

Paul B. Bishop

- • **ANATOMY**
- • **HISTOLOGY**
- • **MECHANOBIOCHEMISTRY**
- • **EFFECTS OF AGING
  AND DEGENERATION**

- • **RECENT ADVANCES IN DISC
  DEGENERATION RESEARCH**
- • **REFERENCES**

For the last several decades, the intervertebral disc has been thought of as playing a central role in the pathogenesis of low back pain. At present however, there is little direct evidence of its exact role in this respect and many fundamental aspects of disc physiology and pathology remain poorly understood (Nachemson, 1975). The gathering of meaningful clinical and basic science data have been hindered by the absence of standardized analytic techniques and investigative procedures. In addition, descriptions of intervertebral disc degeneration have been based chiefly on morphologically defined criteria rather than quantifiable objective findings.

It is now evident that the disc is only one of the mediators of normal spinal mechanics (Kirkaldy-Willis et al., 1978) and that the loss of normal disc function will not necessarily result in a symptomatic patient (Powell et al., 1986). The discogenic component of back pain is most often associated with the end stage of a lengthy degenerative process, and therapeutic intervention at this point has found limited success (Kelsey, 1980). Therefore, recent intervertebral disc research has focused on the early stages of the pathogenesis of disc degeneration, with the aim of providing the opportunity for prevention, early diagnosis, and for more effective forms of treatment.

This chapter reviews the current understanding of the gross and microscopic anatomy of the human intervertebral disc. In addition, a general description of disc ''mechanobiochemistry'' is given to enable the reader to understand more clearly disc physiology and pathology. Finally, some recent advances in disc degeneration research are discussed.

Anatomy

The intervertebral disc is made up of three distinct tissues: (1) the central gelatinous nucleus pulposus (NP); (2) the surrounding fibrous rings called the annulus fibrosus (AF); and (3) the two cartilaginous end plates (CEP) (Fig. 14–1A, B and C), which separate the nucleus and medial annulus from the subchondral bone of the vertebral bodies (Fig. 14–1D).

The disc tissues arise embryologically from the sclerotomes and notochord. During the fourth week of development, the cells of the sclerotomes migrate to the midline to surround the notochord and primitive spinal cord. The formation of the vertebral bodies occurs through fusion of the caudal and cephalic segments of adjacent sclerotomes. Cells from these cephalic segments also give rise to the annulus fibrosus, whereas notochordal cells later differentiate to form the nucleus pulposus. By the tenth week of development, the vertebral bodies develop primary ossification centers and the vertical surfaces become covered with compact bone. At this point, the entire superior and inferior margins of the vertebral bodies are covered with hyaline-like cartilage. At approximately 12 years, ossification centers appear in the outer margins of the cartilage surface and, with cessation of growth (skeletal maturity), they fuse to form a bony ring (Last, 1966; Langham, 1975). The hyaline cartilage held within the ossified ring contains many fine collagenous fibrils (fibrocartilage) and represents the mature end plate.

During fetal development the blood supply to the disc consists of capillary networks supplying the

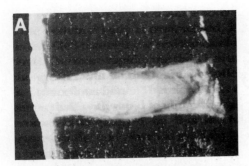

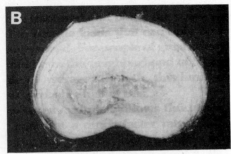

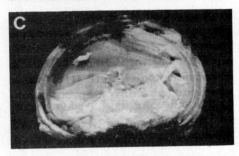

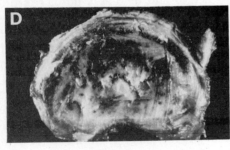

Figure 14–1. Gross anatomy of the healthy intervertebral disc. **(A)** The midsagittal section shows the central bulging nucleus pulposus (NP) surrounded by the annulus fibrosus (AF) and separated from the vertebral bodies by evenly contoured cartilaginous end plates (CEP). Note the slight posterior position (*right*) of the NP and the thick bands of the anterior longitudinal ligament (*left*). **(B)** The disc viewed from above shows the lamellar structure of the AF enclosing the NP, with only thin margins of AF present on the posterior (*bottom*) and posterolateral margins. **(C)** With the AF and NP removed, the extent of the CEP can be seen to separate the NP and medial AF from the vertebral body. **(D)** Immediately beneath the CEP is the subchondral bone of the vertebral body.

outer margins of the annulus and the end plates (Brodin, 1955). The capillaries perfusing the annulus are most abundant in the posterolateral regions. The nucleus has no direct blood supply (Schmorl and Junghanns, 1971). By the fourth year, all of these blood vessels have been obliterated. Thus, in the adult, the disc is an avascular structure and receives its nutrient supply and disposes of its metabolic waste products exclusively by diffusion (Hollinshead, 1965). This process is known to occur through capillary beds adjacent to the end plates and lateral annulus (Nachemson et al., 1970). Of these two pathways, passive diffusion through the end plates has been shown to be the most important (Urban et al., 1977). Investigations of canine intervertebral disc nutrition have demonstrated that physiological levels of exercise are important in maintaining disc nutrition (Nachemson, 1985).

In the healthy disc, branches of the sinuvertebral nerves terminate in the posterior surfaces of the annulus (Pedersen et al., 1956), and the ventral rami and gray rami communicantes innervate the lateral margins of the annulus (Bogduk, 1983). The neonatal disc contains unmyelinated nerves, which disappear with maturation (Wyke, 1987). There is no direct nerve supply to the cartilaginous end plates (Jackson, 1966). Nerve endings have been identified in the fissures and clefts of the degenerate disc and are thought to accompany the ingrowth of connective tissue and blood vessels (Vernon-Roberts, 1977).

At the morphological level, the intervertebral disc has been described as a "connective tissue organ," with each disc tissue having different properties to fulfill its mechanical function (Urban and McMullin, 1985). As shown in Figure 14–1B, the annulus fibrosus is a concentrically ringed structure and is made up of approximately 90 sheets of fibrous tissue (Panagiotacopulous and Pope, 1987). The annular fibers are arranged in a helicoid manner and, in adjacent layers, are oriented at 120 degrees to each other (White and Panjabi, 1978). The medial annulus contains obliquely oriented fibers inserting into the end plates, whereas the lateral annulus is chiefly comprised of vertically oriented fibers (Sharpey's fibres) that insert directly into the vertebral bodies (Galante, 1967). The outer portions of the annulus are not readily distinguishable from the anterior and posterior longitudinal ligaments (Fig. 14–1A). The nucleus pulposus has a bulging, translucent appearance and, in the young spine, can readily be distinguished from the annulus (Fig. 14–1B and C). In the lumbar spine the nucleus is located slightly posterior of the midline (Inoue, 1981) and occupies 35 to 50% of the cross-sectional area of the disc (Bijlsna, 1972, White and Panjabi, 1978). The cartilaginous end plates in the healthy disc are evenly contoured and approximately 3 mm thick. They are located on the inferior and superior margins of the vertebral bodies, covering the area immediately above and below the nucleus and medial annulus (Fig. 14–1A and C). Underlying the end plates is the subchondral bone of the vertebral bodies (Fig. 14–1D). It is comprised of an outer ring of dense compact bone and an inner region containing many small perforations that connect with the marrow cavities of the vertebral body (Coventry et al., 1945).

Histology

The individual characteristic of the three disc tissues is further evidenced by their unique histochemical staining properties (Fig. 14–2). These characteristic appearances arise from the different compositions of each tissue's extracellular matrix. As is discussed later in this chapter, the biosynthesis and degradation of the components of the extracellular matrices are critically important factors in the pathogenesis of intervertebral disc degeneration.

The predominantly fibrillar structure of the annulus fibrosus is organized with the collagen fibers tightly and regularly packed in a layered manner and interspersed with other extracellular matrix proteins (e.g., proteoglycan and elastin). Light and electron microscopic studies have demonstrated that the annulus has a more dense fibrillar structure at its periphery than centrally near the nucleus (Buckwalter et al., 1976). Cell densities in the annulus average 9000/mm^3 (Buckwalter, 1980). The cells of the outer annulus resemble those of ligament and tendon, whereas the cells of the inner two-thirds more closely resemble fibrocartilage with clusters of chondrocytes seen embedded in the extracellular matrix (Pritzker, 1977). The collagen-producing cells located in the annulus are biconvex in shape with elongated nuclei and are distributed along the collagenous fibrils. This gives rise to a meshwork-like structure that restricts the diffusion of large molecules and acts as a permeability barrier to control the transport of extracellular substances (Kramer, 1973). The outer cells contain large numbers of cytoplasmic organelles (Golgi apparatus, mitochondria, and rough endoplasmic reticulum), suggesting that active protein (or glycoprotein) biosynthesis is occurring. The chondrocyte-like cells of the inner annulus are also rich in the organelles associated with protein biosynthesis and are surrounded by a distinct, Alcian blue staining matrix (See Fig. 14–2B).

In the healthy disc, the nucleus pulposus contains a matrix that stains intensely with Alcian blue (Fig. 14–2A and B), and is virtually acellular (average cell density of 4000/mm^3) (Pritzker, 1977; Buckwal-

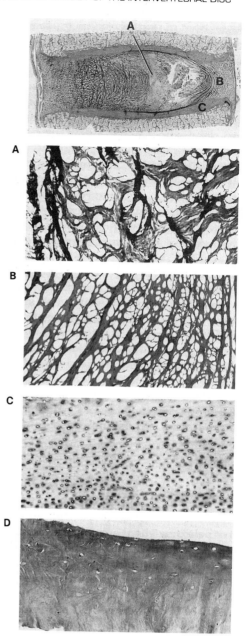

Figure 14–2. Microscopic anatomy of the intervertebral disc. (*Top*) The sagittal section of the intervertebral disc (X64) visualized with contrast histological staining. **(A)** The nucleus pulposus (NP) (X128) has the appearance of a randomly organized collagenous network, whereas **(B)** the anus fibrosus (AF) (X128) has a lamellar structure of tightly layered collagen fibers. **(C)** The cartilaginous end plate (CEP) (X128) has many darkly staining chondrocyte nuclei reflecting the high cell density. **(D)** A higher magnification of the CEP (X640) shows a lower cell density near the surface of the tissue (i.e., adjacent to the vertebral body) with many lacunae.

ter, 1980; Lipson and Muir, 1981). Unlike the dense, lamellar organization of the collagenous network in the annulus, the collagenous fibrils in the nucleus are sparse and oriented in a random manner. Many large noncollagenous matrix proteins are scattered among, and attached to, the fibrils (Inoue, 1971). Electron microscopic examination of the cells in the human nucleus pulposus has shown many vacuoles and glycogen granules, but relatively few organelles (Buckwalter, 1980). Studies conducted using murine discs have shown only poorly developed Golgi complexes in the nucleus, unlikely to be capable of producing a rich proteoglycan matrix (Higuchi et al., 1980).

Hematoxylin and eosin (H&E) staining of the cartilaginous end plate delineates a pink matrix from the blue stain (Alcian blue) of the many chondrocytes (Fig. 14–2C) (Donisch and Trapp, 1971). The end plate cartilage is hyaline in appearance, but at skeletal maturity contains many fine collagenous fibrils (Bernick and Caillet, 1982). The end plates do not have firm attachments to their adjacent vertebral bodies. Scanning electron microscopic studies have shown that there are no fibrillar connections between the end plates and the subchondral bone, thus rendering the end plate vulnerable to horizontal shearing forces (Inoue, 1981). The subchondral bone is trabecular in the central regions (Fig. 14–2C) and is similar to that found in the marrow cavity of the vertebral body. As illustrated by Figure 14–2C, the end plate has a high density of chondrocytes (15,000/mm³), which contain well-developed Golgi complexes (Higuchi et al., 1982a,b). It has been suggested that the cells of the end plate are the main source of the extracellular matrix components for all disc tissues (Bishop and Pearce, 1988).

Mechanobiochemistry

In the mature, nondegenerate state, the intervertebral disc tissues have relatively low cell densities (Eyring, 1969). Therefore, it is the properties of the extracellular matrix that are responsible for the functional capacity of the disc in vivo (Urban and Maroudas, 1980). The extracellular matrices of the disc tissues consist chiefly of collagenous fibers embedded in a semifluid gel of proteoglycan (and small amounts of other proteins) and water. The collagen of the human intervertebral disc is almost entirely type II. In the annulus and end plate, type I collagen is also found; type II predominates in the inner lamellae and type I in the outer layers (Eyre and Muir, 1977; Eyre, 1980). From a biomechanical point of view, the primary roles of the collagenous fiber meshwork are to retain the highly hydrated proteoglycan molecules and to limit the swelling of the tissue (Eyre, 1980). Thus, the ability of the healthy

disc to absorb compressive loads and to redistribute mechanical forces effectively results from the fluidity and noncompressibility of the aqueous gel containing the proteoglycan molecules (Spilker, 1980; Maroudas et al., 1986). The water content of the individual tissues of healthy discs has been reported as 90% in the nucleus pulposus, 78% in the annulus fibrosus (Naylor and Horton, 1955; Panagiotacopulous et al., 1987), and 75% in the cartilaginous end plates (Bishop, 1988).

Experiments conducted using a needle probe attached to a manometer have measured substantial hydrostatic pressures inside the nucleus pulposus (Nachemson, 1975). The high swelling pressure exhibited by the nucleus, which is balanced by the compressive load on the spine, is due to the unique properties of large, negatively charged glycoproteins called proteoglycans (Urban, 1977; Urban and McMullin, 1988). Proteoglycans are now thought to be the chief cellular indicators of disc functional capacity and appear to be the key to understanding the pathogenesis of disc degeneration (Bishop, 1988). Electron microscopic studies have shown that intervertebral disc proteoglycans have a bottle brush-like structure (Fig. 14–3) (Rosenberg et al., 1970). They

Proteoglycan Monomer

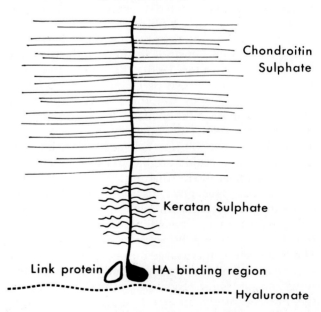

Chondroitin Sulphate

Keratan Sulphate

Link protein   HA-binding region

Hyaluronate

Figure 14–3. The proteoglycan monomer. The bottle brush-like structure of a proteoglycan monomer consists of a central protein core with a globular region at the amino terminus called the hyaluronic acid (HA)-binding region. This specialized region (with the link protein) facilitates binding the monomer to a long polysaccharide chain of hyaluronate. Attached to the protein core in distinct regions are many long-chain polysaccharides called glycosaminoglycans, which are negatively charged in vivo. The two most commonly found glycosaminoglycans in the intervertebral disc are chondroitin sulfate (ChS) and keratan sulfate (KS).

are made up of varying numbers, sizes, and types of polyanionic sulfated polysaccharide chains (glycosaminoglycans) covalently attached to a shared protein core (Kuettner and Kimura, 1985). The glycosaminoglycans are polysaccharides comprised of disaccharide repeating units. Each unit consists of an amino sugar linked by a glycosidic bond to a non-nitrogenous sugar (Bayliss et al., 1978). The amino sugar or hexosamine may be either D-glucosamine or D-galactosamine and the nonnitrogenous sugar either D-glucuronic acid and/or L-iduronic acid or, in the case of keratan sulfate, D-galactose (Fig. 14–4). Each disaccharide unit (except in hyaluronate) may also contain one or more ester sulfate groups. At physiological pH, the sulfate ester groups hold a negative charge. This results in a molecule containing long chains of polyanions that attract counter-

ions in Donnan equilibrium and contributes to the tissue's tendency to bind water and swell (Maroudas, 1973). As shown in Figure 14–5, proteoglycan molecules can align themselves along a chain of hyaluronic acid (HA) at intervals of approximately 30 to 40 disaccharide units through a noncovalent interaction between their HA binding region (HABR) and a section of the HA chain at least 10 disaccharides long (Pedrini and Ponseti, 1973; Hascall and Heinegard, 1974). This gives rise to extremely large aggregates having molecular weights of approximately 200 million daltons (Buckwalter et al., 1985). The interaction between the specialized terminus of the core protein (HABR) and the HA chain is facilitated and stabilized by a globular polypeptide termed a link protein (Hardingham, 1979).

Studies of the proteoglycan composition of the

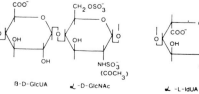

Figure 14–4. The glycosaminoglycans found in the intervertebral disc. Note that the sulfate ester and carboxyl groups are negatively charged at physiological pH. The abbreviations used are: β-D-GlcNAc (β-D-N-acetylglucosamine), β-D-GalNAc (β-D-N-acetylgalactosamine), β-D-G1cUA (β-D-glucuranic acid), β-D Gal (β-D-galactose), α-L-IdUA (α-L-iduronic acid), α-D-GlcNAC (α-D-N-acetylglucosamine).

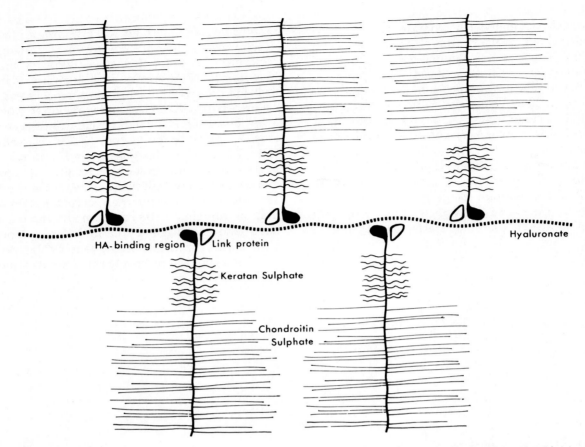

Figure 14–5. The proteoglycan aggregate. Proteoglycan monomers are aligned along chains of hyaluronate at intervals of 30 to 40 disaccharide units through a noncovalent interaction between the hyaluronate (HA) binding site and a section of the hyaluronate chain at least 10 disaccharide units long. This gives rise to extremely large aggregates (and

disc tissues in the human infant demonstrated that: (1) the aggregating and nonaggregating molecules in the nucleus pulposus resemble those found in the end plate; (2) the nucleus contains a large population of small aggregates; and (3) the average length of the disc monomers is similar. These findings are consistent with the hypothesis that proteoglycan biosynthesis is centered (and controlled) at a single site, possibly in the cartilaginous end plates.

Effects of Aging and Degeneration

A detailed morphological study of degenerative changes in 100 lumbar spines conducted by Vernon-Roberts has produced a systematic description of intervertebral disc degeneration (Vernon-Roberts, 1981). The first morphologically identifiable events in this process are the appearance of splits and clefts in the nucleus pulposes (Fig. 14–6A and B). These clefts increase in size and number to coalesce eventually and extend into the annulus fibrosus. The poste-

rior and posterolateral regions of the annulus are favored locations for this process to occur because, as previously described, the annulus is thinner on its posterior aspect and the posterolateral regions have been weakened by the obliterated blood vessels present in the fetal disc. These changes are often accompanied by circumferential clefts between the layers of the annulus. As these tears enlarge, they predispose the disc to additional injury, particularly through torsion strain, which will in turn further enlarge the gaps in the annulus, eventually leading to disc herniation (Kirkaldy-Willis et al., 1978). Other clefts can occur in the nucleus at right angles to the plane of the disc, extending into the end plate to produce eventually herniation into the vertebral bodies (Schmorl's nodes). The net effect of these changes is to reduce the height of the disc and thereby significantly alter the biomechanical equilibrium that exists in the healthy motion segment.

The earliest microscopic changes that take place in the disc with aging and degeneration occur in the cartilaginous end plates (Pritzker, 1977). Cell death

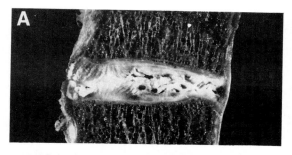

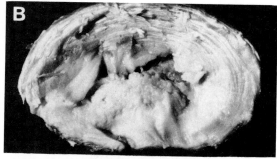

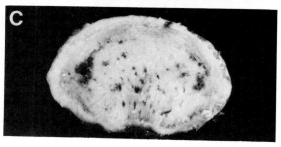

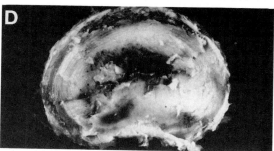

Figure 14-6. Gross anatomy of the degenerate intervertebral disc. **(A)** The midsagittal section shows marked loss of disc height, many fissures and clefts in the annulus fibrosus (AF) and the nucleus pulposus (NP) and numerous focal defects in the cartilaginous end plates (CEP). Osteophyte formation is evident on the anterior margins (*left*) of the vertebral bodies. **(B)** The disc viewed from above shows that the larger clefts are in the NP and medial AF and are extending into the posterolateral margins of the disc. **(C)** The CEP has an irregular appearance with many small defects present that penetrate to the underlying subchondral bone. **(D)** With the CEP removed, the subchondral bone contains regions of calcification, resulting in a pitted appearance.

and metachromasia are seen in the superficial layers and are accompanied by the loss of the normal-ordered array of tissue chondrocytes. These changes have been likened to those seen in osteoarthritic cartilage and are thought to represent an attempt by the tissue to repair itself (Pritzker, 1977; Buckwalter, 1980). In moderately degenerate discs, fissuring and fibrillation of the superficial layers of the end plate are seen. These changes coincide with calcification and replacement of the deeper layers by endochondral ossification (Fig. 14–6C and D). With more advanced aging and/or degeneration, marked thinning of the end plate occurs and focal defects appear. The subchondral bone becomes irregular and eventually leads to sclerotic change (Vernon-Roberts, 1977).

With age, the matrix of the nucleus pulposus changes its histochemical staining characteristics and becomes less distinguishable from the matrix of the annulus. After age 30, large chondroid cells appear in increasing numbers in the nucleus (Pritzker, 1977). The fibrocytes in the annulus produce an Alcian blue matrix that separates the collagen fibers surrounding each cell. This process (annular cell metaplasia) begins in the transition zone (TZ) between the annulus and nucleus. At the same time, fraying and splitting of the innermost annular fibers are seen, and the large chondroid cells seen in the nucleus begin to appear in the TZ. In the advanced stages of degeneration, large pools of Alcian blue matrix appear between the annular fibers. The histological features of end plate age-related change are typically first evident in the third decade (Herbert, 1975). Cell death and focal loss of metachromasia are seen in the superficial layers with disorganization and clumping of the chondrocytes also appearing in the central portion of the end plate (Aoki et al., 1987). In the early stages of degeneration, regenerative changes such as increased metachromasia of territorial matrix may be seen. In advanced degeneration, the deeper cartilage cells become calcified, preventing the remaining CEP cells from receiving nutrition and leading to end plate destruction. A decrease in the supply of nutrients to the end plate also has severe consequences for the maintenance of the annulus (Higuchi and Abe, 1987) and is thought to lead directly to degeneration of the nucleus (Pritzker, 1977).

At the molecular level, the most notable changes that occur in the disc proteoglycans with aging and degeneration are reduction in the total proteoglycan and water content with a concomitant relative increase in collagen (Adams and Muir, 1986). These changes are most prominent in the nucleus pulposus (Urban and McMullin, 1988). The proportion of aggregating proteoglycan in the disc decreases with aging, whereas the proportion of nonaggregating proteoglycan increases (Adams and Muir, 1976). These changes are likely due to a decrease in the length of the protein core, because the chain lengths of the predominant glycosaminoglycans (ChS and KS) remain unchanged (Pedrini-Mille et al., 1980). Other investigators have reported a higher proportion of aggregated proteoglycan, a higher ratio of glucosamine to galactosamine (KS to ChS), and a higher proportion of chondroitin 6-sulfate relative to chondroitin 4-sulfate in the nucleus of degenerate discs (Lyons et al., 1981). These observations may be complicated by the apparent ability of the intervertebral disc to respond to degenerative change by activating proteoglycan biosynthesis (McDevitt et al., 1981). Studies using artificially induced herniation of rabbit nucleus and chemonucleolysis of dog nucleus have shown evidence of an initiated repair mechanism (Lipson and Muir, 1981; Bradford et al., 1984). This response is perhaps similar to that observed in osteoarthritic knee cartilage, where the proteoglycans isolated from degenerate tissue contain regions with larger chondroitin sulfate chains than in normal tissue (Cox et al., 1985).

Recent Advances in Disc Degeneration Research

The interpretation of many early studies investigating changes in the intervertebral disc with aging and degeneration has been made difficult because: (1) degenerate discs collected surgically have been compared with control discs collected postmortem; (2) the state of degeneration has been ill defined; and (3) few specimens have been examined (Bishop, 1988).

Recent research has resulted in two significant advances that show promise in overcoming these difficulties. First, magnetic resonance imaging (MRI) has provided investigators with an accurate in vivo method of imaging the spine and its associated soft tissues. This technique offers immediate clinical and scientific relevance to the study of degeneration, as it has allowed the correlation of morphological, chemical, mechanical, radiological, and epidemiological data with a standard reference. Magnetic resource imaging signal changes have been shown to be associated with degenerative disc disease, disc herniation, infection, and surgical intervention (Chaffetz et al., 1983; Han et al., 1983; Modic, 1983; Modic et al., 1984; Aguila et al., 1985; Maravilla et al., 1985; Pech and Haughton, 1985).

Figures 14–7 and 14–8 compare the gross morphology and magnetic resonance images of lumbar spines containing healthy (Fig. 14–7) and degenerate discs (Fig. 14–8). It is readily apparent that MRI is capable of discerning subtle changes in disc morphol-

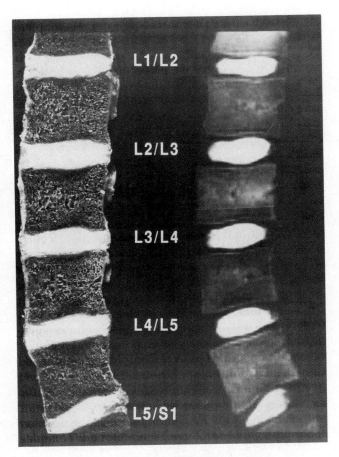

Figure 14–7. Gross morphology and magnetic resonance image (MRI) of the midsagittal section of a lumbar spine containing healthy discs. The L1-2 to L5-S1 discs of a 16-year-old boy are shown. The gross morphology (*left*) illustrates the appearance of healthy intervertebral discs, with a gelatinous nucleus pulposus readily distinguishable from the fibrous annulus. The cartilaginous end plates are smooth with a slight concave contour. The margins of the vertebral bodies are smooth and rounded. The MRI (*right*) has a homogeneous and bright signal in the region of the nucleus revealing a clear demarcation between annulus and nucleus. The region of the CEP appears as a single dark line, which clearly demarcates the vertebral body from the nucleus. The contour of the vertebral body margin is smooth and rounded with no projections.

ogy. The uniform high intensity signal from the nucleus present in healthy discs can be seen to develop a region of decreased signal intensity centrally in degenerate discs. This region of decreased signal parallels the vertebral end plates (Aquila et al., 1985). Further degenerative change results in diminution of the high-intensity signal from the nucleus, and the sharp difference in the signal intensities between the nucleus and the annulus can no longer be distinguished.

Magnetic resonance imaging has several advantages over plain film radiography in the assessment of disc status. The chief limitations of plain film radi-

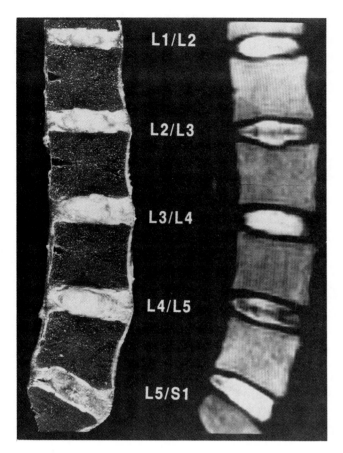

Figure 14-8. Gross morphology and magnetic resonance image (MRI) of a midsagittal section of a lumbar spine containing degenerated discs. The L1-2 to L5-S1 discs of a 47-year-old man are shown. The gross morphology (*left*) of the L4-5 and L5-S1 discs shows a consolidated nucleus pulposus containing mucinous material. The demarcation between annulus and nucleus is indistinct, and focal gaps and defects are present in both the annulus and nucleus. A relative widening of the annular zone is apparent. There is thinning of the cartilaginous end plates and the contour of the subchondral plate is undulating. Cartilaginous or compact bony lipping of the margins of the vertebral bodies can be seen. The MRI (*right*) has an overall diminished signal intensity (*light gray*) with a stippled appearance of brighter and darker signals (L4-5). Distinct gray horizontal bands are seen within the nuclear zone (L2-3). Areas of dark signal intensity within the annulus can be seen where it meets the end plate (L2-3). The margins of the vertebral bodies are tapered and slightly pointed and projections from the vertebral body are present.

ography are that the observed changes reflect more severe and/or advanced stages of degeneration (i.e., early changes are not seen). Figure 14–9 compares a plain film radiograph with an MRI of a degenerate disc in the lower lumbar spine. This comparison demonstrates that what appears as relatively mild degenerative changes on x-ray, are seen to coincide with substantial loss of MRI signal, reflecting marked changes in disc morphology.

The basis of the second advancement in the understanding of disc degeneration pathogenesis has arisen from studies relating changes in disc biochemistry to changes in disc morphology and, more recently, to changes in the MRI of the disc. A number of earlier investigations have established that degenerative changes in the intervertebral disc are intimately related to changes in proteoglycan content (Pearce and Grimmer, 1976). It has now been established that a systemic depletion of proteoglycan from the entire lumbar spine predisposes all the lumbar intervertebral discs to degeneration (Pearce et al., 1987). Thus, the low proteoglycan concentration seen in degenerate discs appears to induce, rather than result from, degeneration.

Other investigations have shown that aging and degeneration of the intervertebral disc are distinct processes, because each affects a different category of proteoglycan (with different glycosaminoglycan compositions) (McDevitt, 1981). In addition, other studies have linked degenerative changes in connective tissues to a lack of sufficient turnover of aging matrix molecules (Poole, 1986). Several investigators have also reported the presence of proteoglycan-specific degradative enzyme activity in osteoarthritic knee cartilage (Sokoloff, 1987). Studies of changes in the proteoglycan composition of end plate with human lumbar disc degeneration have identified alterations in the distribution of selective proteoglycan subspecies (Bishop and Pearce, 1988). Recent investigations have also suggested that proteoglycan content may be an important determinant of disc MRI signal intensity. It has been demonstrated that early changes in nucleus pulposus MRI coincide with loss of proteoglycan content (Thompson et al., 1988).

From these observations a model describing the earliest events of the degenerative process has been hypothesized. It suggests that a previously unknown class of proteolytic enzymes (metalloproteases) is activated and selectively digests specific proteoglycan subspecies so that a different population of proteoglycans are affected by degeneration than by aging. Furthermore, the proteases involved in the degenerative process have degradative activities much greater than agents involved with disc aging. The disc then attempts to repair itself by maximally activating proteoglycan biosynthesis, but the rate of replacement is inadequate to balance the rate of degradation. With continued degradation, the size of the proteoglycan molecules decreases to the point where they are able to diffuse through the holes in the enclosing collagen meshwork and are then lost from the tissue. Thus, the ability of the tissue to imbibe water is substantially decreased, compressibility is markedly diminished, and functional capacity greatly reduced.

X-RAY   NMR

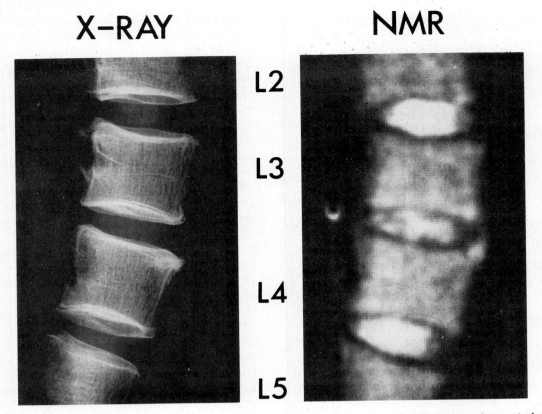

Figure 14-9. Plain film radiography and nuclear magnetic resonance (NMR) image or MRI of the lateral aspect of a lumbar spine. The x-ray of the lumbar spine shows evidence of osteophyte formation on the anterior superior margin of the L-4 vertebral body, and there is evidence of mild disc thinning. These findings represent the early radiological signs of a degenerating disc at the L3-4 level. The NMR image of the same disc illustrates that the L3-4 disc differs significantly from the adjacent discs and has undergone marked degenerative change.

As diagnostic techniques capable of recognizing degenerative change at the molecular level are developed and the characteristics of these metalloproteases become better understood, it will then become possible to devise therapeutic strategies to inhibit or eliminate their degradative actions and thereby greatly reduce the contribution of intervertebral disc degeneration to the pathogenesis of back pain.

References

Adams P, and Muir H. Qualitative changes with age of human lumbar discs. *Ann Rheum Dis* 1976;35:289.

Adams P, and Muir H. Quantitative changes with age of proteoglycans of human lumbar discs. *Ann Rheum Dis* 1976;35:284–296.

Aguila LA, Pirdino DW, and Modic MT, et al. The intranuclear cleft of the intervertebral disc. *Radiology* 1985;155:155–158.

Aoki J, Yamamoto I, and Kitamura N, et al. End-plate of the discovertebral joint: Degenerative change in the elderly adult. *Radiology* 1987;164:411–414.

Bayliss MT, Ridgway GD, and Ali SY. Age related changes in the composition and structure of human articular cartilage proteoglycans. *Biochem J* 1978;176–683.

Bernick S, and Caillet R. Vertebral end-plate changes with ageing of human vertebrae. *Spine* 1982;7:97–102.

Bijlsna F. The ageing pattern of the human intervertebral disc. *Gerontologia* 1972;18:157–167.

Bishop PB. Proteoglycans and degenerative spondylosis. *J Manip Phys Ther* 1988;36–39.

Bishop PB, and Pearce RH. Changes in the proteoglycans of the human intervertebral disc cartilaginous end-plate with ageing and degeneration. *Trans Orthop Res Soc* 1988;13:152.

Bogduk N. The innervation of the lumbar spine. *Spine* 1983;8:286.

Bradford DS, Oegema T, and Cooper K, et al. Chymopapain, chemonucleolysis and nucleus pulposus regeneration. A biochemical and biomechanical study. *Spine* 1984;9:135.

Brodin H. Path of nutrition in articular cartilage and the intervertebral disc. *Acta Orthop Scand* 1955;24:177.

Buckwalter JA, Pedrini-Mille A, Pedrini V, and Tudisco C. Proteoglycans of human infant intervertebral disc. *J Bone Joint Surg* 1985; 67-A:284–294.

Buckwalter JA, Cooper RR, and Maynard JA. Elastic fibres in human intervertebral discs. *J Bone Joint Surg* 1976;58-A:73–76.

Buckwalter JA. Fine structures of the human intervertebral disc. In Kelsey J, White A, and Mosby CV, eds. *American Academy of Orthopaedic Surgeons Symposium on Low Back Pain.* Philadelphia: 1980.

Coventry MB, Ghormley RK, and Kernohan JW. The intervertebral disc: its microscopic anatomy and pathology. Part I: Anatomy, development and physiology. *J Bone and Joint Surg* 1945;27:105–112.

Cox JM, McDevitt CA, Arnoczky SP, and Warren RF. Changes in the chondroitin sulphate-rich region of proteoglycans in experimental osteoarthritis. *Biochim Biophys Acta* 1985;850:228.

Chaffetz NI, Genant HK, Moon KL, et al. Recognition of lumbar disc herniation with NMR. *Am J Radiol* 1983;141.

Donisch EW, and Trapp W. The cartilage end-plates of the human vertebral column. Some considerations of postnatal development. *Anat Rec* 1971;169:705–716.

Eyre D, and Muir H. Quantitative analysis of types I and II collagens in human intervertebral discs at various ages. *Biochim Biophys Acta* 1977;492:29–42.

Eyre D. Biochemistry of the intervertebral disc. *Int Rev Connect Tissue Res* 1980;8:227.

Eyring EJ. The biochemistry and physiology of the intervertebral disc. *Clin Orthop* 1969;67:16–28.

Galante J. Tensile properties of the human lumbar annulus fibrosus. *Acta Orthop Scand* (Suppl) 1967;100.

Han JS, Kaufman B, and El Yousef SJ, et al. NMR imaging of the spine. *Am J Rad* 1983;141:1137–1145.

Hardingham TE. The role of link protein in the structure of cartilage proteoglycan aggregates. *Biochem J* 1979;177:237.

Hascall V, and Heinegard D. Aggregation of proteoglycans. I. The role of hyaluronic acid. *J Biol Chem* 1974;249:4232.

Herbert CM, Lindberg KA, Jayson MIV, and Bailey AJ. Intervertebral disc collagen in degenerative disc disease. *Ann Rheum Dis* 1975; 34:467.

Higuchi M, Kaneda K, and Abe K. Age-related changes in the nucleus pulposus of the intervertebral disc in mice: An electronmicroscopic study. *J Jpn Orthop Assoc* 1980;22:184–192.

Higuchi M, Kaneda K, and Kazuhiro A. Postnatal histiogenesis of the cartilage plate of the spinal column: electron microscopic observations. *Spine* 1982a;7:89–96.

Higuchi M, Kaneda K, and Abe K. Postnatal histiogenesis of the cartilage plate of the spinal column. *Spine* 1982b;7:89–96.

Higuchi M, and Abe K. Postmortem changes in ultrastructures of the mouse intervertebral disc. *Spine* 1987;12:48.

Hollinshead WH. Anatomy of the spine: Points of interest to orthopaedic surgeons. *J Bone Joint Surg* 1965;47-A:209.

Inoue H, and Takeda T. Three-dimensional observations of collagen framework of lumbar intervertebral discs. *Acta Orthop Scand* 1975;46:949–956.

Inoue H. Three-dimensional architecture of lumbar intervertebral discs. *Spine* 1981;6:139–146.

Jackson HC. Nerve endings in the human lumbar spinal column and related structures. *J Bone Joint Surg* 1966;48A:1272.

Kelsey JL. *Epidemiology of low back pain.* American Academy of Orthopaedic Surgeons Symposium on Low Back Pain. Philadelphia: C.V. Mosby;1980.

Kirkaldy-Willis WH, Wedge JT, Yong-Hing, and Reilly J. Pathology and pathogenesis of lumbar spondylosis and stenosis. *Spine* 1978;3:319.

Kramer MS. Clinical biostatistics LIV. The biostatistics of concordance. *Clin Pharmacol Ther* 1973;29:111–123.

Kuettner KE and Kimura JH. Proteoglycans: An overview. *J Cell Biochem* 1985;27:327.

Langham J. *Medical Embryology.* Baltimore: Williams and Wilkins;1975.

Last J: *Anatomy.* Toronto: Lea & Febiger: 1966.

Lipson SJ, and Muir H. Proteoglycans in experimental disc degeneration. *Spine* 1981;6:194–210.

Lyons G, Eisenstein SM, and Sweet MBE. Biochemical changes in intervertebral disc degeneration. *Biochim Biophys Acta* 1981; 673:443–453.

McDevitt CA, Billingham M, and Muir H. In vivo metabolism of proteoglycans in experimental osteoarthritic and normal canine articular cartilage and the intervertebral disc. *Semin Arthritis Rheum* 1981;11:17.

McDevitt CA. The proteoglycans of cartilage and the intervertebral disc in ageing and osteoarthritis. Tissue repair and Regeneration. *Handbook of Inflammation* 1981;3:111–143.

Maravilla KR, Lesh P, and Weinreb JC, et al. Magnetic resonance imaging of the limbar spine with CT correlation. *Am J Neuroradiol* 1985;6:237–245.

Maroudas A. Physiochemical properties of articular cartilage. In Freeman MAR, ed. *Human articular cartilage,* 1st edition. London: Pitman Med Pub Co; 1973:131–170.

Maroudas A, Mizrahi J, and Katz EP, et al. Physiochemical properties and functional behavior of normal and osteoarthritic human cartilage. In Kuettner K, Schleyerbach R, and Hascall V, eds. *Articular Cartilage Biochemistry,* 1st edition. New York: Raven Press 1986;311–326.

Modic MT, Weinstein MA, and Pavlicek W, et al. Magnetic resonance imaging of the cervical spine. *Am J Radiol* 1983;141:1129–1136.

Modic MT, Paulicek W, and Weinstein MA, et al. Magnetic resonance imaging of intervertebral disc disease. *Radiology* 1984;152:103–111.

Nachemson AF, Lewin T, Maroudas A, and Freeman MAR: In vitro diffusion of dye through the end-plate and the annulus fibrosus of human lumbar intervertebral discs. *Acta Orthop Scand* 1970;41:589–607.

Nachemson AF. The role of degenerative disc disease in low back pain. *Spine* 1975;1:59.

Nachemson, AF. Advances in low back pain. *Clin Orthop Rel Res* 1985;200:267–278.

Naylor A, and Horton WG: The hydrophilic properties of the nucleus pulposus of the intervertebral disc. *Rheumatism* 1955; 11:32–35.

Panagiotacopulous ND, Pope MH, Krag MH, and Block R. Water content in human intervertebral discs. Part I. Measurement by magnetic resonance imaging. *Spine* 1987;12:912–917.

Panagiotacopulous ND, and Pope MH. Water content in human intervertebral discs. Part II. Viscoelastic behavior. *Spine* 1987;12:918–924.

Pearce RH, and Grimmer BJ. The chemical composition of the proteoglycans of human intervertebral disc. *Biochem J* 1976;157:753–763.

Pearce RH, and Grimmer BJ, and Adams ME. Degeneration and the chemical composition of the human lumbar intervertebral disc. *J Orthop Res.* 1987;5:198–205.

Pech P, and Haughton VM. Lumbar intervertebral disc: Correlative MR and anatomic study. *Radiol.* 1985;156:699–701.

Pedersen HE, Blunck CFJ, and Gardner E. The anatomy of lumbosacral posterior rami and meningeal branches of spinal nerves: With an experimental study of their functions. *J Bone Joint Surg* 1956;38-A:377.

Pedrini VA, and Ponseti IV: Glycosaminoglycans of the intervertebral disc. *J Lab Clin Med* 1973;82:938–950.

Pedrini-Mille A, Pedrini V, O'Connor R, and Tudisco C: Age related changes in the proteoglycans of human intervertebral disc. *Orthop Trans* 1980;4:221.

Poole, AR. Changes in the collagen and proteoglycan of articular cartilage in arthritis. *Rheumatology* 1986;10:316–371.

Powell MC, Wilson M, Szypryt P, et al. Prevalence of lumbar disc degeneration observed by magnetic resonance in symptomless women. *Lancet* 1986;1:1367.

Pritzker K. Ageing and degeneration in the lumbar intervertebral disc. Symposium on the lumbar spine. *Orthop Clin North Am* 1977; 8:265–277.

Rosenberg L, Hellman W, and Kleinschmidt AK. Macromolecular models of protein-polysaccharide from bovine nasal cartilage based on electron microscopic studies. *J Biol Chem* 1970; 245:4123.

Schmorl G, and Junghanns H. Development, growth, anatomy and function of the spine. In *The Human Spine in Health and Disease.* New York: Grune & Stratton: 1971.

Sokoloff L.Osteoarthritis as a remodelling process. *J Rheum* 1987; 14:7–11.

Spilker RL. Mechanical behavior of a simple model of an intervertebral disc under compressive loading. *J Biomech* 1980;13:895–901.

Thompson JP, Pearce RH, and Ho B. Correlation of gross morphology and chemical composition with magnetic resonance images of human lumbar intervertebral discs. *Trans Orthop Res Soc* 1988;13:276.

Urban JP, and McMullin JF. Swelling pressure of the intervertebral disc: Influence of proteoglycan and collagen contents. *Biorheology* 1985;22:145–157.

Urban JPG, Holm S, Maroudas A, and Nachemson A. Nutrition of the intervertebral disc: An in vivo study of solute transport. *Clin Orthop and Related Res* 1977;129:101–114.

Urban J, and Maroudas A. The chemistry of the intervertebral disc in relation to its physiological function. *Clin Rheum Dis* 1980; 6:51.

Urban JPG, and McMullin JF. Swelling pressure of the lumbar in-

tervertebral discs: Influence of age, spinal level, composition and degeneration. *Spine* 1988;13:179–187.

Vernon Roberts B. Degenerative changes in intervertebral discs. *Rheum Rehab* 1977;16:13.

Vernon-Roberts B. Pathology of intervertebral disc disease. In Jayson MIV, ed. *The Lumbar Spine and Back Pain,* 3rd edition. London: Pitman Medical; 1981.

White AA, and Panjabi MM. Physical properties and functional biomechanics of the spine. In *Clinical Biomechanics of the Spine.* Toronto: Lippincott;1978.

Wyke B. The neurology of low back pain. In Jayson MIV, ed. *The Lumbar Spine and Back Pain.* New York: Churchill-Livingstone; 1987.

The Pathophysiology of Zygapophyseal Joints

Lynton G.F. Giles

- **ANATOMY OF THE ZYGAPOPHYSEAL JOINTS**
  Articular Cartilage
  Joint Capsule
  Synovial Membrane
  Innervation of the Zygapophyseal Joints
  Innervation of the Synovial Folds
- **PATHOLOGY OF THE ZYGAPOPHYSEAL JOINTS**
  Overview of Joint Pathophysiology
  Osteoarthritis

  Ligamenta Flava
  Synovial Fold Entrapment
- **EFFECT OF LEG LENGTH INEQUALITY ON LUMBOSACRAL ZYGAPOPHYSEAL JOINTS**
- **CLINICAL PRESENTATION OF ZYGAPOPHYSEAL JOINT FACET SYNDROME**
- **CONCLUSION**
- **REFERENCES**

There are normally 5 lumbar, 12 thoracic, and 7 cervical vertebrae, that are unfused, as well as 5 sacral and 4 coccygeal vertebrae, that are fused. Each vertebra consists of two principal parts; i.e., the anterior vertebral body, which is composed of spongy bone covered by a thin layer of compact bone, and the posterior vertebral arch with its processes (Koreska et al., 1977). Adjacent mobile vertebrae articulate by means of the "articular triad" (Hirsch et al., 1963); i.e., the intervertebral joint anteriorly and the paired zygapophyseal synovial joints posteriorly. This chapter deals specifically with zygapophyseal joints. In general terms, the anatomy of all the synovial zygapophyseal joints (posterior "facet" joints; interlaminar joints) is similar, but they vary in shape and orientation depending on their position within the spine (Maigne, 1972; Rickenbacher et al., 1982). The orientation and angulation to the horizontal for typical lumbar, thoracic, and cervical vertebrae are shown schematically in Figure 15–1.

The laminae, spinous processes, and transverse processes are connected by ligamenta flava; interspinous, supraspinous, and intertrasverse ligaments; and the ligamentum nuchae, respectively, (depending on the spinal level), which can all be regarded as accessory ligaments of these joints (Williams and Warwick, 1980). The articular capsule of zygapophyseal joints contains intra-articular syno-

vial folds, which are normal structures found in almost all the zygapophyseal joints (Tondury, 1972).

The lumbar zygapophyseal joints are described in greater detail than their thoracic and cervical counterparts, as the lumbar zygapophyseal joints have been the subject of extensive research in an attempt to understand their function and pathology in relation to the costly and debilitating condition of low back pain, with or without sciatica. These lumbar zygapophyseal joints are described with regard to (1) their anatomy, (2) their pathology and resulting pain, and (3) the clinical presentation of zygapophyseal joint "facet" syndrome.

Anatomy of the Zygapophyseal Joints

The lumbar zygapophyseal joints are synovial joints that are formed by the convex, laterally facing, inferior articular process of the upper vertebra and the

The financial support provided for the histological studies by the Foundation for Chiropractic Education and Research (U.S.A.) and the Australian Spinal Research Foundation Ltd. (Australia), is gratefully acknowledged. The assistance of the clinical and technical staff at the Institute of Forensic Pathology, Brisbane, Australia, is gratefully acknowledged.

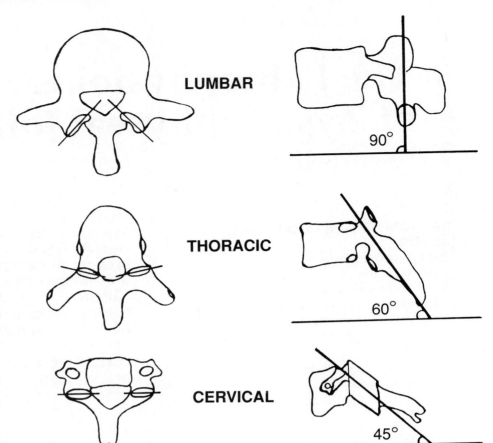

Figure 15–1. Orientation of zygapophyseal joint facets. The approximate horizontal orientation (black lines) of the zygapophyseal joint facets is shown for lumbar, thoracic, and cervical spines. The approximate inclination of the respective facet surfaces to the horizontal is shown in degrees. Both the horizontal orientation and the facet inclination vary according to the specific spinal level for a given vertebral segment.

concave, medially facing, superior articular process of the lower vertebra (Hadley, 1961). These joints lie posterolateral to the lumbar spinal canal and posterior to the intervertebral foramina or "canals" (Baddeley, 1976). The lumbar zygapophyseal joints, which are originally orientated in the coronal plane, assume their final form and orientation in childhood (Lutz, 1967). In the upper lumbar spine these joints are approximately sagittally orientated, but they gradually become more coronally orientated as they reach the lumbosacral junction (Pheasant, 1975). They are "biplanar" joints, with both coronal and more sagittally orientated planes present in each joint (Taylor and Twomey, 1986). Their articular facets have a smooth hyaline articular cartilage surface averaging 10 × 8 mm in adults (Weinstein et al., 1977).

The zygapophyseal joint is a true diarthrodial joint, complete with a joint capsule and a synovial lining (Keim, 1973). The posterolateral and posteromedial parts of the capsule are fibrous and resemble the fibrous capsule of other synovial joints. However, the medial part of the capsule is formed by the ligamentum flavum (Hirsch et al., 1963) (Fig. 15–2).

Articular Cartilage

Hyaline articular cartilage lines all sliding joint surfaces (Rhodin, 1974). The cartilage surface is devoid of perichondrium (Junqueira et al., 1986), and it has a special shock-absorbing property, which may be explained by the interaction between collagen, proteoglycans, and the extracellular fluid as a response to loading (Christensen, 1985). Normal adult hyaline articular cartilage is aneural and avascular (Ham and Cormack, 1979) and is composed of approximately 75% water and 25% solids (Serafini-Fracassini and Smith, 1974). Its histological zones are shown in Figure 15–3.

Hyaline articular cartilage cell density and chemical content vary in different parts of the same joint and at different depths of the tissue (Stockwell, 1979). The cartilage has a dense extracellular matrix populated by a sparse, diffuse population of chondrocytes (von der Mark and Conrad, 1979). The main components of the matrix are long fibers of collagen, which form a meshwork, and proteoglycans filling the interstices of this meshwork. The arcade arrangement of the collagen fibers, in which fibers orientated perpendicular to the subchondral bone plate arch around to become tangential to the articu-

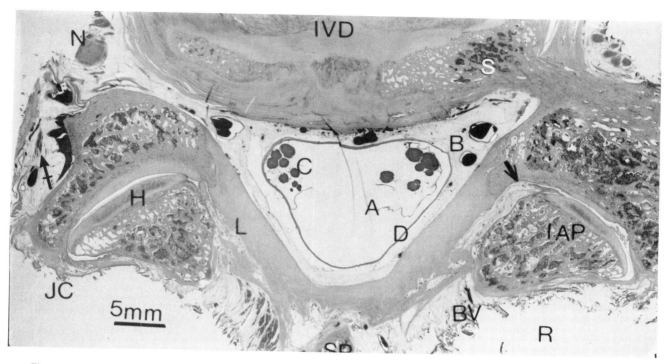

Figure 15–2. A 100-μm-thick horizontal section of the lumbosacral zygapophyseal joints at the level of the inferior joint recesses from a 54-year-old man. (The plane of the section is slightly oblique.) A = arachnoid membrane; B = Batson's venous plexus; C = cauda equina; D = dura mater; H = hyaline articular cartilage; IVD = intervertebral disc; JC = posterolateral fibrous capsule; L = ligamentum flavum; N = spinal ganglion; R = right side; S = sacrum; Sp = base of trimmed off spinous process. The intra-articular synovial fold inclusion is shown by an arrow (→). Arrow (➡) shows a neurovascular bundle. (Ehrlich's hematoxylin stain with light green counterstain.) (*Reprinted by permission from the Bulletin of the Hospital for Joint Diseases Orthopaedic Institute, 42: 1982, p. 251.*)

lar cartilage surface, was described by Benninghoff (1925) (Fig. 15–3). Normal human adult hyaline articular cartilage contains only type II collagen (Goldwasser et al., 1978), which (1) protects the chondrocytes, (2) provides attachment for proteoglycans, (3) anchors the cartilage to the subchondral bone, and (4) resists the tensile stresses produced by compression (MacConaill, 1951; Kempson et al., 1968; Weightman, 1976).

Hyaline articular cartilage thickness varies in different parts of the same joint (Gardner, 1978), but it is usually thicker at the periphery of concave surfaces and at the center of convex surfaces (Bullough, 1979). However, this is not usually the case in lumbar zygapophyseal joints, where the cartilage may be thicker at the center of concave surfaces (Giles, 1989). Across the center of lumbar zygapophyseal joints, the combined thickness of both hyaline articular cartilages is approximately 2 to 2.4 mm (Giles and Taylor, 1984).

Hyaline articular cartilage transmits loads and allows repetitive joint motion without breakdown (Edwards and Chrisman, 1979) and its elastic properties permit normal joint function. The cartilage's ability to deform under load enables greater congruency to occur between opposing surfaces of the joint,

thereby spreading a load over a larger surface area (McCutchen, 1962; Malemud and Muskowitz, 1981).

Joint Capsule

The zygapophyseal joint capsule is unique in having a fibrous capsule posterolaterally and posteromedially, whereas the ligamentum flavum forms the anteromedial capsule (Hirsch et al., 1963; Reilly et al., 1978). The fibrous capsule is relatively loose above and below where it forms superior and inferior recesses, which contain small synovial fat pads (Lewin et al., 1961). The capsule contains mainly fibrocytes or fibroblasts with little gr ound substance, and its fibers are mainly white collagenous fibers, which are arranged in parallel bundles having a diameter of 0.3 to 0.5 μm. The relatively poor blood supply only allows slow healing once the capsule is damaged (Barnett et al., 1961). A tendon of the multifidus muscle is attached to the fibrous capsule as the multifidus muscle crosses the joint to attach to the mamillary process and the posterior part of the joint capsule (Cyron and Hutton, 1981; Giles, 1989).

The ligamenta flava are interlaminar ligaments that are located within the spinal canal and cover most of the posterior bony wall of the spinal canal

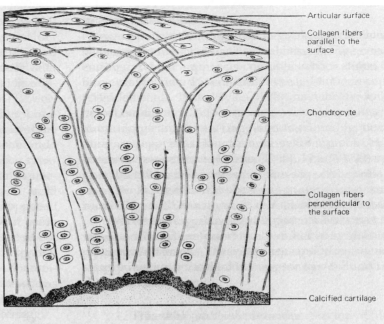

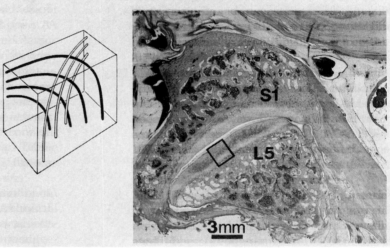

Figure 15-3. A. A 100-μm-thick horizontal section from the left lumbosacral zygapophyseal joint of a 54-year-old man. The articular facets of the superior articular process of the sacrum (S1) and the inferior articular process of the fifth lumbar vertebra (L5) are lined with hyaline articular cartilage. The rectangle on the L-5 inferior articular process is represented in the lower diagram **B.** shows the histological zones of hyaline articular cartilage. The collagen fibers in the deeper zones are perpendicular to the cartilage surface, then they become parallel to the surface in the more superfical zones; see also the lower left schematic diagram **C.** The deeper chondrocytes are more spherical and are arranged in approximately vertical rows, whereas the superficial chondrocytes are flattened and are randomly located. (*Adapted from Junqueira, et al. p. 162, and Giles, p. 44–45.*)

(Rolander, 1966; Dommisse, 1975). These ligaments consist of fibers of yellow elastic tissue that extend from the articular capsule to the midline where the laminae fuse to form the spinous process (Williams and Warwick, 1980). The fiber direction is slightly oblique in the capsular portion and is essentially perpendicular in the medial interlaminar portion. The anteromedial border of the ligament passes around the zygapophyseal joint, skirts the posterior edge of the intervertebral canal, forming its roof. Then it blends with the fibrous capsule (Brown, 1938; Naffziger et al., 1938; Ramsey, 1966).

The ligamentum flavum provides a smooth covering for the posterior part of the spinal canal and acts as (1) a fibrous capsule on the ventral part of the zygapophyseal joint, (2) an elastic band keeping the spinal nerves free from compression when passing

through the intervertebral canal, and (3) as a check ligament to prevent hyperflexion (Hirsch et al., 1963; Rolander, 1966; Weinstein et al., 1977). These ligaments are generally thin, but broad and long in the neck, thicker in the thoracic region, and thickest at lumbar levels, (Williams and Warwick, 1980) where their thickness ranges from 2 to 10 mm depending on where it is measured (Horwitz, 1939; Herzog, 1950; Reilly et al., 1978; Giles and Taylor, 1984). According to Farfan (1973), the average thickness for the ligamentum flavum in the lumbar spine is 3 mm, although this may vary with the health of the adjacent joints. The height of the ligamentum flavum ranges from 1.0 to 2.0 cm (Herzog, 1950). In the adult, the ligamenta flava consist of yellow elastic fibers (80%), collagen fibers (20%) interspersed between the elastic fibers and a few spindle-shaped fibrocytes

(Ramsey, 1966; Kirkaldy-Willis, 1984), with only a few irregularly dispersed blood vessels (Ramsey, 1966; Giles, 1989).

Synovial Membrane

The synovial membrane is a complex lining tissue that is the conduit for the exchange of nutrients and waste products between blood and the joint tissues. The cells of the synovial lining membrane synthesize and secrete the proteins and proteoglycans that are necessary for normal joint lubrication (Simkin, 1979; Hasselbacher, 1981). The synovial membrane consists of two parts; i.e., a *synovial lining layer* (or synovial intima), which is predominantly cellular, and a *subsynovial layer* (or synovial subintima), which is formed by loose fibrous connective tissue rich in blood vessels, lymphatics, and adipose tissue (Davies, 1950; Ghadially and Roy, 1969; Giles et al., 1986).

The synovial membrane lines the inner surface of the zygapophyseal joint capsule and the fat pads in the joint recesses forming synovial folds, which are normally present in almost all zygapophyseal joints (Tondury, 1972; Giles, 1986; Singer et al., 1990). An example of a lumbosacral intra-articular synovial fold is shown in Figure 15–4. The synovial membrane also lines the intracapsular parts of bone that are not covered by articular cartilage (Collins, 1949; Dieppe and Calvert, 1983), and it overlaps the nonarticular margins of the cartilage where it terminates without a clear line of demarcation (Barnett et

al., 1961). Small diameter (0.2 to 1.2 μm) nerve fibers have been found in the synovial lining and subsynovial layers of lumbar zygapophyseal joints (Giles, 1989), and it is reasonable to assume that synovial folds in all zygapophyseal joints have a similar innervation.

The synovial lining layer has a smooth, moist, and glistening surface with small villi (Paget and Bullough, 1980; Giles and Taylor, 1982). The synovial lining layer cells (secreting fibroblasts) form a meshwork between the joint cavity and the subsynovial tissue (Barland et al., 1962; Giles, 1989) (Fig. 15–5). The synovial lining cells do not form a continuous compact layer as with true epithelium, but form a layer that varies in depth and that can have minute gaps between the synovial cells (Ghadially and Roy, 1969; Hadler, 1981). The synovial lining cells are of two types, A and B cells. The A cells have a phagocytic function, whereas the B cells probably represent different functional stages of the same cell type (Schumacher, 1975; Junqueira et al., 1986).

The subsynovial layer of the synovial membrane can be areolar, areolar-adipose, fibrous or fibroareolar. This layer is rich in blood vessels, and it has a plentiful supply of elastic fibers, which impart a function of elastic recoil during joint movement (Castor, 1960; Rhodin, 1974; Giles, 1988). The zygapophyseal joint intra-articular synovial folds have two common types of subsynovial tissue, fibrous and adipose (Giles and Taylor, 1982). The

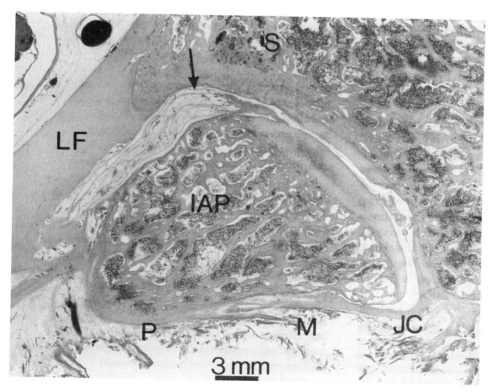

Figure 15–4. Horizontal section of the right lumbosacral zygapophyseal joint of a 54-year-old man. IAP = inferior articular process of L-5; JC = posterolateral fibrous joint capsule; LF = ligamentum flavum; M = multifidus muscle fibers; P = periosteum; S = sacral superior articular process. The arrow points to intra-articular synovial fold inclusion. (Ehrlich's hematoxylin stain with light green counterstain.) *(Adapted from Giles et al., 1986, p. 110a.)*

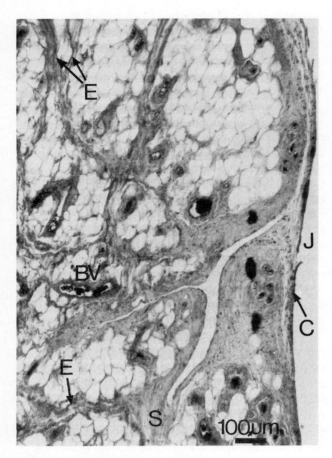

Figure 15-5. A 30-μm-thick section showing part of a synovial fold from the lumbosacral zygapophyseal joint of a 45-year-old woman. Note the synovial lining cells (C) in the synovial lining (intimal) layer. BV = blood vessel containing blood cells; E = elastic fibers; J = joint cavity; S = interlocular fibrous septum in the subsynovial (subintimal) layer. There is a rich blood supply. (Modified Schofield's silver impregnation and Verhoeff's hematoxylin counterstain.) *(Adapted from Giles, p. 121.)*

intra-articular synovial folds consist of various shapes and sizes and are described in almost all the zygapophyseal joints (Tondury, 1940, 1972; Hadley, 1961; Kos, 1969; Giles, 1986). Some controversy exists on the subject of zygapophyseal joint "synovial folds" and "menisci." Authors refer to "true" mesenchymal intra-articular menisci (Lewin et al., 1961) as semilunar fibrous structures, that remotely resemble menisci (Engel and Bogduk, 1980, 1982), or as "meniscoid inclusions" (Bourdillon, 1973). According to Tondury (1972), however, no "true" menisci are found in zygapophyseal joints, a finding that is confirmed by this author.

The free irregular margins of the synovial folds may be quite long and thin and may project between the articulating surfaces; they are often fibrous at their tips (Keller, 1959; Giles and Taylor, 1982;

Kirkaldy-Willis, 1984: Giles, 1986). The principal functions of the intra-articular synovial folds are (1) to fill space between peripheral noncongruent parts of the articular surfaces (Tondury, 1972); and (2) to secrete synovial fluid (a dialysate of plasma and hyaluronate protein), which acts as a lubricant and allows nutrients to flow through it from the capillaries in the synovial fold and the capillary bed surrounding the joint cavity (Simkin, 1979; Paget and Bullough, 1980; Knight and Levick, 1983).

Innervation of Zygapophyseal Joints

Spinal nerves divide into anterior and posterior primary rami. The anterior primary rami form the cervical, brachial and lumbosacral plexuses, whereas in the thoracic region they remain segmental as intercostal nerves (Chusid, 1985). The posterior primary rami provide innervation for the zygapophyseal joints. The distribution of the posterior primary ramus is shown in Figure 15–6.

Each lumbar posterior primary ramus, which has a diameter of 2 mm or less, divides into a medial branch, which has a diameter of less than 1 mm, and a lateral branch (Sunderland, 1975; Bradley, 1980). The medial branch descends beneath the mamillo-accessory ligament, then gives branches to the fibrous capsule as it passes to lie directly superficial to the communication between the fat-filled inferior recess of the joint and the synovial cavity (Lewin et al, 1961; Giles, 1988). The nerves ramify diffusely within the capsule and contain sensory fibers (Wyke, 1981). According to Wyke (1980, 1981) and Paris (1983), a zygapophyseal joint is innervated by no less than three adjacent posterior primary rami. Most authors, however, found each joint to be supplied by only two spinal nerves (Pedersen et al., 1956; Bradley, 1974; Sunderland, 1975; Bogduk, 1976; Reilly et al., 1978; Giles, 1989): one spinal nerve supplying the superior aspect of the zygapophyseal joint one segment caudad, and the other supplying the zygapophyseal joint capsule in the region of the inferior recess at the same level at which the spinal nerve leaves the spinal cord.

The innervation of the fibrous joint capsule consists of both myelinated and unmyelinated fibers, with a full triad of nerve endings, i.e., fine free fibers, complex unencapsulated endings, and small encapsulated endings (Hirsch et al., 1963). Some of these nerve endings have been classified as "pain sensitive" on the basis of their histological appearance (Ikari, 1954; Pedersen et al., 1956). Fine free nerve fibers and endings, which are considered to be nociceptive, have been described on the outermost posterior surface of the ligamentum flavum (Pedersen et al., 1956; Hirsch et al., 1963), but not in its deeper regions (Hirsch et al., 1963; Jackson et al.,

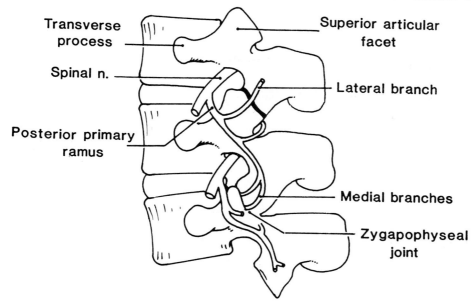

Transverse process

Spinal n.

Posterior primary ramus

Superior articular facet

Lateral branch

Medial branches

Zygapophyseal joint

Figure 15–6. Diagram of two lumbar nerves with some of their branches. (*From Moore, KL. Clinically Oriented Anatomy, ed. 2, William & Wilkins Co., Baltimore, 1985, p. 649, with permission.*)

1966; Reilly et al., 1978; Giles, 1988), although Bridge (1959) claimed that the ligamentum flavum contained many nerves in its deep region in thoracolumbar specimens. However, no immunoreactivity to substance P antibody was found in small pieces of ligamentum flavum by Korkala (1985) and Giles and Harvey (1987), indicating that no nociceptive-type nerves were present in this ligament.

Innervation of the Synovial Folds

Historically, the synovial folds have been found to have no innervation (Gardner, 1950; Hadley, 1976; Wyke, 1972, 1981; B.D. Wyke, personal communication, 1983) and, therefore, have been considered not to be involved in zygapophyseal joint pain (Wyke, 1981). Recent histological studies by Giles and co-workers (Giles et al., 1986; Giles and Taylor, 1987a, b; Giles and Harvey, 1987; Giles, 1988), however, have shown that lumbar zygapophyseal joint synovial folds contain both paravascular and non-paravascular nerve fibers (Fig. 15–7). These range in diameter from 0.5 to 1.2 μm in the synovial lining layer. Nerve fiber and/or fasciculus diameters range in diameter from 0.2 to 13 μm in the subsynovial layer. Substance P antibody immunofluorescent nerves were demonstrated in the synovial folds by Giles and Harvey (1987), and these were considered to have a putative function of nociception, as substance P has been closely identified with nociception (Henry, 1982; Liesi, 1983). It should be noted that nerve fibers are also seen in the cancellous bone of the vertebral arches (Hovelacque, 1925; Roofe, 1940) and the paraspinal muscles (Lim et al., 1961) such as the multifidus, which is closely associated with the fibrous joint capsule.

Pathology of the Zygapophyseal Joints

Overview of Joint Pathophysiology

It is important to note that spinal pain may have a multifactorial etiology and that there may be several types of back pain that closely mimic each other, each with its own unique pathophysiological etiology (Haldeman, 1977, 1980). With this in mind, the pathology of zygapophyseal joints is considered now.

The bony articular processes of the zygapophyseal joints are susceptible to all the disorders that affect bone, the main disorders being infections, benign and malignant tumors, endocrine disorders such as osteoporosis, congenital abnormalities, and fractures. The synovial zygapophyseal joints are also affected by disorders of the large synovial joints, for example, osteoarthritis, rheumatoid arthritis, and ankylosing spondylitis. These pathological processes are not discussed in this chapter, apart from osteoarthritis.

It should be emphasized that, because of the articular triad, consisting of the fibrocartilaginous intervertebral joint and the two synovial zygapophyseal joints (Lewin et al., 1961), structural abnormalities in the intervertebral disk are always accompanied by osteoarthritis changes in the zygapophyseal joints (Vernon-Roberts, 1980). With this in mind, specific functional and "degenerative" joint disease (osteoarthritis) conditions affecting the various components of a zygapophyseal joint are considered now.

Osteoarthritis

Osteoarthritis is said to be *primary* when no etiologic factors can be discerned and *secondary* when an iden-

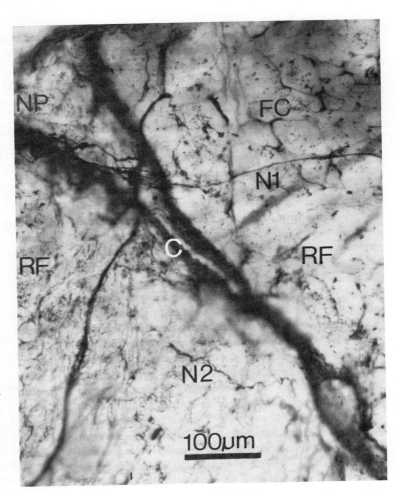

Figure 15-7. Part of a whole mount, silver-impregnated synovial fold from a 40-year-old man. Note the extensive paravascular nerve plexus (NP) on the capillary (C) and the synovial fold fat cells (FC). A single nerve fiber (N1) with an average diameter of 1.7 μm traverses the synovial fold; it is not associated with any blood vessels. The silver-stained structure (N2) consists of one or two nerve fibers. Also note the reticular fibers (RF) adjacent to the fat cells. (*From Giles et al., pp. 44–45, with permission.*)

tifiable cause is found (Dick, 1972), such as previous injury to a joint (Huskisson and Hart, 1978). According to Bland (1983), there are four theories of the pathogenesis of osteoarthritis: (1) the initial event occurs in cartilage, due to a change in the microenvironment of the chondrocytes (a view held by most investigators); (2) the initial event occurs in subchondral bone with mechanical factors being the primary cause; (3) micro-osteonecrosis occurs in the subchondral bone due to vascular disease; and (4) a proteolytic enzyme from type A synovial cells that is normally neutralized by an inhibitor from type B synovial cells digests the protein core of chondroitin sulfate if the inhibitor is absent (Glynn, 1977).

Whatever the mechanics, osteoarthritis of zygapophyseal joints leads to bone proliferation at the edges of the facets with some degree of encroachment on the spinal and intervertebral canals (McRae, 1977). Large osteophytes can project from the margins of zygapophyseal joint articular surfaces anteriorly into the intervertebral canal, or medially into the spinal canal. Osteophytes projecting into the intervertebral canal from the margins of osteoarthritic

zygapophyseal joints may cause pressure on the spinal nerve (Vernon-Roberts, 1980) and, in a small spinal canal, osteophytes can contribute to neurological symptoms and signs (McRae, 1977) due to spinal stenosis. Furthermore, in the cervical spine, osteophytes from the zygapophyseal joints, as well as from the joints of von Luschka, may compress the vertebral artery, interfering with brainstem and posterior fossa circulation (Bland, 1987). Although osteoarthritis occurs in the thoracic spine, it is almost always asymptomatic, which is probably due to this area being minimally mobile (Bland, 1987).

The articular surface of zygapophyseal joints usually retains an intact covering of hyaline articular cartilage even when large osteophytes have formed and there is dense sclerosis of subchondral bone (Fig. 15–8). These joints may, however, show the classic changes of severe osteoarthritis (Vernon-Roberts, 1980). Occasionally, zygapophyseal joints exhibit a subchondral bone cyst. The impacted cartilage in the articular process of Figure 15–8 probably represents traumatic herniation of hyaline articular cartilage and an early stage of subchondral bone cyst formation.

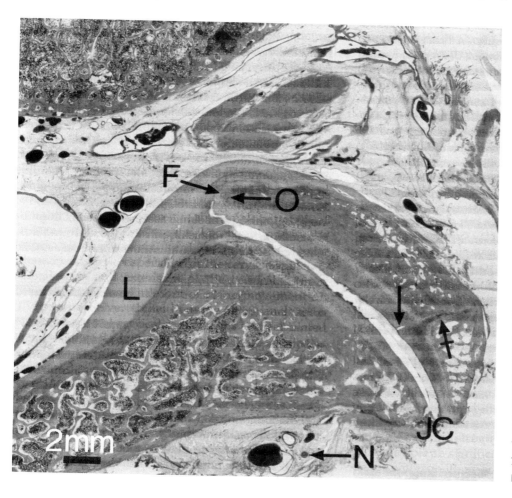

Figure 15–8. A 100-μm-thick horizontal section through the right L-5 to S-1 zygapophyseal joint of a 54-year-old man. Note the early osteophyte (O) with subchondral sclerosis and a fibrocartilage "bumper" (F). Some areas of the hyaline articular cartilage show other early osteoarthritic changes; e.g., early fibrillation and clustering of the chondrocytes. Also note the fissure in the cartilage and the defect in the subchondral bone plate with hyaline articular cartilage impacted in the articular process. JC = posterolateral fibrous joint capsule; L = ligamentum flavum; N = neurovascular bundle nerve.

Facet osteoarthritis is considered to be a relatively important cause of intractable back pain in young and middle-aged adults (Eisenstein and Parry, 1987). The painful symptoms of osteoarthritic zygapophyseal joints are due partly to (1) joint wear (involving cartilage degeneration with loss of joint space, formation of osteophytes and loose bodies, and joint capsule fibrosis); (2) episodes of synovial fold inflammation; and (3) inflammation, fraying, and degeneration of ligaments around the joints (Golding, 1970). Venostasis may occur in the adjacent bone marrow, resulting in hypertension (Arnoldi, 1976; Bland, 1983), which may cause pain due to pressure on small nerves in the bone (Arnoldi, 1976). Osteoarthritis can also lead to swelling of the joint capsules (McRae, 1977), which are well innervated.

Ligamenta Flava

Swollen ligamenta flava can encroach upon the spinal canal, and they are a contributory factor in spinal pain syndromes (Bland, 1987). Referred pain syndromes can occur in the presence of swollen ligamenta flava in association with a small lumbar spinal canal, and may even cause sciatica in some patients who have normal-sized spinal canals (McRae, 1977). Thickened ligamenta flava (which have no true hypertrophy, but thickening and fibrosis (Dockerty and Love, 1940) can buckle inward, depressed by enlarged laminae, or they can become incorporated into zygapophyseal joint osteophytes at the site of attachment of the ligamentum flavum to the zygapophyseal joint capsule (Weinstein et al., 1977). Spurs in the ligamentum flavum may displace the ligament, causing encroachment on the intervertebral canal and distortion of the spinal nerve (Hadley, 1964).

Thickening of the ligamenta flava can, in conjunction with zygapophyseal joint facet subluxation and disk thinning, compromise the nerve root in the intervertebral canal (Hadley, 1951). As the ligamentum flavum extends far laterally (Fig. 15–8) to blend with the fibrous joint capsule on the roof of the lateral recess and intervertebral canal, minimal thickening may cause dorsal root compression (Weinstein, 1977).

Synovial Fold Entrapment

The innervated synovial folds (Giles and Harvey, 1987; Giles, 1988) may interfere mechanically with joint movement (Lewit, 1968), causing pain and muscle spasm. Pain also may result from entrapment of the synovial folds between the facet surfaces. Two main mechanisms by which pain may arise due to synovial fold pinching are (1) *traction* on pain-sensitive tissues such as the synovial fold and the fibrous joint capsule, and (2) synovial fold *traumatic synovitis* with associated tissue damage and cell rupture. The latter condition may cause the release of pain-producing substances such as histamine, substance P, bradykinin, and potassium ions, all of which cause nociceptive nerve impulses, and ischemia, with resultant ischemic pain due to an accumulation of metabolic products (e.g., lactic acid).

Two other zygapophyseal joint pathologies, that can cause spinal pain with radiculitis and that have been identified histologically are (1) a synovial cyst (Bland and Schmidek, 1985) and (2) an intra-articular lipoma (Husson et al., 1987).

Effect of Leg Length Inequality on Lumbosacral Zygapophyseal Joints

The clinical findings of Rush and Steiner (1946), Giles and Taylor (1981), Friberg (1983), and Gofton (1985) indicate that there is a strong correlation between leg length inequality of 1 cm or more and low back pain. It has been found that the zygapophyseal joints carry a proportion of the incumbent body weight (Farfan, 1973; Hutton and Adams, 1980) varying from 16 to 40% of the total compressive load on the spine (Hakim and King, 1976; Hutton and Adams, 1980). In cases where leg length inequality of 1 cm or more is present with pelvic obliquity, a marked postural scoliosis may be present (Fig. 15–9).

Carefully standardized erect posture radiographs can be used to measure accurately leg length inequality, pelvic obliquity, and the associated postural scoliosis by using a wire plumb line between the patient and the cassette as a reference line (Giles and Taylor, 1981). Patients with unleveling of the left and right pubic rami were excluded from the clinical study by Giles and Taylor (1981) as this unleveling could be due to sacroiliac joint subluxation.

A method for measuring the left and right lumbosacral zygapophyseal joint facet angles from erect posture oblique radiographs (Giles, 1981) is shown graphically in Figure 15–10. The plumb line, between the bucky and the cassette, gives a true vertical reference line on the radiograph, as in the case of anteroposterior pelvis–lumbar spine radiographs. This

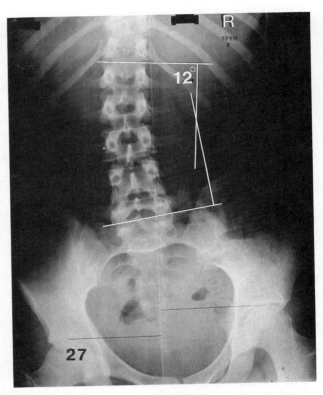

Figure 15–9. An erect posture radiograph, taken using the method of Giles and Taylor, of a 19-year-old woman with a left leg length deficiency of 27 mm, pelvic obliquity, and a postural scoliosis of 12 degrees. The postural scoliosis was measured using Cobb's method; i.e., the angle of curvature is measured by drawing lines parallel to the superior surface of the uppermost vertebral body of the curvature and to the inferior surface of the lowest vertebra of the curvature. (Radiograph viewed in the posteroanterior position.)

line is used as a reference point to draw a horizontal line at right angles to it on the radiograph. A line is then drawn through the plane of each lumbosacral zygapophyseal joint to bisect the horizontal line so that the inclination of the facet surfaces to the horizontal can be measured using a perspex protractor (Giles, 1981). It has been shown that there is a statistically significant difference between paired left and right lumbosacral zygapophyseal joint facet angles with the horizontal ($7.1 \pm 4.4°$) in patients with leg length inequality and pelvic obliquity, whereas in cases with equal leg lengths, the left and right angles are virtually the same ($1.8 \pm 1.6°$) (Giles, 1981). The difference in angles associated with leg length inequality and pelvic obliquity implies that asymmetrical biomechanical loads will be borne by the paired lumbosacral zygapophyseal joints in cases where leg length inequality of 1 cm or more and pelvic obliquity are present.

Indeed, Giles and Taylor (1984) found that leg length inequality of 1 cm or more is associated with a

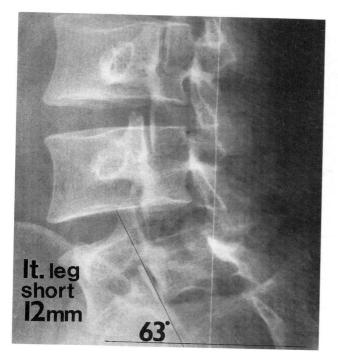
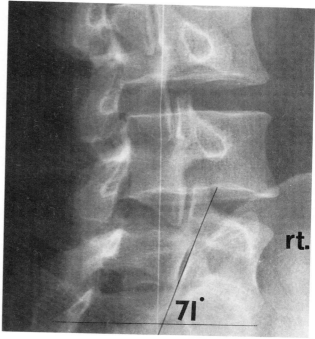

Figure 15–10. Measurement of right and left lumbosacral zygapophyseal joint facet angles in a patient with a left leg length deficiency of 12 mm.

tendency toward asymmetrical changes in zyga-pophyseal mid-joint cartilage thickness and sub-chondral bone thickness in postural scoliosis. In cases of leg length inequality of 1 cm or more with pelvic obliquity and postural scoliosis, the zyga-pophyseal joint facets are probably no longer con-gruous and, consequently, increased friction may occur at some point of the gliding movement (Cailliet, 1968). Abnormally shaped or positioned zygapophyseal joint facet surfaces appear to be a cause of osteoarthritis (Huskisson and Hart, 1978; Giles, 1987), which is not a disease but is an expres-sion of the morphological consequences of stresses applied to the zygapophyseal joints (Bogduk and Twomey, 1987). Preliminary data suggest a tendency toward a larger area of bumper-fibrocartilage in the lumbosacral zygapophyseal joints of cadavers with a leg length inequality of 1 cm or more and a postural scoliosis of 4 degrees or more (Giles, 1989). The data indicate that, in such a postural scoliosis, there is probably a greater sideways "thrusting" of the lat-eral margins of the facets of the zygapophyseal joints against the innervated synovial lining layer. This condition could cause pain of zygapophyseal joint origin, as the synovial lining membrane and sub-synovial tissue have small diameter nerves that have been shown to have substance P antibody positive profiles and are, therefore, considered to have a pu-tative function of nociception.

Finally, the mechanisms by which leg length in-equality may produce low back pain must involve (1) some lumbar spine pathology, whether structural or functional; (2) possible sacroiliac joint dysfunction; (3) possible pelvic–lumbar muscle dysfunction; or (4) a combination of these factors.

Clinical Presentation of Zygapophyseal Joint Facet Syndrome

Zygapophyseal joint facet syndrome is common but, because it is usually not demonstrable radiographi-cally, it is frequently overlooked (Bernard and Kirkaldy-Willis, 1987). It is known that in this syn-drome lumbar zygapophyseal joints may produce re-ferred pain in the legs (Farfan, 1977; Kirkaldy-Willis and Cassidy, 1984) and that the course of this re-ferred pain may be to the buttock, over the greater trochanter, down the back of the thigh to the knee, and sometimes down the posterior or outer calf to the ankle, but rarely to the foot or toes (Kirkaldy-Willis, 1983). Patients with radicular pain due to os-teoarthritis zygapophyseal joints causing stenosis of the intervertebral or spinal canals will on occasion, report pain of a "claudicant" character that is precip-itated, aggravated and progressively intensified by walking. This pain differs however, from the claudicant calf pain of peripheral vascular insufficiency in that the pain is experienced first, and most severely, proximally in the limb, and the patient typically has to sit or lie down to get relief (Macnab, 1977). Thus, zygapophyseal joint dysfunction does not necessarily give rise to pain locally in the joint; it may give rise to pain at any place that shares a common nerve supply with the affected joint (Mennell, 1960). The injection of normal zygapophyseal joints with contrast material (Conray 60) followed by 1 to 3 mL of 5% hypertonic saline, under fluoroscopic control, caused a pain referral pattern in the typical locations of "lumbago and sciatica" (Mooney and Robertson, 1976). Furthermore, it caused marked myoelectric activity in the hamstring muscles of two patients with chronic low back pain and sciatica, and straight leg raising was diminished to 70 degrees in these patients. In three patients in whom depressed tendon reflexes were present, facet block injection (2 to 5 mL of 1% Xylocaine) obliterated the referred pain and the clinical signs of diminished straight leg raising and depressed tendon reflexes within 5 min.

Conclusion

Although this chapter has stressed zygapophyseal joint anatomy and pathology, the multifactorial etiology of spinal pain, with or without radiculitis, must always be considered in differential diagnosis. Some examples of other causes of low back pain, with or without referred pain, are considered in other chapters of this book.

References

Arnoldi CC. Intraosseous hypertension. *Clin Orthop* 1976;115:30–34.

Baddeley H. Radiology of lumbar spinal stenosis. In Jayson M, ed. *The Lumbar Spine and Back Pain*. London: Sector Pub. Ltd; 1976:151–172.

Barland P, Novikoff AB, and Hamerman D. Electron microscopy of the human synovial membrane. *J Cell Biology* 1962;14:207–220.

Barnett CH, Davies DV, and MacConaill MA. *Synovial Joints: Their Structure and Mechanics*. London: Longmans;1961:25, 48–51, 56.

Benninghoff A. Form und Bau der Gelenk-knorpel in ihren Beziehungen zur Funktion. *Z Anat Entwicklungsgesch* 1925; 76:43.

Bernard TN, and Kirkaldy-Willis WH. Recognizing specific characteristics of nonspecific low back pain. *Clin Orthop* 1987; 217:266–280.

Bland JH. The reversibility of osteoarthritis: a review. *Am J Med* 1983;74:16–26.

Bland JH. *Disorders of the Cervical Spine*. Philadelphia: W.B. Saunders Company;1987:71, 73.

Bland JH, and Schmidek HH. Symptomatic intraspinal synovial cyst in a 66 year old marathon runner. *J Rheumatol* 1985;12:1006–1010.

Bogduk N. The Anatomy of the lumbar intervertebral disc syndrome. *Med J Aust* 1976;1:878–881.

Bogduk N, and Twomey LT. *Clinical Anatomy of the Lumbar Spine*. Melbourne: Churchill-Livingstone; 1987:129.

Bourdillon JF. *Spinal Manipulation* 2nd ed. London: William Heinemann Medical Books Ltd.; 1973:22–23.

Bradley KC. The anatomy of backache. *Aust N Z J Surg* 1974; 44:227–232.

Bradley KC. The posterior primary rami of segmental nerves. In Dewhurst D, Glasgow EF, Tahan P, Ward AR, and Idczak RM, eds. *Aspects of Manipulative Therapy, Proceedings of a Multidisciplinary International Conference in Manipulative Therapy*. Melbourne: Ramsay Ware Stockland Pty Ltd.; 1980:56–59.

Bridge, CJ. Innervation of spinal meninges and epidural structures. *Anat Rec* 1959;133:553–561.

Brown HA. Enlargement of the ligamentum flavum. *J Bone Joint Surg* 1938;20:325–338.

Bullough PG. Pathologic changes associated with the common arthritides and their treatment. *Pathol Ann* 1979;2:14, 69–83.

Cailliet R. Low Back Pain Syndrome, 2nd ed. Philadelphia: F.A. Davis; 1968.

Castor CW. The microscopic structure of normal human synovial tissue. *Arthritis Rheum* 1960;3:140.

Christensen SB. Osteoarthrosis. *Acta Orthop Scand* 214, 1985;56:1–43.

Chusid JG. *Correlative Neuroanatomy and Functional Neurology*, 19th ed. California: Lange Medical Publications; 1985:134.

Cobb JR. Outline for the study of scoliosis. Instructional course lectures. *Am Acad Orthop Surg* 1948;5:261–275.

Collins DH. *The Pathology of Articular and Spinal Diseases*. London: Edward Arnold, 1949.

Cyron BM, and Hutton WC. The tensile strength of the capsular ligaments of the apophyseal joints. *J Anat* 1981;132:145–150.

Davies DV. Structure and function of synovial membrane. *Br Med J* 1950;1:92–95.

Dick WC. *An Introduction to Clinical Rheumatology*. London: Churchill Livingstone; 1972.

Dieppe P, and Clavert P. *Crystals and Joint Disease*. London: Chapman and Hall; 1983:14.

Dockerty MB, and Love JG. Thickening and fibrosis (so-called hypertrophy) of the ligamentum flavum. A pathological study of fifty cases. *Proc Staff Meet Mayo Clinic* 1940;15:161–166.

Dommisse GF. Morphological aspects of the lumbar spine and lumbosacral region. *Ortho Clin North Am* 1975;6:163–175.

Edwards CC, and Chrisman OD. Articular cartilage. In Albright JA, and Brand RA, eds. *The Scientific Basis of Orthopaedics*. New York: Appleton-Century-Crofts; 1979:315–347.

Eisenstein SM, and Parry CR. The lumbar facet arthrosis syndrome. Clinical presentation and articular surface changes. *J Bone Joint Surg* 1987;69(B):3–7.

Engel RM, and Bogduk N. *The Menisci of the Lumbar Zygapophyseal Joints*. Anatomical Society of Australia and New Zealand, 18th Annual Conference, 1980.

Engel RM, and Bogduk N. The menisci of the lumbar zygapophyseal joints. *J Anat* 1982;135:795–809.

Farfan HF. *Mechanical Disorders of the Low Back*. Philadelphia: Lea & Febiger; 1973:21, 31, 145.

Farfan HF. A reorientation in the surgical approach to degenerative lumbar intervertebral joint disease. *Orthop Clin Nth Am* 1977;8:9–21.

Friberg O. Clinical symptoms and biomechanics of lumbar spine and hip joint in leg length inequality. *Spine* 1983;8:643–651.

Gardner DL. Structure and function of connective tissue and joints. In Scott JT, ed. *Copeman's Textbook of the Rheumatic Diseases*, 5th ed. London: Churchill Livingstone; 1978;78–124.

Gardner E. Physiology of movable joints. *Physiol Rev* 1950;30:127–176.

Ghadially FN, and Roy S. *Ultrastructure of Synovial Joints in Health and Disease*. London: Butterworths; 1969;1–48.

Giles LGF. Lumbosacral facetal "joint angles" associated with leg length inequality. *Rheumatol Rehab* 1981;20:233–238.

Giles LGF. Lumbosacral and cervical zygapophyseal joint inclusions. *Manual Med* 1986;2:89–92.

Giles LGF. Lumbosacral zygapophyseal joint tropism and its effect on hyaline cartilage. *Clin Biomechanics* 1987;2:2–6.

Giles LGF. *Anatomical Basis of Low Back Pain.* Baltimore: Williams and Wilkins; 1989.

Giles LGF. Human lumbar zygapophyseal joint inferior recess synovial folds: A light microscope examination. *Anatomical Rec* 1988;220:117–124.

Giles LGF, and Harvey AR. Immunohistochemical demonstration of nociceptors in the capsule and synovial folds of human zygapophyseal joints. *Bri J Rheumatol* 1987;26:362–364.

Giles LGF, and Taylor JR. Low-back pain associated with leg length inequality. *Spine* 1981;6:510–521.

Giles LGF, and Taylor JR. Intra-articular synovial protrusions in the lower lumbar apophyseal joints. *Bull Hospital Joint Dis Orthopaedic Inst* 1982;XLII:248–255.

Giles LGF, and Taylor JR. The effect of postural scoliosis on lumbar apophyseal joints. *Scand J Rheumatol* 1984;13:209–220.

Giles LGF, and Taylor JR. Human zygapophyseal joint capsule and synovial fold innervation. *Bri J Rheumatol* 1987(a);26:993–98.

Giles LGF, and Taylor JR. Innervation of human lumbar zygapophyseal joint synovial folds. *Acta Orthopaedica Scand* 1987(b);58:43–46.

Giles LGF, Taylor JR, and Cockson A. Human zygapophyseal joint synovial folds. *Acta Anatomica* 1986;126:110–114.

Glynn LE. Primary lesion in osteoarthrosis. *Lancet* 1977; 1:574–575.

Gofton JP. Persistent low back pain and leg length disparity. *J Rheumatol* 1985;12:747–750.

Golding D. *General Management of Osteoarthritis. Joints and Their Disease.* London: British Medical Association;1970:95–102.

Goldwasser M, van der Rest M, and Glorieux FH. *The Collagen Composition in Osteoarthritic Human Cartilage.* Transactives of the 24th Annual Meeting: Orthopaedic Research Society, Vol 3, 1978; 139.

Hadler NM. The biology of the extracellular space. *Clin Rheumatic Dis* 1981;7:71–97.

Hadley LA. Intervertebral joint subluxation, bony impingement and foramen encroachment with nerve root changes. *Am J Roentgenol* 1951;65:377.

Hadley LA. Anatomico-roentgenographic studies of the posterior spinal articulations. *Am J Roentgenol* 1961;86:270–276.

Hadley LA. *Anatomico-Roentgenographic Studies of the Spine.* Springfield, Ill: Thomas; 1964:181.

Hadley LA. Anatomico-Roentgenographic Studies of the Spine. Springfield, Ill: Thomas; 1976:186, 189, 190.

Hakim NS, and King AI. Static and dynamic articular facet loads. In *Proceedings, 20th Stapp Car Crash Conference*, Philadelphia, Society of Automotive Engineers, Warrendale; 1976:609–637.

Haldeman S. Why one cause of back pain? In Buerger AA, and Tobis TS, eds. *Approaches to the Validation of Manipulation Therapy.* Springfield, Ill: Thomas, 1977:187–197.

Haldeman S. The neurophysiology of spinal pain syndromes. In Haldeman S, ed. *Modern Developments in the Principles and Practice of Chiropractic.* New York: Appleton-Century-Crofts; 1980: 119–142.

Ham AW, and Cormack DH. *Histology*, 8th ed. Philadelphia: J.B. Lippincott Co; 1979:476, 642.

Hasselbacher P. Structure of the synovial membrane. *Clin Rheumatic Dis* 1981;7:57–69.

Henry JL. Relation of substance P to pain transmission: neurophysiological evidence. In Porter R, and O'Connor M, eds. *Substance P in the Nervous System.* Ciba Foundation Symposium. London: Pitman Co.; 1982:206–224.

Herzog W. Morphologie und pathologie des ligamentum flavum. *Frankfurter Zeitschrift fur Pathologie* 1950;61:250–267.

Hirsch C, Ingelmark BE, and Miller M. The anatomical basis for low back pain. *Acta Orthop Scand* 1963;33:1–17.

Horwitz T. Lesions of the intervertebral disc and ligamentum flavum of the lumbar vertebrae: anatomic study of 75 human cadavers. *Surgery* 1939;6:410–425.

Hovelacque A. Le nerf sinuvertebral. *Ann d'Anat Path* 1925;5:435–443.

Huskisson EC, and Hart FD. *Joint Disease: All the Arthropathies*, ed 3. Bristol: John Wright and Sons Ltd.; 1978:89.

Husson JL, Chales G, and Lancien G, et al. True intra-articular lipoma of the lumbar spine. *Spine* 1987;12:820–822.

Hutton WC, and Adams NA. The forces acting on the neural arch and their relevance to low back pain. In *Engineering Aspects of the Spine.* London: Mechanical Engineering Pub. Ltd.; 1980:49–55.

Ikari C. A study of the mechanism of low back pain. The neurohistological examination of the disease. *J Bone Joint Surg* 1954; 36A:1272–1281.

Jackson HC, Winklemann RK, and Bickel WH. Nerve endings in the human lumbar spinal column and related structures. *J Bone Joint Surg* 1966;48A:1272–1281.

Junqueira LC, Carneiro J, and Long JA. *Basic Histology*, 5th ed. California: Lange Medical Publications; 1986:201–203.

Keim HA. Low back pain. *Ciba Clinical Symposia* 1973; 25:4, 9.

Keller G. Die Arthrose der Wirbelgelenke in ihrer Beziehung zum Ruckenschmerz. *Zeitschrift fur Orthopadie* 1959;91:538–550.

Kempson GE, Fregman MAR, and Sevanson SAV. Tensile properties of articular cartilage. *Nature* 1968;220:1127.

Kirkaldy-Willis WH. The perception of pain. In Kirkaldy-Willis WH, ed. *Managing Low Back Pain.* New York: Churchill Livingstone; 1983:45–49.

Kirkaldy-Willis WH. The relationship of structural pathology to the nerve root. *Spine* 1984;9:49–52.

Kirkaldy-Willis WH, and Cassidy JD. Toward a more precise diagnosis of low back pain. In Genant HK ed. *Spine Update 1984. Perspectives in Radiology, Orthopaedic Surgery, and Neurosurgery.* San Francisco: Radiology Research and Education Foundation; 1984:5–16.

Knight AD, and Levick Jr. The density and distribution of capillaries around a synovial cavity. *Quart J Exper Physiol* 1983;68:629–644.

Koreska J. Biomechanics of the lumbar spine and its clinical significance. *Orthop Clin North Am* 1977;8:121–133.

Korkala O, Gronblad M, Liesi P, and Karaharju E. Immunohistochemical demonstration of nociceptors in the ligamentous structures of the lumbar spine. *Spine* 1985;10:156–157.

Kos J. Contribution a l'etude de l'anatomie et de la vascularisation des articulations intervertebrales. *Bull Assoc Anat Berlin* 1969; 142:1.088–1.105.

Lewin T, Moffett B, and Viidik A. The morphology of the lumbar synovial intervertebral arches. *Acta Morphol Neerlando-Scandinavica* 1961;4:299–319.

Lewit K. Beitrag zur reversiblen Gelenksblockierung. *Zeitschr Orthop* 1968;105:150.

Liesi P, Gronblad M, and Korkala O, et al. Substance P: neuropeptide involved in low back pain. *Lancet* 1983;1:1328–1329.

Lim RKS, Guzman F, and Rodgers DW. Note on the muscle receptors concerned with pain. In Barker D, ed. *Symposium on Muscle Receptors.* Hong Kong: Hong Kong University Press; 1961.

Lutz G. Die Entwicklung der kleinen Wirbelgelenke. *Z Orthop* 1967;104:19–28.

MacConaill MA. The movement of bones and joints 7. The mechanical structure of articulating cartilage. *J Bone Joint Surg* 1951; 33B:251.

Macnab I. *Backache.* Baltimore: Williams and Wilkins Co.; 1977:198.

Maigne R. *Orthopaedic Medicine: A New Approach to Vertebral Manipulations.* Springfield, Ill: Thomas;1972:9.

Malemud CJ, and Moskowitz RW. Physiology of the articular cartilage. *Clin Rheumatic Dis* 1981;7:29–55.

McCutchen CW. Animal joints and weeping lubrication. *New Scientist* 1962;15:412.

McRae DL. Radiology of the lumbar spinal canal. In Weinstein PR, Ehni G, and Wilson CB eds. *Lumbar Spondylosis. Diagnosis, Management and Surgical Treatment.* Chicago: Year Book Med. Pub. Inc.; 1977;92–114.

Mennell JMcM. *Back Pain. Diagnosis and Treatment using Manipulative Techniques,* ed 1. Boston: Little Brown and Co; 1960;111.

Mooney V, and Robertson J. The facet syndrome. *Clin Orthop* 1976;115:149–156.

Naffziger HC, Inman V, and Saunders JBdeCM. Lesions of the intervertebral disc and ligamenta flava. *Surg Gynec Obstet* 1938; 66:288–299.

Paget S, and Bullough PG. Synovium and synovial fluid. In Owen R, Goodfellow J, and Bullough P eds. *Scientific Foundations of Orthopaedics and Traumatology.* London: William Heinemann Med. Books Ltd.: 1980;18–22.

Paris SV. Anatomy as related to function and pain. *Orthop Clin North Am.* 1983;14:475–489.

Pedersen HE, Blunck CFJ, and Gardner E. The anatomy of lumbosacral posterior rami and meningeal branches of spinal nerves (sinu-vertebral nerves) with an experimental study of their function. *J Bone Joint Surg* 1956;38A:377–391.

Pheasant HC. Sources of failure in laminectomies. *Orthop Clin North Am* 1975;6:319–329.

Ramsey RH. The anatomy of the ligamenta flava. *Clin Orthop* 1966;44:129–140.

Reilly J, Yong-Hing K., MacKay RW, and Kirkaldy-Willis WH. Pathological anatomy of the lumbar spine. In Helfet AJ, and Gruebel DM, eds. *Disorders of the Lumbar Spine.* Philadelphia: J.B. Lippincott; 1978:26–50.

Rhodin JAG. *Histology:A Text and Atlas.* London: Oxford University Press; 1974:200, 340–362.

Rickenbacher J, Landolt AM, and Theiler K. *Applied Anatomy of the Back.* Berlin: Springer-Verlag, 1982;30.

Rolander SD. Motion of the lumbar spine with special reference to the stabilizing effect of posterior fusion. *Acta Orthop Scand* 1966;90.

Roofe PG. Innervation of annulus fibrosus and posterior longitudinal ligament. *Arch Neurol Psychiat* 1940;44:100–103.

Rush WA, and Steiner HA. A study of lower extremity length inequality. *Am J Roentgenol* 1946;56:616–623.

Schumacher HR: Ultrastructure of the synovial membrane. *Ann Clin Lab Sci* 1975;5:489–498.

Serafini-Fracassini MD, and Smith JW. *The Structure and Biochemistry of Cartilage.* Edinburgh: Churchill-Livingstone;1974:21.

Simkin PA. Synovial physiology. In McCarthy DJ, ed. *Arthritis and Allied Conditions,* 9th ed. Philadelphia: Lea & Febiger; 1979: 167–178.

Singer KP, Giles LGF, and Day RE. Intra-articular synovial folds of thoracolumbar junction zygapophyseal joints. *Anatomical Record* 1990;226;147–152.

Stockwell RA. *Biology of Cartilage Cells.* Cambridge: Cambridge University Press;1979;1.

Sunderland S. Anatomical perivertebral influences on the intervertebral foramen. In Goldstein M, ed. *The Research Status of Spinal Manipulative Theory.* NINCDS Monograph 15. Bethesda, Md; 1975;129–140.

Taylor J, and Twomey L. Age changes in lumbar zygapophyseal joints: observations on structure and function. *Spine* 1986; 11:739–745.

Tondury G. Anatomie fonctionelle des petites articulations de rachis. *Ann Med Physique* 1972;15:173–191.

Tondury G. Beitrag zur Kenntniss der kleinen Wirbelgelenke. *Z Anat Entw Gesch* 1940;110:568–575.

Vernon-Roberts B. The pathology and interrelation of intervertebral disc lesions, osteoarthrosis of the apophyseal joints, lumbar spondylosis and low back pain. In Jayson MIV, ed. *The Lumbar Spine and Back Pain,* ed 2. Kent, U.K.: Pitman Medical; 1980:83–114.

von der Mark K, and Conrad G. Cartilage cell differentiation. *Clin Orthop* 1979;139:185–205.

Weightman B. Tensile fatigue of human articular cartilage. *J Biomech* 1976;9:133.

Weinstein PR. Pathology of lumbar stenosis and spondylosis. In Weinstein PR, Ehni G, and Wilson CB, eds. *Lumbar Spondylosis. Diagnosis, Management and Surgical Treatment.* Chicago: Year Book Med Pub.; 1977;43–91.

Weinstein PR, Ehni G, and Wilson CB. Clinical features of lumbar spondylosis and stenosis. In Weinstein PR, Ehni G, and Wilson CB, eds. *Lumbar Spondylosis, Diagnosis, Management and Surgical Treatment.* Chicago: Year Book Med. Pub.; 1977;115–133.

Williams PL, and Warwick T. *Grays Anatomy,* 36th ed. London: Churchill-Livingstone; 1980:271, 427, 445, 545.

Wyke BD. Articular neurology: A review. *Physiotherapy* 1972;58: 94–99.

Wyke BD. The neurology of low back pain. In Jayson MIV, ed. *The Lumbar Spine and Back Pain,* 2nd ed. Kent: Pitman Medical; 1980:265–339.

Wyke BD. The neurology of joints. A review of general principles. *Clin Rheumatic Dis* 1981;7:223–239.

chapter 16

Pathophysiology of the Sacroiliac Joint

J. David Cassidy
Dale R. Mierau

- **ANATOMY OF THE SACROILIAC JOINT**
- **BIOMECHANICS OF THE SACROILIAC JOINT**
- **PATHOGENESIS OF SACROILIAC SYNDROME**
- **DIAGNOSIS OF SACROILIAC JOINT SYNDROME**
- **TREATMENT OF SACROILIAC JOINT SYNDROME**
- **CONCLUSION**
- **REFERENCES**

Although the sacroiliac joint may very well be a common source of mechanical low pack pain, there is little objective evidence available to substantiate this view. The diagnosis of sacroiliac syndrome or dysfunction is based on subjective clinical findings, and a reliable method of measuring this dysfunction has not yet been developed. Nevertheless, clinicians involved in the nonoperative treatment of low back pain often direct treatment toward this joint, providing relief for their patients. The purpose of this chapter is to review what is known about the sacroiliac joint and its possible role in the pathogenesis of low back pain.

Anatomy of the Sacroiliac Joint

The sacroiliac joint is usually auricular or C-shaped, with the convex contour facing anterior and slightly inferior (Fig. 16–1). There can be marked variations in the size, shape, contour, and relative lengths of the cephalad and caudal limbs of the joint. In humans, the caudal limb is usually longer than the cephalad limb (Cassidy and Townsend, 1985). The vertically oriented auricular surface lies obliquely at an angle to the sagittal plane. Along with the symphysis pubis, the sacroiliac joints impart a limited degree of flexibility to the pelvic ring.

The sacroiliac joint is a weight-bearing joint, that is stabilized by a series of very strong ligaments. These include the sacrospinous and sacrotuberous ligaments, attaching from the anterior and posterior surface of the sacrum and running to the ischial spine and tuberosity, respectively. The massive interosseous ligament (Fig. 16–2) binds the sacrum to the ilium and forms the posterior joint margin. The thin posterior sacroiliac ligament overlies the interosseous ligament, and is separated from it by the dorsal rami of the sacral nerves and vessels. The anterior sacroiliac ligament is little more than a thickening of the joint capsule. These ligaments serve to bind the sacrum tightly between the two ilia.

As with the synovial facet joints of the lumbar spine, the sacroiliac joints are contained by a fibrous joint capsule. This capsule is well-developed anteriorly, but poorly developed posteriorly, where fasciculi of the interosseous ligament can extend into the joint and appear to be intra-articular. This phenomenon might account for the intra-articular ligament described by Illi (1951).

Wyke has reported that the sacroiliac joint capsule contains a dense plexus of unmyelinated nerve fibers indicative of a nociceptive receptor system analogous to other synovial joints (Wyke, 1982). According to Duckworth (1970), segmental derivation of this nerve supply can range from as high as L-2 to as low as S-4. In a dissection study by Solonen

Acknowledgments

The authors would like to acknowledge the assistance of David Geary and Shirley Stacey, for the illustrations; Bob Van den Buecken and John Junior, for the pathology photographs; and David Mandeville, Robin Currie, and Beverly Parent, for general photography.

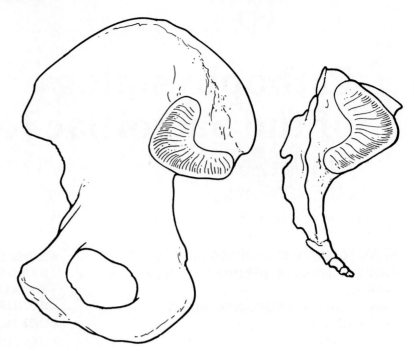

Figure 16–1. The auricular-shaped adult sacro-iliac joint. Note the central elevation of the iliac surface (left) that fits into a corresponding sacral depression (right).

(1957), the anterior aspect of the joint was most frequently innervated by the L-4 and L-5 levels, whereas the dorsal aspect of the joint most commonly received its innervation from the S-1 and S-2 levels. This wide range of segmental innervation could account for the large spectrum of somatic referred pain patterns attributed to sacroiliac disorders.

Up until the mid-1960s, the sacroiliac joint was commonly classified as an amphiarthrosis: two hyaline cartilage-covered articular surfaces joined by fibrocartilage, or a synarthrosis: articular surfaces joined by fibrous tissue (Lavignolle et al., 1983). Only recently have anatomists agreed that the sacroiliac joint is a true diarthroidial articulation. This confusion was largely due to the nature of the cartilage surfaces and age-related intra-articular changes (Bowen and Cassidy, 1981). Most of the early studies on sacroiliac joint anatomy were restricted to cadaver

and autopsy material from older age groups. Older joints characteristically show marked degenerative changes, including fibrous adhesions across the joint space. The situation was further confused by the appearance of fibrocartilage on the iliac side of the joint. These findings invariably led to the conclusion that the joint was a relatively immobile amphiarthrosis or synarthrosis.

Currently, there is general agreement that the joint is an atypical synovial articulation with a well-defined joint space and two opposing cartilage surfaces. It is atypical because one surface, the iliac surface, has the appearance of fibrocartilage rather than hyaline cartilage. Moreover, the joint often undergoes degenerative changes at an early age, giving it the appearance of an amphiarthrosis in the later years of life (Bowen and Cassidy, 1981).

The unusual makeup of the cartilage surfaces of

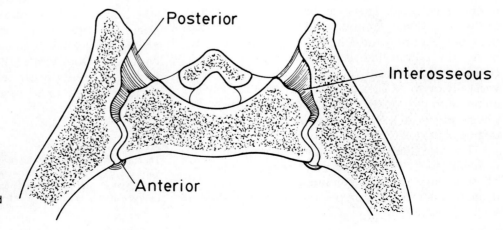

Figure 16–2. Horizontal section illustrating the obliquely positioned sacroiliac joints and their intrinsic ligaments: the anterior, interosseous, and posterior ligaments.

the sacroiliac joint results from its unique developmental anatomy. Cavitation (formation) of the joint space begins between 10 and 12 weeks' gestation in a mass of mesenchymal cells interposed between the primitive ilium and sacrum (Schunke, 1938). At this stage in development, the ilium has ossified and the sacrum is formed in hyaline cartilage. From this point onward, the two sides develop quite differently.

On the sacral side, a hyaline cartilage surface is present immediately at cavitation. With further development, the sacral cartilage anlage undergoes central enchondral ossification, leaving a peripheral hyaline cartilage cap at the articular surface at the sacroiliac joint. On the iliac side, there is a layer of dense mesenchymal cells overlying the already ossified ilium at the stage of cavitation. With further development and definition of the joint space, a small nest of chondrocytes develops underneath this mesenchyme. These cells develop into pallisading columns beneath and increasingly thinner layer of mesenchymal tissue. At birth, the sacral side is covered by a thick cap of hyaline cartilage, whereas the iliac side is covered by a thin layer of stacked chondrocytes, which in turn are covered by a thinner layer of mesenchymal tissue (Bowen and Cassidy, 1981). During infancy, the mesenchymal layer thins and slowly disappears, leaving a thin articular surface that has the appearance of fibrocartilage (Fig. 16–3).

The histological appearance of the adult sacroiliac joint is unique (Fig. 16–4). On the sacral side there is normal articular cartilage. Chondrocytes are paired together or occur alone in lacunae that are evenly dispersed throughout a homogeneous matrix. However, the iliac side appears quite different.

Chondrocytes form stacks (palisades) and tend to clump together into groups (chondrons) separated by distinct bundles of collagen fibers oriented at right angles to the joint surface. This appearance is more compatible with fibrocartilage than hyaline cartilage (Bowen and Cassidy, 1981; Walker, 1986). It should be noted, however, that biochemical analysis of sacroiliac cartilage has failed to show any difference between the two sides (Paquin et al., 1983). Both sides contain type II collagen, typical of hyaline cartilage. Type I collagen, which is typical of fibrocartilage, has not been found in the iliac cartilage. Nevertheless, the iliac cartilage has the appearance of fibrocartilage.

The gross anatomic appearance of the young sacroiliac joint reflects its unique histological makeup (Fig. 16–5). The sacral side appears smooth and creamy white, typical of articular cartilage. The iliac side is strikingly different. Its surface is rough and blue in color. This is the result of the friable nature of the fibrocartilage surface and the blue color of the trabecular bone beneath the thin transparent layer of fibrocartilage. This difference in the gross appearance of the joint is maintained throughout life (Bowen and Cassidy, 1981).

The surface topography of the sacroiliac joint changes considerably with increasing age (Bowen and Cassidy, 1981). Before puberty, the joint surfaces are flat. In young isolated autopsy specimens of the joint, it is possible to elicit small movements in any direction. After puberty, the surface topography begins a slow and dramatic transition. In the pubescent joint, a crescent-shaped ridge begins to develop along the entire length of the iliac surface. A corresponding depression develops on the sacral side (see

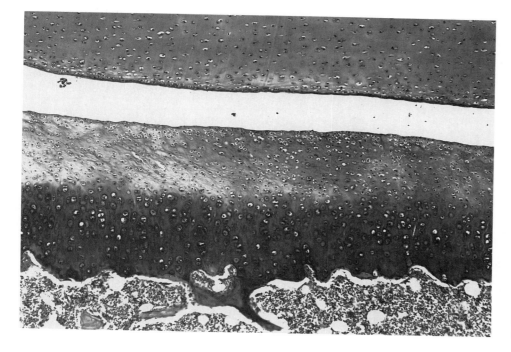

Figure 16–3. Histological section through a 1-year-old sacroiliac joint. The sacral surface (above) has the appearance of hyaline cartilage, whereas the iliac surface (below) has the appearance of fibrocartilage. (safranin O, X96)

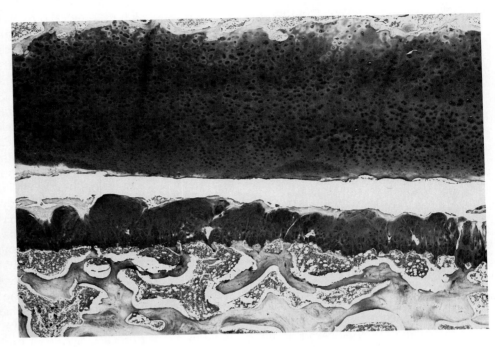

Figure 16–4. Histological section through the sacroiliac joint of a 20-year-old man. There is considerable fibrillation, crevice formation, and clumping of chondrocytes on the iliac side of the joint (below). There is no evidence of osteoarthrosis on the sacral side of the joint (above). (safranin O, X38)

Figs. 16–1 and 2). By the third decade of life, this interdigitation is well developed and limits the direction of motion in isolated autopsy specimens to a posterosuperior–anteroinferior nodding, also described as x-axis rotation or sacral nutation (Bowen and Cassidy, 1981). With increasing age, the surface irregularities become more prominent (Fig. 16–6). By middle age, each joint has an unique surface topography, with the male joints showing a greater degree of irregularity. All of these changes are highly variable both within and between subjects (Weisl, 1954).

One constant feature of the sacroiliac joint is its tendency to develop osteoarthrosis early in life (Resnick et al., 1975). It is not uncommon to see fibrillation, crevice formation, and clumping of chondrocytes on the iliac side of the joint by the third decade of life in men and soon after in women (MacDonald and Hunt, 1952; Bowen and Cassidy, 1981).

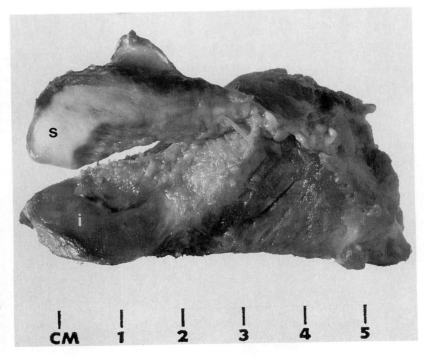

Figure 16–5. Gross anatomy of a sacroiliac joint of a 2-year-old boy. The articular surfaces are relatively flat. The sacral sides have a smooth creamy-white appearance, whereas the iliac side appears dark and corrugated (i).

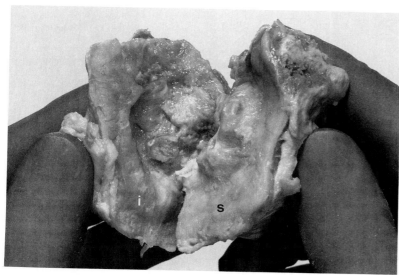

Figure 16–6. Gross anatomy of a sacroiliac joint of a 56-year-old man. The iliac (i) elevation and corresponding sacral (s) depression fit together like a tram rail.

In fresh autopsy specimens, the iliac surface often appears roughened and coated by fibrous plaques in some locations. In older specimens, the cartilage becomes thin with areas of deep erosions. The iliac subchondral bone is often sclerotic.

Similar changes do not generally affect the sacral cartilage until the fourth or fifth decades of life. On this side of the joint, the cartilage usually remains thick and the subchondral bone appears normal. Surface irregularities, such as fibrillation and crevice formation, do occur, but not to the extent seen on the iliac side of the joint. On occasion, the joint undergoes chondroid or bony ankylosis later in life. Of over 120 autopsy specimens of all ages examined at our center, only three were ankylosed, and all of these occurred in men over 50 years of age. Higher fusion rates are present in studies confined to older specimens (Brooke, 1924; Sashin, 1930; Resnick et al., 1975). Certainly, fibrous adhesions are more common in middle-aged and elderly joints, but these can also be observed in younger specimens, particularly in men (Walker, 1986).

In summary, the sacroiliac joint has an unique anatomy that changes with increasing age. The cartilage surfaces have a different histological makeup from fetal life onward. The iliac cartilage has the appearance of fibrocartilage, and is prone to premature osteoarthrosis. The joint surfaces become increasingly irregular during adult life.

Biomechanics of the Sacroiliac Joint

Although many attempts have been made to describe and measure motion in the sacroiliac joint, its biomechanical function remains largely unknown.

The joint is surrounded by some of the largest and most powerful muscles in the body, but none of these cross the joint or are known to have a direct influence on joint motion. However, contraction of any of the adjacent muscles, such as the erector spinae, psoas, quadratus lumborum, piriformis, abdominal obliques, and glutei muscles, will place shear and moment loads on these joints in proportion to their contraction forces (Miller, 1985). Such factors as the dense strong ligamentous complex, the irregular interlocking joint surface topography, and the great magnitude of force required to disrupt the joint suggest that the sacroiliac joint is very stable and capable of only minimal movement. Nevertheless, the joint probably plays some limited, yet still undefined, role in biomechanics of the lumbosacral spine.

Both in vitro and vivo kinematic studies have shown a variable degree of mobility in the sacroiliac joints (Table 16–1). There is general agreement that the joints move, but the exact nature of this motion and the function of these joints is largely unknown. In general, these studies have shown a variable degree of motion using different methods of measurement. However, the following trends have emerged:

1. The range of motion is small and decreases with increasing age.
2. The range of motion is greater in women and increased during pregnancy.
3. The motions are coupled and dependent on some degree of joint separation.
4. The predominant motion is x-axis rotation coupled with some degree of z-axis translation (Fig. 16–7).

These findings are in agreement with those predicted on an anatomic basis (Bowen and Cassidy,

TABLE 16-1.   BIOMECHANICAL STUDIES OF THE SACROILIAC JOINT

Method of Study	Findings
Manual stressing of 200 cadaveric specimens	Mobility increased in women & during pregnancy, decreased with increasing age
Radiographic measurements on 27 men & 30 women volunteers	5.6 mm of ventral sacral movement between standing and recumbency
	No sex difference
Pins inserted into the iliac spines of 12 volunteers	5 mm of movement with flexion while standing
Stereoradiographic measurements during hip flexion in a single cadaver and volunteer	Change between ilia: up to 15 mm in vitro & 26 mm in vivo
Stereoradiographic measurements in 3 women & one man	Two degrees of x-axis rotation of sacrum in various postures
Topographical study of 11 cadaveric specimens	Rotation is coupled with separation & translation
Stereophotographs of 21 subjects during standing hip flexion	1–16 mm of motion seen between ilia
Stereoradiographic measurements on 5 young adults	10–12 degrees of x-axis rotation coupled with 6 mm z-axis translation
Stereophotographic measurements in 20 young scoliotics	1.6 degrees of x-axis rotation of ilium about sacrum
Stereoradiographic measurements on 25 low back pain patients	Mean x-axis rotation of 2.5 degrees with 0.7 mm translation

1981). The interlocking surfaces of the adult sacroiliac joint result in a tram-rail-like arrangement, with the motion occurring along a roughly circular pathway (Fig. 16–8). This would place the axial center of rotation behind the joint surface in the vicinity of an extracapsular iliac tubercle, which Bakland and Hansen (1984) have described as the axial sacroiliac joint.

The sacroiliac joints are weight bearing and must resist downward shear loads in the range of 300 to 1750 N in daily activities (Miller, 1985). In relaxed standing, the lumbar discs are subjected to a compression load of about 1000 N. Therefore, under the same circumstance, each sacroiliac joint would resist about 500 N of downward shear as well as a flexion

moment of about 20 Nm. During lifting tasks, maximal compression loads at the L-3 level have been estimated at 3500 N (Nachemson, 1976). Therefore, the shear on each sacroiliac joint would rise to about 1750 N during lifting. Gunterberg et al. (1976) demonstrated a mean downward shear strength of 4865 N for both joints in cadaver specimens.

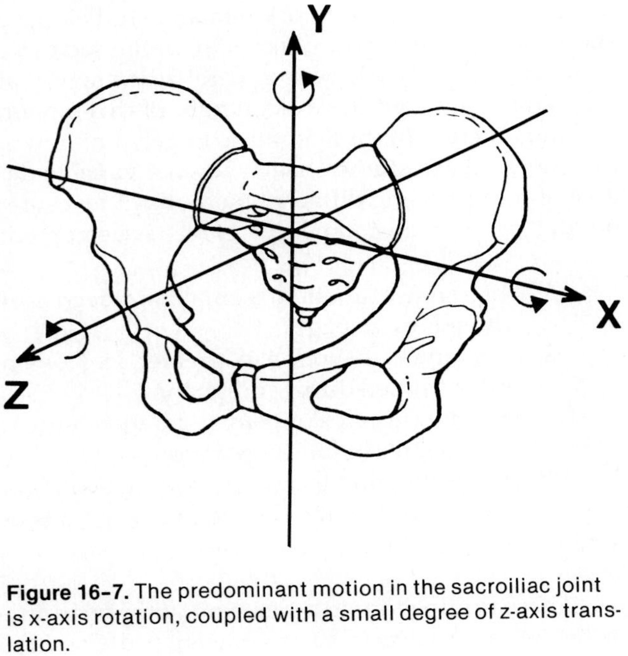

In a recent study, Miller et al. (1987) compared the mechanical properties of the sacroiliac joint with that of a lumbar motion segment. Their results showed that the sacroiliac joint is able to withstand about six times as much medially directed force (lateral shear on a lumbar motion segment) and seven times as much lateral bending force. Conversely, the lumbar motion segment is able to withstand about 20 times as much axial compression and nearly twice as much axial torsion as the sacroiliac joint. Based on this information, it seems more likely that sacroiliac strain would result from some combination of axial compression and torsion that would place stress on the weaker anterior sacroiliac ligament. Forward bending, twisting, and lifting are most likely the main activities responsible for strains to this joint. Further biomechanical studies will help to delineate fully the role of the sacroiliac joint in low back pain.

Figure 16-7. The predominant motion in the sacroiliac joint is x-axis rotation, coupled with a small degree of z-axis translation.

Pathogenesis of Sacroiliac Syndrome

Sacroiliac syndrome is a collection of symptoms and signs that result from mechanical irritation of the sacroiliac joint (Kirkaldy-Willis and Hill, 1979). As with other causes of mechanical low back pain, the pathogenesis and pathology of this syndrome are not well understood. In many cases, experts in the field of low back pain deny that the joint plays any role in

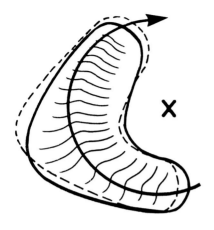 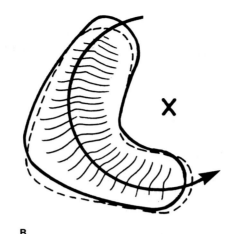

B

Figure 16–8. The motion at the sacroiliac joint is dictated by its surface topography. The interlocking surfaces allow sacral nutation or negative (**A**) and positive (**B**) rotation about the x-axis. The axial center of rotation is located just behind the joint (x).

the pathogenesis of low back pain (Currey et al., 1979). On the other hand, others believe that this joint is responsible for a large proportion of mechanical backache (Bernard and Kirkaldy-Willis, 1987).

The popularity of the sacroiliac joint as a cause for mechanical backache has been subject to considerable historical variation. Before the discovery of the herniated intervertebral disc by Mixter and Barr in 1943, the sacroiliac joint was thought to be a primary source of low back pain. The accepted theory was that sciatica develops as a result of joint subluxation and subsequent irritation of the lumbosacral plexus as it traverses the sacroiliac joint (Cox, 1927). After 1934, the focus of attention switched to the intervertebral disc and sciatica became an indication for disc excision. Over the next 40 years, almost all low back pain was attributed to mechanical derangement of the intervertebral disc.

Over the last decade there has been much renewed interest in the sacroiliac joint as a cause of low back and leg pain. This is partially due to the poor results of indiscriminate surgical treatment of back pain and sciatica by discectomy and/or fusion and better diagnostic criteria for the diagnosis of disc herniation. We now know that less than 10% of general practice patients suffering from back pain have an intervertebral disc herniation (Dillane et al., 1966; Roland, 1983). Unfortunately, similar statistics are not available for the prevalence of sacroiliac syndrome. Although myelography, computerized tomography, and magnetic resonance imaging can reliably demonstrate a disc herniation, they have not been found to be useful in the diagnosis of sacroiliac syndrome. At present, there is no known objective method of demonstrating sacroiliac syndrome.

Despite the lack of objective diagnostic criteria, there have been some reports on the prevalence of sacroiliac syndrome, based on subjective clinical findings. In our own University Hospital Back Pain Clinic, a retrospective review of 1,293 patients with low back pain treated over a 12-year period revealed that chronic sacroiliac dysfunction was the primary diagnosis in 23% of cases (Bernard and Kirkaldy-Willis, 1987). Other studies have implicated the sacroiliac joint as the main problem in as many as 50 to 70% of adults with low back pain (Barbor, 1978; Bourne, 1979). Children might also be affected, and a survey of a primary and secondary school in the city of Saskatoon found a surprisingly high percentage of children with a history of low back pain and associated clinical evidence of sacroiliac dysfunction (Mierau et al., 1984).

There is evidence that sacroiliac disorders are more common in women (Cassidy et al., 1985). They are particularly prone to this problem during menstruation, pregnancy, and after childbirth (Grieve, 1976; Potter and Cassidy, 1979). Hormonal influences during these periods result in relaxation of the pelvic ligaments, predisposing the sacroiliac joints to mechanical strain. Sacroiliac disturbances have also been reported to occur after gynecologic surgery in about 10% of women (Novotny and Dvorak, 1971).

A recent study of women with low back pain found that 40% had scintigraphic evidence of sacroiliac disease, but no other evidence of inflammatory arthritis (Davis and Lentle, 1978). Similar findings have been reported in men (Chisin, 1984). A yet unpublished study, just completed at our center, suggests that the bone scan might prove to be the first objective test for the diagnosis of sacroiliac syndrome (Mierau, 1989). These results show that small increases in radionuclide uptake occur on the side of the symptomatic sacroiliac joint. This suggests that sacroiliac syndrome is associated with a chronic low-grade inflammation. Furthermore, whenever two or more sacroiliac stress tests were positive (Figs. 16–9 and 10), the bone scan invariably showed increased uptake over that joint.

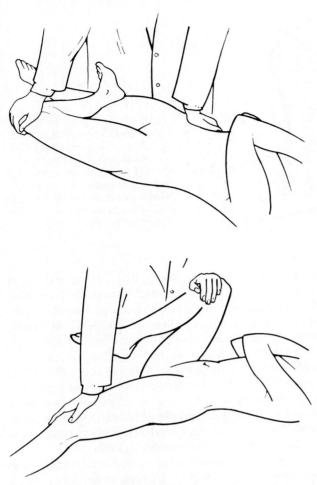

Figure 16-9. Faber Patrick's test (above) stresses the hip and the sacroiliac joint through flexion, abduction, and external rotation of the hip. A positive test will produce posterior buttock or groin pain in the absence of hip joint pathology. Gaenslen's test (below) counter-rotates the two sacroiliac joints, stressing them at their end range of motion. It can aggravate the symptoms of sacroiliac syndrome on either side.

There has been a great deal of speculation regarding the pathological causes of mechanical sacroiliac syndrome or dysfunction. Osteoarthrosis occurs at a young age in this joint. However, there is a poor correlation between pain and the presence of osteoarthrosis elsewhere in the spine (Magora and Schwartz, 1976; Witt et al., 1984). This, too, is probably true for the sacroiliac joints, as it is not uncommon to see radiographic evidence of degenerative changes in patients with no symptoms. Generally speaking, degenerative changes in the spine are positively correlated to increasing age.

Many clinicians still believe that subluxation or small displacements of the sacroiliac joint are responsible for the symptoms (Greenman, 1986; Bourdillon, 1987). This notion has been further perpetuated by the success of manipulation in the treatment of sacroiliac syndrome. In fact, many manipulative techniques require precise direction of force to reduce different types of displacements. However, sacroiliac subluxation has never been confirmed radiographically, despite many attempts to do so. Furthermore, there is now overwhelming evidence that manipulation does not reduce subluxation, but rather exerts its effect by increasing mobility and reducing pain through proprioceptive reflex stimulation (Terrett and Vernon, 1984; Kirkaldy-Willis and Cassidy, 1985, Mierau et al., 1988). The notion that manipulation reduces sacroiliac subluxation is popular, but unsubstantiated.

Altered mobility or dysfunction of the sacroiliac joint has been implicated as the main pathology in sacroiliac syndrome. The term implies a malfunction of the normal mechanics of the joint causing either too much motion (hypermobility) or too little motion (hypomobility or fixation). The obvious problem with this approach is that the normal biomechanics of the joint are not well understood, and the movements of the joint are so slight that they are difficult to detect. Furthermore, variations in the normal range of motion have yet to be defined.

Nevertheless, some clinicians believe that the injured sacroiliac joint is unstable and treatment might include a trochanteric belt or sclerosant injections to the sacroiliac ligaments (Macnab, 1977; Grieve, 1983). Others maintain that the symptomatic joint is stiff or fixed (Gitelman, 1980). This might explain why patients with sacroiliac syndrome respond to manipulation of the joint (Cassidy et al., 1985). In the lumbar spine, reduced mobility is common in patients with low back pain, and an increase in mobility is positively correlated to an improvement in symptoms (Mayer et al., 1984; Mellin, 1985). Perhaps the same is true for the sacroiliac joint. However, as appealing as these theories might be, there is no objective evidence to support them. In fact, a recent stereoradiographic study failed to demonstrate any difference in mobility between symptomatic and asymptomatic joints (Sturesson et al., 1989). Until more precise and reliable methods of measuring sacroiliac mobility are developed, the exact role of altered mobility in the pathogenesis of this disorder will remain unknown.

Diagnosis of Sacroiliac Joint Syndrome

The diagnosis of sacroiliac syndrome is based almost entirely on the history and clinical examination. The history is that of mechanical backache with or without referred pain into the lower extremity. Many

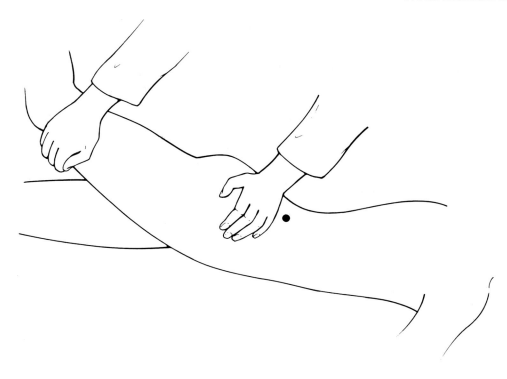

Figure 16–10. The extension test (Yeoman's test) rotates the ilium at the sacroiliac joint. A positive test will produce pain over the posterior sacroiliac ligament. This test also extends the lumbosacral spine and stretches the femoral nerve.

times the patient is a young woman with a history of dysmenorrhea, recent pregnancy, or delivery (Potter and Cassidy, 1979). This syndrome has been described in persons with altered gait due to hip, knee, ankle, or foot disorders and place undue postural stress onto one or both of the sacroiliac joints (Solonen, 1957). Activity-related sacroiliac syndrome has been reported in ballet dancers, skaters, and military recruits (Ayres et al., 1981; Chisin et al., 1984). In some cases, the back pain associated with spondylolisthesis may be partially due to sacroiliac dysfunction (Mierau et al., 1987). Persistent back pain after hip surgery has been attributed to the sacroiliac joint (Pap et al., 1987). Sacroiliac manipulation has been employed successfully to treat low back pain after discectomy and spinal fusion. (Diakow and Cassidy, 1983; McGregor and Cassidy, 1983).

Most often the pain of sacroiliac syndrome is localized over the posterosuperior iliac spine and buttock. It may be referred into the groin and lower extremity in a nondermatomal pattern. Rarely, this syndrome can present as lower quadrant abdominal pain and be confused with urologic disease and appendicitis (Norman, 1968). Groin, trochanteric, and knee pain can occur in both sacroiliac syndrome and hip disorders. On occasion, treatment has been erroneously directed toward the sacroiliac joint when the pain is from hip joint disease (Kitchen et al., 1988; Quon et al., 1989). Because the sacroiliac joint

receives its innervation from such a wide range of spinal levels, referred pain from this joint can cause some diagnostic confusion.

On examination, the patient might present with a slight limp due to difficulty in bearing weight on the affected side (Robinson et al., 1987). There is usually tenderness over the posterosuperior iliac spine and the posterior sacroiliac ligament. Unilateral lumbar paraspinal muscle spasm and gluteal trigger points often accompany this syndrome. Midline lumbar tenderness and decreased lumbar range of motion occur when there is associated lumbar dysfunction. Straight-leg raising can be reduced by the associated back pain and hamstring tightness. Signs of nerve root tension and neurological deficit do not occur in sacroiliac syndrome. The patient may complain of paresthesias or subjective decrease in light touch sensation in the lower limb, but there is preservation of temperature, pain, and position sense. Any loss of muscle power in the lower extremities is due to pain rather than neurological deficit. A portion of the examination should be directed toward excluding other causes for low back pain, both mechanical and pathological.

There are several clinical tests available that place stress on the sacroiliac joints and elicit pain in sacroiliac syndrome. Gaenslen's, Faber-Patrick's, and the extension tests are the most useful (Figs. 16–9 and 10). All of these provocation tests place equal stress on the hip joint, and hip joint pathology must be ruled out before their interpretation. In most cases, two of these three tests are positive in sacroiliac syndrome.

There are numerous clinical tests that attempt to assess sacroiliac mobility. The most popular is the test first described by Gillet (1979). This test attempts to measure x-axis rotation at the sacroiliac joint when the subject flexes the hip joint (Fig. 16–11). This small amount of rotation is amplified at the posterosuperior iliac spine because of its location dorsal to the axial center of rotation (Fig. 16–12). In an abnormal test, the motion is lacking, and this is one indication for manipulation. Although the test appears to be reliable, its validity remains to be proven (Herzog et al., 1989). For example, in cases of lumbar paravertebral muscle spasm the Gillet test can appear to be positive (Fig. 16–13).

The differential diagnosis of sacroiliac syndrome can be problematic. On occasion the joint can be the site of serious disease, and the examiner must be aware of the possibility of infection, inflammatory arthropathy, and neoplasm. In suspicious cases, there should be an adequate radiographic examination of the lumbar spine, sacroiliac, and hip joints. This may need to be supplemented by laboratory examination of blood (including sedimentation rate, HLA B27 antigen, antinuclear antibodies, and rheumatoid factor) and urinalysis. Radionuclide bone scanning should be considered in cases of suspected sacroiliitis or neoplasm of the spine. In the majority of cases of sacroiliac syndrome, the x-rays are unremarkable.

Some spinal disorders can present with symptoms that are difficult to distinguish from sacroiliac syndrome. Disorders of the lower lumbar facet joints can result in somatic referred pain, which is similar to the pain from sacroiliac syndrome (Mooney and Robertson, 1976; McCall et al., 1979). Thoracolumbar facet syndrome (Maigne's syndrome) and small tho-

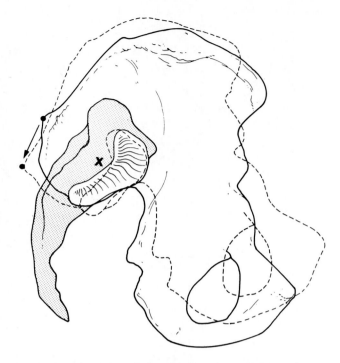

Figure 16–12. Gillet's test measures x-axis rotation at the sacroiliac joint in the clinical setting. The small amount of rotation at the joint is amplified at the PSIS (*arrow*) that is some distance posterior to the center of rotation (x).

racolumbar compression fractures are often confused with sacroiliac syndrome because of referred pain along the course of the cluneal nerve at the iliac crest overlying the sacroiliac joint (Proctor et al., 1985). Sacroiliac syndrome has been known to simulate intervertebral disc syndrome (Norman and May, 1956). Lateral nerve entrapment often refers pain to the buttock and down the leg in a similar fashion to the sacroiliac joint (Kirkaldy-Willis and Hill, 1979). Ankylosing spondylitis, rheumatoid arthritis, Reiter's syndrome, psoriasis, and inflammatory

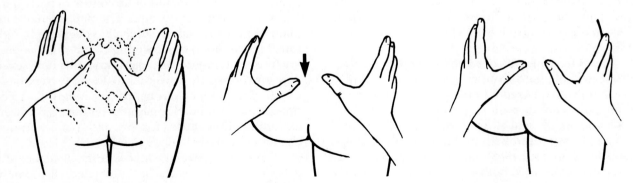

Figure 16–11. Gillet's test for sacroiliac motion requires palpation of the relationship between the posterior superior iliac spine (PSIS) and the second sacral spinous process (SSSP), left illustration. Normally, when the patient raises his or her knee, the PSIS drops at the end of hip flexion, middle illustration. If the joint is fixed (stiff), the small amount of iliac rotation that occurs after hip flexion is absent and the PSIS remains level to the SSSP, right illustration.

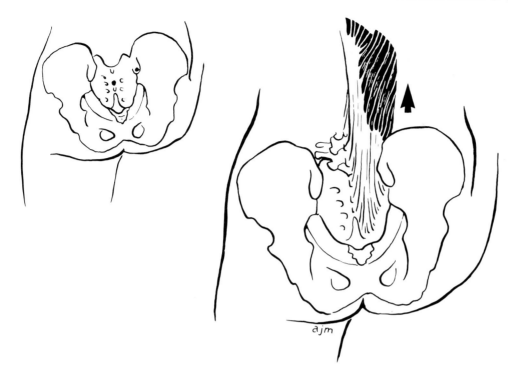

Figure 16–13. Rotation of the ilium at the sacroiliac joint can be limited by lumbosacral paravertebral muscle spasm (on the right) as well as sacroiliac joint fixation (on the left). Therefore, Gillet's test can be positive in acute low back pain due to other causes than sacroiliac joint syndrome. (*From J of Canadian Chiropractic Assn, Vol. 24, No. 2, p 73, June 1980, with permission.*)

bowel disease can lead to sacroiliitis, which can be confused with sacroiliac syndrome in the initial stages of the disease. Pelvic metastases have been known to mimic sacroiliac syndrome in the early stages (LaFrance et al., 1987). The astute clinician will consider all these possibilities before diagnosing sacroiliac syndrome.

Treatment of Sacroiliac Joint Syndrome

In most cases, acute sacroiliac syndrome is a benign, self-limiting disorder. After a short period of rest, most patients will return to their normal activities without consulting a physician or chiropractor. Unfortunately, there is a high risk of recurrence, and about 60% of these patients will suffer a second episode of back pain over the next 2 years (Bergquist-Ullman and Larsson, 1970; Nachemson, 1982). If the pain persists, limits daily activities, or becomes recurrent, the patient should undergo an initial investigation to rule out serious pathology and then a regimen of treatment.

At our center, the first line of treatment for sacroiliac syndrome is a regimen of manipulation. In a prospective clinical study at our hospital, over 90% of patients disabled by chronic sacroiliac syndrome responded to a 2- to 3-week regimen of daily sacroiliac manipulation (Cassidy et al., 1985). Similar results have been reported in other studies of manipu-

lation (Riches, 1930; Zhiming, 1984). Successful treatment with manipulation does not prevent recurrence of the problem. We also recommend attendance at our Back School and postural exercises to rehabilitate the patient (Kirkaldy-Willis, 1988). Increasing physical fitness through activity is the only effective method known to prevent recurrent back pain (Cady et al., 1979).

There are many different techniques available to manipulate the sacroiliac joint. We have found the side-posture method the most effective (Figs. 16–14 and 15). The manipulative thrust is delivered to the posterosuperior iliac spine or the ischial tuberosity. This results in a cracking sound, which is the result of intra-articular cavitation of synovial carbon dioxide (Unsworth et al., 1971; Mierau et al., 1988). The goal of this form of treatment is to mobilize a stiff or fixed joint and not to reduce a misalignment. The method of manipulation should vary according to patient tolerance. Care should be taken to avoid injury to the lumbar spine in patients with associated spondylolisthesis, disc herniation, or other co-existing lesions in the lumbar spine (Cassidy and Kirkaldy-Willis, 1988). In the case of postoperative back pain, sacroiliac manipulation should not be attempted until the patient has made a complete recovery from his or her operation (McGregor and Cassidy, 1983). It is important to limit the force of the manipulation in the elderly and in pregnant women.

Injection of local anesthetic into the painful sacroiliac joint is another treatment option. It is not al-

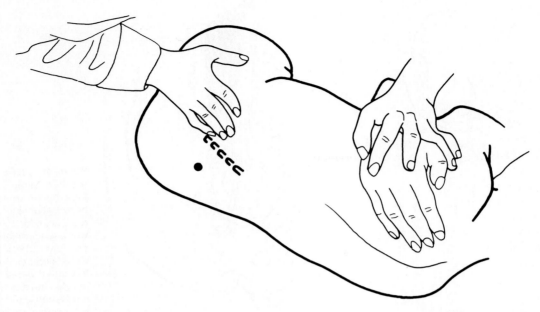

Figure 16–14. The superior sacroiliac manipulation is accomplished by contacting the PSIS and thrusting the ilium into flexion (positive x-axis rotation). (*From J of Man and Physio Thera, 6 (1), March 1983, with permission.*)

ways possible to infiltrate the joint space because of the inaccessibility of the obliquely oriented interlocking articular surfaces. Nevertheless, good results have been obtained with injection of a mixture of local anesthetic and corticosteroid into the posterior and interosseous ligaments (Bourne, 1979; Schuchmann and Cannon, 1986). We find this procedure particularly useful in cases that do not initially respond to manipulation (Bernard and Kirkaldy-Willis, 1987). In some difficult cases, we combine injection with manipulation. In addition, sacroiliac injection

can be useful in differentiating groin pain that originates from sacroiliac or hip disorders.

Other treatments have been advocated for sacroiliac instability. The use of a trochanteric belt has been advocated by Macnab (1977). Although there are no studies on the efficacy of this treatment, it might be useful in the management of postpartum sacroiliac dysfunction. Surgical fusion of the sacroiliac joint has been advocated in the past (Solonen, 1957). A more recent study of sacroiliac arthrodesis for chronic back pain reported 50% satisfactory re-

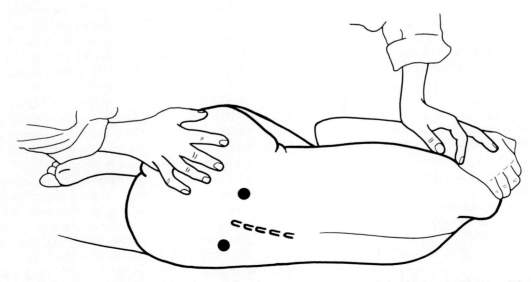

Figure 16–15. The inferior sacroiliac manipulation is accomplished by contacting the ischial tuberosity and thrusting the ilium into extension (negative x-axis rotation). (*From J of Man and Physio Thera, 6 (1), March 1983, with permission.*)

sults (Waisbrod et al., 1987). In our opinion, sacroiliac instability or hypermobility is uncommon and joint arthrodesis is rarely indicated.

Conclusion

Although the basic anatomic structure of the sacroiliac joint has been thoroughly investigated, its biomechanical function is not certain. The joint does possess a small range of motion that serves to give the pelvic ring a degree of elasticity. In addition, the role that this joint plays in the pathogenesis of low back pain is not entirely clear. Nevertheless, manipulation of the painful sacroiliac joint is successful in the majority of cases. There is an obvious need for more research into the role of the sacroiliac joint in low back pain.

References

Ayres J, Hilson AJW, and Maisey MN, et al. An improved method for sacro-iliac joint imaging: a study of normal subjects, patients with sacroiliitis and patients with low back pain. *Clin Radiol* 1981;32:441.

Bakland O, and Hansen JH. The "axial sacroiliac joint." *Anat Clin* 1984;6:29.

Barbor R. Back pain. *Br Med J* 1978;ii:566.

Bernard TN, and Kirkaldy-Willis WH. Non-specific low back pain. *Clin Orthop* 1987;217:266.

Bergquist-Ullman M, and Larsson U. Acute low back pain in industry. *Acta Orthop Scand* (Suppl) 1970;170:1–110.

Bourdillon JF. A torsion-free approach to the pelvis. *Manual Medicine* 1987;3:20.

Bourne IHJ. Treatment of backache with local injections. *Practitioner* 1979;222:708.

Bowen V, and Cassidy JD. Macroscopic and microscopic anatomy of the sacroiliac joint from embryonic life until the eighth decade. *Spine* 1981;6:620.

Brooke R. The sacroiliac joint. *J Anat* 1924;58:299.

Cady LD, Bischoff DP, and O'Connell ER, et al. Strength and fitness and subsequent back injuries in firefighters. *J Occup Med* 1979;21:269.

Cassidy JD, and Kirkaldy-Willis WH. Manipulation. In Kirkaldy-Willis WH, ed. *Managing Low Back Pain.* New York: Churchill-Livingstone; 1988.

Cassidy JD, Kirkaldy-Willis WH, and McGregor M. Spinal manipulation for the treatment of chronic low back and leg pain: an observational study. In Buerger AA, and Greenman PE, eds. *Empirical Approaches to the Validation of Manipulative Therapy.* Springfield, Ill: Thomas; 1985.

Cassidy JD, and Townsend HGG. Sacroiliac joint strain as a cause of back and leg pain in man—implications for the horse. *Proc Am Assoc Equine Practr* 1985;31:317.

Chisin R, Milgrom C, and Margulies J, et al. Unilateral sacroiliac overuse syndrome in military recruits. *Br Med J* 1984;289:590.

Colachis SC, Wardin RE, Bechtol CO, and Strohm BR. Movement of the sacroiliac joint in the adult male: a preliminary report. *Arch Phys Med Rehabil* 1963;44:490.

Cox HH. Sacroiliac subluxation as a cause of backache. *Surg Gynec Obstet* 1927;45:637.

Currey HLF, Greenwood RM, Lloyd GG, and Murray RS. A prospective study of low back pain. *Rheumatol Rehabil* 1979;18:94.

Davis P, and Lentle BC. Evidence for sacroiliac disease as a common cause of low backache in women. *Lancet* 1978;ii:496.

Diakow P, Cassidy JD, and de Korompay V. Post-surgical sacroiliac syndrome: A case study. *J Can Chiropr Assoc* 1983;27:19.

Dillane JB, Fry J, and Kalton G. Acute back syndrome—a study from general practice. *Br Med J* 1966;ii:82.

Drerup B, and Hierholzer E. Movement of the human pelvis and displacement of related anatomical landmarks on the body surface. *J Biomech* 1987;20:971.

Duckworth JWA. The anatomy and movements of the sacroiliac joints. In Wolf-Trier HD, ed. *Manuelle Medizin und ihre Wissenschaftlichen Grundlagen.* Heidelberg: Verlag fur physikalische Medizin; 1970.

Egund N, Olsson TH, Schmid H, and Selvik G. Movements in the sacroiliac joints demonstrated with roentgen stereophotogrammetry. *Acta Radiol Diagn* 1978;19:833.

Frigerio NA, Stowe RR, and Howe JW. Movement of the sacroiliac joint. *Clin Orthop* 1974;100:340.

Gillet H, and Lieken M. *Belgian Chiropractic Research Notes.* Brussels: 1979.

Gitelman R. A chiropractic approach to biomechanical disorders of the lumbar spine and pelvis. In Haldeman S., ed. *Principles and Practice of Chiropractic.* New York: Appleton-Century-Crofts; 1980.

Greenman PE. Innominate shear dysfunction in the sacroiliac syndrome. *Manual Medicine* 1986;2:114.

Grieve E. Lumbo-pelvic rhythm and mechanic dysfunction of the sacroiliac joint. *Physiotherapy* 1981;67:171.

Grieve EFM. Mechanical dysfunction of the sacroiliac joint. *Int Rehabil Med* 1983;5:46.

Grieve GP. The sacroiliac joint. *Physiotherapy* 1976; 62:384.

Gunterberg B, Romanus B, and Stener B. Pelvic strength after major amputation of the sacrum. An experimental study. *Acta Orthop Scand* 1976;47:635.

Herzog W, Read LJ, and Conway JW, et al. Reliability of motion palpation procedures to detect sacroiliac fixations. *J Manipulative Physiol Ther* 1989;12:86.

Illi FW. *The Vertebral Column: Life Line of the Body.* Chicago: National College of Chiropractic; 1951.

Kitchen RG, Mierau D, Cassidy D, and Dupuis P. Congenital dislocation of the hip and adult low back pain: A report of three cases. *J Can Chiropr Assoc* 1988;32:11.

Kirkaldy-Willis WH. *Managing Low Back Pain.* New York: Churchill-Livingstone; 1988.

Kirkaldy-Willis WH, and Cassidy JD. Spinal manipulation in the treatment of low-back pain. *Can Fam Physician* 1985;31:535.

Kirkaldy-Willis WH, and Hill R. A more precise diagnosis for low back pain. *Spine* 1979;4:102.

LaFrance LJ, Cassidy JD, Nykoliation JW, and Mierau DR. Back pain and spinal metastases: A case study. *J Can Chiropr Assoc* 1987;31:79.

Lavignolle B, Vital JM, and Senegas J, et al. An approach to the functional anatomy of the sacroiliac joints in vivo. *Anat Clin* 1983;5:169.

MacDonald GR, and Hunt TE. Sacroiliac joints: Observations on the gross and histological changes in the various age groups. *Can Med Assoc J* 1952;66:157.

Macnab I. Lesions of the sacroiliac joints. In Macnab I, ed. *Backache.* Baltimore: Williams and Wilkins; 1977.

Magora A, and Schwartz A. Relation between the low back pain syndrome and x-ray findings. 1. degenerative osteoarthritis. *Scand J Rehab Med* 1976;8:115.

Mayer TG, Tencer AF, Kristoferson S, and Mooney V. Use of noninvasive techniques for quantification of spinal range-of-motion in normal subjects and chronic low-back dysfunction patients. *Spine* 1984; 9:588.

McCall IW, Park WM, and O'Brien JP. Induced pain referral from posterior lumbar elements in normal subjects. *Spine* 1979;4:441.

McGregor M, and Cassidy JD. Post-surgical sacroiliac joint syndrome. *J Manipulative Physiol Ther* 1983;6:1.

Mellin G. Physical therapy for chronic low back pain: Correlations between spinal mobility and treatment outcome. *Scand J Rehab Med* 1985;17:163.

Mierau DR. Radionuclide scanning of sacroiliac joint syndrome. Presented at Orthopaedic Rounds. Saskatoon, 1989.

Mierau DR, Cassidy JD, and Bowen V, et al. Manipulation and mobilization of the third metacarpophalangeal joint: A quantitative radiographic and range of motion study. *Manual Medicine* 1988; 3:135.

Mierau DR, Cassidy JD, Hamin T, and Milne RA. Sacroiliac joint dysfunction and low back pain in school aged children. *J Manipulative Physiol Ther* 1984;7:81.

Mierau D, Cassidy JD, McGregor M, and Kirkaldy-Willis WH. A comparison of the effectiveness of spinal manipulative therapy for low back pain patients with and without spondylolisthesis. *J Manipulative Physiol Ther* 1987;10:49.

Miller J. The biomechanics of the lumbar posterior elements and sacroiliac joints. In Buerger AA, and Greenman PE, eds. *Empirical Approaches to the Validation of Spinal Manipulation.* Springfield, Ill: Thomas; 1985.

Miller JAA, Schultz AB, and Andersson GBJ. Load-displacement behavior of sacroiliac joints. *J Orthop Res* 1987;5:92.

Mixter WJ, and Barr JS. Rupture of the intervertebral disc with involvement of the spinal canal. *New Engl J Med* 1934;211:210.

Mooney V, and Robertson J. The facet syndrome. *Clin Orthop* 1976;115:149.

Nachemson A. The lumbar spine: An orthopaedic challenge. *Spine* 1976;1:59.

Nachemson AL. The natural course of low back pain. In White AA, and Gordon SL eds. *American Academy of Orthopaedic Surgeons Symposium on Idiopathic Low Back Pain.* St Louis: CV Mosby; 1982.

Norman GF. Sacroiliac disease and its relationship to lower abdominal pain. *Am J Surg* 1968;116:54.

Norman GF, and May A. Sacroiliac conditions simulating intervertebral disc syndrome. *West J Surg* 1956;64:461.

Novotny A, and Dvorak V. Functional disturbances of the vertebral column after gynaecological operations. *Manual Medicine* 1971; 3:65.

Pap A, Maager M, and Kolarz G. Functional impairment of the sacroiliac joint after total hip replacement. *Int Rehabil Med* 1987;8:145.

Paquin JD, van der Rest M, and Maire PJ, et al. Biochemical and morphologic studies of cartilage from the adult human sacroiliac joint. *Arthritis Rheum* 1983;26:887.

Potter GE, and Cassidy JD. Diagnosis and manipulative management of post-partum back pain: A case study. *J Manipulative Physiol Ther* 1979;2:99.

Proctor D, Dupuis P, and Cassidy JD. Thoracolumbar syndrome as a cause of low-back pain: A report of two cases. *J Can Chiropr Assoc* 1985;29:71.

Quon JA, Burns SH, and O'Connor SM, et al. Slipped capital femoral epiphysis: A report of two cases. *J Can Chirop Assoc* 1989;in press.

Resnick D, Niwayama G, and Goergen TG. Degenerative disease of the sacroiliac joint. *Invest Radiol* 1975;10:608.

Riches RW. End results of manipulation of the back. *Lancet* 1930;i:957.

Robinson RO, Herzog W, and Nigg BM. Use of force platform variables to quantify the effects of chiropractic manipulation on gait symmetry. *J Manipulative Physiol Ther* 1987;10:172.

Roland MO. The natural history of back pain. *Practitioner* 1983; 227:1119.

Sashin D. A critical analysis of the anatomy and the pathological changes of the scroiliac joints. *J Bone Joint Surg* 1930;53A:69.

Schuchmann JA, and Cannon CL. Sacroiliac strain syndrome: Diagnosis and treatment. *Tex Med* 1986;82:33.

Schunke BG. The anatomy and development of the sacroiliac joint. *Anat Rec* 1938;72:313.

Solonen KA. The sacroiliac joint in the light of anatomical, roentgenological and clinical studies. *Acta Orthop Scand* (Suppl) 1957;27:1.

Sturesson B, Selvik G, and Uden A. Movements of the sacroiliac joints: A roentgen stereophotogrammetric analysis. *Spine* 1989; 14:162.

Terrett ACJ, and Vernon H. Manipulation and pain tolerance: a controlled study of the effect of spinal manipulation on paraspinal cutaneous pain tolerance levels. *Am J Phys Med* 1984;63:217.

Unsworth A, Dowson D, and Wright V. Cracking joints: a bioengineering study of cavitation in the metacarpophalangeal joint. *Ann Rheum Dis* 1971;30:348.

Waisbrod H, Krainick J-U, and Gerbershagen HU. Sacroiliac joint arthrodesis for chronic lower back pain. *Arch Orthop Trauma Surg* 1987;106:238.

Walker JM. Age-related differences in the human sacroiliac joint: a histological study; implications for therapy. *J Orthop Sports Physical Ther* 1986;7:325.

Weisl H. The articular surfaces of the sacro-iliac joint and their relation to the movements of the sacrum. *Acta Anat* 1954;22:1.

Weisl H. The movements of the sacroiliac joint. *Acta Anat* 1955;23:80.

Wilder DG, Pope MH, and Frymoyer JW. The functional topography of the sacroiliac joint. *Spine* 1980;5:575.

Witt I, Vestergaard A, and Rosenklint A. A comparative analysis of x-ray findings of the lumbar spine in patients with and without lumbar pain. *Spine* 1984;9:298.

Wyke B. Receptor systems in lumbosacral tissues in relation to the production of low back pain. In White AA, and Gordon SL eds. *American Academy of Orthopaedic Surgeons Symposium on Idiopathic Low Back Pain.* St. Louis: CV Mosby; 1982.

Zhiming M. Manipulative treatment of subluxation of the sacroiliac joint. *J Traditional Chin Med* 1984;4:33.

chapter 17

Interaction of Spinal Biomechanics and Physiology

John J. Triano

- **BASIC BIOMECHANICAL CONCEPTS**
- **MAJOR MUSCULOSKELETAL TISSUE PROPERTIES**
  Bone
  Articular Cartilage
  Synovial Fluid Joint Lubrication
  Intervertebral Discs
  Ligaments, Tendons, and Fascia
  Muscle
  Nerve

- **KINEMATICS AND KINETICS OF MOTION SEGMENTS**
  Kinematics of Intervertebral Foramina
  Motion Segment Behavior
- **LOAD DISTRIBUTION IN THE FUNCTIONAL SPINAL UNITS**
  Subluxation Hypotheses
  Effects of Subluxation
- **CONCLUSION**
- **REFERENCES**

Recognition of costs from spine-related impairments has recently been given by the National Institutes of Occupational Safety and Health (Millar, 1986). Mechanical factors are involved in both the onset and treatment for many of these disorders. Traditional and modern theories of chiropractic practice tenaciously hold to beliefs that spinal lesions manifest themselves primarily in two ways: mechanically and neurologically. Appearing independently or as coexisting components, the clinical presentation of patients is commonly seen as a varying mixture of the two. There are good reasons, then, to study the mechanics of the human trunk and spine as prevention and intervention strategies for spinal disorders are sought. For that reason, the study of spine impairments ought begin with an understanding for what is known about the mechanics of motion segments and the tissues that attach to them. Mechanical properties and behavior of tissues are related to their structure. They may ultimately be explained in terms of the networks of collagen and elastin fibers, muscle, ground substance, interstitial fluids, and their properties. Moreover, the behavior of organs that they constitute depends on their tissues, on their geometry, and their relationship to neighboring organs (Fung, 1987).

Basic Biomechanical Concepts

The clinician uses his or her perceptions of motion segment behavior to make therapeutic decisions. Many impressions are derived from auditory, palpatory, or visual cues collected during a manual examination. At the outset, then, a review of the principal concepts and terms that describe mechanical qualities may be helpful. It is these perceived qualities that give rise to clinical notions about the patient's condition.

Mechanical qualities can be separated into categories based on whether the tissue acts primarily like a solid, a fluid, or a mixture of the two. Solids are described according to their elasticity, strength, hardness, and stiffness (Table 17–1). Energy used in deforming a solid body is stored, ready to be returned in ways described by these expressions. Bone, tendon, and ligament are body tissues that act primarily like elastic solids under most circumstances. Fluids, on the other hand, possess the quality of viscosity, which allows them to flow, as with cerebrospinal fluid and blood. Once energy has been used to cause a fluid to flow, that energy is dissipated and cannot be returned. Finally, some tissues

TABLE 17–1. PHYSICAL PROPERTIES USED TO DESCRIBE CHARACTERISTICS OF SOLID TISSUES

Compliance. The distance moved under the influence of a unit load. The inverse of stiffness.

Creep. Gradual continued deformation of a structure after the initial change of shape when loaded.

Deformation. The change of shape from loads applied to a material or structure.

Elastic. A property of the stress–strain relationship where energy of deformation is stored and released as the body returns to its unstressed shape.

Force. Influence on a body that deforms it or causes it to accelerate.

Hardness. The tendency of a surface to resist deformation.

Hysteresis. Rate of recovery from deformation. Rate of restoration to original shape is often slower than the rate of deformation.

Moment. A force acting at some distance from the point of interest. Moments tend to deform a body by twisting it or accelerating it in a spin.

Stiffness. The ratio of stress to strain or force to deformation. The amount of load needed to move a unit distance.

Stress. Force distributed across a surface area. Axial stress: Force perpendicular to the surface. Shear stress: Force parallel to the surface.

Strain. Deformation caused by stressing a body. Usually expressed as a change per unit length for each unit length. A strain of 2 mm $\neq$ 100 mm length is 0.02.

Ultimate strength. Amplitude of load that will cause physical separation or fracturing of a material.

Yield strength. Amplitude of load at which a body looses its elastic properties and ability to regain its unstressed shape.

and their by-products, as with cartilage and synovial fluid, are viscoelastic, displaying attributes of both solids and fluids.

The manual examination of joint structure evaluates their performance under prescribed circumstances. Assessment of joint efficiency at carrying out assigned tasks to the limits of pain tolerance is made by studying the motions or forces that are involved. The field of mechanics that describes motion, velocity, and acceleration is called kinematics. A vertebra may undergo six methods of motion (Fig. 17–1). Evaluation of intersegmental kinematics can be conducted, for example, through manual palpation, by stress radiographs, or by optoelectronic monitoring, yielding qualitative or quantitative information, respectively, about movement behavior.

Kinetics is the study of the forces that arise as motions change. Forces on the body are sometimes measured directly through isometric, isokinetic, isotonic, or isoinertial means. Computer-based biomechanical models now available to estimate joint loads may be used to predict jobs that are potentially harmful to some but acceptable to others. For example, a worker may be counseled to change his or her lifting posture or speed to avert the development of detrimental compressive forces on a damaged disc. Other clinical measurements include testing the passive resistance of vertebral segments at their extremes of motion: a characteristic called "end feel" or "joint play." The relative resistance to a manually applied load and the apparent displacement that occurs are regarded as evidence of disturbed joint function.

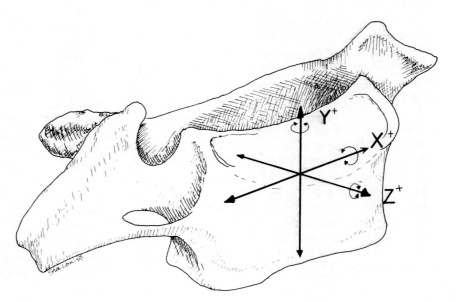

Figure 17–1. Cervical vertebra with an orthogonal reference showing six possible ranges of vertebral motion.

Major Musculoskeletal Tissue Properties

Bone

Bone has three basic functions: (1) to provide structural support, (2) to protect softer internal organs, and (3) to act as lever arms for activation of movement and locomotion.

Despite its image as a hard and inflexible member, the demands placed on an osseous structure require a wide range of strengths and flexibilities. Bone elasticity can be illustrated by the action of the vertebral lamina during lumbar spine extension. Figure 17–2A represents a motion segment in a neutral rest position. The angle (θ_n) indicates the orientation of a line from the facet contact center to the vertebral body centers. The bar over the lamina area implies a rigid structure that will not bend. During extension movement, if the upper vertebra were rigid as portrayed, the contact of the facet surfaces would tend to halt further displacement. Continued exten-

sion could arise only by a pivoting action at the facet contact, as depicted in Figure 17–2B or by a large sliding motion of one facet across the other. In either case, strain at the disc and the capsular ligaments are likely to arise if the total range of intersegmental rotation observed clinically is achieved.

For example, suppose an 8-degree (Plamondon et al., 1988; Hayes et al., 1989) extension of the intervertebral segment occurs. Using a typical distance from the facet centroid to the anterior disc fibers, a 7-mm stretch at the front of the disc can be predicted. Similarly, the posterior disc margin would be compressed 2 mm and a very small vertebral body translation of only 0.16 mm would occur. In vitro testing of intact motion segments shows realistic compressions less than 1 mm (Hirsch and Nachemson, 1954; Reuber et al., 1982) under physiological loading conditions.

In contrast, however, if an axis of rotation for extension is located approximately 40% of the disc anteroposterior diameter from the posterior disc mar-

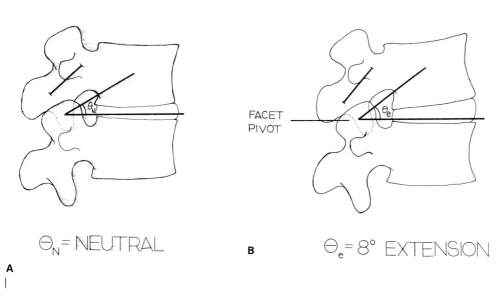

θ_N = NEUTRAL

A

FACET PIVOT

B θ_e = 8° EXTENSION

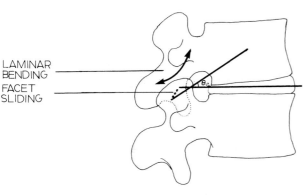

LAMINAR BENDING
FACET SLIDING

θ_e = 8° EXTENSION

C

Figure 17–2. A. θ_n defines the neutral resting position of the top vertebra. Rigidity of the lamina is represented by the bold black bar. **B.** With a hypothetical pivoting action at the facet by an extension (θ_e), large tensile loading of the disc fibers would occur. **C.** Actual extension (θ_e) causes a sliding of the facets and bending of the lamina that reduces the tensile loading of the disc fibers.

gin, as is commonly assumed, a more reasonable explanation of the mechanical behavior can be made (Panjabi and White, 1978). Figure 17–2C depicts a combined facet sliding action with an elastic bending of the lamina. Here, the anterior margin is stretched only 2.1 mm and the translation of the vertebra posteriorly is 2.5 mm. Although the facets do tend to slide across one another, bending of the lamina is necessary to permit an 8-degree rotational movement without disrupting the joint capsule. Displacements of this kind agree more closely with biomechanical observations.

Bone does not have the same capacity to absorb loads in all directions (a property called anisotropy). This nonuniform load capacity is largely attributable to the trabeculation that occurs in cancellous bone in response to Wolf's law, which governs local density of bone. That is, stress molding of the bone causes dense trabecular development in the path of maximum stress transmission. The price paid is a relative weakness to stresses from other directions. Table 17–2 shows the ultimate strength of human bone to compressive and tensile loads from different directions (Reilley and Burnstein, 1975). Clearly, bone is best able to absorb compressive loads along the direction of the bone diaphysis. Transverse tensile loads or shearing are less well absorbed.

Obviously, the vertebrae of the spine are under progressively higher loads from the neck down to the pelvis. It should not be surprising, then, that bone from each region demonstrates its own characteristic strength and size. Figure 17–3 shows the average compressive force needed to fracture the vertebral body for each region of the spine (Pintar, 1986). Despite the apparent differences from one part of the spine to the other, deformation of intact bones before they fracture is quite consistent. Pintar's data (1986) show that overall, vertebra will compress about 6 mm (0.25 in.). The decreasing vertebral size, not a change in bone properties, explains the differing strengths seen at each region.

Once bone has exceeded its failure strength and fractures, the amount of permanent distortion that remains is a function of three factors: (1) treatment applied to unload the damaged segment, (2) inher-

TABLE 17–2. ULTIMATE STRENGTH OF COMPACT BONE TISSUE IN TENSION AND COMPRESSION FROM VARIOUS DIRECTIONS

Load Type	Load Direction	
	Axial	**Transverse**
Compressive	193 MPa	133 MPa
Tensile	133 MPa	51 MPa
Shear	—	68 MPa

MPa = 1,000,000 pascal units
Pascal units - Newton/cm^2 = .0348 lb/in^2
[Adapted from Reilly and Burnstein, 1975, p. 398.]

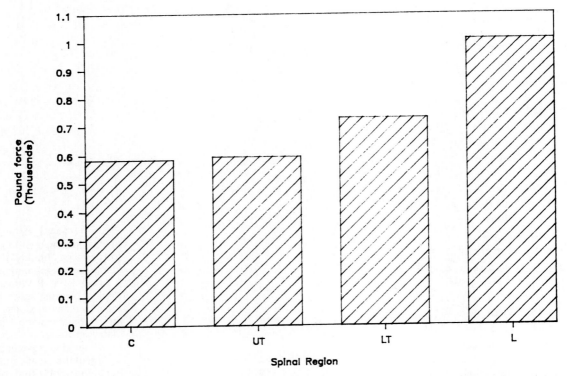

Figure 17–3. Mean values of compressive force or failure of intact vertebrae from different spinal regions. A loading rate of 0.1/second is represented. (*Adapted from Pintar, 1986, p. 47.*)

ent resilience of bone, and (3) the extent to which healing mechanisms fill in any residual gaps. The mechanical resilience of compressed vertebrae was studied by Ugale and colleagues (1987). In their study, the average force required to produce structural failure was 1074 pounds. The load was removed, and the amount of recovery in vertebral body height was measured and expressed in terms of a percentage of the original body height. A clear relationship was observed between the degree of compression and the ability to recover original height after unloading. If compressed 50%, an approximate 80% recovery was observed, most of it occurring within 3 minutes. A small additional improvement was noted over the next 24 hours. On the other hand, a deformity of 15% or less was followed by a 98% restoration of original height. It would seem that both the severity of damage and the speed with which the segment is unloaded have a large role in the residual effects of compressive fracture.

Bone is both stiffer and stronger than other tissues at higher strain rates (Carter and Hayes, 1976), whereas the sensitivity of other tissues to the rate of loading is negligible. A 300-fold increase in the rate of load application will not significantly alter the deformation of muscle or ligament. However, a similar change in strain rate for bone will result in approximately a 30% difference in both stress and strain levels. This is the basis for injury sometimes arising in the bone and other times in the connecting soft tissues from the same apparent loads. The strain rate to which bone is normally subjected varies as much as 1000% in normal activities, for example, between slow walking (0.001/sec) and vigorous exertion (0.01/sec). As a consequence, the elasticity of bone will differ as much as 15% (Cowin et al., 1987).

On first impression, knowing about vertebral strengths may seem rather academic. However, information of this kind is highly valuable as an aid to managing work-related injuries and industrial health practices. The best predictor currently available to estimate the relative risk of individual injury from specific job tasks comes from studies on the compressive strength of the vertebra. As was noted previously, an individual's vertebrae increase in strength from the top of the spine downward. Although relative strength is a complex function of age, sex, height, weight, muscular strength, and activity level (Chaffin and Andersson, 1984), it is now well established that most individuals can safely undertake lifts that generate a peak of 770 pounds of compressive load at L-5–S-1 (NIOSH, 1981). Furthermore, the majority of workers cannot tolerate work lifts that lead to compressive loads greater than 1540 pounds. Recent clinical developments in functional capacity assessment for injured workers or for pre-

employment selection use a personal computer to make the determination of spinal load estimates a simple and quick process (Mayer and Gatchel, 1988).

Articular Cartilage

Biomechanical properties of cartilage will be considered only in so far as they are relevant to amphiarthrodial or diarthrodial articulations of the spinal column. Other structural roles for fibrous or elastic cartilage are beyond the scope of this chapter.

Articular cartilage has been studied primarily for its elastic and viscoelastic properties. When articular cartilage is damaged, joint mechanical characteristics can be significantly altered. The hyaline cartilage covering most fully movable joints offers a tough, resilient, and glistening smooth surface to protect the end of the bone and to ensure minimal resistance to motion. Joint surface interactions are remarkably frictionless. A lubricated cartilaginous interface has a coefficient of friction* of 0.002. By way of comparison, ice-on-ice has a coefficient of friction of .03, and steel surfaces (such as in car engines with oil lubricants) have a much higher friction coefficient of about 0.2 (Chaffin and Andersson, 1984).

Mature cartilage has limited regenerative ability but still maintains a wear life often lasting more than seven decades. Under ideal conditions in laboratory animals (Mow, 1980); (Salter, et al., 1980), continuous passive motion has been able to stimulate generation of near normal cartilage tissue in 1-mm defects after 4 weeks. This contrasts with the formation of adhesions and absence of healing when the joints were immobilized. Intermittent voluntary activity with weight bearing prevents adhesions but does not appear to stimulate healing.

Articular cartilage is fashioned from only 20% porous tissue mass and 80% by interstitial fluid (Mow et al., 1980; Fung, 1981). It is rarely over 2 mm thick. Articular cartilage is visoelastic in character. Under stress, fluid moves in when the tissue is dilated and out when it is compressed. The mechanical properties of articular cartilage change with the fluid content. Movement of fluid is also a principal way in which the chondrocytes are nourished, because cartilage is largely avascular. Thus the stress–strain history of a joint is important to the function and well-being of its cartilage (Fung, 1981; Vudik, 1980).

Constitutive properties of hyaline cartilage are highly nonlinear, showing an ability to undergo large deformations while still being able to return to the original shape and dimension. The traditional engineering view of elasticity described by a single

---

*Coefficient of friction is a ratio of the force needed to make a body glide across a surface compared with the weight or force holding the two surfaces in contact.

Young's modulus* is inadequate (Woo, 1987). Under tensile testing, for example, linear materials will lengthen elastically in the direction of stretch and shrink a very small percentage in the direction perpendicular to the stretch. As tension continues to pull the tissue apart, it will fail. For articular cartilage, on the other hand, the stretching distance is quite large and the perpendicular contraction is nearly as great. Tests of fresh tissue material show that the amount of transverse contraction are as much as 50% of the longitudinal lengthening distance produced (Woo, 1987). Ultimate strength ranges between 1451 to 2465 lb/in² (10 to 17 MN/m²). The rate at which the interstitial fluid moves in or out of articular cartilage is dependent on the amplitude and, to a much smaller extent, the rate of the load application. Two other important and related mechanical features arise from interstitial fluid movement: creep deformity and stress relaxation. Under a constant load, the cartilage surface will indent as fluid is pushed out. Fluid extrusion is complete with just 3 minutes of constant load. If the surface forces persist, a gradual continued compression, called creep, will develop. Reaching equilibrium can take as much as 16 minutes (Mow, 1980). Upon unloading, imbibition of fluid occurs. Recovery occurs in two phases, immediate and delayed. The early rebound of tissue height reflects the solid elastic properties of the tissue medium. Then fluid begins to be

*Young's modulus is a numerical description of the relationship between the amount of stress a tissue undergoes and the deformation that results. Mathematically, it is the slope of the stress–strain response graph for a given structure.

slowly resorbed, swelling the matrix back to its initial dimension. Final recovery, however, occurs somewhat more slowly than the original creep deformity.

Stress relaxation describes the behavior of the internal forces on the matrix as the load is applied and is left in place. Figure 17–4 depicts the stress that the chondrocytes undergo from a hypothetical compressive force. Notice the rapid increase to a maximum that corresponds to the instant immediately after applying the surface load. The stresses then begin to dissipate as the internal microstructure deforms by creeping. This finally reaches a balance asymptotically where no further deformity will occur and the internal stresses have been minimized. The time necessary to reach full relaxation effects may be prolonged. Measurements have been carried out as long as 100 minutes (Fung, 1981). A schematic relating the microscopic fluid and matrix motions is shown in Figure 17–5.

Dynamic loading also causes shifting of the fluid equilibrium within the tissue matrix. But because of the intermittent surface forces that arise (during running, for example), both creep deformity and stress relaxation occur, but in cyclical fashion. Because each application of load is transient, neither full equilibrium from squeezing out interstitial fluids nor recovery from imbibition may happen with each cycle. Figure 17–6 portrays the combined dynamic creep and stress relaxation effects on cartilage. A steady-state cyclic response is eventually reached. Running on a constant slope and at a fixed speed, for instance, the hyaline cartilage will reach a steady state in about 10 load cycles.

Observations of mechanical performance of car-

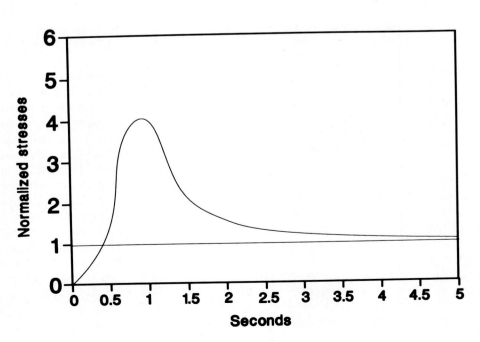

Figure 17-4. Normalized stress values for articular cartilage placed under constant compressive loading. Equilibrium is often reached in 1 to 5 seconds. (*Adapted from Mow et al., 1980.*)

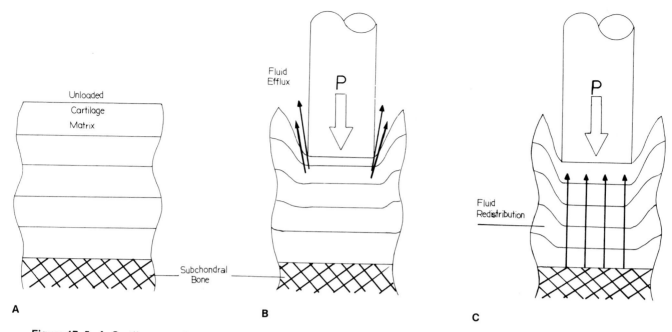

Figure 17–5. **A.** Cartilage matrix with evenly distributed fluid is represented by the evenly spaced intervals. **B.** Load applied to the surface first squeezes fluid out of the upper most layers of the matrix. **C.** As the load remains constant, fluid redistributes itself evenly through the layers.

tilage will play an important role in understanding the theoretical basis for joint dysfunction by synovial tags or ''blocking'' mechanisms that are described under the section on subluxation hypotheses. With aging, typical degenerative changes occur (Taylor and Twomey, 1986) that may be related to the kinds of stresses that arise in the joint cartilage over the years. Curved facet surfaces are exposed to different kinds of forces depending on the part under study.

The more sagittally oriented portion of the facet, exposed to higher shearing forces, thins. A fibrocartilaginous meniscoid tag may develop inward from the joint capsule. The anterior more coronal portion tends to thicken and undergo fibrillation perpendicular to the bone cortex because of the compressive forces. These events set up the mechanical environment that is believed to be responsible for some patient's pain.

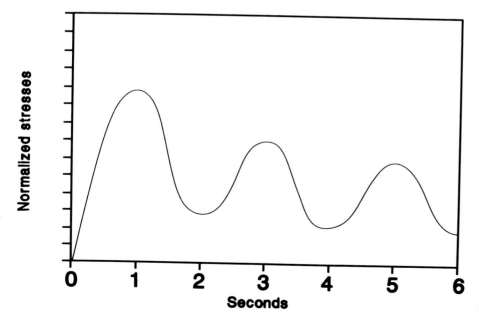

Figure 17–6. Stress relaxation from redistribution of fluids is observed dynamically with cyclic loads as in running. Full cartilage deformation and minimization of stress is reached in as few as 10 steps.

Synovial Fluid Joint Lubrication

As noted earlier, the surfaces of freely movable joints are nearly frictionless under usual circumstances. A change of environmental factors, for example, prolonged static postures or local inflammation, can tangibly alter the coefficient of friction between joint surfaces (Fung, 1981). If a joint is held still, as when squatting for a time to work in the garden, it will become stiff. However, as soon as it is moved, it quickly loosens up. This characteristic arises from two properties of snyovial fluid. They are, the ability of synovial fluid to move interchangeably between the articular cartilage matrix and the joint cavity as well as the rheological properties of the fluid itself.

The composition of synovial fluid is nearly the same as blood plasma, but with a decreased total protein content and a higher concentration of hyaluronic acid (Gibbs et al., 1968, Ogston and Stamler, 1953). Although there is less total protein, synovial fluid is much more viscous than blood owing to the mechanical molecular interactions of hyaluronic acid. The long mucopolysaccharide chains in healthy joint fluid exist as a continuous tangle of molecular branches that occupy the entire volume of articular space. Viscoelastic behavior results that permits the fluid to act as both a cushion and a lubricant to the cartilage. On sudden loading of the joint, the interlocked molecules act like coiled springs to absorb some of the shock. When a steady shearing force occurs with movement, the chains tend to straighten, disengaging from each other and allowing fluid flow. High viscosity draws the fluid between the sliding joint surfaces and minimizes direct cartilage contact.

Friction is very low when the cartilage matrix is filled with a normal amount of fluid material. As load is applied, fluid is extruded to the surface and the joint becomes progressively stiffer as local friction builds up (Malcom, 1976) at the contact zone (Figs. 17–7 and 17–8). As noted earlier, it takes only about 3 min of static load to squeeze all of the fluid out of the articular cartilage.

Intervertebral Discs

Disc cartilage differs substantially in its biomechanical behavior from that of articular cartilage. It is neither fibrocartilage nor hyaline cartilage, but retains some biomechanical features of both. In terms of weight bearing, water is the most important constituent of disc cartilage. The proportion of water decreases with age, beginning at about 88% at birth and declining to 70% in the eighth decade.

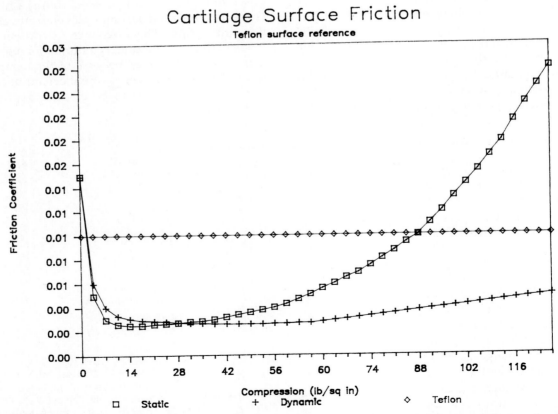

Figure 17–7. Changes in the relative amount of cartilage surface friction with increasing compressive loads under static and dynamic conditions. The coefficient of friction for Teflon is used as a reference standard.

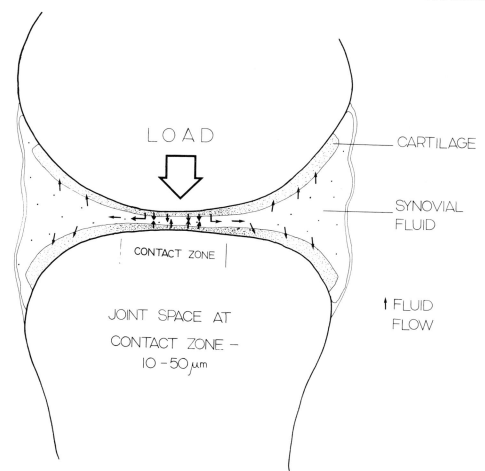

LOAD

CARTILAGE

SYNOVIAL
FLUID

CONTACT ZONE

JOINT SPACE AT
CONTACT ZONE –
10 – 50 μm

↑ FLUID
FLOW

Figure 17–8. Fluid moves out of the cartilage matrix at the contact zone and is resorbed by unloaded areas of the surface.

Approximately one-third of the spinal column is occupied by intervertebral discs. Their biomechanical characteristics, in large measure, account for the behavior of the spine as a whole during the performance of normal tasks. Generally, the direction of vertebral motions are governed by the loading of the intervertebral discs and the plane of the articular facets (Dumas, 1988). The magnitude of motions, however, are limited primarily by the disc. Consequently, the stiffness properties of discs are important for understanding normal disc function as well as disc pathomechanics.

The primary function of intervertebral discs is to facilitate bending motion and to limit translational movement. As can be seen in patients who have suffered a serious vertebral fracture or internal derangement of a disc, relatively large displacements resulting from instability of the vertebra can occur. The spinal cord and emerging nerve roots are exposed to substantial risk under these circumstances. Yet, normal physical activities require wide swings in position of the body as a whole that are permitted by the discs acting similar to a ball-and-socket joint mechanism. Each disc contributes a small part to the total

spinal flexibility. Disc tissue properties reflect limiting boundary conditions through stiffnesses that are quite different depending on the kind of load that the spine experiences. Table 17–3 lists the angular and translational displacements of vertebra under physiologic loads from a single direction (Barkson et al., 1979; Schultz et al., 1979; Moroney et al., 1988). The hierarchy of stiffnesses demonstrates preferential resistance to loads from specific directions. Compression and lateral shearing are opposed primarily by the disc. Anteroposterior motions, however, are constrained by the articular pillars through facet contact and capsule integrity. The disc bears very little moment load. That is, larger angular displacements arise with quite small torques applied. The spine is guarded particularly against long axis torsion by both the disc and by the facets. Factors of disc stiffness play an intricate role in one newer theory of intervertebral joint disorder called buckling, to be discussed later.

The high flexibility of the disc to bending is a function of the combined properties of elasticity in the annulus and relative incompressibility of the healthy nucleus pulposus. Making up about 40% of

TABLE 17-3. MECHANICAL PROPERTIES OF LUMBAR AND CERVICAL MOTION SEGMENTS

Load	Lumbar Segments		Cervical Segments	
	Facets Intact	Facets Removed	Facets Intact	Facets Removed
Compression [No preload]	0.18 mm[a]	0.19 mm[a]	0.10 mm	0.20 mm
Compression	0.51 mm[b]	0.50 mm[b]	—	—
Posterior shearing	0.80 mm[a]	1.24 mm[a]	1.10 mm[c]	0.30 mm[d]
Anterior shearing	1.21 mm[a]	1.42 mm[a]	0.40 mm[a]	0.30 mm[d]
Lateral shearing	1.00 mm[a]	1.11 mm[a]	0.40 mm[a]	0.20 mm[d]
Flexion	5.51°	5.93°	6.10°[e]	6.90°[f]
Extension	2.99°	—	3.50°[e]	5.20°[f]
Lateral flexion	4.90°	4.68°	4.90[e]	4.30°[f]
Torsion	1.50°	2.28°	2.10°[e]	3.50°[f]

[a] Axial loads = 32.5 lb [145 N] force without preload.
[b] Axial loads = 89.9 lb [400 N] force as an upper body weight equivalent.
[c] Axial loads = 35.2 lb [157 N] force.
[d] Axial loads = 4.6 lb [16 N] force.
[e] Bending loads = [2.2 Nm].
[f] Bending loads = [0.22 Nm].
Bending loads = 0.73 ft lb [10.6 Nm].
[Adapted from Berkson et al., Schultz et al. Moroney et al.]

the cross-sectional disc area, the nucleus pulposus is a loose mesh of collagen fibers and mucoprotein gel. The proteoglycans within the gel are hydrophilic and adsorb almost nine times their volume of water. Mechanically, then, the nucleus exerts an outwardly directed pressure against the lamina of the constraining annular ring and vertebral end plates. Hydraulic systems spread pressures equally in all directions. Consequently, the compressive forces acting on a healthy disc are nearly even in distribution across the cartilaginous (Kulak et al., 1975) end plates. In a reclining position, where the effects of weight bearing on the disc are minimized, the hydraulic pressure measured in the disc (Nachemson, 1965) reach 50 lb/in. (343.2 KN/m²). Acting together, the healthy annulus and nucleus supply the classic ball-and-socket action, permitting high angular mobility without concentrating stresses at any local point.

Under the influence of weight bearing and acceleration from body movement, the compressive forces on the disc are transformed into pressures directed radially against the annulus. In this way, the high strength of collagen fibers can be put to good use and reinforce the toughness of the spine as a flexible rod. Figure 17-9A displays the four components of stress that are transmitted by the disc. The outward pressure against the layered annular wall causes a slight circumferential bulging of the disc. The amount of bulge is not evenly distributed, because the nucleus is not situated exactly at the center. Different regions around the disc have thicker fibrous reinforcement from the annulus. When the annulus weakens and tears, the stress transmitted by pure compression is increased (Fig. 17-9B), whereas the radial, tensile, and circumferential hoop stresses that tend to contain the nucleus are significantly reduced. The result is a tendency for increased lateral bulging at the periphery, particularly to the posterolateral region occupying one wall of the lateral recess. Table 17-4 shows the magnitude of bulging measured in normal and degenerative disc specimens from the lumbar spine (Reuber, 1982).

TABLE 17-4. CIRCUMFERENTIAL BULGING OF NORMAL AND DEGENERATED DISCS TESTED UNDER SIMULATED TASKS GENERATING 90 LB [400 N] AND 180 LB [800 N] COMPRESSIVE LOADS, RESPECTIVELY

Disc type	Simulated tasks	
	Standing [400 N]	Bending [800 N]
Normal		
Lateral bulge	0.41 mm	0.55 mm
Postlateral bulge	0.19 mm	0.34 mm
Degenerated		
Lateral bulge	0.62 mm	0.80 mm
Postlateral bulge	0.62 mm	0.78 mm

[Adapted from Reuber et al.]

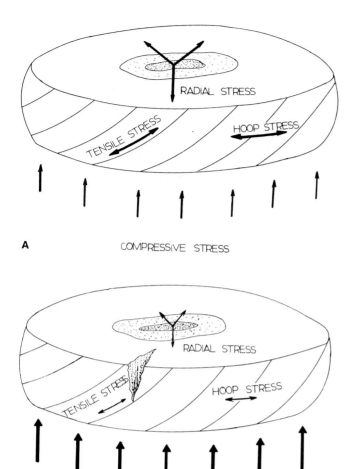

A   COMPRESSIVE STRESS

B   COMPRESSIVE STRESS

Figure 17–9. A. Four kinds of stress experienced by the healthy, loaded intervertebral disc are portrayed. The relative amount for each is given by the length and boldness of the arrows. **B.** Radial tearing results in decrease in radial, tensile, and hoop stresses whereas compressive stress increases.

Prolapse of a disc may occur rapidly in association with a traumatic or forcefully applied load. On the other hand, gradual disc bulging and herniation may also occur and probably represents a fatigue failure of the annular rings (Adams and Hutton, 1985).

Younger individuals are more susceptible to gradual failure over a period of months. Less viscous discs in older individuals are more likely to have sudden onset massive ruptures not requiring any preceding bulge.

Ligaments, Tendons, and Fascia

Probably the most important physiological characteristics of ligaments, tendons, and fascia are their cable properties; that is, the transmission of directed loads along a straight line from one attachment point to another. Tendons precisely transmit forces from muscle to bone to execute movements, whereas ligaments limit that motion and provide joint stability. To achieve this, bundles of parallel fibers are suspended in an amorphous ground substance, making up a noncellular matrix that performs the work of the tissue. The difference between connective tissues of this kind can be attributed primarily to the density of these fibers, the amount of elastin they contain, and the extent to which the bundles are oriented in the same direction. Fascia, for example, is typically a thin sheet with more collagen bundles deposited in different orientations. An arrangement such as this permits the tissue to bear loads from multiple directions in the fascial plane. Some ligaments, notably the ligamentum flavum of the spine, have a higher proportion of elastin fibers that contribute to an elastic preload of the motion segment even when it is in a neutral position. Finally, tendon is the most acellular tissue, showing a high degree of densely packed, parallel oriented fibers. Such a composition lends itself well to cable functions of transmitting only tensile forces along the tendon axis. Three biomechanical properties of these connective tissues have great importance in the study of musculoskeletal disorders: (1) properties of tensile strengths, (2) creep deformation at physiological loads, and (3) response of tissues to immobilization and injury.

The physiological working range of tendons, ligaments, and fascia is not well established. Table 17–5 compares the ultimate tensile strengths of human tendons, fascia, and ligaments with their strain properties (Yamada, 1970). As would be expected, the elastic ligamentum nuchae has the greatest ca-

TABLE 17–5. COMPARISON OF ULTIMATE TENSILE STRENGTH AND STRAIN PROPERTIES FOR HUMAN CONNECTIVE TISSUES

Connective Tissue Type	Ultimate Strength	Percent Elongation
Tendon	60 [8702]	10%
Fascia	15 [2176]	117%
Ligamentum Nuchae	2.5 [348]	125%

Units are pounds per square inch [Newtons ≠ cm^2] and strain in percent elongation.
[Adapted from Yamada.]

pacity to deform under tension but has the weakest ultimate strength before physical separation. Contrast the elasticity of the ligament to that of the tendon, which is 24 times stronger but 12 times less extensible. Table 17–6 shows the maximum percent elongation of spinal ligaments tested under physiological conditions by Panjabi and colleagues (Panjabi et al., 1982).

Evidence exists to suggest that, like Wolf's Law for bone remodeling, connective tissue also responds to increased tissue stresses. For instance, there is a strong correlation between the cross-sectional area of a tendon and the force the corresponding muscles are able to generate (Viidik, 1987). Maximum strength is estimated to be about four times the load created by maximum isometric tension of the corresponding muscle (Harkness, 1968). Thus, there is good reason to encourage a slow, progressive buildup in exertion for persons beginning exercise and fitness routines. A sufficient adaptation time is required for the soft tissues and bone to develop ability to handle the newly developing muscular tension that they must transmit.

The array of collagen fibers in a nearly parallel orientation is the basis for the strength of tendons and ligaments. Under microscopic examination, the fiber bundles appear undulating or wavy when in a relaxed condition. The absence of perfect fiber alignment and the presence of occasional elastic fibers in some structures accounts for this.

When a tendon or ligament comes under tension, its response is viscoelastic. There is a gradual straightening out of the lax fibers as the load is progressively distributed to them all. This is achieved by fiber bundles sliding along their longitudinal axis and shifting fluid from the matrix between fibers. If the load remains in place for any length of time, the total length of the connective tissue will increase slightly due to creep deformity. Since more of the collagen fibers are engaged directly in bearing the tensile loads, the ligament also is able to withstand higher stresses after it has been preconditioned in this way. This mechanism may account for some of the beneficial effects of an athlete's preliminary stretch routines (Viidik, 1987). When the load is removed, the mechanism is reversed and the healthy structure is restored. Continued exercise to the end of a joint's range of motion can bring about a functional lengthening of about 10% in the ligaments (Chaffin and Andersson, 1985). Persistence of greater flexibility requires continued use.

Viscoelastic and creep properties additionally explain the rate-dependent effects in both accidental and nonaccidental injury. Single-applied loads can result in tearing the tendon or avulsing a piece of the bone at the tendonous insertion. An excess load slowly applied will engage all of the tendon fibers and result in failure of the bone first. Rapid-acting loads do not allow sufficient time for the viscoelastic changes, and failure of tendon occurs. Even at lower intensity, detrimental effects can be seen. For example, prolonged static exertion or repetitive effort at the extremes of joint range for the wrist is associated with a high incidence of carpal tunnel syndrome. Chronic irritation and inflammation arise when sufficient recovery and rest of the tissues is not allowed. Physiological stressing of the tissues by encouraging normal flexibility is decisive in preventing excessive shortening during recovery. These mechanisms probably play a similar role in other cumulative trauma or ''overuse'' syndromes.

Even short intervals of immobilization have profound effects on periarticular connective tissues. That inactivity results in shortened fibrous tissue elements is well known. However, the time frame under which these changes occur and their clinical implications are not always emphasized. Experimental immobilization for repeated periods of short duration are as harmful as prolonged immobilization for 3 months. Review of immobilization effects was published by Videman (1987). A cascade of mechanical events is initiated by the physical shortening of the collagen fibers within the ligaments and a periarticular fibrosis. Capsular tension increases, and the joint cartilage is placed under high compression stress. Higher joint compressions were found to persist in rabbit models for up to 7 weeks. Fibrillation and atrophy of the articular cartilage began to occur as early as 4 weeks. These changes were only partially reversible when mobility was restored. Surprisingly, similar cumulative effects were obtained with repeated intervals of immobilization as little as 4 days in a 10-day cycle.

Muscle

Skeletal muscle is a biomechanically intricate structure often taken for granted by health professionals. Although the list of known pathology that invades

TABLE 17–6. MAXIMUM PERCENT ELONGATION FOR SEVEN INTRINSIC SPINAL LIGAMENTS FROM A 11 LB FT (15 Nm) MOMENT

Ligament	Percent Elongation
Anterior longitudinal	113%
Posterior longitudinal	113%
Transverse	126%
Ligamentum flavum	116%
Capsule	119%
Interspinous	128%
Supraspinous	132%

[Adapted from Panjabi et al.]

muscle tissue is astonishingly small, the mechanisms of action and neurological control of normal muscle functions still daunt investigators. Interest in muscle mechanics focuses on the effects produced by tensile forces transmitted along the long axis of muscle fibers. The direction of force transmission within a muscle belly will depend on the degree of pennation and angle of insertion into tendon or aponeuroses. Tangible effects include: (1) initiation and control of locomotion, (2) co-contraction stabilization of joints, and (3) modification of the loads on joint structures. The outcome of muscle activation depends on the number of muscles engaged, the relative cross-sectional area of each, and the intensity with which they are individually activated. Consequently, most exertion and task performance do not have a unique combination of elements. Efficiency, in turn, is dependent on such factors as the posture from which a given effort is attempted and the degree of motivation behind it.

Even limiting the discussion to physical force transmission through the muscle, all factors become involved. Tension can be exerted passively through the elastic muscle components alone or actively through myoelectric contraction-coupling and sarcomere shortening. These elements of performance are the primary bases for the remaining description for muscle mechanics.

The muscle organ is a composite tissue. The tendon and muscle fiber cross-bridges play important roles as series elastic elements (Huxley, 1974) in supplying an undamped spring action during locomotion. The horse and kangaroo, for example, have long and compliant muscles whose tendons traverse the distal joint of the leg. Passive stretching during galloping or jumping stores energy in the elastic components, which is recovered during the release of tension at push-off (Huxley and Simmons, 1971) as the fibers snap back. The tension from cross-bridge action and contraction-coupling initiated by the action potential release of calcium is called developed tension (McMahon, 1987). Both elastic series and developed tensions summate to give the total tension that is responsible for whatever work is done. Analogous action occurs in the human triceps surae group.

Clinical emphasis on strength measurement is described in more detail in the section (Chapter 20) on instrumentation. In that context, developed tension is considered under four general categories: (1) isometric, where the muscle length is held constant; (2) isotonic, where tension is constant but muscle length changes; (3) isokinetic, where velocity of movement is held constant; and (4) isoinertial, where torque developed around the joint is held constant. Table 17–7 relates the factors of muscle length, posture, velocity, and torque under ideal conditions for each kind of tension.

The maximum developed tension that can be achieved at any instant is a function of both the length of the muscle sarcomere and the velocity at which it is contracting. Obviously, analysis of any individual exertion can be quite complex because the nervous system, through the muscle spindle reflex mechanisms, can independently alter sarcomere length. That is, muscle tone adjustments are only partially dependent on the distance between insertional attachment points that are determined by posture. This interaction is described by the length–tension curve depicted in Figure 17–10. The biceps muscle is stretched, for instance, as the included angle of the elbow is increased. When the joint passes 90 degrees, competitive effects emerge. The elastic elements are engaged increasingly, whereas the degree of muscle fiber overlap and cross-bridge interaction begins to decrease. Load transmission is transferred from primary developed tension to elastic tension as the muscle elongates. The differences in distribution based on the muscle length has clinical implications during physical examination. As illustrated below, a muscle under tension also exhibits a proportional surface hardness. Interpreting the meaning of a hard muscle examined by palpation (e.g., palpation of spasm) needs to be made in the context of the posture under which it is examined and the relative activation normally to be expected. Passive elongation or stretching at end-range joint position and developed tension from myoelectric activation are alternate explanations for perceived surface hardness that need to be weighed.

How fast a muscle contracts has a profound influence on its ability to generate tension. There is a

TABLE 17–7. RELATIONSHIP OF MUSCLE PARAMETERS FOR COMMON CLINICAL TESTS OF MUSCLE STRENGTH

Condition	Length	Tension	Velocity	Torque
Isometric	C	V	O	V
Isotonic	V	C	V	V
Isokinetic	V	V	C	V
Isoinertial	V	V	V	C

C = constant; V = variable; O = no change.

Length Tension Curve

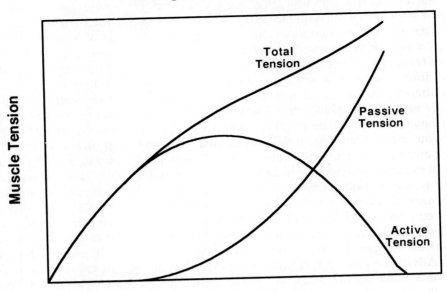

Figure 17–10. Total tension in the muscle results from the summation of passive tension of the elastic elements and active tension from muscle fiber contraction. The contribution of each component changes with muscle length.

distinct trade-off between the ability to generate mechanical power output from a muscle and the speed at which the force is developed. The optimal speeds for maximum power output and minimal variation ranges between 20 and 40% of the maximum velocity (McMahon, 1987). Figure 17–11 displays the force-velocity relationship for voluntary muscle expressed as a percentage of maximum velocity on the x-axis and maximum isometric tension on the y-axis. Positive values of velocity indicate concentric shortening, whereas negative units are for eccentric contraction seen during resisted muscle elongation.

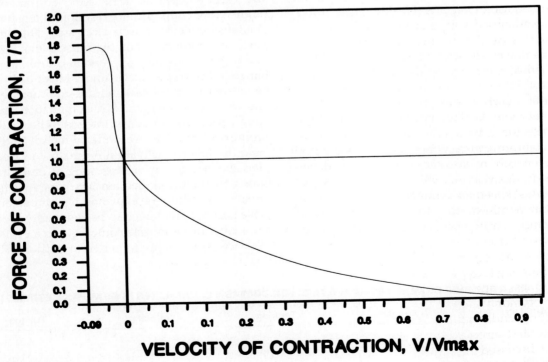

Figure 17–11. Force–velocity relationship of fiber contraction as derived from the classic Hill equation. Tension (T) and velocity (V) are normalized by expressing them as ratios of the maximum isometric tension (T_0) and maximum velocity (V_{max}), respectively. (*McMahon, 1987*).

Clearly, the developed tension from concentric contraction is responsible for most of the total force. Rapid shortening decreases the possible force that can be generated. For lengthening contractions, small velocities are associated with a rise in developed tension six times steeper than small shortening velocities. However, the effect is short lived. At a lengthening velocity that is only 5 to 10% of maximum velocity value, the muscle force suddenly reaches a plateau and soon falls off dramatically. The plateau and sudden drop in force is termed "yielding" and can be illustrated quite readily with use of a quick exertion against an extremity held in position with isometric contraction. At moderate velocities, the measured force will be well below the maximum isometric tension. These results are independent of neurological control and represent the limits of normal, healthy muscle mechanics.

Advances in musculoskeletal biomechanics over the past two decades have relied heavily on the relationship between myoelectric activity and developed tension. During any postural task or activity of daily living, the body bears stresses from the effects of body weight, the accelerations of movement and external loads that are being carried. All of these loads cause moments to occur about the various joints, including the spine. For humans to remain upright and successfully accomplish daily tasks, muscle action must offset the joint moments. Unfortunately for joint structures, while the muscle action allows us to remain erect, it also increases the internal compressive joint forces substantially. As discussed earlier in this chapter, it is the compressive joint loading at the lumbar spine that can be used successfully to predict the likelihood of injury for a given effort (NIOSH, 1981).

Isometric muscle tension consistent with common daily exertions increases in direct relationship to its myoelectric activity. Along with computer models, this information has been used to estimate activity-related job or recreational stress on the spine. Unfortunately, under very heavy exertion or moderate-to-fast speed movements, the relationship becomes quite nonlinear and models prove less reliable. Estimation errors range from 25 to 100% as speed increases (Kromodiharjo and Mital, 1986).

In practice, the assessment of muscular health is made by comparing four parameters: bulk, strength, surface hardness, and electrical activation. Four judgments commonly are recognized: normal tone, spasm, atrophy, and swelling. Evaluation by electrical activation and direct strength assessment measures will be discussed in Chapter 20.

Muscle spasm, particularly in the trunk muscles, is appraised by bulk and the relative firmness of the muscle belly. However, the spasm–pain–spasm cycle has been largely discredited (Ahern et al., 1988, Cohen et al., 1986). Clinical wisdom that pain and spinal disorders are associated with local spasm is an oversimplification. In populations of low back pain patients, greater muscle tension has been found by some investigators (Sherman, 1985; Triano and Schultz, 1987; Hoyt et al., 1981; Cram and Steeger, 1983, Triano, 1989), however, others report no difference or a decrease (Basmajian, 1981; Wolf and Basmajian, 1979; Collins et al., 1982). The circumstances under which either condition can be expected are hard to settle because of the lack of comparable information available from each report. Trunk muscle activity associated with pain from specific shearing stress of the L-3 facet joint has been measured (Triano et al., 1989). Figure 17–12 demonstrates that increasing joint pain from prolonged static loads is associated with a decline in paraspinal muscle activation. Interpretation is made even more difficult by the appearance of compartment syndromes in the lumbar spine (Styf and Lysell, 1987), for example, with an accumulation of intramuscular pressures, surface hardness, and tenderness. Figure 17–13 shows the relationship between surface hardness and muscle activation from applied joint torques at the low back (Triano et al., 1988; Styf, 1987). Although the apparently simple relationship looks promising, the ability to use surface hardness as an indicator of muscle activity reliably requires standardizing posture and avoiding positions or activity that introduce confounding postural factors including fatigue or muscle stretching. Extreme joint positions, for instance, that stretch the muscle to maximum length also markedly increase its surface hardness. Probably, palpatory examination should be conducted in more than one functional posture and results compared with expected values. Paraspinal assessment requires the use of recumbent, sitting, and standing positions to arrive at clinically meaningful interpretations. Even then, an underlying compartment syndrome and swelling responsible for the perceived hardness to palpation can not be fully ruled out. Only magnetic resonance imaging (MRI), intramuscular cannulation for pressure measurement, or electromyographic (EMG) measures calibrated to the relative muscle tensions are likely to finally settle the question.

Nerve

The enclosure of the spinal cord and exit of segmental nerves from the vertebral column requires a remarkable mechanical design. A high degree of mobility must be accommodated while offering full protection to the sensitive neural elements. Historically, chiropractic has focused on the potential risks from mechanical interactions at this site. For the

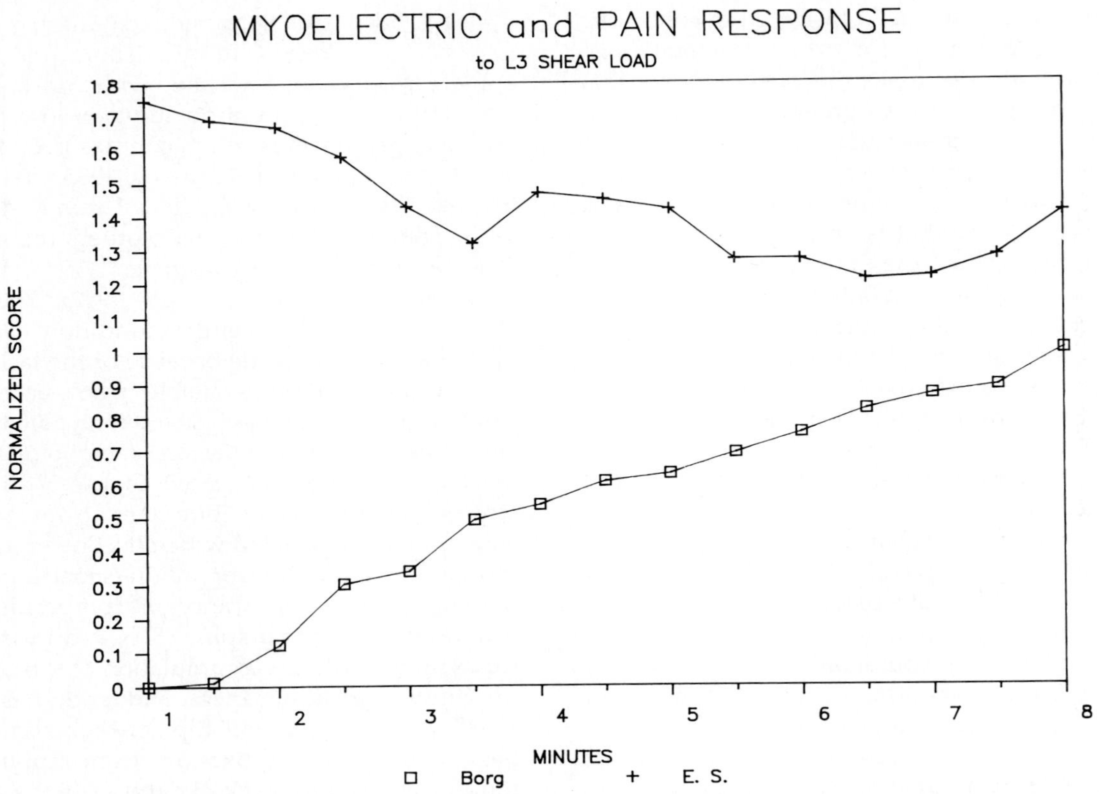

MYOELECTRIC and PAIN RESPONSE
to L3 SHEAR LOAD

Figure 17–12. Myoelectric and pain response to L-3 shear load. Active muscle response of the erector spinae (E.S.) and amount of back pain (Borg pain scale) from posteroanterior shear loading of the spine at L-3 are plotted over time. Response is the same for healthy and low back pain subjects. (*Adapted from Triano et al., 1989*)

healthy spinal column, there is little chance that detrimental interactions will arise. Where congenital or degenerative factors or trauma interrupt normal kinematics and distort anatomic dimensions, latent hazards can be awakened. Obvious somatic symptoms of sciatic or median nerve involvement, for example, can be accompanied by far-reaching central nervous system and peripheral effects (Luttges et al., 1986; Nathan, 1987). To make matters more complex, overt clinical changes are rarely consistent with the devastating histological picture of Wallerian degeneration seen with experimental lesions. Instead, symptoms more closely resemble signs thought to represent augmented nerve function.

Internal forces that act on nerves tend to compress, stretch, and twist them. The range of potential stresses may run from small loads that promote healthy tissue stimulation to those that result in irritation, inflammation, and degradation. Understanding the relative risks from various anomalies and pathologies requires some way of gauging when an increasingly strong perturbation becomes a noxious stimulus. It makes little sense, for example, for physicians to concern themselves with small degrees of tension on a nerve trunk that are less than those that might arise in the course of normal, healthy motions.

Structurally, the peripheral nerves are encased in a tough protective covering of their own. Epineural sheaths are fibrous elements that invaginate and separate the nerve into bundles and split the bundles into fascicles. Progressively smaller collections of nerve fibers are encased to the level immediately outside of the myelin-coated axons. Glycoproteins are the predominant biochemical constituents that give tensile mechanical strength. The epineurium is the thickest and toughest protective element. It should be no surprise, then, that nerve roots having much less glycoprotein content (Luttges and Grosswald, 1976) are more susceptible to injury by mechanical forces (Panjabi et al., 1983) than are nerve trunks. It takes up to 13 times the tensile force that would damage a nerve root to permanently damage the peripheral trunk. Table 17–8 shows the upper limit of nerve stretch reported by Luttges and colleagues (Luttges et al., 1986) for samples of mouse nerve root and trunks. Mouse nerve was used because of its close biochemical resemblance to human nerves.

Nerves are surprisingly strong under experimental stretch conditions. Their resistance comes from two sources that are reminiscent of the way that tendons absorb loads. The undulating course of

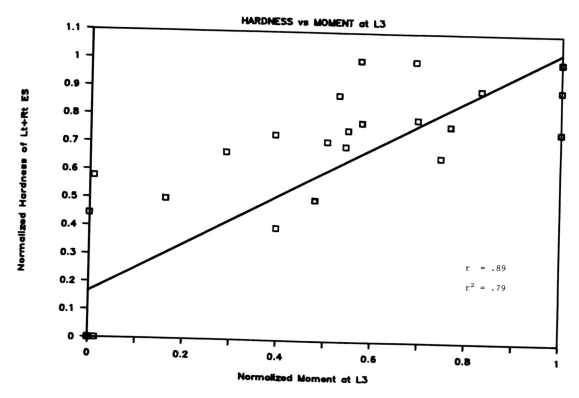

Figure 17-13. Hardness of combined left and right erector spinae (hardness vs moment at L-3). Hardness of combined left and right erector spinae muscles (hardness vs moment at L-3). Surface hardness and muscle tension increases in direct proportion to the bending moment carried by the vertebra (r = Pearson correlation coefficient, r² = coefficient of determination).

axons at resting length gives a reserve that permits some straightening before the elements are put under any notable stress. Parallel epineural or perineural elements then are engaged to shunt forces along their length and avoid nerve damage. Load sharing by these means allows more than 40% elongation before nerve integrity is disrupted. Although nerve roots lack the added reinforcing glycoproteins, their ability to lengthen and slide in the intervertebral foramina allows a wide variety of spinal movements without risk.

Compression stress is countered by mechanisms quite different from those opposing tensile stretching. A nerve fascicle that is cut open bulges outward, indicating that an inner pressure exists (MacGregor et al., 1975). A nerve begins to deform when an outside force exceeds the nerve's balancing hydrostatic pressure. The point at which compression block develops with physical deformation is related to an axon's diameter. Larger fibers (proprioceptive, touch, and motor) are affected first. In experimental studies (Sharpless, 1974), complete compression block of nerve trunk conduction requires 150 mm Hg pressure. Roots reach block at only 30 mm Hg; a value only slightly above normal interstitial pressure, which is approximately 18 mm Hg.

A graded reduction in nerve function from in-

TABLE 17-8. UPPER LIMIT STRESS AND STRAIN VALUES FOR MOUSE NERVE ROOT AND TRUNK

	Stretch Load		Compressive Load (mmHg)
	Stress (lb/in²)	Strain (%)	
Nerve root	13	42	
Nerve trunk	471	45	30
			150

Stress expressed as pounds per square inch, strain as % elongation. Column three gives the compressive pressures necessary to achieve complete conduction block. [From Luttgess and Grosswald, 1976, and Sharpless, 1974]

creasing pressures applied clinically is not as evident as experimentation would suggest. That is, functional anomalies can arise that are measurable but are not associated with evident signs or symptoms. Electrodiagnostic abnormalities thought to reflect subclinical compressive disorders across the carpal tunnel, for instance, have been described (Neary et al., 1975). However, a clear correlation between compression and degree of clinical impairments is not apparent (Friberg, 1939; Gill and White, 1955; Tanzer, 1962). This disparity may be an indication of the significance that active inflammatory reactions play in intermittent nerve insult rather than as passive responses to mechanical perturbations.

Nerves rest in fascial clefts protected from external pressures by surrounding soft tissue or bone. Although generally constrained to remain in the cleft between muscles, where internal pressures are probably more uniform, the nerve has freedom to glide across a surprisingly large distance. The median nerve, for instance, will slide longitudinally in its bed up to 4 cm (McLellin and Swash, 1976). Similar translations through the intervertebral foramen of less than 1 cm have been described (Breig and Troup, 1979). A slip of epineurium attaching the nerve to the intervertebral foramen is often present and may serve as strain relief for the more sensitive root structures. Dural ligaments have been identified that affix the dura and nerve roots at their exit from the main dural sac to the posterior longitudinal ligament and vertebral body. The overall arrangement tends to hold the nerve forward in the canal (Spencer et al., 1983). Coupled with 40% elasticity of the nerve tissue, direct root and cord tensions are unlikely.

Effects of partial occlusion of the nerve bed, such as those that might occur with disc herniation, foraminal stenosis, or spinal instability, have been investigated (Triano and Luttges, 1982). Dynamic perturbations of the nerve rubbing across a partial obstruction give rise to inflammatory responses. Physiological changes are more consistent with clinical findings of pain, spasm, and paresthesia than hyporeflexia, flaccidity, and anesthesia that are associated with Wallerian degeneration. Because the mechanical stimulant is intermittent and dependent largely on the degree of patient activity, the nerve may not be able to readily accommodate. Figure 17–14 is a display from a mouse sciatic nerve that has undergone intermittent mechanical irritation for more than 30 days. Under healthy conditions, the second action potential should be much smaller than the first, owing to the physiological refractoriness of axons. Normal nerves would respond at the second stimulus with 50 to 70% amplitude of response one. With intermittent mechanical irritation, a facilitation effect can be seen. It is not yet known how potent

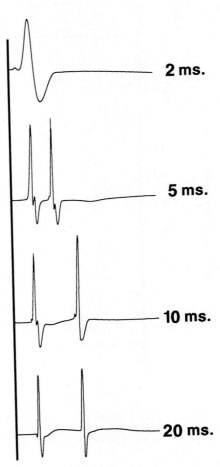

Figure 17–14. Response of mouse sciatic nerve to double-pulse stimulation after 30 days of intermittent mechanical irritation. Pulses are separated by progressively longer intervals and displayed at sweep speeds given to the right of each trace in milliseconds per centimeter of sweep.

these kinds of irritation are or under what circumstances they will subside. Although similar study of roots has not been conducted, all evidence suggests that they would respond similarly, but to relatively mild forces.

Kinematics and Kinetics of Motion Segments

Kinematics of Intervertebral Foramina

The frequency of direct nerve irritation from mechanical disorders of the spine and the circumstances under which they arise are unknown. An early step toward understanding the importance of these mechanisms was begun with studies of nerve sensitivity to subtle mechanical perturbations discussed in the section just above. However, demonstrating the feasibility to cause physiological and inflammatory changes is not the same as proving that mechanical intervertebral dysfunctions cause them. Much more information about how spines work is needed before the stages involved in the pathomechanics can be predicted.

Intervertebral foramina (IVF) dimensions can be affected by pathology at a number of sites along its course. Some causes include degenerative joint disease of the facets, adhesion formation, or disc degeneration and herniation (Goddard and Reid, 1965; Epstein, 1980). The cross-sectional area of the nerve itself takes up less than 50% of the available space and is situated generally toward the upper half of the foramen. With adverse movement or degenerative disease, mechanical perturbation and compression may occur. At least for overriding facets (Panjabo et al., 1983) and lateral recess entrapments (Ciric, 1980; Verbeist, 1954), impingements such as these have been observed. For most common complaints of back pain, however, overt evidence of pathology cannot be found and unequivocal findings of movement abnormality are not yet agreed on.

Based on anatomic measurements, Panjabi and colleagues (Panjabi et al., 1983) have used computer models to evaluate changes in IVF morphology from motion in healthy and degenerative intervertebral units. Table 17-9 gives the dimensions for space around the nerve predicted for a typical lumbar IVF during upright postures. Figure 17-15 depicts the changes in shape that occur for flexion and extension, lateral bending, and rotation. The maximum decrease in size of the foramen occurs during extension, with a loss estimated at 20%. In healthy motion segments, approximately 74 mm² remains available for extraneural contents. Degenerative discs collapse this area to about 5 mm². It is unlikely that intact motion segments can cause direct foraminal impingement on the emitting nerve. On the other hand, degenerative changes or fibrous adhesions in the area may be a chronic source of mechanical irritation and inflammation. No clinical information is available about altered neural activity at the cord segment level from nerve perturbation or anomalous proprioception that might be present.

Motion Segment Behavior

Health status of a functional spinal unit (FSU) or motion segment is judged from findings collected during the examination. The number of component structures recruited during activity permits a great variability in how tasks may be accomplished. Conclusions about spinal function are obtained from summation of behavior from each region and each motion segment sequentially. For example, forward bending of the healthy spine and pelvis follows a normal lumbopelvic rhythm. Motion begins with the upper lumbar vertebra and progresses down the spine. By the time the trunk has reached 40 to 70 degrees inclination from the vertical (Schultz et al., 1985), all FSUs have been fully engaged. At that point flexion–relaxation occurs (that is, activity of the paraspinal muscles suddenly ceases) and the axis of bending shifts to the femur heads, where the gluteal and hamstring muscles lower the body the remaining distance. Yet, it is quite common to observe full regional bending flexibility in postoperative patients with one or more segments fused. Adjustment in task strategies forces the redistribution of movement at an earlier stage. Most of the effort comes from an increased range of motion about the femur heads and added strain on the discs adjacent to the fused area.

During the course of examining a patient, it is necessary to critically distinguish regional and subregional kinematic strategies that a patient uses. Factors of recruitment timing, quality and intensity, range and velocity with which each part is used can be helpful. Figure 17-16 shows tangible evidence of shifting load shares from the spinal ligaments to the muscle by loss of normal flexion–relaxation in a patient with debilitating low back disorder. At the tissue level, normal lumbopelvic rhythm translates into a mechanical loading of the ligaments when flexion–relaxation occurs. That is, when the muscles become electrically silent, the spine is literally hanging by its ligaments. In the illustration, muscle activity of a healthy individual contrasts with that of a chronic, recurrent back pain patient while both achieve a full 90-degree forward bend. Altered distribution of spinal loads is evident from the persistence of muscle action (Hoyt, et al., 1981; Schultz, et al., 1985; Triano

TABLE 17-9.   MEAN VALUES OF INTERVERTEBRAL FORAMINAL DIMENSIONS PREDICTED FOR MIDPOSITION OF PHYSIOLOGICAL MOVEMENTS UP TO 5 DEGREES IN HEALTHY AND DEGENERATIVE MOTION SEGMENTS

	Healthy Disc	Degenerated Disc
Height (mm)	20.9	15.2
Width (mm)	10.2	7.7
Area (mm²)	185.2	108.0

[Adapted from Panjabi et al., 1983]

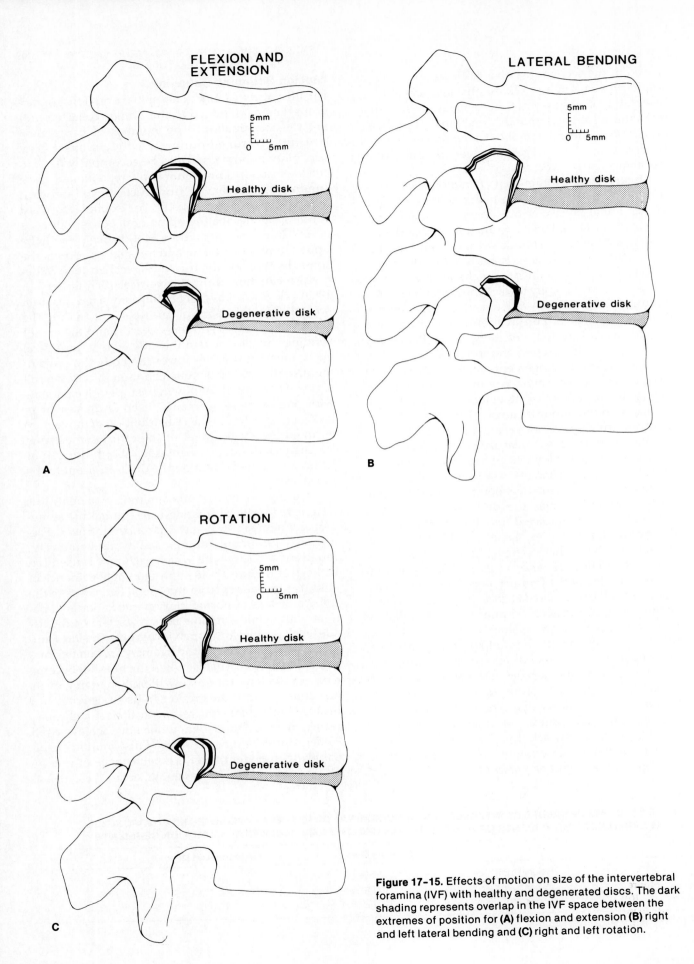

FLEXION AND EXTENSION

5mm

0   5mm

Healthy disk

Degenerative disk

A

LATERAL BENDING

5mm

0   5mm

Healthy disk

Degenerative disk

B

ROTATION

5mm

0   5mm

Healthy disk

Degenerative disk

C

Figure 17-15. Effects of motion on size of the intervertebral foramina (IVF) with healthy and degenerated discs. The dark shading represents overlap in the IVF space between the extremes of position for **(A)** flexion and extension **(B)** right and left lateral bending and **(C)** right and left rotation.

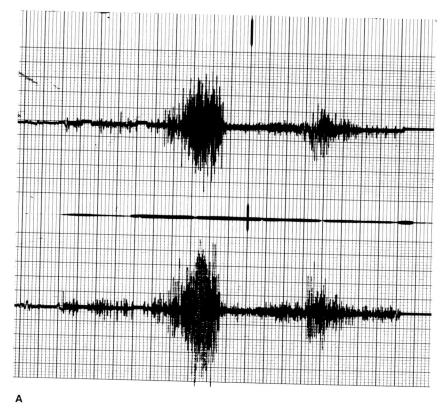

A

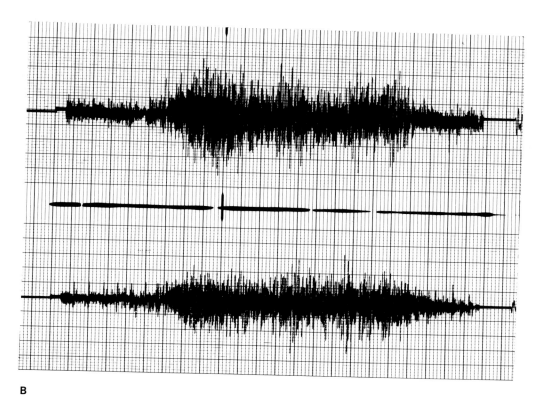

B

Figure 17–16. A. Paraspinal surface myoelectric recording during full forward bending of the torso in a healthy subject. The top represents the left side of the spine, the bottom trace the right side. **B**. Muscle action with full forward bending in a patient having moderate disability noted in activity of daily living from low back pain. Note the absence of flexion–relaxation.

and Schultz 1987) throughout the range. Unfortunately, no good objective tools are yet available to quantify subregional function. Even surface EMG, as that used to produce Figure 17–16, although promising, lacks sufficient discriminability in all but limited clinical circumstances.

Each vertebra can move in translation and rotation about all three coordinate axes. Motion is initiated and guided by a balance between gravitational pull, muscle action, and joint geometries. Physiological movement is limited by the strains of the ligaments and the plane of the facet joints. Many studies have been conducted (Bean, et al., 1989; An, et al.; Schultz et al., 1982) trying to determine the basis by which the body may choose a given strategy in accomplishing a given task. No compelling proof yet exists to accept any set of assumptions as being definitive. However, there is strong evidence to suggest that the body will select the combination of lowest muscle energies that will simultaneously keep the compressive and shearing forces of the spine at a minimum. When these loads become excessive, damage to disc, facet, ligament, and muscle can be expected.

Although the spine has numerous connections to the functional spinal units, each FSU plays a limited role in protecting the spine. Collectively, the elements are capable of sustaining loads as high as five times body weight. For the simple main motions of flexion, extension, and rotation the relative importance of major structures has been determined. The ligaments situated furthest from the center of rotation for any instant will undergo the largest strain (Panjabi et al., 1982). However, the relative contribution in maintaining joint integrity will be based on those structures that offset the largest loads. For flexion, the supraspinous ligament may undergo the largest strain. But, it is the capsular ligaments that are the first line of defense for joint integrity. Transection studies (Adams et al., 1980; Posner et al., 1982) have found a gradually increasing tension in the ligaments as flexion progresses. The joint capsules ultimately peak at an average 39% of the load at end range. The disc resistance peak is an additional 29%, with the ligamentum flavum and the supraspinous–interspinous pair contributing another 13%

and 19%, respectively. Extension is limited primarily by the anterior longitudinal ligament and contact between the posterior articulations. (Normal values of displacement for intact FSUs undergoing flexion are 1.7 mm ± 0.6 mm and 6 ± 4 degrees. Extension values are 2.1 mm ± 0.7 mm and 16 ± 10 degrees, respectively (Posner et al., 1982). Rotational motion in the intact segment is largely limited by the orientation of the facet joints followed next by the disc lamina. For that reason, rotation is much more evident in the thoracic spine than in the lumbar region. The importance of the facet and capsular ligaments in contributing to stability during sagittal plane motion and axial rotation has been elegantly displayed (Panjabi et al., 1988; Adams and Hutton, 1981). A 3-Nm moment was used to load a motion segment in vitro. Rotation about all three main axes were tested. The range of motion caused for intact and facetectomized specimens is shown in Table 17–10. Forward flexion and left and right axial twisting movements were significantly increased with varying degrees of facetal excision.

Up to this point, the discussion of motion segment kinematics has been in the simpler terms of main motions that parallel the anatomic reference planes of the body. In most circumstances, description of real movement is more complex. In most voluntary actions, there is a combination of translation and rotation that occurs about all three axes called coupled motions. Some of the first qualitative and empiric characterizations for in vivo spine operation was made by Gillet and Leikens (1985) beginning in 1921. Displacements that arise secondary to main axis motions are much smaller in comparison. These are most readily observed by examining the cervical spine during lateral bending. With a rotation of the vertebra about an axis in the sagittal plane, there are accompanying rotations about the longitudinal and coronal axes. In general, if the patient performs a lateral bend to the right, the spinous process swings to the left and the vertebra flexes partially. In the lumbar spine the pattern is largely reversed.

The amount and direction of coupled movement outside the plane of the primary or main motion varies. Vertebral action appears to be influenced greatly by intersegmental posture and spinal level being ex-

TABLE 17–10. FACET/CAPSULE LIGAMENT IMPACT ON STABILITY OF A MOTION SEGMENT UNDER TORQUE LOADING

	Flexion		Axial Rotation		Lateral Flexion	
Intact	8.2	−4.0	3.3	−3.7	6.7	−5.8
Left total facetectomy	12.4	−5.3	3.7	−5.5	7.3	−6.8
Bilateral total facetectomy	13.7	−6.9	7.9	−7.6	7.7	−7.3

Range of motion in degrees; positive = flexion or left, negative = extension or right. [Adapted from Panjabi et al.]

amined (Panjabi et al., 1988). Figures 17–17 and 17–18 demonstrate these effects during a pure axial twisting of the lumbar spine. Flexion coupling associated with axial rotation applied to L-2 to L-3 while the segment is fully flexed becomes extension coupling while in extended posture. Similarly, associated lateral bending amplitude changes by a factor of one-third. Dramatically, the direction of coupled lateral bending reverses between the upper and lower lumbar regions. At L-1 to L-2, a positive axial rotation causes lateral bending in one direction. The same axial rotation causes an opposite lateral bending at L-5 to S-1.

Effects of coupled actions are present even when considering regional motion. Twenty healthy subjects (Parnianpour et al., 1988) undergoing testing of flexion and extension exhibited an average of 67 degrees sagittal plane motion, 5 degrees coronal, and 4 degrees in the transverse. As they exercised to fatigue, a reduction in the main movement was seen. Simultaneously, increases in the off-axis rotations occurred (Table 17–11). Additional study for the mechanical effects from reduced control of off-axis spine behavior is warranted. Early evidence (McIntyre, 1989) suggests that patients undergoing similar tests have reduced off-axis regional motions.

It has been generally assumed that the relaxed,

TABLE 17–11. EFFECTS OF EXERTION TO FATIGUE ON COUPLED MOVEMENTS OF THE TRUNK IN HEALTHY VOLUNTEERS

Movement	Beginning Range	Fatigue Range
Flexion	67°	60°
Lateral flexion	5°	10°
Rotation	4°	8°

[Adapted from Parnianpour et al., 1988, p. 986.]

upright spinal column adopts a normal and reproducible posture. Many efforts have been made to describe characteristic static configurations. These, it was hoped, could be successfully used to help locate and diagnose spinal lesions. Unfortunately this assumption proves not to be true for either the shape of the spinal column as a whole or the relationships between individual vertebrae (Phillips et al., 1986). Repeated measures of the upright posture throughout the course of a work day, for example, show a significant variation in lordosis and kyphosis. The amount of curvature seems to be related to three distinct factors: (1) time in one posture, (2) weight handled, and (3) fatigue experienced by the individual. Changes such as these may represent an inherent mechanical hysteresis of recovery from loading. Additive effects

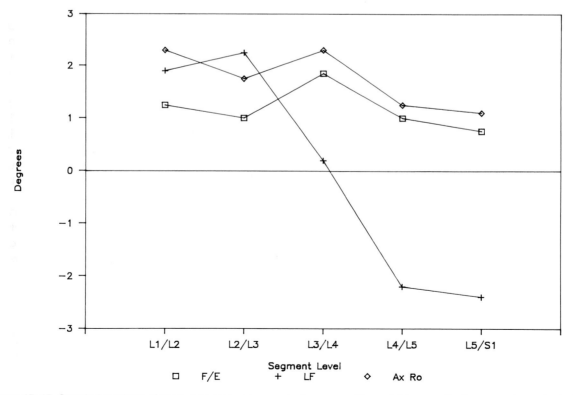

Figure 17–17. Coupled motions of the lumbar spine segments from a positive axial torque. Each segment was tested in a neutral posture. (*From Panjabi et al., (1988) p. 352–353, with permission.*)

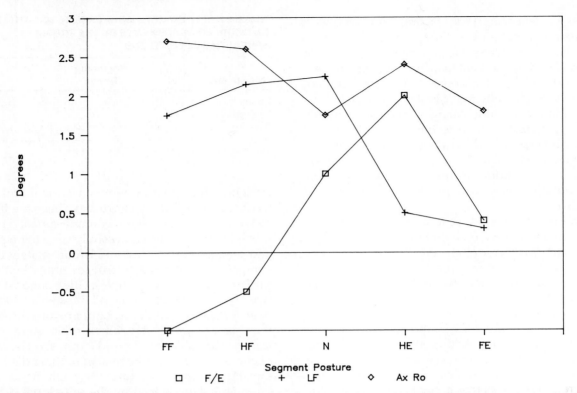

Figure 17–18. Coupled motions of the L-2 – L-3 motion segment from a positive axial torque. The segment was tested with posture varied from full flexion (FF), half flexion (HF), neutral (N), half extension (HE), and full extension (FE). (*From Panjabi et al., 1984, p. 1001, with permission.*)

of viscoelastic properties in the disc, for example, may be responsible for these variations.

Likewise, motion segments do not have a unique rest position. Rather, there is a region to which the vertebra return after the spine is unloaded. This region was named the neutral zone by Panjabi and colleagues (1984). Table 17–12 displays their extent as measured from tests of isolated motion segments. The neutral zone is a highly unstable region where the spine can move readily with a minimum of applied load. Outside of the zone, ligamentous tensions and disc properties begin to oppose actively the joint moments and supply kinematic resistance. It is interesting to note that degeneration of the disc results in relatively large changes in the size of the neutral zone. Unilateral injury of the disc

annulus produces increase in both main and coupled motions up to a factor of two (Panjabi et al., 1984; Goel et al., 1985). Kinematics of FSUs adjacent to the injury with asymmetric movements of the facets have been reported.

Under experimental test conditions, an FSU position can be found such that motion initiated there consists only of main motions and no coupled action. This position is called the balance point (Frymoyer et al., 1990). When the resultant load being carried by the spine is positioned at this point, off-axis motions are eliminated. Located anterior to the disc centroid, the exact position is different for each individual. With so much other information concerning spinal biomechanics, such a small point may easily go unnoticed if not for experimental behavior that may serve as a clue to spinal lesion mechanisms. Under usual test conditions, the application of a load to a motion segment results in predictable displacement and creep based on the tissue stiffness properties. When loaded at the balance point, however, unusually large and sudden deformations can occur. Figure 17–19 illustrates the displacement response of a typical lumbar motion segment under gradually increasing load. The early part of the curve is identical to vertebrae under lifelike loading conditions. Notice that there is a sudden change in the rate

TABLE 17–12. ESTIMATES OF NEUTRAL ZONE RANGE FOR L-5 TO S-1 MOTION SEGMENT

Motions	Angular Range	
	Healthy Disc	*Degenerative Disc*
Flexion/extension	1.8°	3.2°
Lateral flexion	3.2°	2.5°
Rotation	1.6°	3.0°

[Adapted from Panjabi et al., 1984, p. 196.]

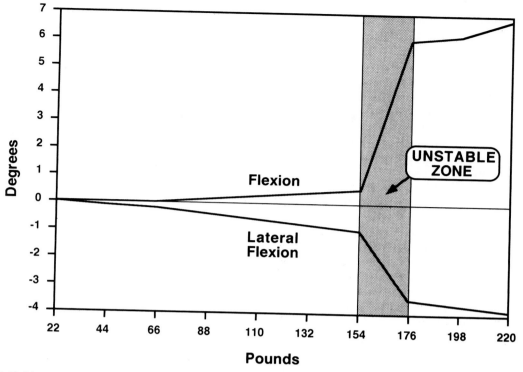

Figure 17–19. Motion segment buckling. Motion segments loaded at the balance point appear to exhibit an unstable zone where small increases in load result in large displacements of the vertebra and an audible "crack." (*From Frymoyer 1990*).

of displacement with no discernable increase in load. Typical deformation behavior is then resumed. The sudden displacement has been associated with an audible cracking sound as if damage had been done to the tissues. Yet, on inspection, no discernible abnormalities have been described.

Summarizing to this point, the dynamic function of the spinal column is initiated by the interaction of loads from outside the FSU. Facet joints act to guide the plane of motion consistent with the curvature of their surfaces when they are engaged. Along with the ligaments and discs, the facet joints supply strong limiting forces to restrain motion within physiologically acceptable limits. When at rest, the configuration of the spine and the position of the vertebrae are dependent on load history. The spine has no unique static configuration; that is, there is no single neutral position for the spine either at regional or subregional levels. Variations in the unloaded positions are large enough to have been confused with early reports of radiographic treatment effects (Triano, 1984) and explain their randomness. Finally, a balance point has been described that permits unusually large displacements to occur. This phenomenon is mechanically analogous to column buckling failure; that is, where the failure is not from destruc-

tion of the tissues, but rather from an unacceptably large deformation.

Load Distribution in the Functional Spinal Units

Mechanisms of support are quite different for most prolonged static postures. Here, with the exception of extreme positions, the interspinal forces are primarily compressive, and the ligaments involve only a small proportion of their strength. Load sharing is divided between the disc anteriorly and the articular pillars posteriorly. As just noted, the relative distribution is posture dependent, and control is reliant on muscle action. Because the disc has such low bending stiffness, the upright spinal column is inherently unstable and will bend fully with as little as a 2.5 kg (5.5 pound) load unless muscle acts to stabilize it.

Some writers have assigned load distributions based on purely geometric reasoning (Ward, 1977; Speiser and Aragona, 1989). Usually, the impetus for their doing so has come from observations of planar x-rays and subjective clinical impressions. Many of these assertions are called into question by more substantive biomechanical studies. For most postures, the healthy lumbar motion segment carries the majority of the compressive load on the disc. In an upright standing posture, the load on the spine is borne by both the disc (82%) and facet articulations (18%). Even with increasing load to the spine in an unchanging posture, measured facet forces remain relatively constant (Lorenz, 1983). This is in contrast to an erect sitting posture where the facets are disengaged and have no contact pressures between them (Adams and Hutton, 1980). With as little as 2 degrees of extension from the neutral anatomic position and extremes of forward flexion, some load begins to be shifted to the facets. Only after creep deformity, say from prolonged static position or very large loads, do the low back facets bear any weight in neutral or flexion postures. Transfer of the load share is readily demonstrated in disc narrowing, where as much as 70% of the intervertebral compressive force crosses the apophyseal joints and risks articular degeneration. Distribution of stresses in the cervical spine is substantially different. Head weight is divided almost equally between a tripod support system consisting of the vertebral body and the articular pillars (Pal and Sherk, 1988).

Shear and rotational loads, generally much smaller than compressive forces, are transmitted differently (Adams and Hutton, 1983; Miller et al., 1987; Jayson, 1987; Shirazi-Adl et al., 1986). In the normal spinal unit, shear forces and torsion are opposed for the most part by the posterior articulations. Excessive strain concentration may occur in extension or rotation tasks that can result in cartilage fracture. Three geometrical features of the motion segment are responsible for individual variation in load sharing between the anterior and posterior elements (Panjabi et al., 1988; Manning et al., 1984): (1) disc height, (2) pedicle length, and (3) facet plane angle. Effects of disc narrowing have been described just above. Reciprocal changes are seen in disc and facet shear stresses with variation in the length of the pedicles. Longer structures tend to decrease shear loading in the form of interfacet pressure while increasing disc load. A 1-cm difference produces a transfer up to 100 N (22 lb). Higher facet inclinations tend to decrease disc load. However, the effect of different angles is only modest at best.

Subluxation Hypotheses

From a scientific perspective, the term subluxation has limited usefulness. Multiple definitions codified by state laws, agency regulation, and professional organizations are circulating. Consequently, each user subscribes to a different meaning. For clarity when discussing mechanical events and their ramifications, the term functional spinal lesion (FSL) is

hereby substituted. It is presumed that an FSL may arise independently or may coexist with organic disease.

Characteristics of the FSLs that allow them to be localized and identified clinically are derived from mechanical test maneuvers. As is currently believed, disorders may involve single or multiple motion segments (Schafer, 1983). Generally, FSLs manifest as aberrations of movement, localized or referred pain, and site tenderness (Lewit, 1987; Paterson and Burn, 1985; Grieve, 1983). At least for chief complaints of the neck, manual assessment of these criteria has proved to be highly accurate (Jull et al., 1986) in identifying the lesioned segment. Music tonus, reflex changes, and neurological signs are less reliable indicators. Their presentation is neither sufficiently consistent or localized (Styf, 1987; Styf and Lysell, 1987; Triano et al., 1988). Anatomic studies for neck pain (Bogduk, 1982) note that these signs tend to involve multiple spine levels. For that reason, they are helpful but not sensitive enough to localize the lesioned segment.

The spine is in a continuous state of balance, either dynamic or static. An FSU undergoing anomalous behavior, must be in one of three circumstances. First, there may be an inappropriate external load causing the motion segment to assume strained paths of motion or position. These could arise from trauma, unsuitable muscle action, or the development of intersegmental adhesions and contracture. Second, there may be an internal blocking of motion such as is supposed in the case of meniscoids or synovial tags. Third, the passive constitutive properties of the tissues may have been altered as with ligamentous tearing, disc buckling, or degeneration. These mechanisms represent supposition based solely on clinical impression. It is probable that no single circumstance is responsible for all cases, and more than one mechanism may operate in any single patient.

Muscle action may be either inappropriately strong or poorly timed when attempting a task. Effects of fatigue on muscle-generated joint torque of the lumbar spine are illustrated in Table 17–11. The loss of motor control and coordination allows an increase in off-axis motions that may alter the normal load sharing between the front and back of the motion segment. Excessive tension may develop, for instance, when a load being carried unexpectedly shifts and offsetting muscles must suddenly engage. If tissues are sufficiently strained, a painful syndrome may follow. At times, a persistent hypertonicity develops to restrict movement temporarily or redistribute loads at the injured part (Hoyt et al., 1981; Triano and Schultz, 1987). Multiple FSUs are affected when superficial back muscles or trunk muscles are recruited in this splinting process. Regional muscle activity would likely limit broad ranges of motion or categories of action such as left bending or flexion. A recent study of patients with low back pain suggests a reduction in secondary axis flexibility that such splinting action would predict (McIntyre, 1989).

Limitations from similar action of intersegmental muscles may be evident only when individual osseous movement is evaluated at end range. Superficial involvement is readily verified by manual examination and surface recording of myoelectric activity. Deep intersegmental muscles are much more difficult to identify and cannot be discriminated by surface electromyography. As a result, confirmation of their participation in persistent FSL remains to be seen.

Internal forces are conceived as arising within the joint. Sources include interarticular adhesions, degenerative joint remodeling, and entrapment of synovial tags or meniscoids. Structural confirmation of each has been given. Acting as mechanical stops, they limit joint flexibility. Unfortunately, there is insufficient information available to settle the degree that each option might play in FSL.

Lewit (1987) reviews a hypothesis for explaining early meniscoid entrapment before degenerative changes enter the picture. With rapid motions, the meniscoid is temporarily pinched between the joint surfaces. Tugging on the joint capsule produces sharp pain and reactive loading from muscle responses. Under prolonged static postures, however, creep deformity and stress relaxation locally deforms the region more than its surroundings. The meniscoid becomes entrapped. Sliding joint action is then converted into a pivoting one over some part of its range. Because there is little space to pivot, the motion is effectively blocked. Only a distraction of the joint can release it. Such a blockage is likely to become apparent only with testing in the specific direction and toward the end of range. Passive flexibility and overpressure clinical tests are based on this model. Passive flexibility is defined as the response of the FSU to perturbation from external forces while it is within its neutral zone. This contrasts with overpressure that stresses the joint at its extreme of voluntary range. Patient response of pain coupled with the examiner's perception of altered stiffness combine to give a positive finding.

Until now, notions about FSLs have been discussed with respect only to a reduced flexibility. Conditions of increased compliance are more easily explained with existing knowledge than fixations or end range restrictions. Larger displacements arise simply by disrupting the normal limiting tissues. Anatomic instability is diagnosed using radiographic criteria (Symposium 1985) and can be reviewed elsewhere.

A third type of kinematic anomaly is manifested by neither an increased nor a decreased range but an altered quality and smoothness of path from one position to another. The path of motion is governed by normal joint geometry, the inherent properties of the tissues, and coordination of muscle-generated joint torques. Altered orientation of facet joints, called trophism, is a relatively common isolated anomaly and is one example of such a mechanism. This anomaly may be developmental or acquired, as in patients with scoliosis or with leg length inequality. The affected FSU is susceptible to high axial torsion and strain to the capsule and disc (Cyron and Hutton, 1980). Biomechanical testing shows asymmetrical motion with a propensity for the vertebral body to rotate toward the more sagittal facet. Higher facet loads on the coronal facing are associated with greater degenerative joint disease on that side. Capsular tearing and adhesion to the adjacent nerve root have been reported (Badgley, 1941).

The literature on injury and alteration of constitutive tissue properties is extensive. Sudden contact injury, as from a fall or other accident, age-related changes, and cumulative trauma, are the main reasons for such tissue alterations. When the tissues are disrupted, their stiffnesses, anatomic dimensions, and ultimate strengths are altered. How well the joint performs under load conditions is likewise affected. Particularly true for cartilage, joint structures are unforgiving, and joint mechanics rarely become fully normal again although routine daily activities may often be resumed. If asymmetrical kinematics persist (for instance, in unilateral disc injury), (Panjabi et al., 1988) unequal sharing of facet loads, degeneration and narrowing of the IVF are likely. Whether from persistent weakness of the recovered part or from habitual abuse of spinal habits and hygiene, recurrence is the rule rather than the exception.

Buckling of FSUs may have important theoretical implications for understanding the spinal lesion. Observation of this phenomenon was accidental. During the course of conducting load–displacement studies of isolated vertebra, the balance point was selected as the load site rather than the geometric center as most investigations have done. Usual small increments of translation and rotation are followed without warning by an audible cracking sound and a sudden large displacement or buckling (Fig. 17–19). Afterward, the FSU returned to more typical linear load–displacement behavior, but from a new extreme position. When buckling occurs within the main body planes, higher compressive loads may result. However, an eccentric buckling might induce motion coupling and damaging axial torsion (Farfan and Gracovetsky, 1984).

The scientific evidence for buckling is intuitively appealing. It may provide clues to the mechanism of injury in some FSLs. The parallel between patient descriptions of sudden onset back pain arising during prolonged quasistatic postures or slow velocity tasks is obvious. Over 52% of spine-related pain, for example, cannot be associated with any significant muscular exertions (Manning, 1984). While sitting at a desk, the patient may lean or shift weight slightly and experience a sudden, sharp back pain accompanied by an audible cracking sound. The incident may or may not subside quickly but often presages more pain within a few days. More studies are needed to determine the clinical relevance of these hypothetical mechanisms.

Effects of Subluxation (FSL)

Little scientific information is presently available to resolve the questions of impact on human health that the FSL may have. Work performed by various clinical investigators has largely settled that therapeutic benefits are achieved through manual treatment of spine pain (Evans et al., 1978; Rasmussen, 1978; Hoehler et al., 1981; Waagen, 1986; Hadler et al., 1987). In an inverse way, data of this sort implicitly acknowledge the functional spinal lesions as a health hazard. Indirect evidence from the fundamentals of biomechanics presented earlier that suggest how health effects may ensue, will now be summarized.

Disorders of joint mobility are of three types: (1) fixation or limitations of range, (2) hypermobility or excessive range, and (3) aberrant paths or rhythms of movement. Both local and distant effects of these disorders are believed to develop. Mechanical deformation and disturbance of normal load sharing on the various components of FSUs are responsible for degenerative and inflammatory changes. Fixation mechanics theory predicts the effects of prolonged static loads that include creep deformity, load transfer from disc to facet, articular cartilage deformation, and joint stiffness. Volitional efforts to move an affected joint appear to cause pain, inflammation, and reactive muscle response. Figure 17–20 summarizes the processes and effects of the development of degenerative joint disease based on current theory (Videman, 1987).

Hypermobility mechanics theory, on the other hand, requires that some congenital or traumatic event alters the properties of restraining tissues to permit excessive joint compliance. Broader ranges of FSU movement are seen, for example, in some patients with disc disease. Pathologically narrowed disc space influences coupled and main motions. Levels L-4 and L-5 correlate with increased coupling,

higher shearing displacement, and generally increased range of motion (Stokes et al., 1981). Intermittent high stresses are transmitted through the motion segment elements, promoting further deterioration. Episodes of inflammatory reaction affecting ligament, facet articulations, and intervertebral foramina contents may result.

Mechanical explanation for altered rhythms of movement allow for either temporary fixation or hypermobility during subregional movements effecting one or more FSUs. Loss of lumbopelvic rhythm and increased off-axis movement during fatigue were described earlier as regional examples. The range for each joint complex is often within normal limits. However, the instantaneous position at any moment during its execution may represent paradoxical positions, momentary decelerations or accelerations. In short, the smoothness of the path is disturbed. Current examination methods are limited to manual assessment. A less well-developed theory than fixation or hypermobility, altered kinematics again implies unnatural load distributions. If restraining tissues have been damaged, the FSU may lose its resistance to combined compression and axial torsion (Panjabi et al., 1984; Adams and Hutton, 1980; Adams and Hutton, 1983; Shirazi-Adl, 1986). Then, even in the absence of new injury, a physiological load may result in large displacements that can become symptomatic. Farfan (1973) proposed this mechanism as an explanation for clinical instability to be discriminated from radiographic instability.

Examples of FSLs coexisting with known pathology are easily found by examining disc herniation. Two alternatives in motion segment behavior have been described. They include fixation and asymmetric motions. In one type, increased flexion accompanies lateral bending at the joint so as to prevent IVF narrowing. In the other type, the joint remains fixed so that no measurable movement occurs. In patients with radiating leg symptoms, main axial torsion and coupled axial torsion may be restricted (Lorenz et al., 1983).

In any case, the physiological consequences of aberrant segmental mechanics can be categorized as nerve impulse and nonimpulse based responses (Gitelman, 1975). Response types include (1) local tissue irritation, (2) biochemical mediator activation, and (3) reflex moderated effects (Will, 1978; Haldeman, 1981; Denslow, 1944; Denslow et al., 1947; Korr, 1978; Terrett and Vernon, 1984). Localized effects are probably responsible for the majority of symptoms from the spine. Excessive physical stimulation results in nociceptor activation with inflammatory swelling at the joint capsule or within disc lamina. In practice, the majority of patients do not

Conceptual Model for Degenerative Joint Disease

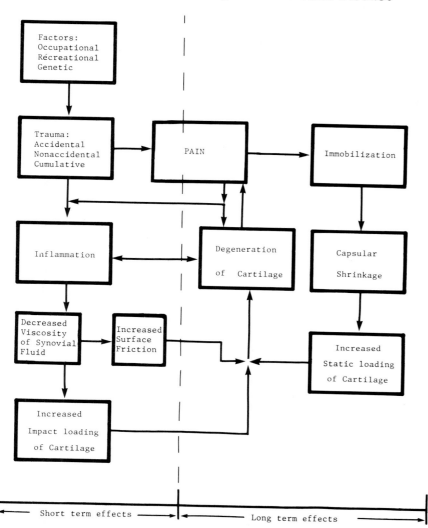

Figure 17–20. Interaction of short- and long-term effects that may contribute to the development of degenerative joint disease.

exhibit the anatomic instability or stenotic narrowing that would be necessary to permit the classically described "pinched nerve." Little clinical or scientific evidence exists to suggest that direct nerve compression plays an important role with FSL. With hypermobility, sufficiently distended capsulitis or foraminal narrowing, intermittent mechanical perturbation of the nerve may occasionally be possible. The onset of inflammatory response initiates a typical biochemical cascade of events. Vasoactive amines are liberated by stimulation of tissues, producing an inflammatory response. A transient vascular constriction is followed by local extreme vascular distention and increased permeability of the blood vessels' basement membrane. Albumin and blood sera leak out of circulation with diaphoresis of leukocytes. Classic signs of swelling, heat, and pain are produced. Spilling of vasoactive substances from torn annular fibers or capsular distention to the associated nerve root is hy-

pothesized as a further means of irritation and onset of inflammation.

Cord mediated changes arise from proprioception (Araki et al., 1984; Kurosawa et al., 1987; Isa et al., 1985; Sato and Schmidt, 1987; Sato and Swenson, 1984) nociception and mechanical stimulus (Goddard and Reid, 1965; Nathan, 1987; Grieve, 1986) of the peripheral nerve. Termed somatosomatic and somatovisceral reflexes, much controversy and interprofessional debate has been stimulated over them. Questions about their relative potency as factors in health and disease and methods to assess them are largely unsettled. Numerous articles have been written concerning the clinical tendency of muscle to undergo tightness and shortening (Janda, 1978; Nouwen et al., 1987; Thabe, 1986) or inhibition and weakness (Triano, 1980; Janda, 1987). Altered motor regulation and performance might be due to disturbances in movement patterns

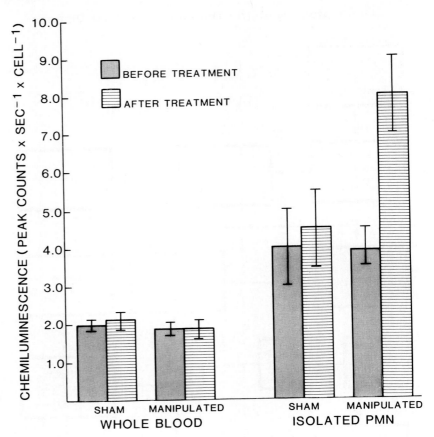

Figure 17–21. Measure of cellular metabolism in polymorphonuclear neutrophils isolated from whole blood of patients undergoing sham and manipulation procedures applied to the thoracic spine. (*Courtesy of Patricia Brennan, PhD, 1987.*)

and afferentation from the symptomatic joints (Humphreys et al., 1989). Similarly, afferent innervation and its effects on visceral functions have been detailed by Sato and colleagues. Stimulation of somatic afferent nerve endings and trunks results in altered functions of blood pressure, heart rate, adrenal secretions, as well as altered bladder and bowel contractions. Sympathetic nerves and ganglia can be directly impinged by osteophytes extending from the spine. As rigid extensions from the vertebrae, a claw spur reaching to the vicinity of the sympathetic chain perturbs it as motion occurs. Clearly, functional spinal lesions feasibly can have neurophysiological effects. Further investigation is necessary to determine the degree to which they are clinically meaningful.

Systemic effects from altered spinal biomechanics have recently been described and are most provocative. Anecdotal stories and clinical impressions relating spinal joint disorders and respiratory infections have occasionally been reported (Wilson, 1946; Facto, 1947; Purse, 1966). Manipulation of the thoracic spine in healthy volunteers has been found to enhance the respiratory bursts of polymorphonuclear neutrophils (Kokjohn et al., 1989) (Fig. 17–21). Cellular response to particulate challenge *in vitro*, measured by chemiluminescence, underwent a burst of activity within 15 minutes after spinal manipulation. Physiological explanation for conversion

of mechanical stimulus to the spine into a systemic circulating response is under examination. Equally intriguing is the fact that early results from ongoing studies suggest that a threshold effect based on the amount of load applied to the joint during manipulation treatment may exist. Although the data are too premature to permit speculation on clinical benefits from any facilitated chemiluminescence, it is obvious that the study of physiological effects from manipulation may lead farther than science had previously envisioned.

Conclusion

Understanding the etiology, pathomechanics, and treatment of functional spinal disorders requires a broad-based knowledge in physics and physiology. Although a great deal of information has been discovered in recent years, future research is likely to reveal many new surprises and new treatment methods as we probe the relations between structure and function.

References

Adams M, and Hutton W. The effect of posture on the role of the apophysial joints in resisting intervertebral compressive forces. *J Bone & Jt Surg* 1980;358–362.

Adams M, and Hutton W. Gradual disc prolapse. *Spine* 1985; 10:524–531.

Adams M, and Hutton W. The mechanical function of the lumbar apophyseal joints. *Spine* 1983;8:327–330.

Adams M, and Hutton W. The relevance of torsion to the mechanical derangement of the lumbar spine. *Spine* 1981;6:241–248.

Adams M, Hutton W, and Stott J. The resistance to flexion of the lumbar intervertebral joint. *Spine* 1980;5:245–253.

Ahern D, Follick M, Council J, et al. Comparison of lumbar paravertebral EMG patterns in chronic low back pain and non-patient controls. *Pain* 1988;34:153–160.

An K, Kwak B, Chao E, and Morrey B. Determination of muscle and joint forces: a new technique to solve the indeterminate problem. *J Biomech Eng* 1985;106:364–367.

Araki T, Ito K, Kurosawa M, and Sato A. Responses of adrenal sympathetic nerve activity and catecholamine secretion to cutaneous stimulation in anesthetic rats. *Neuroscience* 1984;12:289–299.

Badgley C. The articular facets in relationship to low back pain and sciatic radiation. *J Bone Jt Surg* 1941;23:481–496.

Basmajian J: Biofeedback and the placebo effect. *Psychiat Ann* 1981;11:42–49.

Bean J, Chaffin J, and Schultz A. Biomechanical model calculation of muscle contraction forces: A double linear programming method. *J Biomech* 1988;21:59–66.

Berkson M, Nachemson A, and Schultz A. Mechanical properties of human lumbar spine motion segments: II. Responses in compression and shear; influence of gross morphology. *J Biomech Eng* 1979;101:53–57.

Bogduk N. Neck pain: an update. *Australian Fam Phys* 1982;17:75–80.

Breig A, and Troup J. Biomechanical consideration in the straight leg raising test. *Spine* 1979;4:242–250.

Carter D, and Hayes W. Bone compressive strength: The influence of density and strain rate. *Science* 1976;194:1174–1176.

Chaffin D, and Andersson G: *Occupational Biomechanics.* Wiley Interscience, 103–107, 1984.

Chaffin D, and Andersson G. *Occupational Biomechanics,* New York: Wiley Interscience; 1985:87.

Ciric I. The alteral recess syndrome. *J Neurosurg* 1980;53:433–443.

Cohen M, Swanson G, Naliboff B, et al. Comparison of electromyographic response patterns during posture and stress tasks in chronic low back pain patterns and control. *J Psychosom Res* 1986; 30:135–141.

Collins G, Cohen M, Naliboff B, and Schandler S. Comparative analysis of paraspinal and frontalis EMG, heart rate and skin conductance in chronic low back pain patients and normals to various postures and stress. *Scan J Rehab Med* 1982;14:39–46.

Cowin S, Van Burskirk W, and Ashman R. Properties of Bone In Skalak R, and Chien S, eds. *Handbook of Bioengineering.* New York: McGraw Hill; 1987:10.

Cram J, and Steeger J. EMG scanning in the diagnosis of chronic pain. *Biofeedback and Self-Regulation* 1983;8:229–241.

Cyron B, and Hutton W. Articular tropism and stability of the lumbar spine. *Spine* 1980;5:168–172.

Denslow J. Analysis of variability of spinal reflex thresholds. *J Neurophysiol* 1944;7:297–315.

Denslow J, Korr I, and Drems A. Quantitative studies of chronic facilitation in human motoneuron pools. *Am J Physiol* 1947; 150:229–238.

Dumas G. Geometry of spinal facets. In Univ. of Ill, Champaign-Urbana Il. *Biomechanics Proceedings.* American Society of Biomechanics; 1988.

Epstein J. Lumbar nerve root compression at the intravertebral foramen caused by arthritis of the posterior facets. *J Neurosurg* 1980;39:362–369.

Evans D, Burke M, Lloyd K, et al. Lumbar spinal manipulation on trial: Part 1-clinical assessment. *Rheum & Rehab* 1978;17:46–53.

Facto L. The osteopathic therapy of lobar pneumonia. *JAOA* March 1947;46:385–391.

Farfan H. *Mechanical disorders of the low back.* Philadelphia: Lea & Febinger; 1973.

Farfan H, and Gracovetsky S. The nature of instability. *Spine* 1984; 9:714–719.

Friberg S. Studies on spondylolisthesis. *Acta Chiro Scand* 1939;55–58 (suppl):1–140.

Frymoyer J, Pope M, and Wilder D. Segmental instability. In Weinstein J, and Weisel S, eds. *The Lumbar Spine.* Philadelphia: WB Saunders Co., 1990:617.

Fung Y. *Biomechanics, Mechanical Properties of Living Tissues.* New York: Springer-Verlag; 1981;401.

Fung Y. Mechanics of soft tissue. In Skalak R and Chien S, eds. *Handbook of Bioengineering.* New York: McGraw Hill Pub; 1987; 1.1.

Gibbs D, Merrill E, Smith K. Rheology of hyaluronic acid. *Biopolymers* 1968;6:777–791.

Gill G, and Shite H. Mechanisms of nerve root compression and irritation in backache: Surgical decompression in intervertebral disc conditions-spondylolisthesis, spina bifida occult and transitional fifth lumbar vertebra. *Clin Orthop* 1955;5:66–81.

Gillet H, and Leikens M. 1985 Edition of the *Belgian Chiropractic Research Notes,* Huntington Beach, CA: Motion Palpation Institute, 1985:1.

Gitelman R. Spinal manipulation in the relief of pain. Washington DC: NINCDS monograph 15:27–285, (DHEW #NIH 76-998); 1975.

Goddard M, and Reid J. Movements induced by straight leg raising in the lumbosacral roots, nerves and plexus and in the intrapelvic section of the sciatic nerve. *J Neurol Neurosurg Psychiatr* 1965;28:12.

Goel V, Goyal S, Clark C, et al. Kinematics of the whole lumbar spine: effect of discectomy. *Spine* 1985;10:543–554.

Grieve G. *Common vertebral joint problems.* New York: Churchill Livingstone, 1983:159–202.

Grieve G. *Modern manual therapy of the vertebral column.* New York: Churchill-Livingstone, 1986;259–269.

Hadler N, Curtis P, Gillings B, and Stinnett S. A benefit of spinal manipulation as adjunctive therapy for acute low-back pain: a stratified controlled trial. *Spine* 1987;12:703–706.

Haldeman S. Pain physiology as a neurological model for manipulation. *Man Med* 1981;19:5–11.

Harkness R. Mechanical properties of collagenous tissues. In Gould B, ed. *Treatise on Collagen,* Vol 2. New York: Academic Press; 1968:247–310.

Hayes M, Howard T, Guel C, and Kopta J: Roentgenographic evaluation of lumbar spine flexion-extension in asymptomatic individuals. *Spine* 1989;14:327–331.

Hirsch C, and Nachemson A. A new observation on the mechanical behavior of lumbar discs. *Acta Orthop Scand* 1954;23:254–283.

Hoehler F, Tobis J, and Burget A. Spinal manipulation for low back pain. *JAMA* 1981;224:1835–1838.

Hoyt W, Hunt H, DePauw M, et al. Electromyographic assessment of chronic low back pain syndrome. *J Am Osteop Assoc* 1981; 80:728–730.

Humphreys C, Triano J, and Brandl M. Sequential study of H-Reflex alterations in acute idiopathic low back pain patients undergoing conservative treatment. *JMPT* 1989;12:70–78.

Huxley A. Muscular contraction. *J Physiol* 1974;243:1–43.

Isa T, Kurosawa M, Sato A, and Swenson R. Reflex responses evoked in the adrenal sympathetic nerve to electrical stimulation of somatic afferent nerves in the rat. *Neuroscience Res* 1985;3:130–144.

Janda V. Muscle weakness and inhibition (pseudoparesis) in back pain syndromes. In Grieve G, ed. *Modern manual therapy of the vertebral column.* New York: Churchill Livingstone; 1987;19–201.

Janda V. Muscles, central nervous motor regulation and back

problems. In Korr I, ed. *The Neurobiologic Mechanicsms in Manipulative Therapy.* New York: Plenum Press; 1978;27–41.

Jayson M. Compression stresses in the posterior elements and pathologic consequences. *Spine* 1987;8:338–339.

Jull G, Bogduk N, and Marsland A. The accuracy of manual diagnosis for cervical zygapophyseal joint pain syndromes. *Med J of Australia* 1986;148:233–237.

Kokjohn K, Kaltinger C, Lohr G, et al. Enhanced human phagocytic cell respiratory burst following spinal manipulation. Proceedings of Amer Soc Microbiology, New Orleans, 1989.

Korr I. *The neurobiologic mechanisms in manipulative therapy.* New York: Plenum Press; 1978.

Kromodiharjo S, and Mital A. Kinetic analysis of manual lifting activities: part I-development of a three-dimensional computer model. *Inter J Ind Ergo* 1986;1:77–90.

Kulak R, Schultz A, Belytschko T, and Galante J. Biomechanical characteristics of vertebral motion segments and intervertebral discs. The Orthop Clinics of Mo. Amer. WB Saunders; 1975; 121–135.

Kurosawa M, Sato A, Sato Y, and Suzuki H. Undiminished reflex responses of adrenal sympathetic nerve activity to stimulation of baroreceptors and cutaneous mechanoreceptors in aged rats. *Neuroscience Letters* 1987;77:193–198.

Lewit K. *Manipulative therapy in rehabilitation of the motor system.* London: Butterworths; 1987;17–19.

Lewit K. *Manipulative therapy in rehabilitation of the locomotor system.* London: Butterworths; 1987;12–14.

Lorenz M, Patwardhan A, and Venderby R: Load-bearing characteristics of lumbar facets in normal and surgically altered spinal segments. *Spine* 1983;8:122–130.

Luttges M, and Grosswald D. Comparative differences in the proteins of sciatic nerves. Proceedings of the 7th Annual Biomechanics Conference on the Spine. 1976:85–104.

Luttges M, Stodieck L, and Beel J. Postinjury changes in the biomechanics of nerves and roots in mice. *JMPT* 1986:9:89–98.

MacGregor R, Sharpless S, and Luttges M. A pressure vessel model for nerve compression. *J of Neurological Sci* 1975;24:299–304.

Malcom L. Frictional and deformational responses of articular cartilage interfaces to static and dynamic loading. PhD Thesis. San Diego: U of California; 1976.

Manning D, Mitchell R, and Blanchfield L. Body movements and events contributing to accidental and nonaccidental back injuries. *Spine* 1984;9:734–739.

Mayer T, and Gatchel R. *Functional Restoration: A Sports Medicine Approach.* Lea & Febiger; 1988.

McIntyre D. Personal communication. Isotechnologies Inc., 1989.

McLellin D, and Swash M. Longitudinal sliding movements of the median nerve during movements of the upper limb. *J Neurol Neurosurg Psychiatr* 1976;39:566–570.

McMahon T. Muscle mechanics, In Skalak R, and Chien S, eds. *Handbook of Bioengineering.* New York; McGraw Hill, 1987:7.3.

Millar JD. In *Proposed National Strategies for the Prevention of Leading Work-related Diseases and Injuries, Part 1.* Assoc of Schools of Public Health; 1986:vii.

Miller J, Haderspeck K, and Schultz A. Posterior element loads in lumbar motion segments. *Spine* 1987;8:331–337.

Moroney S, Schultz A, Miller J, and Andersson G. Load displacement properties of lower cervical spine motion segments. *J of Biomech* 1988;21:769–779.

Mow V, Kuei S, Lai W, and Armstrong C. Biphasic creep and stress relaxation of articular cartilage in compression: Theory and experiments. *J Biomech Eng.* 1980;102:73–84.

Nachemson A. *In vivo* measurement of intra-discal pressure. *J Bone & Jt Surg* 1965;46AJ:1077.

Nathan H. Osteophytes of the spine compressing the sympathetic trunk and splanchnic nerves in the thorax. *Spine* 1987;12:527–532.

National Institute for Occupational Safety and Health. *A work Practices Guide for Manual Lifting,* Tech Report #81–122. Cincinnati, Oh.: U.S. Dept. of Health and Human Services (NIOSH); 1981.

Neary D, Ochoa J, and Filliatt R. Subclinical entrapment neuropathy in man. *J Neurol Sci* 1975;24:283–298.

Nouwen A, Van Akkerveeken P, and Versloot J. Patterns of muscular activity during movements in patients with chronic low-back pain. *Spine* 1987;12:8.

Ogston A, and Stanier J. The physiological function of hyaluronic acid in synovial fluid; viscous, elastic and lubricant properties. *J Physiol* 1953;119:244–252.

Pal G, and Sherk H. The vertical stability of the cervical spine. *Spine* 1988;13.

Panjabi M, Abumi K, Duranceau J, et al. A Biomechanical Study of Partial and Complete Facetectomies of the Lumbar Spine. Amer Soc of Biomech 12th Annual meeting, September 1988: 163.

Panjabi M, Goel V, and Takata K. Physiologic strains in lumbar spinal ligaments. *Spine* 1982;7:192–203.

Panjabi M, Krag M, and Chung T. Effects of disc injury on mechanical behavior of the human spine. *Spine* 1984; 9:07–713.

Panjabi M, Takata K, and Goel V. Kinematics of lumbar intervertebral foramen. *Spine* 1983;8:348–357.

Panjabi M, and White A. *Clinical Biomechanics of the Spine.* Philadelphia: Lippincott Co.; 1978.

Panjabi M, Yamamoto I, Oxland T, and Crisco J. How does posture affect coupling in the lumbar spine. *Spine* 1988;14:1002–1011.

Parnianpour M, Nordin M, Khanovitz N, and Frankel V. The triaxial coupling of torque generation of trunk muscles during isometric exertions and the effect of fatiguing isoinertial movements on the motor output and movement patterns. *Spine* 1988; 13:982–992.

Paterson J, and Burn L. *An introduction to medical manipulation.* Boston: MTP Press Limited; 1985;32–34.

Phillips R, Frymoyer J, MacPherson B, and Newberg A. Low back pain: a radiographic enigma. *JMPT* Sept. 1986;9:3.

Pintar F. The biomechanics of spinal elements. PhD thesis. Marquette University; 1986.

Plamondon A, Gagnon M, and Maurais G. Application of stereoradiographic method for the study of intervertebral motion. *Spine* 1988;13:9.

Posner I, White A, Edwards W, and Hayes W. A biomechanical analysis of the clinical stability of the lumbar and lumbosacral spine. *Spine* 1982;7:374–389.

Purse F. Manipulation therapy of upper respiratory infections in children. *JAOA* May 1966;65:964–971.

Rasmussen T. Manipulation in treatment of low back pain (a randomized clinical trial) *Man Med,* 1978;8–10.

Reilly D, and Burnstein A. The elastic and ultimate properties of compact bone tissue. *J. Biomech* 1975;8:393–405.

Reuber M, Schultz A, Denis F, and Spencer D. Bulging of lumbar intervertebral disc. *J Biomed Eng* 1982;104:187–192.

Salter RB, Simmonds DR, Malcom BW, Rumble EJ, MacMichael D, Clements N. The biological effect of continuous passive motion in healing of full thickness defects in articular cartilage. *JBJS* 1980;62A,8:1232–1251.

Sato A, and Schmidt R. The modulation of visceral functions by somatic afferent activity. *Jap J of Physiol* 1987;37:1–17.

Sato A, and Swenson R. Sympathetic nervous system response to mechanical stress of the spinal column in rats. JMPT 7, #3:141–147, 1984.

Schafer R. *Clinical biomechanics musculoskeletal actions and reactions.* Baltimore, MD: Williams & Wilkins; 1983;208–219.

Schultz A, Andersson G, Haderspeck K, et al. Analysis and measurement of lumbar trunk loads in tasks involving bends and twists. *J Biomech* 1982;15:669–675.

Schultz A, Haderspeck-Grib K, Sinkora G, and Warwick D. Quantitative studies of the flexion-relaxation phenomenon in back muscles. *J Orthop Res* 1985;3:189–197.

Schultz A, Warwick D, Berkson M, and Nachemson A. Mechanical properties of human spine motion segments: I. Responses in flexion-extension, lateral bending, and rotation. ASME *J Biomed Eng* 1979;101:46–52.

Sharpless S. Neurophysiology of nerve compression and joint fixation. Proceedings of the 5th Annual Biomechanics Conference on the Spine. U of Colorado, Boulder, Co. December 7–8, 1974: 219–278.

Sherman R. Relationships between strength of low back muscle contraction and reported intensity of chronic low back pain. *Am J of Phys Med* 1985;64:190–200.

Shirazi-Adl A, Ahmed A, and Shrivastava S. Mechanical response of a lumbar motion segment in axial torque alone and combined with compression. *Spine* 1986;11:914–927.

Speiser R, and Aragona R. Applied spinal biomechanical engineering methodology utilizing pre and post stress loading roentgenographs and biomechancial physiological rehabilitative spinal maneuvers to restore dynamic function in the lumbar spine. Proceedings of the 1989 International Conference on Spinal Manipulation. Washington, DC, March 1989:75–84.

Spencer D, Irwin G, and Miller J. Anatomy and significance of fixation of the lumbosacral nerve roots in sciatica. *Spine* 1983;6, #6:672–679.

Stokes I, Wilder D, Frymoyer J, and Pope M. Assessment of patients with low-back pain by biplanar radiographic measurement of intervertebral motion. *Spine* 1981;6:233–240.

Styf J. Pressure in the erector spinae muscle during exercise. *Spine* 1987;12:675–677.

Styf J, and Lysell E. Chronic compartment syndrome in the erector spinae muscle. *Spine* 1987;12:680–682.

Symposium on instability of the lumbar spine. *Spine* 1985;10:253–291.

Tanzer R. The carpal tunnel syndrome. *J Bone Joint Surg* 1962; 41A:626–634.

Taylor J, and Twomey L. Age changes in lumbar zygapophyseal joints: Observations on structure and function. *Spine*, 1986;11, 739–745.

Terett A, and Vernon H. Manipulation and pain tolerance. *Am J of Phys Med* 1984;63:217–224.

Thabe H. Electromyography as tool to document diagnostic findings and therapeutic results associated with somatic dysfunctions in the upper cervical spinal joints and sacroiliac joints. *Manual Med* 1986;2:53–58.

Triano J. Accurate determination of motion from plane films. Amer Soc of Biomech, October 1984.

Triano J. (Analysis): Comparison of lumbar paravertebral EMG patterns in chronic LBP and non-patient controls. DC Tracts 1, #3, June 1989.

Triano J. Significant lumbar dyskinesia, *JACA* 1980; 14:S11–S15.

Triano J, and Luttges M. Nerve irritation: A possible model of sciatic neuritis. *Spine* 1982;7:129–136.

Triano J, Prastein R, Papakyriakou M, and Torres B. Estimation of Isometric Muscle Tension from Muscle Hardness. Proceedings from American Society of Biomechanics Annual meeting, Urbana-Champaign, IL, 1988.

Triano J, and Schultz A. Correlation of objective measure of trunk motion and muscle function with low-back disability ratings. *Spine* 1987;12:561–565.

Triano J, Torres B, and Papakyriakou M. Interactions of myoelectric responses and pain from transverse shear loading of the spine. Proceedings of the 1989 International Conference on Spinal Manipulation, Washington, DC. 1989:88–89.

Ugale R, Mykleburst J, Pintar F, et al. Recovery properties of human lumbar vertebrae, abstract. *J. Biomech* 1987;20:888.

Verbeist H. A radicular syndrome from developmental narrowing of the lumbar vertebral canal. *J Bone Jt Surg* 1954;36B:230–237.

Videman T. Experimental models of osteoarthritis: the role of immobilization. *Clinical Biomech* 1987;2:223–229.

Viidik A. Interdependence between structure and function in collagenous tissues. In Viidik A and Vuust J, eds. *Biology of Collagen.* New York: Academic Press; 1980:257–280.

Viidik A. Properties of tendons and ligaments. In Skalak R, and Chien S, eds. *Handbook of Bioengineering.* New York: McGraw-Hill; 1987.

Videman T. Experimental models of osteoarthritis: the role of immobilization. *Clin Biomech* 1987;2:223–229.

Waagen G, Haldeman S, Cook G, et al. Short-term of chiropractic adjustments for relief of chronic low back pain. *Man Med* 1986; 2:63–67.

Ward L. *The Dynamics of Spinal Stress.* Long Beach, CA: O&S Press; 1977.

Will T. The basis of manipulation. *JMPT* 1978;1:155–157.

Wilson P. The osteopathic treatment of asthma. *JAOA:* July 1946; 491–492.

Wolf S, and Basmajian J. Assessment of paraspinal activity in normal subjects and in chronic back pain patients using a muscle biofeedback device. In Asmussen E, Gorgensen J, eds. *International Series on Biomechanics VI-B.* Baltimore: University Park Press; 1979:319–323.

Woo S, Mow V, and Lai W. Biomechanical properties of articular cartilage. In Skalak R, and Chien S, eds. *Handbook of Bioengineering.* New York: McGraw-Hill; 1987;4.13.

Yamada H. Strength of biological materials. In Evans F, ed. Baltimore, MD: Williams and Wilkins; 1970.

III

Spinal Analysis and Diagnostic Methods

From the onset of formalized chiropractic practice and the establishment of licensure and education standards there has been intense discussion as to what qualifies as an acceptable chiropractic physical and spinal examination. Within the chiropractic profession certain schools of thought have proposed a very limited examination. Within this school only the spinal examination is important and this, in turn, was limited only to those parts of the examination necessary to locate and characterize the subluxation or manipulable lesion. Many colleges, however, have taught a much broader scope of diagnostic skills, including a full physical examination, laboratory investigation, and even certain invasive tests. Critics of chiropractic, mainly those within the medical profession, are also split on the matter. They reason that if chiropractors were to be licensed they should be trained and capable of reaching an adequate diagnosis. These critics, at the same time, often frustrate chiropractic education and licensing attempts to access diagnostic procedures and specialists. The legislators in various states and countries have tried to reach rational compromises that seldom satisfied either of these points of view.

Fortunately, chiropractic clinicians and researchers have been evaluating systematically different examination techniques and formulating a basis for an acceptable chiropractic evaluation of a patient before commencing treatment. This has led to the concept of a double or dual diagnosis. Therefore, the chiropractor is expected to reach two distinct diagnoses or conclusions that may or may not interact with each other.

The first conclusion or diagnosis that is made by a chiropractic clinician concerns the general health of the patient. This includes the search for pathology and potential sources of symptomatology. This portion of the examination begins with the history and physical examination as described in Chapter 18 by Sportelli and Tarola. These authors outline the primary examination procedures taught in chiropractic colleges. They describe the significance of certain abnormal findings and how these findings might be interpreted. The use of specific laboratory examination procedures including blood chemistry and hormonal evaluation, urinalysis, electrodiagnostic testing and other instruments to clarify this diagnosis is described by Triano in Chapter 20. Many of these tests can only be performed in certified laboratories and require special training and interpretation, often by a medical specialist. Recent changes in the medical community have made referrals for such testing by chiropractors much easier. The use of radiological and other imaging techniques, such as computed tomography, magnetic resonance imaging, and myelography, are increasingly being used to further the chiropractic diagnostic skills. The use of these tests for pathology recognition are described in Chapter 21 by Howard and Rowe and in Chapter 22 by Howe, Foreman, and Glenn.

The second conclusion or diagnosis that must be made by a chiropractor before treatment is the assessment of spinal function. This aspect of the examination includes the search for an abnormality that is amenable to chiropractic treatment. This abnormality or lesion has been referred to as the subluxation, manipulable lesion, spinal dysfunction, or fixation. The search for more accurate and sensitive means of finding this lesion and determining its clinical significance remains a priority within chiropractic institutions. Traditionally, and still currently, the primary tool of the chiropractor in diagnosing a subluxation or fixation is manual diagnosis or spinal palpation. Faye and Wiles, in Chapter 19, describe the results of research that have been conducted to investigate the reliability of these procedures. They then describe the principles of static and motion palpation with numerous examples. Triano, in Chapter 20, describes the instruments that have been developed with a similar goal, including posture, spinal curvature and motion measuring instruments, thermography, and electrodiagnostic tests. Mick, Phillips, and Breen, in Chapter 23 describe how the x-ray has been used to evaluate spinal function and position as well as its usefulness in defining the characteristics of a subluxation.

As this section demonstrates, the nature and

extent of a chiropractic evaluation is better defined than at any point in its history. Many of the testing and examination procedures require considerable further research to determine reliability, sensitivity, and clinical significance. This research is, however, currently being conducted and the next decade can be expected to lead to an even greater definition of what is expected from a chiropractic examination of a patient and his or her spine.

Scott Haldeman

chapter 18

The History and Physical Examination

Louis Sportelli
Gary A. Tarola

It is as important to know the patient who has the disease as the disease that has the patient.

Sir William Osler

Acknowledgements

The authors would like to express their appreciation to Henry G. West, Jr., D.C., for providing us the opportunity to review and modify the chapter, "Physical and Spinal Examination Procedures Utilized in the Practice of Chiropractic," from the first edition of this text.

A thorough and accurate patient history is said to be the single most important factor in clinical evaluation. The information obtained from a careful history should direct the chiropractic examiner to the specific physical and technological examination procedures necessary to confirm or rule out his or her suspicions of a preliminary diagnosis. A correct diagnosis depends on proper interpretation of clinical findings gathered during physical examination. Accurate interpretation of these findings depends on a thorough knowledge of functional anatomy, physiology, and clinical characteristics common to specific disease states.

Patient Interview and Health History

Observing the patient and the manner in which he or she moves about the office and examination room is an inseparable and important part of history taking. Patients with acute lumbar disc disease, for instance, will often stand and walk about the examination room during the history taking, because sitting may be painful. Observing the patient also enables the examiner to note the patient's current behavior; e.g., hyperactive or depressed.

The interview is an art that must be learned and constantly practiced. During the initial interview, the chiropractic examiner must gain the patient's confidence. The examiner must be articulate and conversant with individuals from every walk of life and recognize various personality types. Every illness ordinarily evokes an emotional response in a patient. An individual may deny having an illness or have a different threshold of pain than another with the same disease state. Whatever the patient's reaction to illness, it is imperative that the clinician present an attitude of understanding and concern. These attitudes encourage the patient's trust, leading to the disclosure of additional information that may be of significant diagnostic importance. It is important, however, that the examiner keep the patient to the point, and discourage irrelevant information. This should be done politely but firmly.

The history is usually taken in an orderly sequence. The questions asked should be easy to understand and should not "lead" the patient. For example, the examiner should not say, "Does this increase your pain"? It would be better to say, "Does this alter your pain in any way"? Because it is irritating to the patient when the examiner too quickly anticipates the patient's response the examiner should ask one question at a time and should receive a complete answer before proceeding (Magee, 1987). The clinician who can combine sensitive insight and understanding with a sensible, objective approach to the patient's problem usually will establish an excellent professional rapport with the patient.

At times, the history must be cut short depending on the chief complaint and its onset. For example, if a patient complains of pain in an area that is directly associated with recent trauma, and the mechanism of injury can be directly related to the patient's complaint, the examiner need not explore much further. Usually, however, acquiring the following information in a sequential manner aids the chiropractic examiner in developing a clinical impression, or suggests specific examination procedures that will efficiently and effectively confirm or rule out a potential diagnosis.

Assessing Sources of Pain

The majority of patients seeking chiropractic health care do so for complaints of a neuromusculoskeletal nature, primarily back and neck pain (ACA, 1989).

1. Determine where the pain was when the problem began and where it is now.
   Ask the patient to point to exactly where the pain was at its onset and where it is now. This practice minimizes misunderstandings that may arise due to a patient's partial or inaccurate verbal description.
2. Determine the type of pain.
   Certain types of pain characteristically originate from certain tissue types. Determining the nature of the patient's pain may, therefore, be useful in reaching a tentative diagnosis. Bone pain tends to be deep. Muscle pain is often dull and aching. Vascular pain tends to be diffuse, aching, and poorly localized. Nerve pain tends to be sharp and burning, and ligament pain is sharp and localized.
3. Determine how the pain originated.
   Was the pain slow or sudden in onset? Was there inciting trauma?
4. Determine the severity of the pain.
   Is the intensity of pain increasing, decreasing, or remaining the same?
5. Determine if the pain is constant, periodic, or occasional.
   The duration and frequency of symptoms help the examiner determine whether the condition is acute or chronic and aid in determining the rapidity of progression. Observing the patient is essential. If the patient appears to move around and shift positions frequently in an attempt to find a comfortable position, the pain may be persistent. Does the patient appear to be losing sleep because of pain?

6. Determine what positions or movements aggravate or relieve the pain.

The examiner should be as specific as possible in ascertaining the precise motions, stress, positions, or activity that aggravate the patient's pain. Is the pain associated with rest or activity, certain postures, visceral function, or time of day? This information is useful in differentiating the etiology of back pain, whether it be viscerogenic, neurogenic, vascular, psychogenic, or mechanical. Viscerogenic back pain produced, for example, by the kidney, gallbladder, or prostate usually is not aggravated by activity or relieved by rest, whereas mechanical back pain may diminish in a recumbent position. Neurogenic back pain from a spinal cord tumor, and pain from a primary or secondary vertebral bone tumor is generally constant, and remains unchanged by postural position. The symptoms of vascular claudication are aggravated by walking and relieved by standing still or resting. Mechanical pain is usually highly reactive to changes in posture, positions, or activity. Morning pain relieved with daily activity is often associated with arthritis.

7. Determine if the pain is in or near a joint, if the joint exhibits locking, unlocking, twinges, instability, or giving way, and the exact movements that cause pain.

In the presence of internal derangement of the knee, for example, pain or locking may occur in flexion one time and in extension another time. If it is due to a loose body joint, the knee may give way with pressure placed on it.

Concomitant Symptoms or Illness

The patient must be carefully questioned about current illnesses, conditions, or diseases. If the patient relates a specific condition or conditions, the examiner should attempt to ascertain the exact diagnosis as well as current and prior treatments, medications, response to treatments, and course of the disease. If the examiner suspects a systemic condition, the following questions may help to identify a possible disorder:

1. Have you been feverish? When and for how long?
   These symptoms may relate to a current or recent infectious process.
2. Have you been nauseated?
   These symptoms may be due to gastrointestinal, gallbladder, or cardiac problems.
3. Have your urinary or bowel habits been altered since the onset of pain?

These symptoms may be due to neurological, intestinal, renal, or urinary tract disorders.

4. Are any of your extremities numb or cold?
   If so, it may be due to subclavian, axillary, iliac, or femoral artery occlusion. Additional vascular analysis may be warranted.
5. Determine if there are any color changes of the limb.
   Circulatory problems may cause trophic changes such as white or brittle skin, loss of hair, and abnormal nails on the hand or foot.
6. Determine the age and sex of the patient.
   Certain conditions are more common in one gender than the other, whereas other conditions occur within certain age ranges.

Patient's Medical History

Determine all accidents, injuries, and occasions of illness in the life of the patient before the current complaint. A description of prior illness or conditions, including their etiology, onset, duration, method of treatment, and response to treatment should be recorded. The results of prior diagnostic procedures (e.g., x-rays and laboratory tests) may be of value if known. Inquire as well about past surgeries and the result of these procedures.

The examiner should know what medications the patient is taking, such as diuretics, steroids, antidepressants, and anticoagulants, to name a few. This information is important to determine whether or not the medication has any relationship to the present complaint. Furthermore, a patient's medication status may contraindicate a specific course of chiropractic treatment, such as spinal manipulation, or suggest caution in undertaking treatment. On occasion, the patient's symptoms may be a reaction to the medication taken. Drug sensitivities and allergic reactions should, therefore, be ascertained.

Systems Review

A review of body systems should include a general statement about the patient's health. This may include any changes in appetite, weight, energy, sleep habits, or general well-being. When indicated, the following may be helpful in identifying certain systemic conditions. Questions may be asked about the head, ears, nose, throat, neck, and skin. Have there been headaches, skin changes, bleeding, recurring sore throat, hoarseness, or difficulty in swallowing? Have there been dizziness, blurred vision, ringing in the ears? Has the patient noticed any masses, stiffness, or changes in the range of motion in the neck?

Questions regarding the presence of cough, hemoptysis, dyspnea, pain, and wheezing may reveal respiratory disease. Questions regarding chest pain, dyspnea, syncope, fatigue, edema, palpitation, cramps, paresthesia, and changes in the color of the hands and feet may indicate disturbance of the cardiovascular system. Problems within the abdomen and genitourinary system may be suspected with questions about the tongue and mouth, dysphasia, appetite, weight loss, bowel habits, stools, jaundice, vomiting, micturition, disurea, retention, and hematuria. Questions and observations regarding unusual appearances in weight, hair distribution, growth, and development could reveal metabolic or endocrine dysfunction. Abnormality of the lymphatic system may result in unusual lumps or bumps.

Questions regarding headaches, vision, diplopia, hearing, tinnitus, vertigo, taste, smell, speech, changes in consciousness, syncope convulsion, involuntary movements, weakness, paresthesia, and sphincter control may indicate nervous system involvement. Inquiries about the blood should include questions concerning the skin color, bleeding of any nature, bruising, and swelling. Information regarding the patient's psychological state may be acquired with questions regarding insomnia, altered behavior, recent changes in the person's life, and emotional stresses from family, jobs, etc.

Lifestyle and Social Background

The course of organic disease and spinal pain is influenced by a patient's lifestyle and social environment. Questioning should be directed into the patient's personal habits such as smoking, use of alcohol, hobbies, recreation, and diet. Social background, including family relationships, emotional adjustments, sexual habits, and occupation, may also directly or indirectly affect a patient's current state of health.

Family Medical History

Hereditary and constitutional factors influence the etiology of certain disease processes such as diabetes mellitus, cancer, hypertension, arteriosclerosis, gout, and coronary artery disease. Questions regarding the deaths or past and present illness of parents, grandparents, and siblings and other family members can, therefore, be important. The chiropractor is particularly interested in the history of musculoskeletal disorders, such as degenerative disc disease, arthritis, and spinal anomalies. A genetic predisposition to certain structural abnormalities can be determined by a careful review of family affliction.

Occupation and Daily Activities

An individual's occupational activities, as well as activities of daily living, may have a significant influence on the musculoskeletal system. The chiroprac-

tic examiner is interested in the patient's physical comfort in the performance of occupational duties, as well as his or her home activities, sports, and recreational habits. The clinician must frequently make recommendations in habit changes to aid in reducing physical stresses from daily activity that may be aggravating the patient's condition.

Supplemental History by Questionnaire

Many chiropractic physicians utilize preprinted questionnaires that contain much of the information stated above. Although questionnaires help to obtain specific information, overreliance on questionnaires minimizes the doctor's opportunity to establish a personal rapport with the patient, and may not provide complete and detailed information about the patient's specific complaints.

The importance of taking an accurate, detailed patient history cannot be overemphasized. As stated previously, the chiropractic examiner should usually be able to make a "preliminary" diagnosis from the history alone. Once the history is completed, the examiner should put the patient at ease by further explaining what will occur during the physical examination.

General Physical Examination

The purpose of physical examination procedures is to add to information previously obtained to identify or confirm a specific disease process or lesion. A thorough patient history, followed by a careful physical examination should lead to an accurate diagnosis. Laboratory examinations, such as myelography and electromyography, should only be used to further substantiate the diagnosis and exclude other ailments (J. Kramer, 1981). The performance of any sophisticated diagnostic procedure should be based on clinical need. It is ill advised to utilize procedures routinely for "screening" purposes alone (Yochum, 1987).

Vital Signs

The patient's height and weight should be vocalized. If the patient challenges the height, it may be a clue to spinal distortion. If the patient remarks about a weight change, the examiner should investigate the cause of the change.

Systolic arterial blood pressure in persons under 40 years of age is usually 110 to 140 mm Hg and the diastolic pressure is 60 to 90 mm Hg (Prior, 1959). Comparison of the blood pressure of both upper extremities should not vary more than 5 to 10%. A difference of 10 to 15 mm Hg suggests arterial compression or obstruction on the low pressure side and may be due to thoracic outlet syndrome or subclavian or axillary artery stenosis. The systolic blood pressure generally increases slightly from recumbency to weight bearing, whereas the diastolic pressure rises slightly. In orthostatic postural hypotension there is a significant drop in the systolic pressure on standing, which may account for fatigue or light headedness.

Causes include drugs, prolonged bedrest, depletion of blood volume, and diseases of the peripheral autonomic nervous system. (Bates, 1983).

Pulse rate varies with age, sex, physical activity, and emotional status, with 72 beats/min being the average. The radial pulse in both upper extremities and the pedal pulse of both lower extremities can be palpated and evaluated for circulatory sufficiency.

The examiner should observe the type, rate, and depth of quiet breathing. In the adult at rest, the normal respiratory rate is 16 to 20 cycles/min and is regular in depth and rhythm. The normal ratio of respiratory rate to pulse rate is 1:4.

Body temperature may be measured with an oral thermometer, and normally does not exceed 37°C.

Systems Examination

After recording the vital signs, the patient's body system status may be examined, taking into account each patient's specific needs. A system review includes examination of the head, cardiovascular system, respiratory system, gastrointestinal system, and genitourinary system (Haldeman, 1980).

The examiner should develop a fairly standard routine so that he or she can examine a patient smoothly and efficiently without forgetting important steps. Failure to follow a systematic procedure may result in overlooking important signs or symptoms. The absence as well as the presence of symptoms and signs should be recorded.

Head. With the patient seated, the clinician should examine the head, hair, scalp, skull, and face of the patient. Of particular interest is the sensitivity of the frontal and paranasal sinuses to palpation. A postnasal discharge, along with a pain response to palpation over the sinus cavities, may be due to sinusitis.

EYES. The alignment of the eyes, eyebrows, and eyelids and the condition of the lacrimal apparatus, conjunctiva and sclera, cornea, iris, and pupils should be noted. Extraocular movements should be noted as well.

EARS. The examiner, where appropriate, should inspect the ear canal and eardrum with an otoscope and check auditory acuity with the ticking of a watch. If acuity is diminished, the examiner should check for lateralization and compare bone conduction with air conduction using a tuning fork. Impacted cerumen, otitis externa, or otitis media may produce hearing loss, pain, or dizziness.

NOSE. The clinician should examine the external nose and, using a nasal speculum, inspect the nares, the mucosa, the septum, and the terminates.

MOUTH AND PHARYNX. Inspect the lips, buccomucosa, gums and teeth, roof of the mouth, tongue, tonsils, and pharynx. Palpating the temporomandibular joint is of particular importance to the chiropractor. Gelb (1977) states that malrelationship of the jaws may have an effect on the entire neuromuscular system.

NECK. Inspect and palpate the cervical nodes, trachea, and thyroid. Deviation of the larynx on deglutition may be indicative of a space-occupying lesion or adhesions. If lymphadenopathy is present, the examiner should look for an infectious source of the lymphatic drainage.

CRANIAL NERVES. The physiological and anatomic implications of disturbed cranial nerve function can be important in the premanipulation, clinical evaluation of the patient. The twelve pairs of cranial nerves should be evaluated in the following manner (Bates 1983).

1. Olfactory Nerve (I). Using a familiar odor, such as menthol, the patient, with eyes shut and one nostril held closed, is asked to identify the test substance. The test is repeated with the other nostril held closed.
2. Optic Nerve (II). Test the visual acuity of each eye, one at a time, with a Snellen eye chart. Examine the fundi with an ophthalmoscope. The normal disc is yellowish-red and flat, with clearly defined margins. If papilledema is present, the optic disc typically is swollen, the margins blurred, and the physiological cup obscured. When papilledema is present, manipulative therapy may be contraindicated and an emergency neurological referral required. The visual fields can be tested by gradually bringing an object, such as a pencil, within the field of vision.
3. Occulomotor, Trochlear, and Abducen Nerves (III, IV, VI). The occulomotor, trochlear, and abducens nerves are checked by asking the patient to follow an object or light with his or her eyes vertically, horizontally, and obliquely to the extremes of movement.

The following short-hand formula identifies the nerves controlling the direction of eye movement:

$$ER_6 (SO_4)3$$

where external rotation (ER) is controlled by cranial nerve VI, superior oblique (SO) movement by cranial nerve IV, and all other eye movements by cranial nerve III. Cranial nerve III is also tested by looking for pupillary constriction when light is shined in the eye.

4. Trigeminal Nerve (V). A blink reflex or corneal stimulation is elicited by touching the cornea from the side with a strand of cotton while the patient is looking upward. The examiner should then stroke the patient's face in the ophthalmic, maxillary, and mandibular distributions of the trigeminal nerve, testing for disturbances of sensation. Motor function of the trigeminal nerve is tested by palpating the contracted masseter and temporalis muscles with the jaws clenched.

5. Facial Nerve (VIII). Control of facial muscles is checked by asking the patient to smile and frown while the examiner observes the patient's face for symmetrical movements.

6. Cochlear Nerve (VIII). The examiner can compare the acuity of hearing in each ear with a ticking watch. Then, the examiner places a vibrating tuning fork on the vertex of the patient's head and asks the patient if he or she senses the vibration equally in both ears. When unilateral hearing loss is due to middle ear disease, the patient reports louder vibration on the diseased side. When there is nerve deafness on one side, the sound will be louder in the normal ear (Weber's test). Next, the examiner should check bone conduction in both ears by using a vibrating tuning fork placed on the mastoid until the patient can no longer detect the vibration. The vibrating tuning fork is then held in front of the ear, in this way testing air conduction. In a normal subject, the patient should be able to detect vibration by air conduction after bone conduction ceases.

7. Glossopharyngeal Nerve (IX). This nerve is tested by the identification of taste over the posterior one-third of the tongue and by the presence of a gag reflex on stimulation of the tonsillar pillars.

8. Vagus Nerve (X). Hoarseness and loss of strength during coughing suggests paralytic involvement of the vagus nerve. The examiner should touch the posterior pharyngeal wall with a tongue depressor to elicit a gag reflex. The examiner should then palpate the larynx for muscle strength of deglutition.

9. Spinal Accessory Nerve (XI). The patient is asked to turn his or her head and shrug his or her shoulders to test the strength of the sternocleidomastoid and trapezius muscles.

10. Hypoglossal Nerve (XII). The patient is asked to stick out his or her tongue. The tongue should be in the midline. If it deviates laterally, the test is positive.

Cardiovascular System. The heart is assessed chiefly by examination through the anterior chest wall by means of inspection, palpation, percussion, and auscultation. The palmar surface of the hand at the base of the fingers is sensitive to vibrations and may detect thrills associated with murmurs.

Percussion is used in evaluating the size of the heart. The first heart sound (S1) and the second heart sound (S2) are identified by listening at the following locations:

1. Aortic area (second right interspace close to the sternum)
2. Pulmonic area (second left interspace close to the sternum)
3. Third interspace close to the sternum where murmurs of both aortic and pulmonic origin may often be heard
4. Tricuspid area (fifth left interspace close to the sternum)
5. Mitral area (fifth left interspace just medial to the midclavical line)

The carotid arteries are examined one at a time by placing the index or middle finger around the medial edge of the sternocleidomastoid muscle. Decreased or absent carotid pulse suggests arterial narrowing or occlusion. Auscultation of the carotid should be performed. Upper cervical manipulation may be contraindicated in the presence of carotid insufficiency.

Respiratory System. The respiratory tract is assessed by examination through the anterior and posterior chest wall by means of inspection, palpation, percussion, and auscultation.

Examination of the posterior thorax and lungs is made with the patient seated. Palpating the chest is useful in identifying areas of tenderness, assessing observed abnormalities such as masses, assessing respiratory excursion from inspiration to expiration, and evaluating vocal or tactile fremitus. Auscultating the lungs is useful in assessing the amount of airflow through the trachial bronchial tree and in evaluating the presence of fluid or a friction rub in the pleura.

Examination of the anterior thorax is made with

the patient supine. The examiner assesses the quality of air flowing through the bronchial tree and lungs for the presence of crepitus, mucus, or fluid. This should be done in a systematic manner covering each lobe of both lungs.

While examining the anterior thorax, a breast examination of the female patient may be performed, noting size, symmetry, and contour with special reference to masses, dimpling, or flattening. With the arms extended over the head, the examiner palpates the axillary lymph nodes. Lymphadenopathy may result from infection or other diseases of the breast or neck. Enlargement of the lymph nodes may also come from habitual use of certain deodorants.

Gastrointestinal System. The abdomen is examined with the patient supine. Inspection of the skin is carried out to determine the presence of scars, dilated veins, the contour and symmetry of the abdomen, and the contour and location of the umbilicus. The abdomen is palpated for any masses of focal tenderness. The abdomen should be examined with superficial and deep palpation. Percussion is useful for general orientation of the abdomen, for measurement of the liver and sometimes of the spleen, and for identification of air in the stomach and bowel. The examiner should auscultate all four quadrants of the abdomen, noting the frequency and character of the sounds of peristaltic movement. A friction rub may be audible with enlargement of the liver or spleen. The examiner can identify the aortic pulsation by deep palpation slightly to the left of the midline. A prominent pulsation with lateral expansion suggests an aortic aneurysm, contraindicating heavy dorsal spinal manipulative therapy, which increases intra-abdominal pressure.

Genitourinary System. With the patient supine, each kidney is examined by deep bimanual palpation. With the patient prone, Murphy's percussion test is made by placing the palm of the hand over the costovertebral angle. The examiner strikes the posterior surface of the hand with the opposite hand. Normally the patient should receive a painless jar or thud; pain suggests kidney infection. A genitourinary examination may include a pelvic examination in women, especially in patients who complain of menstrual cycle-related low back pain. The external genitalia are examined, followed by a bimanual examination, noting the size, shape, consistency, mobility, and tenderness of the uterus, fallopian tubes, and ovaries. In men, examination of the penis and palpation of the testes and scrotum is performed, noting any abnormalities. Both sexes are examined for inguinal and femoral hernia.

No examination of the genitourinary tract is complete without a urinalysis. Because viscerogenic reflexes can cause spinal pain, the chiropractic examiner uses the urinalysis to eliminate urinary tract infection as a cause of referred back pain.

A physical examination may require a rectal examination to be complete. Although the rectum is technically a part of the gastrointestinal system, the rectal examination is more easily performed during examination of the genitourinary system. In men, palpate the prostate to determine size, tenderness, and the presence of nodules.

Principles of Neuromusculoskeletal Evaluation

After a careful case history and appropriate general physical examination, if it has been determined that the etiology of the patient's complaint is of a neuromusculoskeletal origin, the examiner must undertake neuromusculoskeletal evaluation. The majority of neuromusculoskeletal conditions possess static and kinetic components. The chiropractic examiner will need to actively employ his or her knowledge of anatomy, physiology, biomechanics, and kinesiology of the spinal column and extremities before an adequate determination of normal and abnormal function can be made. The purpose of functional testing is to determine objectively the positions or movements that exacerbate the patient's symptomatology. This information will, in most instances, provide the examiner with an understanding of the mechanism of pain production and the specific tissue types involved. When the dysfunction is determined, treatment is directed to return the affected tissues to as near normal a physiological state as possible.

Neurological Examination

Overview. Of all the neuromusculoskeletal conditions treated by doctors of chiropractic, spine and spine-related disorders are the most predominant (ACA, 1989). Many patients with common spinal disorders may present with neurological manifestations in the extremities such as pain, paresthesias, disesthesias, as well as loss of sensation, muscle strength, and/or reflexes. When patients present with evidence of potential neurological deficit, the examiner must first identify the deficit and then identify its etiology.

Nerve compression syndromes often produce symptoms and signs in the extremities according to a specific neurological level. The level can usually be identified clinically because each has its own characteristic pattern of denervation. The levels of the spinal cord with the greatest clinical significance are the

C-5 to T-1 segments innervating the upper extremities and the T-12 to S-4 segments innervating the lower extremities (Leek, et al., 1986). Denervation in the extremities will cause alteration of motor power, sensation, or reflex. Evaluation of the integrity of the neurological levels depends on a knowledge of the dermatomes (areas of sensation on the skin supplied by a single spinal segment), myotomes (groups of muscles innervated by a single spinal segment), and reflexes. Once the neurological level is identified, the astute examiner can often use this information to locate the specific sight of a spinal lesion.

Muscle Testing.   Motor power is evaluated by testing major muscle groups. Muscle testing should be performed against gravity, and when possible, against resistance (Daniels, 1986). Factors to be considered in motor power evaluation are: (1) early muscle fatigue with repetitive muscle contractions, and (2) the ability of the muscles to move a normal joint through its complete range of motion. Muscles in one extremity should always be compared with their counterparts in the opposite limb. If minimal weakness is suspected, repetitive tests of the same muscle group or increased resistance may be necessary to elicit fatigue. Table 18–1 lists a recommended method for grading muscle strength. Grip strength may be tested and graded with a dynamometer, such as the Jaymar or its equivalent (Fig. 18–1). Normally, muscle testing should be repeated on a regular basis to determine whether the level of the lesion has changed and created either further muscular paralysis or improvement.

Circumferential measurements of the major muscle groups of the extremities is often used as part of motor power evaluation. At times, prime movers of a joint may be weak and atrophied, whereas the accessory muscles may be sufficiently strong to fully resist movement of a specific joint, confusing the examiner (Merciew, 1980). Measurement of muscle mass may help identify an area of denervation.

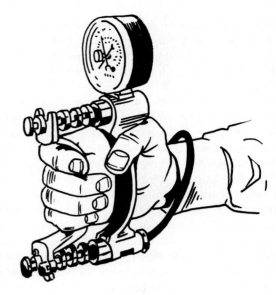

Figure 18–1. Jaymar dynamometer.

Sensory Examination.   The sensory examination is performed by drawing a sharp, sterile instrument along the dermatomal patterns of the upper and lower extremities. Any area of sensory disturbances should be noted. The somatic sensory examination is the most subjective part of the neurological examination because the examiner must rely on findings from the patient's verbal description of sensation. Consistent findings from several sensory examinations gives some assurance of their validity (Lonstein and Hockschuler, 1989). Use of a vibrating tuning fork over bony prominences tests the integrity of the posterior columns of the cord. Diminished vibratory sense is found in posterior column diseases, peripheral neuropathies, and lesions of the midbrain and cerebrum.

Deep Tendon Reflexes.   Deep tendon reflexes (DTR) are obtained by tapping on a muscle tendon and observing the contraction of the muscle. The

TABLE 18–1. GRADING MUSCLE STRENGTH

Muscle Grade	Percent	Description
5: Normal	100	Complete range of motion against gravity with full resistance
4: Good	75	Complete range of motion against gravity with some resistance
3: Fair	50	Complete range of motion against gravity only
2: Poor	25	Complete range on motion with gravity eliminated (a horizontal movement)
1: Trace	10	Evidence of slight contractility; no joint motion
0: Zero	0	No evidence of contractility

A plus (+) or (−) may be used with muscle grades depending on the examiner's judgment of the degree of strength in each grade range. (From Post 1987; Guides to the Evaluation of Permanent Impairment, 2nd ed., AMA 1985; Daniels 1986.)

presence or absence of the reflex enables the examiner to localize peripheral and central neuronal levels. A loss of reflex is associated with interruption of the basic reflex arc; pressure on the nerve root itself may decrease its intensity (hyporeflexia), whereas exaggeration of the deep tendon reflex (hyperreflexia) may be due to lesions involving the pyramidal tract (upper motor neuron lesion), as well as to diseases of the cord, brainstem and cerebral hemispheres. Table 18–2 lists a system of categories used to estimate the degree of reflex muscular contraction.

Common deep tendon reflexes include the biceps reflex (C5-6), triceps reflex (C-7), branchioradialis reflex (C-6), patellar reflex (L-4), and ankle/achilles (S1-2) reflex (Hoppenfield, 1977). Testing should be performed with the patient as relaxed as possible and with the tendon of the tested muscle slightly stretched. Using a reflex hammer, the examiner abruptly and gently taps the tendon. Reflexes are tested bilaterally for comparison. Bilaterally diminished reflexes in the absence of other associated clinical findings are generally insignificant. If a zero reflex is then elicited by reinforcement, the arc is intact although possibly inhibited and may be recorded as 1+. Patient anxiety or an attempt to "help the examiner along" will often produce false grading.

If hyperreflexia with clonus is identified and an upper motor neuron lesion suspected, there are pathologic reflexes that may be utilized to help confirm the suspicion. Babinski's sign, however, is most widely utilized. Scraping the plantar surface of the foot, from the heel and lateral border to the ball of the great toe, normally produces plantar flexion of the toes. When the test elicits dorsi flexion of the great toe with flexion and fanning of the outer toes, the test is positive.

Musculoskeletal Spinal Examination

The adept examiner should be able to determine the specific nature of the patient's musculoskeletal complaint. General structural examination should in-

clude evaluation of posture and gait. Finally the examiner should employ the following procedures localize and assess the nature of chief complaint.

1. Inspection and observation
2. Palpation: soft tissue and hard tissue
3. Range of motion: active and passive
4. Neurological examination: motor power, sensation, reflexes
5. Provocative testing
6. Examination of related areas

Posture Examination

Under ideal conditions, the standing adult exhibits balanced physiological spinal curvature in the lateral plane (Fig 18–2A). The normal spine take-off from a horizontally level pelvis is at a right angle (90 degrees) and ascends in a straight line in the frontal plane (Fig 18–2B). Deviations from normal can cause discomfort and disability. Some common causes of faulty posture are (Cailliet, 1968):

1. Hereditary postures, such as dorsal kyphosis and sway back, as well as postures affected by ligamentous laxity, muscle tone and psychological motor drive
2. Skeletal, muscular, or neurological structural abnormalities, either congenital or acquired, static, or progressive
3. Posture of habit and training

The saying "we stand and we move as we feel" is applicable in the last category. A posture of fatigue (round shoulders, drooped head, sway back, and dull facial expression) is often observable in patients who experience depression and low self-esteem. This posture often causes chronic ligamentous strain because muscular efforts are too feeble to relieve the strain effectively.

In the static, erect position (posture) the body is primarily supported by the ligamentous structures. The relaxed, erect person "leans" on specific ligaments for upright support, including the anterior longitudinal ligament, iliopectineal ligament, and posterior popliteal ligaments with the tensor fascia lata preventing lateral body shift (Cailliet, 1968; White and Panjabi, 1978). Chronic ligament strain is relieved by intermittent small muscular contractions triggered by proprioceptive reflexes of the joints and ligaments. Chronic ligamentous strain can be easily induced with improper posture, prolonged stress positions, or muscle fatigue resulting in pain or discomfort.

In addition to the common causes of faulty posture stated above, the sacral/pelvic angle in the lateral plane and the level pelvis in the frontal plane appear to play a major role in the posture of the entire

TABLE 18–2. DEGREE OF REFLEX MUSCULAR CONTRACTION

Grade	Description
5+	Hyperreflexia with sustained clonus
4+	Hyperreflexia with transient clonus
3+	Hyperreflexia, a brisk response
2+	Normal, normal–sluggish, or normal–brisk response
1+	Hyporeflexia
0	No response, no reflex

[Extrapolated from Van Allen, 1981, p. 55, with permission.]

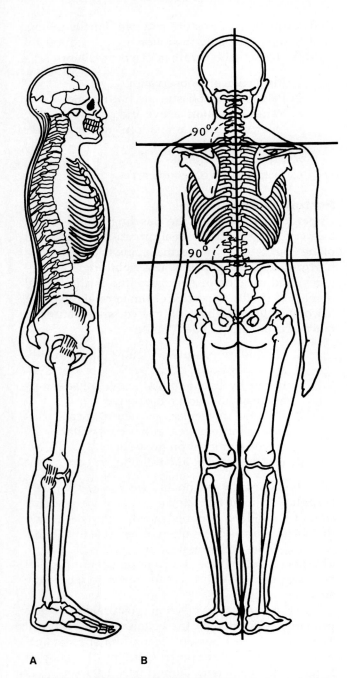

90°

90°

A   B

Figure 18–2. A. Normal lateral spinal curves in the upright individual. **B.** Normal anteroposterior spinal alignment in the upright individual. With a level pelvis and symmetrical bony and soft tissue structures, the spine take-off from the pelvis is at a 90-degree angle, and ascends in a straight line.

spinal column. These two factors determine the angle of lumbar take-off from the sacrum and influence the degree of anterior to posterior and lateral lumbar curvature, which in turn influences the degree of the super incumbent thoracic and cervical curves.

Certain anatomic factors may affect posture, including:

1. Bony contours (e.g., hemivertebra)
2. Laxity of ligamentous structures
3. Fascial and musculotendinous tightness and contracture (e.g., hamstrings, fascia lata, pectoralis, shoulder elevators and depressors, hip flexors)
4. Muscle tonus (e.g., gluteus maximus, abdominals, erector spinae, psoas)
5. Pelvic angle (normal is 30 degrees)
6. Joint position, mobility, and integrity (facets, hip joints, knee, and angle joints)
7. Neurogenic outflow and inflow

Each of the preceding factors may have an effect on the static spine as well as adversely affecting the kinetic spine. These factors may be further enhanced when combined with pathological, traumatic, or congenital states. Common spinal deformities that may result from one or more of the above stated factors are: (Cailliet, 1977, *Scoliosis*)

1. Lordosis: an excessive anterior curvature of the spine
2. Kyphosis: an excessive posterior curvature of the spine
3. Scoliosis: a lateral curvature of the spine

Although posture is thought to reflect primarily the integrity of the structural system of the erect, upright spine, postures in the sitting and recumbent positions may also adversely affect spinal structural integrity and ultimately result in pain or discomfort. When indicated, therefore, evaluation of posture may be carried out with the patient in the standing, sitting, lying (supine and prone), and forward bending positions. Because habitual postures assumed by the patient may increase or alter the patient's symptoms, the patient should be examined in the habitual, relaxed posture that he or she usually adopts.

Standing Posture. A simple tool to aide the clinician in evaluating posture is a double string plumb line. A "T" board is placed on the floor to separate the feet by approximately 3 inches so that the knees do not touch each other. The center of the plumb line should bisect the skull and be superimposed on the spine and the gluteal crease in viewing a normal subject from the rear (Fig. 18–3). The examiner should observe the following:

1. Head tilt. Determine whether the head is in the midline or tilted to one side and/or rotated.
2. Fascial asymmetry
3. Posterior neck line. The muscle bulk of the

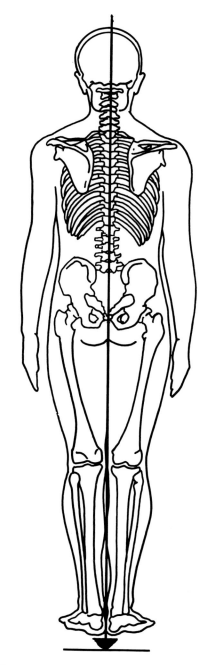

Figure 18–3. Anterorposterior plane plumb line in the normal erect spine. The plumb line falls through the center of the occiput, spine, sacrum, and symphysis pubis, bisecting the space between the legs.

trapezius should be equal and the slope of the muscles should be nearly equal. There is usually a greater slope on the dominant side.

4. Shoulder height. Although the dominant side is generally slightly lower, any discrepancy should be minimal.
5. Clavicles and acromioclavicular joints. Devi-

ations may be due to subluxations, scoliosis, fractures, or dislocations.

6. Cervical and thoracic deviation from the center plumb line
7. Any alteration of the sternum, ribs, or costocartilage
8. Waist angles and distance of the arms from the waist. Discrepancy usually seen in scoliosis
9. Pelvic height. Pelvic obliquity may be due to short leg or muscle spasm.
10. Lumbar spine alignment. (See lumbar spine evaluation for more detail.)
11. Knee position and angulation. (See evaluation of the knee for more detail.)
12. Ankle and foot. Observe the alignment of the medial and lateral malleoli of the ankles and note any pesplanus (flat foot), pescavus (high arch), or other deformity.

Viewed laterally, the spinal curves are eccentrically loaded and balanced one over the other. The plumb line should pass through the mastoid, midway between the back and abdomen, the greater trochanter, and the lateral malleolus (Fig. 18–4). The chiropractic examiner should evaluate the patient from both sides and observe the following:

1. Head position over the body. Off-centering may be due to a specific cervical disorder, such as osteoarthritis, or due to compensation from lower spinal disorders.
2. Cervical, thoracic and lumbar spines. Observe for alterations of the normal lateral spinal curves.
3. Shoulder alignment. Rounded shoulders anterior to the gravity line may be due to excessive thoracic kyphosis or hypertonic anterior shoulder girdle muscles.
4. Tone of the chest, abdominal, and back muscles. Muscle weakness may be a cause of altered spinal posture.
5. Pelvic angle. An increased pelvic angle generally increases the lumbar lordosis and may be implicated in patients with low back pain.
6. Knees. Genu recurvatum may alter pelvic alignment. A fixed knee in flexion may imply a local lesion.

Sitting Posture. With the patient seated on a stool and the patient's back unsupported with his or her feet on the ground, observation is carried out as in the standing position. Any deviations from the standing to the seated position in the frontal, lateral, or posterior views should be noted. In particular, any increase or decrease in the spinal curves should be observed and recorded.

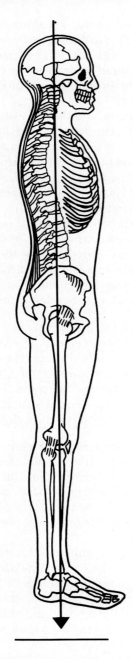

Figure 18–4. Lateral plumb line in the normal erect spine. The plumb line falls through the mastoid process, greater trochanter of the femur, and slightly anterior to the lateral malleolus.

Supine Posture. With the patient supine, the examiner observes head, body, and extremity alignment. It is also important to note any change of contour of the chest and abdomen. Measurement of actual leg length should be performed. It has been common clinical practice to measure from the Anterior Superior Iliac Spine (ASIS) to the medial malleolus on the same side. If true leg length is demonstrated and pelvic obliquity observed in the erect

position, boards of specific thicknesses of 5, 7, 9, 11 mm, etc., should be placed underneath the foot of the short leg until pelvic and lumbar leveling is observed (Cox, 1985). This may aide the examiner in determining appropriate heel or foot lift height if clinically indicated.

Prone Posture. The examiner should evaluate the alignment of the head, trunk, pelvis, and extremities for symmetry. He or she should evaluate the tone of the erector spinae, gluteal, posterior thigh, and calf musculature.

Forward Bending. Observing forward bending is essential to complete the postural evaluation. Forward bending is not solely a function of the lumbar spine, but is a smooth rhythmic movement including lumbar flexion (60 to 65 degrees) and pelvic rotation (20 to 25 degrees). The lumbar curve reversal must be accompanied by a proportionate degree of pelvic rotation, and the reverse must occur upon returning to an erect position (White and Panjabi, 1978). Disturbance of any of the following component parts of the lumbar–pelvic mechanism may destroy proper rhythm and affect posture in any position of forward bending or backward extension (Cailliet, 1968):

1. Extensibility of the longitudinal ligaments
2. Elasticity of the articular capsule
3. Integrity of the disc
4. Elasticity of the muscles
5. Anatomically symmetrical facets. Tropism, scoliosis, or pelvic obliquity may disturb facet alignment that, in turn, may disturb the normal kinetics of the lumbar spine.
6. Adequate synovial linings of the articular surfaces
7. Adequacy of the hip joints to fully rotate in a ball-bearing manner, resilient para-articular tissues of the hip joints, and good muscular control
8. Adequate integrity of the knee and ankle joints

In assessing forward bending, the patient should be asked to bend forward at the hips, with knees straight, in an attempt to touch the fingers to the floor. While in the flexed position, in addition to observing normal lumbar pelvic rhythm, the examiner should observe:

1. The rib cage. A unilateral rib hump may be indicative of structural scoliosis (Adam's sign)
2. Kyphosis
3. Spinal musculature. Evaluate for symmetry
4. The lumbar spine. Evaluate for vertebral ro-

tation (indicative of structural scoliosis) and observe or measure the degree of lumbar spine flexion.

Accurate measurement of lumbar flexion vs. pelvic rotation in forward bending may be desired. Through visualization, the astute examiner can generally describe the coordination and extent of movement observed. The findings should then be recorded, along with the possible mechanical effects causing abnormal movement. For example, ''hyper-lumbar flexion with hypo-pelvic rotation due to tight hamstrings.'' For precise measurement of lumbar flexion vs. pelvic rotation, an inclinometer can be used. This device is currently being advocated for use in impairment rating as described in the *AMA Guides to Permanent Impairment*, 3rd ed. Reference to this text is recommended for information on proper use and application of the inclinometer (Fig. 18–5).

In addition to the above, the examiner may observe and note any abnormal bony or soft tissue contours such as bowing of bones, lumps, or bumps. Although a complete postural evaluation appears extensive, the astute, skilled examiner can usually ''scan'' a patient for abnormalities in posture and record appropriate findings in a very brief period of time. Musculoskeletal spinal evaluation is not complete, however, without evaluation of the patient's gait.

Gait Assessment

The doctor of chiropractic is concerned not only with normal static structure, but kinetic function of the neuromusculoskeletal system. The functions of gait include forward progression, body balance, and support of the body in an upright position during movement. The maintenance of these functions is essential to normal and efficient daily living. Pathology that may affect the lumbar spine and/or lower extremities often manifests itself in abnormalities of gait; therefore, proper evaluation and interpretation

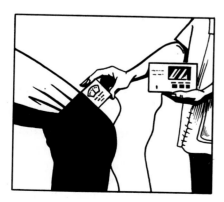

Figure 18–5. Inclinometer, a digital electronic goniometer.

of normal and abnormal gait patterns will enable the examiner to recognize functional and pathological states and effect appropriate treatment.

Normal locomotion patterns tend to be variable and irregular until the age of 7. There are two phases to the normal walking cycle. The stance phase of gait is the interval when the foot is firmly on the ground and prepared to support the upper body weight. This phase includes initial contact (heel strike), load response (foot flat), midstance (single leg stance), terminal stance (heel off), and preswing (toe off). The swing phase of gait is the interval when the leg is moving forward and not bearing weight. This phase includes the initial swing (acceleration), mid-swing and terminal swing (deceleration), and preparation for heel strike in the stance phase (Fig. 18–6). Sixty percent of the normal cycle is spent in the stance phase (25% in double stance with both feet on the ground) and 40% in the swing phase (Hoppenfeld, 1976; Magee, 1987).

Abnormalities in gait can result from central or peripheral neurological dysfunction, neuromuscular pathology, vascular disease, as well as from acquired, developmental, or functional abnormalities of the lumbar spine, hips, knees, ankles, and feet. The following are relatively common gait abnormalities seen in chiropractic practice (Magee, 1987):

1. Antalgic gait. A self-protective method of avoiding a painful component of gait. The pain may be due to nerve root compression in the lumbar spine with painful radiculitis, vascular insufficiency, or pain resulting from injury or pathology to the hip, knee, ankle, foot, or compartments of the leg.
2. Short leg gait. A limp may result from shortening of one lower extremity.
3. Steppage or foot drop gait. The foot often slaps on the ground due to a lack of foot dorsiflexor muscle control.
4. Stiff knee or hip gait. If the hip or knee is stiff or ankylosed, the entire leg is lifted higher than normal to clear the ground.
5. Scissors gait. Due to paralysis or spasm of the hip adductor muscles. The legs are drawn together and the hips are swung forward with great effort.
6. Gluteus maximus gait or lurch. Weakness of the gluteus maximus muscles forces the patient to thrust the thorax posteriorly during the stance phase to maintain hip extension; thus the appearance of lurching forward.
7. Gluteus medius/trendelenberg gait. With a weak gluteus medius muscle, the thorax is thrusted laterally during the swing phase to keep the center of gravity over the stance leg

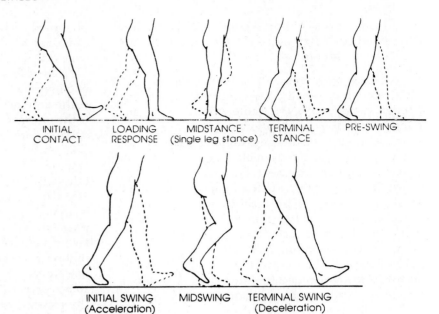

INITIAL CONTACT | LOADING RESPONSE | MIDSTANCE (Single leg stance) | TERMINAL STANCE | PRE-SWING

INITIAL SWING (Acceleration) | MIDSWING | TERMINAL SWING (Deceleration)

Figure 18-6. Phases of gait; Stance phase: initial contact, loading response, midstance, terminal stance, preswing. Swing phase: acceleration, midswing, deceleration. (*Adapted from Magee, D. Orthopedic Physical Assessments. W.B. Saunders Company, Philadelphia, 1987, p. 363–364.*)

and the swinging leg will be thrust laterally and forward through hip and body movement.

8. Ataxic gait. Produces a lurch or stagger with a broad base; all movements exaggerated due to poor sensation or loss of muscle coordination.
9. Parkinsonian gait. Shuffling gait characterized by short, rapid steps. The patient may appear to be leaning forward and walking as though he or she were unable to stop.

Once the chiropractic examiner has assessed the patient's general posture and gait, his or her attention should now be directed to the area of clinical interest, the primary complaint or complaints. Many lesions and disorders of the spine manifest themselves as pain, paresthesia, or functional loss in the extremities. It is imperative that the chiropractic examiner differentiate local extremity lesions from vertebrogenic causes of extremity pain and malfunction. An astute understanding of local extremity lesions is necessary to accurately make this differentiation.

Clinical Evaluation of the Spine and Extremities

Cervical Spine Evaluation

Pain related to the neck, upper thoracic region, and upper extremities may be localized or referred. Unless the examiner is absolutely certain of the location of the lesion, an assessment of all three regions should be carried out (Cyriax, 1978).

Inspection and Observation. If an adequate postural evaluation has been made, this assessment would already have been performed and findings recorded. Briefly, the examiner should note:

1. Head and neck posture. Note evidence of torticollis or scoliosis
2. Should height
3. Muscle spasm or asymmetry
4. Facial expression. The patient's expression should be observed during the entire course of the examination. Different positions causing pain or apprehension may be observed from facial expression.
5. Bony and soft tissue contours
6. Evidence of ischemia in the upper extremity
7. Normal sitting posture. (Described under postural evaluation)

Palpation—Static and Kinetic. In the static position, the bony and soft tissue structures of the posterior, lateral, and anterior aspects of the neck are palpated. The examiner should note the texture of the skin and any tenderness, muscle spasm, unusual nodules, bony prominences, or other signs and symptoms that may indicate the source of pathology. Palpation of the neck is usually best carried out with the patient supine for maximum relaxation of the neck muscles.

Kinetic palpation should always be carried out unless contraindications to movement exist. In case of severe neck trauma or if the patient complains of severe pain, vertigo, or visual disturbances with neck movement, motion palpation should be postponed until further testing confirms the pathology and the patient can tolerate the movement. When permitted, motion palpation will provide the astute, skilled chiropractic examiner with valuable information regarding the functional integrity of the neck. Motion palpation is described in detail in Chapter 19, Manual Examination of the Spine.

Active Range of Motion.
When permitting the patient to carry out active flexion, extension, lateral bending, and rotation of the neck, the examiner should observe differences in range of motion and the patient's willingness to perform the movement. The order of movements should be from least painful to most painful so there will be no residual pain carry over from the previous movement. If limited movement exists, the examiner should determine whether the cause is from pain, spasm, stiffness, or blocking.

It is possible to differentiate between movement, or the lack of it, in the upper and lower cervical spine. During normal flexion, nodding occurs in the upper cervical region and flexion in the lower cervical region. Flexion without nodding indicates restriction in the upper cervical region. Nodding without flexion indicates restriction in the lower cervical region. The following are the general ranges of active cervical motion. *Note:* These ranges represent a wide variation. The ''normal'' range for a specific patient may depend on their body type, age, or internal joint architecture.

1. Flexion: approximately 45 degrees (the patient should be able to touch his or her chin to the chest)
2. Extension: 30 to 40 degrees (the patient should be able to look at the ceiling)
3. Lateral flexion: 30 to 45 degrees per side
4. Rotation: 60 to 90 degrees per side (most patients can rotate the head so that the chin is almost parallel to the shoulder)

Passive Range of Motion.
Testing passive motion should be performed with the patient in the supine position for the greatest relaxation of the neck musculature. The examiner passively moves the neck in flexion, extension, lateral flexion, rotation, and exerts traction force in an anterior, axial, and lateral plane to determine the end feel of each movement.

Performance of passive and active range of motion testing and an understanding of functional anatomy will aide the examiner in differentiating the nature of the lesion. Pain on active movement only may indicate muscle injury (strain). Pain on passive movement only may indicate ligament or joint injury (sprain). Pain and/or restriction with active and passive motion may indicate severe trauma to muscles,

ligaments, and joints, or may be associated with arthritis.

Neurological Examination.
As stated previously in this chapter, many disorders of the cervical spine may manifest themselves in the upper extremities as pain, altered sensation, muscle weakness, and reflex loss. In clinical chiropractic practice, it is common to see patients with arm pain, paresthesia, and weakness with vague or no neck pain at all. These are common characteristics seen in herniated cervical disc lesions or cervical spondylosis. Table 18–3 illustrates common clinical findings in cervical radiculopathy and may aid in identifying the source of the lesion through careful evaluation of neurological signs. When neurological signs are suspected but questionable, electroneuromyography (EMNG) may be useful in identifying the first signs of neurological deficit.

In addition to testing motor power of the upper extremities, muscles supporting the cervical spine may be evaluated for pain or weakness against resistance. Muscles should be tested by the following isometric movements:

1. Neck flexion (often painful and weak after hyperflexion/hyperextension injuries)
2. Neck extension
3. Neck side flexion
4. Neck rotation
5. Shoulder evaluation (C-4 and spinal accessory)

Sensory evaluation of the upper extremities should be performed with a sharp instrument along specific dermatome distributions bilaterally. Hypersensitivity is generally indicative of trauma to the skin or underlying muscles or due to fibromyositis. Decreased sensation over a specific dermatome is generally indicative of nerve root compression or peripheral nerve palsy.

Functional Testing.
All functional maneuvers are designed to reproduce the patient's pain or symptoms by reproducing the abnormal position or movement that causes the pain or symptom. It should be noted that positive findings on certain tests may contraindicate the continued performance of other maneuvers. For example, if the examiner discovers possible occlusion of the carotid or femoral arteries, it would be prudent to avoid other maneuvers that may further constrict the arteries. The following tests may be performed if the examiner feels they are clinically relevant.

DIZZINESS TEST. The patient actively rotates his or her head as far right and left as possible (Fig. 18–7A). After returning the head to midline, the patient then

TABLE 18–3. CERVICAL NERVE ROOT SYNDROMES

Roots	Disc Level	Pain Distribution	Sensory Dysfunction	Reflex Change	Motor Dysfunction
C-5	C4-5	Neck, tip of shoulder, anterior shoulder and upper arm	Deltoid area, lateral arm	Decreased biceps reflex	Spinati, deltoid, biceps and other elbow flexors
C-6	C5-6	Neck, shoulder, medial scapular border, lateral arm, dorsum of forearm, thumb and index finger	Lateral forearm, thumb, and index finger	Decreased biceps and bracioradialis reflex	Elbow flexion, wrist extension
C-7	C6-7	Neck, shoulder, medial scapular border, lateral arm, index and middle finger	Mid forearm, dorsum of hand, and middle finger	Decreased triceps and pectoralis reflex	Pectoralis elbow extension, wrist flexion, finger extension
C-8	C7-T1 uncommon	Neck, medial scapular border, ulnar side of arm and forearm, ring and little finger	Ulnar side of forearm, ring and little fingers	None or decreased finger flexors	Finger flexors and hand intrinsics
T-1	T1-T2 uncommon	Axilla and medial arm	Medial upper arm	None	Hand intrinsics

Data from Batzdorf, 1988; Hoppenfield, 1977; Post, 1987.

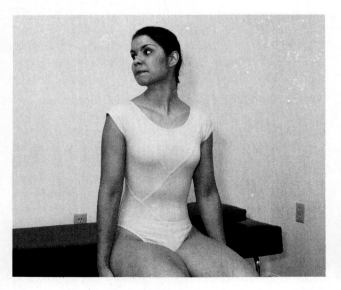
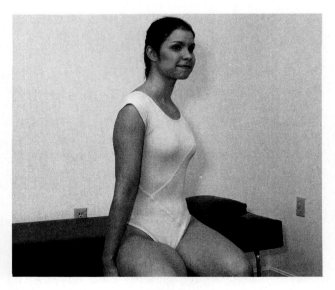

A   **B**

Figure 18–7. A. Dizziness test, part I. **B.** Dizziness test, part II.

rotates his or her shoulders as far right and left as possible while keeping the eyes straight ahead (Fig. 18–7B) (Magee, 1987). Vertigo, dizziness, visual blurring, nausea, faintness, or nystagmus experienced during both maneuvers may indicate vertebralbasilar or carotid artery stenosis or compression. If these symptoms are experienced only when the head is rotated, the problem may lie within the semicircular canals of the inner ear or may be vertebrogenic from stimulation of the cervical spine mechanoreceptors (Ameis, 1986).

PERCUSSION TEST. With the patient seated and head slightly flexed, the examiner percusses the spinous processes, interspinous spaces, and associated musculature of each cervical vertebra with a reflex hammer (Fig. 18–8). When percussion produces acute pain that immediately subsides, it is likely due to traumatic joint pathology. Pain over the musculature is indicative of local muscle injury. Dull pain that slowly disappears suggests fracture, neoplasm, or other bone disease. Pain over the interspinous spaces with radiation in the upper extremities may indicate disc lesion.

CERVICAL COMPRESSION TESTS. With the patient's head facing straight ahead, the examiner exerts a careful downward pressure on the patient's head (Fig. 18–9). Pain in the posterior neck region only indicates injury to the muscles, ligaments, or joints. Radicular pain to one side may indicate a disc lesion (Cipriano, 1985).

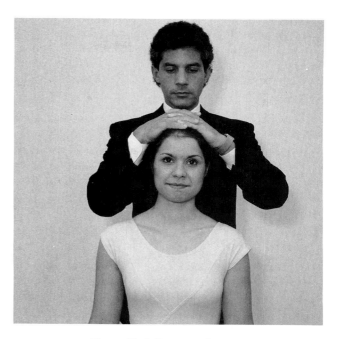

Figure 18–9. Compression test.

FORAMINAL COMPRESSION TEST. The patient laterally flexes the head to one side while the examiner carefully presses straight down on his or her head (Fig. 18–10). Radicular pain or altered sensation into the arm on the side of lateral flexion, indicates nerve root compression. The exact distribution of pain or altered sensation can give some indication as to which nerve root is involved (Cipriano, 1985).

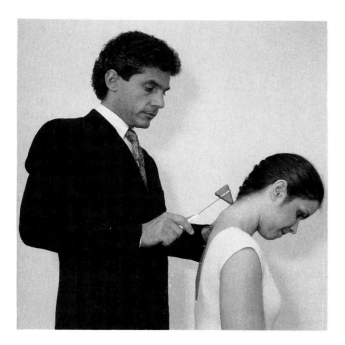

Figure 18–8. Percussion test.

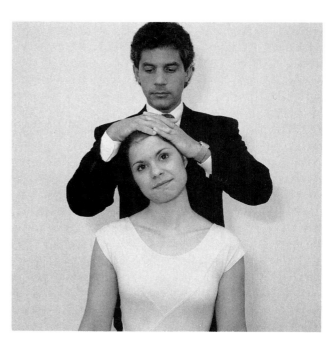

Figure 18–10. Foraminal compression test.

DISTRACTION TEST. With the patient seated, the examiner places one hand under the chin and one under the occiput and exerts upward pressure on the patient's head (Fig. 18–11). The test is positive if the pain is decreased when the head is lifted or distracted. A positive test may indicate nerve root compression or facet capsulitis.

SHOULDER DEPRESSION TEST. With the patient's head slightly flexed to one side, the examiner applies downward pressure on the opposite shoulder (Fig. 18–12). Pain on the side being tested indicates irritation or compression of the neurovascular bundle, foraminal encroachment due to osteophytes, adhesions around the dural sleeve of the nerve and adjacent joint capsule, or shortening of the muscles of the side being tested (Cipriano, 1985).

VALSALVA MANEUVER. The examiner asks the patient to take a deep breath and hold it while bearing down, as if moving the bowels. Increased pain may indicate increased intrathecal pressure that may be due to a space-occupying lesion such as a herniated disc, tumor, or osteophyte (Cipriano, 1985).

SOTO–HALL SIGN. With the patient supine, the examiner applies pressure on the sternum while flexing the patient's neck to his or her chest (Fig. 18–13A). Localized neck pain may be experienced at the level of a lesion, such as a fracture of the spinous tip or vertebral body. Localized pain also may be elicited at the level of a sprain or strain. If during the performance of the Soto–Hall maneuver, the patient devel-

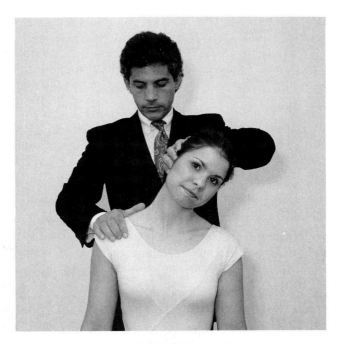

Figure 18–12. Shoulder depression test.

ops a sudden transient electric-like shock spreading down the body and into the upper and lower extremities, the patient is exhibiting a Lhermitte's sign, which is seen in multiple sclerosis, spondylosis, or cervical cord injuries. If the patient flexes both knees when the test is performed (Fig. 18–13B), suspect meningial irritation (Brudzenski's sign). If neck flexion produces low back symptoms (Lidner's sign), there may be a localized vertebrogenic lesion of the low back (Mazion, 1980).

SWALLOWING TEST. The seated patient is instructed to swallow. Pain at the anterior neck region may indicate a space-occupying lesion at the anterior portion of the cervical spine such as a disc protrusion, tumor, or osteophyte or due to a posttraumatic retropharyngeal or retrolaryngeal hematoma (Cipriano, 1985).

ARM ABDUCTION TEST. Ask the patient to fully abduct the arm on the involved side overhead. Relief or diminishing of pain indicates nerve root compression at the side tested.

Thoracic outlet syndromes may also manifest themselves as pain and paresthesia in the upper extremities. Different dynamic, static, congenital, traumatic, and arteriosclerotic factors may compress the subclavian artery and trunks of the brachialplexus as they pass from neck to the arm (Wilbourn and Porter, 1988). The following tests may aid in identifying the specific site of compression:

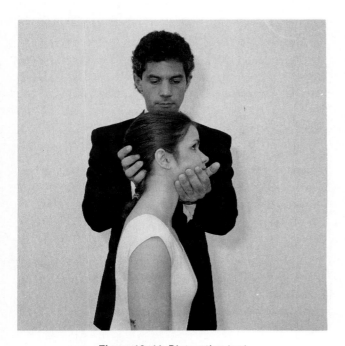

Figure 18–11. Distraction test.

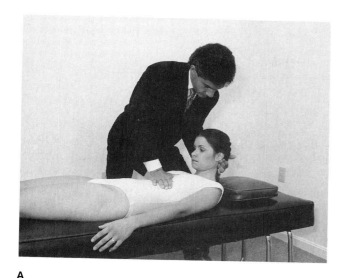

A

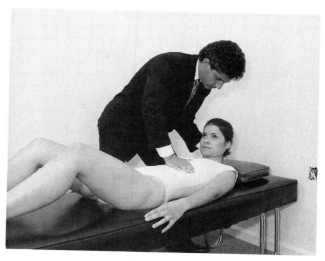

B

Figure 18–13. A. Soto–Hall test. **B.** Brudzenski's sign.

ADSON'S TEST. With the patient seated, the examiner abducts the arm to approximately 30 degrees and assesses the radial pulse. The patient is instructed to rotate his or her head and elevate the chin to the side being tested and then to the opposite side (Fig. 18–14). A decrease or absence of the radial pulse frequently indicates a compression of the vascular component of the neurovascular bundle by the scalenus anterior muscle or the presence of a cervical rib. Paresthesia or radiculopathy in the upper extremity may indicate compression of the neural component of the neurovascular bundle, usually along the ulnar distribution (C-8 to T-1 dermatome levels) (Cipriano, 1985).

COSTOCLAVICULAR TEST. The seated patient is asked to assume an exaggerated military posture, with the shoulders drawn downward and backward and the neck flexed, while the examiner assesses the radial pulses (Fig. 18–15). This maneuver decreases the

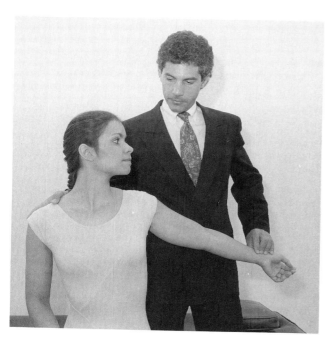

Figure 18–14. Adson's test.

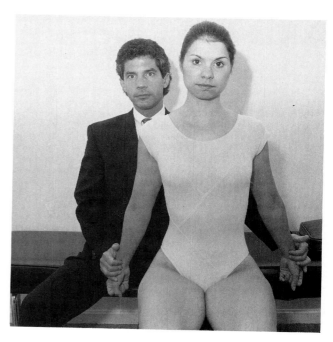

Figure 18–15. Costoclavicular test.

space between the clavicle and the first rib. A decrease or absence of the radial pulse typically indicates a compression of the subclavian artery. Paresthesia or radiculopathy in the upper extremity is indicative of compression of the lower brachial plexus (Cipriano, 1985).

HYPERABDUCTION TEST. With the patient seated, the doctor assesses the radial pulse. The examiner slowly abducts the arm to a position overhead through an arc of 180 degrees (Fig. 18–16). The components of the brachial plexus and the axillary vessels are bent around the coracoid process beneath the pectoralis minor tendon. A decrease or absence of the radial pulse and reproduction of symptoms often indicates a compression of the axillary artery and brachial plexus respectively. Sleeping with the arm overhead is the major offender in this syndrome (Lord, 1971).

If part of the patient's main complaint or complaints is in the upper extremities, the examiner may need to evaluate further the affected extremity to differentiate between a local lesion in the extremity from referred or radicular pain originating in a site more proximal.

Upper Extremities Evaluation

Pain in the region of the shoulder, elbow, wrist, and hand is commonly seen in chiropractic practice and can almost always be accurately diagnosed and effectively treated. A carefully developed history and thorough physical examination will permit an early and accurate diagnosis. Problems of the upper extremities span all ages including young athletes, middle-aged workers, and more sedentary elderly individuals. Patients experiencing upper extremity problems may present with pain, with or without re-

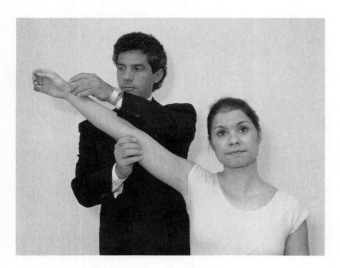

Figure 18–16. Hyperabduction test.

stricted motion. Pain or restricted motion in any of the joints may seriously impair the function of the entire upper extremity.

Shoulders. The shoulder possesses the largest range of motion of any joint in the body. Moreover, it has less stability and less mechanical protection than any other large joint in the body.

INSPECTION AND OBSERVATION. In general inspection of the shoulder, particular attention should be paid to shoulder height, contour, muscle symmetry, and bony prominences. Some observable features and associated disorders are:

1. Local swelling or edema over the shoulder (trauma, acute arthritis, acute calcific bursitis)
2. Changes in contour or color of the hands (systemic form of arthritis, reflex sympathetic dystrophy, thoracic outlet syndrome, vascular occlusion)
3. Atrophy of the deltoid muscles (chronic shoulder pain, axillary nerve paresis)

PALPATION. Bony palpation should include the sternoclavicular joint, clavicle, coracoid process, acromioclavicular articulation, acromion, greater tuberosity of the humerus, bicipital groove, spine of the scapula, and vertebral border of the scapula. Local tenderness over the acromioclavicular joint may indicate advanced degenerative arthritis or acromioclavicular joint subluxation. Swelling lateral to the coracoid process may indicate glenohumeral effusion. Local tenderness over the greater tuberosity often indicates bursitis or rotator cuff lesion. Exquisite tenderness over the bicipital groove may indicate bicipital tendonitis. Pain and tenderness over the midscapular region could result from cervical radiculopathy (usually from a disc lesion or bone spur compression), myofibrositis, or scapulothoracic syndrome.

Soft tissue palpation should include the rotator cuff, the subacromial and subdeltoid bursa, the axilla, and the prominent muscles of the shoulder girdle.

RANGE OF MOTION. The following are normal ranges of shoulder movement:

1. Abduction, 180 degrees
2. Adduction, 45 to 55 degrees
3. Flexion/forward elevation, 180 degrees
4. Extension, 60 degrees
5. Internal rotation, 90 degrees
6. External rotation, 90 degrees

Shoulder pain originating from strain or inflammation is generally more pronounced with abduction. Rotator cuff tendonitis and impingement syndromes usually cause a painful arc of abduction between 60 and 120 degrees. Degenerative or inflammatory conditions of the acromioclavicular joint often causes a high painful arc of abduction between 120 and 180 degrees. Decreased motion in all planes with pain at the extremes of permitted movement is suggestive of a frozen shoulder (Cyriax, 1978).

NEUROLOGICAL EXAMINATION. Neurological examination of the upper extremities should include muscle testing and grading, reflex testing (biceps, triceps, and branchioradialis), and sensory evaluation, if indicated.

PROVOCATIVE TESTING. The examiner should begin provocative testing of the shoulder during the range of motion examination, by applying resistance to each movement. Increased pain at the anterior shoulder region on forward elevation may indicate bicipital tendinitis. Increased pain on resisted abduction suggests supraspinatus tendinitis. Increased pain on internal rotation could be tendinitis of the subscapularis, pectoralis major, latissimus dorsi, or teres major, whereas increased pain on external rotation is suggestive of tendinitis of the infraspinatus or the teres minor.

The "Apley scratch maneuver" can be performed by asking the patient to place the affected hand behind his or her back and attempt to touch the opposite inferior angle of the scapula. Increased shoulder pain may indicate rotator cuff tendinitis, biceps tendinitis, or subacromial bursitis. The patient is then asked to place the affected hand behind his or her head and touch the opposite superior angle of the scapula. The inability to perform this maneuver due to pain may indicate subacromial bursitis or rotator cuff tendinitis. If pain or a snapping sensation is experienced by the patient when returning the hand from overhead to the neutral position, biceps instability or subluxation is suspected (Fig. 18–17).

With subacromial bursitis, there is generally exquisite pain with digital pressure over the involved bursa. With continued pressure over the bursa, the examiner may then passively abduct the arm past 90 degrees, at which point the deltoid muscle covers the bursa (Fig. 18–18). A decrease in tenderness is a positive finding, and confirms subacromial bursitis. In anterior shoulder dislocation, the patient is generally unable to touch the opposite shoulder, and bring the elbow to the chest wall (Fig. 18–19). The ability to do so usually indicates successful reduction of an anterior shoulder dislocation.

Elbow. The elbow functions, to work in concert with the shoulder to place the hand in space, as an essential linkage for the development of the stability

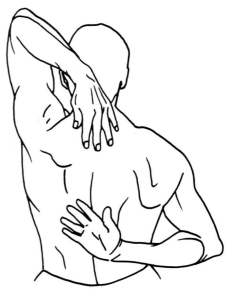

Figure 18–17. Apley scratch maneuver. The left arm is in flexion, external rotation, and abduction, and the right arm is in extension, internal rotation, and adduction. This maneuver can be used to test general range of shoulder movement.

necessary for fine work of the hand, and to supply power to perform work (Conwell, 1969).

INSPECTION AND OBSERVATION. The examiner should inspect for normal axial alignment. When the arm is extended in the anatomic position, the arm generally forms a valgus angle (away from the midline) at the

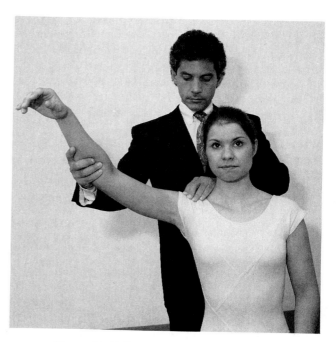

Figure 18–18. Test for subacromial bursitis.

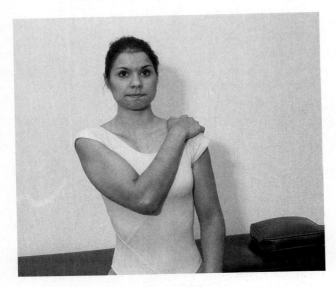

Figure 18–19. Test for anterior shoulder dislocation.

elbow. The normal angle for a man is 5 to 10 degrees and for a woman 10 to 15 degrees (Magee, 1987). Local swelling at the posterior elbow may represent an olecranon bursitis or joint capsule inflammation. Diffuse swelling usually results in the patient holding the elbow in a flexed position (usually around 45 degrees) and may be indicative of supracondylar fracture or crush injuries to the elbow.

PALPATION. Tenderness over the medial or lateral joint margins may indicate medial or lateral epicondylitis, respectively, tendon or ligament injury, or arthritis. Tenderness over the anterior joint region may indicate muscle/tendon strain or nerve or vascular compression syndromes. Pain over the posterior joint region may represent peripheral neuropathies, nerve contusions and, when associated with effusion, olecranon bursitis. Radiating pain from the elbow may be indicative of peripheral nerve compression syndromes or cervical radiculopathy.

RANGE OF MOTION. The following are normal ranges of elbow movement.

1. Flexion, 145 degrees from the zero position. The functional arc of elbow flexion is from 30 to 130 degrees.
2. Extension, 0 to 5 degrees from the zero position
3. Supination, 85 to 90 degrees
4. Pronation, 75 to 90 degrees

NEUROLOGICAL EXAMINATION. If radicular symptoms are present or weakness is suspected, the examination should include evaluation of motor power, sensation, and reflexes of the upper extremities.

FUNCTIONAL TESTING. Pain from muscle strain and tendinitis is generally provoked with active contraction against resistance and/or passive stretch of the involved muscle or tendon. Biceps or triceps tendinitis at their distal insertions is generally painful on action flexion or passive extension and active extension or passive flexion, respectively. The flexors, extensors, pronators, and supinators of the lower arm and wrist have their proximal attachment at the elbow. The wrist flexor/pronator group attach to the medial epicondyle, and the extensor group attaches to the lateral epicondyle. Pain at the lateral epicondyle on resisted wrist extension and/or radial deviation and passive wrist flexion and/or ulnar deviation may indicate lateral epicondylitis/tendinitis. Pain at the region of the medial epicondyle with resisted wrist flexion and/or elbow extension may indicate medial epicondylitis/tendinitis.

The examiner may induce abduction and adduction stress to the joint margins. With abduction stress (Fig. 18–20), increased pain at the medial side of the elbow may indicate medial collateral ligament injury, whereas pain at the lateral joint region may be indicative of radial head or neck fracture or arthritis. With adduction stress (Fig. 18–21), increased pain at the lateral joint region may indicate lateral collateral ligament injury, whereas pain at the medial joint region may indicate degenerative arthritis. If the patient exhibits radicular symptoms along the ulnar distribution of the lower arm and/or hand, the examiner may exert digital pressure and/or percuss the groove between the olecranon process and the medial epicondyle (Fig. 18–22). Hypersensitivity or reproduction of the radicular pain may indicate ulnar neuritis.

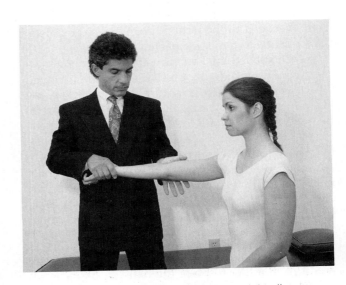

Figure 18–20. Abduction stress test, right elbow.

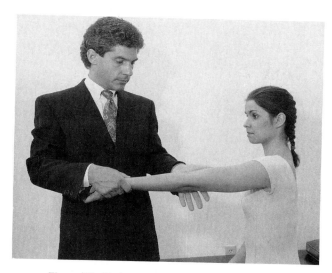

Figure 18-21. Adduction stress test, left elbow.

Wrist and Hand. ''The hand is used by man in many ways—whether for grip or precise pinch, as emphasis of an expression or as tools of communication—hands are finely tuned sensory receptors capable of supplementing or even replacing visual receptors. The vital role that hands play in the ability to function cannot be minimized'' (Leek et al., 1986). Loss of hand function may mean loss of work, play, or ability to care for oneself or family. Many conditions of the hand, if detected early, can be successfully treated by the doctor of chiropractic.

INSPECTION AND OBSERVATION. The examiner should observe the wrist and hands for engorged blood vessels, inflammation, color, fullness, swelling, skin damage, nail changes, and alterations in the palmar and dorsal surfaces. Local inflammation could be in-

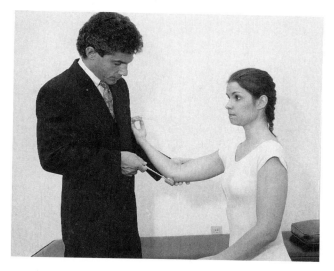

Figure 18-22. Tinel's sign for ulnar neuritis at the elbow.

dicative of trauma, acute sepsis, or arthritis (Calabro, 1986). Color changes of the hand are usually due to vascular occlusion. A lump on the dorsum of the wrist could be indicative of carpal bone dislocation or a ganglion (Conwell, 1970). Deviation of the joints of the fingers can be due to rheumatoid or osteoarthritis, ischemia, or tendon contractures.

PALPATION. Sites of tenderness over the bony and soft tissue structures should be recorded.

RANGE OF MOTION. The following are normal ranges of wrist and hand movement (Hoppenfield, 1976).

1. Wrist
   Flexion, 80 degrees
   Extension, 70 degrees
   Ulnar deviation, 30 degrees
   Radial deviation, 20 degrees
   Supination, 90 degrees
   Pronation, 90 degrees
2. Fingers
   Flexion of metacarpophalangeal (MCP), proximal interphalangeal (PIP), distal interphalangeal (DIP) joints, 90 degrees
   Extension of metacarpophalangeal joints, 30 to 45 degrees
   Extension of proximal interphalangeal and distal interphalangeal joints, 0 to 10 degrees
   Abduction and adduction, 20 degrees
3. Thumb
   Flexion of metacarpophalangeal joint, 50 degrees
   Extension of metacarpophalangeal joint, 0 degrees
   Flexion of interphalangeal (IP) joint, 90 degrees
   Extension of interphalangeal joint, 20 degrees
   Palmar abduction, 70 degrees
   Palmar adduction, 0 degrees

NEUROLOGICAL EXAMINATION. Muscle weakness in the hands may be due to cervical nerve root compression, peripheral neuropathy, median nerve compression within the carpal tunnel, muscle contracture abnormalities, and joint inflammation due to arthritis. Sensory deficit may be due to vascular insufficiency, cervical nerve root compression, peripheral neuropathy, and compression of the median nerve within the carpal tunnel (carpal tunnel syndrome). In the presence of one or more of these symptoms, a neurological examination should be carried out as previously described.

FUNCTIONAL TESTING. Compartment syndromes in the wrist are common clinical findings, compression of the median nerve within the carpal tunnel being the most common (carpal tunnel syndrome). Pain and/or paresthesia in the palmar surface of the hand, thumb, index, and middle finger is characteristic, with use and position exacerbation. The examiner may attempt to reproduce these symptoms by fully flexing (Fig. 18–23), then fully extending the wrists, holding each position for up to 60 seconds (Phalen's test). Pain and/or paresthesia radiating into the hand and fingers may indicate median nerve entrapment within the carpal tunnel. Tapping the median nerve at the location of the carpal tunnel with the finger or reflex hammer (Tinel's sign) may also reproduce the symptoms (Fig. 18–24). Occasionally the ulnar nerve may be entrapped in the palmar surface of the hand as it passes between the pisiform and the hook of the hamate (Guyon's tunnel) and produce pain and/or paresthesia in the ring and little finger. Digital pressure or tapping of the nerve within Guyon's tunnel will usually exacerbate the symptoms when nerve compression exists.

Tenosynovitis of the flexor and extensor tendons of the thumb and fingers is generally exacerbated with contraction against resistance and/or passive stretch of the involved tendon. Tenosynovitis of the abductor pollicis longus and extensor pollicis brevis tendons (de Quervain's disease) produces pain at the base of the thumb at the region of the styloid process of the radius. This can generally be provoked with active thumb abduction and extension and passive thumb adduction and flexion (Fig. 18–25).

If vascular insufficiency is suspected, the examiner can determine the patency of the radial and ulnar arteries with Allen's test. The patient is asked

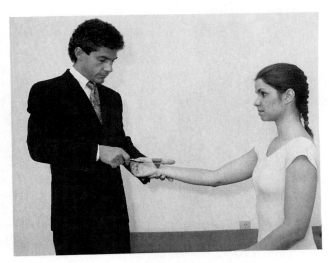

Figure 18-24. Tinel's sign for median nerve irritation due to carpal tunnel syndrome.

to open and close the hands several times and then squeeze the hand tightly in a fist. The examiner's thumbs are firmly placed over the radial and ulnar arteries. The patient then opens the hand while pressure is maintained over the arteries (Fig. 18–26A). One artery is tested by releasing the pressure over the artery to see if the hand flushes. The other artery is tested similarly (Fig. 18–26B). Upon release of arterial pressure, color should return to the tested hand, matching that of the opposite side in 10 seconds or less. Delayed color return may indicate partial block-

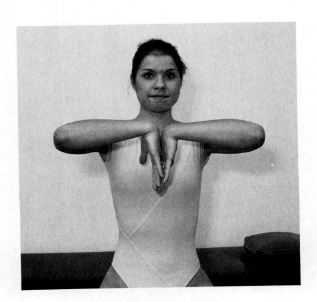

Figure 18-23. Phalen's test.

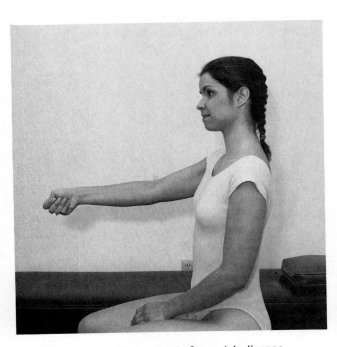

Figure 18-25. Test for de Quervain's disease.

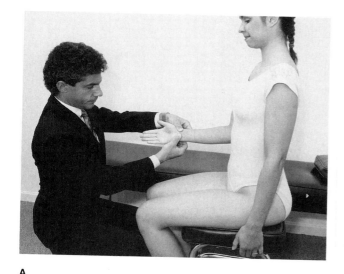

A

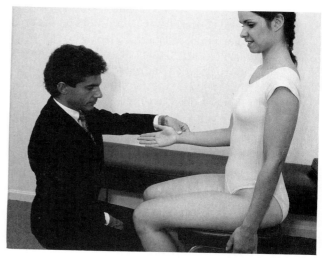

B

Figure 18–26. **A.** Allen's test, part I. **B.** Allen's test, part II.

age, whereas no color return suggests complete blockage of the respective artery.

Thoracic Spine Evaluation

The thoracic spine differs from the cervical and lumbar spines in that it is mechanically stiffer and less mobile. Motion is limited in flexion, extension, and lateral bending. However, most of the rotation possible along the vertebral column below C-2 is obtained in this region. Normally the thoracic spine exhibits a mild kyphosis (posterior curvature). The rib cage, which stiffens and strengthens the thoracic spine, provides additional strength, energy absorbing capacity, and protection to the heart and lungs. Clinically, symptoms can result from major or minor lesions of the soft and hard tissues of the thoracic spine, the ribs, and their attachments. A few common conditions seen in clinical practice are:

1. Fractures of the vertebra and/or ribs
2. Intercostal strain
3. Intercostal neuritis
4. Costotransverse joint syndrome
5. Anterior costal cartilage syndrome
6. Erector spinae strain
7. Middle and lower trapezius strain syndrome
8. Subluxation
9. Disk herniation

Inspection and Observation. When observing the thoracic spine and chest cavity one should note any alterations of overall spinal posture, such as:

1. Kyphosis
2. Dowager's hump

3. Scoliosis. (Scoliosis is classified as one or more lateral curves of the spine and may be structural/pathological/nonflexible or non-structural/functional/flexible.)
4. Chest deformities

The chiropractic examiner should also note alterations in breathing patterns.

Palpation. Depending on the symptoms, the examiner may find need to palpate the posterior, lateral, and anterior chest walls. Tenderness, muscle spasm, temperature alterations, areas of localized or defused swelling and other signs may indicate pathology. Palpation may be performed in the sitting and/or prone position. The following structures should be assessed:

1. Spinous processes and paraspinal musculature
2. Scapula
3. Ribs and costocartilage
4. Abdomen

Range of Motion. The thoracic spine permits the greatest amount of rotation of the trunk below the level of C-2. Although the remaining movements are limited due to the rib cage, slight movement does exist. The following are average ranges of thoracic spine movement (Magee, 1987).

1. Forward flexion, 20 to 45 degrees. The examiner should note any increased or decreased kyphosis. Although the patient is flexed, the examiner can observe the spine for structural or nonstructural scoliosis.

2. Extension, 25 to 45 degrees. During extension, the thoracic spine could curve slightly backward or at least straighten.
3. Lateral flexion, 20 to 40 degrees
4. Rotation, 35 to 50 degrees
5. Costovertebral expansion/chest expansion, 2 in. men; 1½ in., women

Motion palpation of the thoracic spine should be carried out for detection of segmental hypermobility, hypomobility, or fixation.

Neurological Examination. Pathology in the thoracic spine such as space-occupying lesions from disc herniation or tumor can affect the deep tendon reflexes in the lower extremities. Therefore, the patellar, hamstring, and ankle reflexes may need to be assessed. The abdominal/superficial reflexes are mediated through peripheral and sensory pathways, primarily through the corticospinal tract and based on cutaneous stimulation (Van Allen, 1981). The examiner uses an applicator stick and lightly and quickly strokes the skin in all four quadrants of the abdomen (Fig. 18-27). Normally, the umbilicus will be deflected toward the side of stimulus. An absence of the response is indicative of an upper motor neuron lesion such as an ipsilateral cord disease or contralateral cerebral disease and is common in multiple sclerosis. Absent abdominal reflexes are usually associated with hyperreflexia of the lower extremities and a present Babinski sign. The examiner may then ask the patient to raise his or her head and shoulder from the table. A positive finding (Beevor's sign) is when the umbilicus deviates from the midline in any direction (Fig. 18-28). This would indicate muscle weakness or paralysis of those in the

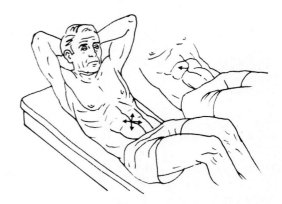

Figure 18-28. Beevor's sign.

opposing direction and could be indicative of a space-occupying lesion.

Sensory evaluation of the thoracic spine is different because there is a great deal of overlap in dermatomes. The absence of just one dermatome, therefore, may produce no noticeable loss of sensation. Specific dermatomal landmarks include nipple line (T-4), xyphoid (T-7), umbilicus (T10-11) and groin (T-12).

Although muscle testing of the thoracic spine is difficult due to limited movement, muscle testing of forward flexion, extension, lateral flexion, and rotation can be carried out to some degree in the sitting position, or against gravity.

Functional Testing. Muscle strains are generally exacerbated with active contraction and passive stretch. Therefore, during the range of motion examination, paraspinal and intercostal muscle strains can generally be assessed. The pain is usually further provoked at the site of lesion on forward bending, and contralateral side bending. The examiner may attempt to provoke the pain further in the thoracic spine by passively flexing the patient's neck, approximating the patient's chin to the chest (Soto–Hall). A pulling pain in the thoracic spine is indicative of strain and sprain. Acute localized pain in the upper thoracic spine may be due to fracture of the spinous process or vertebral body. If this procedure is performed in the supine position, and the patient involuntarily flexes both knees while performing this maneuver (Brudzinski's sign), meningeal irritation is suspected. If there is suspicion of rib fracture, the examiner may exert downward pressure on the sternum. Localized pain at the site of lesion is strongly suggestive of rib fracture.

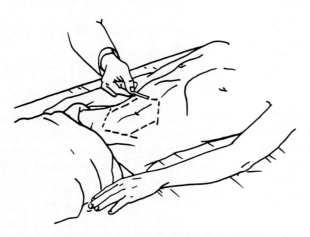

Figure 18-27. Superficial abdominal reflexes. The examiner lightly strokes the abdomen in the directions indicated. A normal response would elicit contraction of the muscles stroked.

Lumbar Spine and Pelvis Evaluation

Pain in the lumbar spine or pelvis can be due to a local pathology or referred from the thoracic and cervical spines or from pathology of other body systems. When evaluating a patient presenting with low back pain or discomfort, unless the examiner is certain that a local lesion exists, he or she must first eliminate the possibility of the pain resulting from fracture, metastatic disease, metabolic disease, or diseases of the viscera. These can be identified or ruled out through the case history and general physical examination and imaging procedures, such as x-ray, CT scans, or MRI. The lumbar spine is called upon to support the greatest load of any other spinal region. It furnishes support for the upper body and transmits weight of the upper body to the pelvis and lower limb. Unless there is a definitive history of trauma, it is often difficult to determine whether pain in the lumbar spine originates in the lumbar spine, sacroiliac joints, or hip joints; therefore, all three should be assessed in a systematic manner.

Inspection and Observation. The examiner may observe the method by which the patient walks into the examination room (gait, described in detail earlier in this chapter). He or she should note if there is a limp or list and if it appears to be due to deformity or pain. At the same time, the examiner can note the patient's body type (ectomorphic, mesomorphic, endormorphic). Next, the patient's posture should be assessed in the upright position and observed anteriorly, laterally, and posteriorly. Although postural evaluation is described in detail earlier in this chapter, the examiner should pay particular attention to the assessment of the following characteristics in the patient presenting with low back pain.

From the anterior and posterior view, the head, shoulders, and hips should be level and the spine straight. Pelvic unleveling may be associated with pelvic obliquity, leg strength discrepancy (Friberg, 1987), acute muscle spasm, lower extremity deformities, scoliosis, and acute lumbar disc lesions. Spinal deviation from the midline may be structural, due to scoliosis or congenital anomalies, or functional due to leg length discrepancies, vertebral subluxation, or muscle spasm.

Acute low back pain is often characterized by a sharp, angular deviation due to involuntary protective muscle spasm (antalgic posture). The deviation is created by reflex muscle spasm in the body's attempt to reposition the injured body part to a safer, less painful position (the principle is similar for torticollis in the cervical spine). The patient may present in a position of flexion antalgia where the lumbar lordosis has been either straightened or reversed and is usually associated with a central disc protrusion or facet joint syndrome or muscle strain. The degree of local pain and/or radiculitis is usually associated

with the severity of the pathology. Flexion antalgia that is associated with a body list to the right or left may indicate unilateral facet joint syndrome or posterolateral disc protrusion or prolapse (Bernard and Kirkaldy-Willis, 1987).

An acute body list associated with sciatic radiculopathy is usually indicative of disc disease. A body list toward the side of sciatic radiculopathy is most likely due to a disc protrusion or prolapse on the medial side of the nerve root. A body list away from the side of local pain and/or radiculopathy is probably due to a disc protrusion or prolapse on the lateral side of the nerve root (Fig. 18–29). If the examiner is uncertain whether a lateral list is present, he or she may ask the patient to bend forward. This maneuver will stretch the nerve roots around an existing disc protrusion resulting in antalgic deviation of the body at some point in the forward bend movement (Kramer, 1981). The examiner can then correlate the side of deviation to the side of pain and/or radiculopathy, thereby identifying a medial versus lateral protrusion.

From the side, the examiner may look for exaggerated or decreased curvature. Increased lumbar lordosis may be due to anterior pelvic tilting with associated increase to the pelvic and sacral angles, often associated with hip flexion contracture deformities, degenerative disc disease, and weak abdominal muscles. Decreased lordosis in the absence of acute pain may indicate advancing degeneration or stenosis (Liyang, 1989). The examiner can also observe the ribs, hips, knees, ankles, and feet for alignment, areas of swelling, and abnormal bony or soft tissue contours. He or she can also observe any skin markings such as café-au-lait spots associated with neurofibromatosis, an unusual hair growth such as Faun's beard associated with spina bifida or syringomyelia. A step deformity in the lumbar spine may be indicative of spondylolisthesis.

Palpation. The lumbar spine should be palpated from the anterior and posterior aspects. Any tenderness, altered temperature, muscle spasm, swelling, altered position or movement, and other signs and symptoms that may indicate the source of pathology should be noted. The examiner may need to assess the following structures:

1. Spinous processes, interspinous spaces, and paraspinal musculature
2. Sacrum, sacroiliac joints and coccyx
3. Iliac crest, ischial tuberocity, hip joint, and sciatic nerve
4. Symphysis pubis
5. Inguinal area. The inguinal region may be palpated for hernia, infection (lymph nodes), abscess, and femoral artery patency.

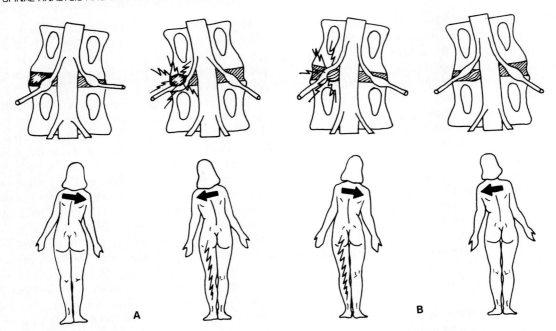

Figure 18–29. Patients with disc protrusion or herniation may present with antalgic posture, listing to one side or the other. This may be due to a voluntary or involuntary mechanism to alleviate nerve root irritation. This list may also occur, however, in patients with mechanical back pain of different origins. With disc lesions, however, it is hypothesized that, when the protrusion is lateral to the nerve root (**A**), the list is toward the contralateral side of pain. When the protrusion is medial to the nerve root (**B**), the list is toward the ipsilateral side of pain. In either case, it is believed that the list is an attempt of the body to reduce nerve root pressure and pain. (*Adapted from White AA, and Panjabi MN. Clinical Biomechanics of the Spine. J.B. Lippincott Company, Philadelphia, 1978, p. 299.*)

6. The abdomen. When indicated, the abdominal aorta should be palpated and auscultated. Abdominal aortic aneurysms are prevalent in men over 50 with a history of arteriosclerosis.

Range of Motion. Passive range of motion in the lumbar spine is difficult to assess because of body weight. During active range of motion, the examiner should assess limitations of movement and its possible causes, such as pain, spasm, stiffness, or blocking. The following are the active movements and ranges of the lumbar spine:

1. Forward flexion, 40 to 60 degrees. Flexion of the lumbar spine is usually permitted just beyond reversal of the normal lumbar lordosis. On forward bending, a simultaneous movement of pelvic rotation (25 to 30 degrees) is necessary to reach the floor with the fingers (lumbar pelvic rhythm) (White and Panjabi, 1978). Flexion is usually limited and painful in lumbar strain/sprain syndromes and blocked with disc lesions. Pain on reextension from the flexed position may indicate lumbosacral facet instability (Kirkaldy-Willis, 1983).
2. Extension, 20 to 35 degrees. Acute disc pro-

trusions generally block lumbar extension. When extension is permitted to some degree and local or radicular pain is produced, the examiner may suspect facet joint irritation, lumbosacral instability due to disc degeneration, or lateral spinal stenosis.

3. Lateral flexion, left and right, 15 to 20 degrees. Lateral bending that elicits pain in the lumbar paraspinal musculature is usually indicative of erector spinae strain or spasm. Lateral bending may be blocked toward the side of the pain (lateral disc protrusion) or to the contralateral side (medial disc protrusion).
4. Rotation, right and left, 30 to 40 degrees. Although this is a primary function of the thoracic spine, rotation causes shearing stress in the posterior facet articulations. Painful rotation is usually indicative of facet joint syndrome.

Motion of the sacroiliac joints should be assessed in all patients with low back pain (Fig. 18–30). Acute or chronic low back pain may have its origin within the sacroiliac joints. This joint is stabilized in the pelvic ring by a narrow ear-shaped articulation, supported by strong ligaments and provides limited

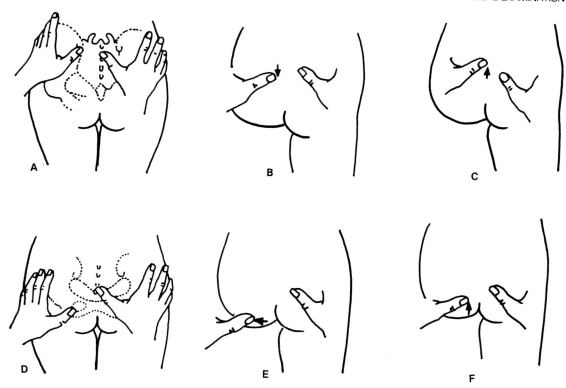

Figure 18–30. Motion palpation of the left sacroiliac joint. **A.** The examiner places the right thumb over the second sacral tubercle and the left thumb over the posterior superior iliac spine (PSIS) and the patient is asked to raise the left knee toward the chest. This tests the motion of the upper part of the joint. **B.** Normal movement; the PSIS moves downward. **C.** Abnormal movement; the PSIS moves upward. **D.** The examiner then places the right thumb over the apex of the sacrum and the left thumb over the ischial tuberosity and the patient is again asked to raise the knee toward the chest. This tests the motion of the lower part of the joint. **E.** Normal movement; the ischial tuberosity moves laterally. **F.** Abnormal movement; the ischial tuberosity moves in a superior direction.

movement. These joints are subject to stress with excessive lifting, bending, stooping, or sitting. Degeneration of the lower lumbar spinal segments and pregnancy also transfers stress to the sacroiliac joints (McGill, 1978). Sacroiliac strain or subluxation generally causes local joint pain with referred pain to the groin and anterior thigh or buttocks and posterior thigh.

The examiner may also find it necessary to evaluate the range of motion of the hip joints, knees, and ankles, depending on clinical need. (The hip, knee, and ankle examination will be addressed later in this chapter.)

Neurological Examination. Nerve root compression syndromes may manifest themselves in the lower extremities as pain, altered sensation, motor power deficit, and/or reflex loss.

Anatomically, the lumbar nerve roots, as they descend in the cauda equina exit at their respective intervertebral foramen above their corresponding disc level (Sidman, 1965). Compression of a specific nerve root by protruded disc material is typically from the disc level above the numbered neurological

level within the spinal canal involved (L-4 disc compresses L-5 nerve root, L-5 disc compresses S-1 nerve root, etc.). Disk lesions, therefore, causing neurological deficit can usually be clinically localized if the examiner can isolate its effect on pain distribution, motor power, sensation, and/or reflex changes. Table 18–4 illustrates common clinical findings associated with nerve entrapment syndromes in the lumbar spine.

Generally, in nerve root compression syndromes, the smaller muscle groups of the ankle, foot, and toes show the first signs of muscle weakness. Sensation of the lower extremities is best tested bilaterally using a sharp instrument. Hypersensitivity generally indicates myofibrosis. Decreased sensation over a specific dermatome may indicate nerve root compression or peripheral nerve palsy. When neurological signs are questionable, electroneuromyography may be a useful adjunct, and reveal the first objective evidence of neurological involvement.

Functional Testing. Mechanical low back pain (in the absence of definitive neurological signs) is usually associated with positions or activities that

TABLE 18–4. LUMBAR NERVE ROOT SYNDROMES

Roots	Disc Level	Pain Distribution	Sensory Dysfunction	Reflex Change	Motor Dysfunction
L-1	T12-L1 Rare	Lumbar, hip and groin	Iliac crest and groin	None	None
L-2	L1-2	Lumbar, hip, groin, anterior thigh	Front to thigh to knee	None	Psoas, hip adduction
L-3	L2-3	Lumbar, upper buttock, anterior thigh and knee	Front of thigh and medial knee	Decrease in patellar reflex	Psoas, quadriceps (forward leg elevation)
L-4	L3-4	Low lumbar, buttock, groin, medial leg, dorsum, of foot and big toe	Medial calf and dorsum of foot and big toe	Decrease in patellar reflex	Tibialis anterior and extensor hallucis longus
L-5	L4-5 common	Low lumbar, buttock, posterior and lateral thigh, Lateral calf, dorsum of foot	Lateral calf, dorsum of foot, medial three toes	Usually none, may see decrease in ankle reflex	Extensor hallucis, ankle dorsiflexors (foot drop), gluteus medius
S-1	L5-S1 most common	Low lumbar, posterior thigh and calf, lateral border of foot	Posterior thigh and calf, lateral border of foot, lateral two toes	Decrease or absent ankle reflex	Ankle plantar flexors and everters, calf and hamstrings, gluteal wasting

Data from Lonstein and Hochschuler, 1989; Hoppenfield, 1977.

load the spine or that stress the injured tissue and is relieved in positions of reduced load (Lonstein and Huchshuler, 1989). Therefore, clinical diagnosis of mechanical low back pain may be solely dependent on the details of the case history, the distribution of pain, and the skill of the examiner in his or her ability to reproduce and/or reduce symptoms by appropriate functional maneuvers. When necessary, the following maneuvers may aid the examiner in identifying the site of lesion and particular tissues involved.

STRAIGHT LEG RAISE TEST (SLR). With the patient supine and the knee extended, the examiner (1) raises the leg until the patient complains of pain or tightness, and (2) establishes its exact location (low back, leg, or both (Fig. 18–31A). If there is a question as to the degree of pain, the examiner may passively flex the patient's chin to his or her chest (Fig. 18–31B). This maneuver places greater traction on the spinal cord and nerve roots and may bring out grade pain in space-occupying lesions. With the SLR maneuver, there is slack in the sciatic nerve root from 0 to 35 degrees. Angular deformation of the sciatic roots begins at 35 degrees and diminishes at around 70 degrees with no further root deformation (Magee, 1987). With disc lesions, central protrusions tend to cause pain in the back, lateral protrusions tend to cause pain in the lower extremity, and intermediate/medial protrusions cause both. Also, the size of

the disc protrusion usually correlates directly with the degree at which the SLR test becomes positive (Shiging, et al., 1987). Dull posterior thigh pain usually indicates tight hamstring muscles. Dull low back pain may indicate a local lumbar strain or sprain and usually occurs when the SLR is over 70 degrees. If the patient complains of pain on the opposite side of straight leg raise, it may indicate a medial disc herniation (Well leg raise test/Fajersztajn test). The examiner may then perform a straight leg raise with the hip internally and externally rotated (Fig. 18–31C). If pain is elicited with internal rotation and relieved with external rotation, a piriformis muscle strain is suspected. Straight leg raise may also be performed in the sitting position (Bechterew's test).

PRONE KNEE BENDING TEST/FEMORAL STRETCH TEST/ NACHLAS TEST/ELY TEST. With the patient prone, the examiner passively flexes the knee to approximate the heel to the buttock while stabilizing the pelvis with the opposite hand to prevent hip rotation (Fig. 18–32). Pain in the gluteal region may reveal sacroiliac joint lesion. Pain in the lumbar region may indicate lumbar disc syndrome or facet joint syndrome. Tension at the anterior thigh may reveal tightness of the quadricep muscles or femoral nerve irritation. Passive elevation of the ipsilateral hip may indicate hip flexion contracture of the iliopsoas muscle.

SIGN OF THE BUTTOCK. The examiner performs a unilateral straight leg raise test to the point of pain, then

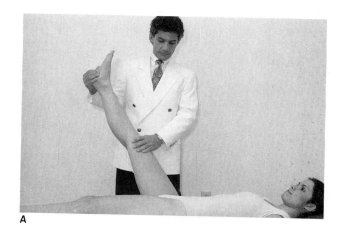

A

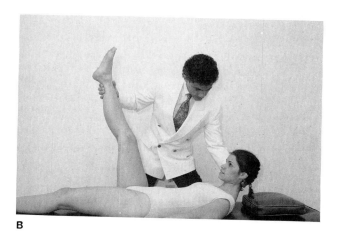

B

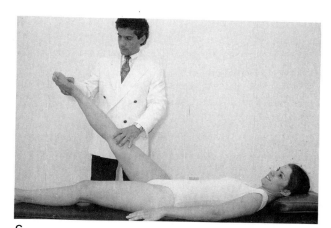

C

Figure 18-31. A. Straight leg raise test (SLR). **B.** SLR with neck flexion. **C.** SLR with hip rotation.

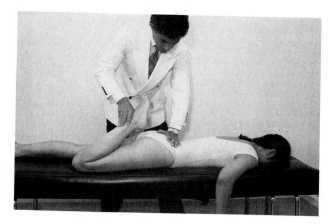

Figure 18-32. Femoral stretch test.

croiliac or hip joints. If hip flexion increases and pain decreases, the test is negative and indicative of a problem in the lumbar spine (Forst, 1981).

BOWSTRING SIGN. With the patient supine, the examiner places the patient's extended leg on top of his or her shoulder. The examiner exerts thumb pressure over the upper hamstring muscles. If pain is not elicited, the examiner then applies thumb pressure into the popiteal fossa (Mazion, 1980). Pain in the lumbar region or radiculitis may indicate nerve root compression.

MINOR'S SIGN. When observing the patient rise from a sitting position, low back pain may increase and the patient may need to assist him or herself by pushing up on the arms of the chair or walking up the legs with the hands to reduce pain. The sign may indicate disc protrusion and/or sciatic radiculopathy.

KEMP'S TEST. With the patient seated or standing, (Fig. 18-33) the examiner stands behind the patient,

flexes the patient's knee and hip, approximating the knee to the chest. If greater pain and/or blocking is experienced on knee/hip flexion, it is a positive sign of the buttock and indicates disease in the buttocks, such as bursitis, tumor, abscess, or lesions in the sa-

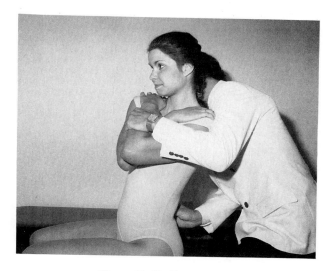

Figure 18-33. Kemp's test.

grasps him or her around the chest with one arm and supports the lumbosacral region with the opposite hand. The examiner then bends the patient obliquely backward (Cox, 1985). Pain on the concave side accompanied by radiculopathy on the same side may indicate lateral disc protrusion. Pain on the convex side accompanied by radiculopathy may indicate medial disc protrusion.

DEJERINE'S TRIAD. If the patient describes an increase in low back and/or leg pain when he or she coughs, sneezes, laughs, or bears down as if straining at stool (Valsalva's maneuver), there may be an increase in intrathecal pressure, most likely induced by a space-occupying lesion such as a disc protrusion, tumor, or osteophyte.

MILGRAM'S TEST. With the patient supine, instruct him or her to raise the legs from the table approximately 3 to 6 in. If it is difficult, or the patient is unable to elevate his or her legs from the table due to increased pain in the low back and/or leg, it is a positive test indicative of disc protrusion.

YEOMAN'S TEST. With the patient prone, the examiner flexes the patient's knee, places one hand under the knee, and the other stabilizes the pelvis. The examiner then extends the hip (Fig. 18–34). Deep sacroiliac pain indicates a sprain of the anterior sacroiliac ligaments. Pain in the lumbar spine may indicate lumbar involvement.

GAENSLEN'S TEST. With the patient supine and the affected side toward the edge of the table, the patient is instructed by approximate the knee of the unaffected side to his or her chest and to drop the affected leg off the side of the table (Fig. 18–35). The examiner then places pressure on both legs in a scissors fashion. Pain in the sacroiliac joint may indicate a sacroiliac sprain or subluxation.

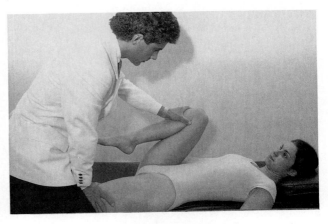

Figure 18–35. Gaenslen's test.

MENNELL'S TEST. With the patient prone, the examiner exerts inward pressure with the hands over the sacroiliac joints bilaterally as if to press them together. Pain in one or both sacroiliac joints may indicate sacroiliac lesion. The examiner then exerts outward pressure on both sacroiliac joints bilaterally. Pain in the sacroiliac region may indicate sacroiliac lesion; pain in the lumbosacral region may indicate lumbar involvement.

HIP JOINT STRESS TEST. The hip joints should be stressed through passive range of motion in all directions while ascertaining the patient's reaction. Pain in the sacroiliac joint may indicate sacroiliac joint lesion; pain in the hip joint may indicate hip joint lesion.

TRENDELENBURG TEST. The standing patient flexes one knee and hip in an attempt to approximate the knee to the chest. Normally, the pelvis on the raised leg side will elevate. A positive sign occurs when the pelvis on the raised leg side depresses, indicating weakness of the gluteus medius muscle with failure to abduct the hip on the opposite side.

HEEL WALKING AND TOE WALKING. With the patient standing, usually during evaluation of gait, the patient is instructed to walk across the examination room on his or her heels and then on his or her toes. An inability to maintain elevation of the toes during heel walking may indicate weakness of ankle and/or toe dorsiflexors and may be due to compression of the L-4 and/or L-5 nerve root. Inability of the patient to maintain elevation of the heels during toe walking may indicate weakness of the foot and ankle plantar flexors due to compression of the S-1 nerve root. If weakness is questionable, the examiner may ask the patient to stand on one leg and repetitively rise up and down on the toes and then on the heels. Early fatigue of one side compared with the other is indicative of weakness.

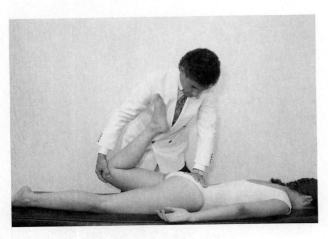

Figure 18–34. Yeoman's test.

If the examiner fails to identify lumbar pathology in the patient with low back pain or suspects that more distal abnormalities may be contributing to the patient's symptoms, the examiner should proceed to the areas of the lower extremity as dictated by clinical need and judgment.

Lower Extremities Evaluation

Hip. The hip joint is one of the largest and most stable joints in the body. If it is injured or diseased, pain is usually perceptible during walking (Aegerter et al., 1975). Pain from the hip can be referred to the sacroiliac joint, the lumbar spine groin, thigh, or knee (Rosse, 1980). If the examiner suspects hip joint disease, these related areas may need to be examined. Diagnosis of hip joint injury or pathology can be made with a careful history and thorough physical examination, supplemented by radiologic and laboratory evaluations as needed.

INSPECTION AND OBSERVATION. Gait should first be evaluated when the patient walks into the examination room. The examiner should detect any limp, deformity, or leg length discrepancy. The examiner can inspect the skin of birth marks, discoloration, abrasions, and areas of swelling. Posture and stance are usually affected in hip joint pathology. The examiner may detect changes in the position of the pelvis, trunk and lumbar spine, such as pelvic obliquity and lumbar spine take-off in the frontal and lateral plane. Hip flexion contracture may lead to an increased lumbar lordosis due to an anterior inferior tilting of the pelvis (a common finding in degenerative hip disease). Differences in bony and soft tissue contours should be noted.

PALPATION. The examiner may palpate the bony prominences of the anterior and posterior aspect of the pelvis, hips, sacroiliac joints, and upper legs. Tenderness over the greater trochanter with swelling may indicate trochanteric bursitis. General soreness along the lateral border of the pelvis and upper leg may result from myofibrositis of the tensor fascia lata muscle, common in chronic low back pain syndromes and degenerative hip joint disease. Pain over the sacroiliac joint may indicate a local lesion. Sciatic nerve tenderness may be due to a herniated lumbar disc, piriformis muscle spasm, or direct trauma to the nerve. The inguinal region may also be evaluated for hernia and femoral artery patency.

RANGE OF MOTION. Active movements of the hip joint are as follows (Magee, 1987):

1. Flexion, 110 to 120 degrees
2. Extension, 10 to 15 degrees
3. Abduction, 30 to 50 degrees
4. Adduction, 30 degrees
5. Lateral/external rotation, 40 to 60 degrees
6. Medial/internal rotation, 30 to 40 degrees

Passive range of motion and joint play should be tested to evaluate the end feel of the hip joint capsule. Restriction may indicate muscle or ligament contracture or degenerative hip disease.

NEUROLOGICAL EXAMINATION. When necessary, all of the muscles affecting hip joint motion should be evaluated against resistance and graded. Weakness associated with pain suggests a local muscle or joint lesion. Weakness without pain may indicate neurological deficit and should be investigated as previously outlined in this chapter. If distal symptoms are present, lower extremity sensation, motor power, and reflexes should be assessed.

FUNCTIONAL TESTING. Local hip joint lesions are generally exacerbated with prolonged standing and walking. Clinically, pain can usually be provoked by gently stressing the joint at the extremes of all permitted motions. The examiner may begin functional testing of the hip during the range-of-motion examination by exerting gentle, passive stretch to the joint, slightly past its active range. For example, flexion may be tested with the patient supine, asking the patient to perform a knee–chest maneuver. The examiner may then place additional pressure on the patient's leg inducing passive stress to the hip joint in flexion (Fig. 18–36). Pain or restriction of movement in the hip joint may indicate local joint inflammation or degenerative joint disease. Pain in the sacroiliac joint may indicate local lesion. Involuntary flexion of the opposite hip during this maneuver may indicate hip flexion contracture (Rosse, 1980). Additional stress to the joint can be applied by asking the patient to cross one leg, placing the foot to the opposite knee (Patrick's test) (Fig. 18–37). The ex-

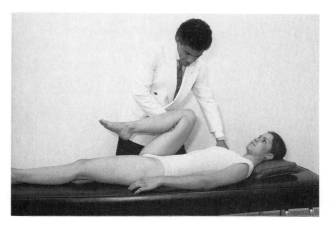

Figure 18–36. Hip flexion test.

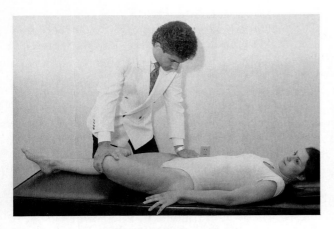

Figure 18-37. Patrick's test.

aminer then stabilizes the opposite anterior superior iliac spine (ASIS) and presses down on the knee of the leg being tested. This induces passive flexion, abduction and external rotation, and extension (Fabere sign). Pain or restriction of the hip joint may indicate joint inflammation or degenerative joint disease. With the patient prone, the examiner can passively extend the hip by stabilizing the pelvis with one hand and elevating the leg with the opposite hand (Yeoman's test, see lumbar evaluation). Pain or restrictive movement in the hip joint may indicate local lesion. Pain in or around the sacroiliac joint may reveal a sacroiliac lesion. Pain at the anterior thigh suggests quadriceps contracture or femoral nerve irritation. Resisted motion with this maneuver associated with groin pain may indicate hip flexion contracture.

The examiner may also need to assess abduction and adduction contractures about the hip. This can be ascertained by having the patient lie supine with the ASIS level. The examiner then forms an imaginary angle of the lower extremities with the line joining the two ASISs. An angle less than 90 degrees may indicate adduction contracture. An angle greater than 90 degrees may indicate abduction contracture. If the examiner attempts to shift the affected leg to a 90-degree angle, the pelvis will shift instead of the leg (Fig. 18–38). Joint play movements including joint compression, lateral distraction, and caudal glide can be assessed with stress maneuvers in the respective directions, comparing the amount of available movement on both sides. Pain and/or restriction may indicate joint inflammation, contracture, or degenerative joint disease.

Hip joint pathology is often the result of uneven loading or biomechanical alteration from pelvic obliquity and/or leg length discrepancy. Clinically, true leg length is measured with the patient supine and legs 15 to 20 cm apart and parallel. If one hip is fixed in abduction or adduction, the good hip should be abducted or adducted an equal amount. Measurement is made from the ASIS to the medial or lateral malleolus, and comparative measurement is made on the opposite leg (Fig. 18–39). The examiner may then wish to differentiate femoral from tibial shortening. Femoral measurement is from the greater trochanter of the femur to the lateral knee joint line. Tibial shortening is measured from the medial knee joint line to the medial malleolus. General clinical assessment of femoral versus tibial shortening can be obtained with the patient supine, both knees flexed to 90 degrees, and the feet flat on the table and parallel (Fig. 18–40A and B). If the knee is short and posterior on the affected side, a decreased femoral length or posterior displacement of the femoral head is suspected. If the knee is short and anterior on the affected side, decreased tibial length is indicated. If the knee is long and anterior on the affected side, it indicates anterior displacement of the femoral head or increased length of the femur.

Figure 18-38. Abduction contracture testing. With fixed adduction contracture of the hip (**A**), and attempt to bring the legs to a parallel position will result in a "hiking" or shifting of the pelvis to an oblique position (**B**). The reverse occurs with abduction contracture. (*Adapted from The American Orthopedic Association; Manual of Orthopedic Surgery. Chicago, 1972, p. 45.*)

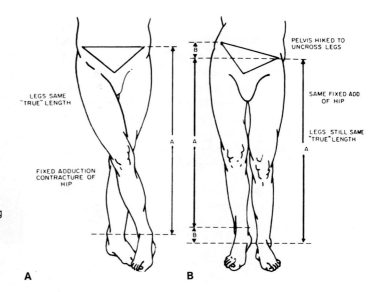

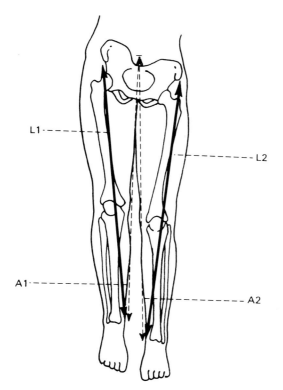

Figure 18-39. True leg length (L-1 and L-2) versus apparent leg length (A1 and A2). True leg length is measured from the ASIS to the medial malleolus. Apparent leg length is measured from the umbilicus to the medial malleolus. In the case illustrated, the right leg appears shorter due to pelvic tilt and A1 is less than A2, but true leg lengths are equal (L-1 equals L-2). (*Adapted from Rosse, C. Clawson, D. The Musculoskeletal System in Health and Disease. Harper & Row, Cambridge, 1980, p. 267.*)

Knee. The knee joint is the largest, strongest, most superficial and most vulnerable joint in the human body. Pathology and injuries of the knee represent an extremely common problem in chiropractic practice. Direct trauma can result from competitive athletics as well as activities of daily living (Torg, 1987). An accurate diagnosis is dependent on a thorough knowledge of regional anatomy, a sound understanding of biomechanics, a careful case history disclosing the mechanism of injury, and a thorough clinical examination.

INSPECTION AND OBSERVATION. The examiner can inspect for areas of localized or defused swelling. Muscles should be inspected for symmetry of contours and visible atrophy. The relative position of the patella to the femur can be observed and abnormal bony contours or joint positions noted. For example, genu recurvatum is usually a normal variant in people with lax ligaments. Fixed, flexed knees, however, indicate joint pathology. Enlargement of the knee with associated valgus (windswept) deformity usually indicates rheumatoid arthritis, whereas a varus (Gunstock) deformity may indicate osteoarthritis (Post, 1987).

PALPATION. Palpation should include both the bony and soft tissue structures of the knee and surrounding areas. Gaps above or below the patella may indicate ruptures of the quadriceps or infrapatellar tendon, respectively. Palpable effusion over the patella is indicative of prepatellar bursitis. Point tenderness over the medial or lateral joint lines indicates meniscus fragmentation, whereas collateral ligament injury usually causes pain at their insertion, slightly above or below the joint line. A painful palpable lump in the popliteal fossa may be indicative of a ''Baker's cyst.''

RANGE OF MOTION. Typical ranges of motion for the knee joint are as follows:

1. Flexion, 135 degrees
2. Extension, 0 to 5 degrees
3. Internal/external rotation, 10 degrees each

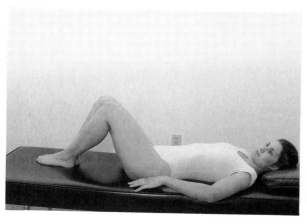

A

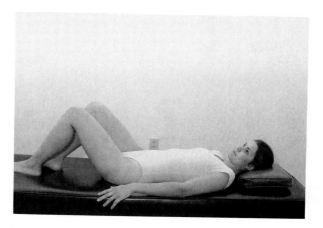

B

Figure 18-40. A. Decreased femoral length. **B.** Decreased tibial length.

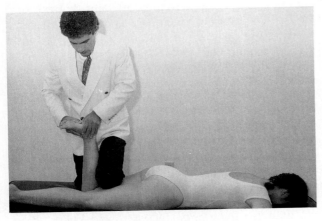

Figure 18-41. Apley's compression test.

The examiner may also ask the patient to squat in a deep knee bend. Both knees should be able to flex symmetrically. The patient can then be instructed to stand up from a squatting position. The examiner should note whether the patient is able to stand straight with knees in full extension or whether one leg is relied on more than the other during the procedure.

FUNCTIONAL TESTING

Apley's Compression Test. With the patient prone, (Fig. 18–41) the examiner flexes the patient's knee to 90 degrees. The examiner places one knee on the patient's posterior thigh for stability. Downward pressure on the patient's heel is applied while internally and externally rotating the foot. Pain on either side of the knee may indicate a torn meniscus on the respective side.

McMurray's Test. With the patient supine and knee completely flexed, (Fig. 18–42A) first the

examiner medially rotates the tibia and gradually extends the knee. A loose fragment of the lateral meniscus may cause an audible or palpable snap or click associated with pain. The examiner then repeats the procedure with lateral rotation of the tibia (Fig. 18–42B). A palpable or audible snap or click associated with pain at the medial joint margin may indicate medial meniscus fragmentation.

Drawer's Sign. With the patient supine, the knee is flexed and the foot placed flat on the table. The examiner grasps behind the knee and draws the tibia anteriorly then pushes it posteriorly (Fig. 18–43A and B). Normal movement is approximately 6 mm. Anterior or posterior movement of the tibia more than 6 mm may indicate rupture of the anterior and posterior cruciate ligaments, respectively.

Adduction Stress Test [Varus Stress]. With the patient supine, (Fig. 18–44) the examiner places one hand over the medial knee joint and the opposite hand over the lateral ankle. The examiner then pushes the knee laterally. Pain on the lateral aspect of the knee may indicate lateral collateral ligament instability.

Abduction Stress Test [Valgus Stress]. With the patient supine, (Fig. 18–45) the examiner places one hand over the lateral knee joint and the opposite hand over the medial ankle. The examiner then pushes the knee joint medially. Pain at the medial aspect of the knee may indicate medial collateral ligament instability.

Patellar Ballottement Test. With the patient supine, the examiner applies a slight tap or pressure with his or her fingers over the patella in an attempt to push the patella against the femur. If fluid or effusion is present, a floating of the patella will be felt. When

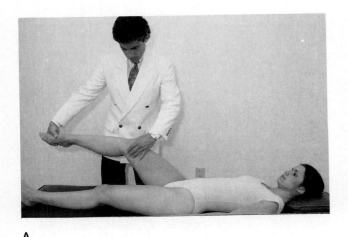

A

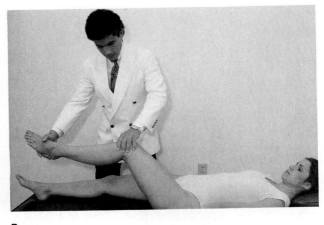

B

Figure 18-42. A. McMurray's test, medial rotation, right knee. **B.** McMurray's test, lateral rotation, left knee.

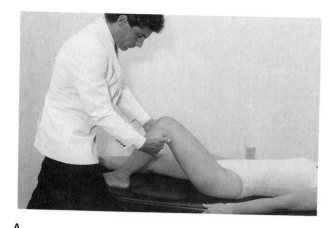

A

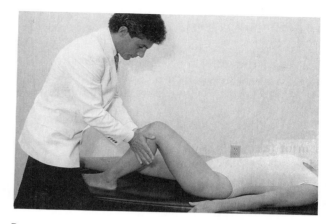

B

Figure 18–43. A. Drawer's sign, anterior. **B.** Drawer's sign, posterior.

the patella is pushed down, it may strike the femur with a palpable tap. When it is released, it will elevate. This may indicate infrapatellar bursitis or acute inflammation of the patellofemoral articulation.

Patellar Grinding Test. With the patient supine and knee extended, the examiner places hand pressure over the patella and moves it medially, laterally, superiorly, and inferiorly over the femur. Pain in the knee joint may indicate either condromalacia or retropatella arthritis.

Ankle and Foot. Approximately 80% of people today have foot problems that can be corrected with proper assessment, treatment, and personal care. The chiropractic clinician should be concerned with lesions of the ankle and foot because they can alter the mechanics of gait, resulting in stress and pathology of the lower limb joints, hip joints, sacroiliac joints, and lumbar spine. The foot and ankle are the focal points to which the total body

weight is transmitted during ambulation, and both are capable of adjustments necessary for fine balance on a variety of terrain. This concentrated stress often results in injury and deformity. The foot is also highly affected by a number of general systemic conditions such as rheumatoid arthritis and diabetes (Hamilton, 1985).

INSPECTION AND OBSERVATION. Observation should include gait, toe in/toe out, and varus or valgus deformities of the foot, ankle, and toes. Locations of corns and calluses illustrate areas of friction or mechanical stress. The examiner should inspect for the general appearance of the feet and anatomic position in weight bearing and nonweight bearing. Areas of swelling, deformity, color changes in weight bearing and nonweight bearing can be assessed. Unilateral localized swelling is usually indicative of sprain. Generalized swelling is usually secondary to massive trauma (Mosely, 1965). Bilateral swelling over

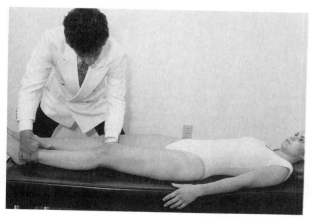

Figure 18–44. Adduction stress test.

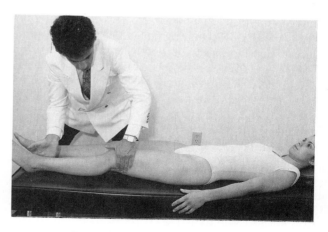

Figure 18–45. Abduction stress test.

the malleoli may indicate cardiac or lymphatic problems or an obstruction of venus return.

PALPATION. The examiner may palpate the bony and soft tissue structures of the ankle and foot to detect areas of altered temperature, tenderness, and swelling. Deformities, such as claw toes, hammer toes, mallot toes, valgus, varus and cavus foot deformities, should be assessed (weight bearing and non-weight bearing).

RANGE OF MOTION. Typical ranges of motion for the foot and ankle are as follows (Hoppenfield, 1976):

1. Ankle
   Dorsiflexion, 20 degrees
   Plantar flexion, 50 degrees
   Supination, 45 to 60 degrees
   Pronation, 15 to 30 degrees
2. Subtalor joint
   Inversion, 5 degrees
   Eversion, 5 degrees
3. Forefoot
   Adduction, 20 degrees
   Abduction, 10 degrees
4. Great toe flexion
   Metatorsophalangeal joint, 45 degrees
   Interphalangeal joint, 90 degrees
5. Great toe extension
   Metatarsophalangeal joint, 70 degrees
   Interphalangeal joint, minimal
6. Lesser toe flexion
   Metatarsophalangeal joint, 40 degrees
   Proximal interphalangeal joint, 30 degrees
   Distal interphalangeal joint, 60 degrees
7. Lesser toe extension
   Metatarsophalangeal joint, 40 degrees
   Proximal interphalangeal joint, 30 degrees
   Distal interphalangeal joint, negligible

FUNCTIONAL TESTING. Ankle sprains are a common malady of people of all ages. Sprain, depending on its severity, generally results in pain, inflammation, and ligamentous instability. Inversion sprain is the most common, resulting in pain and/or edema and/or hematoma at the anterolateral joint region. This can generally be diagnosed through observation and an accurate assessment of the mechanism of injury (inversion). When observable signs are not present, and the mechanism is unclear, the examiner may need to stress the joint in various directions to bring about the pain. With the patient supine, the examiner can induce lateral stress by grasping the foot and passively inverting it (Fig. 18–46). Pain or gapping is indicative of sprain or tear of the anterior talofibular and/or calcaneal fibular ligament (inversion sprain). Medial stress is induced when the ex-

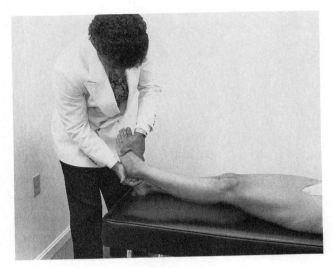

Figure 18–46. Lateral stress test.

aminer grasps the foot and passively everts it (Fig. 18–47). Pain or gapping may indicate sprain or tear of the deltoid ligament (eversion sprain). Posterior stress is induced when the examiner grasps the dorsum of the foot with one hand, and the posterior distal tibia with the other, and exerts a pulling pressure on the tibia (Fig. 18–48). Pain or gapping with this maneuver may indicate a posterior talofibular ligament tear. Anterior stress is induced when the examiner places one hand on the heel and the other on the anterior distal tibia and pushes the tibia posteriorly (Fig. 18–49). Pain or gapping with this maneuver may indicate a tear in the anterior talofibular ligament.

Compartment syndromes about the ankle are a

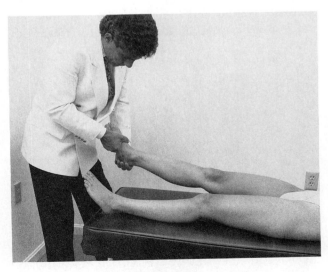

Figure 18–47. Medial stress test.

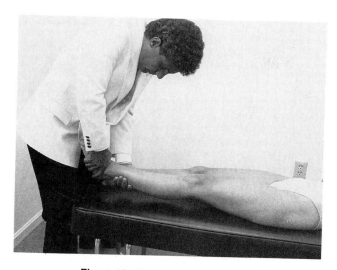

Figure 18–48. Posterior stress test.

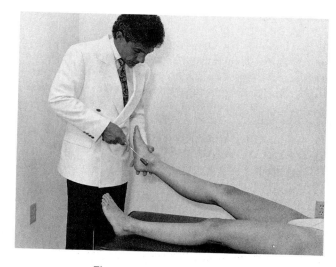

Figure 18–50. Tinel's foot sign.

common clinical finding, the most common being tarsal tunnel syndrome. This syndrome is associated with compression of the posterior tibial nerve as it passes along with the flexor tendons inferior to the medial malleolus and underneath the flexor retinaculum. Compression is usually due to chronic joint inflammation, joint degeneration, or chronic foot pronation. The patient generally experiences pain at the medial heel region, with radiation to the first, second, and third toes. The examiner can usually reproduce the pain or paresthesia with digital pressure over the posterior tibial nerve, just inferior to the medial malleolus, or by tapping it with a reflex hammer (Tinel's foot sign) (Fig. 18–50).

With posterior heel pain or weak plantar flexion, the examiner may squeeze the calf muscles against the tibia and fibula and observe foot movement. A loss of plantar flexion of the foot may indicate a ruptured Achilles tendon. Tenderness in the calf, however, with generalized foot paresthesia and/or temperature changes may be associated with thrombophlebitis. Pain associated with thrombophlebitis can generally be provoked by placing the patient supine, dorsiflexing the patient's foot, and squeezing the calf muscles (Fig. 18–51). Pain or pressure about the plantar or lateral aspect of the heel may indicate plantar fascitis or painful heel syndrome.

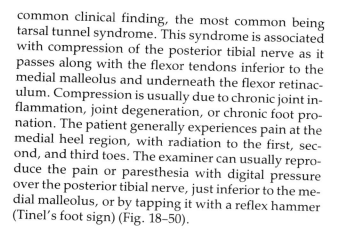

Figure 18–49. Anterior stress test.

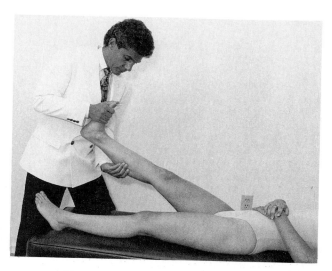

Figure 18–51. Test for thrombophlebitis.

Conclusion

The purpose of the case history and physical examination is to determine the cause of the patient's health problem. A thorough patient history will generally direct the chiropractic examiner to the area or areas requiring physical examination assessment and suggest the extent to which each area must be examined. The results obtained from the physical examination should lead the chiropractor to a clinical impression regarding the etiology and severity of the patient's health problem. Furthermore, the examiner can ascertain whether the patient's condition will be amenable to chiropractic care, or whether the services of another health care provider may be necessary. If the patient agrees to begin chiropractic care, periodic reexamination and evaluation will enable the clinician to determine whether the patient is improving, or whether the patient's condition is static or deteriorating. Periodic reassessment of the patient's health problem during a course of treatment will provide the doctor of chiropractic direction for future treatment and/or referral for specialty care based on clinical need.

References

ACA Membership Survey. Matthew Brennen (Pub.), 1990.

Aegerter E, and Kirkpatrick JA. *Orthopedic Diseases*. Philadelphia: W.B. Saunders Company; 1975.

Ameis A, Cervical whiplash: considerations in the rehabilitation of cervical myofascial injury. *Canadian Family Physician* September 1986;32.

Bates B. *A Guide to Physical Examination*. Philadelphia: J.B. Lippencott Co., 1983.

Batzdorf U., *Spine: State of the Art Reviews—Differential Diagnosis of Arm and Thoracic Radicular Pain and Sensory Disturbance*. Philadelphia: Hanley & Belfus, Inc.; September 1988;2:4.

Bernard TN, and Kirkaldy-Willis WH. Recognizing Specific Characteristics of Nonspecific Low Back Pain. *Clinical Orthopedics and Related Research* April 1987; 217.

Cailliet R. *Low Back Pain Syndrome*. Philadelphia: F.A. Davis Company; 1968.

Cailliet R. *Soft Tissue Pain and Disability*, Philadelphia: F.A. Davis Company; 1977.

Cailliet R. *Scoliosis: Diagnosis and Management*. Philadelphia: F.A. Davis Company; 1977.

Calabro JJ. Clinical Symposia. *Rheumatoid Arthritis: Diagnosis and Management*. New Jersey: Ciba-Geigy Corp.; 1986.

Cipriano JJ. *Regional Orthopedic Tests*, Maryland: William & Wilkins; 1985.

Conwell HE. Clinical Symposia. *Injuries to the Wrist*. New Jersey: Ciba-Geigy Corp.; 1970

Conwell HE. Clinical Symposia. *Injuries to the Elbow*. New Jersey: Ciba-Geigy Corp.; 1969.

Cox JM. *Low Back Pain: Mechanism, Diagnosis and Management*, 4th ed. Baltimore: Williams & Wilkins; 1985.

Cyriax J. *Textbook of Orthopaedic Medicine*. Great Britain: Spottiswoode Ballantyne Ltd.; 1978.

Daniels L, and Worthingham C, *Muscle Testing*, 5th ed. Philadelphia: W.B. Saunders, Inc.; 1986.

Forst JJ. *Contributions a l'etude Clinique de la Sciatique*. Paris: These; 1981:33.

Friberg O. The statics of postural pelvis tilt scoliosis; a radiographic study on 288 consecutive chronic LBP patients. *Clinical Biomechanics* 1987;2:211–219.

Gelb HG. *Clinical Management of Head, Neck and TMJ Pain and Dysfunction*. Philadelphia: W.B. Saunders Company; 1977.

Guides to the Evaluation of Permanent Impairment, 2nd ed., A.M.A., 1985.

Guides to the Evaluation of Permanent Impairment, 3rd ed., A.M.A., 1988.

Haldman S. *Modern Developments in the Principles and Practice of Chiropractic*. New York: Appleton-Century-Crofts; 1980.

Hamilton WG. Clinical Symposia. *Surgical Anatomy of the Foot and Ankle*. New Jersey: Ciba-Geigy Corp.; 1985.

Hoppenfield S. *Orthopaedic Neurology*. Philadelphia: J.B. Lippincott Company; 1977.

Hoppenfield S. *Physical Examination of the Spine and Extremities*. New York: Appleton-Century-Crofts; 1976.

Kirkaldy-Willis WH. *Managing Low Back Pain*. New York: Churchill-Livingston; 1983.

Kramer, J. *Intervertebral Disc Diseases*, trans. IF Goldie. West Germany: Druckerei Karl Grammlich; 1981.

Leek JC, Gershwin ME, and Fowler WM. *Principles of Physical Medicine and Rehabilitation in the Musculoskeletal Diseases*. New York: Grune & Stratton, Inc.; 1986.

Liying D, Yinkan X, Wenming Z, and Zhilha Z. The effect of flexion extension motion of the lumbar spine on the capacity of the spinal canal; an experimental study. *Spine* 1989;14:523–525.

Lonstein M, and Hochschuler S. *Spine: State of the Art Reviews-Differential Diagnosis of Lumbar Disc Disease*. Philadelphia: Hanley and Belfus, Inc.; January 1989;3:1.

Lord JW, and Rosati LM. Clinical Symposia. *Thoracic Outlet Syndromes*. New Jersey: Ciba-Geigy Corp., 1971.

Magee DJ. *Orthopedic Physical Assessment*. Philadelphia: W.B. Saunders Co.; 1987.

Mazion JM. *Illustrated Manual of Orthopedic Signs/Tests/Maneuvers for Office Procedure*. Orlando: Daniels Publishing Company; 1980.

McGill SM. A Biomechanical Perspective of Sacro-Iliac Pain. *Clinical Biomechanics* 1987; 2:145–151.

Merciew LR, and Pettid FJ. *Practical Orthopedics*. Chicago: Year Book Medical Publishers, Inc.; 1980.

Mosely HF. Clinical Symposia. *Traumatic Disorders of the Ankle and Foot*. New Jersey: Ciba-Geigy Corp.; 1965.

Post M. *Physical Examination of the Musculoskeletal System*. Year Book Medical Publishers, Inc.; Chicago-London; 1987.

Prior JA, Silberstein JS. *Physical Diagnosis*. St. Louis: Mosby; 1959.

Rosse C, and Clawson D. *The Musculoskeletal System in Health and Disease*. Philadelphia: Harper & Row; 1980.

Shiging X, Quanzhi Z and Dehao F. Significance of the straight leg raising test in the diagnosis and clinical evaluation of lower lumbar intervertebral disc protrusion. *J of Bone and Joint Surg* 1987; 69-A:517–521.

Sidman, RL, and Sidman M. *Neuroanatomy*. Great Britain: Churchill-Livingston; 1965.

Torg JS, Vegso JJ, and Torg E. *Rehabilitation of Athletic Injuries: An Atlas of Therapeutic Exercise*. Chicago: Year Book Medical Publishers, Inc.; 1987.

Van Allen MW, and Rodnitzky RL. *Pictorial Manual of Neurologic Tests*, 2nd ed. Chicago: Year Book Medical Publishers, Inc.; 1981.

Wilbourn, A, and Porter J. *Thoracic Outlet Syndromes—Spine: State of the Art Reviews*. Philadelphia: W.B. Saunders Company; September 1988:2; 4.

White, AA, and Panjabi MM. *Clinical Biomechanics of the Spine*. Philadelphia: J.B. Lippincott Company; 1978.

Yochum TR, and Rowe LJ. *Essentials of Skeletal Radiology*. Baltimore: Williams and Wilkins; 1987;I, II.

chapter 19

Manual Examination of the Spine

Leonard John Faye
Michael R. Wiles

History and Evolution of Spinal Analysis

The Hippocratic school of spinal manipulation maintained a "static" concept of spinal analysis, basing manipulation procedures on notions of misalignment, spinal curvature, and other deformities. D. D. Palmer's early chiropractic concepts were similarly based. Manipulation was considered to be indicated in the presence of spinal misalignment or "subluxation," a term originally used by Hippocrates. Palmer's static conceptualization of manipulable lesions provided the foundation for early chiropractic practice.

Static palpatory methods are still recognized as an important means of gathering information about the tissues overlying and adjacent to the manipulable lesion. Observation and palpation of the spine form half of the classic tetrad of any physical examination: observation, palpation, percussion, and auscultation. The static examination reveals information about tissue texture, inflammation, static alignment, muscle spasm, and even the state of local vascular function. Manipulative therapy, however, is a dynamic and kinetic process, and it seems logical that it should be supported by a dynamic and kinetic diagnostic procedure. This reasoning is the basis for the development of the various motion palpation techniques.

The idea of the subluxation as a kinetic pathophysiological phenomenon was first mentioned as far back as 1906 (Smith (et al., 1906). In a textbook called *Modernized Chiropractic,* loss of segmental mobility was considered an important component of the subluxation. The authors wrote, "A simple subluxated vertebra differs from a normal vertebra only in its field of motion and the center of its field of motion; because of being subluxated its varying positions of rest are differently located than when it was a normal vertebra . . . its field of motion may be too great in some directions and too small in others." Little emphasis, however, was placed on the dynamic phenomena associated with the subluxation until the work of Gillet, Mennell, and Illi.

In Belgium, in the late 1930s, Gillet and his associate Liekens jointly developed what would become the science of motion palpation (Gillet, 1984). In a review of his own research (Gillet, 1983), Gillet states that he was motivated by frustration with the static model, which maintained that spinal subluxations were static entities representing "bones out of place," and which were corrected "back into alignment" by an adjustment. Gillet successfully generated interest in the idea of motion palpation of the spine, and he produced one of the earliest regular chiropractic publications, which became the ancestor of the *European Journal of Chiropractic.*

As often happens in the process of innovation, Gillet came into collaborative contact during the 1930s with Fred Illi of Switzerland. Illi was involved in early x-ray studies of the erect spine. At that time, the practice of chiropractic was illegal in Belgium, and it was difficult for Gillet to become involved in x-ray research. Consequently, Gillet continued to work on palpatory techniques that were particularly important to chiropractors practicing without x-rays. Illi later spent time at the National College of Chiropractic where his work continued under Joseph Janse's encouragement and culminated in the publication of his now classic text on the dynamics of the spine and pelvis (Illi, 1951).

As with the development of chiropractic methods, traditional medicine's thoughts on manipulation were based on the idea of subluxations as a static entity. The medical writings of the 1930s and 1940s are very similar to chiropractic work of the same period in that both refer to bony subluxations as simple misalignments (Weiant and Goldschmidt, 1966). During the 1930s and 1940s, Cyriax probably dominated the field of manipulative medicine in London. His concepts of motion palpation were largely based on the idea of "end-feel" (Cyriax, 1982). End-feel was described as the subjective sensation felt by the palpator at the end of the passive range of motion of a joint. Cyriax defined a "soft end-feel" and a "hard end-feel," both of which were thought to be palpa-

ble at the vertebral levels of disc protrusion. Soft end-feel was the sensation perceived at the site of a soft protrusion of a nucleus pulposus. The use of the word "soft" is coincidental in this case. A hard end-feel was the sensation felt at the site of a "hard" disc lesion; that is, the partial herniation of a fragment of hardened nucleus pulposus through a fissure in the annular fibers. This subjective sensation of joint "play" at the end of the normal passive range of motion was a key concept in the practice of manipulation as taught by Cyriax.

Paralleling Cyriax's model was the work of Mennell. As with Cyriax, Mennell appears to have learned about the spine and manipulation from his father, also a physician. After practicing in Britain for a short time, he came to the United States where his work continued and culminated in the publication of his classic triad, *Back Pain* (Mennell, 1960), *Joint Pain* (Mennell, 1964), and *Foot Pain* (Mennell, 1964). Mennell's basic idea of motion palpation was that a normal joint possessed a characteristic "joint play," which he defined as the involuntary motion that was possible at the end of the normal range of passive motion. Normal joint function was evidenced by normal joint play. A student of Mennell's, Bourdillon (1970), became somewhat more eclectic in his concepts of palpation. Not strictly adhering to the joint play concept, he described restricted movement and excess muscle tension as indicators for manipulative therapy.

Among the other contributors to the development of motion palpation, Robert Maigne (Maigne, 1960) discussed reversible "intervertebral derangement," which could be detected by, among other means, passive and active motion testing. Maigne is perhaps best known for his concept of manipulation into the direction of no pain. Others in the field of medical manipulative therapy, such as Lewit (1985), Crisp (1960), and Dvorak (1984), also contributed varying concepts of motion palpation. In summary, our current understanding of motion palpation developed from the work of Gillet, with contributions from Illi (pelvic and sacroiliac motion), Mennell (loss of joint play), and Cyriax (hard and soft end-feels).

One of Gillett's major contributions was his insistence that bones did not physically "subluxate" in the sense implied by the original static concepts of Palmer. Rather, he noted that most frequently spinal joints would be found to lack the proper subjective degree of motion. Thus, he coined the term "fixation" to describe these palpatory sensations. Gillet intended to distinguish the static misalignment (subluxation) from the kinetic dysfunction (fixation), the latter being more commonly found than the former. Because soft tissues also can be involved in spinal dysfunction, Gillet further divided fixations into muscular, ligamentous, articular, and bony subcategories.

Muscular fixations are at one end of the "fixation continuum," and these represent a disturbance of vertebral motion that occurs in the presence of muscular hypertonicities without structural changes (such as ligamentous shortening). At the end of the passive range of motion of a joint with a muscular fixation, a soft "rubbery" sensation is palpated (Faye and Shafer, 1989). A chronic muscular fixation may lead, in turn, to shortening of related ligaments (probably due to a chronic state of hypokinesia). These, when palpated at the end of the normal passive range of motion, produce a more abrupt (or "hard") sensation. Such a fixation represents the "ligamentous fixation" in Gillet's continuum. Next in this continuum is the articular fixation, the most common type of joint dysfunction, that is said to occur after chronic joint hypokinesia and ligamentous shortening. The nature of intra-articular blockage or fixation is not entirely understood, and may represent a functional state, or may be associated with a structural lesion such as an intra-articular fat mass. Finally, to complete the continuum, Gillet described the "bony fixation" that, in essence, is ankylosis. This type of lesion is not amenable to manipulation therapy and is primarily of diagnostic importance before any other anticipated manipulative therapy.

Motion Palpation Research

Research into palpation methods can be divided into three groups.

1. Spinal palpation and findings in patients with visceral complaints (Nicholas et al., 1985; Rosero et al., 1987; Tarr et al., 1987, are examples).
2. Spinal palpation and findings in patients with somatic complaints (Brunarski, 1982; Thabe, 1986; Jull et al., 1988, are examples).
3. Palpation itself, in terms of interexaminer and intraexaminer reliability, sensitivity, and specificity. This is the area of study that is discussed below.

There are various questions that arise from research into motion palpation of the spine. First, to what extent do palpation methods exhibit specificity; that is, how accurate are they at determining what a normal spine is? Second, to what extent is motion palpation sensitive; that is, able to determine a manipulable lesion. Unfortunately, the specificity of motion palpation has not been clearly established. Wiles (1980)

found sacroiliac motion palpation testing to have high specificity using student subjects. But Brunarski (1982) later found this not to be the case using subjects with low back pain, although his findings do suggest a high degree of sensitivity. Possible differences in the palpation techniques of individual practitioners may account for the differences in results, because the same kind of conflicting results have been found in regards to interexaminer correlation.

Interexaminer correlation is the degree that results correspond between one examiner and another, using the same patient. It is important that the appropriate statistical method is used if a correlational study is being done. Some studies have determined high levels of interexaminer agreement, but this does not necessarily imply high levels of correlation. For example, two examiners may agree 60% of the time. The 40% of disagreements, however, may be extreme differences, thus resulting in a very low overall correlation. Coefficient of correlation, rather than percent agreement is a much better measure of the degree of relationship between two variables. Wiles (1980), Carmichael (1987), Johnston (1976, 1983), and Bergstom (1986) have all demonstrated significant levels of interexaminer correlation, whereas Love and Brodeur (1987) failed to demonstrate significant correlation levels. Love and Brodeur did, however, find significant intraexaminer correlation in their study, and they commented that these findings may indicate differences in individual palpation techniques. Carmichael (1987) also found motion palpation techniques to have significant intraexaminer reliability. In a physiotherapy study of motion examination of the lumbar spine, Jull and Bullock (1987) found high levels of reliability in the lumbar spine. However, others such as Keating, Boline, and Mootz have not found this level of confidence in reliability (Boline et al., 1988; Keating and Boline, 1988; Keating, 1989; Mootz et al., 1989).

The importance of individual technique (the "art" of motion palpation) as an interfering variable in research, or as a factor influencing the reliability of findings has been mentioned (Wiles, 1980; Love and Brodeur, 1987; Jull et al., 1988). This factor further clouds research efforts into these methods and demonstrates the great difficulty of using scientific methods to study a diagnostic method that is highly dependent on a practitioner's experience and technique. Although Keating has rightly indicated the paucity of scientific endorsement of motion palpation, nevertheless, there remains numerous data implying the usefulness and reliability of this type of examination in manipulation science (Jull and Bullock, 1987; Carmichael, 1987; Boline et al., 1988)

Some further interesting issues have arisen from

studies into palpation techniques. There is some indication that static evaluation of the spine may be more reliable than motion evaluation (Johnston, 1983; DeBoer et al., 1985) This is perhaps not surprising given the less complete palpatory cues resulting from static analysis and the easier standardization of static palpation protocol. Furthermore, DeBoer et al., (1985) found that static palpation was more reliable in an area of the spine (midcervical) where motion palpation was found not to be reliable. Also, the reliability of static palpation was not found to be as experience dependent (Johnston et al., 1983) as motion palpation. In summary, research findings can be found to show that motion palpation is sensitive; that it is specific (although some controversy exists); that it demonstrates inter- and intraexaminer reliability; that experience may be important; and that adding static analysis to a motion examination may yield more significantly reliable findings.

As more research is done in this area, we will likely be able to determine exactly how best to examine manually the motion of vertebral segments to reliably determine the need for manipulation. The ''art forms'' of palpation will have to be addressed in future research in this area. There are currently so many variables and so many conflicting results in the study of motion palpation that each new study seems to only complicate our understanding of these methods. Perhaps, as Mootz (1989) suggested, we should determine which techniques possess the most desirable characteristics and pursue these techniques further, to refine them and thereby provide future researchers with examination techniques as close to a gold standard as science applied to art can produce.

Definition and Classification of Palpation Techniques

Palpation is the use of the tactile senses to determine variations in tissue consistence to recognize whether these variations are normal or abnormal. During palpation, the practitioner senses variations in temperature, shape and contour, textures, resistance, and motion. Palpation is usually conducted with a light, medium, or deep touch, using the pads of the fingertips. The patient is observed for facial winces, questioned as to the presence of pain, and if pain is severe, is heard reacting. The latter being the most severe ''audibilized pain.''

There are two basic classifications of manual palpation, static and dynamic. Static palpation reveals both objective and subjective information. The examiner must be proficient in identifying bony landmarks, the origin and insertion of palpable muscles and tendons, and the region of a ligament or meniscus. Static palpation determines abnormal texture, temperature, contour, and tenderness of the tissues in question.

Static examination of the spine begins as the examiner glides his or her hands over the patient's bare skin from occiput to sacrum, noting any warm spots or swellings, hard nodules, raised areas of muscles in spasm, cold moist areas, or any other abnormal signs. This examination can be conducted with the patient sitting or prone on the examination table. With the patient prone, the following muscles can be palpated:

1. Suboccipital muscles
2. Posterior cervical muscles
3. Trapezius muscles
4. Shoulder girdle muscles
5. Thoracic paraspinal muscles, especially near the rib heads
6. Lumbar paraspinal muscles, especially near the quadratus lumborum, making sure to follow both bundles
7. Multifidus and other posterior lumbosacral muscles, including the posterior pelvic musculature over the hip joint

The location and significance of trigger points are fully discussed elsewhere in this text. However, one should make special notation of hyperesthetic spinous processes during the overall screening of the posterior spinal musculature.

The anterior cervical musculature is best palpated with the patient sitting or supine. The examiner supports the supine patient's neck and head with one hand while gliding the thumb down the sternocleidomastoideus muscle, scalenus muscle, and other anterior cervical muscles from superior to inferior, making note of painful, spastic areas.

Palpation of resistance is conducted for different purposes and, therefore, different techniques are employed. The prone springing tests are a variation of basic orthopedic tests. The examiner stands to one side of the prone patient and, using the thumbs, pushes the spinous processes laterally away from the midline. This normal capsular end-feel is ''springy'' and painless. Two findings are possible. First, very painful foraminal compression may occur on the near side, with increased radiation of radicular pain. Second, marked resistance to lateral movement may occur with local sharp pain that does not linger after the pressure is relieved. The first response may indicate a neurological compromise and/or an inflamed joint. The second response may indicate a joint dysfunction fixation.

The classic method of static palpation attempts

to determine if the spinous process is to the right or left of the vertebral midline. Motion palpation, on the other hand, is employed to determine:

1. Normal active range of motion
2. Hypermobile or aberrant motion
3. Capsular end-feel

Strictly speaking, motion palpation techniques only encompass the first two purposes. Determining capsular end-feel is properly designated as fixation palpation. The clinical significance of capsular end-feel is important enough that most examiners using motion palpation include it in practice.

Motion palpation methods are well described by Grice and his colleagues. Their method of upper cervical palpation is also shown in a text by Vernon. Fixation palpation was described originally by Gillet and Leikens, and motion palpation of the extremities was very well described by J. Mennell, M.D. More recently, a complete text of motion palpation of the spine and extremities has been authored by Faye and Schafer (1989).

Motion palpation methods are used to determine the joints in dysfunction and the specific direction of motion loss. The level of joint dysfunction and the direction in which the joint fails to function determine the level of the manipulation and the line of drive of a manipulation force. The manipulation is usually directed into the resistance. It is essential, therefore, to predetermine if the resistive segment is amendable to manipulation and that the resistance is not due to a pathology that would be further exacerbated by the adjustive force. As a general rule, if pressing into the resistance causes pain that disappears immediately after the pressure is released, then a manipulation is likely to be safe. (Faye and Schafer, 1989) If pain persists for a minute or so after removing the pressure of palpation, then the examiner should consider the existence of pathology that warrants further diagnostic work-up.

Description of Palpation Techniques

Initially, a quick scan of the whole spine and pelvis is performed to determine which spinal levels require a thorough specific examination. A quick scan can be conducted with the patient sitting on a stool or on the examination table, with the examiner sitting behind the patient. (Fig. 19–1) The examiner's left hand and elbow rests gently across the patient's shoulders and holds the patient in a neutral sitting posture. This elbow, hand contact is used to guide the patient from neutral into slight flexion and extension during

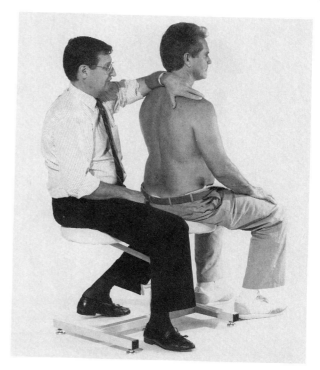

Figure 19–1. The classic motion palpation position with the stabilizing arm clasping the patient's shoulder girdle. (*Courtesy L. J. Faye and M.P.I.*)

the scan. The examiner coordinates the use of the back of his or her hand to gently and rhythmically jiggle the patient into alternate mild flexion and extension to determine the levels of fixation or resistance. In a normal spine all levels jiggle from neutral to a very slight extension and back to neutral and forward to a very slight flexion easily. Figures 19–2, 19–3, and 19–4 demonstrate the hand position for springing the sacrum and the sacroiliac joints. Figures 19–5, 19–6, 19–7, and 19–8 show the hand position for the palpation quick scan of the lumbar and thoracic motion units. Figure 19–8 is specific for the upper thoracic area. Figure 19–9 shows the cervical quick scan position of the examiner's hands. The patient can also be placed prone on the table, and the palm of the examiner's hand used to spring the spine from the sacroiliac joints up to the base of the cervical spine. Then, using the thumb and index finger, the examiner palpates the cervical region to determine where there is marked resistance to the springing movement. These nonspecific methods are very useful in quickly pinpointing levels of fixation. These areas of fixation do not necessarily coincide with the levels of the inflamed joints that are causing the patient's symptoms.

More recently, the development of passive motion chiropractic adjusting tables have made it possible to quickly scan spinal motion while the patient is

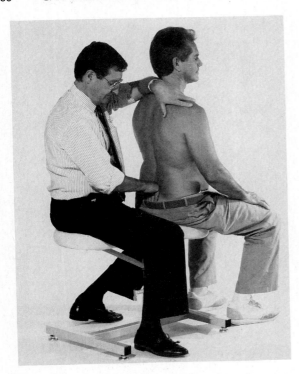

Figure 19-2. Technique for springing the sacrum. (*Courtesy L. J. Faye and M.P.I.*)

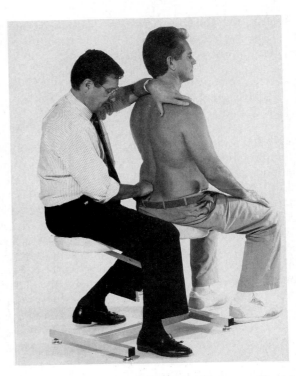

Figure 19-4. Technique for springing the left sacroiliac joint. (*Courtesy L. J. Faye and M.P.I.*)

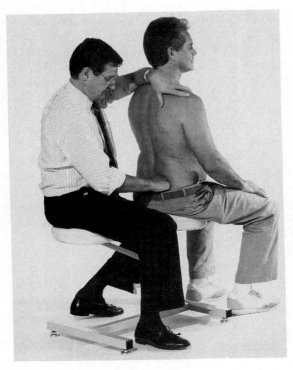

Figure 19-3. Technique for springing the right sacroiliac joint. (*Courtesy L. J. Faye and M.P.I.*)

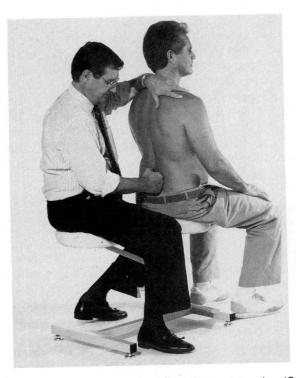

Figure 19-5. Technique for springing the lumbar spine. (*Courtesy L. J. Faye and M.P.I.*)

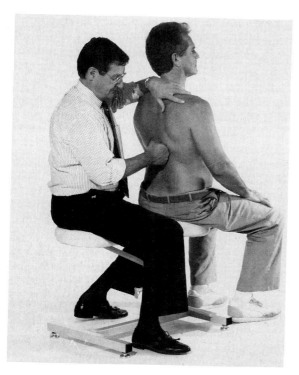

Figure 19-6. Technique for springing the thoracolumbar junction. (*Courtesy L. J. Faye and M.P.I.*)

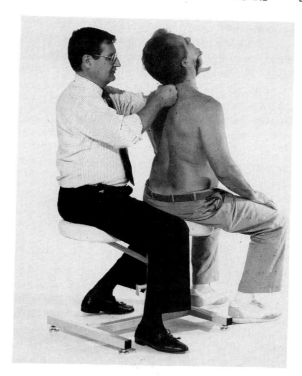

Figure 19-8. Technique for springing the upper thoracic spine. (*Courtesy L. J. Faye and M.P.I.*)

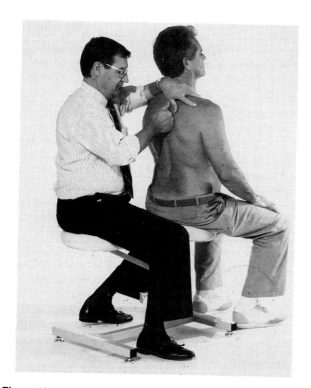

Figure 19-7. Technique for springing the midthoracic spine. (*Courtesy L. J. Faye and M.P.I.*)

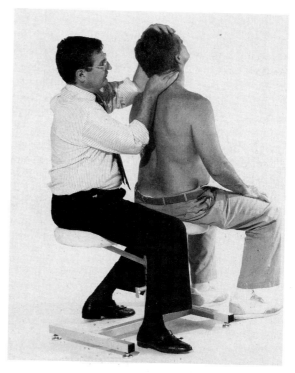

Figure 19-9. Technique for springing the cervical spine. (*Courtesy L. J. Faye and M.P.I.*)

being mechanically distracted through the flexion of the pelvis and legs. During the down-stroke of these tables the spine is elongating intersegmentally along its Y-axis. The examiner can then spring the spine with the palm of his or her hand to see if there is freedom of movement. The interspinous spaces can also be palpated during this action to determine whether or not they are widening during the Y-axis distraction. Once the areas of dysfunction are determined it is then necessary to carry out specific palpation procedures.

Sacroiliac Palpation

The examiner sits behind the standing patient who is able to steady him or herself by placing one hand on a window sill or chair back. Next, the examiner palpates the right or left posterior superior iliac spine (PSIS) and the first sacral tubercle. These are palpation points used to determine motion in the upper sacroiliac joints. To determine if there is motion in the right upper sacroiliac joint, the examiner's left thumb is placed on the first tubercle of the sacrum and the right thumb on the right PSIS. The patient is then asked to raise his or her right leg while bending the knee so the thigh is horizontal to the floor (Faye and Schafer, 1989). During the knee-raising motion (especially at the end range of motion of full flexion of the hip joint) the examiner's right thumb should travel inferior as it follows the right PSIS. There should be very little motion of the sacrum during this action. The examiner then places his or her left thumb on the patient's left PSIS and the right thumb on the first tubercle of the sacrum. The patient is then asked to raise his or her bent left leg while flexing the hip until the thigh is parallel with the floor. The left PSIS should travel much more inferiorly than the first spinous process of the sacrum. If the examiner's thumb on the patient's left PSIS does not move considerably inferior to the examiner's thumb on the first tubercle during this hip flexion action, then it may be assumed that the gliding motion of the innominate bone of the sacrum has not occurred and a fixation is present. By way of comparison, normal motion causes the PSIS to become much more prominent as hip flexion is occurring.

To determine if the innominate bone can extend freely against the sacrum, the examiner palpates the right PSIS and the first tubercle of the sacrum as the patient swings his or her right leg posteriorly. During this action the PSIS becomes much less prominent as the examiner's thumb travels anteriorly with the PSIS. Innominate bone extension can also be determined by having the patient flex his or her left leg while the examiner palpates the right PSIS and the

first sacral tubercle. In this case as the left hip flexes, there should be little movement of the sacrum until the thigh becomes parallel with the floor. At that point, there should be a very slight inferior motion of the first sacral tubercle, indicating proper flexion gliding of the sacrum against the stationary weight-bearing innominate bone.

These tests are repeated on the left side. Tests of both sides must be conducted for the upper sacroiliac joint to be considered free to consequentially participate with the hip flexion and extension that occurs during ambulation.

Similar tests are used to detect gliding motion and extension of the lower portion of the sacroiliac joint. The examiner's right thumb is placed on the most inferior part of the right innominate bone, just opposite the sacroiliac joint, and the left thumb is placed on the sacrum just opposite the most inferior part of the right sacroiliac joint. The patient is asked to flex the right knee until the thigh is parallel with the floor. The examiner's right thumb should move inferiorly with the most inferior part of the right innominate bone. The patient is then asked to either extend the left leg to allow palpation of extension or the patient is asked to lift the left leg to see whether or not there is sacral movement against the right innominate bone as the left thigh becomes parallel to the floor. Once again, the thumbs are moved so that the left thumb is on the left innominate bone just opposite the most inferior border of the sacroiliac joint, and the right thumb is moved over to the sacrum, just opposite the most inferior border of the left sacroiliac joint. The patient is then asked to flex his or her left knee to determine if the left lower joint can move during hip flexion. Extension of the lower portion of the sacroiliac joint is checked on the left side either by having the the patient extend his or her left leg or by flexing his or her right hip.

To determine if there is sacroiliac joint play movement, the patient rests on his or her right side while flexing the left hip so that the left foot is behind the right knee. To palpate the left sacroiliac joint, the examiner places his or her right index or middle finger over the left sacroiliac joint space and using the left hand, presses the patient's left knee toward the floor. If this knee pressure leverage causes a slight palpable separation and widening of the left sacroiliac joint space, then there is normal joint play movement. This process is reversed to test the right sacroiliac joint, with the patient lying on his or her left side while flexing the right hip so that the right foot is behind the left knee, with the left leg out straight. The examiner's left index or middle finger is placed over the right sacroiliac joint space. Using the right hand, the examiner pushes the right knee toward the floor to see whether or not the right sacroiliac joint space gaps or separates, as it should when there is normal joint play.

It should be noted that these two techniques are a combination of motion palpation and fixation palpation. The standing procedure determines whether or not the innominate bone is gliding on the sacrum during flexion and extension of the hip joint and whether or not the sacrum is gliding against the innominate bone on the opposite side. The recumbent procedure is used to determine whether or not there is truly fixation of the joint, specifically the loss of joint play.

A third method of sacroiliac palpation that is becoming quite popular is conducted while the patient lies prone on a continuous passive motion motorized adjusting table. During Y-axis distraction of the pelvic flexion phase, the examiner palpates the sacroiliac joint space to see whether or not motion is occurring. This joint can also be palpated during the action phase of the mechanical table, when lateral flexion of the trunk has been introduced. This gives information as to whether or not there is sacroiliac joint separation occurring as a result of the trunk movement.

Motion Palpation of the Lumbar Spine

The lumbar spine can rotate around all three axes. These movements are referred to as forward flexion, backward extension, right lateral flexion, left lateral flexion, left body rotation, and right body rotation. During these actions there are accompanying coupled and translation motions. The lumbar spine can be placed at the limit of each of these ranges of motion and then sprung or pushed to detect whether or not there is a springy end-feel. It is not possible to determine whether it is the lack of coupled motion or the lack of rotation that is the cause of the loss of motion. However, if manipulative forces are applied in the direction of the loss of motion, the restricting factor will be diminished and increased ranges of motion will occur.

Lumbar Flexion Palpation

To palpate flexion in the lumbar spine, the examiner sits behind the patient (also seated) with his or her left elbow over the patient's left shoulder and the forearm extended so that the left hand can clasp the patient's right trapezius musculature (Fig. 19–10). The patient is asked to flex forward and is guided into full forward flexion. The examiner's right thumb is placed between the lumbar spinous processes to determine whether or not the interspinous space is widening as the spinous processes separate. Using this technique, the examiner systematically palpates

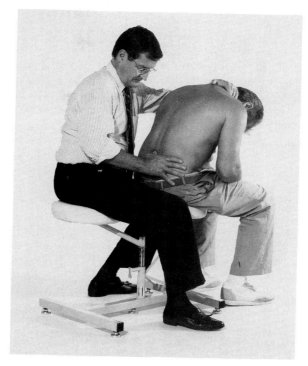

Figure 19–10. Lumbar motion palpation of interspinous separation during flexion. (*Courtesy L. J. Faye and M.P.I.*)

between the spinous processes, with the patient flexing forward each time on each occasion the examiner's thumb pushes against the superior spinous process of the motion unit being palpated. This spinous "push" is used to determine if there is a springy end-feel. It is important to center the flexion at the motion unit being palpated. This testing procedure not only determines if the interspinous soft tissue is allowing the interspinous space to separate, but also determines whether the superior facet is gliding on the inferior facet during flexion of the lumbar spine.

Lumbar Extension Palpation

Extension of the lumbar spine occurs with two distinct motions. First, compress or telescope together the zygopophyseal joints in extension (Fig. 19–11). Once this has occurred, a fulcrum is formed, and further hyperextension occurs because of opening of the disc spaces anteriorly. The lumbar bodies separate because they are not restricted by the anterior ligaments and other soft tissues. For this reason, palpation of the lumbar spinal extension occurs in two separate sequences. To palpate zygopophyseal extension, the thumb at the palpating hand is placed beside the spinous process (Fig. 19–11). Using an elbow placed over the patient's shoulder, the patient is drawn backward into extension. The palpating thumb, pushing toward the anterior, should not

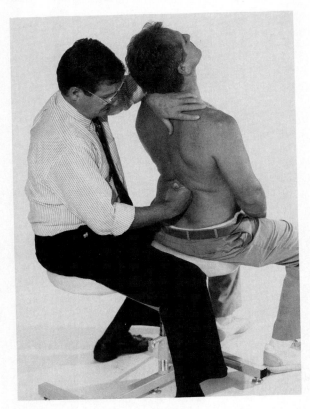

Figure 19–11. Lumbar hyperextension palpation showing thumb reinforcement. (*Courtesy L. J. Faye and M.P.I.*)

meet a restrictive resistance. It should be able to spring easily into the lumbar spine. Although the palpating thumb is a couple of inches away from the zygopophyseal joint, joint movement can be easily determined. The same action is repeated on the other side of the spinous process. Once this early motion component is palpated, the patient's spine is guided into hyperextension, and pushed with greater force to see whether or not the intervertebral joint space will open anteriorly. The second phase of extension palpation is conducted like the first, however, the thumb supports the index and middle finger as it presses over the interspinous space. These reinforced fingers act as a fulcrum for this movement.

Lumbar Rotation Palpation
While sitting behind the seated patient, the examiner places his or her left elbow over the patient's left shoulder and clasps the patient's right trapezius muscle with his or her left hand. Next, the examiner rotates the patient to the left, trying to produce as little lateral flexion of the spine as possible (Fig. 19–12). Lumbar spinal rotation to the left may be reinforced by using the right thumb to press against the left side of the spinous process or to push anteriorly against

the right side. In either case, the examiner palpates for a springy end-feel at the limit of left spinal rotation. This left-rotation procedure is repeated for each lumbar segment.

Next, right lumbar spinal rotation is tested. The examiner reverses position, placing his or her right elbow over the patient's right shoulder while grasping the patient's left trapezius with his or her left hand. The patient is guided in rotation to the right, and the examiner uses his or her left thumb to reinforce lumbar spinal rotation by pressing against the right side of the spinous process or by pushing anteriorly on the left. Again, the examiner palpates for springy end-feel of each lumbar segment tested.

Lumbar Lateral Flexion Palpation
To palpate left lateral flexion, the examiner's left elbow is placed on the patient's left shoulder while clasping the patient's right trapezius muscle with his or her left hand. The examiner places the pad of his or her right thumb against the spinous process, with the body of the thumb *pointing toward the patient's head*. The examiner's fingers are pointed to the right side of the spine, *parallel with the floor*. Using the right thumb as a fulcrum, the examiner bends the patient's trunk laterally to the left without rotation; centering the force at the level of the thumb and spinous process of the motion unit that is being palpated (Fig. 19–13). At full left lateral flexion, the ex-

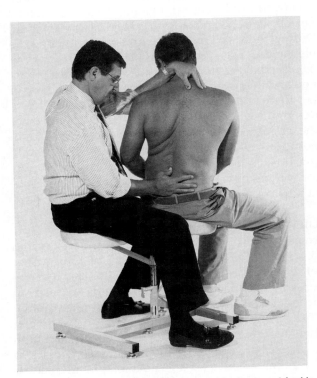

Figure 19–12. Lumbar rotation palpation. Springy end-feel is tested from this point. (*Courtesy L. J. Faye and M.P.I.*)

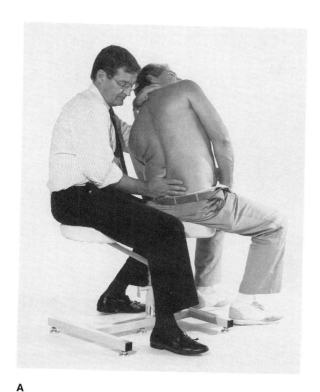

A

Figure 19–13. A. Left lateral flexion palpation of the lumbar spine. Both motion palpation and spring end-feel are determined by this technique. (*Courtesy L. J. Faye and M.P.I.*) **B.** Leander mechanical traction treatment table.

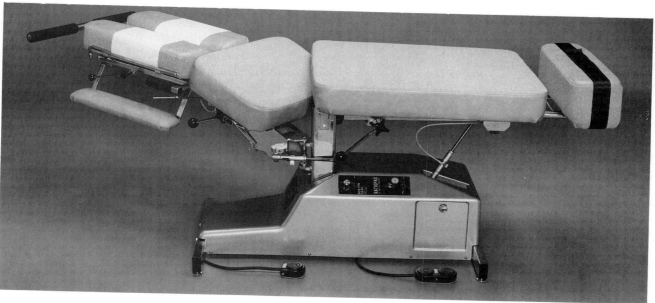

B

aminer pushes with his or her thumb on the spinous process to determine whether or not the motion unit has a springy end-feel.

Next, right lateral flexion is tested. The examiner places his or her right elbow on the patient's right shoulder while clasping the patient's left trapezius muscle with his or her right hand. This time the pad of the left thumb palpates the right side of the spinous process of the lumbar vertebra being challenged. The examiner flexes the patient's trunk laterally to the right, making sure there is no spinal rotation. At the end of right lateral flexion, the left thumb actively pushes against the spinous process to determine whether or not there is a springy end-feel. The Leander mechanical traction treatment table (Fig. 19–13B) has a laterally flexing head and torso unit

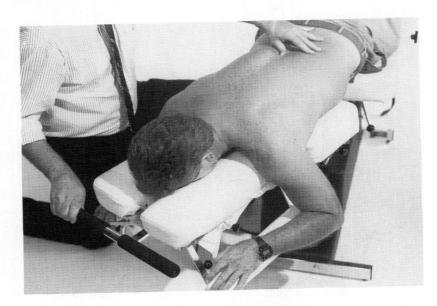

Figure 19–14. Motion palpation in the prone position during right lateral flexion. The spinous process should move to the left and have a springy end-feel. (*Courtesy L. J. Faye and M.P.I.*)

and is an excellent tool for palpating lateral flexion dysfunction (Faye and Schafer, 1989). While the patient is lying prone on this table and the pelvis and leg piece is producing distraction by flexing, it is possible to flex simultaneously and laterally the torso while trapping the spinous process with the thumb or index finger of the palpating hand.

Motion Palpation Y-Axis Distraction on a Mobile Adjusting Table

With the use of a mobile adjusting table, Dr. Leander Eckard has demonstrated during lectures that many low back conditions are complicated by failure of the disc spaces to separate. Motion x-ray studies during Y-axis distraction show disc spaces separating and an examiner's palpating index finger or thumb can actually make a deeper impression between the spinous processes. In the case of Y-axis distraction fixation, x-ray motion studies show two vertebrae locked together without any movement of the joint space. This loss of movement can be palpated as a failure of the interspinous space to separate while the table is applying distraction (Fig. 19–15).

These mobile adjusting tables make it possible to palpate rotation, lateral flexion, and Y-axis translation. It should be noted, however, that because the patient is prone, lateral flexion causes the spinous process to rotate toward the convexity, not toward the concavity as it does in sitting motion palpation.

Motion Palpation of the Thoracic Spine

The thoracic spine is more complicated to palpate than the lumbar spine. At some levels there are costotransverse joints and costovertebral joints, as well as the zygopophyseal joints. For thoracic motion units to move in their normal ranges of flexion, extension, right and left lateral flexion, and right and left body rotation, it is necessary for the costotransverse joints to be fully mobile. The costovertebral joints are rarely in dysfunction and would appear to seldom interfere with the thoracic motion unit. Because the costotransverse joints are commonly involved in thoracic motion unit dysfunction, the examiner should pay particular attention to these joints during the motion palpation routine of the thoracic spine. It is extremely important that the palpator recognize the natural resistance due to the stabilizing factor of the ribs and the costotransverse joints. This increased stiffness of the thorax often leads to palpation errors that are not made in the cervical or lumbar regions.

From a clinical point of view the upper thoracic spine may also be the cause of biomechanical insults to the lower and midcervical spine. The lower thoracic spine, especially the thoracolumbar junction, may be the cause of lower lumbar biomechanical insult. It is for these reasons that full motion palpation examination of the sacroiliac, lumbar, thoracic, and cervical areas of the spine should be conducted in the initial workup of a patient, even if the patient is complaining of pain in only one area of the spine.

Thoracic Flexion Palpation

To palpate flexion of a thoracic motion unit, the examiner sits behind the patient with one arm draped over the patient's shoulder and with the thumb of the palpating hand placed between the spinous processes. Controlling and centering flexion at the level of the thumb between the spinous processes, the examiner draws the patient's spine through a series of short flexion movements. By continually raising the

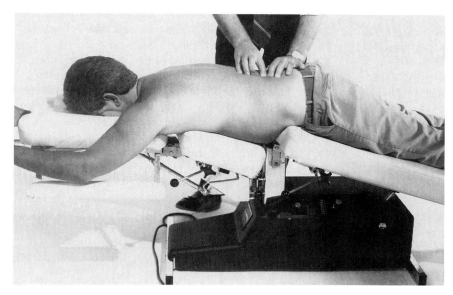

Figure 19-15. Y-axis distraction palpation. The interspinous space opens and closes with each stroke of the motorized table. Note the lumbar spine is in its normal lordosis due to dropped abdominal section. (*Courtesy L. J. Faye and M.P.I.*)

level at which flexion occurs, it is possible to determine whether or not the interspinous space is enlarging as the spinous processes separate on flexion. These actions are repeated from the interspinous space between L-1 and T-12 up to the space between T1-2. As noted earlier, it may be difficult to mechanically stress or push on the spine to elicit springy endfeel at all levels.

Thoracic Extension Palpation

To palpate thoracic extension the examiner's arm is draped over the patient's shoulder while sitting behind the seated patient. The patient's back is pushed in a series of extension moves from neutral to extension using the back of the palpating hand. Specifically, the examiner presses his or her thumb first to the right side and then to the left side of the spinous process while guiding the patient into extension. To determine if there is anterior separation of the thoracic motion units the patient is placed into hyperextension by using more force. This is achieved by pushing against a thoracic spinous process with the fingers supported by the thumb (Fig. 19–16). To get sufficient leverage for these maneuvers in the upper thoracic region, the patient is asked to interlock his or her fingers behind the neck and place the elbows close together in front of the chin. Using the non-palpating hand placed under both elbows, the examiner raises and lowers the patient's elbows like a pump handle (Fig. 19–16). With the palpating hand, the examiner determines whether or not extension is occurring at the posterior joints.

Thoracic Rotation Palpation

Assuming the standard palpating position, (see Fig. 19–1), the patient is rotated to the right and then to

the left using the thumb of the palpation hand either to spring the spinous processes into further rotation or to palpate laterally to the spinous process while pushing forward. It is important to prevent lateral flexion of the thoracic spine.

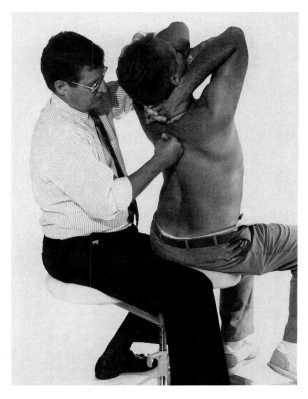

Figure 19-16. Motion palpation of the thoracic spine showing extra leverage using patient's arm. (*Courtesy L. J. Faye and M.P.I.*)

Costotransverse Joint Palpation

During motion palpation of the costotransverse joints, the examiner slides his or her palpating hand laterally away from the spinous process until it contacts the tubercle of the rib (Fig. 19–17). The examiner reaches around the front of the patient with the nonpalpating arm, resting the biceps in front of the patient's shoulder, and grasps behind the contralateral shoulder to rotate the patient's thorax. Because of the double leverage this position affords, the examiner can introduce extreme rotation to the thoracic spine. At the end of rotation, the palpating thumb springs the rib. If the rib has not glided at the costotransverse joint, the rib palpates as much more prominent than a mobile rib, and the challenging motion is usually extremely painful to the patient. This pain is typical in that it does not linger once the challenge has been relieved.

Starting from the lowest of the costotransverse joints, the examiner systematically palpates each rib up to the second rib. The examiner then reverses position, systematically palpating the opposite ribs from inferior to superior.

To palpate the right first costotransverse joint, the examiner places his or her right index finger into the triangular space just in front of the trapezius muscle and just behind the clavicle to make contact

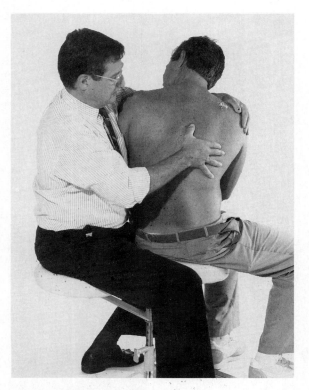

Figure 19–17. Right costotransverse joint motion palpation showing shoulder leverage for controlling thoracic rotation. (*Courtesy L. J. Faye and M.P.I.*)

with the first rib. Once this contact is established, the examiner guides the patient's head through extension, and contralateral (left) rotation with the nonpalpating hand. At the end of this cervical motion, it should be extremely difficult to palpate the first rib. If the first rib remains palpable, springing this rib will elicit a nonspringy, hard end-feel, and typically the patient will experience great discomfort.

Costovertebral Joint Palpation

Currently there is no method of palpating the costovertebral joint. Costovertebral joint dysfunction typically produces a deep thoracic pain. This pain usually subsides after manipulation of the thoracic spine along the long axis of the rib at the affected level. It is assumed that this manipulation facilitates costovertebral joint mobility.

Y-Axis Translation Thoracic Spine Palpation

To palpate the Y-axis thoracic translation, it is necessary to use a mobile treatment table that causes distraction. As with the lumbar spine, the examiner palpates the interspinous separation in the thoracic region as the table is in the downstroke (Fig. 19–18).

Motion Palpation of the Cervical Spine

Motion palpation of the cervical spine is divided into two procedures. The first procedure tests the biomechanics of the upper cervical region, which consists of the joints between the atlas and the occiput and the atlas and the axis. The second procedure of cervical palpation is used to examine the mid and lower cervical joints. The joints of luschka influence lateral cervical flexion and may also influence anterior-to-posterior cervical rotation and flexion. These poorly understood joints will not be covered further here, but one must assume that they do get manipulated during cervical manipulation.

Upper Cervical Palpation

The upper cervical spine is palpated to determine if there is atlanto-occipital joint movement. Sitting behind the patient, as in Figure 19–19, the examiner's thumb and index finger of the palpating hand are placed under the right and left rims of the occiput, putting pressure on the suboccipital musculature. With the stabilizing hand placed on the patient's forehead, the examiner guides the patient's head to produce cervical flexion, extension, lateral flexion, and rotation. During these movements, the examiner senses whether or not there is freedom of motion or tension in the suboccipital region. Often, this

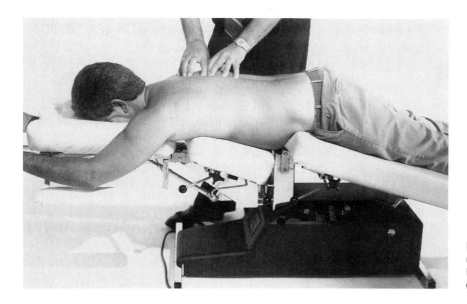

Figure 19-18. Y-axis translation of thoracic spine is palpated during neutral long axis extension on motorized table. (*Courtesy L. J. Faye and M.P.I.*)

general scan of the upper cervical region will produce great discomfort to the patient and evoke referred pain in the head, ears, behind the eyes or into the neck. More specifically, the examiner palpates to determine if there is anterior-to-posterior and posterior-to-anterior rotation of the occiput on the atlas. The examiner should also palpate anterior and posterior occipital glide on the masses (Fig. 19–20) and whether or not there is a springy joint play

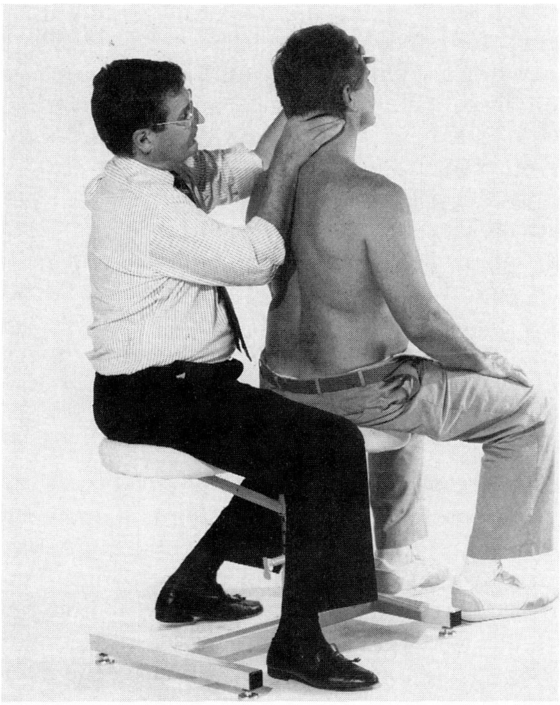

Figure 19-19. Motion palpation of the upper cervical region, general appreciation. (*Courtesy L. J. Faye and M.P.I.*)

movement or lateral flexion of the occiput on the atlas.

Upper Cervical Rotation Palpation. Gillet reported a sequence of events that should occur. The examiner places the palpating middle finger on the tip of the transverse process of the atlas and the palpating index finger on the anterior of the mastoid process and rotates the head from posterior to anterior on the side of palpation. If the occiput rotates freely on the atlas, the mastoid will displace the palpating finger from the tip of the transverse process, and maintaining palpation of the tip of the transverse process becomes very difficult. Upon rotating the patient's head from anterior to posterior on the side of palpation, the mandible makes it difficult to continue palpation of the tip of the transverse process of the atlas at the end of the normal range of rotation. Consequently, if on palpating the tip of the transverse process of the atlas during rotation from neutral to anterior or from neutral to posterior, the tip of the transverse process remains palpable, there is a fixation between the atlas and the occiput. This procedure. is conducted both on the left and right sides.

Anterior Glide Palpation—Occiput on Atlas. For this palpation procedure the examiner sits behind the seated patient and places the palpating index or middle finger on the tip of the transverse process very slightly anteriorly (Fig. 19–20). The examiner places the nonpalpating hand with the fingers on top of the head and the palm of the hand over the occiput. The examiner uses the nonpalpating hand to push the cranium forward, making sure that the patient's chin does not rise or lower,

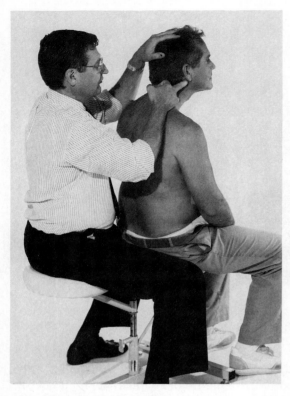

Figure 19–20. Anterior glide movement of occiput on atlas showing chin horizontal. Palpate motion with right finger and end resistance with left hand pushing forward. (*Courtesy L. J. Faye and M.P.I.*)

but travels forward parallel to the floor. The palpating finger should feel the space increase between the anterior tip of the transverse process of the atlas and the mandible. As part of this palpation procedure, it is also important to determine if there is a springy end-feel, which can be detected by the hand pushing on the occiput anteriorly. To summarize, there is a double palpatory finding using this method. The first detects the space widening in front of the tip of the transverse process and the second detects the springy end-feel of the condyle as it travels anteriorly on the atlas. This procedure is conducted on the right and left sides.

Cervical Lateral Flexion Palpation. Although it is questionable whether there is lateral flexion motion of the occiput on the atlas, it is our clinical experience that the joint-play movement of lateral flexion can be very important. To palpate occipital flexion on the atlas, the examiner's palpating finger is placed on the tip of the transverse process of the atlas and the nonpalpating hand is placed on the contralateral side on top of the head. With very gentle lateral flexion of the cranium centered at the palpating finger, the examiner should be able to

evoke either a pain-free springy end-feel of lateral flexion or a clinically significant very painful blocked end-feel. This procedure is repeated on the other side.

Cervical Flexion–Extension Palpation. The anterior glide maneuver previously described is sufficient to determine if flexion and extension is occurring in the atlanto-occipital joints. If one needs further confirmation, the following procedure can be used. With the patient supine, the examiner cups the patient's occiput in both hands with the fingers along the rim of the occiput and guides the patient's chin into full flexion and then full extension. At the end of each range of motion, the examiner senses for a springy end-feel.

Once the atlanto-occipital joints have been palpated, the posterior arch of the atlas is contacted posterolaterly under the rim of the occiput. The palm of the palpating hand faces forward, with the pad of the middle finger positioned under the rim of the occiput and on the posterior arch of the atlas. The examiner's nonpalpating hand cradles the patient's forehead (Fig. 19–21). From this position, the examiner guides the upper cervical region through extension, lateral flexion to the ipsilateral side, and rotation from posterior to anterior. At the end of each range of motion the atlantoaxial joint is palpated for normal springy end-play (see Fig. 19–19).

To palpate for flexion and anterior-to-posterior rotation, the palm of the palpating hand is turned toward the ceiling and the palpating middle finger is slid up in front of the sternocleid-to-mastoid muscle, contacting the anterior tip of the atlas. The examiner then flexes the upper cervical spine by lowering the patient's chin and gently springing posteriorly on the tip of the transverse process. Next, the examiner rotates the patient's head from anterior to posterior on the ipsilateral side, once again springing the tip of the transverse process at the end range of motion. Although this palpation is always likely to produce some pain, when there is a loss of movement in flexion and anterior to posterior rotation, the palpation will produce considerably more pain and no springy end-feel will be noted.

Mid and Lower Cervical Palpation

The mid and lower cervical spine is palpated with the examiner sitting behind the seated patient in the classic fashion. The palm of the palpating hand is turned facing the patient's neck, but is inverted so that the thumb is pointing toward the floor (Fig. 19–21). Palpating from this position uses the tendons for recording resistance, instead of relying only on compression on the pads of the fingers. Cervical motion is guided by the nonpalpating hand, which

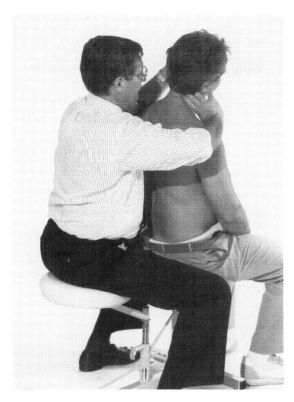

Figure 19–21. Midcervical lateral flexion palpation showing palpation hand, palm forward. (*Courtesy L. J. Faye and M.P.I.*)

gently clasps the patient's forehead. Care should be taken to produce pure movements, as it is very easy to introduce an undesired secondary motion. Two rotations around each axis as well as intersegmental long-axis extension are tested. Rotations around the x-axis are flexion and extension, for example.

Cervical Rotation Palpation—Posterior to Anterior. The palpating middle finger is placed on the articular pillar of C-2. When palpating with the right hand, the left hand turns the patient's head to the left. At the end-range of rotation the examiner pushes the articular pillar forward into further rotation to determine the springy end-feel. Hard, blocked end-feel is an indicator for rotary manipulation at this level. The examiner continues by advancing the palpating finger down one joint at a time, always in line with the articular pillars. Each joint is challenged by repeating the guided rotation first and then pushing further into rotation. Once the lowest cervical level has been tested, the examiner reverses hand positions and repeats the process on the other side.

Cervical Lateral Flexion Palpation. With the patient seated, the examiner assumes the midlower cervical palpation position described earlier as shown in Figure 19–21. Starting on the right articular

pillar at C-2, the examiners' left hand guides the patient's head and neck into lateral flexion, toward the palpating right hand. The palpating hand forms a fulcrum that centers the lateral flexion at the palpation level. The examiner tests end-feel at the limit of lateral flexion. Loss of lateral flexion motion is of great clinical significance. Many of the classic cervical manipulations are aimed at restoring cervical lateral flexion dysfunction. The procedure is repeated at each cervical level and on the other side after the examiner reverses his or her hands.

Cervical Extension Palpation. The same midlower cervical palpation position is used (see Fig. 19–21), only this time the examiner guides the patient's head and neck into extension. The examiner's palpating hand is placed posteriorly on the articular pillar and acts as a fulcrum to assure that extension is centered at the palpation level. Once again, the examiner palpates down the articular pillar at each cervical joint level, challenging each level for springy end-feel. Then, reversing hand positions, the examiner palpates the other side. Cervical extension fixations can be either unilateral or bilateral as with all cervical fixations of a motion unit.

Cervical Flexion Palpation. Palpating for the lack of cervical flexion and the loss of springy end-feel is accomplished with a very light touch. Contrary to the previous midlower cervical palpation procedures, the palpation hand is turned with the palm toward the palpator with the thumb pointing up. Starting at C-2, the examiner slides the pad of the middle finger from the anterior midline until the anterior of the transverse process is contacted. As the examiner's nonpalpating hand guides the patient's head and neck into flexion, the apex of flexion is centered at the palpating finger. Using very gentle pressure, the examiner then pulls backward and superiorly. If flexion is restricted and a hard end-feel is present, a pseudo-doorbell sign may be elicited. The true doorbell sign may not be present when the neck is palpated in the neutral position. As before, flexion palpation should be repeated at each cervical motion unit. The hand positions are then reversed to palpate the other side.

Cervical Rotation Palpation—Anterior to Posterior. The positioning of the patient and the examiner's palpating hand is the same as for flexion palpation. This time, however, the patient's head is rotated from anterior to posterior on the palpating side. The examiner's palpating finger follows the transverse process posteriorly and very gently pulls posteriorly, creating more anterior-to-posterior rotation. On occasions when hard end-feel is detected, the patient will typically experience quite severe pain. The patient may also feel disoriented or nauseous, experience heart palpitations, dyspnea, or other cervical syndrome symptoms. If any of these reactions are elicited, the examiner should not repeat the test on the same side, as it may cause facilitation and irritation of the sympathetic ganglion chain. The examiner should, however, palpate both sides of the neck by reversing the palpation and guiding hands.

Cervical Y-Axis Translation Palpation. The examiner sits at the head of the stationary table with the patient lying supine. The palms of the hands are placed on each side of the patient's neck. With the fingers meeting in the midline, palpate between the spinous processes, from C-7 to C-1 while exerting gentle Y-axis distraction in the cervical spine. If the interspinous space fails to separate, a fixation is present. A very tender interspinous nodule usually is associated with this dysfunction.

Conclusion

Motion palpation is a diagnostic art and subject to many limitations. It should always be a part of a complete spinal analysis and its findings interpreted in the light of all the pertinent facts. Motion palpation skills are refined with experience; only the basic concepts and elementary skills can be learned during chiropractic training. These skills, however, are essential to determine the motion unit to be manipulated, and the direction of a manipulative thrust (Faye and Schafer, 1989).

References

Bergstrom E, and Courtis G. An inter- and intra-examiner reliability study of motion palpation of the lumbar spine in lateral flexion in the seated position. *Europ J Chiropractic* 1986;34:121–141.

Boline PD, Keating J, Brist J, and Denver G. Interexaminer reliability of palpatory evaluations of the lumbar spine. *Am J Chiropractic Med* 1988;1:5–11.

Bourdillon J. *Spinal Manipulation.* New York: Appleton Lange; 1987.

Brunarski D. Chiropractic biomechanical evaluations: validity in myofascial low back pain. *J Manipulative Physiol Ther* 1982; 5:155–161.

Carmichael JC. Inter- and intraexaminer reliability of palpation for sacro-iliac dysfunction. *J Manipulative Physiol Ther* 1987;10:164–171.

Crisp E. Manipulation of the spine. In Licht S, ed. *Massage, Manipulation and Traction.* New York: Krieger; 1960.

Cyriax J. *Textbook of Orthopedic Medicine*, Volume 1, *Diagnosis of Soft Tissue Lesions.* London: Bailliere Tindall; 1982.

DeBoer K, Harmon R, Tuttle C, and Wallace H. Reliability study of detection of somatic dysfunction in the cervical spine. *J Manipulative Physiol Ther* 1985;8:9–15.

Dvorak J, and Dvorak V. *Manual Medicine Diagnostics.* Stuttgart: George Thieme; 1984.

Eckard L. Video and personal correspondence. Port Orchard (Washington): Leander Mfg and Research; date unspecified.

Faye L, and Schafer R. *Motion Palpation and Chiropractic Technic.* Huntington Beach; Motion Palpation Institute; 1989.

Faye L. Video Series, Chiropractic Technique, Dynaspine Inc. Los Angeles.

Gillet H. The history of motion palpation. *European J Chiropractic* 1983;31:196–201.

Gillet H, and Liekens M. *Belgian Chiropractic Research Notes.* Huntington Beach: Motion Palpation Institute; 1984.

Illi F. *The Vertebral Column, Lifeline of the Body.* Chicago: National College of Chiropractic, 1951.

Jirout J. Pattern of changes in the cervical spine in lateroflexion. *Neuroradiol* 1971;1:164.

Johnston WL. Interexaminer reliability in palpation. *JAOA* 1976;76:286–287.

Johnston WL, Allan BR, Hendra JL, et al. Interexaminer study of palpation in detecting the location of spinal segmental dysfunction. *JAOA* 1983;82:839–845.

Jull G, and Bullock M. A motion profile of the lumbarspine in an aging population assessed by manual examination. *Physiotherapy Practice* 1987;3:70–81.

Jull G, Bogduk N, and Marsland A. The accuracy of manual diagnosis for cervical zygapophyseal joint pain. *Med J Australia* 1988; 148:233–236.

Keating JC, and Boline PD: Letter to the editor. *J Manipulative Physiol Ther* 1988;11:443–444.

Keating JC. Interexaminer reliability of motion palpation of the lumbar spine: a review of quantitative literature. *Am J Chiropractic Med* 1989;3:107–110.

Lewit K. *Manipulative Therapy in Rehabilitation of the Motor System.* London: Butterworths; 1985.

Love RM, and Brodeur RR: Inter- and intraexaminer reliability of motion palpation for the thoracolumbar spine. *J Manipulative Physiol Ther* 1987;10:1–4.

Maigne R. *Orthopedic Medicine: A New Approach to Vertebral Manipulations.* Springfield, Il: Charles C. Thomas; 1972.

Mennell JM. *Back Pain.* Boston: Little Brown; 1960.

Mennell JM. *Foot Pain.* Boston: Little Brown; 1964.

Mennell JM. *Joint Pain.* Boston: Little Brown; 1964.

Mootz RD, Keating JC, and Kontz H. Intra- and interobserver reliability of passive motion palpation of the lumbar spine. *J Manipulative Physiol Ther* 1989;12:440–445.

Nicholas AS, DeBias DA, and Ebrenfeuchter W. Somatic component of myocardial infarction. *Br Med J* 1985;291:13–17.

Pauc RA. *The Osseous Anatomy of the Cervical Spine.* Ashford Press; 1982: 78.

Rosero HO, Greene CH, and DeBias DA. Correlation of palpatory observations with the anatomic locus of acute myocardial infarction. *JAOA* 1987;87:118–122.

Sandoz R. Some physical mechanisms and effects of spinal adjustments. *Ann Swiss Chiropractors Assoc* 1976;6:91.

Smith O. *Modernized Chiropractic*, place and publisher unknown, 1906.

Tarr RS, Feely RA, Richardson DL, et al. A controlled study of palpatory diagnostic procedures: assessment of sensitivity and specificity. *JAOA* 1987;87:296–301.

Thabe H. Electromyography as a tool to document diagnostic findings and therapeutic results associated with somatic dysfunctions in the upper cervical spine and sacroiliac joints. *Manual Med* 1986;2:53–58.

Weiant C, and Goldschmidt S. *Medicine and Chiropractic.* New York: J Augustin; 1966.

Wiles MR. Reproducibility and interexaminer correlation of motion palpation findings of the sacro-iliac joint. *J Can Chiropractic Assoc* 1980;24:59–69.

chapter 20

The Use of Instrumentation and Laboratory Examination Procedures by the Chiropractor

John J. Triano
Dennis R. Skogsbergh
Matthew H. Kowalski

In the conduct of patient assessment, the term *instrument* has been used to mean more than laboratory apparatus or hardware devices. Fundamentally, an instrument is a clinical tool that yields a measure. As such it may take on various forms. The intent of this chapter is to portray the essence and utility of different modes of assessment in overview fashion: from questionnaires to research equipment, and from historical implements to the recent technological advances in clinical instrumentation.

Three kinds of measurements give relevant information about patient status or response to treatment. In general, they are: (1) perceptual measurements (e.g., reports of pain severity, satisfaction with lifestyle), (2) functional measurements (e.g., range of motion, strength, activities of daily living) and, (3) physiological measurements (e.g., neurological assessment, serological changes). In clinical practice various instruments can collect information about any of these measurement variables.

Clinical testing has as its primary purpose, the identification and quantification of body structure

319

and function. In elementary fashion, the physician's hands and eyes are the initial testing instruments used to define tissue characteristics, appraise surface contours, recognize landmarks, and estimate temperature. By these same means the examiner judges strength, defines position, and evaluates movements.

The case history coupled with a discerning physical examination typically supplies most of the information from which a diagnosis and prognosis is based. Occasionally, the chief complaint cannot be fully understood by these means alone, and the nature of the disorder is narrowed to three or four possibilities. Alternatively, the patient is placed in a nonspecific diagnostic category. In fact, a specific anatomic cause for spine-related complaints commonly remains unidentified (Bigos and Battie, 1987). In these situations, additional diagnostic efforts are necessary to trim the differential listing and to understand more fully the nature of the involvement. Instrumentation, when properly used, facilitates the confirmation of clinical impressions and helps establish a definitive diagnosis upon which an appropriate treatment plan can be organized.

Instrumentation also can provide evidence of abnormal body function and patient performance that may not coincide with distinguishable morphological lesions. The mere presence of a structural or radiographic abnormality does not necessarily relate it to the cause of the patient's impairment. For example, about half of the asymptomatic population has disk pathology as noted on lumbar computed tomographic (CT) scans (Weisel et al., 1984). There seems to be about an equal prevalence of disc thinning Splithoff, 1953; Lawrence, 1969) and congenital anomalies (Fullenlove and Williams, 1957; Frymoyer et al., 1984) in symptomatic and asymptomatic groups. Circumstances like these create the need for cautious clinical interpretation and correlation of findings.

The principal value of instrumentation lies in its ability to focus on the patient's functional capacity and not on symptoms. It is often possible to quantify some of these parameters and their physiological and biomechanical effects on the body, regardless of the exact nature of the anatomic lesion.

Evaluating Instruments

The test characteristics that determine the clinical utility of any instrument are listed in Table 20–1. Each quality is distinct, but there can be significant interdependence. Focusing on these points simplifies the task of evaluating a prospective device and averts the need to rely on marketing claims and sales representatives for making selections.

Validity is the most clinically important test char-

TABLE 20–1. TEST CHARACTERISTICS DETERMINING CLINICAL USEFULNESS

Validity
Accuracy and precision
Reliability
Discriminability

acteristic. A test is valid when it measures the desired function, and when that function is pertinent to the patient's complaint. For example, it would be invalid to use electromyography (EMG) or thermographic measurements to quantify a patient's pain and suffering, because pain is not measured by them.

The *accuracy* of a measure or test is determined by comparison to a known value. For instance, a weight scale can be checked for accuracy by measuring a known mass and observing how closely the resulting value compares. Repeated use of some devices and the simple effects of passing time may cause loss of calibration. Maintaining accuracy, therefore, depends on regular calibration. The accuracy of an instrument, however, cannot be adjusted beyond its inherent precision.

Precision describes the repeatability of a measure across the range over which it will be used (Fig. 20–1). Accuracy and precision are two key factors that may change over the extent of possible test circumstances (Sirohi and Krishna, 1983; Holma, 1984). To illustrate this concept, consider digitizing an x-ray to determine the degree of scoliosis. If the instrument is only capable of an accurate measure of vertebral motion to within 5 degrees, and the expected intersegmental movement is 7 to 10 degrees, the system will have little clinical value (Triano et al., unpublished data).

The *reliability* of a measure depends not only on the accuracy of the instrument but also the characteristics of the variable being measured. Measurement of human attributes is subject to a large number of error sources. Instrument errors and the specifications under which the results are meaningful should be known. Different instruments are accurate to a greater or lesser degree depending on the range over which they are used, or on the population to be tested. Certainly, the performance characteristics of an instrument determine the range and conditions under which the results they provide can be relied upon. Operator proficiency and judgment, and observer skill or dexterity are other features that may play a decisive role in the reliability of a measurement. As an example, the application of spinal goniometric measurements is no longer considered appropriate for the calculation of physical impairment,

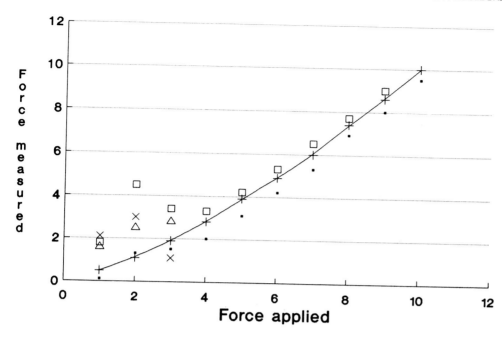

Figure 20–1. A hypothetical plot of force measurements from an instrument that has greater precision for values above 5, which defines its useful range. Multiple measurements for values less than 5 show greater variability and are, therefore, less precise.

because a better instrument, the inclinometer, is now the standard of reliability (Engelberg, 1988).

Inherent errors in instruments are always present. Whether they are important depends on the error behavior and its size in comparison with the magnitude of the function being tested. Two kinds of inherent errors, constant and proportional, are common variables each time a measurement is made, and they depend on how the testing unit is engineered. *Constant errors* remain consistent over the range of the unit's capabilities. As Figure 20–2 shows, the percentage of the measure that is uncer-

tain gets smaller as the size of the measured variable increases. On the other hand, some instruments are constructed with the error being a percentage of the measure, i.e., a *proportional error* (Fig. 20–3). Under these conditions, the area of uncertainty gets larger as the amplitude of the measured variable gets larger.

Does the information obtained from an instrument allow one to distinguish between healthy and unhealthy patients? This characteristic, known as *discrimination*, is determined by referring to a normative data base consisting of studies of people from

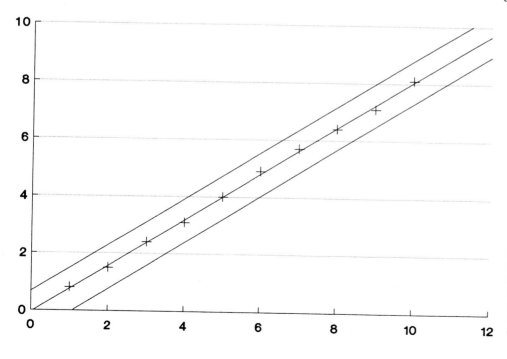

Figure 20–2. Solid lines represent the boundaries of uncertainty for a measurement using an instrument design with a constant range of error. As the measurement value increases, the error percentage decreases.

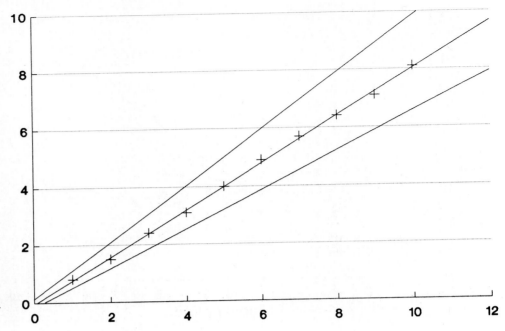

Figure 20–3. Boundaries of uncertainty for a measurement using an instrument design that allows for a fixed error percentage.

both groups. The relative frequency of false-positive (i.e., healthy persons who test positive) and false-negative tests (i.e., unhealthy persons who test negative) occurring for each group also helps to define the test's discriminability. Figure 20–4 shows a hypothetical distribution of test results from healthy and unhealthy subject samples. The cut-off value (X_C) represents the reference point from which clinical judgment is made between healthy and unhealthy subjects. Ideally, a highly discriminating test would have few false-positive and false-negative results.

Finally, it is worth emphasizing that the in-tended application of the test measure determines validity and discriminability. As an example, people who have significant scoliosis tend to have increased paraspinal myoelectric activity on the convex side. However, it would be inappropriate to use measurements of myoelectric activity as a diagnostic indicator of scoliosis for the following reasons. First, the degree of myoelectric activity is extremely posture sensitive. Indeed, patients without curvature may assume postures that myoelectrically resemble those having scoliosis. Second, the amount of activity difference between the left and right sides at the apex is

POSSIBLE OUTCOME CATEGORIES

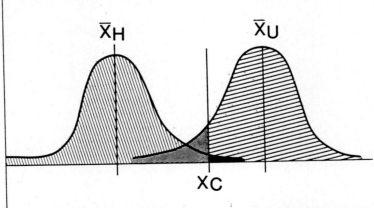

Figure 20–4. A test's discriminability is portrayed by separating test results into healthy (X_H) or unhealthy (X_U) groups. A cut-off value (X_C) is selected to minimize instances of false-negative and false-positive results.

■ PATIENT VALUE > X_C, PATIENT HEALTHY, "FALSE POSITIVE"

▨ PATIENT VALUE < X_C, PATIENT HEALTHY, "NEGATIVE"

▤ PATIENT VALUE > X_C, PATIENT SICK, "POSITIVE"

▦ PATIENT VALUE < X_C, PATIENT SICK, "FALSE NEGATIVE"

reliable only at higher visually obvious degrees of curvature. Therefore, use of paraspinal EMG, although valid in its own right as a comparison of relative muscle activities, is not discriminating in this context and has no clinical value in the diagnosis and management of scoliosis.

Patient Motivation

Test results should be interpreted in conjunction with observations made while the test is performed. A common mistake is to assume that a single measurement reflects the patient's legitimate performance capability. Several factors underlying patient motivation can confound the outcome of any test. These sources of error include misunderstood instructions, apprehension of the test setting, fear of pain arising from the test, and questions of secondary gain.

Two approaches can be used as examples of how to judge whether a patient's test results reflect an organic lesion, or are influenced by patient motivation. They are: (1) the use of repeated measurement, and (2) the use of related tests to examine the same function.

Repeated measurements of key indicators taken at one sitting are useful in assessing motivation. This strategy is based on the assumption that a person who is holding back, or attempting to influence a test outcome, usually cannot produce comparable results on repeated efforts. The hypothesis has been studied and verified specifically during muscle strength testing by Hazard and colleagues (1988). They conducted strength tests and concealed the results from the subjects. Sincere efforts produced results that differed less than 15% across repetitions. Some instruments automatically make mathematical comparisons between consecutive test results and report the outcome as a coefficient of variation. Acceptable ranges of variation are between 10 and 15%.

A second method of evaluation checks for internal consistency of the results between different tests that focus on the same variable. The *related-test* approach is routinely employed during physical and psychological examinations. This is much akin to the kinds of observations that clinicians routinely make when comparing unguarded patient activities to those observed under more formal circumstances of the examination. The malingering patient may easily flex to put on footwear in contrast to a severely limited forward bending during the actual physical examination. To achieve this same kind of observation while using a test instrument, it is necessary to compare the consistency of results from several tests that are procedurally or sequentially different, yet evaluate the same functions (Deutsch, 1989; Triano et al., 1991). For example, a patient undergoing strength

testing may be asked to exert at two different levels of effort, say 50 and 25% of maximum. A short time later they will be asked to do so again, but in reverse order. Patients who are insincere have difficulty in giving the same performance when the sequence is interchanged.

Perceptual Measurements

Questionnaires as Instruments

Physical signs can be rather insensitive measures of a patient's disability (Roland and Morris, 1983a,b). This is especially true for patients suffering from chronic musculoskeletal disorders (Vallfors, 1985). Furthermore, independent and direct measurement of the degree to which an illness affects a patient is not possible. Standardized rating scales and questionnaires afford a simple means of appraising many aspects of patient life and health (Barlow et al., 1984). Some also allow for the recounting of objective circumstances. Those commonly used in the chiropractic community assess pain, activities of daily living (ADL), somatization, depression, and anxiety (Table 20–2). Moreover, many questionnaires have the advantage of being *self-normalizing*. That is, they ask the patient to rate his or her current ability or comfort in comparison to his or her own status when healthy.

Questionnaire selection and clinical yield depend on several factors including the type of infor-

TABLE 20–2. RELIABLE AND VALIDATED QUESTIONNAIRES

Outcome Variable	Questionnaire
Pain	Low Back Pain Scale [Leavitt et al., 1980]
	McGill Pain Score [Turner, 1988]
	Visual Analog Scale [VAS] [Huskisson, 1974, 1982] [Bergquist-Ullman and Larsson, 1977] [Coxhead et al., 1981]
Disability	Illness Behavior Questionnaire [Pilowsky and Spense, 1983]
	Million Subjective Index [Million et al., 1982] [Mayer et al., 1987]
	Oswestry Disability Score [Fairbanks et al., 1980]
	Pain Disability Index [Tait et al., 1987]
	Roland-Morris Disability Scale [Roland and Morris et al., 1983] [Hadler et al., 1987]
	Sickness Impact Profile [Bergner et al., 1981] [Deyo et al., 1986]

mation to be obtained, their reliability and validity, and the application protocol. For instance, disability questionnaires are *more discriminating* indicators of outcome than pain-rating scales. And, some models are more useful as predictors of *good outcomes* than of poor outcomes.

To provide information on treatment outcomes, a questionnaire must be administered *both* before and after a treatment plan. Pain analogue scales should be used frequently (Coxhead et al., 1981), and linked to separate subjective variables whenever possible (Million et al., 1982).

Generally, questionnaires may be divided into two categories, self-reporting and physician administered. There are advantages and disadvantages of all instruments and the benefits of each are debated.

Self-reporting questionnaires offer the advantage of being self-normalizing. In addition, they serve as the only means to gain a measure of the patient's perception of how his or her own condition impacts upon him or her. Self-normalizing instruments are more open to being manipulated by patients who are seeking to amplify or suppress the severity of their symptoms. The reliability of a patient's responses can be estimated by using two related questionnaires that test for the same categories of information. Consistency between the two sets of answers would be expected to help confirm the reliability of a patient's responses, although the underlying assumptions of this approach have not been fully studied.

Patient reactivity, however, is the primary disadvantage of the self-reporting questionnaire. "Reactivity" is manifest as an unintentional change in the patient's response on repeated use of the questions that assess a single parameter. It may be caused in part by the patient reinterpreting the questions as he or she is exposed to them repeatedly. This phenomenon also may be attributable to the progressive amount of attention that the questionnaire draws to a subject discussed by a series of questions (Barlow et al., 1984).

Physician-administered questionnaires ask for essentially the same information with the attending clinician asking the questions directly in interview format and recording the patient's responses. One advantage of a physician-administered questionnaire is that patients who are manipulating their responses tend to be inconsistent in responding to different forms of the same question. Sensing this, the doctor can direct the flow of the interview or ask alternative questions. An additional advantage of physician administration is the benefit derived from the involvement of a trained observer whose skill can help in interpreting the patient's response.

The results of both formats are open to several response variables and forms of manipulation by the patient. Carelessness in execution (lack of patient motivation), acquiescence (tendency to agree with positively worded items), and social desirability (motivated by the need for approval, the patient chooses a socially acceptable answer) are examples (Topf, 1986). The physician should, therefore, become acquainted with the testing instruments, their strengths and weaknesses, and not be cavalier in adopting them for use. When necessary, supplemental testing can be done and the results compared for inconsistencies.

Functional Measurements

Measurement of Position

Posture. Historically, the assessment of posture has received superficial treatment in the literature. This is also true of the strategies that have been developed to change it. But, we know from studies in ergonomics that trunk and head positions adopted during work can be used as an objective index of the intensity of work stress, concentration, or manual dexterity (Ayoub, 1990). Also, habitually poor posture may apply stresses to specific areas of the body that contribute to the longevity of the patient's condition (Kvalseth, 1983).

Most tasks are posture specific. The choice of a particular position might be considered the most important factor contributing to whether an attempted physical activity is risky or safe. Therefore, it is important to be able to evaluate static posture in both the occupational consultation and clinical practice. Clinical and historical understanding must be correlated with static posture analysis and functional assessment to determine the significance in each case.

Plumbline Analysis. The plumbline was one of the first tools to be used in chiropractic to analyze posture. The plumbline provides a visual frame of reference for the line of action of the centers of gravity from each body segment, enabling the clinician to detect postural deviation, asymmetry, and suspect areas of postural stress (Fig. 20–5). Patients are observed in the anterior, posterior, and lateral stances, and assessed for alignment abnormality.

Scoliometry. Various forms of instruments are available to quantify the physical signs of scoliosis. The *scoliometer*, developed by Fipps in 1906, provided a grid system for actual plotting of spinal deformity and postural changes. Later the device was modified by attaching a plumbline to a static frame device that standardized the position of the patient by means of a foot plate (Fig. 20–6). Movable cords were stretched between the upright supports and

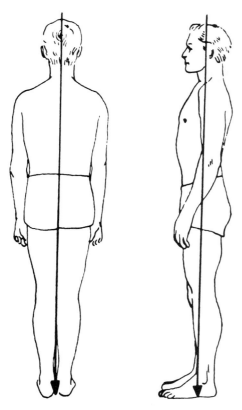

Figure 20–5. Gravity line of reference through normal surface landmarks, anteroposterior and lateral views. For females, the gravity line will pass anterior to the acetabulum.

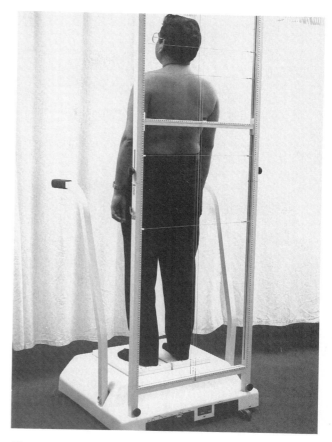

Figure 20–6. Postural analysis performed with a modern plumbline. In this case, the positioning foot plates are load cells under the feet that measure bilateral weight distribution.

placed parallel to shoulder and pelvic levels as an aid to visual inspection.

The most important measurement quantifies the deformity of the rib cage associated with axial rotation of the vertebrae. The prominence of the rib hump correlates with the severity of the curvature and may presage its progression (Roaf, 1966). The differences from side to side are measured in millimeters or in degrees of deformity. Measures can be made with a simple inclinometer and millimeter ruler or by a bubble-level scoliometer (Fig. 20–7). Bubble-level scoliometers also are used to quantify unleveling of the shoulder and pelvic girdles, in combination with a vertical centimeter rule to quantify the shoulder or pelvic height above the horizontal line.

Moiré Topography. Moiré topography is a photographic technique that highlights body contours (Moreland, 1981). The relative number of resulting concentric contour lines on a Moiré photograph are proportional to the distance that symmetric anatomic landmarks project from a purely flat surface (Fig. 20–8). The contour shadows are produced by using a grid placed between an angled light source and the subject. The clinician

stands directly in line behind both the subject and grid. From this vantage point the interference or fringe patterns created are viewed or photographed. Patterns are created by the visual superposition of the shadow cast by the grid, and the grid itself.

Patient positioning is very important with this method of postural analysis, as the grid-to-patient distance relationship must be kept constant to achieve accurate follow-up evaluation.

Moiré topography continues to have some usefulness as an investigational procedure, but its clinical utility has not been demonstrated. It is performed quickly and is reproducible, but the results are difficult to quantify and no good correlation to physical findings exists. Adequate interpretation is, therefore, lacking.

Bilateral Weight Distribution. Asymmetric posture should not automatically imply unbalanced loading at the spinal base or of the extremities. Shifts in upper body segments can be offset by changes in

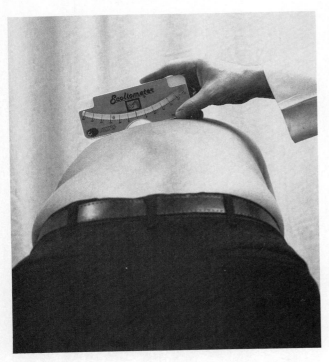

Figure 20-7. Rib hump measurement in a scoliotic patient using a scoliometer made from a ball bearing in a fluid-filled track. Deformity is measured in the number of degrees the back varies from the horizontal.

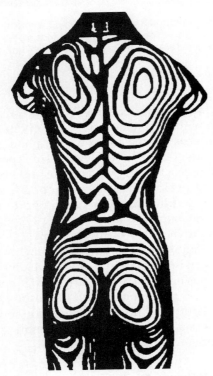

Figure 20-8. Contour analysis pattern seen with Moiré topography. Outlines are an optical effect produced by a grid superimposed on its own shadow created by an angled light source.

lower body segments. The simplest means employed to determine if the loads transmitted throughout the skeleton are asymmetric is through the use of bilateral scales or load cells (Hoppenfeld, 1967; Coggins, 1975; Vernon and Grice, 1984). With the patient standing, each foot on a separate load cell (see Fig. 20–6), The clinician can directly record unilateral loads on the pelvis.

Asymmetric weight bearing has been proposed as a contributing feature in the development of degenerative joint disease, sacroiliac instability, chronic lumbar strain, and other conditions (Illi, 1965; Mitchell, 1971; Coggins, 1975; Fisk, 1977; Hildebrandt, 1977). Although this is empirically and intellectually appealing, its validity remains to be demonstrated.

Measuring Leg-Length Inequality. Considerable interest and controversy exist regarding leg-length inequality. Throughout the history of chiropractic, significant concern has been focused on anatomic and functional leg-length discrepancies. All the various schools of thought have, at one time or another, considered this area of inquiry. In concert with the concerns of other disciplines that have addressed the issue, a number of questions remain controversial. What is the consequence of leg-length inequality? Does it cause or aggravate spinal complaints? What degree of discrepancy is necessary? How effective are therapeutic measures of correction?

Judovich and Bates (1954), in a fluoroscopic study of leg length, concluded that a leg-length deficiency of 3/8 in. or more could cause chronic back pain, and that correcting the deficiency would worsen the pain. Stoddard (1969) and Nichols (1960) agreed that roughly 10 mm of asymmetry was necessary to induce symptoms. Seeman's study (1978), representing the consensus of one group within the profession, suggested that 3.25 mm was adequate to cause back pain or, at least, be an aggravating component of symptoms. Logan (Coggins, 1975), Bailey (1978), Fisk (1977), and Rothenberg (1988) feel that the pelvis and leg length should be balanced to achieve relief of structural strain and resulting symptoms. Cleveland and associates (1988) state that the amount of leg-length discrepancy that is clinically meaningful has not been established. Hellsing (1988) found no correlation at all between leg-length inequality and back pain.

An extensive survey of length inequality was performed by Bailey and Beckwith as long ago as 1937. Using carefully positioned 14 × 17 in. pelvic radiographic evaluations, they examined a series of 432 subjects with asymmetric leg lengths. They found about equal distribution of shortened right (47%) and left (53%) legs. The average discrepancy noted was 8.8 mm. Associated asymmetry of standing spinal mechanics was carefully noted. In 88% of the cases the innominate ipsilateral to the short leg was found to be low, as was the sacrum 72% of the time. Such a clear correlation was not seen, however, in convexity of any lumbar curvature that may have developed. In 45% of the cases, convexity was directed to the short leg side, and in 32% of the cases to the long leg side. No lateral deviation occurred in the remaining cases (23%). These findings suggest that the principal mechanisms of accommodation to a short leg are as dependent on lumbar mechanics as on the attitude of the pelvis. In a recent study, Hoikka and co-workers (1989) found good correlation with pelvic tilt, moderate correlation with sacral tilt but, again, poor correlation with any lumbar scoliosis.

Several methods of measuring vertical symmetry of the lower extremities have been used (Horsfield and Jones, 1986). They include physical and radiographic measures. Clarke (1972) did a reliability study on two of the more commonly used methods. He compared results in palpation and leg measurement to those of a standing 14 × 17 in. radiograph with the central ray positioned at the level of the femoral heads. He considered agreement to exist between methods of measurement when the system being evaluated yielded a value within a generous tolerance of 5 mm of the x-ray findings. On this basis he determined that palpation of the femoral trochanter agreed 32% of the time and the measurement of the iliac crest internal malleolus distance was accurate in 40% of the measurements. Such poor performance as this is unacceptable when the standard used to determine accuracy of technique allows for a variance equaling 50% of the 10-mm maximum deficiency considered by many to be clinically significant. Friberg et al. (1988) concluded that clinical methods are inaccurate and highly imprecise.

Clinically, both improvement and aggravation of symptoms have been seen on trying to correct leg-length deficiency. This would seem to suggest that more rigid criteria are needed to determine the patient needing correction, versus the one that would be best left alone. For example, a study was done by Schuit et al. (1989) to determine the effect of heel lifts on ground reaction force patterns in subjects with structural leg-length asymmetry. In this investigation it was found that although heel lifts help achieve pelvic leveling, ground reaction forces increase and such may cause potentially harmful increased joint stresses within the lower extremities. Earlier work by Triano (1983) attempted to examine trunk muscular function as a means of evaluating beneficial effects from use of heel lift therapy as an alternative to radiographic assessment. Although the results were

promising, much more needs to be done before such methods are able to be broadly used clinically.

In summary, there are two principal situations for determining leg length. In the adult, the modified Chamberlain's view is used to quantify the degree of any leg-length variation. In the child, a scanogram (Fig. 20–9) is used to quantify the variance, locate the source of that variance, and to search for evidence of possible underlying pathology. Scanograms are also useful in predicting the severity of deficit at skeletal maturity (Mosley, 1978). In this way conservative management can be appropriately maintained until the patient nears skeletal maturity. Surgical intervention may be indicated when the ultimate difference is likely to exceed 2.5 cm.

Automated Measurements of Posture.

Quantifying position in three-dimensional space has been used as a research tool for several years. Several methods of spatial measurement are available including sonic, magnetic, photoelectric, and electrogoniometric systems that locate the position of a point in space with respect to an arbitrary fixed refer-

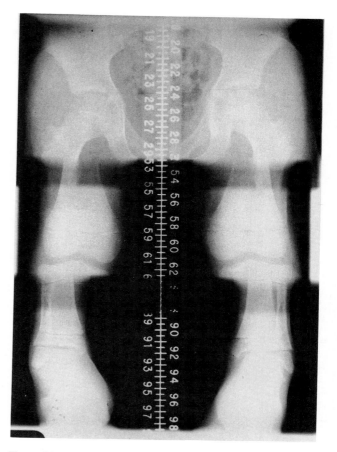

Figure 20–9. Scanogram. A radiopaque rule incorporated to the film image permits direct measurement of bone length with accuracy up to 1 mm.

ence point. Discussion of each is beyond the scope of this chapter primarily because they are not available for, or useful in, general practice.

One commercially available electrogoniometric system (Fig. 20–10) is promoted as a means to evaluate posture, spinal curvature, leg-length asymmetry, and regional and intervertebral flexibility (Gosselin, 1987). A marker probe is positioned on the body at key landmarks, and sensors located in the probe's armature determine three-dimentional position. The patient must hold a constant posture while all anatomic sites are recorded. A second position can be assumed and differences between them can be compared. Calculations are then made to deduce the various parameters of posture and flexibility.

Measurement of spinal curvature with this equipment (labeled as Cobb's angle) uses digitization of points on the spinous processes. The posterior deformity in this manner is similar to true Cobb angles determined from standard radiographs (Herzenberger et al., 1989), but underestimates the actual measure up to 26%. Consequently, the reliability of measure from test to test, important in de-

termining the need for therapeutic intervention, is highly questionable.

The high level of electronic accuracy for systems like this can easily convey a false sense of reliability. It is easy for the unwary operator to forget about the much larger human sources of error, for example, as in the accuracy of locating reliable anatomic landmarks. The evidence of this was noted in the section on leg-length measurements where an error up to 2.5 cm was seen in finding landmarks. Such errors adversely influence the validity, reliability, and accuracy of automated measurements. Four specific factors can confound such measurements: (1) interexaminer reliability in landmark identification, (2) amplitude of postural sway or stability during recording of multiple landmark positions, (3) magnification of measurement error by the mathematics of automated mathematics (Panjabi, 1982), and (4) use of new methods of analysis before being validated as clinically useful and discriminable.

In the instance of the first two cases, the errors caused by the manual inaccuracies are larger than the inherent instrument errors by several orders of magnitude. This makes the promoted benefit of the machine accuracy and precision significantly less important. When measurements including error are used during automated processing, as in surface marker estimates of Cobb angles or in digitizing x-rays, for instance, the size of the errors is magnified algebraically with each step of the analysis. Finally, with the onset of the technology boom in spine assessment equipment, there is an accompanying proliferation of new and innovative methods that simply lack sufficient fundamental research to understand how to use the information they generate.

Measurement of Range of Motion

In the general course of patient care, range of motion is examined using goniometers or inclinometers. Most devices quantify the regional movement of a part and express it as an angular displacement about some center of rotation.

Goniometers. Essentially, a *goniometer* is a 180 or 360-degree protractor joined to a mobile arm (Fig. 20–11). One arm is aligned proximal to the joint being evaluated, whereas the other is aligned with the bone distal to the articulation. The degree of joint movement can be measured throughout active or passive ranges. This type of instrument has been in common usage and is available in several sizes to accommodate different regions of the body. Its usefulness is greatest in the extremities, particularly the small joints of the hands and feet.

Inclinometers. Inclinometers use the constant vertical direction of gravity as a reference and require

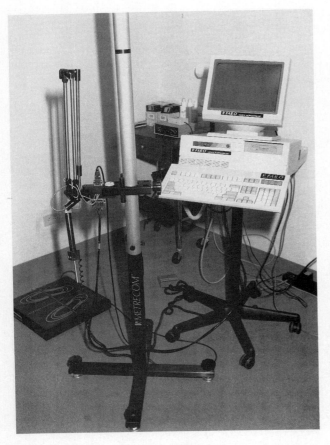

Figure 20–10. A spatial digitizing system used to quantify body landmark locations in different postures. (*Courtesy of James Filberth, D.C.*)

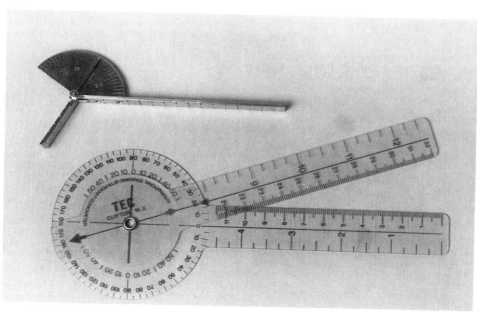

Figure 20–11. Different sizes of goniometers allow range-of-motion measurements of small joints (*above*) and larger joints (*below*).

only that a side rest against the body segment surface. Digital or analogue, and mechanical or electronic versions are available (Fig. 20–12).

Where applicable, inclinometric measurements have proved to be more accurate than the goniometer. This is because it is difficult to align the central axis with the joint center and its arms with the body segment link axis. The range of error for the goniometer is 10 to 15 degrees whereas the range of error for an inclinometer is conservatively estimated to be within 5 degrees (Chaffin and Andersson, 1984; Mayer and Gatchel, 1988).

One advantage of electronic inclinometers is that the number of measurement values that must be handled by the examiner is reduced by automatically calculating the ranges of motion, rather than reporting just the end positions. The intrinsic value of range-of-motion measurements is further enhanced by the ability of the electronic inclinometer to measure movements of multiple body locations quickly and to compute the relative movement between them. For example, whereas a goniometer can yield an estimate of upper body movement during flexion or extension, an electronic inclinometer can partition

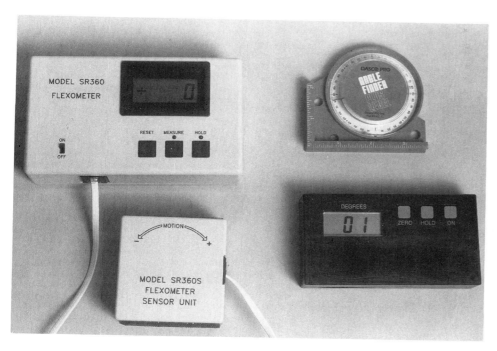

Figure 20–12. Some inclinometers automate the necessary calculations whereas others require this to be done by the physician.

the same motion into its pelvic and lumbar components.

Regardless of measurement method, several patient features may affect the reliability of range-of-motion measurements. These factors include age, level of regular activity, sex, and weight. Children are capable of the greatest ranges of motion. By adolescence, however, joint flexibility is reduced by about 10%; and it generally remains stable into the seventh decade. Gender differences also are observed, with women having up to 15% greater range than men. For either sex, regular exercise can increase and maintain a person's joint flexibility by about 10% (Chaffin and Andersson, 1984). Extra body mass acts as a physical obstacle to bending of a joint simply by blocking movement. Finally, patient attention and motivation affect range-of-motion measurements. There is a tenfold variance in rated impairment between professionals for the same injury (Mayer et al., 1985).

Optoelectronic measurement systems have been used in research for some time, but clinical applications are becoming more readily available. Probably the most prevalent clinical use of optoelectronic systems is in conjunction with the use of force plates to assess gait abnormalities. Video-based systems are available for other applications including analysis of foot and spinal biomechanics. Figure 20–13 illustrates the output from one of these systems measuring cervical rotation (Motion Analysis, Inc.). The position of lightweight markers attached to the body surface are detected by computer and digitized to

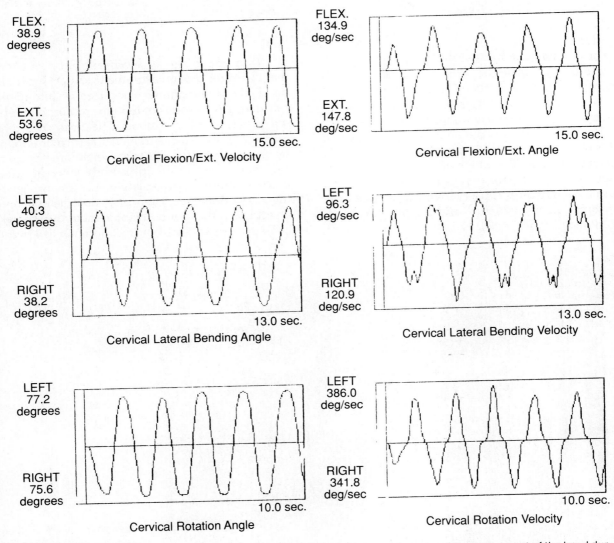

Figure 20–13. Output from a computerized optoelectronic recording system that quantifies movement of the head during flexion and extension, lateral bending, and rotation. Velocity is computed by numerically differentiating the position data. Note the reproducibility of the motions. (*Data gathered by Spinetrack software from Motion Analysis, Inc.*)

supply planar position coordinates. The raw position data may then be processed to yield information on the three-dimensional ranges and speed of movements.

Although less sophisticated analysis are used, video monitoring is often used in industrial practice to capture the salient features and at least semiquantify motions and postures at the work stations.

Measurement of Strength

The term *strength* is open to various interpretations, but in this context it denotes the capacity for active development of muscle tension, and through the resulting muscle force, to generate joint torque. The mode by which the muscle is tested provides only an indirect estimate of the ability of muscle groups to develop force. It should be understood that the actual quality that is tested is the action of the machine or instrument caused by the patient's exertion. Computerized muscle dynamometer systems quantify more variables that the average physician can properly interpret (Sapega, 1990).

For the interpretation of changes in a subject's test results to be meaningful, the reliability and validity of the procedures used must be high. The most effective means to ensure reliability is through test standardization and close attention to the correspondence of test conditions to those of the actual demands that the patient's lifestyle makes on his or her performance.

Manual muscle strength grading performed in a clinical examination setting provides only a rough approximation and its use is limited. The ability of even skilled clinicians to determine strength differ-

ential is rather restricted (Beasley, 1956; Watkins et al., 1984). Relative muscle strength is judged more on the basis of total force and duration of effort that the examiner uses to overcome the patient, than on the actual force generated by the patient (Sapega, 1990). Examiners contrasting the relative strengths of symmetric muscle groups identify the stronger limb as being the weaker of the two as much as 20% of the time when differences are small (Saraniti et al., 1980). Accuracy in manual assessment requires differences in strength of 35% or more (Sapega, 1990). Since the introduction of hand-held dynamometers (Fig. 20–14), while not eliminating all the problems of manual testing, greater degrees of accuracy (Bohannon, 1989) and reliability have been demonstrated (Bohannon, 1986; Byl, 1988; Silverman, 1989).

Even more sophisticated strength testing methods are available to quantify the patient's performance capacity. It is important to remember that the clinical utility of these various assessments is primarily confined to one of three circumstances. The test clearly must be relevant to the individual's activities that have been impaired, or to normative data, and can clearly discriminate healthy from unhealthy people. In the case of employment-related tests, the evaluation must closely simulate critical job tasks (Ayoub, 1983).

Generally, instrumented strength testing equipment can be used both as a diagnostic measure, and as a therapeutic modality for training and rehabilitation. Both have a significant impact on clinical practice, but the following review primarily relates to its use in assessment.

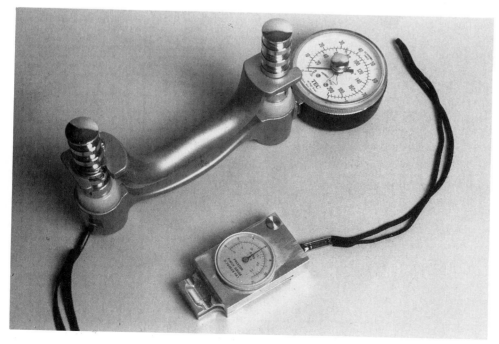

Figure 20–14. Dynamometers for evaluating grip and pinch strength.

Diagnostic assessment naturally falls into three categories: (1) preventative evaluation (as in employee job matching), (2) postinjury evaluation, and (3) outcome monitoring when treatment would normally have ended. The notion of preventative evaluation is particularly useful for preseason athletic counseling and for considering the relative risk to workers entering a physically demanding job. The thoughtful choice of employees whose physical capacity exceeds job demands, including a margin of safety, may be the best means now available to control liability associated with strenuous work (Ayoub, 1983). Caution is necessary in constructing relevant tests to ensure that persons who are physically handicapped are not discriminated against.

Postinjury assessment is a highly promoted area for the use of strength evaluation. It has two primary objectives: the quantification of ongoing impairment and disability, and the determination of a baseline clinical status so that measurable therapeutic goals can be set for rehabilitation. Significant clinical information can be obtained toward these objectives, but careless interpretation of test data can result in inappropriate clinical decisions. Sapega (1990) reviewed the details of the common underlying assumptions and has recommended guidelines for interpreting imbalances in strength for bilateral muscle groups. Table 20–3 summarizes these recommendations for unilateral injuries and emphasizes that a real difference in performance between the left and right sides is not necessarily an abnormal difference. Factors including sports activity, lifestyle, and previous injury also must be considered. In a healthy population, the average discrepancy may easily be as much as 12%. For evaluating an individual's performance, differences of 20% or more may be needed to discriminate abnormalities.

In the case of testing strength function of the axial skeleton, there are few satisfactory intrinsic standards of reference available. Under these conditions it is best to have normative data on the specific population of persons who are active in the same way as the patient being evaluated before he or she was injured. Moreover the data needs to be specific for the mode of testing to be used. Finally, it is important to recognize that it is inappropriate to evaluate patients for strength when they are still in the acute stage of injury.

A patient who progresses past the acute stage can be assessed to establish short-range and quantitative therapeutic goals for continued treatment, including rehabilitation. Outcome monitoring is then carried out to discern if the patient's performance is moving toward the treatment goals, or if maximum therapeutic benefit has been reached.

Mayer and Gatchel (1988) have coined the term *deconditioning syndrome* to describe the development of progressive debilitation in chronic and susceptible postinjured cases. Deconditioning is progressive and arises from inactivity adopted by the patient as a mechanism of coping with the injury, as well as from inappropriately prolonged activity restrictions that may be imposed by the treating physician. The patient not only becomes weaker physically, but generally is fearful of physical activity. Approximately 30% of cases with limitations because of pain that lasts longer than 30 days are likely to suffer from deconditioning syndrome. Upon trying to return to normal activity, these patients tend to undergo new injury. Strength evaluation can be tailored to the critical features of the patient's preinjury activity.

Although there are limited uses for strength measures as valid predictors of risk, their ability to monitor performance changes from treatment programs has strong proponents (Triano and Schultz, 1987; Beimborn and Morrissey, 1988; Mayer and Gatchel, 1988; Seeds et al., 1988; Hazard et al., 1989; Parnianpour et al., 1989; Pollock et al., 1989; Sapega, 1990, Sherman et al., 1987).

Strength Testing Methods. The emphasis on computerized muscle-dynamometry systems has overshadowed earlier isometric and psychophysical testing methods. No single method of strength evaluation is decidedly superior or more valid for measuring muscular strength (Sapega, 1990).

Several methods of strength quantification are in common use (Table 20–4). The differences be-

TABLE 20–3. SUMMARY RECOMMENDATIONS FOR UNILATERAL INJURIES

Group	Imbalance	Interpretation
Healthy	<10%	Normal
	10–20%	Possibly abnormal
	>20%	Probably abnormal
Prior injury (or disuse)	10–20%	Probably abnormal
	>20%	Abnormal
Return to preinjury activity	10–20%	Return to full activity
	>20%	Restrict activity

From Sapega, 1990, p. 1569.

TABLE 20–4. MUSCLE STRENGTH TESTING METHODS AND EXAMPLES OF TESTING DEVICES

Test Method	Device
Isometric	Hand dynamometer
	Pinch gauge
	Dynatron
	Ergometrics
	Promatron
Iskinetic	Biodex
	Cybex
	Lido
Isoinertial	Isostation B-200
	Merac
Dynamic variable resistance	Free weights
	Kaypro
	Nautilus

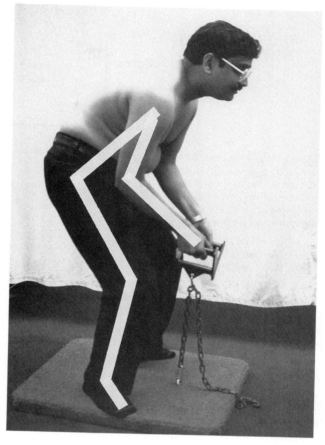

Figure 20–15. Isometric lift strength test. The patient assumes his common life posture and exerts an isometric lift effort. Joint centers are connected to create body segment angles used to quantify the lift posture.

tween them are based on the variable of muscle contraction that is independently defined and controlled by the examiner during the test. Each method uses different measurement parameters and, with one exception, the results produced by dissimilar strength-testing methods may correlate, but they cannot be related directly to one another quantitatively. Each method also has a number of advantages and disadvantages. For valid interpretation of test results, the unique characteristics of each must be kept in mind.

ISOMETRIC TESTING. Isometric strength testing is performed by having the patient assume a specified posture and exert force against an unyielding resistance (Fig. 20–15). Although the muscle contraction causes a significant rise in muscular tension and some internal fiber shortening, no joint motion occurs.

There are several technical concerns in the performance of strength tests: (1) the inertial effects at the onset of the test, (2) patient fatigue, (3) patient posture, and (4) patient motivation. The objective of the test is to identify and record the maximum voluntary contraction force that can be sustained. Chaffin and Andersson (1984) have proposed standardized minimum criteria for sustained effort of 2 seconds to define stability. To meet that goal, the maximum value plateau of the recording is used. Figure 20–16 is a stylized schematic representing an isometric strength measurement. The test should be conducted without any jerking motions as this tends to cause spiking of the recording from inertial effects that represent unsustainable force.

Repeated performance of near maximal efforts can cause *fatigue*. To avoid these effects, a 30-second rest period should be permitted between repetitions. If more that three repetitions are to be used, the rest interval should be increased to a full 2 minutes.

The patient's *motivation* to supply a maximum

effort during isometric testing is a key feature. It is not possible, however, to know with certainty that any effort, no matter how impressive, is the patient's true maximum. Several strategies to approximate more closely the maximum load have been devised. Khalil et al. (1987) reported an acceptable maximum effort approach that attempts to find a maximum voluntary contraction that a patient recovering from spinal pain can perform without inducing unacceptable discomfort. The researchers used verbal coaxing after an isometric attempt reached an apparent plateau. Generally, patients are able to supply two or three increments of additional force, amounting to as much as a 240% increase, without added risk. Triano et al. (1991) have proposed a scheme of adding visual feedback of strength levels that seems to achieve an additional 9 to 19% increase in performance during isometric testing of trunk muscles.

Motivation during isometric measurements of grip strength has been studied using repeated measurements (Niebuhr and Marion, 1987; Smith et al.,

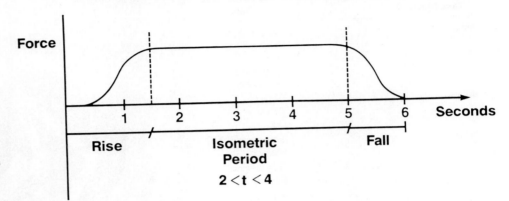

Figure 20–16. Schematic of an ideal isometric strength curve. A 1-second rise to maximum is followed by a minimum 2-second plateau that is used for taking the measurement.

1989). Any variation greater that 10 to 15% between trials suggests voluntary holding back in performance. Several instruments automatically make comparisons of this kind and may report the difference between repeated exertions as a *coefficient of variation* (CV). This helps one discern between different levels of cooperation with the test instructions. Although with this application, the term is not used in the same rigorous sense as implied.

Finally, the patient's posture can substantially affect the results from strength testing (Williams and Stutzman, 1959), and the loads transmitted to the joint structures (Chaffin and Andersson, 1984). Posture of the trunk and extremities must be precisely reproducible between test sessions for results to be compared reliably (Sapega, 1990). The use of static photographs permits an explicit quantification of body posture during the exertion that can be used later for testing in the same posture. Even subtle changes in joint angle can cause significant differences in strength measures.

Measures of absolute strength are probably not very important because they are affected greatly by the exertional level of daily activities and routine exercise. A 10% side-to-side disparity in strength is common (Gleim et al., 1978). Variation in strength up to 20% or more may be needed to exceed two standard deviations of average discrepancy (Gleim et al., 1978; Mira et al., 1980; Wyatt and Edwards 1981; Lakomy and Williams, 1984). Therefore, clinical judgments based on values less than 15 to 20% change in performance should be made very cautiously.

Sports medicine research suggests that healthy joint function bears some relationship to a relative balance of opposing muscle groups (Kibler et al., 1989). Studies of patients with low back pain complaints often demonstrate abnormalities in these ratios with a tendency for loss of strength in the extensor muscles (McNeill et al., 1980; Triano and Schultz,

1987). A prospective study, however, examining the predictive value of such measures has not been done. For isometric trunk strengths, the normal reciprocal ratios obtained in upright test postures are listed in Table 20–5.

Knowledge of the force generated during an isometric test, coupled with quantification of the patient's posture photographically, allows computation of the stress on the spine (Fig. 20–17). using biomechanical computer models. The quantification of the subject's posture is critical to obtain accurate results (see Fig. 20–15). Changes in posture by only a few degrees can make as much as 25 to 30% difference in back loads. For sagittally symmetrical tasks, the calculation has an accuracy within 15% (Chaffin and Andersson, 1984). About 70% of manual materials-handling jobs can be modeled adequately with sagittally symmetric tests.

Although not able to define *work* or *power*, the measurement of isometric strengths may bear a stronger predictive capacity than has been previously believed (Whitley and Smith, 1963; Nelson and Fahrney, 1965). Data also can be collected at multiple points in an arc of active range to create a strength curve very similar to those generated on the isokinetic systems (Kulig et al., 1984).

ISOKINETIC TESTING. *Isokinetic* contraction is the dynamic muscular exertion through range of motion where the velocity of joint movement is held constant (Thistle et al ., 1967). The velocity variable is set on the testing instrument by the examiner, and con-

TABLE 20–5. MEAN TRUNK STRENGTH RATIOS

Extension/flexion	1.3
Side bending	1.0
Rotation	1.0

Adapted from Beimborn and Morrissey, 1989, p. 658.

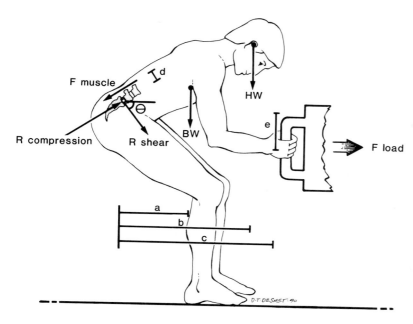

$$R \text{ shear} = (F \text{ load})\text{Cos}\Theta + (BW)\text{Sin}\Theta + (HW)\text{Sin}\Theta$$

$$R \text{ compression} = (F \text{ load})\text{Sin}\Theta - (BW)\text{Cos}\Theta - (HW)\text{Cos}\Theta - (F \text{ muscle})$$

$$F \text{ muscle} = \frac{1}{d}\left[(F \text{ load})e - (BW)a - (HW)b\right]$$

Figure 20–17. Computerized mathematical model of lift test used to estimate spinal compressive loads under isometric conditions. Accurate postural information allows the computer to scale the moment arms (*a,b,c,d,e*) so that the estimates are within 15% of actual spinal stresses.

trol over movement is exerted only when the body part attains or exceeds a preset value of angular motion. The primary measurement obtained is the *torque* generated during the controlled part of motion, and is only valid during the controlled part of the motion. In principle, the resistance offered by the machine (Fig. 20–18) is equivalent to the applied muscle torque over the entire range of movement. This represents the patient's muscular capacity. The maximum voluntary effort will coincide with the greatest mechanical advantage of the joint for the motion that is being attempted (Baltzopoulos and Brodie, 1989).

There are two sources of error in isokinetic measurements that should be taken into account during evaluation; one is extrinsically produced and the other is inherent to the machine. The first error results from the effect of gravity on a body moving in space with some speed. In its raw form, the torque measured does not represent the muscular torque alone. Rather it is the combined effect of the muscular torque and the changing effect of gravitational forces as the center of mass of the body part moves through space. Although gravity certainly does not change its line of action, the change in limb orientation alters the amount of torque registered by the machine through the range of measurement. Error from this effect ranges from −6.5 to 26% (Baltzopoulos and Brodie, 1989). Some isokinetic

systems can be upgraded to compensate automatically for this inertial error, and it is important to do so if comparisons of performance between persons are to be made.

The second error, a machine artifact that arises from the inertial effect of motion as the preset velocity is achieved, is known as *torque overshoot*. The torque output during isokinetic movements consists of a prominent initial spike that resembles the jerking sometimes seen in isometric tests. This results from the dynamometer control unit overcoming the accelerating limb-lever system to limit its final speed. As the body part accelerates, it picks up momentum and reaches the preset threshold, at which point the control system is initiated. By that time, the instantaneous acceleration of the part is still rising and must be countered (Fig. 20–19). This is achieved by initially exerting a higher counterpressure to stabilize the limb speed to the set value.

To eliminate this artifact, machines have built-in filters or damper systems. The settings are controlled by the examiner at one of several optional levels. The effect of the damper not only results in suppressing the artifact, but it also delays the torque response curve and reduces its amplitude. The effect is to alter the clinical impression for location of maximum mechanical advantage, and to underestimate the generated muscular torque. This effect can be accounted

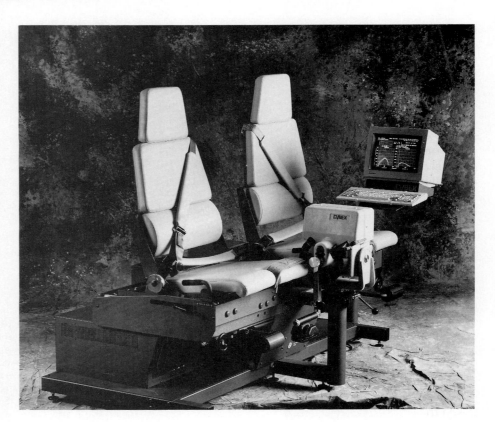

Figure 20–18. A computerized isokinetic system configured for evaluating the lower extremity. *(Courtesy of Cybex, Division of Lumex, Ronkonkoma, NY.)*

for electronically, or by ensuring that repeated testing is performed at the same damper setting so that machine artifacts are constant. In this way, follow-up tests can be compared for possible clinical improvements, but lost information will not be recovered.

In general, higher movement velocities are associated with a decreased torque development. This is felt to reflect a change in neurological strategy in activating the muscle fibers (Barnes, 1980). Standard isokinetic measurements are commonly taken at increments of 30 degrees/sec using two to six repeti-

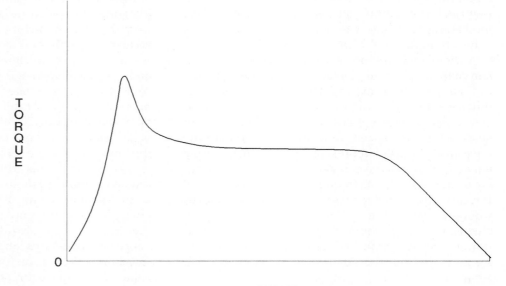

Figure 20–19. Torque overshoot. The initial peak is an artifact of instrumentation. Useful clinical measurements are obtained from the stable velocity shown here as the plateau of the curve.

tions. The maximum single torque value produced is used as the measure of performance. Surprisingly, averaging should not be done because each exertion carries information about both the maximum torque and the location in the range of motion where greatest mechanical advantage occurred. In a diseased limb, for example, both may vary. Averaging is likely to result in loss of information on joint location.

From 0 (isometric) to 60 degrees/sec, the torque produced remains quite stable. Because of this, there is an ability to relate the outcome of isokinetic measurements with isometric results. Beimborn and Morrissey (1988) reported an extensive survey of the literature on reciprocal ratios of trunk muscles. For these slower speed isokinetic measures, the normal flexion–extension trunk ratio is the same as for isometric exertions. Several investigators have observed isokinetically antagonist–agonist reciprocal ratios in low back pain patients. As with isometric evaluation, the ratio falls when impairment is present (Thorstensson and Arvidson, 1982; Langrana et al., 1984; Mayer et al., 1985, 1986; Triano and Schultz, 1987).

Little data are available from which to define a statistical or functional significance to abnormal ratios in the extremities, and the values of these ratios vary greatly among healthy individuals. When there is symmetry of strength, however, it is generally expected that the ratios also will be symmetrical. Therefore, the absolute value of the ratios has no documented inferential merit, but Kannus (1988) and Nunn and Mayhew (1988) feel the side-to-side balance has some importance.

Patient motivation is just as important a concern here, as with isometric evaluation. The most valuable means of assessing sincerity of the patient's effort is through repeated measurement. A minimum variation of 10 to 15% again suggests good cooperation (Hazard et al., 1989).

ISOINERTIAL TESTING. Isoinertial strength testing requires the control of torque values that the patient will be permitted to use during movement. Although no testing method yet devised allows an assessment of free dynamic motion such as would occur at a work site or in sports, isoinertial equipment may come closer than others. Several authors have examined the ability to predict performance by setting torque (Kroemer, 1983, 1985; Jiang et al., 1986a,b; Jacobs et al., 1988; Parnianpour et al., 1989; Stevenson et al., 1989). Characteristic qualities of both isokinetic and isoinertial measurements are depicted in Figure 20–20. Contrasts in the system measures are apparent, showing that it is impossible to relate directly the two kinds of results.

The advantage of evaluating all three planes of

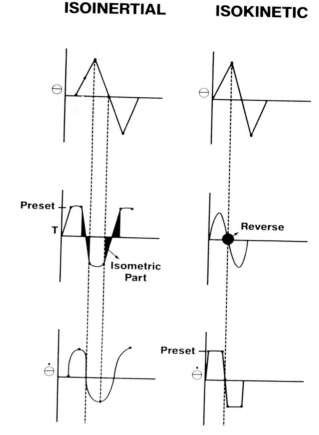

Figure 20–20. Schematic of an angular position (Θ), trunk-generated torque (T), and movement of angular velocity (Θ̇). Characteristics of isokinetic and isoinertial systems are compared in both left and right rotations. Preset levels indicate operator-controlled functions.

spinal motion (Fig. 20–21) would be obvious from the ability to stimulate more closely healthy, isolated spinal actions once a large pool of normative data for various kinds of lifestyles becomes available. For example, just recently there are data reported on people who are sedentary (Gomez et al., 1991). Isoinertial systems can be made capable of monitoring position, velocity, and torque simultaneously while they independently vary. Measures of regional coupled motions appear to hold promise in discriminating fatigue effects from healthy movement (Parnianpour et al., 1989). Likewise, velocity measurements appear to be sensitive to lumbar spine disorders. With such a high degree of versatility and options for test combinations, checks for internal consistency between measures can be made easily. Deutsch (1989) has proposed a protocol for testing spinal function that reports high levels of discriminability between healthy and low back pain patients. Independent corroboration of these results has not yet appeared in the scientific literature.

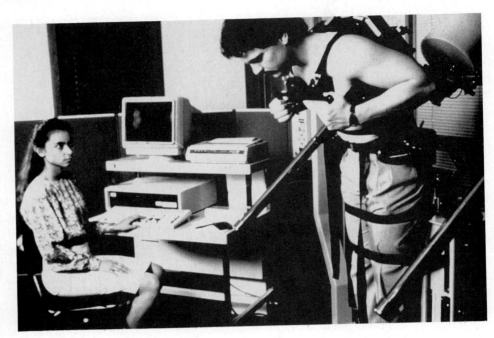

Figure 20–21. Computer-monitored triaxial testing (Isotechnologies, Inc.) is carried out by setting torque resistances for all three axes independently.

Conclusions. There are a number of systems available to perform assessments for prevention, postinjury, and treatment outcome. It probably does not matter which system is selected to carry out the evaluation, provided the constraints relevant to each are kept in mind as clinical judgments are made. When necessary, each can be used to establish a patient's baseline, and each can be used to determine improvement or failure to improve. Under very rigorous test circumstances, some of them can be used to estimate risk of injury from heavy exertion.

More reliable data results when attention is paid to careful positioning and stabilization, and when strict adherence to the technique of testing is used. But, all systems share a common weakness. There is no proof that any one testing mode or any system has a greater inferential capacity with respect to human function. It has yet to be shown conclusively that testing can clearly predict that a patient returned to a certain activity level will have less risk of reinjury under actual functional conditions. Only continued research and development of broader normative data bases than are now available will finally test the underlying assumptions currently used in these clinical applications.

Physiologic Measurements

Thermographic Recordings

Temperature Regulation and Heat Loss. Body heat loss to the environment takes place passively by convection, conduction, and radiation. Evaporation is an active source of heat loss, that is controlled directly by the body. A complex internal thermoregulatory mechanism holds the core body temperature constant despite marked variations in metabolic rate and ambient environmental temperature. Regulation involves primary physiological responses designed to adjust the metabolism, increase the secretion of sweat that allows evaporative heat loss to the environment, and augments the peripheral blood flow. Figure 20–22 demonstrates a model of skin similar to that proposed by Atkins and Wyndham (1969) for the study of heat transmission.

More specifically, regional body temperature is governed by the interaction of central autonomic control mechanisms (Ruch et al., 1965) and multisegmental spinal vasomotor reflexes (Fuhrer, 1975). The hypothalamus contains two reciprocally acting thermoregulatory centers that coordinate and integrate neural discharges to the various structures that are involved with temperature control. Vasoconstrictive sympathetic actions for both upper and lower extremities have been measured (Fuhrer, 1975).

Regional variations of sympathetic thermoregulation produce a complex pattern of temperature distribution. These interactions are important elements in the ability to obtain reliable and repeatable thermographic examinations. First, the body is complex in form, and that form changes with gross movement and psychophysiological alteration. Second, it has a nonuniform internal structure. Normal body temperature varies locally with this complexity, as well as in a cephalocaudal pattern. The mean temperature of the forehead is 34.8°C, whereas the mean temperature at the feet is 31.6°C.

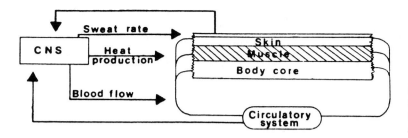

Figure 20–22. Schematic model of heat loss through the skin. Accuracy depends on skin thickness and thermal conductivity variables. (*After Atkins and Wyndham, 1960; p. 106.*)

Halberg (1969) observed circulatory changes in both skin and core temperatures that cycle regularly on 24-hour, 7-day, 30-day, and annual periods (*circadian cycles*). Desynchronization of normal temperature cycles may be seen in the mentally retarded and in chronically ill patient (Halberg, 1960).

The skin has been described as a thermal *black body* that neither gives up, nor absorbs heat at normal environmental temperatures. However, with skin reflectance of roughly 5%, any mean radiant temperature that is substantially different from the skin temperature will give noticeable error in thermographic measurements (Stolwijk, 1975). No corrective thermoregulatory response will be elicited by an unclothed body if the mean ambient temperature is kept at a level between 33.5° to 34°C (Houdas and Guieu, 1974).

Thermosensitive Instruments. Measurements of skin temperature and the amount of heat radiated from anatomically symmetrical regions yields useful information about the relative circulatory volume to each part. The principles of conduction and radiant emission of heat energy from the body have been employed to develop measuring instruments of varying sensitivity. Thermocouple devices detect skin temperature by conduction; and infrared emission (representing 66% of the heat loss) has been measured by several methods (DeBois, 1937).

Several thermocouple devices have been marketed to be used for the manual determination of local paraspinal temperature variations. Having either unilateral or bilateral probes, these devices all operate similarly. The Nervoscope (Electronic Development Laboratories) is an example of a hand-held, dual-probe thermocouple unit. Historically, this device provided a limited, bilateral evaluation of skin temperature (Trott et al., 1972; Pullella, 1974). With the patient seated, the probes were placed astride the spinous processes and allowed to equilibrate to the skin temperature for 5 seconds. Then, with a smooth gliding motion, the clinician scanned the length of the spine. The detected temperature differentials were displayed by a calibrated galvanometer, the needle of which indicated the relatively warmer side.

Sample plottings from the Nervoscope of an asymptomatic patient and one with spine pain are shown in Figure 20–23. Sharp deflections were interpreted as indicative of lesions causing localized changes in vasoconstriction or vasodilation. Although sometimes still used, these types of paraspinal measures have not been shown to have good discriminability, and their reliability of measurement is highly doubtful (Trott, 1972).

THERMOGRAPHY. The measurement of temperature differentials across the torso, the extremities, and the head has been proposed as a means of evaluating

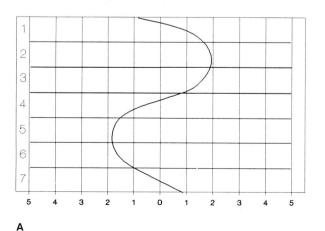

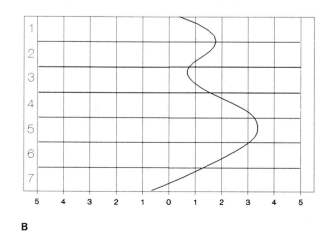

A

B

Figure 20–23. Plotted N thermocouple skin readings from an asymptomatic (**A**), and symptomatic (**B**) patient.

functional changes resulting from somatic lesions. Areas of increased cutaneous temperature have been ascribed to vasodilation occurring during a migraine headache (Walshe, 1973), inflammation (Kimmel, 1966; Agarwal et al., 1970; Duensing et al., 1973; Owen et al., 1973; Huskisson et al., 1973), or muscle spasm (Cooper, 1959; Karpman et al., 1970; Dudley, 1978). Decreased cutaneous temperature may reflect vasoconstriction, vascular obstruction, or fibrous and fatty replacement (Jones, 1974).

An abundance of literature is available documenting employment or thermography in the screening for breast cancer, detection of deep vein thrombosis, identification of allergic reactions (Baillie, 1990), qualification of vascular phenomena, and the identification of pain (Pochaczevsky, 1987; Sherman et al., 1987). The clinical value of the data, however, remains uncertain. Current literature indicates that thermography lacks sensitivity, specificity, and prognostic significance for breast cancer and has largely been abandoned (Ciatto et al. 1987; Handelsman, 1989; Mustacchi et al., 1990; Williams et al., 1990). Thermography has a rather high sensitivity to deep vein thrombosis, but the specificity remains quite low; the test results are likely to reflect a high percentage of false positives. It might be useful as a screening procedure (Jonker et al., 1986; Hoffman, 1989; Holmgren, 1990).

Pain and the effect of its severity cannot be measured, but thermography offers a means of qualifying vasomotor changes at the region of a patient's complaint that are thought to be associated with pain, and may be useful in the detection of malingering (Sherman, 1987). Judovich and Bates 1954) investigated skin temperatures associated with tender areas and found as much as 3°C reduction from normal. They attributed this to vasoconstriction and felt this to be objective evidence of the patient's complaints.

Infrared thermography measures the radiant heat loss of the body that occurs in the infrared radiation range. DeBois (1937) determined infrared body emissions to be from 5 to 20 microns with an average of approximately 9 microns. The advantage of this technique is that it uses infrared-sensitive film and simultaneous evaluation of all areas of the spine can be made.

Accurate and repeatable thermographic examinations are rather time consuming and dependent on standardized procedures. Typically, the examination room must be windowless, draft free, and maintained at a temperature of 20° ± 1°C (Jones, 1974). As the patient disrobes, an abrupt drop in skin temperature results. An adaptive period averaging 8 minutes is needed for warmer environments (Fig. 20–24). To ensure a sufficiently representative steady

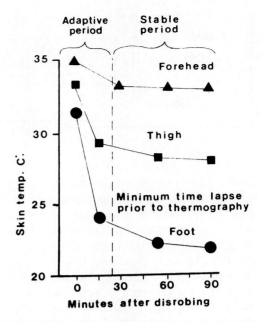

Figure 20-24. Effect of ambient room temperature on skin temperature of unclothed subjects. (*After Houdas and Guieu, 1974, p. 162.*)

state for skin temperature, an arbitrary stabilizing period three times the adaptive period before recording has been proposed (Houdas and Guieu, 1974).

Because the body temperature varies according to several time cycles, the patient needs to establish constant patterns of work and rest. The peak body temperature in the average individual working on a regular day shift schedule occurs at approximately 3 to 4 PM (Reinberg, 1975). Follow-up evaluations, then, need to be conducted at the same time of day as the initial test.

Fairly characteristic patterns have been described (Goldberg, 1966; Edeiken et al., 1968; Raskin, 1976; Dudley, 1978) that provide a reliable and objective method for clinical evaluation of musculoligamentous injuries. There is some disagreement, however, about the constituency of a normal thermogram of the spine (Heinz, 1964; Lebkowski et al., 1973; Jenness, 1975). Several authors have presented findings that appear to provide a basis for clinical use. The erect posture thermogram presents three bilaterally symmetrical areas of increased thermal emission in the lumbar region of the spine and is represented in Figure 20–25. Dudley (1978) observed that it is uncommon to find perfect symmetry in the pattern, and thus integration of all clinical findings is important. However, basic symmetry can be expected in the healthy subject.

The results of comparative studies of thermography and other diagnostic procedures for nerve root entrapments are quite varied. Raskin (1976) reported

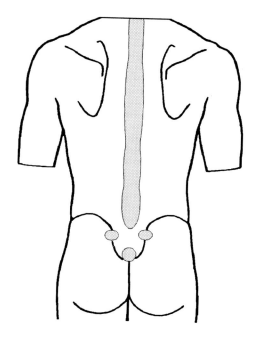

Figure 20–25. Schematic distribution depicting heat areas expected on a normal thermogram of the lumbar spine.

a comparative study between the results of myelography and thermography in 76 patients (Table 20–6). Of the patients with surgically verified disc compression of the nerve root, 88% demonstrated a positive myelogram and 71% demonstrated a positive thermogram. This suggests that a positive thermogram is a reliable noninvasive method of evaluating compression nerve injury, whereas a negative thermogram is inconclusive (Duensing, 1973; Raskin, 1976; Gerow et al., 1990).

More recent studies do not settle the problem. Where some studies claim that thermography has little diagnostic and uncertain prognostic value in the evaluation of low back pain and radiculopathy (Mills et al., 1986; So et al., 1989), others praise its sensitivity and positive predictive value (Chafetz, 1988; Uematsu, 1988). Ash (1986) concluded that the positive thermographic findings in patients with radicular symptoms, do not follow a sensory dermatomal pattern.

Edeiken and colleagues demonstrated that central herniation of an L4-5 disc produces a bilaterally warm region between the normal lower lumbar and sacroiliac areas, whereas lateral herniation caused a unilateral area of heat (Edeiken et al., 1968). At the lumbosacral region, a centrally placed disc, obliterates the normally cool region at the lumbosacral area. Lateral position at this level causes a focal area of warmth at the level of, and slightly medial to, the normal sacroiliac area.

Thermographic studies of strain and sprain injuries show that the diffuse areas of spasm and heat associated with these lesions are quite large and persist longer than the thermographic patterns associated with disc lesions. Although both sprain and strain, and disc disorders, could mimic the pattern of a sacroiliitis or a spondylitis, the correlation should be adequate to give a differential diagnosis.

Thermographic images have been used in the diagnosis of myofascial pain syndromes and their respective pain referral zones. There has been a high correlation between the thermographically defined referral zones and those as described in the literature. Additional zones, not previously identified, have also been recognized. (Diakow, 1988)

Others have presented studies showing that ankylosing spondylitis present patterns different from intervertebral disc herniation (Connel et al., 1964; Agarwal et al., 1970; Owen et al., 1973).

On balance, then, thermography remains a promising procedure for which clear clinical consensus as to appropriate use remains to be developed.

Electrophysiologic Recordings

Although clinical electrocardiography began in 1901 and electromyography in 1938, the potential of electrophysiologic recording of various excitable tissues as a clinical technique within the chiropractic profession has hardly been approached. In fact, these studies may offer valuable and reliable objective evidence of neural dysfunction accompanying motion segment disorders.

Essentially, the basis of all electrophysiologic recording studies consists of the measuring of action potentials generated by muscles or nerves. The gen-

TABLE 20–6. POSITIVE MYELOGRAMS VERSUS POSITIVE THERMOGRAMS IN SURGICALLY CONFIRMED CASES OF LUMBAR DISC HERNIATION

Number of Patients	Positive Myelogram [%]	Positive Thermogram [%]
Surgically treated [38]	31–79	20–46
Confirmed disk [24]	21–88	17–71
Confirmed spinal stenosis [14]	10–71	3–21

From Raskin [1959]

eration of all membrane action potentials, regardless of the type of cell, is based on a transmembrane electrochemical gradient, theoretically described by the Goldman equation (Ruch et al., 1965).

Transmission characteristics of the impulse leading to propagation are defined by the cable properties of long thin cells. A potential electrical charge difference as great as 90 mV exists between the external and internal aspect of the cell membrane. This is termed the *resting membrane potential*, and it represents a potential gradient for the movement of potassium and sodium ions across the membrane. The resistance produced by a high length to diameter ratio allows for a "leakage" of current into the surrounding less resistant interstices. Once stimulated (*depolarization*) current flow can move (*propagation*) from one section into the next by virtue of the potential difference between the excited and resting segments. This leakage or flow, called volume conduction (Fig. 20–26), can be sensed by an appropriately located electrode. The compared potentials will appear as a biphasic deflection indicating the approach and recession of an impulse relative to the recording electrode (Fig. 20–27). By choosing various procedures of measurement, a pattern of pathophysiological changes may be defined that sheds light on the location and nature of underlying pathology.

Several variables affect all electrophysiologic recordings: (1) the size and location of the recording electrode, (2) the configuration of the electrode position relative to the structure being recorded, (3) characteristic resistance of the tissues, (4) the pathophysiology of the patient's problem, and (5) artifacts. In the field of electrocardiography, some of these variables have been controlled by the use of multiple locations for a more precise interpretation of the findings. The optimal location for electrode positioning for electrocardiography, electroencephalography, electromyography, and electroneurography are well described in standard clinical handbooks on each topic.

Electrodiagnosis. Several specialized procedures are available to evaluate select neuromuscular func-

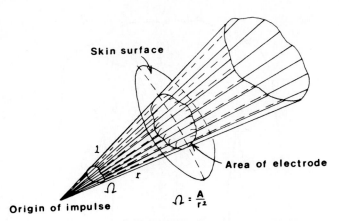

Figure 20–26. The surface potential recorded is proportional to the amplitudes of the membrane potential and the solid angle formed at the surface. (*From Ruch et al., 1965.*)

tions. These include measures of myoelectric activity during muscular loading, fatigue studies, conduction velocity tests, H-wave and F-wave responses, and evoked potentials. Some of the potential uses for electrodiagnosis within the scope of chiropractic practice are tabulated in Table 20–7. Generally these studies can be simply grouped as: (1) stimulation studies and (2) electromyographic (EMG) studies (Cohen, 1976). The clinical procedures are sometimes divided according to whether needle or surface electrodes are used.

Surface electrode studies incorporate an artificial electrical stimulation of the nerve trunk or sensory fibers, applied through an electrode secured to, or just beneath, the skin to elicit responses. This technique spares a patient the discomfort of needle placement, but the benefit may be offset by the greater stimulus impulse intensity necessary to penetrate through soft tissues (Brown, 1984). Surface electrodes may be used in many cases, but are traditionally applied to the examination of nerve conduction velocities, reflex studies, and kinesiological evaluations (Ludin, 1980).

The use of an intramuscularly introduced *needle electrode* is classically termed electromyography. This

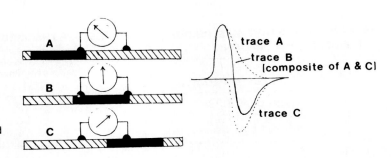

Figure 20–27. Mechanism of polarity change produced by an action potential passing a bipolar recording electrode. (*From Ruch et al., 1965.*)

TABLE 20–7. BASIC ELECTROMYOGRAPHIC TEST PROCEDURES WITH INDICATIONS FOR TESTING

Test	Structure Tested	Indication
Muscle loading	Descending pathways, peripheral nerve—afferent and efferent; myoneural junction muscle	Suspected hypertonicity, hypotonicity, dyskinetic patterning, low-back pain, myogenic and neurogenic atrophy
Fatigue studies	Descending pathways, peripheral nerve—afferent and efferent; myoneural junction muscle	Myesthenia gravis; low-back pain, dyskinetic patterning
Conduction velocity	Motor nerve integrity	Acute nerve injury, neuritis, compression neuropathy
H reflex	Afferent, efferent nerves; homologous neuronal pool	Excitability curves, suspected descending pathway lesions; potential use in subluxation undetermined
F reflex	Afferent nerve and motor neuron	Excitability curves, suspected descending pathway lesions; potential use in subluxation undetermined

technique may be used in all varieties of electromyographic studies, but it is required to detect denervation, myoneural junction disorders, cerebellar and brainstem tremors, anterior cord disease, and motor unit potentials.

All electrophysiological recordings are prone to artifactual interference. An artifact that occurs during both surface and needle electrode readings is *cross-talk.* This is the result of contamination and mixing of signals between muscles because interstitial fluids conduct electric potentials so well. Up to 16% of the surface recordings from the upper leg muscles is from such *co-contraction* activity (Dowling et al., 1989). For this reason, very little can be gleaned regarding the activity of muscles distant from the electrodes.

NERVE STIMULATION STUDIES. Nerve stimulation studies can be performed using either surface or needle electrodes. Basic information may be gained about the neuromuscular sensory and motor conduction velocity and reflex responses of the nerve (i.e., H reflex and F waves). Practically, this information may be used to evaluate the nerve trunk integrity and significant compression, or temporal dispersion from metabolic neuropathy.

Both sensory and motor studies permit analysis of waveform, amplitude, and duration of the impulse (Jabre, 1983). Motor velocities can only be measured orthodromically (i.e., proximal to distal) as the nerve causes a muscle twitch response. The sensory measurements may be made either orthodromically or antidromically (i.e., distal to proximal) as the nerve action potential itself is maintained (Thompson, 1981).

Nerve conduction velocity (NCV) determinations

provide information about the speed at which a nerve impulse travels along a motor or sensory fiber. The time (latency) for a supramaximal stimulus to travel a known distance can be measured. If the nerve is stimulated at two different points, two latencies can be obtained and a velocity calculated. The following equation is used: $NCV = D/(L_{proximal} - L_{distal})$. The distance in millimeters (D) between the two electrodes divided by the difference in latency time in milliseconds (L) equals the velocity in meters per second (NCV).

Determined nerve conduction values are then compared with a known set of velocities for the specific nerve segment. The velocity differs as the nerve courses distally, due to tortuosity and decreasing diameter of the fibers. Measurements may be made at several points along the nerve to enable the identification and location of a lesion (Table 20–8). Eisen (1977) has shown how compression by disc lesions can be monitored through evaluation of nerve conduction velocity.

F-wave responses are considered to be the antidromic excitation of anterior horn cells after a maximal peripheral nerve stimulation. The F wave consists of the time required for the evoked potential to ascend antidromically to the anterior horn cells, and for the resultant action potential to descend orthodromically to the muscle fibers (Thompson, 1981). They are of a similar latency as the H reflex, but require stronger stimulation. The amplitude of response may indicate the facilitated status of motor neurons (Simpson, 1973). The F wave is used, although rarely (Cohen, 1976), to locate lesions in the proximal portion of the pathway, including the roots, plexuses, and peripheral nerves.

H reflexes result from minimal stimulation to the

TABLE 20–8. CONDUCTION TIMES BETWEEN KNEE AND ANKLE MEASURED BY M AND F RESPONSES (MSEC – MEAN +/– 2.5 SD)

	Latency; stimulating at ankle	Latency; stimulating at knee	Difference: conduction time between knee and ankle
Posterior tibial nerve (n = 60)			
M response	5.85 ± 0.9	13.15 ± 1.5	7.3 ± 1.05
F response	47.4 ± 3.3	39.7 ± 2.95	7.6 ± 1.8
Peroneal nerve (n = 41)			
M response	5.2 ± 0.8	11.65 ± 1.2	6.4 ± 0.9
F response	44.6 ± 3.6	38.2 ± 3.1	6.3 ± 1.8

IA afferent fibers of nerve trunks to evoke a monosynaptic homologous muscle contraction. The H reflex travels at a combined average efferent and afferent conduction velocity of 46 m/sec after peripheral stimulation. They may be used as an index of cord segment facilitation (Humphreys et al., 1989), and an index of proximal segment nerve compression. The electrode positioning and mechanisms of these measurements in humans are shown schematically in Figure 20–28. Actual latencies will vary depending on the nerve being tested and the site of the electrodes.

The most common area to elicit the H reflex in the adult is at the soleus muscle, mediated through the tibial nerve. Most other areas of the body, with the exception of the median nerve, loose the response by 18 months of age during normal neurological development. The H reflex is, therefore, useful in the diagnosis of S-1 and C-7 nerve root lesions, and in studies of proximal nerve segments in either proximal or peripheral neuropathies. In the absence of motor deficit, the H reflex may be abolished by nerve lesions and, therefore, used to evaluate impairment of the sensory division (Cohen, 1976).

Humphreys et al. (1989) reported the first evidence in humans that acute onset functional motion segment disorders are associated with changes in neuronal pool sensitivity, at least for the lower lumbar spine. Using the relationship in size between the maximum recorded H wave and the directly evoked twitch of the muscle (M wave), and H:M ratio was constructed to examine the relative sensitivity at the cord level. Figure 20–29 shows the kind of changes in waveforms observed. H:M ratios were elevated in the acute low back pain subjects but not in the controls. Increase in the response to stimulus was seen to subside over time as the patient's clinical course improved. Subsequent ongoing study of this phenomenon confirms these findings (Cramer et al., 1991). In patients with compressive neuropathy, increased latency and suppression of the H wave are observed. Unfortunately, this measure does not appear to be responsive enough to changes to be used as an outcome measure for individual patients.

Monosynaptic reflexes in patients with L-5 to S-1 nerve compression were studied by Deschuytere and Rosselle (1973). Using the extensor digitorum longus for S-1 and the triceps surae for L-5 nerve roots, differences in latencies for the responses were seen. Up to 10-msec delay occurred in the affected limb as opposed to the normal limb. This led the investigators to conclude that a 2-msec difference in latency is evidence of chronic compression. Triano and Humphreys (1987) reported a case study of F-wave

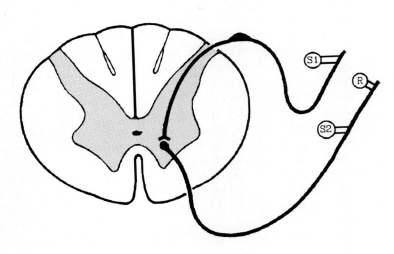

Figure 20–28. Diagram of nerve stimulation testing of H reflex and F wave. S1, stimulation transmitted through monosynaptic pathways to be recorded at R. S2, stimulation transmitted antidromically to motor neurone and returned to be recorded at R.

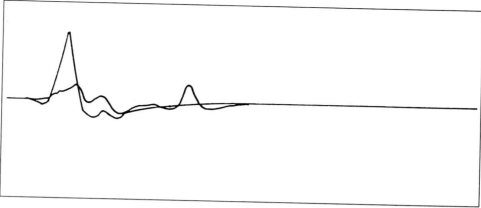

A

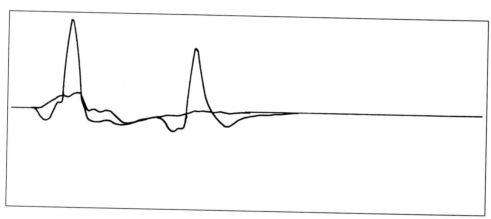

B

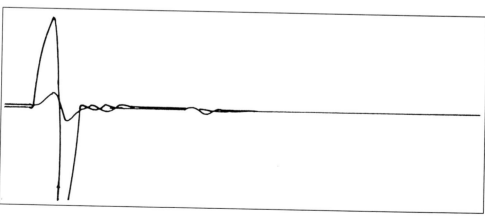

C

Figure 20-29. A. Superimposed H and M traces created by stimulating a healthy peroneal nerve and recording the monosynaptic H reflex from the triceps surae. The ratio of maximum H amplitude to maximum M amplitude (H/M max) is 0.3. **B**. Superimposed H and M traces from a patient with acute mechanical low back pain. The H/M max is 0.63. Note that there is no increased time latency in the appearance of the H wave. **C**. Superimposed H and M traces from a patient with compressive neuropathy at L5-S1. Note the suppression of the H wave and the time delay in its appearance. (*Courtesy of Electrodiagnosis Laboratory, National College of Chiropractic.*)

changes of this kind in the ulnar nerve that were clinically associated with aggravation from manipulative treatment. This response was interpreted as early evidence of nerve irritation. The patient had been under successful manipulative care previously when he aggravated the condition by painting his ceiling. F-wave latency returned to normal after a change of therapy to other conservative methods.

ELECTROMYOGRAPHY. At rest, muscles should be electrically silent. The measurement of muscle activity at rest and during contraction can provide the examiner with information pertaining to the functional status of the neuromuscular junction and pathway. Both surface and needle electrodes can be employed and are used as sensors, rather than impulse transmitters. To obtain accurate information about single motor units, needle electrodes are necessary. Because the potentials recorded by surface electrodes represent the entire muscle activity, these measurements are preferred when the objective is to determine the electric potentials generated by the whole muscle or the motor conduction velocity, and assessing conduction block (Brown, 1984). These principles are applied in NCV and in kinesiologic studies evaluating of dyskinetic movement patterns.

Kinesiologic Studies. Surface electrode muscle loading and fatigue studies may be useful to evaluate muscular recruitment and gauge the relative activity as the muscles act on spinal structures. The fundamental hypothesis underlying these measures is that motion segment disorders are associated with alterations in the intensity of local muscle activity. These methods are current areas of intense investigation and are quite controversial. Clinical applications of these measurements have been proposed under the heading of surface paraspinal EMG scanning. At the current state of knowledge, however, the clinical usefulness remains low because the discriminability of these procedures is poor.

A surface measurement that monitors the intrinsic myoelectric volitional responses can be used to examine superficial layer muscle recruitment and fatigue. When calibrated against known exertional efforts, biomechanical estimates of muscle tensions for simple isometric tasks can be made (Bean et al., 1988). Predictions of muscle tension, at least for surface muscles, seem to deteriorate as exertions near maximum effort are achieved.

A sample setup for bilateral recording of paraspinal musculature is shown in Figure 20–30 that depicts the principles of recording and display consistent to all electrophysiologic monitoring. Especially with myoelectric surface monitoring, many variations or adaptations may be made to meet the individual testing needs as long as the fundamental limitations of the procedure are kept in mind.

Although the sample area is small and only a portion of the cumulative muscle action is recorded, it is considered representative of the whole muscle. The overlapping and interdigitating organization of neuromuscular motor units throughout the muscle belly allows this to be true. Each motor unit consists of a single motor nerve and up to 200 separate muscle fibers that are interposed between fibers from other motor units.

Quantification of muscular performance is much more reliable when some procedure such as integration of the responses is used. The integral of

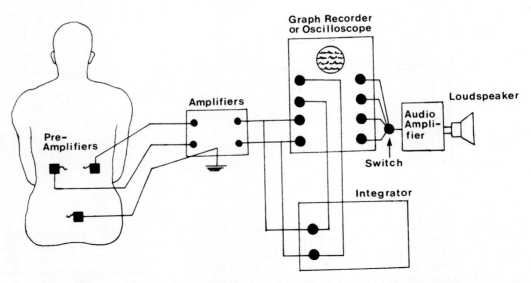

Figure 20–30. Sample electrode and recording configuration for bilateral recording of paraspinal muscles.

recruitment and frequency of muscle fiber activation is directly proportional to the isometric force exerted. Use of the muscle through a range of motion, however, causes a curvilinear relationship that is less well defined (Eason, 1960; Missiuro et al., 1962; Basmajian, 1985).

Simple testing of myoelectric activity during routine tasks, such as sitting, standing, and bending, provide an adequate load on postural muscles to record significant changes in as short as 6 minutes. Triano and Luttges (1985) reported evidence that an ensemble of flexion and postural tasks might discriminate healthy subjects from unhealthy patients, whereas single postures alone were insufficient. Triano and Schultz (1987) further examined the relationship of paraspinal muscle behavior during forward bending to the amount of disability registered on the Oswestry self-reporting questionnaire. Significant muscle recruitment abnormality was observed in patients with higher degrees of limitation in activities of daily living. This was evidenced by loss of the normal silence of muscle activity that is found after 70 degrees of trunk inclination, termed *flexion–relaxation* (Fig. 20–31). However, more information on the sensitivity and specificity of these measures is needed before they can be fully evaluated as outcome measures. Dynamic measurements of this kind hold some hope for future applications of myoelectric monitoring.

Muscle activities in static postures are examined for relative differences in right and left myoelectric amplitudes. The core validity of these comparisons is in doubt. Under static postural conditions, acute spinal symptoms may be associated with alterations in muscular tone (e.g., hypotonus, hypertonus, spasm). However, the meaning of measurements associated with them is uncertain and do not significantly contribute to therapeutic decision making.

In chronic back pain, matters are even worse. The literature is replete with efforts to quantify a relationship between muscle myoelectric activity and low back pain. Results are currently split. For static postures, no compelling evidence that the spasm–pain–spasm cycle exists (Ahern et al., 1988). Even when surface EMG amplitudes have been reduced by biofeedback, no reduction in symptoms has been reported (Nouwen, 1983). Therefore, common clinical assumptions about physical findings of "hypersensitivity" need to be reexamined.

A survey of recent literature on the topic shows that seven groups of investigators were unable to identify reliably increased myoelectric behaviors that correlated to the diagnosis or severity of low back pain (Collins et al., 1982; Corlett et al., 1983; Nouwen and Bush, 1984; Miller, 1985; Sherman, 1985; Cohen et al., 1986; Ahern et al., 1988). In static

postures, Ahern and colleagues (1988) showed that healthy people have as much relative difference in the paraspinal myoelectric activity as do chronic low back pain patients.

Similarly, the total amount of activity was not different between samples (Fig. 20–32). Six other groups have found differences based on more complex spine loading tasks and multiple testing procedures (Chapman and Troup, 1969; Kravitz et al., 1981; Nouwen, 1983; Soderberg and Barr, 1983; Triano and Luttges, 1985; Triano and Schultz, 1987).

Dyskinetic movement patterns. The works of Vannerson and Nimmo (1973), Janda (1969, 1974, 1978), Janda and Stara (1971), and Stary et al. (1965) form a body of clinical myoelectric evidence that describes the dependence of joint stability and integrity on the quality of movement patterns and the functional efficacy of cortical and spinal control systems. Poor movement pattern established by muscular coordination is thought to exist in conjunction with joint dysfunction and may be responsible for its onset or persistence.

Stary et al. (1965) and Grice (1974) suggest evidence that a significant relationship exists between major EMG asymmetries and functional disorders of the spine. Triano and Davis (1976a,b) have presented myoelectric evidence of the loss of normal coordination between antagonistic muscle groups that logically would result in aberrant joint control and protection. Jayasinghe et al. (1978) found that patients with low back pain demonstrate an imbalance of the lumbar spine while standing. Simultaneous recording of muscles suspected of contributing to joint dyskinesia may be fruitful by helping the clinician establish a rehabilitation program that will correct the disturbed joint movement and thus relieve the patient's discomfort.

Obviously, this system of evaluation is too time consuming to be used routinely. However, in patients who have responded unsatisfactorily to previous therapy, future myoelectric monitoring procedures may ultimately be found to discriminate deep-seated functional disturbances of the locomotor mechanisms.

Motor Unit Potentials. A motor unit consists of the anterior horn cell, its axon, and all the muscle fibers innervated by its branches (Jabre, 1983). Needle electrode EMG is used to measure single motor unit potentials. The examination is performed in several steps. First, upon needle insertion any degree of spontaneous activity is measured after the insertional activity has equilibrated. Both visual and acoustic monitoring is available; the latter recommended as being superior (Ludin, 1980).

Second, the patient is instructed to provide a

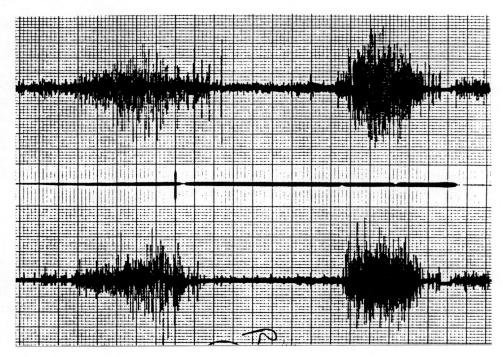

A

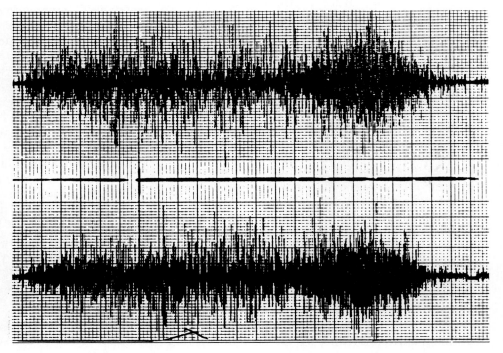

B

Figure 20–31. A. Normal pattern of reduced myoelectric activity during the latter part of full forward bend followed by renewed activity on rising to an upright posture. **B.** Absence of flexion–relaxation in a patient with significant restriction in activities of daily living.

muscle contraction of varying degrees of intensity while the motor unit potentials are simultaneously measured. The characteristics of the duration, amplitude, and phases of the action potential are examined for abnormalities suggesting disease.

Phenomena associated with neurological disorders include synchronization for motor unit potentials, fibrillation potentials, positive sharp waves, and fasciculation (Table 20–9). Myopathies, regardless of cause, have similar EMG abnormalities. The most characteristic is a diminished mean duration of action potentials. Other findings include

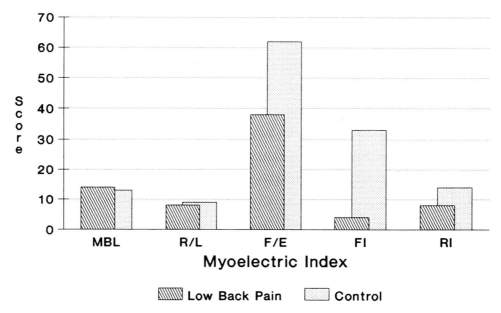

Figure 20-32. Comparison of paraspinal myoelectric activities in low back pain patients and control volunteers for both static and dynamic measurements. Static upright posture: MBL = mean bilateral sum; R/L = difference between right and left paraspinal muscles. Dynamic bending or rotational tasks: F/E = difference between maximum and minimum activity, full forward bending; FI = flexion index (average F/E); RI = rotation index, difference between right and left at full rotation. (*Adapted from Ahern et al. 1988, p. 157*).

all types of spontaneous activity, increased polyphasic potentials, and reduced motor unit field (Taylor, 1962; Simpson, 1973; Smorto and Basmajian 1985). There is no evidence to date that suggests that these types of findings are seen as a consequence of the kinds of spinal lesions that chiropractors usually treat.

Traditional interpretation techniques are designed to elicit evidence of organic myopathy or neural degeneration. Both frequency and morphology of motor unit action potentials recorded by needle electrodes may show alterations. Innervation ratio of muscle fibers may widen (Coers and Woolf, 1959) and the action potential may become polyphasic (Fig. 20-33) (Buchthal, 1977).

The evaluation by Johnson and Melvin (1971) of 314 patients with lumbar radiculopathy concluded that management and prognostic decisions may well be made based on the presence or absence of sharp waves within 7 to 10 days and disagreement between clinical and EMG findings at 14 to 21 days. If the pain persists but the EMG findings show im-

TABLE 20-9. PATHOLOGIC ELECTROMYOGRAPHIC FINDINGS OF NERVE DEGENERATION

Types of Activity	Peripheral Nerve	Anterior-Horn Cell	Descending Tracts
Spontaneous activity of short duration: 1) fibrillation potentials; 2) positive sharp waves	+	Spontaneous activity during sleep, infantile muscular atrophy	—
Fasciculations	Benign	Malignant	—
Patterns of maximal effort	Discrete activity; amplitude: acute stage—diminished < 1.5 mV [normal 2–4 mV]; chronic stage—increased < 4 mV]	Discrete activity; amplitude > 6mV	Possibly discrete activity; amplitude normal or decreased
Motor duration potentials [mean]	+30%	>30%	Normal [± 20%]
Incidence of polyphasic potentials	Acute stage—normal [≤ 12%]; chronic stage—> 12%	>12%	Normal [≤ 12%]
Maximum amplitude	Acute stage—normal [± 30%]; chronic stage—increased [< 30%]	≥ + 500% giant waves	Normal [± 30%]

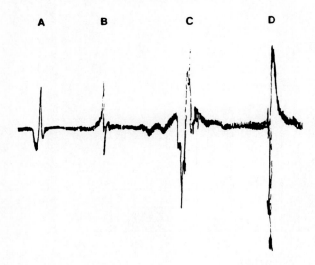

Figure 20-33. Action potentials from voluntary motor units. (A) normal, (B) myopathy, (C) polyneuritis, and (D) motor neurone disease. (*From Simpson, 1973.*)

provement, radical surgical approach can usually be avoided as the case is not likely to be an irreversible disk lesion. When present, changes in surface recordings (for example, F wave and H reflexes) appear as soon as 48 hours after injury.

Electrocardiography. The term electrocardiology is used to describe the recording of the electrical action potentials generated during the contraction of heart muscle. These recordings are plotted as a function of time and vertical deviations from the horizontal plane and indicate the relative amount of myocardial depolarization and repolarization. Cardiac muscle contraction is normally initiated in the sinoatrial node (*pacemaker*) located in the right atrium. The impulse first depolarizes the atria and continues to initiate a wave of depolarization through the ventricular tissues by exciting the atrioventricular node. Atrioventricular nodal impulses continue through the Purkinje fibers rapidly to innervate the entire ventricular structure. The atrioventricular node does have an inherent automaticity, but the normally functioning sinoatrial node governs its pace. The electrical activity of these impulses was first recorded by William Einthoven using a string galvanometer electrocardiogram (ECG) in 1901.

Einthoven used three bipolar surface "limb leads" to examine myocardial electric potentials. These are placed at sites remote from the heart; one on each arm and the third on the left leg, forming a triangle with the heart roughly centered. By examining the action potentials between each lead, the axis and direction of electrical activity can be defined. The diagnostic ability was further enhanced by addition of the six precordial leads of Wilson. By combining the recordings from all the leads, the wave of propagation can be examined from multiple viewpoints. This allows for determination the location of a lesion within the conduction system. Common pathologies have characteristic waveforms, and comparison enables lesion grading.

At rest the normal cardiac muscle is polarized at -90 mV until an impulse is received through the conduction system. It is the depolarization of cardiac muscle that is responsible for the QRS complex seen on the normal ECG, whereas repolarization results in the T wave. Atrial depolarization is represented by the P wave (Fig. 20-34). During depolarization, the ECG shows a deflection until the maximum potential is reached ($+30$ mV), when repolarization commences. Figure 20-35 illustrates the changes seen in the ECG pattern depending on the net direction of the electrical activity, and the axis as it travels through the myocardium. These variations form the basis for the multilead ECG used in clinical diagnosis. The electrode positions and lead directions used in the standard electrocardiogram are shown in Figures 20-36 and 20-37.

Extensive study of the electrical activity generated by the heart has been underway since first discovered. Today, a significant degree of understanding of the meaning of various graphic patterns has been provided. The ECG is very useful in the diagnosis of various heart diseases and the differentiation of noncardiac disorders such as thyroid, renal, pulmonary, and electrode disorders (Table 20-10).

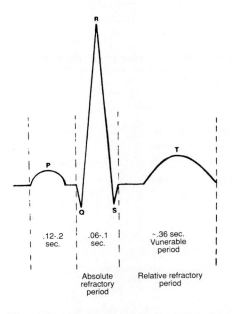

Figure 20-34. Stylized schematic of an ECG depolarization.

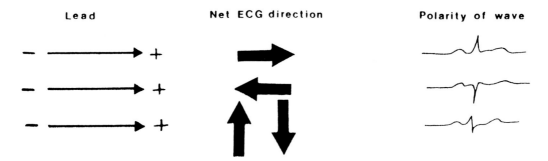

Lead   **Net ECG direction**   **Polarity of wave**

Figure 20–35. Relationship of ECG lead direction and polarity of waveform deflection. Used to determine the axis of electrical activity from which vector analysis may be derived.

Chiropractors use ECG examinations as an adjunct to the diagnosis of suspected cardiac disorders (Wicks, 1991). Although few actually have the instrument, access can be readily gained through diagnostic referral.

Haldeman (1978) has listed the sources claiming efficacy for manipulative therapy in treatment of cardiovascular disease. As he has noted, most of these claims are based on case studies and noncontrolled evaluations. Specific disorders for which manipulative therapy has been advocated include congestive heart failure (Howell and Kappler, 1973; Triano, 1973), ischemic heart disease (Tilley, 1975; Rogers and Rogers, 1976), hypertension (Norris, 1964; Fichera, 1969; Hood, 1974; Tran and Kirby, 1977; Yates et al., 1988), and certain arrhythmias (Egli, 1962; Triano and Ziegler, 1977).

Over the years several researchers within the chiropractic profession have attempted to identify specific vertebral levels of lesion that are consistently found in association with heart disease (Loban, 1928; Janse, 1947; Egli, 1962). Rogers and Rogers (1976) and Triano and Ziegler (1977) have separately reported finding specific spinal patterns of lesions at multiple vertebral levels that seem to be found consistently in patients suffering from heart disorders. Anecdotal and uncontrolled reports have been provided by many researchers and clinicians about improvement within patients having both ischemic and arrhythmic disorders of the heart after correction of spinal lesions.

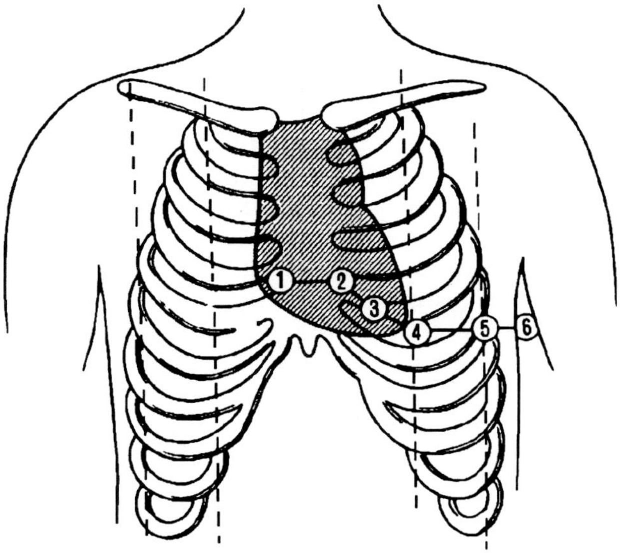

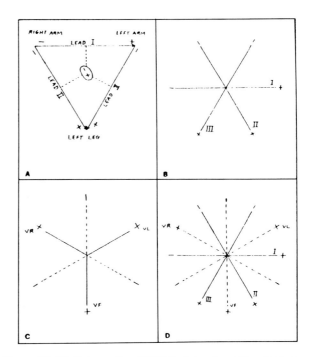

Figure 20–37. Schematic of ECG limb lead position and polarity. The myocardium is visualized at the center of each. **A.** Einthoven's triangular reference frame; **B.** transposition of legs of triangle to cross at center; **C.** orientation of unipolar leads, and **D.** superimposition of both to produce hexaxial reference frame. Normal deflection of lead II at right.

Figure 20–36. Position of unipolar chest leads for standard recording.

TABLE 20–10. CLASSIC ECG PATTERN CHANGES ASSOCIATED WITH PATHOLOGIC CONDITIONS

		Appearance	Interpretation
P wave		>0.12 sec, > 3 mm high	Right atrial enlargement
		>0.12 sec, > 3 mm high	Left atrial enlargement
QRS segment		>0.12 sec	Bizarre complex of premature ventricular contraction
			Acute injury
		>0.04 sec, >1/3 of QRS height	Infarct
		M pattern in V$_1$ and V$_2$, >0.12 sec	Right bundle branch block
		M pattern in V$_5$ and V$_6$, > 0.12 sec	Left bundle branch block
T wave		Leads I, II, V$_2$–V$_6$	Ischemia
		Leads V$_4$–V$_6$	Left ventricular strain
		Leads V$_1$–V$_4$	Right ventricular strain

The influence of the autonomic nervous system on the myocardium is well known. The effect of abnormal neurological activity on the production of arrhythmia is also well established, and it has been suspected to play a role in atherosclerotic (Gutstein et al., 1978) and congestive heart disease (Triano, 1973). However, no firm evidence is available at this time that would suggest the mechanism by which a spinal lesion would result in these cardiovascular abnormalities. Many authors have presented a theoretical basis for somatic involvement with cardiac and other internal diseases, and have provided laboratory evidence to support their arguments (Bollier, 1961; Homewood, 1962; Phillips, 1974; Miller, 1975; Sato, 1975; Tilley, 1975). Referred pain, somatovisceral reflexes, nerve encroachment, altered proprioception, nerve root inflammation, and fibrosis are some of the supposed possibilities. Certainly, combinations of these also might be possible. However, good correlation of these effects has not been found in humans (Prinzmetal, 1959; Demany et al., 1968; Levy, 1971; Dhurandhar et al., 1972; Yasue et al., 1974; Maseri et al., 1975).

Clinical Laboratory Procedures

Chiropractors use laboratory procedures primarily for the same purposes as clinicians in the other healing professions. For the present purposes, laboratory procedures will be arbitrarily sectioned into three hierarchial concerns: (1) the differential diagnosis of symptoms produced by somatic lesions from referred symptoms, (2) testing for contraindications to manipulative therapy, and (3) nutritional evaluation and monitoring.

Differential Diagnosis of Somatic and Referred Symptoms. The literature is replete with refer-

ences to referred pain and somatic changes where objective findings do not obviously rule out visceral involvement in somatic disorders, or somatic involvement with visceral disorders. In addition, the clinical picture presented by the patient may be complicated by coexistence of separate pathologies, symptomatic or not. It is both legally and morally obligatory that the clinician identify the nature of the lesion from which a patient is suffering.

Disorders with somatic reference of pain in the spinal region include peptic ulcer, aneurysm, pylorospasm, colitis, diverticulitis, abdominal carcinoma, prostatic carcinoma, and obstructive uropathy, among others. All may initiate back pain as their first symptom (Braunwald et al., 1987). Laboratory procedures encompassing the full gamut of standard tests and profiles included in hematology, serology, and urinalysis, are helpful in making these differentiations (Kieffer, 1965; Wicks, 1990).

Contraindications to Manipulative Treatment. Of special concern to the chiropractor is the identification of conditions specifically contraindicating certain types of manual therapy. Under certain pathological circumstances undue manipulative force may result in increased joint irritation, nerve compression, vertebral collapse, or hemorrhage. There exists a mild controversy over those conditions defined as being detrimentally affected by the manipulative approach. Stoddard (1969) and Jaquet (1976) attempted to rectify this discrepancy by defining classifications as "relative" or "absolute." It is doubtful that absolute contraindications would be disagreed upon by many. They include vertebral malignancy, tuberculosis, osteomyelitis, infectious arthritis, acute vertebral fracture, extreme osteoporosis, and extensive disc prolapse with evidence of severe nerve damage (Mennell, 1960; Stoddard, 1969; Jaquet, 1976). Relative contraindications may include some cases of osteoarthritis, disk prolapse, spondylolisthesis, hypermobility, severe scoliosis, and vertebrobasilar insufficiencies. Candidates for this category also might include hemangioma of the vertebral bodies, metabolic bone disease, and diabetic neuropathy. About these, there is likely to be much disagreement. Stoddard's attempt to settle this dispute was to suggest that only "experienced" manipulative practitioners attempt to manage these patients. No prospective studies exist that give compelling evidence to reconcile differences in clinical judgment often reflected in these kinds of listings.

More common tests used for these conditions include serum calcium and phosphorus, Ca:P ratio, alkaline phosphatase, acid phosphatase, complete blood count, erythrocyte sedimentation rate, urinalysis, protein electrophoresis, and immunoelectrophoresis (Fisk, 1977; Schafer, 1977). Laboratory results are interpreted in combination with results from clinical findings. Obviously, radiographic analysis also should be pursued where suspected diagnosis could be clarified by that procedure.

Nutritional Evaluation and Monitoring.

Throughout the course of its history the chiropractic profession has been vitally interested in the clinical usefulness of nutrition and the rational approach of nutritional counseling as therapy for malnutrition, chronic undernutrition (Busse et al., 1978), overnutrition (Schneider et al., 1977), functional disease, and some organic disorders. This represents some attitudes and approaches within the profession and is not a specific claim.

Nutritional science today is controversial. Concepts of relative versus absolute deficiency, validity of the recommended daily allowance (RDA), type A lunch programs (Cichoke, 1972; Head et al., 1973; Sims and Morris, 1974; Caliendo et al., 1977; Frank et al., 1977; Ziegler et al., 1977; Albanese, 1978; Busse et al., 1978; Kohrs et al., 1978; Munro and Young, 1978; Sawyer, 1991), and variances of individual nutritional needs are hotly contested issues. In these concerns the profession has long been immersed.

Americans appear to be more susceptible to overnutrition or chronic undernutrition rather than frank malnutrition. Obvious segments of the population affected by nutritional problems are those with low incomes, children during rapid growth periods, and the elderly affected by psychosocial problems and chronic diseases. Often, for patients in these categories, clinical symptoms and laboratory findings are nonspecific. Diagnosis, then, must rely on a careful patient history and the absence of other conditions likely to be responsible for the patient's complaints. Periodic laboratory testing becomes very

TABLE 20–11. STANDARD TESTS AVAILABLE FOR DIRECTING NUTRITIONAL EVALUATION

Nutrient	Test
Vitamin A and carotene	Plasma vitamin A, plasma carotenoids, response to 200,000 IU vitamin A
Vitamin D	Serum Ca, serum P, serum alkaline phosphatase
Vitamin C	Whole blood, buffy coat
Protein	Plasma total protein, serum albumin, plasma essential amino acid/total amino acid
Riboflavin	Plasma flavin adenine dinucleotide, urinary riboflavin
Thiamine	Blood lactate, plasma pyruvate transketolase [TK] RBC, thiamine pyrophosphate effect on TK, urinary thiamine
Pyridoxine	Urinary xanthurenic acid after 10 g D/L-tryptophane
Vitamin B_{12}	Plasma-B12 level [*Euglena gracilis* in serum]
Pantothenic acid	Serum pantothenic acid
Iron	Serum iron, serum iron-binding capacity
Folic acid	Serum level [*L, casei*], forminimino glutamic acid after 20 g 1-histidine HCl p.o.
Magnesium	Serum Mg
Zinc	Plasma Zn
Copper	Serum Copper
Vitamin K	Plasma prothrombine time
Sodium	Serum Na
Tocopherol	Plasma Tocopherol
Potassium	Serum K

valuable as a means of monitoring patient response and affirming diagnosis.

Standard biochemical tests for specific nutritional deficiencies are listed in Table 20–11. Tests for specific organ malfunction are often equally as important and informative.

The outcome of nutritional and pharmaceutical therapies prescribed for certain conditions are monitored by laboratory analysis. These include infection, cardiovascular disease, arteriosclerosis, anemia, osteoporosis, renal disease, and diabetes (Robinson, 1965; Goldman, 1967; Hollen, 1969; Forshee, 1971; Palmateer and Hollen, 1971; Pressman, 1971; Born, 1972; Dudley, 1972; Schroeder, 1975; Wozny, 1975; Dold, 1976; Jowsey, 1976; Schneider et al., 1977; Kritchevsky, 1978; Jamison, 1987, 1990). Careful observation of the physiological response is critical so that modifications in the treatment may be made.

Functional disorders are often misunderstood and misdiagnosed entities. A few of these have been found to have measurable biochemical alterations that allow easier diagnosis and monitoring but remain poorly described. Examples of the types of functional disorders for which laboratory evaluation is found to be useful include hypoglycemia, carbohydrate malabsorption, hypothyroid, and functional hypoadrenia (Jessen, 1967; Hollen, 1969; Buehler, 1971; Sisson, 1976; Walther, 1976). There remains a good deal of room for validation study and statistical analysis.

The only reliable means of determining the presence of functional hypoglycemia or malabsorption of carbohydrates is by using an oral glucose tolerance test. A typical 3-hour response to glucose loading is shown in Figure 20–38. Clinical differentiation of hypoglycemia can be perplexing and easily confused with anxiety, thyroid disorders, hypoadrenia, anemia, undernutrition, chronic inflammatory disease, Addison's disease, insomnia, and other problems that may cause chronic fatigue. The suspicion of the alert clinician often can be clarified by testing.

Other Instruments

Several other types of examining instruments have been or are still being used within the chiropractic profession. As none of these are widespread, only the fundamentals of their use will be described.

Plethysmography. The plethysmograph is an instrument that records the changes in size of a body part resulting from alterations in vascular flow. Blood volume can be measured directly as a result of pressure–volume changes accompanying constriction or dilation of the blood vessels.

This method has been used successfully by Figar and Krausova (1965) and Figar et al. (1967) to portray improvement after manipulation in 32 of 44 previously determined abnormal finger plethysmograms of patients with radicular syndromes involving the sixth to eighth cervical segments.

Further use of this instrument should be encouraged particularly in specific neurocirculatory disturbances and also may prove useful in radicular syndromes involving the extremities.

Spirometry. Estimation of vital capacity, total lung capacity, expiratory flow rate, maximum voluntary ventilation, and forced expiratory volume are important in the evaluation and clinical follow-up of lung disorders. After a full inspiratory effort the patient expels into the mouthpiece of the spirometer. Automated instrumentation then quantifies the various pulmonary function values and expresses them as percentages relative to the patient's somatotype (Freedman, 1983; Conrad, 1984).

The detrimental influence of scoliosis and restricted chest expansion on cardiopulmonary function is well documented (Davis, 1950; O'Donovan, 1951; Bergofsky et al., 1965; Bjure et al., 1970; Weber et al., 1975). These sources have reported asthmatic patients whose symptoms were relieved after treatment of thoracic scoliosis or radiculitis of the spine. Goldman (1972) further listed a high incidence of spinal lesions involving third to fifth thoracic vertebrae in such patients, but no statistical significance was given or effect of treatment described. Wilson (1946) concurred with the location of spinal lesion but also listed the need of ''freeing'' the fourth and fifth ribs bilaterally during the therapeutic process. In addition, he stressed the value of the patient's responsibilities for rest, diet breathing exercise, and avoidance of allergens.

Purse (1966) reported a study of 4600 cases of respiratory infection. Treatment of these cases was through spinal manipulation alone. He concluded that patients so treated not only recovered from the primary infection but also showed an apparent reduction in the frequency of complications compared with those treated by other means.

The types of spirometric findings associated with these conditions are divided into two main categories: obstructive findings and restrictive findings (Ayres, 1972; Braunwald et al., 1987). The air trap-

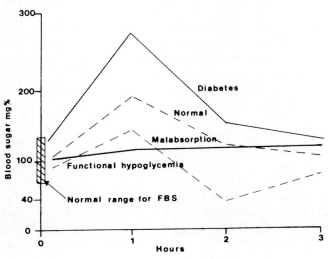

Figure 20–38. Typical responses seen with various conditions during 3-hour oral glucose tolerance test.

ping mechanisms of inflamed bronchi result in characteristic obstructive signs that are summarized by reduction in forced expiratory flow and forced mid-expiratory flow rate with evidence of "stair stepping" of maximal voluntary ventilation.

Disorders causing reduced expansion, such as scoliosis, are considered restrictive diseases and are characterized by reduced vital capacity, increased forced expiratory volume, and normal flow rates. Reports providing description of changes in these more objective parameters have not been found in the literature.

Good controlled studies are needed to evaluate the nature of manipulative therapy for these conditions.

Conclusion

A wide range of instruments with varying degrees of sensitivity and specificity are available to assist the chiropractic physician in clinical decision making. Their acceptance and usefulness vary significantly. Some are generally accepted, well established, and widely used. Others have general acceptance but have limited use. Still others have no proven value or are developmental in nature.

As in many other branches of health care, the technology is developing faster than the capacity for the average clinician to keep pace. As a result, it is not surprising that each new procedure or tool is embraced enthusiastically by some and soundly rejected by others.

The main features of any instrument that can be evaluated to ascertain clinical utility can be summarized on the basis of discriminability and normative data. If each practicing physician insists on high quality studies leading to the substantiation of these characteristics for every instrument they use, the common state of uncertainty and confusion about validity and appropriate uses will rapidly decline.

References

Agarwal A, Lloyd KN, and Dovey P. Thermography of the spine and sacroiliac joints in spondylitis. *Rheum Phys Med* 1970; 10:349.

Ahern DK, Follick MJ, and Council JR, et al. Comparison of lumbar paravertebral EMG patterns in chronic low back pain patients and non-patient controls. *Pain* 1988;34:153.

Albanese AA. Calcium nutrition in the elderly: Maintaining bone health to minimize fracture risk. *Postgrad Med* 1978;63:167.

Ash CJ, Shealy CN, Young PA, and Van Beaumont W. Thermography and the sensory dermatome. *Skeletal Radiol* 1986;15:40.

Atkins AR, and Wyndham CH. A Study of temperature regulation in the human body with the aid of an analog computer. *Pfleugers Arch* 1969;307:104.

Ayoub MA. Design of a pre-employment screening program. In Kvalseth TO, ed. *Ergonomics of Workstation Design*. London: Butterworths;1983: 152–8.

Ayoub MA. Ergonomic deficiencies. I. pain at work. *J Occup Med* 1990;32:52.

Ayres SM. Pulmonary function studies. In Holman CW, and Muschenheim C eds. *Bronchopulmonary Diseases and Related Disorders*. Hagerstown: Harper & Row; 1972.

Bailey HW. Theoretical significance of postural imbalance especially the "short leg." *J Am Osteopath Assoc* 1978;77:452.

Bailey HW, and Beckwith DO. Short leg and spinal anomalies. *J Am Osteopath Assoc* 1937;13:4.

Baillie AJ, Biagioni PA, Forsyth A, and Garioch JJ. Thermographic assessment of patch-test responses. *Br J Dermatol* 1990;122:351.

Baltzopoulos V, and Brodie DA. Isokinetic dynamometry applications and limitations. *Sports Med* 1989;8:101.

Barlow DH, Hayes S, and Nelson R. *The Scientist Practitioner: Research and Accountability in Clinical and Educational Settings*. New York: Pergamon Press; 1984;112, 124.

Barnes WS. The relationship of motor unit activation to isokinetic muscular contraction at different contractile velocities. *Phys Ther* 1980;60:1152.

Basmajian JV, and DeLuca CJ. *Muscles Alive: Their Function Revealed by Electromyography*, 5th ed. Baltimore: Williams & Wilkins; 1985.

Bean JC, Chaffin DB, and Schultz AB: Biomechanical model calculation of muscle contraction forces: A double linear programming method. *J Biomech* 1988;21:59.

Beasley WC. Influence of method on estimates of normal knee extensor force among normal and postpolio children. *Phys Ther Rev* 1956;36:21.

Beimborn DS, and Morrissey MC. A review of the literature related to trunk muscle performance. *Spine* 1988;13:655.

Bergner M, Bobbitt RA, Carter WB, and Gilson BS. The Sickness Impact Profile: Development and final revision of a health status measure. *Med Care* 1981;19:787.

Bergofsky EH, Turnio GM, and Fishman AP. Cardiorespiratory failure in kyphoscoliosis. *Medicine* 1965;38:263.

Bergquist-Ullman M, and Larsson U. Acute low back pain in industry—A controlled prospective study with special reference to therapy and confounding factors. *Acta Orthop Scand* (Suppl) 1977;170:1.

Bigos SJ, and Battie MC. Acute care to prevent back disability. Ten years of progress. *Clin Orthop* 1987;221:121.

Bjure J, Grimby G, and Kasalicky J, et al. Respiratory impairment and airway closure in patients with untreated idiopathic scoliosis. *Thorax* 1970;25:451.

Bohannan RW. Hand-held dynamometry; Stability of muscle strength over multiple measurements. *Clinical Biomech* 1986;2:74.

Bohannan RW, and Andrews AW. Accuracy of spring and strain gauge hand-held dynamometers. *J Orthop Sports Phys Ther* 1989; 10:323.

Bollier W. Spine and internal disease. *Ann Swiss Chiropr Assoc* 1961;2:167.

Born BA. Nutritional aspects in the prevention and treatment of arteriosclerosis. *ACA J Chiropr* 1972;9:S53.

Braunwald E, Isselbacher KJ, and Petersdorf RG, et al., eds. *Harrison's Principles of Internal Medicine*. New York: McGraw-Hill; 1987.

Brown WF. *The Physiological and Technical Basis of Electromyography*. Boston: Butterworths; 1984.

Buchthal F. Diagnostic significance of the myopathic EMG. In Rowland F, ed. *Pathogenesis of Human Muscular Dystrophies*. Amsterdam: Exerpta Medica; 1977.

Buehler MT. The hypoglycemic state. *ACA J Chiropr* 1971; 8:S33.

Busse EW. How mind, body, and environment influence nutrition in the elderly. *Postgrad Med* 1978;63:118.

Byl NN, Richards S, and Asturias J. Intrarater and interrater reliability of strength measurements of the biceps and deltoid using a hand held dynamometer. *J Orthop Sports Phys Ther* 1988;9:399.

Caliendo MA, Sanjur D, Wright J, and Cummings G. Nutritional status of preschool children. *J Am Diet Assoc* 1977;71:20.

Chafetz N, Wexler CE, and Kaiser JA. Neuromuscular thermography of the lumbar spine with CT correlation. *Spine* 1988;13:922.

Chaffin DB, and Andersson GBJ. *Occupational Biomechanics.* New York: Wiley Publishers; 1984.

Chapman AE, and Troup JDG. The effect of increased maximal strength on the integrated electrical activity of lumbar erectores spine. *Electromyography* 1969;9:263.

Ciatto S, Palli D, Rosselli del Turco M, and Catarzi S. Diagnostic and prognostic role of infrared thermography. *Radiol Med* 1987; 74:312.

Cichoke AJ. Protein malnutrition and introduction of low-cost protein-rich supplements. *ACA J Chiropr* 1972;9:S11.

Clarke GR. Unequal leg length—An accurate method of detection and some clinical results. *Rheum Phys Med* 1972;11:385.

Cleveland RH, Kushner DC, and Ogden MC, et al. Determination of leg length discrepancy. A comparison of weight-bearing and supine imaging. *Invest Radiol* 1988;23:301.

Coers C, and Woolf AL. *The Innervation of Muscle—A Biopsy Study.* Springfield, Ill: Thomas; 1959.

Coggins WN. *Basic Techniques and Systems of Body Mechanics.* Florrissant, Elco, 1975

Cohen HL, and Brumlik JD: *Manual of Electroneuromyography,* 2nd ed, Hagerstown: Harper & Row; 1976.

Cohen MJ, Swanson GA, and Naliboff BD, et al. Comparison of electromyographic response patterns during posture and stress tasks in chronic low back pain patterns and control. *J Psychosom Res* 1986;30:135.

Collins GA, Cohen MJ, Naliboff BD, and Schandler SL. Comparative analysis of paraspinal and frontalis EMG, heart rate and skin conductance in chronic low back pain patients and normals to various postures and stress. *Scand J Rehab Med* 1982;14:39.

Connell JF Jr, Morgan E, and Rousselot LM. Thermography in trauma. *Ann N Y Acad Sci* 1964;121:171.

Conrad SA. Pulmonary function testing equipment. In Conrad SA, Kinasewitz GT, and George RB, eds. *Pulmonary Function Testing—Principles and Practice.* New York: Churchill-Livingstone, 1984.

Cooper P, Randall WC, and Hertzman AB. Vascular convection of heat from active muscle to overlying skin. *J Appl Physiol* 1959;14:207.

Corlett E, Manecica I, and Guillau P. The relationship between EMG activity of the sacrospinalis and reported back discomfort. *Euro J Applied Physiol.* 1983;50:213.

Coxhead CE, Inskip H, and Meade TW, et al. Multicentre trial of physiotherapy in the management of sciatic symptoms. *Lancet* 1981;1:1065.

Cramer G, Humphreys C, Triano J, and Hondras M. The H/M ratio as an outcome measure of chiropractic treatment efficacy in acute low back pain. *Proceedings ICSM,* 1990.

Davis D. Respiratory manifestations of dorsal spine radiculitis simulating cardiac asthma. *Ann Intern Med* 1950;32:954.

DeBois EF. *The Mechanism of Heat Loss and Temperature Regulation.* Stanford: Stanford University Press; 1937.

Demany MA, Tambe A, and Zimmerman HA. Coronary arterial spasm. *Dis Chest* 1968;53:714.

Deschuytere J, and Rosselle N. Diagnostic use of monosynaptic reflexes in L5 and S1 root compression. In Desmedt JE, ed. *New Developments in Electromyography and Clinical Neurophysiology,* vol. 3. Basel: S. Karger; 1973.

Deutsch S. *B-200 Back Evaluation System.* Hillsborough: Isotechnologies; 1989–90.

Deyo RA, Diehl AK, and Rosenthal M. How many days of bed rest for acute low back pain? a randomized clinical trail. *New Engl J Med* 1986;315:1064.

Dhurandhar RW, Watt DL, and Silver MD, et al. Prinzmetal's variant form of angina with arteriographic evidence of coronary arterial spasm. *Am J Cardiol* 1972;30:902.

Diakow PR. Thermographic imaging of myofascial trigger points. *J Manipulative Physiol Ther* 1988;11:114.

Dold WR. Anemia investigation and classification. *ACA J Chiropr* 1976;13:S35.

Dowling JJ, and Kennedy SR. The quantitative assessment of EMG crosstalk in human soleus and gastrocnemius muscles. Thirteenth annual meeting of the American Society of Biomechanics. Vermont: August 1989.

Dudley WN. Triglycerides and sucrose. *ACA J Chiropr* 1972;9:S79.

Dudley WN. Preliminary findings in thermography of the back. *ACA J Chiropr* 1978;15:S83.

Duensing F, Becker P, and Rittmeyer K. Thermographic findings in lumbar disc protrusions. *Arch Psychiatr Nervenkr* 1973;217:53.

Eason RG. Electromyographic study of local and generalized muscular impairment. *J Appl Physiol* 1960;15:479.

Edeiken J, Wallace JD, Curley RF, and Lee S. Thermography and herniated lumbar discs. *Am J Roentgenol* 1968;102:790.

Egli A. Spine and heart vertebrogenic cardia syndromes. *Ass Swiss Chiropr Assoc* 1962;6:95.

Eisen A, Schomer D, and Melmed C. An electrophysiological method for examining lumbosacral root compression. *Can J Neurol Sci* 1977;4:117.

Engelberg AL, ed. *Guides to the Evaluation of Permanent Impairment,* 3rd ed. Chicago: American Medical Association; 1988.

Fairbanks JCT, Davies JB, Mbaot JC, and O'Brien JP. The Oswestry low back pain disability questionnaire. *Physiotherapy* 1980;66:271.

Fichera AP, and Celander DR. Effect of osteopathic manipulative therapy on autonomic tone as evidenced by blood pressure changes and activity of the fibrinolytic system. *J Am Osteopath Assoc* 1969;68:1036.

Figar S, and Krausova L. A plethysmographic study of the effects of chiropractic treatment in vertebrogenic syndromes. *ACTA Univ Carol Med* (Suppl) 1965;21:84.

Figar S, Krausova L, and Levit K. Plethysmographic examination following treatment of vertebrogenic disorders by manipulation. *ACTA Neuroveg* 1967;29:618.

Fisk JW. *A Practical Guide to Management of the Painful Neck and Back—Diagnosis, Manipulation, Exercises, Prevention.* Springfield, Ill: Charles C. Thomas; 1977;10.

Forshee GK. Arterio and atherosclerosis with relation to vitamin D. *ACA J Chiropr* 1971;8:S81.

Frank GC, Voors AW, Schilling PE, and Berenson GS. Dietary studies of rural school children in a cardiovascular survey. *J Am Diet Assoc* 1977;71:31.

Freedman S. Design of respiratory circuits and spirometry. In Laszlo G, and Sudlow MF, eds. *Measurement in Clinical Respiratory Physiology.* London: Academic Press; 1983.

Friberg O, Nurminen M, and Korhonen K, et al. Accuracy and precision of clinical estimation of leg length inequality and lumbar scoliosis: Comparison of clinical and radiological measurements. *Internat Disabil Studies* 1988;10:49.

Frymoyer JW, Newberg A, and Pope MH, et al. Spine radiographs in patients with low-back pain. An epidemiological study in men. *J Bone Joint Surg* 1984;66A:1048.

Fuhrer MJ. Effects of stimulus site on the pattern of skin conductance responses evoked from spinal man. *J Neurol Neurosurg Phychiatr* 1975;38:749.

Fullenlove TM, and Williams AJ. Comparative roentgen findings in symptomatic and asymptomatic backs. *Radiology* 1957;68:572.

Gerow G, Callton M, and Meyer JJ, et al. Thermographic evaluation of rats with complete sciatic nerve transection. *J Manipulative Physiol Ther* 1990;13:257.

Gleim GW, Nicholas JA, and Webb JN. Isokinetic evaluation following leg injuries. *Phys Sportsmed* 1978;68:74.

Goldberg HI, Heinz ER, and Taveras JM. Thermography in neurologic patients: Preliminary experiences. *Acta Radiol* 1966;5:786.

Goldman SR. Pathogenesis of the diabetic syndrome. *ACA J Chiropr* 1967;4:S22.

Goldman SR. A structural approach to bronchial asthma. *Bull Eur Chiropr Union* 1972;21:66.

Gomez T, Beach G, and Cooke C, et al. Normative database for trunk range of motion, strength, velocity, and endurance with the isostation B-200 lumbar dynamometer. *Spine* 1991;16:15.

Gosselin G. Diagnostic tools for the sports chiropractor. *SOMA* October 1987;23.

Grice AS. Muscle tonus change following manipulation. *J Can Chiropr Assoc* 1974;18:29.

Gutstein WH, Harrison J, and Parl F, et al. Neural factors contribute to atherogenesis. *Science* 1978;199:449.

Hadler NM, Curtis P, and Gillings DB. A benefit of spinal manipulation as adjunctive therapy for acute low-back pain: A stratified controlled trial. *Spine* 1987;12:703.

Halberg F. Temporal coordination of physiologic function. *Cold Spring Harb Symp Quant Biol* 1960;25:289.

Halberg F. Chronobiology. *Annu Rev Physiol* 1969;31:675.

Haldeman S. Clinical basis for discussion of mechanisms of manipulative therapy. In Korr IM, ed. *The Neurobiologic Mechanisms in Manipulative Therapy*. New York: Plenum Press; 1978: 53–76.

Handelsman H. Thermography for indications other than breast lesions. *Health Technology Assessment Reports* 1989;2:1.

Hazard RG, Fenwick JW, and Kalisch SM, et al. Functional restoration with behavioral support—A one-year prospective study of patients with chronic low-back pain. *Spine* 1989;14:157.

Hazard RG, Reid S, Fenwick J, and Reeves V. Isokinetic trunk and lifting strength measurements: Variability as an indicator of effort. *Spine* 1988;13:54.

Head MK, Weeks RJ, and Gibbs E. Major nutrients in the type A lunch. *J Am Diet Assoc* 1973;63:620.

Heinz ER, Goldberg HI, and Taveras J. Experiences with thermography in neurologic patients. *Ann N Y Acad Sci* 1964;121:171.

Hellsing AL. Leg length inequality. A prospective study of young men during their military service. *Upsala J Med Sci* 1988; 93:245.

Herzenberger JE, Waanders NA, and Closkey RA, et al. Spinous process angle versus Cobb angle in adolescent idiopathic scoliosis—Relationship of the anterior and posterior deformities. Proceedings of the Scoliosis Research Society, Amsterdam: September 1989.

Hildebrandt RW. *Chiropractic Spinography—A Manual of Technology and Interpretation*. Des Plains: Hilmark Publication; 1977.

Hoffmann R, Largiadèr F, and Brutsch HP. Liquid crystal contact thermography—A new screening procedure in the diagnosis of deep venous thrombosis. *Helv Chir Acta* 1989;56:45.

Hoikka V, Ylikoski M, and Tallroth K. Leg-length inequality has poor correlation with lumbar scoliosis. A radiological study of 100 patients with chronic low-back pain. *Arch Orthop Trauma Surg* 1989;108:173.

Hollen WV. Clinical carbohydrate evaluation. *ACA J Chiropr* 1969;6:S73.

Holma J. *Experimental Methods for Engineers*. New York: McGraw-Hill, pg 44–63, 1984

Holmgren K, Jacobsson H, Johnsson H, and Lofsjogard-Nilsson E. Thermography and plethysmography, a non-invasive alternative to venography in the diagnosis of deep vein thrombosis. *J Int Med* 1990;228:29.

Homewood AE. *The Neurodynamics of the Vertebral Subluxation*. Ontario, Chiropractic Publishers; 1962.

Hood RP. Blood pressure. Results in 75 abnormal cases. *Dig Chiropr Econ* 1974;16:36.

Hoppenfeld S. *Scoliosis: A Manual of Concept and Treatment*. Philadelphia: Lippincott; 1967.

Horsfield D, and Jones SN. Assessment of inequality in length of the lower limb. *Radiography* 1986;52:223.

Houdas Y, and Guieu JD. Environmental factors affecting skin temperatures. *Bibl Radiol* 1974;6:157.

Howell RK, and Kappler RE. The influence of osteopathic manipulative therapy on a patient with advanced cardiopulmonary disease. *J Am Osteopath Assoc* 1973;73:322.

Humphreys CR, Triano JJ, and Brandl MJ. Sensitivity study of H-reflex alterations in idiopathic low back pain patients vs. a healthy population. *J Manipulative Physiol Ther* 1989;12:71.

Huskisson EC. Measurement of pain. *Lancet* 1974;2:1127.

Huskisson EC. Measurement of pain. *J Rheumatol* 1982; 9:768.

Huskisson EC, Berry H, Browett J, and Wykeham Balme H. Measurement of inflammation. *Ann Rheum Dis* 1973;32:99.

Illi FW. The phylogenesis and clinical import of the sacroiliac mechanism. *J Can Chiropr Assoc* 1965;9:9.

Jabre JF, and Hackett ER. *EMG Manual*. Springfield, Ill; Thomas; 1983.

Jacobs I, Bell DG, and Pope J. Comparison of isokinetic and isoinertial lifting tests as predictors of maximal lifting capacity. *Europ J Appl Physiol Occup Physiol* 1988;57:146.

Jamison JR. Dietary control of mild essential hypertension. *J Manipulative Phys Ther* 1987;10:101.

Jamison JR. Dietary intervention in the clinical prevention of ischemic heart disease. *J Manipulative Phys Ther* 1990;13:247.

Janda V. Postural and phasic muscles in the pathogenesis of low back pain. Proceedings of the 11th Congress of the International Society of Rehabilitation of the Disabled. Dublin: 1969.

Janda V. Muscle and joint correlation. Proceedings of the 4th Congress of the International Federation of Manipulative Medicine. Prague: 1973–4.

Janda V. Muscles, central nervous motor regulation and back problems. In Korr IM, ed. *The Neurobiologic Mechanisms in Manipulative Therapy* (pp. 27–42). New York: Plenum Press; 1977.

Janda V, and Stara B. Comparison of movement in healthy and spastic children. Proceedings of the 2nd International Symposium—Cerebral Palsy. Prague: 1971.

Janse J, Houser RH, and Wells BF. *Chiropractic Principles and Technique*. Chicago: National College of Chiropractic; 1947.

Jaquet P. *An Introduction to Clinical Chiropractic*. Geneva: Jaquet and Grinard; 1976.

Jayasinghe WJ, Harding RH, Anderson JAD, and Sweetman BJ. An electromyographic investigation of postural fatigue in low back pain—A preliminary study. *Electromyogr Clin Neurophysiol* 1978;18:191.

Jenness ME. The role of thermography and postural measurement in structural diagnosis. In Goldstein M, ed. *Research Status of Spinal Manipulative Therapy*, NINCDS Monograph No. 15. Washington: U.S. DHEW; 1975:255.

Jessen AR. Diagnosis of thyroid dysfunction. *ACA J Chiropr* 1967;4:S49.

Jiang BC, Smith JL, and Ayoub MM. Psychophysical modeling of manual materials-handling capacities using isoinertial strength variables. *Hum Factors* 1986a;28:691.

Jiang BC, Smith JL, and Ayoub MM. Psychophysical modelling for combined manual materials-handling activities. *Ergonomics* 1986b;29:1173.

Johnson EW, and Melvin JL. Value of electromyography in lumbar radiculopathy. *Arch Phys Med Rehabil* 1971;52:239.

Jones CH. Physical aspects of thermography in relation to clinical techniques. *Bibl Radiol* 1974;6:1.

Jonker JJ, Sing AK, de Boer AC, and den Ottolander GJ. The value of adding thermographic leg scanning to impedance plethysmography in the detection of deep vein thrombosis. *Thromb Res* 1986;42:681.

Jowsey J. Osteoporosis. *Postgrad Med* 1976;60:75.

Judovich B, and Bates W. *Pain Syndromes—Diagnosis and Treatment*, 4th ed. Philadelphia: F.A. Davis; 1954.

Kannus P. Ratio of hamstring to quadriceps femoris muscles' strength in the anterior cruciate ligament insufficient knee. Relationship to long-term recovery. *Phys Ther* 1988;68:961.

Karpman HL, Knebel A, Semel CJ, and Cooper J. Clinical studies in thermography: II. application of thermography in evaluating musculoligamentous injuries of the spine—A preliminary report. *Arch Environ Health* 1970;20:412.

Kieffer JD. Laboratory procedures in the low back syndrome. *ACA J Chiropr* 1965;2:17.

Khalil TM, Goldberg ML, and Asfour SS, et al. Acceptable maximum effort (AME) a psychophysical measure of strength in back pain patients. *Spine* 1987;12:372.

Kibler WB, Chandler TJ, Uhl T, and Maddux RE. A musculoskeletal approach to the preparticipation physical examination. Preventing injury and improving performance. *Am J Sports Med* 1989;17:525.

Kimmel E. Electro-analytical instrumentation. *ACA J Chiropr* April 1966a;3:9.

Kimmel E. Electro-analytical instrumentation. *ACA J Chiropr* May 1966b;3:9.

Kimmel E. Electro-analytical instrumentation. *ACA J Chiropr* June 1966c;3:11.

Kohrs MB, O'Neil R, and Preston A, et al. Nutritional status of elderly residents in Missouri. *Am J Clin Nutri* 1978;31:2186.

Kravitz E, Moore ME, and Glaros A. Paralumbar muscle activity in chronic low back pain. *Arch Phys Med Rehabil* 1981;62:172.

Kritchevsky D. How aging affects cholesterol metabolism. *Postgrad Med* 1978;63:133.

Kroemer KHE. An isoinertial technique to assess individual capacity. *Hum Factors* 1983;25:493.

Kroemer K. Testing individual capability to lift materials. Repeatability of a dynamic test compared with static testing. *J Safety Res* 1985;16:1.

Kulig K, Andrews JG, and Hay JG. Human strength curves. In Terjung RL, ed. *Exercise in Sport Sciences Reviews*. New York: MacMillan; 1984:12:417.

Kvalseth TO, ed. *Ergonomics of Workstation Design* London: Butterworths; 1983.

Lakomy HKA, and Williams C. Measurement of isokinetic concentric and eccentric muscle imbalance. *Int J Sports Med* (Suppl) 1984;5:40.

Langrana NA, Lee CK, Alexander H, and Mayott CW. Quantitative assessment of back strength using isokinetic testing. *Spine* 1984;9:287.

Lawrence JS. Disc degeneration. Its frequency and relationship to symptoms. *Ann Rheum Dis* 1969;28:121.

Leavitt F, Garron DC, Whisler WW, and D'Angelo CM. A comparison of patients treated by chymopapain and laminectomy for low back pain using a multidimensional pain scale. *Clin Orthop* 1980;146:136.

Lebkowski J, Polocki B, and Borucki A, et al. Determination of the level of prolapsed intervertebral disc ischialgia by means of electric thermometer. *Pol Tyg Lek* 1973;28:907.

Levy MN. Sympathetic–parasympathetic interactions in the heart. *Circ Res* 1971;29:437.

Loban JM. *Technic and Practice of Chiropractic*, 4th ed. Denver: Bunn-Loban; 1928.

Ludin HP. *Electromyography in Practice*. Stuttgart: Georg Thieme Verlag; 1980.

Maseri A, Nimmo R, and Chierchia S, et al. Coronary artery spasm as a cause of acute myocardial ischemia in man. *Chest* 1975;68:625.

Mayer TG, and Gatchel RJ. *Functional Restoration for Spinal Disorders: The Sports Medicine Approach*. Philadelphia: Lea & Febiger; 1988: 208.

Mayer TG, Gatchel RJ, and Kishino N, et al. A prospective short-term study of chronic low back pain patients utilizing novel objective functional measurement. *Pain* 1986;25:53.

Mayer TG, Gatchel RJ, and Maher H. et al. A prospective two year study of functional restoration in industrial low back injury. An objective assessment procedure. *JAMA* 1987;258:1763.

Mayer TG, Smit SS, Keeley J, and Mooney V. Quantification of lumbar function. part 2: sagittal plane trunk strength in chronic low-back pain patients. *Spine* 1985;10:765.

McNeill T, Warwick D, Andersson G, and Schultz A. Trunk strengths in attempted flexion, extension, and lateral bending in healthy subjects and patients with low-back disorders. *Spine* 1980;5:529.

Mennell J McM. *Back Pain—Diagnosis and Treatment Using Manipulative Techniques*. Boston: Little Brown; 1960.

Miller DJ. Comparison of electromyographic activity in the lumbar paraspinal muscles of subjects with and without chronic low back pain. *Phys Ther* 1985;65:1347.

Miller WD. Treatment of visceral disorders by manipulative therapy. In Goldstein M, ed. *The Research Status of Spinal Manipulative Therapy*, NINCDS Monograph No. 15. Washington: DHEW; 1975; 29.

Million R, Hall W, and Nilsen KH, et al. Assessment of the progress of the back-pain patient. *Spine* 1982;7:204.

Mills GH, Davies GK, Getty CJ, and Conway J. The evaluation of liquid crystal thermography in the investigation of nerve root compression due to lumbosacral lateral spinal stenosis. *Spine* 1986;11:427.

Mira AJ, Markley K, Greer RB III. A critical analysis of quadriceps function after femoral shaft fracture in adults. *J Bone Joint Surg* 1980;62A:61.

Missiuro W, Kirschner H, and Kozlowski S. Electromyographic manifestations of fatigue during work of different intensity. *ACTA Physiol Pol* 1962;13:11.

Mitchell FL, and Pruzzo NL. Investigation of voluntary and primary respiratory mechanisms. *J Am Osteopath Assoc* 1971; 70:1109.

Moreland MS, Pope MH, and Armstrong GWD, eds. *Moire Fringe Topography and Spinal Deformity*. New York: Pergamon Press; 1981.

Mosley CF. A straight line graph for leg length discrepancies. *Clin Orthop* 1978;136:33.

Munro HN, and Young VR. Protein metabolism in the elderly: Observations relating to dietary needs. *Postgrad Med* 1978; 63:143.

Mustacchi G, Milani S. and Ciatto S, et al. Observer variation in mammary thermography: Results of a teaching file test carried out in four different centers. *Tumori* 1990;76:29.

Nelson RC, and Fahrney RA. Relationship between strength and speed of elbow flexion. *Res Quart* 1965;36:455.

Nichols PJR. The short leg syndrome. *Br Med J* 1960; 1:1863.

Niebuhr BR, and Marion R. Detecting sincerity of effort when measuring grip strength. *Am J Phys Med* 1987;66:16.

Norris T. The study of the effect of manipulation on blood pressure. *Acad Appl Osteopath Yearbook*, Carmel, CA: The Academy of Applied Osteopathy; 1964.

Nouwen A. EMG biofeedback used to reduce standing levels of paraspinal muscle tension in chronic low back pain. *Pain* 1983; 17:353.

Nouwen A, and Bush C. The relationship between paraspinal EMG and chronic low back pain. *Pain* 1984;20:109.

Nunn KD, and Mayhew JL. Comparison of three methods of assessing strength imbalances at the knee. *J Orthop Sports Phys Ther*, 1988;10: 134.

O'Donovan D. The possible significance of scoliosis of the spine in the causation of asthma and allied allergic conditions. *Ann Allergy* 1951;9:184.

Owen E, and Holt GA. *Thermographic Patterns in Sacroiliitis and An-*

kylosing Spondylitis. New York: American Thermographic Society, 1973.

Palmateer DC, and Hollen WV. Urinary tract calculi diagnosis and treatment. *ACA J Chiropr* 1971;8:S25.

Panjabi MM, Goel VK, and Walter SD. Errors in kinematic parameters of a planar joint: Guidelines for optimal experimental design. *J Biomechanics* 1982;15:537.

Parnianpour M, Li F, Nordin M, and Kahanovitz N. A database of isoinertial strength tests against three resistance levels in sagittal, frontal, and transverse planes in normal male subjects. *Spine* 1989;14:409.

Phillips RB. The irritable reflex mechanism. *J Can Chiropr Assoc* 1974;18:22.

Pilowsky I, and Spence ND. *Manual for the Illness Behavior Questionnaire* (IBQ), 2nd ed. Adelaide, Australia: University of Adelaide; 1983.

Pochaczevsky R. Thermography in posttraumatic pain. *Am J Sports Med* 1987;15:243.

Pollock ML, Leggett SH, and Graves JE, et al. Effect of resistance training on lumbar extension strength. *Am J Sports Med* 1989; 17:624.

Pressman R. Calcium and neglected minerals. *ACA J Chiropr* 1971;8:S45.

Prinzmetal M, Kennamer R, and Merliss R. et al. Angina pectoris I. a variant form of angina pectoris—Preliminary report. *Am J Med* 1959;7:375.

Pullella SF, Andre J, and Bell L, et al. Correlative study of various instruments and procedures in chiropractic. *ACA J Chiropr* 1974;11:S197.

Purse FM. Manipulative therapy of upper respiratory infections in children. *J Am Osteopath Assoc* 1966;65:964.

Raskin M. *Thermography in Low Back Diseases. Medical Thermography: Theory and Clinical Applications.* Los Angeles: Brentwood; 1976.

Reinberg A. Circadian changes in the temperature of human beings. *Bibl Radiol* 1975;6:128.

Roaf R. *Scoliosis.* Baltimore: Williams & Wilkins; 1966.

Robinson R. Calcium and vitamins C and D in nutrition of bone, muscle, and nerve. *ACA J Chiropr* 1965;2:14.

Rogers JT, and Rogers JC. The role of osteopathic manipulative therapy in the treatment of coronary artery disease. *J Am Osteopath Assoc* 1976;76:21.

Roland M, and Morris R. A study of the natural history of back pain, Part I: Development of a reliable and sensitive measure of disability in low-back pain. *Spine* 1983a;8:141.

Roland M, and Morris R. A study of the natural history of low-back pain, Part II: development of guidelines for trials of treatment in primary care. *Spine* 1983b;8:145.

Rothenberg RJ. Rheumatic disease aspects of leg length inequality. *Semin Arthritis Rheum* 1988;17:196.

Ruch TC, Patton HD, Woodbury JW, and Towe AL. *Neurophysiology.* Philadelphia: Saunders; 1965.

Sapega AA. Muscle performance evaluation in orthopaedic practice. *J Bone Joint Surg* 1990;72A:1562.

Saraniti AJ, Gleim GW, Melvin M, and Nicholas JA. The relationship between subjective and objective measurements of strength. *J Orthop Sports Phys Ther* 1980;2:15.

Sato A. The somatosympathetic reflexes: their physiological and clinical significance. In Goldstein M, ed. *The Research Status of Spinal Manipulative Therapy,* NINCDS Monograph No. 15. Washington: DHEW; 1975, 163–173.

Sawyer CE. Nutritional disorders. In Lawrence D, ed. *Fundamentals of Chiropractic Diagnosis and Management.* Baltimore: Williams & Wilkins; 1991.

Schafer RE, ed. *Basic Chiropractic Procedural Manual.* DesMoines: American Chiropractic Association; 1977.

Schneider HA, Anderson CE, and Coursin DB: *Nutritional Support of Medical Practice.* Hagerstown: Harper & Row; 1977.

Schroeder RM. Diseases related to the pathologic biochemistry of calcium, phosphorus, and alkaline phosphatase metabolism. *ACA J Chiropr* 1975;12:S13.

Schuit D, Adrian M, and Pidcoe P. Effect of heel lifts on ground reaction force patterns in subjects with structural leg-length discrepancies. *Phys Ther* 1989;69:663.

Seeds RH, Levene JA, and Goldberg HM. Abnormal patient data for the isostation B100. *J Orthop Sports Phys Ther* 1988;10:121.

Seeman DC. C1 subluxations: Short leg and pelvic distortions. *The Upper Cervical Monograph* Monroe, MI: The National Upper Cervical Chiropractic Association, Inc. Ralph R. Gregory, D.C., 1978;2:5, 1.

Sherman RA. Relationships between strength of low back muscle contraction and reported intensity of chronic low back pain. *Am J Phys Med* 1985;64:190.

Sherman RA, Barja RH, and Bruno GM. Thermographic correlates of chronic pain: analysis of 125 patients incorporating evaluations by a blind panel. *Arch Phys Med Rehabil* 1987;68:273.

Silverman JL, Rodriquez AA, and Agre JC. Reliability of a hand-held dynamometer in neck strength testing. *Arch Phys Med Rehabil* (Suppl) 1989;70:94.

Simpson JA. Neuromuscular diseases. In Remond A, ed. *Handbook of Electroencephalography and Clinical Neurophysiology.* Amsterdam: Elsevier; 1973, 27.

Sims LS, and Morris PM. Nutritional status of preschoolers. *J Am Diet Assoc* 1974;64:492.

Sirohi RS, and Krishna HLR. *Mechanical Measurements,* 2nd ed. New York: Halstead Press: 1983: 36–58.

Sisson JA. *Handbook of Clinical Pathology.* Philadelphia: JB Lippincott; 1976.

Smith GA, Nelson RC, Sadoff SJ, and Dadoff AM. Assessing sincerity of effort in maximal grip strength tests. *Am J Phys Med Rehabil* 1989;68:73.

Smorto MP, and Basmajian JV. *Electrodiagnosis: A Handbook for Neurologists.* New York: Harper & Row; 1977.

So YT, Aminoff MJ, and Olney RK. The role of thermography in the evaluation of lumbosacral radiculopathy. *Neurology* 1989; 39:1154.

Soderberg GL, and Barr JO. Muscular function in chronic low back dysfunction. *Spine* 1983;8:79.

Splithoff CA. Lumbosacral junction. Roentgenographic comparison of patients with and without backache. *JAMA* 1953; 152:1610.

Stary O, O'Brda K, Pfieffer J, and Barankova M. Polyelectromyographic studies of proprioceptive analysis disorders during the initial phases of vertebrogenic disorders in children. *Acta Univ Carol Med (Suppl)* 1965;21:21.

Stevenson JM, Andrew GM, and Bryant JT, et al. Isoinertial tests to predict lifting performance. *Ergonomics* 1989;32:157.

Stoddard A. *Manual of Osteopathic Practice.* New York: Harper & Row; 1969.

Stolwijk JAJ. Heat exchanges between body and environment. *Bibl Radiol* 1975;6:144.

Tait RC, Pollard CA, and Margolis RB, et al. The pain disability index: Psychometric and validity data. *Arch Phys Med Rehabil* 1987;68:438.

Taylor A. The significance of grouping motor unit activity. *J Physiol* 1962;162:259.

Thistle HG, Hislop HJ, Moffroid M, and Lowman EW. Isokinetic contraction: A new concept of resistive exercise. *Arch Phys Med Rehabil* 1967;48:279.

Thompson LL. *The Electromyographer's Handbook.* Boston: Little Brown; 1981.

Thorstensson A, and Arvidson A. Trunk muscle strength and low back pain. *Scand J Rehabil Med* 1982;14:69.

Tilley RM. The somatic component in heart disease. In *Clinical Review Series—Osteopathic Medicine* Eli H. Stark (ed.) Acton, MA: Publishing Sciences Group: 1975, 129–136.

Topf M. Response sets in questionnaire research. *Nursing Res* 1986;35:119.

Tran TA, and Kirby JD. The effect of upper cervical adjustment upon the normal physiology of the heart. *ACA J Chiropr* 1977; 14:S58.

Triano JJ. The pathophysiology of congestive heart failure. *Chiropr Econ* March/April 1973;72.

Triano J. Objective electromyographic evidence for the use and effects of lift therapy. *J Manipulative Physiol Ther* 1983;6:13.

Triano J, Baker J, McGregor M, and Torres B. Optimizing measures on maximum voluntary contraction. *Spine* (submitted for publication with revisions), 1991.

Triano JJ, and Davis BP. Experimental characterization of the reactive muscle phenomenon. *Chiropr Econ* Sept/Oct 1976a;44.

Triano JJ, and Davis BP. Reactive muscles: reciprocal and crossed reciprocal innervation phenomenon. Proceedings of 7th Annual Biomechanics Conference on the Spine. Boulder: University of Colorado, 1976b.

Triano JJ, and Humphreys CR. Patient monitoring in the conservative management of cervical radiculopathy. *J Manipulative Phys Ther* 1987;10:94.

Triano JJ, and Luttges M. Myoelectric paraspinal response to spinal loads: Potential for monitoring low back pain. *J Manipulative Phys Ther* 1985;8:137.

Triano JJ, and Schultz AB. Correlation of objective measure of trunk motion and muscle function with low-back disability ratings. *Spine* 1987;12:561.

Triano J, and Ziegler C. Typical spinal pattern of nineteen cardiopulmonary patients treated chiropractically. *Chiropractic Journal* 1977.

Trott PH, Maitland GD, and Gerrard B. The neurocalometer: A survey to assess its value as a diagnostic instrument. *Med J Aus* 1972;1:464.

Turner JA, and Clancy S. Comparison of operant behavioral and cognitive–behavioral group treatment for chronic low back pain. *J Consult Clin Psychol* 1988;56:261.

Uematsu S, Jankel WR, and Edwin DH, et al. Quantification of thermal asymmetry. Part 2. Application in low-back pain and sciatica. *J Neurosurg* 1988;69:556.

Vallfors B. Acute, subacute and chronic low back pain. Clinical symptoms, absenteeism and working environment. *Scand J Rehabil Med* (Suppl) 1985;185:1.

Vannerson JF, and Nimmo RL. Specificity and the law of facilitation in the nervous system. *ACA J Chiropr* 1973;10:S17.

Vernon H, and Grice A. The four quadrant weight scale: A technical and procedural review. *J Manipulative Phys Ther* 1984;3:165.

Walshe FMR. *Diseases of the Nervous System Described for Practitioners and Students*, 10th ed. Baltimore; Williams & Wilkins, 1973.

Walther DS: *Applied Kinesiology—The Advanced Approach in Chiropractic*. Pueblo, CO: Pueblo Systems, D.D. 1976.

Watkins MP, Harris BA, and Kozlowski BA. Isokinetic testing in patients with hemiparesis. A pilot study. *Phys Ther* 1984; 64:184.

Weber B, Smith JP, and Briscoe WA, et al. Pulmonary function in asymptomatic adolescents with idiopathic scoliosis. *Am Rev Respir Dis* 1975;111:389.

Weisel SW, Tsourmas N, and Feffer HL, et al. A study of computer-assisted tomography. I. The incidence of positive CAT scans in an asymptomatic group of patients. *Spine* 1984;9:549.

Whitley JD, and Smith LE. Velocity curves and static strength-action strength correlations in relation to the mass moved by the arm. *Res Quart* 1963;34:379.

Wicks D. Laboratory evaluation. In Cox JM, ed. *Low Back Pain—Mechanism, Diagnosis and Treatment*, 5th ed. Baltimore: Williams & Wilkins, 1990.

Wicks D, Cardiovascular disorders in ambulatory patients. In Lawrence D, ed. *Fundamentals of Chiropractic Diagnosis and Management*. Baltimore: Williams & Wilkins; 1991, 221–264.

Williams KL, Phillips BH, and Jones PA, et al. Thermography in screening for breast cancer. *J Epidemiol Community Health* 1990;44:112.

Williams M, and Stutzman L. Strength variation through the range of joint motion. *Phys Ther Rev* 1959;39:145.

Wilson PT. The osteopathic treatment of asthma. *J Am Osteopath Assoc* 1946;45:491.

Wozny PJ. Iron and anemias. *ACA J Chiropr* 1975;12:S135.

Wyatt MP, and Edwards AM. Comparison of quadriceps and hamstring torque values during isokinetic exercise. *J Orthop Sports Phys Ther* 1981;3:48.

Yasue H, Touyama M, and Shimamoto M, et al. Role of autonomic nervous system in the pathogenesis of Prinzmetal's variant form of angina. *Circulation* 1974;50:534.

Yates RG, Lamping DL, Abram NL, and Wright C: Effects of chiropractic treatment on blood pressure and anxiety: A randomized, controlled trial. *J Manipulative Phys Ther* 1988;11:484.

Ziegler EE, O'Donnel AM, and Stearns G, et al. Nitrogen balance studies with normal children. *Am J Clin Nutr* 1977;30:939.

Spinal X-Rays

Brian A. Howard
Lindsay J. Rowe

During the last 15 years, technological advances in the field of diagnostic radiology have provided the clinician with a wide variety of imaging modalities to visualize the spinal column (Table 21–1). Clinicians often have not been able to keep abreast of these advances. The major difficulty confronting the clinician today is deciding if imaging is necessary and which imaging modality will provide the most relevant information quickly, inexpensively, and the least invasively. This chapter discusses the relative indications for imaging and the principles of plain film interpretation.

Indications for Spinal Imaging

The role of any medical imaging modality is to provide the most accurate depiction possible of anatomicopathological changes. Accurate interpreta-

tion of a medical image requires correlation of the imaging findings with the clinical information previously obtained from the patient history, physical examination, and laboratory reports. Frequently, imaging provides definitive information regarding the underlying disorder responsible for the patient's presenting signs and symptoms, and also provides a template for effectively managing the patient's progress. Finally, the presenting clinical features, physical findings, and previous imaging results help guide the clinician's decision for further imaging studies. But this decision should also depend on the availability and the degree of invasiveness of the chosen imaging modality.

Regional anatomic evaluations or skeletal screenings constitute the major types of imaging studies performed. The rationales for undertaking these studies are listed in Table 21–2. Table 21–3 lists

TABLE 21-1. IMAGING MODALITIES

Noninvasive
  Ultrasound
  Radiography
  Xeroradiography
  Scintigraphy
  Computed axial tomography [CT]
  Magnetic resonance imaging [MRI]
Invasive
  Myelography
  Arthrography
  Radiculography
  Discography
  Epidural venography
  Spinal arteriography
  Percutaneous biopsy
  Chemonucleolysis
  Discotomy

some of the more important clinical indications for spinal imaging before manual treatment.

Age

The aged patient is at greater risk of neoplastic, degenerative, metabolic, and postsurgical changes involving the spine (Deyo, 1986; Kelen, 1986; Waddell, 1982; Kirkaldy-Willis et al., 1978). In the younger patient, imaging may be necessary to exclude congenital abnormalities. Younger patients, however, are at greater risk of the adverse effects of ionizing radiation because they live longer and they have a higher cellular mitotic rate.

Trauma

A history of recent or remote physical trauma is a very important indication for regional imaging examination to demonstrate potentially altered anatomy.

Previous Spinal Surgery

Previous spinal surgery may cause postoperative sepsis, recurrent discal pathology, failed fusion, per-

TABLE 21-2. RATIONALES FOR SPINAL IMAGING

Clinical assessment
  Biomechanical assessment
  Pathologic assessment
    Surgical/nonsurgical
Clinical progression
  Response to treatment
  Disease progression
  Complications
Litigation considerations
  Accidents
  Preemployment
  Workers compensation
Research
  Diagnostic imaging
  Therapeutic efficacy

TABLE 21-3. CLINICAL INDICATIONS FOR SPINAL IMAGING

Patient history
  Over 50 years of age
  Recent trauma or remote significant trauma
  Previous spinal surgery
  Fever
  Night pain
  Previous cancer
  Nonremitting and worsening pain
  Deformity and stiffness
  Steroid therapy
  Drug and alcohol abuse
  Inflammatory rheumatologic symptoms
  Unexplained loss of weight and change in bowel habits
  Diabetes and/or hypertension
Physical findings
  Dermopathy [psoriasis, melanoma]
  Cachexia
  Deformity and immobility
  Scars [surgical, accidental]
  Lymphadenopathy
  Localized pain, tenderness, spasm
  Motor or sensory neurodeficit
  Elevated erythrocyte sedimentation rate, alkaline or acid phosphatase
  Rheumatoid factor positive with significant titer
  HLA B 27 positive
  Serum gammopathy

Adapted from Deyo 1986 and Kelen, 1986.

sistent lateral stenosis, and meningeal scarring or ossification. The presence of instrumentation in the spine adds to the diagnostic problem because of the potential of component failure, disengagement at sites of attachment, or vertebral fracture at sites of attachment.

Sweating and Pyrexia

Sweating, pyrexia, and spinal pain should alert the clinician to the possibility of sepsis; however, this nonspecific clinical picture is also seen in carcinomatoses, lymphoreticular disorders, and systemic inflammatory arthropathies, conditions indicating clinical imaging (Deyo, 1986).

Pain

Persistent pain and pain that interferes with work, hobbies, and sleep should not go unheeded. Sophisticated imaging may be necessary to identify the underlying pathology (Gehweiler, 1983).

Drug and Alcohol Abuse

Intravenous drug abusers are at increased risk of septic arthritis (Holtzman 1971). Alcoholics frequently suffer from chronic pancreatitis, which may present with referred visceral back pain. Or the pain may be the result of associated medullary infarcts of which there is an increased frequency in this disorder (Sarles and Sahel, 1976).

Steroid and Other Drug Use

Patients receiving long-term steroid therapy are at increased risk of osteopenia, avascular necrosis, insufficiency fractures, and infections (Curtiss et al., 1954; Madell and Freeman, 1969). Patients on heparin or warfarin are at increased risk of spontaneous epidural hemorrhage (Dabbert, 1970). The use of nonsteroidal anti-inflammatory drugs may be associated with aggressive patterns of degenerative arthritis (Newman and Ling, 1985). The use of anticonvulsants is often associated with osteomalacia, which may give rise to spinal pain secondary to mechanical failure (Genuth et al., 1972; Richens and Rowe, 1970).

History of Cancer

Spinal pain in cancer patients should be considered evidence of metastasis until proved otherwise. Usually, a total-body radioisotopic bone scan with technetium-99m MDP is indicated. Previous radiotherapy and/or chemotherapy may be associated with osteonecrosis or a second malignancy, especially in patients with long-term survival. Scintigraphy, computed tomography (CT) scanning, or magnetic resonance imaging (MRI) are most helpful in evaluating these patients.

Neurologic Deficit

Sensory and/or motor neurodeficits suggest nerve entrapment centrally or in the lateral recess, and are indications for more sophisticated transaxial imaging or myelography depending on what is available in the community.

Other Indications for Imaging Studies

Unexplained loss of weight, change in bowel or bladder habits, a history of chronic smoking, regional lymphadenopathy, and unexplained anemia are the warning signs of cancer and its potentially destructive effects on the spine. Abnormal laboratory values can give clues to underlying Paget's disease, prostatic cancer metastases, myeloma, carcinomatoses, metabolic bone disease, and inflammatory arthropathies that may afflict the spine.

All of the previously cited considerations are regarded as indications for routine radiography as well as for further imaging modalities such as scintigraphy, CT scanning and/or MRI to further define detected abnormalities. Reevaluation is indicated, either with the same modality or with more sensitive sophisticated imaging modalities, if signs and symptoms persist or worsen.

Routine Spinal Radiography

Radiography is the most commonly used imaging modality (Whitehouse, 1986; Sherman, 1986). This is an integral component of any clinical assessment of the musculoskeletal system, especially when manual treatment is anticipated. (Inglis et al., 1979; Grigg, 1965; Kelner et al., 1980). Advances in x-ray beam generation and the appropriate use of beam filtering, grids, bucky diaphragms, and screen–film combinations have reduced the radiation dose to the patient (Sherman and Bauer, 1982). Although this imaging modality is readily available, reliable, and noninvasive, other modalities may have to be used to further elucidate the underlying nature of the detected abnormality.

Routine spinal radiography requires the use of an x-ray unit capable of generating a minimum of 300 mA and 125 Vp and preferably having both an upright and recumbent bucky. At least two views in the frontal and lateral projection should be obtained (Rowe and Yochum, 1987; Schmorl and Junghanns, 1971). Further views are obtained as necessary to define suspected pathology. Recumbent films are more likely to exclude pathology as they are technically superior. If after the initial evaluation biomechanical derangements such as fixed or dynamic instabilities are suspected, then dynamic and upright films can be obtained (Nash and Moe, 1969). The patient should stand erect for at least 1 hour before performing the upright imaging study (Young et al., 1970; Lawrence, 1985; Fineman et al., 1963; Lowe et al., 1976) to allow the effect of gravity to accentuate the abnormal spinal curvature, instability, or vertebral body slippage (Friberg, 1987; Hadley, 1951; Howe, 1973). Supplementary views, such as oblique views, allow a second look at the vertebral body, its cortical margins, and adjacent viscera, as well as visualization of the neural arch. Calcified walls of an aortic aneurysm are sometimes best seen on the oblique views. Specialized views (e.g., Pillar view or Swimmers view) have been devised to view the more difficult anatomic regions.

Full Spinal Projections

Three-foot full spinal x-rays provide a general view of spinal curvature. When taken upright, postural effects on spinal curvature can also be assessed. The use of graduated filters rather than split screens is recommended. Radiation protection for the patient's thyroid, breasts, pelvis, and extrapelvic gonads should be considered. Patients should not be subjected to serial full spinal projections over extended periods. Structural details are poorly visualized on these examinations, and significant pathologies are easily overlooked. For these reasons, full spinal projections should be used only to provide information used to determine subsequent regional views.

Dynamic Studies

Static images of the limits of spinal range of motion in either the coronal or sagittal planes may be helpful in determining motion segment instability (Brown et al., 1976; Keeson et al., 1984). Alternative procedures such as cineradiography and videofluoroscopic recording are possible, but the radiation exposure to the bone marrow and gonads is excessive (Fielding, 1957; Reynolds, 1938; Pennal et al., 1972; Sandoz, 1971; Rich, 1964; Davis, 1945; Knutson, 1944). In some research centers, evaluation with biplanar imaging with fixed reference points allows three-dimensional computerized assessment (Pearcy et al., 1984). The use of ultrafast rare earth screen–film combination systems is recommended in this situation. The role of digital imaging in dynamic studies and scoliosis studies is yet to be defined.

Motion segments may show increased, decreased, or normal motion. Abnormal motion such as excessive translation, rocking, or eccentric rotation is possible but may not be demonstrable (Sandoz, 1965, Cassidy, 1976; Cassidy and Potter, 1979; Dupuis et al., 1985; Jackson, 1977; Walheim and Selvick, 1984). The greater the amplitude of intersegmental hypermobility the greater the chance that central and/or lateral nerve root canal encroachment may occur (Jirout, 1956; van Akkerveeken et al., 1979; Weitz, 1981).

Careful preoperative selective anesthesia of the involved interfacetal joints, pars defects, and recurrent sinu vertebral nerves may confirm the source of the patient's symptoms in motion segments where instability is demonstrated.

Sequential Studies

Interval follow-up studies employing standardized views are used to help ascertain changes in the condition of patients with scolioses, and healing fractures and are also used to monitor the outcome of therapies such as surgical fusion. Follow-up imaging of arthritic patients allows determination of disease control, progression, or the development of complications.

Interpretation of Routine Spinal Radiographs

General Guidelines

Technical Evaluation. Are the films dark and overexposed or light and underexposed? Exposure affects the appreciation of altered bone density. Has the patient been positioned properly and are the views orthogonal? Obliquity of projections causes untold number of suspicious lesions. If there is any doubt films should be repeated with appropriate technical corrections.

Anatomic Evaluation. Assessment of the cortical margins and overall contour of the vertebral body and neural arch is most important. Awareness of and familiarity with the numerous anatomic variants and congenital anomalies provide the sound diagnostic base needed to avoid misinterpretation of a radiographic image.

Radiologic Densities. Knowledge of the five basic radiographic densities constituting the shadows seen on radiographs is essential. In increasing order of radio-opacity these shadows are due to air, fat, water, bone, and metal.

Sensitivity. Detection of significant early bone loss is unreliable with plain film radiography. A 5-cm lesion of the vertebral body can be missed if there is no cortical loss of bone (Borak, 1942). Loss of more than 45% of vertebral body volume is necessary for reliable detection (Lachman, 1955; Ardran, 1951). There is also a radiographic lag period of up to 3 weeks before bone destruction or reactive periosteal changes can be detected in acute inflammatory conditions.

Interpretative Methodology

Overview. The film should be approached as though it were the patient and analyzed in such a fashion that the primary areas of origin of spinal pain are carefully evaluated. Start by establishing the patient's name, sex, age, and race. Obvious abnormalities should be recognized. Then, a systematic assessment of bone alignment, density, and contour should be completed, followed by an assessment of joint spacing and soft tissues in the paraarticular compartment and in the adjacent visceral compartment. Assessment of the soft tissues is necessary to exclude renal masses and aortic aneurysms. The evaluation of the osseous structures for pathology should be structured, and a categorical approach to this evaluative process is suggested. Finally, a review of the osseous walls of the spinal canal should be performed to detect possible secondary effects of space-occupying lesions within the spinal canal and/or lateral nerve root canal. Film corners and complex anatomic sites should again be carefully reviewed and bright-lighted as necessary.

Radiological Discriminators. The characteristic features and the extent of the detected abnormality should be ascertained. Multifocal lesions, polyostotic distribution, and multisystem involvement are key factors. Specific lesional characteristics such as location in the vertebra, shape, margin, pattern of osseous destruction or production, internal calcification, ossification, septation, cortical periosteal new bone formation, and adjacent soft tissue changes are important. The routine radiograph information can be supplemented by scintigraphy, CT scanning and MRI. Only the histopathologist can give an unqualified tissue diagnosis. Today, percutaneous biopsy is being performed more frequently under fluoroscopic or CT scan control so as to obtain histopathological correlation (Ayala and Zornosa, 1983; El-Khoury et al., 1983; Murphy, 1983). Once all this information has been ascertained and considered then categorization of the lesion should be attempted. Once recognized, an abnormality should be analyzed with the following radiological discriminators in mind (Rowe and Yochum, 1987).

Categorical Approach to Interpretation

Recognition of the multiplicity of pathological changes that can affect the osseous spine is facilitated by following a simple, systematic method of categorization. There are seven basic categories of bone disease: congenital, traumatic, arthritic, tumor, infection, hematologic, and nutritional–metabolic–endocrine.

Congenital Spinal Anomalies. Numerous congenital spinal anomalies (Table 21-4) are well documented in major reference texts. Spinal anomalies are deviations from what is regarded as normal. Normal variants are anomalies considered to have no clinical significance as determined by retrospective

TABLE 21-4. CONGENITAL SPINAL ANOMALIES

Cervical spine
  Craniocervical junction   Platybasia, occipitalization,
                            paramastoid process, spina bifida,
                            or agenesis of the neural arch
                            Agenesis of the dens or nonfusion
                            with axis
Cervical, thoracic, and lumbar spine
  Vertebral body maldevelopment resulting in block motion
    segments, butterfly vertebrae, or hemivertebrae in both
    coronal and sagittal planes
  Neural arch abnormalities consisting of incomplete fusion or
    agenesis of one or all components—pedicle, articular facet,
    lamina, or spinous process
  Transitional segments at the lumbosacral junction possibly
    involving body and/or neural arch
Sacrum
  This consists of five fused vertebral segments. Dysraphic
    changes can affect the anterior or posterior components.
    Partial or total agenesis can occur as part of the caudal
    regression syndrome and is associated with maternal
    diabetes.

anatomic and clinical studies (Guebert et al., 1987). There is, however, now an increasing awareness of the so-called symptomatic variant.

VATER is a useful mnemonic reminding the clinician that congenital osseous spinal anomalies are frequently associated with anorectal anomalies, tracheoesophageal fistulas, and renal and radial anomalies. Diffuse spinal changes can be seen in the various inherited spondylocostal or spondyloepiphyseal dysplasias. Craniocervical instability is commonly seen in Down's syndrome but has been reported in other congenital syndromes. The finding of disordered growth is a potential discriminator for congenital etiology; however, any insult in the neonatal period may result in deranged growth and compensatory overgrowth in the adjacent unaffected regions. The vertebral body and neural arch can be involved together or separately. Figure 21–1 demonstrates these features.

Spinal Trauma. Spinal fractures and fracture dislocations tend to occur at predictable sites because of the biomechanical configuration of the spinal curves. Simple or burst compression fractures are the most common, and tend to occur at the thoracolumbar junction. Caused by flexion and axial loading forces, compression fractures are characterized by a loss of anterior vertebral body height with angular deformity of the anterior vertebral cortex (step sign) (Fig. 21–2). Vertebral endplate definition may be lost and is associated with a line of sclerosis resulting from impaction of the vertical trabeculae.

Assessment of the posterior vertebral body height as compared with vertebral levels above and below is imperative. Loss of height typically indicates that the anterior wall of the spinal canal has been breached and that possible spinal canal encroachment has to be excluded. The fracture is now considered a burst-type fracture and is unstable until proved otherwise. Vertebral instability means potential for progressive deformity, either acute or chronic, which may result in further canal encroachment and progressive neurodeficit. Significant loss of vertebral body height raises the question of other vertebral pathology such as osteoporosis, myeloma, or metastatic carcinoma.

A clinical history of trauma in the presence of point tenderness and osteoporosis may require further imaging using scintigraphy, CT scanning, or MRI to exclude significant traumatic insult. Care must be taken in the presence of Scheuermann's disease of the lower thoracic spine, which is often mistaken for multiple acute compressional fractures (Alexander, 1977; Fon et al., 1980).

Spinal Arthritic Disorders. The spine is a composite of motion segments, with each segment con-

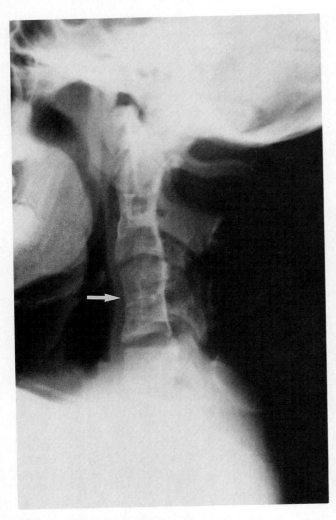

Figure 21–1. Multiple congenital block vertebrae, C2–4 and C–C6. Congenital synostosis (fusion) is present at multiple levels. Observe the characteristic hypoplastic vertebral bodies and intervertebral disc. The anterior contour is notably concave, with the apex of the curve at the level of the disc (*arrow*). The posterior elements are also fused. Note the hypoplastic posterior arch of atlas. Multiple congenital block vertebrae in the cervical spine constitute a radiologic hallmark of Klippel–Feil syndrome. The combination of hypoplasia and fusion tends to exclude fusion secondary to trauma, infection, and surgery. (*Courtesy of Douglas L. Herron, D.C.*)

thologies (Fig. 21–3). Loss of discal height, subchondral sclerosis, vacuum phenomenon, traction osteophytes, and marginal osteophytes in association with malalignment, are typical findings. Anterolisthesis or posterolisthesis is most common at C6–7 and L4–5 motion segment levels (Heithoff, 1984). There also occurs degenerative osteoarthrosis of the interfacetal joints with craniocaudal subluxation and lateral nerve root entrapment. This is best appreciated with either CT scanning or MRI in the sagittal median and paramedian planes which dem-

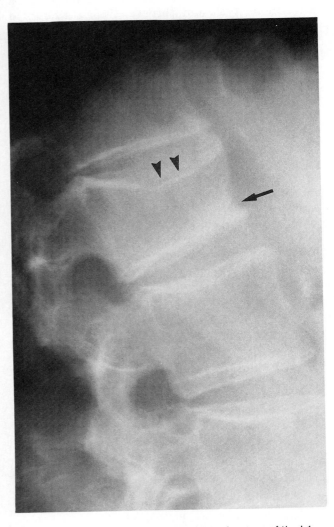

Figure 21–2. Posttraumatic compression fracture of the L1 vertebral body. Loss of the anterior vertebral body height (*arrow*) and depression of the superior endplate (*arrowheads*) are characteristic findings of this condition. Also observe the slight retrolisthesis of the vertebral body, suggestive of discoligamentous damage. Preservation of the posterior vertebral body height is an important differentiating feature. Posterior involvement could indicate a burst component to the fracture with canal encroachment. Loss of trabecular continuity could raise the question of a pathologic fracture caused by metabolic bone disease or the presence of a neoplastic process.

sisting of at least three major joints—the discal symphysis and the two synovial interfacetal joints. As might be expected, arthritic disease is a common affliction of the vertebral column. In his description of degenerative diseases of the spine, Resnick (1985) demonstrated that there are two basic patterns of discal abnormality: (1) intervertebral osteochondrosis resulting from involvement of the nucleus pulposis, and (2) spondylosis deformans resulting from degeneration of the annulus fibrosus.

Commonly, there may be a mixture of these pa-

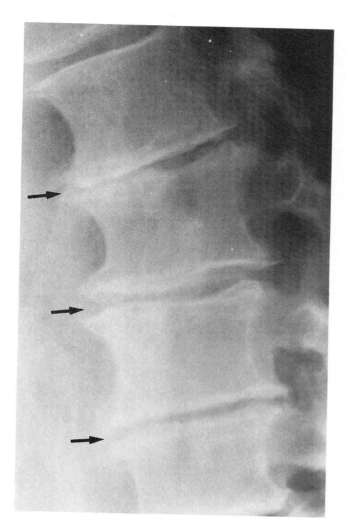

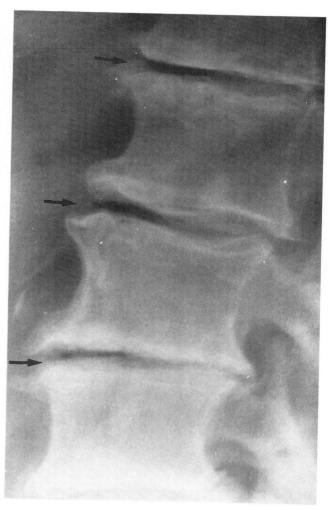

A

B

Figure 21-3. Degenerative disc disease of the lumbar spine. (**A**) Flexion view demonstrates disc space narrowing at multiple levels with claw osteophyte formation *(arrows).* (**B**) Extension view demonstrates linear radiolucencies induced at the previously identified narrowed disc spaces (vacuum phenomenon). On extension, nitrogen gas accumulates in radial discal fissures *(arrows).* Flexion and extension radiographs are useful in determining the presence and degree of segmental instability. The presence of vacuum phenomenon is compatible with motion at these segmental levels.

onstrates effacement of epidural and perineural fat planes (Ciric et al., 1980).

Spondylosis deformans usually occurs segmentally. Flowing anterolateral shields of ossification form as the result of an idiopathic ossifying diathesis of the anterior longitudinal ligament and associated prevertebral soft tissue. This condition is termed DISH (for diffuse idiopathic skeletal hyperostoses) and can also affect the posterior longitudinal ligament, causing compressive myelopathy (Alenghat et al., 1982). The discal space, interfacetal joints, and the synovial portion of the sacroiliac joints usually remain unaffected, characteristics that differentiate

DISH from the "bamboo spine" or ankylosing spondylitis (Ogryzlo and Rosen, 1969).

Inflammatory spondyloarthropathies can be either seropositive or seronegative (Yochum and Rowe 1979). Ankylosing spondylitis is a seronegative spondyloarthropathy characterized by bilateral sacroiliitis and inflammatory enthesopathy of the outer annular fibers and inflammatory synovial changes in the interfacetal joints. This condition causes the formation of bridging syndesmophytes of the discovertebral juncture and fusion of the interfacetal joints. "Carrot stick" fractures may then occur through the fused discal space, giving rise to a pseudoarthrosis of the spine. Other seronegative spondyloarthropathies, psoriasis and Reiter's syndrome, differ from ankylosing spondylitis in that bulky paravertebral ossification occurs in asymmetric, skiplike fashion with bilateral but asymmetric sacroiliitis.

Seropositive rheumatoid disease has a predilection for the upper cervical motion segments (Bland et al., 1967). The inflammatory pannus causes erosion of the occipitoatlantoidal joints as well as the median and lateral atlantoaxial joints. With loss of substance to the articular facets, there is cranial settling with pseudobasilar invagination. More commonly, median erosive disease is associated with ligamentous disruption of the transverse ligament as seen in Figure 21-4. Instability occurs with increased motion between the anterior tubercle of C1 and the dens and between the clivus and the dens (Bland et al., 1967). Disruption of the transverse ligament is seen in up to 50% of rheumatoid patients, 45% of psoriatic patients, and 15% of ankylosing spondylitis patients (Isdale and Conlon, 1971; Sharp and Purser, 1961; Killebrew et al., 1973). This may be associated with compromise of the brain stem and its vasculature by both the mechanical effect of the instability and by the mass effect of the inflammatory pannus.

Erosive disease of the apophyseal joints can be associated with involvement of the discovertebral junction with loss of disc height, irregular destruction of the vertebral endplates, and mild paraspinal soft tissue swelling. This is reminiscent of infectious discitis. The diagnosis, with the exception of infection, is made by percutaneous aspiration and or biopsy or open surgical biopsy of the discovertebral junction. The resultant instability may require fusion.

Spinal Tumors. Spinal tumors are conveniently broken down into those that involve the vertebral body, neural arch, and contents of the spinal canal. Spinal tumors may be benign or malignant. Malignant tumors have the ability to metastasize and are frequently fatal. Because of the extensive vascular network supplying the red marrow of the spine and ribs, most malignant lesions of the spine are the result of metastases from either melanomas or carcinomas of the thyroid, breast, bronchus, kidney, prostate, or colon (Vider et al., 1977). Destruction of a vertebral segment generally tends to start in the vertebral body and extends into the neural arch. Lesions may be focally lytic or diffusely infiltrative as in carcinomatoses where infiltration of the bone marrow by neoplastic cells produces signs of generalized osteopenia on routine radiography and a ''super scan'' with scintigraphy. The loss of the cortical margin is the most telling radiographic sign for detecting the

presence of tumor. This is well exemplified by loss of the pediculate cortical margin. Blastic metastases cause increased density, which may be focal or diffuse, giving the ''ivory vertebra'' appearance. This sign is seen particularly with mucin-secreting adenocarcinomas, lymphoreticular neoplasms, and tumors that secrete biogenic amines (carcinoids).

Of the principal spinal malignancies, multiple myeloma is the most common. This condition may present as nonspecific osteopenia, or multiple punched-out lytic defects, or as a solitary lytic lesion.

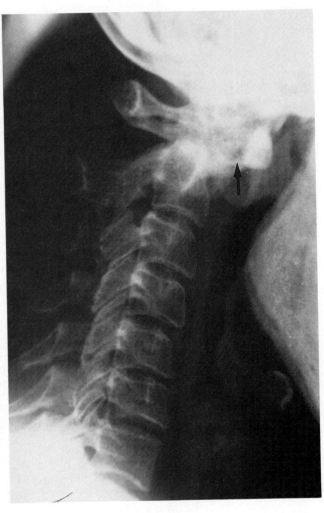

Figure 21-4. Atlantoaxial subluxation in rheumatoid arthritis of the cervical spine. Flexion of the cervical spine demonstrates anterior translation of the atlas with widening of the atlantodental interspace (ADI) measuring 10 mm *(arrow)*. Atlantoaxial instability is secondary to partial or complete disruption of the transverse ligament of the atlas. The most common cause of ligament disruption is a noninfectious inflammatory process associated with systemic arthropathies such as rheumatoid arthritis, psoriasis, ankylosing spondylitis, and Reiter's syndrome. Congenital atlantoaxial instability is seen in disorders such as Down's syndrome. (*Courtesy of C. William Kusiar, D.C.*)

In 3% of cases there is a sclerotic form of myeloma, which may be associated with organomegaly, peripheral neuropathy, and endocrinopathy (Woolfenden et al., 1980).

Hemangioma is the most common form of benign spinal tumor (Mohan et al., 1980). Ten percent of hemangiomas extend into the pedicle, are associated with epidural involvement, and are commonly symptomatic. The thoracolumbar spine is the most common region of occurrence. The plain film hallmark of the hemangioma is the altered trabecular pattern of the affected vertebra, resulting in accentuation of the vertical primary stress trabeculae, usually without expansion of the vertebral body (Fig. 21–5).

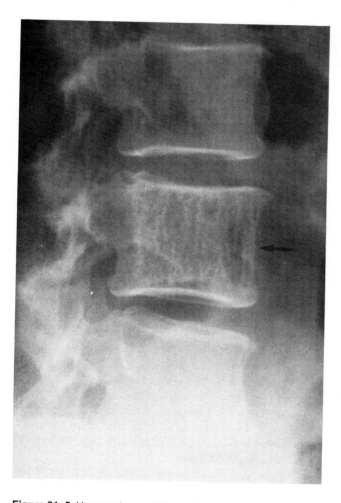

Figure 21–5. Hemangioma of the lumbar spine, identified by the prominent, coarse vertical trabeculae within the vertebral body *(arrow)*. This condition is the most common benign neoplasm of the spine. Note the lack of bony expansion and the cortical thickening characteristic of Paget's disease. Involvement of the posterior neural arch is seen more commonly in the symptomatic variety and suggests involvement of the epidural tissue, which is best demonstrated with intravenous enhanced CT or MRI.

This must be differentiated from Paget's disease. Solitary sclerotic endosteal-based islands of cortical bone are also a common finding, and have to be differentiated from isolated sclerotic metastases and isolated osteoid osteomas and osteoblastomas known to cause painful scolioses (Gamba et al., 1984). The latter tend to occur in younger patients. Sixty percent of osteoid osteomas occur in the lumbar spine with a predilection for the neural arch. Nocturnal pain relieved with aspirin ingestion is the classic scenario. The lesion occurs on the concave side of the scoliosis. A central lucent nidus with or without a sclerotic central focus surrounded by reactive sclerosis in the pedicle is the classic description, and the imaging modality of choice is scintigraphy which shows a focal region of marked activity. Giant cell tumors and aneurysmal bone cysts also involve the posterior neural arch. These usually result in a radiolucent expansile, thinly corticated lesion and may be confused with osteoblastomas. Other tumorlike lesions such as fibrous dysplasia and eosinophilic granuloma are also seen.

Intraspinal tumors are usually, but not exclusively, primary neoplasms within the cord (intramedullary), within the dural space (intradural extramedullary), and in the epidural space (extradural). Intraspinal tumors are usually best visualized by CT scanning following myelography or by MRI. The plain film clues of intraspinal tumors are scalloping of the segmental posterior vertebral body and erosion of the medial cortical pediculate margins with apparent widening of the interpediculate distance, the Elseberg–Dyke sign (Elseberg and Dyke, 1934). Most commonly occurring at the thoracolumbar junction, intramedullary lesions are usually due to expendymomas and astrocytomas of the cord and filum terminale. Intradural extramedullary lesions are mostly due to neurofibromas or meningiomas. These lesions tend to cause scalloping of adjacent cortical margins with thinning of the pedicle and enlargement of the nerve root canal. Extradural lesions are most commonly due to metastatic lesions of the vertebral body with associated soft tissue extension.

Spinal Infections. Spinal infections usually are manifested as either discitis or vertebral body osteomyelitis with discitis. Spinal infections occur most frequently in children and in the elderly. Diagnosis of this type of infection in a young, otherwise healthy adult raises the question of intravenous drug abuse (Holtzman and Bishko, 1971). Urinary, gastrointestinal, respiratory tract, and endocardial infections are the common primary sites of infection that may seed the discovertebral junction. Infections may also occur after spinal surgery and discal chemonucleolysis.

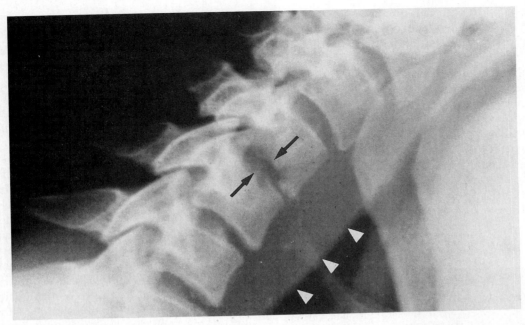

Figure 21-6. Discovertebral infection of C4–5. Note the decrease in disc height with associated loss in the cortication of the adjacent vertebral endplates *(arrows)*. Anterior extension of the inflammatory process has thickened the retropharyngeal soft tissues *(arrowheads)*. This constellation of findings is characteristic of spinal infection. These infections may occur by hematogenous dissemination, as seen with intravenous drug abusers, and may also occur by mechanical implantation following chemonucleolysis, surgery, and less often myelography.

The classical radiographic features are irregular destruction of the vertebral endplates, loss of discal height, associated paraspinal abscess, and angular kyphosis (Fig. 21–6). Epidural abscess formation may occur, and this is a neurosurgical emergency. Spinal infections may spread contiguously in all directions, and can extend beneath the longitudinal ligament, producing scattered gougelike defects in the anterior vertebral body margins. This is most commonly seen with tuberculosis. Punctate calcification of the caseation necrosis may occur in the later stages. Other granulomatous processes, such as mycotic infections, can give the same early destructive picture.

The presence of gas in the soft tissues alerts the physician to anaerobic gas-forming infections. Scintigraphy and MRI are the most sensitive modalities in the earlier stages of inflammatory spinal infections. Conventional tomography and CT scans can help quantify the bony destruction, while MRI and CT scans demonstrate the soft tissue changes and associated abscesses.

Percutaneous aspiration, or biopsy will help isolate the organism for appropriate antibiotic therapy and percutaneous drainage of abscess can be performed on occasion; however, surgical debridement and fusion are more common. Postsurgical spinal sepsis is extremely difficult to diagnose when in the subacute stage. Combined scintigraphy with diphosphonate, gallium, and indium is helpful. MRI with intravenous paramagnetic enhancement will likely be more sensitive in the earlier stages but is relatively nonspecific (Mountford et al., 1983, Fletcher et al., 1984).

Hematological Diseases. Spinal manifestations of hematological diseases are infrequent and usually seen only in patients with severe blood dyscrasias. Chronic hemolytic anemias such as thalassemia and sickle cell disease cause expansion of the red marrow myeloid factory, rarefaction of the trabeculae, and slight accentuation of the primary stress vertical trabeculae. These disease processes result in an osteopenic, slightly enlarged vertebral body with a coarse trabecular pattern. In lymphoreticular diseases such as leukemia and lymphoma, congenital storage diseases such as Gaucher's, and the mucopolysaccharoidoses this nonspecific pattern may be associated with visceromegaly.

Diffuse patchy sclerosis can be seen in myeloid diseases such as myelofibrosis, myelosclerosis, and mastocytosis. The weakened bone in all of these entities allows discal ballooning, loss of vertebral body height as a result of infraction of the vertebral endplates, and the development of Schmorl's nodes and wedge fractures (Schmorl and Junghanns, 1971). Ischemic necrosis of the vertebral endplates gives rise to the classical ''H'' vertebral bodies. Histiocytoses such as eosinophilic granuloma are tumor-

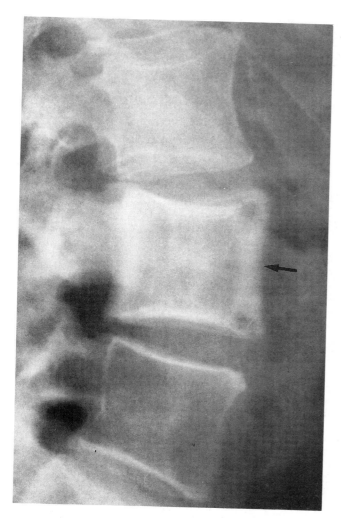

Figure 21-7. Paget's disease of the third lumbar vertebra. The overall density and size of the vertebral body are increased and the cortex is thickened *(arrow)*. Note extension into the pedicle. This appearance is often mimicked by osteoblastic metastases, especially from prostatic adenocarcinoma. This is easily differentiated from a classic appearing hemangioma. Involvement of the neural arch predisposed to central canal stenosis.

lucent, with accentuation of the cortical margins and remaining compressile vertical trabeculae. Fatty marrow replacement of the red marrow also occurs. Weakening of the vertebral body may result in wedge fractures, ballooning of the endplates, and (occasionally) complete vertebral collapse with compromise of the canal contents because of the burst component (Lourie, 1982). Osteopenic fractures associated with hypercallosity raise the question of steriod-induced osteopenia. Fractures may occur with the development of an intravertebral vacuum. These are associated with ischemic necrosis of the vertebral body by a mechanism that is not understood (Maldeque et al., 1978).

Osteomalacia tends to demonstrate an ill-defined coarsening of the trabeculae with osteopenia, as well as the characteristic pseudofractures in the more severe presentations. Renal osteodystrophy causes both a diffuse ill-defined increase in bone density (chalkiness) and the classic "rugger jersey" appearance of the spine with sclerosis of the vertebral endplates and intervening relative lucency of the midvertebral body.

Paget's disease has been included under metabolic bone disorders because of the disordered remodeling of bone that is characteristic of its active phase. The spine is a common site of presentation and has a variety of appearances dependent on the phase of evolution of the disease (Frame and Marel, 1981). The main radiographic feature is the disorganized trabecular pattern with sclerosis and expansion (Fig. 21-7). The main differential diagnosis includes hemangiomas and osteoblastic metastases, especially from adenocarcinoma of the prostate. Vertebral body expansion occurs in all directions and may encroach on the spinal canal, leading to central or lateral spinal stenosis. Malignant transformation of Pagetic bone has been reported but is exceedingly rare in the spine (Patel et al., 1984).

Special Radiographic Procedures

Discography

A well-established adjuvant imaging modality, discography is used to evaluate discal integrity and to identify symptomatic levels when CT scans and myelography are equivocal. Discography is typically performed in conjunction with chemonucleolysis. Using either a midline transdural or extradural posterolateral approach to the discal surface, a small-needle puncture of the disc is made, in a diagnostic study, and approximately 1 to 2 mL of aqueous non-inonic contrast medium is injected. Spot views and/or CT scans are subsequently obtained (Collins, 1975; McCulloch and Macnab, 1983). Recently, per-

like conditions that lead to focal or diffuse marrow replacement by a proliferative small cell granulomatous process. Histiocytoses have a variety of clinical presentations. With extensive vertebral body involvement, complete collapse of the vertebral body can occur, often after trivial trauma, producing the radiographic picture called "vertebra plana."

Metabolic Disorders. Disorders of metabolism, whether focal or systemic, may be reflected in the appearance and density of the vertebral body. Osteoporosis, the most common metabolic bone disease, is characterized by loss of trabecular bone and cortical thinning. The vertebral body becomes increasingly

cutaneous discotomy under general anesthesia has been performed on contained discal protrusions via the same approaches. Contrast extending to the periphery of the disc is abnormal. This can be focal or diffuse in nature. Leakage through the center or periphery of the vertebral endplate is consistent with a central or marginal Schmorl's node.

Arthography

The intraarticular facet block is both diagnostic and therapeutic, and is used in patients with low back pain with normal spinal imaging, in postsurgical patients, and in patients with facetal osteoarthritis. Under fluoroscopic control facetal puncture is made and radiographic nonionic contrast, long-acting anesthetic, and steriods are injected. The normal facetal arthrogram is smooth. Irregular filling defects and communication through a pars defect into the superior facet are the major abnormalities. Filling defects are commonly due to synechiae, synovial hyperplasia, and facetal pad enlargements (Carrera, 1980; Destouet et al., 1982).

Radiculography

Radiculography with selective nerve block is used to identify symptomatic levels of previously identified but equivocal abnormalities. Under local anesthesia with fluoroscopic control the nerve root sheath is impinged with a small spinal needle. This is confirmed by the patient's aggravated symptoms. Contrast medium and local anesthetic are injected. The induced anesthesia relieves the patient's symptoms, thus confirming the symptomatic level, and allows limited assessment of the extraforaminal root sheath to the level of the dorsal nerve root ganglion (Stockley et al., 1988).

Ultrasound

The use of reflected high-frequency sound waves integrated in space and time to give real-time images allows depiction of soft tissue planes and fluid collections. Solid tissues depict a homogeneous echogenic picture depending on the internal structure of the tissue. Fluid accumulation gives little impedance to the passage of the sound wave and therefore is an echo-poor or sonolucent area. Ultrasonography plays an immensely important role in evaluating the prenatal spine. It is also used intraoperatively to evaluate the spinal cord and the structures anterior to it (neurosonography) (Quencer et al., 1984).

Xeroradiography

Limited availability and excessive radiation exposure for the slight increase in visualization of soft tissue planes, as a result of edge enhancement, have restricted the use of this modality to mammography.

References

Alenghat JP, Hallett M, and Kido DK. Spinal cord compression in diffuse idiopathic skeletal hyperostosis. *Radiology* 1982; 142:119–120.

Alexander CJ. Scheuermann's disease: A traumatic spondylodystrophy. *Skel Radiol* 1977;1:209.

Adran GM. Bone destruction not demonstrable by radiography. *Br J Radiol* 1951;24:107.

Ayala AG and Zornosa J. Primary bone tumors: Percutaneous needle biopsy: Radiologic–pathologic study of 222 biopsies. *Radiology* 1983;149:675–679.

Bland JH, Buskirk FW, Davis PH, et al. Rheumatoid arthritis of the cervical spine. *Arthritis Rheum* 1967;5:637.

Borak J. Relationship between the clinical and roentgenological findings in bone metastases. *Surg Gynecol Obstet* 1942;75:599.

Brown RH, Burstein AH, Nash CL, and Schock CC. Spinal analysis using three dimensional radiographic technique. *J Biomechanics* 1976;9:355.

Carrera GF. Lumbar facet joint injection in low back pain and sciatica: Description of Technique. *Radiology* 1980;137:661–664.

Cassidy JD. Roentgenological examination of the functional mechanics of the lumbar spine in lateral flexion. *J Can Chiropractic Assoc* 1976;July: 13.

Cassidy JD and Potter GE. Motion examination of the lumbar spine. *J Manipulative Physiol Ther* 1979;2(3):151.

Ciric I, Mikhael MA, and Tarkington JA, et al. The lateral recess syndrome: A variant of spinal stenosis. *J Neurosurg* 1980;53:433–443.

Collins HR. An evaluation of cervical and lumbar discography. *Clin Orthop* 1975;134:133–138.

Curtiss PH, Clark WS, and Herndon CH. Vertebral fractures resulting from prolonged cortisone & corticotropin therapy. *JAMA* 1954; 156:467.

Dabbert O. Spinal meningeal hematoma, warfarin therapy and chiropractic adjustment. *JAMA* 1970;214:11.

Davis AG. Injuries of the cervical spine. *JAMA* 1945; 127(3):149.

Destouet JM, Gilula LA, and Murphy WA, et al. Lumbar facet joint injection: Indication, technique, clinical correlation, and preliminary results. *Radiology* 1982;145:321–325.

Deyo R. Lumbar spine films in primary care. *J Gen Intern Med* 1986;1:20.

Dupuis PR, Yong-Hing K, Cassidy JD, and Kirkaldy-Willis WH. Radiologic diagnosis of degenerative lumbar spinal instability. *Spine* 1985;10(3):262.

El-Khoury GY, Terepka RH, Mickelson MR, et al. Fine-needle aspiration biopsy of bone. *J Bone Joint Surg* [Am] 1983;65:522–525.

Elseberg CA and Dyke CG. Diagnosis & localization of tumors of spinal cord by means of measurements made on x-ray films of vertebrae, and correlation of clinical and x-ray findings. *Bull Neurol Inst NY* 1934;3:359.

Fielding JW. Cineroentgenography of the normal cervical spine. *J Bone Joint Surg* [Am] 1957;39(6):1280.

Fineman S, Borrelli FJ, and Rubenstein BM, et al. The cervical spine: Transformation of the normal lordotic pattern into a linear pattern in the neutral posture. A roentgenographic depiction. *J Bone Joint Surg* [AM] 1963;45:1179.

Fletcher BD, Scoles PV, and Nelson AD. Osteomyelitis in children. Detection by magnetic resonance: Work in progress. *Radiology* 1984;150:57–60.

Fon GT, Pitt MJ, and Thies AC. Thoracic kyphosis. Range in normal subjects. *AJR* 1980;134:979.

Friberg O. Lumbar instability: A dynamic approach by traction-compression radiography. *Spine* 1987;12(2):119.

Frame B and Marel GM. Paget disease: A review of current knowledge. *Radiology* 1981;141:21–24.

Gamba JL, Martinez S, and Apple J, et al. Computed tomography of axial skeletal osteoid osteomas. *AJR* 1984;142:769.

Gehweiler J: Low back pain: The controversy of radiologic evaluation. *AJR* 1983;140:109.

Genuth SM, Klein L, and Rabinovitch S, et al. Osteomatacia accompanying chronic anticonvulsant therapy. *J Clin Endocrinol Metabol* 1972;35:378.

Grigg ERN. *The Trail of the Invisible Light,* Springfield, Ill: Thomas; 1965.

Guebert GM, Yochum TR, and Rowe LJ. Congenital anomalies and normal skeletal variants. In Yochum TR and Rowe LJ, eds. *Essentials of Skeletal Radiology.* Baltimore, Md: Williams & Wilkins; 1987: Ch. 2, p. 95.

Hadley LA. Intervertebral joint subluxation, bony impingement & foraminal encroachment, with nerve root changes. *AJR* 1951; 65:377.

Heithoff KB. High resolution computed tomography and stenosis: An evaluation of the causes and cures of the failed back syndrome. In *Computed Tomography of the Spine.* Baltimore, Md: Williams & Wilkins; 1984.

Hotzman RS and Bishko F. Osteomyelitis in heroin addicts. *Am Intern Med* 1971;75:693.

Howe JW. The chiropractic concept of subluxation and its roentgenological manifestations. *J Clin Chiropractic* 1973;Sept : 64.

Inglis BD, Fraser B, and Penfold BR. *Chiropractic in New Zealand Report. Commission of Inquiry into Chiropractic.* Government Printer, New Zealand; 1979:84.

Isdale IC and Conlon PW. Atlanto-axial subluxation. A six year follow up report. *Ann Rheum Dis* 1971;30:387.

Jackson R. *The Cervical Syndrome,* 4th ed. Springfield, Ill: CC Thomas; 1977: 40–41.

Jirout J. Studies of the dynamics of the spine. *Acta Radiol* 1956;46:55.

Keeson W, During J, and Beeker TW, et al. Recordings of the movement at the intervertebral segment L5–S1. *Spine* 1984; 9:83.

Kelen G. Guidelines for the use of lumbar radiography. *Ann Emerg Med* 1986;15(3):245.

Kelner M, Hall O, and Coulter I. *Chiropractors—Do They Help?* Fitzhenry & Whiteside; 1980.

Killebrew K, Gold RH, and Scholkoff SD. Psoriatic spondylitis. *Radiology* 1973;108:9.

Kirkaldy-Willis WH, Wedge JH, and Yong-Hing K, et al., Pathology and pathogenesis of lumbar spondylosis and stenosis. *Spine* 1978;3(4):319.

Knutson F. The instability associated with disc degeneration in the lumbar spine. *Acta Radiol* 1944;25:593.

Krishnamurthy GT, Tubis M, and Hiss J, et al. Distribution pattern of metastatic bone disease. A need for total body skeletal image. *JAMA* 1977;237:2504–2506.

Lachman E. Osteoporosis: The potentialities and limitations of its roentgenologic diagnosis. *AJR* 1955;74:712.

Lourie H. Spontaneous osteoporotic fracture of the sacrum: An unrecognized syndrome of the elderly. *JAMA* 1982;248:715–717.

Lowe RW, Hayes TD, Kaye J, et al. Standing roentgenograms in spondylolisthesis. *Clin Orthop* 1976;117:80.

Madell SH and Freeman LM. Avascular necrosis of bone in Cushing's syndrome. *Radiology* 1969;83:1068.

Maldeque B, Noel H, and Malgem J. The intravertebral vacuum cleft: A sign of ischemic vertebral collapse. *Radiology* 1978; 129:23.

McCulloch JA and Macnab I. *Sciatica and Chymopapain.* Baltimore, Md: Williams and Wilkins; 1983.

Mohan V, Gupta SK, and Tuli SM, et al. Symptomatic vertebral hemangeomas. *Clin Radiol* 1980;31:575.

Mountford PJ, Coakley AJ, Hall FM, et al. Dual radionuclide subtraction imaging of vertebral disc infection using an 111 In-labeled leukocyte scan and a 99m Tc-tin colloid scan. *Eur J Nucl Med* 1983;8:557–558.

Murphy WA. Radiologically guided percutaneous musculoskeletal biopsy. *Orthop Clin North Am* 1983;14:233–241.

Nash CL and Moe JH. A study of vertebral rotation. *J Bone Joint Surg [Am]* 1969;5(2):223.

Newman NM and Ling RSM. Acetabular bone destruction related to non-steroidal anti-inflammatory drugs. *Lancet* 1985:11–13.

Ogryzlo MA and Rosen PS. Ankylosing (Marie-Strumpell) spondylitis. *Postgrad Med J* 1969;45:182.

Patel DV, Hammer RA, and Levin B, et al. Primary osteogenic sarcoma of the spine. *Skel Radiol* 1984;12:276–279.

Pearcy M, Portek I, and Shepherd J. Three dimensional x-ray analysis of normal movement in the lumbar spine. *Spine* 1984; 9:294.

Pennal GF, Conn GS, and McDonald G, et al. Motion study of the lumbar spine—A preliminary report. *J Bone Joint Surg [Br]* 1972;54:442.

Quencer RM, Montalvo BM, Green BA, and Eismont FJ. Intraoperative spinal sonography of soft-tissue masses of the spinal cord and spinal canal. *AJR* 1984;143:1307–1315.

Resnick D. Degenerative diseases of the vertebral column. *Radiology* 1985;156:3–14.

Reynolds RJ. Cineradiography by the indirect method. *Radiology* 1938;31:177.

Rich EA. Observations noted in 11,000 feet of experimental cineroentgenography film. *J Am Chiropractic Assoc* 1964;1(3).

Richens A and Rowe DJF. Disturbance of calcium metabolism by anticonvulsant drugs. *Br Med J* 1970;4:73.

Rowe LJ and Yochum TR. Principles of radiological interpretation. In Yochum TR and Rowe LT, ed *Essentials of Skeletal Radiology,* Baltimore, Md: Williams & Wilkins; 1987.

Sandoz RW. Technique & interpretation of functional radiography of the lumbar spine. *Ann Swiss Chiropractic Assoc* 1965:66.

Sandoz RW. Newer trends in the pathogenesis of spinal disorders. A tentative classification of the functional disorders of the intervertebral motor unit. *Ann Swiss Chiropractic Assoc* 1971:93.

Sarles H and Sahel J. Pathology of chronic calcifying pancreatitis. *Am J Gastroenterol* 1976;66:117.

Schmorl G and Junghanns H. *The Human Spine in Health and Disease,* 2nd ed. Besemann EF, trans. New York: Grune & Stratton; 1971.

Sharp J and Purser DW. Spontaneous atlantoaxial dislocation in ankylosing spondylitis & rheumatoid arthritis. *Ann Rheum Dis* 1961;20:47.

Sherman R. Chiropractic x-ray rationale. *J Can Chiropractic Assoc* 1986;30(1):33.

Sherman R and Bauer F. *X-ray X-pertise—From A to X.* Fort Worth, Tex: Parker Chiropractic Research Foundation; 1982.

Stockley I, Getty CJM, and Dixon AK, et al. Lumbar lateral canal entrapment: Clinical, radiculographic and computed tomographic findings. *Clin Radiol* 1988;39:144–149.

van Akkerveeken PF, Obrien JP, and Park WM. Experimentally induced hypermobility in the lumbar spine. *Spine* 1979;4:236.

Vider M, Maruyama Y, and Navarez R. Significance of the vertebral venous (Batson's) plexus in metastatic carcinoma. *Cancer* 1977; 40:67–71.

Waddell G. An approach to backache. *Br J Hosp Med* 1982; Sept: 187.

Walheim GG and Selvick G. Mobility of the pubic symphysis. *Clin Orthop Relat Res* 1984;191:129.

Weitz EM. The lateral bending sign. *Spine* 1981;6(4):388.

Whitehouse GH. New imaging techniques in rheumatology. *Br J Rheumatol* 1986;25(2):217.

Woolfenden JM Pitt MJ, and Durie BGM, et al. Comparison of bone scintigraphy and radiography in multiple myeloma. *Radiology* 1980;134:723–728.

Yochum TR and Rowe LJ. Arthritides of the upper cervical complex. In *Aspects of Manipulative Therapy,* 2nd ed. New York: Churchill-Livingstone; 1979;ch. 3.

Young LW, Oestrich AE, and Goldstein LA. Roentgenology in scoliosis: Contribution to evaluation and management. *AJR* 1970; 108:778.

chapter 22

Advanced Imaging Modalities

Joseph Howe
Stephen M. Foreman
William V. Glenn, Jr.

- **ADVANCED IMAGING MODALITIES**
  Computerized Tomography
  Magnetic Resonance Imaging
  Computerized Tomography Versus
  Magnetic Resonance Imaging
- **ADJUNCT SPINAL IMAGING**
  MODALITIES

  Myelography
  Radionuclide Scintigraphy
- **CLINICAL INDICATIONS FOR**
  ADVANCED IMAGING
- **CONCLUSION**
- **REFERENCES**

The use of diagnostic imaging, primarily plain film radiography, has been an integral part of the practice of chiropractic for decades. Plain film radiographs are used for biomechanical analysis and for diagnosis of pathological conditions that may contraindicate chiropractic care. Although useful for evaluating pathology, plain film radiographs have their limitations in the clinical setting. Plain film radiographs poorly visualize nondisplaced fractures, soft tissue structures such as the intervertebral discs and spinal cord, and early bone destruction and repair. The advent of the advanced imaging techniques has supplemented the chiropractor's diagnostic armamentarium. The following sections introduce and discuss the practical use of these modalities by the practicing doctor of chiropractic.

Advanced Imaging Modalities

Computerized Tomography

Body section radiography, variously called laminography, planigraphy, and most recently tomography, has been used since 1914 to produce radiographic images of specific thin planes of the body. Plain film tomography is accomplished by moving the x-ray tube and receptor synchronously in opposite directions (Andrews, 1946). Tomographic technology developed slowly until 1973, when Godfrey N. Hounsfield introduced a new technique that combined the principle of plain film tomography with a computer to produce the first diagnostic axial cross-

sectional images of the body. Computerized axial tomography (CAT) uses the differential absorption of x-rays as they pass through the body to form digital matrices, which the computer converts into a cross-sectional image. Prior to this innovation, the cross-sectional radiographic presentation of anatomy was poorly understood and rarely used in the clinical setting. Since that time, however, this radiological procedure, which was initially termed computerized axial tomography, has become a sophisticated and mature imaging technology, one that is firmly entrenched in radiological practice and occupies a principal role in diagnostic imaging of the human body. As computer software was developed to reformat the data from which axial images are produced into sagittal, coronal, oblique, curved coronal, and curved oblique images (Fig. 22–1), and even into shaded three-dimensional images (Fig. 22–2), the axial designation was dropped and the procedure is now called computerized tomography (CT). Although it is important to understand, the mechanism of producing CT images is well described in numerous publications (Andre and Resnick, 1988; Howe et al., 1987; Brooks and DiChiro, 1975) and will not be detailed in this chapter.

Computerized tomography has both advantages and disadvantages in the clinical setting. The major disadvantages of this imaging modality are its use of ionizing radiation and its relative insensitivity to small differences in the x-ray absorption characteristics of many tissues. The latter disadvantage makes it difficult to differentiate similar soft tissue struc-

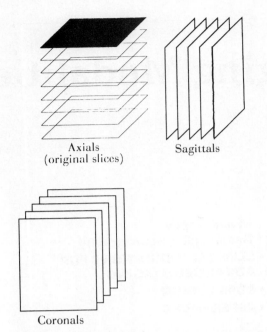

Axials
(original slices)

Sagittals

Coronals

Figure 22–1. Multiplanar reformatting of CT images. The original matrix of numbers from which the image is formed can be sorted in the other planes and images can be formed in whatever plane is desired.

tures without the use of contrast medium. The radiation exposure to the patient from a CT study is now comparable to or only slightly greater than that incurred from multiple plain film views of the part of the body examined (Evans and Mettler, 1985; Rothman and Glenn, 1985). This improved dose rate is possible because the individual axial sections are tightly collimated so that only a very thin section of the body is exposed for each axial section. Also, the x-ray energies used are usually at or above 120 kVp, so that the milliampere seconds per axial section are as low as possible to achieve the desired image.

One of the great advantages of CT is its ability to manipulate the data acquired from a single axial imaging mode and reformat or reprocess it into other planes or points of orientation such as coronal or sagittal views. The resulting images can also be displayed with differing contrast levels (Fig. 22–3). For example, the data from the visualization of soft tissues, e.g., spinal cord or brain, may be optimized, and is termed a *soft tissue window*. The technician may also emphasize the osseous structures with bone window images. Each window is desirable for a complete assessment of the area. In addition, the observer can manipulate the window widths and levels via the computer to vary contrast.

The proper use of bone and soft tissue windows is important as they, along with axial, sagittal, and coronal reconstruction views, can often eliminate the need for supplemental administration of contrast me-

dium during the CT scan. The use of spinal contrast is common in some imaging centers. Some radiologists use contrast medium with every examination and others use it only when attempting to visualize soft tissue structures. This creates a problem for the practicing chiropractor. Patients may develop an allergic reaction to the contrast material, the chiropractor would not be able to properly follow the patient during this time, and care would have to be turned over to a medical physician. In our experience the use of contrast is greatly limited in studies that use both the bone and soft tissue windows and combine the axial, coronal, and sagittal views. In this way the spine is viewed from three different perspectives and two different contrast settings for maximum clinical information. It also allows the patient to avoid the use of contrast and the potential complications of intrathecal injection as described under Myelography.

Another advantage of CT is its spatial resolution which, because of the geometry of the system, can alter image sizes but maintain exact contours. This capability makes it possible to reformat the image of a structure to actual life size if desired, to enlarge or reduce it if advantageous, or, as noted earlier, to construct three-dimensional images (Howe et al., 1987; Andre and Resnick, 1988; Rothman and Glenn, 1985; Pate et al., 1988). This three-dimensional technology can even be used to produce models of the scanned part that differ within a very small tolerance from the actual structure. This has been used to create exact prosthetic replacements for structures such as mandibles and a hips.

Magnetic Resonance Imaging

Magnetic resonance imaging (MRI) is another technology that produces tomographic thin-section images of anatomy and employs a computer. In 1946, Bloch and Purcell, et al. discovered the phenomenon known as magnetic resonance, and shortly thereafter its use in chemistry became commonplace to determine chemical composition and structure of complex molecules. In 1973, Lauterbur showed that images could be constructed from the magnetic resonance signal. Hinshaw and his colleagues produced the first magnetic resonance (MR) images of a human wrist in 1979, and since that time the technologic advances have been multiplying.

Although MR images generally resemble those produced by CT, they are acquired by a different process and differ in their clinical application. MR images are not based on information gathered from the transmission of energy through the imaged structure. Instead, imaging information is gathered by detecting the energy released by hydrogen atoms within the body when these are subjected to strong magnetic fields. Each hydrogen atom has a north

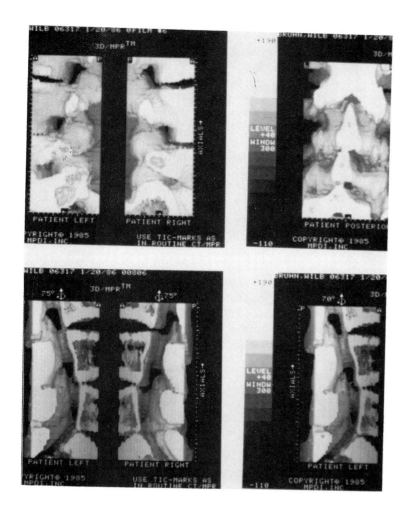

Figure 22–2. Three-dimensional shaded images from a CT scan. By electronically removing part of the structures (*bottom*), the contours of the spinal canal, lateral recesses, and nerve root canals can be seen in detail. The major advantage is in localizing fracture fragments that might cause neurologic damage.

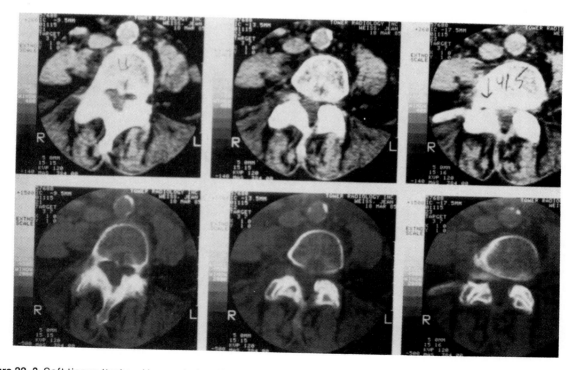

Figure 22–3. Soft tissue (*top*) and bone window (*bottom*) images from a CT scan of the lumbosacral spine. The same data are enhanced to display bone or soft tissue characteristics. These illustrate severe facet joint disease resulting in spinal canal and lateral recess stenosis.

and south pole constituting the axis around which its electrons precess or spin. These axes have random orientation under usual conditions, but when the body is placed in a very strong magnetic field the magnetic axes line up in a new position, either with or opposite to the magnetic field. When a specific radio frequency (RF), the Larmor frequency, is introduced counter to the magnetic field, the atomic axes rotate and change their orientation according to the characteristics of the RF introduced. In many cases, the new alignment of the atoms is 90°, or at right angles, to their position which was determined by the strong magnetic field. When the RF is turned off the atoms return to the original orientation. In doing so they release energy, which is the MR signal picked up by antennas in the MR scanner. This weak signal emanating from the individual atoms is converted to the MR image. More detailed information on the physics of MR is available in other dissertations by Murphy (1988), Young (1988), Elster et al. (1986), Partain et al. (1984), and Harms et al. (1984).

Magnetic resonance imaging has a great advantage in that it does not use ionizing radiation. To date, considerable data have shown no adverse biologic effects from the magnetic fields used. There are, however, a few contraindications to the use of MR, mainly the presence of ferromagnetic materials in the body, such as ferromagnetic vascular clips in the brain, or the presence of a pacemaker, the function of which would be altered by the magnetic field (New et al., 1983; Mesgarzadek et al., 1985; Laakman et al., 1985).

Magnetic resonance imaging differentiates tissues according to their concentration of hydrogen ions rather than their radiodensity. Thus, structures containing relatively large quantities of hydrogen ions, such as soft tissue and fluid-filled compartments, will produce images having a contrast and resolution exceeding those produced by standard ra-

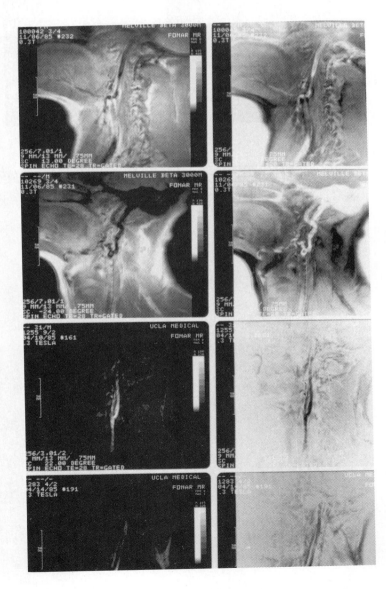

Figure 22–4. Blood vessels demonstrated by MRI. Moving blood does generate a signal allowing demonstration of vessels without the need for injecting a contrast medium. This illustration shows the carotid arteries in several modes by manipulation of the MRI data to produce the desired image characteristics.

diographic techniques. Cortical bone, in contrast, has a relatively low concentration of hydrogen as it is composed primarily of calcium and thus produces a very low MR signal and an image with little detail. But bone marrow, which is rich in fat and hydrogen, yields a signal that allows depiction of osseous structures, although presently not as good as can be achieved with CT.

Other structures may be indirectly visualized with MR. Moving blood, for example, produces a null MR signal, which allows vessels to be differentiated sharply from surrounding tissues (Fig. 22–4). Hemorrhage, where blood is stagnant, can also be differentiated from adjacent tissues. Likewise, edema produces a different signal than surrounding materials and can be imaged as well (Fig. 22–5). MRI has its most significant utility in spinal imaging because of its ability to visualize soft tissues and to differentiate various tissues within the spinal canal as well as those adjacent to the vertebrae. For example, cerebrospinal fluid (CSF) can be made to appear bright

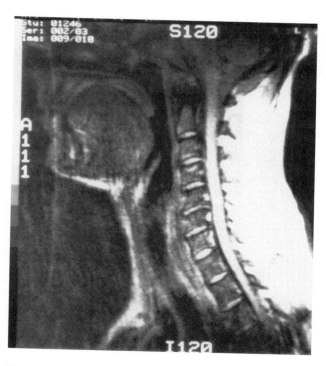

Figure 22–6. Midsagittal, T2-weighted MRI scan of the cervical spine. The cerebrospinal fluid produces a characteristically bright signal sometimes called the ''myelogram effect.'' Note also the bright signal in the disc spaces on T2 weighting.

and simulate a myelogram or, by using a different pulse sequence, can be made less bright so that the spinal cord can be seen surrounded by CSF within the thecal tube (Fig. 22–6). T1-weighted images, often used to provide optimum visualization of vertebral bodies and facet joints, show fat as the brightest signal (''fat scan''), whereas on T2-weighted images water (CSF) is brighter (''water scan'') (Fig. 22–7). The T2-weighted images are often used to image structures such as intervertebral discs and nerve roots. The use of both T1 and T2 settings is required for a complete study of many areas.

Unlike CT, MRI techniques do not involve reformatting the one set of data to create images of different body planes and to enhance differences in contrast. Rather, MRI allows multiple parallel planes to be imaged simultaneously, and contrast is varied by employing different pulse sequences and reading echoes at different time intervals. Continuing development of imaging parameters is allowing shorter data acquisition times, enabling a greater use of MRI (Frahm et al., 1986; Utz et al., 1986). Procedures for CSF gating to reduce pulsation artifacts are also allowing improved MR images, particularly in the cervical spine (Perkins and Wehrli, 1986). The use of surface coils, which allow reception of signals very close to specific body areas, has also brought about a better signal-to-noise ratio, resulting in enhanced detail and shortened scanning time and/or better spatial resolution in areas such as the

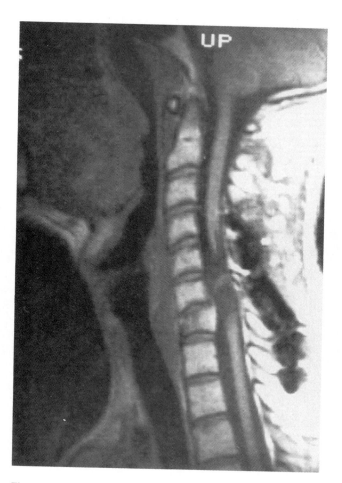

Figure 22–5. This T1-weighted MR image shows transection of the spinal cord from a fracture of C7 with displacement into the spinal canal. The altered signal in the cord shows the extent of damage and the posterior soft tissue edema is shown by the large area of low signal intensity.

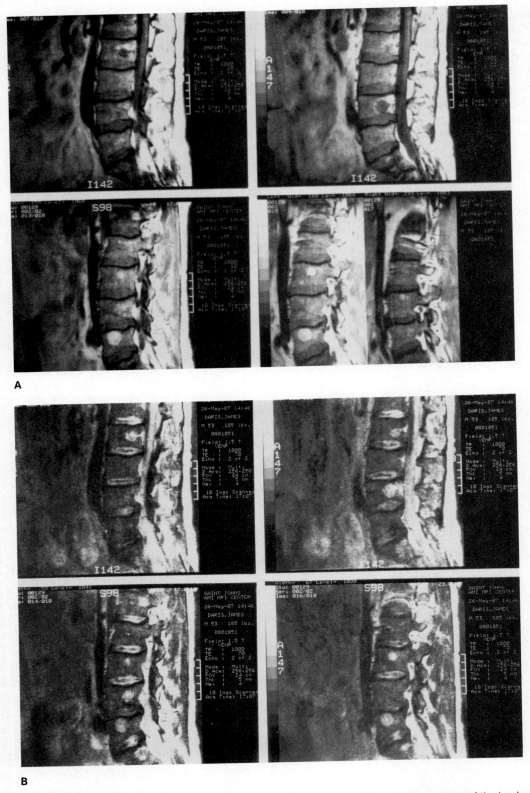

Figure 22–7. (A) Sagittal T1-weighted MRI sequence. **(B)** Similar T2-weighted images. **(C)** Coronal sequence of the lumbar spine of this patient who has several vertebral body lesions that were not evident from plain film radiography. The round lesions in the L3 and L5 vertebral bodies seen on the lower images of A and B have high signal intensity on the T1-weighted sequence and more moderate intensity with T2 weighting. The lesion in the L4 vertebral body seen on the upper sagittal images has relatively low signal intensity with T1 weighting and becomes bright on the T2 sequence. These lesions are hemangiomas and fatty foci in the vertebral bodies. They are also well demonstrated on the coronal images. (*Continues next page*)

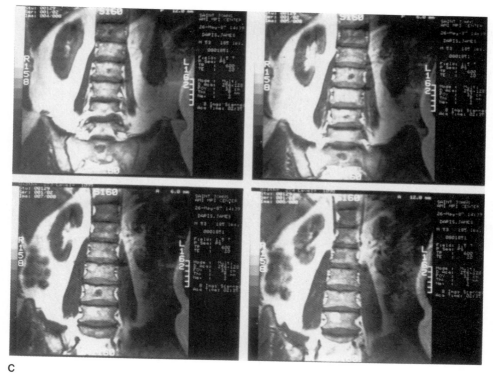

C

Figure 22–7. *Continued.*

shoulder and knee (Murphy, 1988; Kneeland et al., 1986; Edelman et al., 1985).

Computerized Tomography Versus Magnetic Resonance Imaging

Both CT and MRI have significant roles to play in spinal imaging. CT is used to best advantage to see bone; MRI produces better images of soft tissues, but has some advantages in imaging certain bone pathologies. CT is able to show calcification, which is poorly seen, if at all, on MR images. CT reveals spurs, endplate ridging, and the confines of bony canals to best advantage (see Fig. 22–3), hence its use to depict suspected degenerative joint disease or fractures. To see spinal cord injury or disease, the CSF in the subarachnoid space, other neurologic abnormalities, and the paraspinal soft tissue structures, MRI is the best imaging choice (Fig. 22–8). Both CT and MRI adequately illustrate disc herniation, but MRI has an advantage, at least theoretically, in that it can show diminished water content in discs as an indication of degenerative disc disease (Fig. 22–9). Some clinical problems, such as cervical trauma, may need the consideration of both modalities. In general, use CT for bone and MRI for soft tissue. When both areas require visualization, use both as too much information is never a bad thing in the clinical setting (Foreman and Croft, 1988).

At the present time a water-soluble myelographic contrast medium is used during CT scans to visualize suspected cervical disc herniation (Fig. 22–10), but some inaccuracies have been shown to occur when this procedure is used in patients with cer-

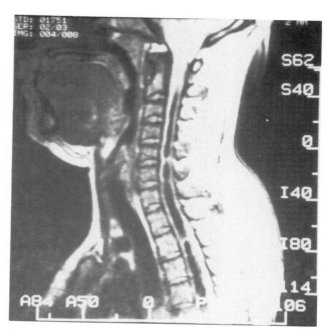

Figure 22–8. Syrinx cavities in the spinal cord demonstrated by MRI. Three long cavities extend from the lower portion of C2 to the lower aspect of T4. Note also the low position of the cerebellum entering the upper portion of the spinal canal, demonstrating the Arnold–Chiari phenomenon.

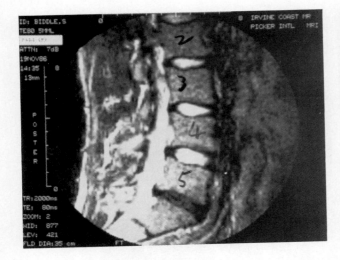

A

B

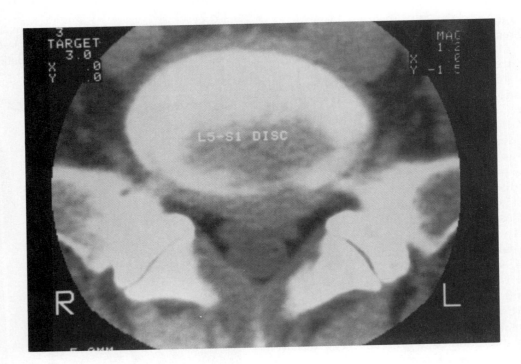

C

Figure 22-9. (A,B) Relatively midsagittal T2-weighted MR images from two different patients. Both show decreased signal intensity in the L5/S1 disc interspace in contrast to the high signal in the other interspaces. This is evidence of loss of hydration of the disc, which accompanies degeneration of the nucleus pulposus. In B, a large herniation of disc material into the spinal canal is obvious at the degenerated L5 disc level. **(C)** Axial CT image demonstrating a diffuse posterior disc bulge with central focal herniation, which slightly effaces the anterior of the thecal sac and slightly displaces the left nerve root as it exits the sac.

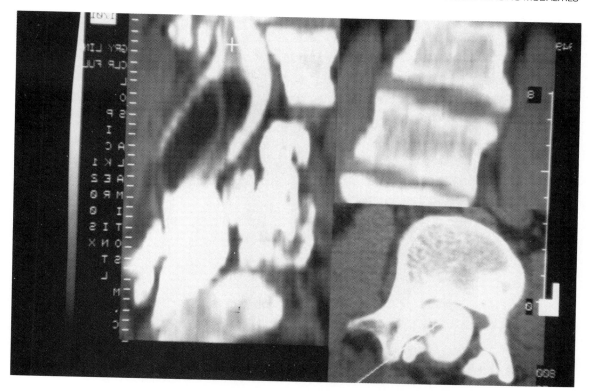

Figure 22-10. An axial image from a CT scan in which myelographic medium had been injected into the subarachnoid space is shown on the lower right. The picture on the upper right is a coronally reformatted image through the vertebral body/disc region at the same level. The image on the left is a reformatted sagittal image that shows a lipomeningocele deforming the thecal sac. The scoliosis and eccentricity of the spine associated with this anomaly account for the inability to discern the vertebrae in usual fashion on the sagittal image. The injection of subarachnoid contrast medium to obtain myelographic studies has been a helpful diagnostic tool in the past, but this invasive procedure is increasingly less necessary as the cord and intraspinal structures become better demonstrated by improved MRI sequences.

vical radiculopathy (Leeds et al., 1988). As further advances in MRI overcome or further minimize artifacts from CSF pulsations, the advantages of MRI will probably supercede those of CT for these specific imaging applications. As a mature technology, CT has probably peaked in its variety of uses in spine imaging. As MRI technology continues to evolve, its use to image blood vessels and to depict chemical shift phenomena and other physiological processes will surely increase.

Adjunct Spinal Imaging Modalities

Myelography

Myelography, fluoroscopy, and radiography following the injection of contrast medium into the thecal sac have been in use since the early 1920s (Shapiro, 1984), but are increasingly being supplanted by MRI and CT.

The procedure is accomplished by first placing a spinal tap needle in the spinal canal. Some CSF is usually removed initially to allow for laboratory anal-

ysis. The contrast medium, for example, iopamidol or iohexol, is then injected into the thecal sac. This allows the neurological structures to be covered in conrast medium and visualized on plain films. The contrast medium is then moved to other parts of the spine by tilting the table and allowing gravity to move the injected liquid with change of position. This entire process is observed under fluroscopy by the radiologist and spot films are taken with the patient in various positions. Additional films may be taken by the technician.

Myelography allows the thecal sac to be visualized, but does not clearly visualize the spinal cord or cauda equina, this despite the lesser opacity afforded by the nonionic contrast media that have become the criteria for the procedure. As the contrast medium is contained entirely inside the thecal sac, the contents of the spinal canal outside the thecal sac cannot be seen except by displacement of the myelographic column by extraneous structures. This major disadvantage of myelography has resulted in the non-visualization of a variety of extrathecal problems for years. For example, canal stenosis is not as well de-

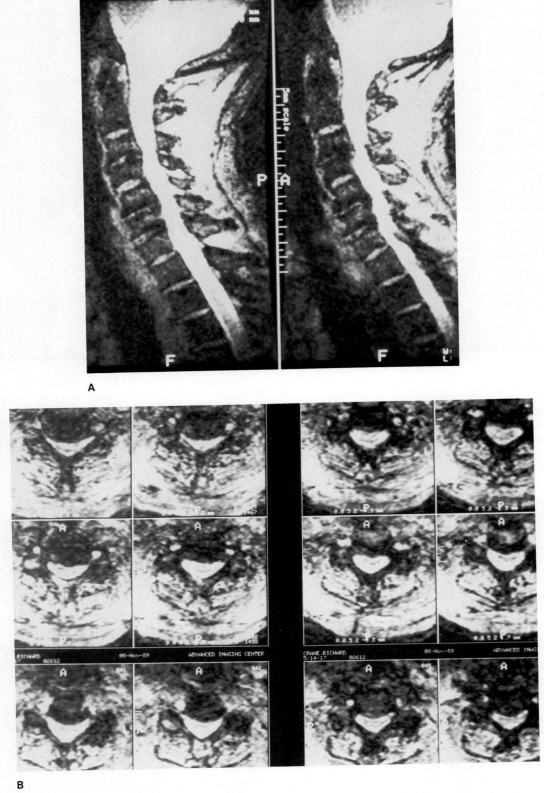

Figure 22–11. T2-weighted sagittal and axial images of a cervical spine with severe spinal canal stenosis. The midsagittal image, although showing the narrowing of the spinal canal, cannot depict the extent and severity of such narrowing as well as axial depiction. The left upper axial images and the lowest right image demonstrate the canal narrowing and distortion at those levels that can be compared with the larger canal at other levels seen on the other axial images.

picted by myelography as by CT or especially MRI (Fig. 22–11). Lateral disc herniations or other space-occupying lesions that do not impinge on the thecal sac are not visualized by myelography, whereas both CT and MRI show such abnormalities well. The use of small amounts of myelographic medium in conjunction with CT, termed a *minimyelogram,* has been advocated by several authors (DiChiro and Shellinger, 1976; Kieffer, 1985; Meyer et al., 1982; Seibert et al., 1981), and is especially helpful in visualizing cervical and thoracic spinal areas. CT following routine myelography is also employed in some circumstances.

Other disadvantages of myelography arise from the invasive nature of the procedure. Needle insertion injuries, although uncommon, do occur as does allergic reaction to the contrast medium. This allergic side effect is now less common with the nonionic contrast media used today, but some risk is still present. Postmyelographic headaches and long-term arachnoiditis are also problems to be encountered and dealt with by physicians employing this diagnostic test.

Given the noninvasive qualities of CT and MRI and their ability to visualize beyond the anatomical constraints of the thecal sac, we believe the newer imaging methods are superior to myelography in most respects. It is the opinion of the authors that myelography is an outmoded imaging mechanism and should rarely if ever be employed when high-quality CT or especially MRI is available.

Radionuclide Scintigraphy

Radionuclide scintigraphy is an imaging modality that has definite advantages in certain circumstances. Because this chapter deals with spinal imaging, only bone scintigraphy will be discussed. Radionuclides bonded to elements that seek certain tissues give diagnostic information that may be of great value.

Technetium-99*m*-labeled polyphosphates are the most widely used of the bone-seeking radiotracers (Alazraki, 1988; Mandell, 1988). Fifteen to twenty millicuries (mCi) is intravenously injected into the patient. During the 2-to 3-hour waiting period after the injection, the radionuclides are transported through the vascular system to areas of bone repair or building. The radionuclides accumulate near the areas of increased bone metabolism, resulting in a "hot" area on the film in such areas as tumors, infections, fractures, reactive bone formation secondary to arthritis, and generalized periostitis.

The radiation dose to the patient, in the past, was quite high and the procedure was usually limited to patients with known malignant tumors. The

information obtained during these early scans was used to stage the tumors and to search for areas of osteolytic destruction via metastasis. This is no longer true as the techniques have improved as a result of the use of a combination of short-lived radiopharmaceuticals and lower-energy pharmaceuticals and the improved focusing of imaging equipment that takes advantage of these improvements. The absorbed body dose, after the radionuclides have been excreted by the kidneys, is approximately 0.009 rad/mCi.

In the clinical setting, the entire skeleton is scanned when metastatic carcinoma is sought (Fig. 22–12). The spine and pelvis are scanned from the anterior and from the posterior and, on rare occasions, obliquely or laterally. Scans of specific areas may be done when information on localized lesions is desired. Dynamic bones scans, using a three-phase technique, may also be done. The first phase consists of an immediate radionuclide angiogram taken as the radionuclide is being transported through the vascular system. The second phase is a blood pool scan when the tracer is largely in the extracellular spaces surrounding the bones. The final

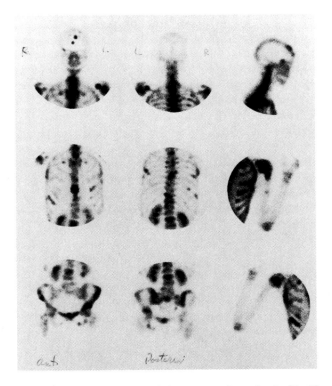

Figure 22–12. Scintigraphic bone scans of a patient with diffuse metastatic bone carcinoma. Note the increased uptake of the radionuclide in several ribs, in the skull, in one upper humerus, and in one hip joint area. The radionuclide is concentrated in foci of increased bone production or metabolic activity.

phase, a delayed scan (approximately 3 hours postinjection) when the radionuclide more optimally images the bones, may be used to evaluate bone tumors or infections (Mandell, 1988). Other variations of scintigraphy, such as single-photon-emission computed tomography (SPECT), make possible the visualization of the spine transaxially, coronally, or sagitally (Keyes, 1982). Although this procedure is more time consuming and expensive than other bone scanning techniques, it has the advantage of being able to much more closely identify discrete lesions.

Radionuclide bone scans are very sensitive in detecting bone disease, but are nonspecific. Whereas it takes from 30 to 50% or greater medullary bone destruction to be adequately seen on plain film radiographs, radioscintigraphy will show such lesions at 4 to 7% destruction. Any malignant bone tumor is capable of producing an active bone scan (Mandell, 1988). Benign tumors or tumorlike lesions may also yield a positive bone scan if bone destruction or production is occurring. Whenever there is increased metabolic bone activity, a "hot" scan with increased radioactivity will be demonstrated. Occasionally, the distribution of disease is so widespread and relatively uniform that an abnormal bone scan may be misinterpreted as negative. This phenomenon, termed a *superscan*, occurs in widespread metastasis, renal osteodystrophy, myelofibrosis, and, occasionally, Paget's disease and fibrous dysplasia (Alazraki et al., 1988; Mandell, 1988). It is usually accompanied by relatively diminished uptake in the urinary tract, which in the usual scans is well seen because of excretion of the radionuclide. Photopenic or "cold" scintigraphic foci may also be found when there is bone destruction or replacement that does not excite repair or other osteoproductive activity (Alazraki et al., 1988; Mandell, 1988; Mettler and Guiborteau, 1983).

Radioscintigraphy is especially helpful in early detection of infection or inflammatory disease in the spine, sacroiliac joints, and paraspinal tissues. If such disease is suspected, and a technetium scan is negative, a gallium scan may be done (Alazraki, 1988; Mandell, 1988; Mettler and Guiborteau, 1983). Gallium may be used initially if the suspicion of infection is very high. The detection of stress fractures or of subtle fractures when radiographic findings are equivocal is a particularly useful application of bone scanning. This may have particular application in early detection of pars intraarticularis stress fractures, which result in spondylolysis and/or spondylolisthesis.

Although radioscintigraphy in spinal imaging is not used as extensively as other imaging modalities, it has a definite role and deserves consideration when metastasis, infection, inflammatory disease, metabolic disease, stress fracture, and other conditions that alter bone production or metabolism are suspected, especially if routine radiography is inconclusive.

Clinical Indications for Advanced Imaging

The practicing chiropractor has a variety of diagnostic needs that cannot be met with the use of plain film radiographs alone. First, because of the high percentage of trauma cases encountered, chiropractors need to completely evaluate patients for the presence of small, nondisplaced fractures in the spine. These fractures are often difficult to localize on plain films. Of similar concern is the detection of intraspinal problems of osseous origin, such as facet arthrosis, central spinal stenosis, and lateral recess stenosis, each of which can cause nerve root ischemia and associated clinical problems (Foreman, 1985). The proper detection of these problems will have an obvious effect on the form, duration, and outcome of care.

Computerized tomography has the unique ability to visualize the surface and interior of osseous structures with a high level of detail by using a "bone window" and to inspect the injured area from any number of angles through the use of multiplanar reconstruction (Fig. 22–13). Combine these assets with the ability to collimate the scan thickness to 1 mm, and the usefulness of this instrument in meeting the needs of the practicing chiropractor can easily be appreciated. Perhaps the most effective use of CT in chiropractic practice is to assess the patency of the spinal canal and the intervertebral foramen. These areas are frequently compromised by the osteophytes associated with the degenerative processes of the spine and are a common problem in the elderly. Many patients with a combination of degenerative disease and nonresolving symptoms are at least candidates for spinal CT.

The second clinical need that is poorly met by plain film radiography is the visualization of soft tissue structures such as intervertebral discs, the spinal cord, and the brain. Without the use of radiographic contrast medium, plain films poorly detect pathology in these areas. Detecting intervertebral disc disease can be particularly challenging. The intervertebral discs are well known for their ability to swell, herniate, and fragment, all of which can produce marked pain and disability in a patient. The type of treatment and the overall effect of care depend on the accurate identification of the location and sever-

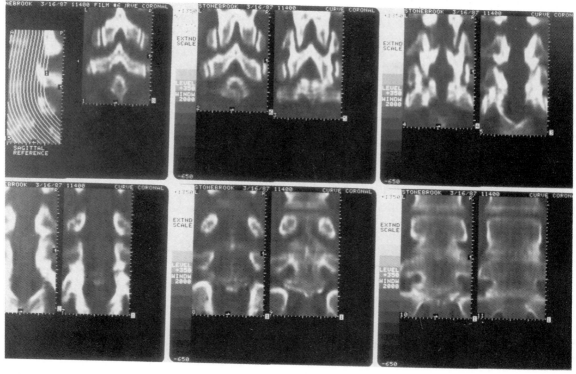

Figure 22–13. Curved coronal reformatting of CT scans. The image on the upper left shows the specific matrices of data displayed in the images. The spine is shown as a sequence of tomographic sections (*left to right, top to bottom*) from spinous processes anteriorly to the vertebral bodies.

ity of the disc problem. Spinal cord pressure and the resultant myelopathy are also serious clinical problems that require accurate diagnosis if function is to be preserved. Plain film radiographs only reveal end stage in spinal cord pathology, if at all. The detection of brain pathology by plain films is limited to the detection of intracranial calcifications, abnormal shifting of these structures, and signs of increased intracranial pressure such as enlargement of the sella turcica.

The use of MRI to visualize the spinal cord has added new clinical options for both the chiropractor and the patient. In the past, the main option was myelography with its potential complications of adhesive arachnoiditis and postlumbar puncture headaches. The use of CT improved the diagnostic process a great deal, but contrast media were still needed in many cases for the diagnosis of soft tissue lesions. MRI has increased this visualization as never before and greatly reduced the need for contrast medium. Brain imaging with MRI has also revolutionized the fields of neuroradiology. MRI can visualize brain anatomy and greatly aid the chiropractor in the detection of intracranial pathology.

Finally, the doctor of chiropractic may need to completely evaluate pathology of the osseous system. Subtle problems, such as metastases, can cause pain and weaken the affected osseous structures. Other subtle conditions may include occult fractures and osteomyelitis. Any of these disorders can affect the type of care to be rendered, and proper detection of such conditions at an early stage can prevent catastrophic complications. Plain film x-rays will reveal osseous pathology only after loss of 30 to 50% of the stored calcium in the affected bone. Scintigraphy, however, will be positive after only 4 to 7% bone loss, making it a much more sensitive indicator of ongoing osseous pathology.

Conclusion

Plain film radiography is still the gold standard for the practicing doctor of chiropractic; it is readily available, is cost effective, and reveals major bone pathology. The limitations of plain film radiography are a lack of sensitivity in revealing small, nondisplaced fractures; poor soft tissue visualization; and poor ability to demonstrate early bone loss. The modalities of CT, MRI, and scintigraphy are increasingly being used by doctors of chiropractic in their practices to better serve and diagnose their patients.

These tests are not to be used in every case, however. It should be understood that, as with x-rays and any other test, the patient must have the clinical criteria that would indicate the use of the test. Otherwise, the test would be considered to be unreasonable and unnecessary. The following points should serve as a guide to the use of advanced imaging modalities.

1. *The imaging modality should be used to confirm the diagnosis indicated by both the history and the clinical findings on physical examination.* For example, ''back pain'' alone is insufficient to justify a CT or MRI study. But if back pain is combined with the history of sudden onset while lifting, physical examination findings of nerve root tension signs, and an antalgic posture, the doctor has more than sufficient cause to consider the MRI scan.

2. *The modality should be aimed at a specific anatomic problem.* In imaging there is no such thing as a ''one trick pony.'' Use CT for bone, MRI for soft tissue, and scintigraphy for metabolic bone disease. In this way the examination will reveal the most information possible.

3. *The test should not be ordered without an adequate understanding of the procedure.* Chiropractors should attend an approved postgraduate seminar or review the available literature on the subject and consult with their radiologist before using these procedures.

4. *The result of the test should potentially change the direction of care.* Why perform a test if the chiropractor will treat the patient the same whether the result is positive or negative? If a positive test result will not change the care, the test is probably unreasonable and unnecessary and may be considered excessive by the state board of examiners.

References

Alazraki N. Radionuclide techniques. In Resnick D and Niwayama G, eds. *Diagnosis of Bone and Joint Disorders*, 2nd ed. Philadelphia: WB Saunders; 1988.

Andre M and Resnick D. Computed tomography. In Resnick D and Niwayama G, eds. *Diagnosis of Bone and Joint Disorders*, 2nd ed. Philadelphia: WB Saunders; 1988.

Andrews JR. Planigraphy: Introduction and history. *AJR* 1936;36:575–587.

Bloch F. Nuclear induction. *Phys Rev* 1946;70:460–474.

Brooks RA and DiChiro G. Theory of image reconstruction in computed tomography. *Radiology* 1975;117:561.

DiChiro G and Shellinger D. Computed tomography of spinal cord after lumbar intrathecal introduction of metrizamide (computed assisted myelography). *Radiology* 1976;120:101–104.

Edelman RR, Shoukimas GM, and Stark DD, et al. High resolution surface-coil imaging of lumbar disk disease. *AJR* 1985;144:1123–1129.

Elster AD, Handel SF, and Goldman AM. *Magnetic Resonance Imaging: Reference and Atlas.* Philadelphia: JB Lippincott; 1986.

Evans RJ and Mettler FA. National CT use and radiation exposure, United States 1983. *AJR* 1985;144:1077–1081.

Foreman S. Nerve root ischemia and pain secondary to spinal stenosis syndrome. Technical and clinical considerations. *J Manipulative Physiol Ther* 1985;8(2):81–85.

Foreman, S. and Croft A. MRI and CT imaging of the cervical spine after trauma: An algorithm. *J Chiropractic* 1988;24(11):65–68.

Frahm J, Hasse A, and Matthaire D. Rapid NMR imaging of dynamic processes using the FLASH technique. *Magn Reson Med* 1986;3:321–327.

Harms SE, Morgan TJ, and Yamanshi WS, et al. Principles of nuclear magnetic resonance imaging. *Radiographics* 1984;4(spec ed):26–43.

Hinshaw WS, Andrew ER, and Bottomley PA, et al. An in vivo study of the forearm and hand by thin section NMR imaging. *Br J Radiol* 1979;52:36.

Hounsfield GN. Computerized transverse axial scanning (tomography). *Br J Radiol* 1973;46:1016–1022.

Howe JW, Yochum TR, and Rowe LJ. Diagnostic imaging of spinal stenosis and intervertebral disc disease. In Yochum TR, ed. *Essentials of Skeletal Radiology.* Baltimore, Md: Williams & Wilkins; 1987.

Keyes JW Jr. Perspectives on tomography. *J Nucl Med* 1982;23:633–640.

Kieffer SA. Post-operative spine: CT and CT myelography. In *Diseases of the Spine.* NE Chase, H Firooznia, and II Kricheff (eds). New York: New York University Medical Center; 1985.

Kneeland JB, Jesmanowicz A, and Froncisz W, et al. High resolution MR imaging using loop-gap resonators. *Radiology* 1986;158:247–250.

Laakman RW, Kaufman B, and Hans JS, et al. MR imaging in patients with metal implants. *Radiology* 1985;157:711.

Lauterbur PC. Image formation by induced local interactions: Examples by employing nuclear magnetic resonance. *Nature* 1973;242:190–191.

Leeds NE, Elkin CM, and Leon E, et al. Myelography. In *Imaging Modalities in Spinal Disorders.* ME Krichun (ed). Philadelphia:WB Saunders; 1988.

Mandell G. Radionuclide imaging. In: *Imaging Modalities in Spinal Disorders.* Philadelphia:WB Saunders; 1988.

Mesgarzadek M, Revesz G, Bonakdarpour A, Betz RR. The effect on medical metal implants by magnetic fields of magnetic resonance imaging. *Skel Radiol* 1985;14:205.

Mettler FA Jr and Guiborteau MJ. *Essentials of Nuclear Medicine.* New York: Grune & Stratton; 1983.

Meyer JD, Latchaw RE, and Roppolo HM, et al. Computed tomography and myelography of the post-operative spine. *AJNR* 1982;3:223–228.

Murphy WA. Magnetic resonance imaging. In Resnick D and Niwayama G, eds. *Diagnosis of Bone and Joint Disorders*, 2nd ed. Philadelphia:WB Saunders; 1988.

New PFJ, Rosen BR, and Brady TJ, et al. Potential hazards and artefacts of ferromagnetic surgical and dental materials and devices in nuclear magnetic resonance imaging. *Radiology* 1983;147:139.

Partain CL, Price RR, and Patton JA, et al. Nuclear magnetic resonance imaging. *Radiographics* 1984;4(spec ed):5–25.

Pate D, Resnick D, Andre M, and Sartoris D. Three dimensional computed tomography. In *Imaging Modalities in Spinal Disorders* ME Kricun (ed). Philadelphia:WB Saunders; 1988.

Perkins GP and Wehrli FW. CSF enhancement in short gradient echo images. *Magn Reson Imaging* 1986;4:465–467.

Purcell EM, Torrey HC, and Pound RV. Resonance absorption by nuclear magnetic monents in solids. *Phys Rev* 1946;69:37–38.

Rothman SLG and Glenn WV Jr: *Multiplanar CT of the Spine*. Baltimore, Md: University Park Press; 1985:ch. 1.

Seibert CE, Barnes JE, and Dreisbach JN, et al. Accurate CT measurement of the spinal cord using metrizamide: Physical factors. *AJNR* 1981;2:75–78.

Shapiro R. *Myelography,* 4th ed. Chicago: Year Book Medical; 1984.

Utz JA, Herfkens MD, Glover GH, and Pele N. Three second clinical NMR images using a gradient recall acquisition in steady state mode (GRASS). [Abstract] *Magn Reson Imaging* 1986;4:106.

Young SW. *Magnetic Resonance Imaging: Basic Principles,* 2nd ed. New York: Raven Press; 1988.

Spinal Imaging and Spinal Biomechanics

Timothy Mick
Reed B. Phillips
Alan Breen

Chiropractic is known for its use of spinal imaging to investigate biomechanics and pathology. In some respects chiropractic has been isolated by this practice, although other allied disciplines, in particular orthopedics and bioengineering, now pay greater attention to the diagnostic and research potential of spinal imaging (Begg and Falconer, 1949; Benson et al., 1976; Bhalla and Simmons, 1969; Brown et al., 1976). Of particular interest to the chiropractor, however, has been the pursuit of objective measurements with which to compare findings obtained using a highly developed palpation sense. Historically, this interest has been dominated by static studies of symmetry and regularity in intervertebral position, especially in relation to mechanical advantage in static weight bearing. Nevertheless, motion has assumed increasing importance as a more integrated expression of the biomechanics of the spinal segments. Although the desire for information about the mechanics of joints is not completely satisfied by the available technology, such information as can be obtained from imaging is often decisive in clinical manage-

ment. In some instances, the information may correlate well with findings from the prior clinical examination. In other cases, biomechanical findings derived from spinal imaging may fail to support previous clinical findings, presenting a challenging dilemma to the chiropractor. In still other situations, abnormal biomechanics (e.g., instability) first manifested on x-rays or other imaging may contraindicate spinal manipulative therapy (SMT).

This chapter focuses on the radiographic manifestations of normal and abnormal spinal biomechanics. Where appropriate, brief descriptions of the pertinent gross anatomy are given. The discussion of biomechanics individually addresses each spinal region. Because of the complexity of the cervical and lumbar spine and the relatively few works related to the thoracic spine (outside of the vast literature on scoliosis), our discussion is limited to the cervical and lumbar regions. For thorough coverage of the topic of scoliosis and related biomechanics of the thoracic spine, the reader is referred to the excellent text by Bradford et al. (1987).

Biomechanical Imaging Techniques

The amount of biomechanical information obtained in each individual case will vary with the type of imaging employed. Plain film radiography is generally the initial imaging modality of choice. Standard x-ray series provide static information only, capturing the structural status of the spine at a finite moment. Static films are supplemented by "functional" plain radiographs exposed with the patient at the extreme of one of several ranges of motion. Flexion, extension, lateral bending, and rotation views are often obtained. Although individual segmental movement cannot be assessed, aberrant motion may be identified as restricted or increased mobility or as abnormal vertebral alignment at the end of a given range of motion. Biomechanical information obtained from either static or "functional" radiographs must always be evaluated in the light of clinical findings.

In addition to the basic plain film examination, more sophisticated (and more expensive) imaging modalities are available. Such techniques include biplanar orthogonal radiography (Brown et al., 1976; Frymoyer et al., 1979a, 1979b; Matteri et al., 1976; Pearcy, 1985; Pearcy et al., 1984, 1985; Pope et al., 1977; Stokes et al., 1981), cineradiography (Buonocore et al., 1966; Fielding, 1957, 1963, 1964; Howe, 1970, 1974; Jones, 1960a,b, 1962a,b, 1967; Rich, 1966; Woesner and Mittis, 1972), dynamic computed tomography (CT) (Dvorak, 1985; Dvorak et al., 1987a,b; Penning and Wilmink, 1987), and even dynamic magnetic resonance imaging (MRI) (Rothman, 1980). Although these modalities are not generally available in the chiropractor's office, the information obtained from these studies is useful. Knowledge gained from them can increase the understanding of abnormalities seen on plain films.

The remaining discussion is directed toward findings on upright postural examinations, which are generally advocated whenever possible over recumbent films because of the biomechanical information they may provide. For patients who cannot remain motionless and for heavy individuals, recumbent films can be used. Recumbency may reduce the amount of biomechanical information, but this limitation may not always be as significant as might be assumed (Saraste et al., 1985). Furthermore, the benefit in terms of radiation dose to the patient and diminished motion artifact may outweigh this limitation.

Upper Cervical Spine Biomechanics

Static Biomechanical Analysis of the Upper Cervical Spine

Sagittal Alignment. There is a wide range of normal static alignments of the upper cervical spine in the neutral posture. The relationship of the occiput to C-1 and C-1 to C-2 on the neutral lateral film correlates roughly with the characteristics of the lower cervical curve. For example, individuals with a hypolordotic or kyphotic lower cervical spine generally demonstrate relative extension of C-1 on C-2 and occiput on C-1, producing what has been described as a biphasic cervical configuration. Individuals with a hyperlordotic cervical spine tend to show relative flexion of the occiput on C-1 and of C-1 on C-2. Although this condition could be related to changes in the tone of postural muscles, it probably represents an adaptive mechanism necessary to keep the line of vision of an individual parallel to the horizon (Howe, 1988, personal communication).

The relationship of the occiput to C-1 is evaluated radiographically using several measurements (Powers et al., 1979; Yochum and Rowe, 1987). The incidence of occipitoatlantal subluxation or dislocation seen outside of an emergency room setting is very low because of the severity of trauma necessary to cause such a lesion (Powers et al., 1979; Woodring et al., 1981). Thus, these measurements have little practicality for the chiropractic practitioner.

Of more general importance is the relationship between C-1 and C-2 as seen on the lateral film. Atlantoaxial subluxation (AAS) or dislocation, particularly anterior AAS, is much more common and may result from a variety of etiologies, including trauma (Garber, 1964; Resnick and Niwayama, 1988; Yochum and Rowe, 1985, 1987). Anterior AAS will generally produce an increase in the anterior atlantodental interspace (ADI) seen on lateral cervical neutral and flexion films. The ADI, measured at the midpoint of the interspace, should not exceed 3.0 mm in adults and 4.5 to 5.0 mm in children (Cattell and Filzer, 1965; Hinck and Hopkins, 1960; Yochum and Rowe, 1987).

There are two varieties of pseudosubluxation occurring as normal variants in the upper cervical spine; both are most apparent on the flexion lateral view. The first is a V-shaped appearance to the ADI which, by speculation, has been related to a normal cephalocaudal increase in the strength of the transverse ligament of the atlas (Bohrer et al., 1985). The second occurs in children and, occasionally, in young adults at C2–3 (Harrison et al., 1980; Jacobson and Beeckler, 1959; Swischuck, 1977). Younger individuals may possess a general physiologic ligamentous laxity, demonstrating disproportionately greater motion at C2–3, unlike most adults, who show the greatest flexion/extension motion at C4–5 or C5–6. On flexion, C-2 appears to subluxate several millimeters anteriorly, but maintenance of a normal alignment of the spinolaminar line of C-2 relative to C-1 and C-3 indicates that this change is simply due to the great degree of flexion occurring at C2–3. This same phenomenon may occur at C-3 on C-4 as well (Fig. 23–1). The V-shaped

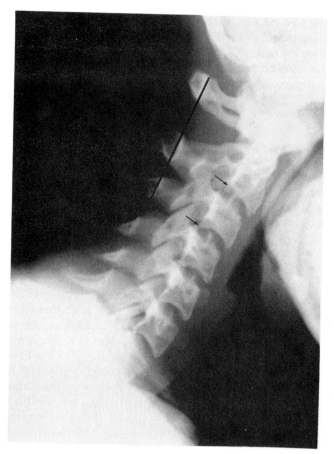

A

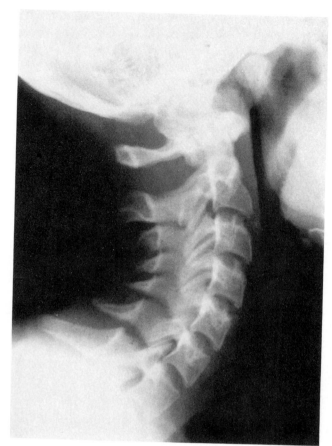

B

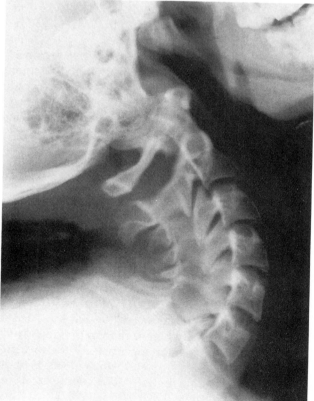

C

Figure 23-1. (A) Pseudosubluxation of C-2 on C-3 and C-3 on C-4 in a 15-year-old female patient with history of minor trauma. Physiologic ligamentous laxity allows an apparent 1- to 2-mm anterolisthesis (*arrows*) because of the disproportionately greater flexion in this region. Maintenance of a normal relationship at the upper cervical spinolaminar junction lines and absence of other radiographic abnormalities on **(B)** neutral and **(C)** extension films help to rule out true ligamentous injury.

ADI and the pseudosubluxation of C-2 are not considered contraindications to SMT.

Coronal Alignment. The normal coronal relationship of C-1 to C-2, viewed on the anteroposterior (A-P) open-mouth radiograph, is present when there is bilateral symmetry of the C-1 lateral masses and the lateral ADIs, with the dens and spinous process of C-2 centrally located (van Damme et al., 1979). The lateral masses of C-1 should be situated directly above the superior articular surfaces of C-2, and the lateral C1–2 joint spaces should appear equal. All of these statements presuppose a carefully positioned film without rotation or lateral flexion of the head. Even slight degrees of rotation or lateral flexion will produce a false impression of rotation of C-1 relative to C-2. This is manifested as an apparent increase in the medial-lateral width of the more anterior lateral mass and a corresponding decrease in the adjacent lateral ADI. Meanwhile, the contralateral lateral mass and lateral ADI show precisely the opposite findings (Fielding, 1957; Werne, 1957) (Fig. 23–2).

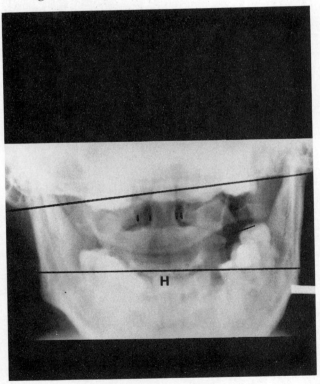

Figure 23–2. Anteroposterior open-mouth view demonstrating the effect of lateral flexion and rotation on the position of the head. Observe the relationship between the upper line connecting the mastoid tips and the lower horizontal line (H), showing the presence of right lateral flexion. Right head rotation is seen as slight right deviation of the central incisors relative to the dens. There is an apparent offset of the left C1 lateral mass relative to C-2 and alterations in the lateral atlantodental interspaces (cf. paired markers) and the widths of the lateral masses. The true position of C-1 relative to C-2 is difficult to determine when such positioning errors are present.

The findings consequent to this positioning error may mimic a fixed rotatory subluxation of C-1 or lateral listhesis of C-1 seen following tearing of the alar ligament (Lee, 1986; Reich and Dvorak, 1986). Occasionally, A-P open-mouth films with lateral flexion or cineradiography have been necessary to distinguish positional distortion from true abnormality in alignment (Fielding, 1977; Hohl and Baker, 1964; Jacobson and Adler, 1956; Paul and Moir, 1949; Wortzman and Dewar, 1968). So much variability and asymmetry exist in the static coronal alignment of C-1 on C-2 that some workers have been prompted to conclude that such asymmetries should be considered normal variations that correlate poorly with clinical findings (Hohl and Baker, 1964; Lee, 1986; Paul and Moir, 1949).

Other nonpathologic factors besides positioning errors may alter the symmetric C1–2 relationship. A variety of congenital anomalies of the craniovertebral junction may occur, all of which may alter this relationship (McRae and Barnum, 1953; McRae, 1971; Shapiro and Robinson, 1976). Additionally, the normal discrepancy in the rate of growth of C-1 and C-2 during childhood can produce a lateral offset of the lateral masses of C-1 and C-2, simulating a Jefferson fracture (Suss et al., 1983). Although this finding does not contraindicate the use of SMT, the radiographic findings must be correlated with the clinical presentation. When there is reason to strongly suspect a fracture, advanced imaging is required to definitively exclude this possibility.

Kinematic Studies of the Upper Cervical Spine

Kinematic studies of the upper cervical region attempt to delineate the types and amounts of motion occurring in this region. The first qualitative study appeared in 1957 (Werne, 1957). The most accurate study was done by Panjabi and colleagues in 1988, using stereophotogrammetry (measurements derived from three-dimensional photographs) on fresh cadavers to quantify upper cervical motions to an accuracy of 0.5°. Their findings agreed closely with the results of earlier studies using radiographic measurements (Clark et al., 1986; Dvorak, 1985; Dvorak et al., 1987a,b; Penning, 1978; Penning and Wilmink, 1987; Werne, 1957). The convex occipital condyles and the concave superior articular surfaces of the C-1 lateral masses allow approximately 20° of extension of the occiput on C-1 but only an average of about 3.5° of flexion. Approximately 7° of axial rotation and 5.5° of lateral flexion occur to each side. These figures for rotation are higher than in previous studies because of the greater sensitivity of the measuring device (Clark et al., 1986; Dvorak, 1985; Dvorak et al., 1987a,b; Panjabi et al., 1988; Penning, 1978; Penning and Wilmink, 1987; Werne, 1957).

The convex configuration of the C-1 inferior articular surfaces and the C-2 superior articular surfaces and their relatively loose joint capsules allows more motion than at occiput–C-1 (Panjabi et al., 1988; Werne, 1957). Brav (1936) reported a case of an individual who could displace his atlas laterally on axis for financial gain, without apparent ill effects. Flexion and extension at C1–2 are approximately equal, with an average of 11° of extension and 11.5° of flexion. Approximately 6.5° of lateral flexion to each side occurs at C1–2, whereas nearly 40° of axial rotation occurs in each direction (Panjabi et al., 1988). Thus, at least 50% of the entire cervical spine rotation occurs at C1–2 (Fielding, 1957; Panjabi et al., 1988).

An occasional lateral listhesis of C-1 on C-2 has been reported. This appears to be complex synkinetic ''coupled'' motion occurring only as a function of lateral flexion and rotation of C-1. Therefore, quantification of this motion cannot be accurately performed (Hohl and Baker, 1964). This does explain, however, the apparent offset of the lateral masses of C-1 on C-2 often seen on the A-P open-mouth projection that is almost invariably related to lateral flexion and rotation of the head.

Lower Cervical Spine Biomechanics

Static Biomechanical Analysis of the Lower Cervical Spine

Sagittal Alignment. Biomechanical assessment of the lower cervical spine begins with an observation of static relationships. The normal sagittal cervical configuration is generally considered to be lordotic, with an average curve of approximately 40° (range 35–45°). The simplest method of quantifying the cervical curve is by evaluating the Cobb angle, as if measuring a scoliosis. A horizontal line drawn on the lateral cervical neutral film through C-1 and a second line paralleling the inferior endplate of C-7 should intersect to form this angle (Yochum and Rowe, 1987) (Fig. 23–3). Other more complex methods of evaluations the cervical lordosis have also been described (Borden et al., 1960; Jochumsen, 1970; Yochum and Rowe, 1987).

Trauma and degenerative disc disease in the cervical spine will decrease or even reverse the cervical lordosis (Borden et al., 1960; Davis, 1945; Fineman et al., 1963; Frymoyer et al., 1986; Hohl and Baker, 1964; Jackson, 1977; Juhl et al., 1962; Rechtman et al., 1961). The former apparently does so because of posttraumatic muscle hypertonicity; the latter results in the loss of the normal posteriorly wedged configuration of the cervical disc. There is a poor correlation between the neutral lateral cervical configu-

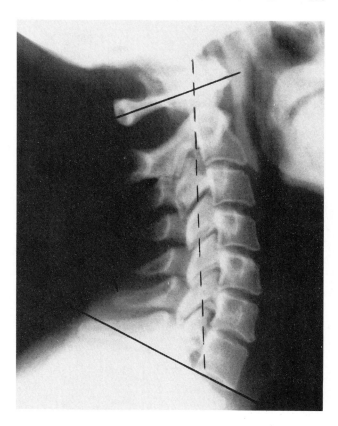

Figure 23–3. Lateral cervical neutral film showing (**A**) the method of measuring the neutral cervical lordosis and (**B**) the cervical gravity line. Despite a normal cervical curve of 45°, the gravity line (broken line) is shifted posteriorly, a condition thought to place greater compressive forces on the posterior joints.

ration and clinical findings. Hypolordosis and even kyphosis in the cervical spine are often seen even in asymptomatic individuals with no history of trauma and no evidence of degenerative disease in the cervical spine. Elevation or lowering of the chin at the time of the radiographic examination will increase or decrease the cervical lordosis on the neutral lateral film (Fineman et al., 1963; Juhl et al., 1962).

The static relationship of the head and upper cervical complex relative to the cervicothoracic junction is observed by drawing a vertical line inferiorly from the center of the odontoid process of C-2. This line, termed the *cervical gravity line,* should pass through the anterior aspect of the C-7 vertebral body (Fox and Young, 1954) (see Fig. 23–3). Alterations of this position represent either anterior or posterior carriage of the head. Studies to evaluate the clinical significance of such alterations have not been performed.

Jackson (1977) described the position of greatest stress in the cervical spine on lateral flexion and extension films by drawing a line paralleling the posterior aspect of the C-2 vertebral body and a second line paralleling the posterior aspect of the C-7 verte-

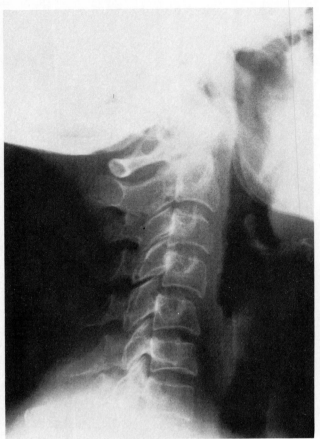

A

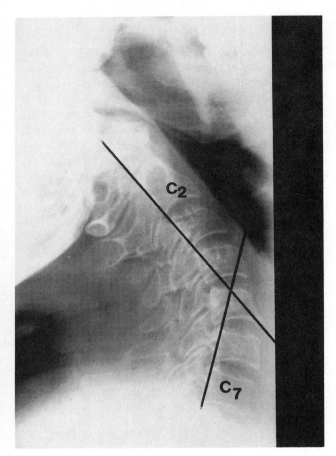

B

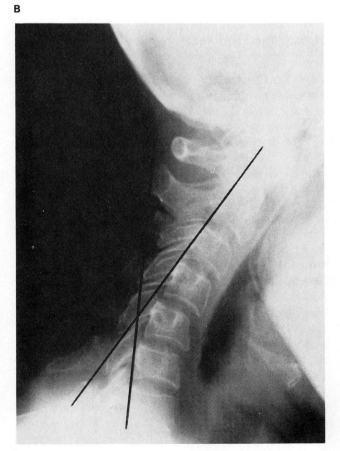

C

Figure 23-4. Jackson's lines of stress. Despite mild reversal of the cervical lordosis on (**A**) the neutral film, the stress lines intersect at their normal location on both the (**B**) extension and (**C**) flexion films.

bral body. These lines should normally intersect at the C4–5 level on extension and at C5–6 on flexion. Presumably, muscle hypertonicity, joint dysfunction, and degenerative changes in the cervical spine may alter the position of these lines, producing abnormal stresses (Fig. 23–4).

The posterior cervical vertebral body lines below C-1 (George's line) help evaluate for subluxation, dislocation, or instability in the cervical spine (George, 1919; Litterer, 1983). Combined anteroposterior displacement of George's line exceeding 3.5 mm at a given level relative to the vertebra below occurring at the extremes of flexion and extension is considered to indicate instability (White et al., 1975, 1976). This same measurement may be applied in evaluation of lumbar spine instability.

Anterior displacement of George's line up to 50% following trauma is seen in unilateral facet dislocations, whereas bilateral facet dislocations may produce greater than 50% displacement (Beatson, 1963; White et al., 1976). These situations generally represent contraindications to cervical SMT. Rotation during exposure of the lateral radiographs can give a false impression of alteration in George's line. A double cortical shadow at the posterior vertebral body is often misinterpreted as antero- or retrolisthesis. This is true in the lumbar spine as well.

The posterior cervical line or spinolaminar junction line has already been mentioned as a means of confirming atlantoaxial subluxation. The line may also be altered in displaced fractures of the dens and in posttraumatic or degenerative instability in the lower cervical spine (Swischuck, 1977; Yochum and Rowe, 1987).

Coronal Alignment. On frontal radiographs of the lower cervical spine, the spinous processes should be in alignment, with no abrupt lateral deviations and no increase in the interspinous distance at a given level. Either finding should be correlated with the lateral film and may indicate ligamentous disruption and a contraindication to SMT (Gehweiler et al., 1980; Harris, 1978).

Kinematic Studies of the Lower Cervical Spine

Cervical spine motion has been discussed in studies using plain film radiography and cineradiography (Buonocore et al., 1966; Howe, 1970, 1974; Jones, 1960a,b, 1962a,b, 1967; Rich, 1966; Woesner and Mittis, 1972). Dimnet and Pasquet have addressed the fundamental challenges of documenting cervical spine kinematics. The ultimate goal is to derive information that is accurate diagnostically and clinically useful. Increasing the amount of information extracted, however, increases the radiation dose to the

patient (Dimnet et al., 1982). This fact becomes especially important when one considers that investigational tools such as cineradiography (whose clinical application has not yet been thoroughly documented) may result in patient radiation doses of 3.5 to 6.0 rad/min for an average 4-minute cervical examination (Fielding, 1957; Jones, 1960b). This is approximately 15 to 20 times the dose received from a seven-view, plain film cervical exam (Davis series) (Gofman and O'Connor, 1985).

Efforts to develop alternative methods for imaging cervical spine kinematics continue in order to reach a compromise between the low cost/low dose/low yield of the standard plain film examination and the high dose/high cost/higher yield of biplanar radiography and cineradiography (Dimnet et al., 1982). A new innovative method uses multiple midsagittal magnetic resonance (MR) images taken at various stages of cervical flexion and extension and viewed in rapid sequence to produce a type of "motion picture" of the spine (Rothman, 1989). This method is expensive but generally does not present any known hazard to the patient (Partain et al., 1988). A second promising method uses digitization of the information found on stress radiographs of the spine to develop kinematic models of symptomatic subjects (Breen et al., 1988a,b). This is discussed in greater depth later in the chapter.

Lateral bending plain films have been used to a limited extent in the cervical spine. Jirout demonstrated normal coupled rotation in the cervical spine (spinous processes deviate toward convexity), and also described a concomitant "ventral and dorsal tilting" of the vertebrae during this motion. He recognized "compensatory hypermobility" adjacent to levels affected by congenital nonsegmentation ("blocked" vertebrae) or degenerative disc disease (Fig. 23–5). He also described hypomobility secondary to degenerative disc disease, labeling this a "static block" and any hypomobility at apparently normal discs a "dynamic block," he concluded that this finding heralds the onset of degenerative disc disease. Unfortunately, quantitative studies and controlled clinical trials have not been performed to verify his conclusions (Jirout, 1971, 1972a,b, 1974, 1979).

Flexion/extension studies have received much greater attention, and several different methods for quantitative evaluation of intersegmental motion, along with normal values, have appeared (Aho et al., 1955a,b; 1955; Arlen, 1978; Bhalla and Simmons, 1969; Buetti-Bauml, 1954; Colachis and Strohm, 1965; Dunsker et al., 1978; Kottke and Mundale, 1959; Penning, 1960, 1978). A detailed description of the specific methods of evaluating cervical flexion and extension cannot be presented here, but most

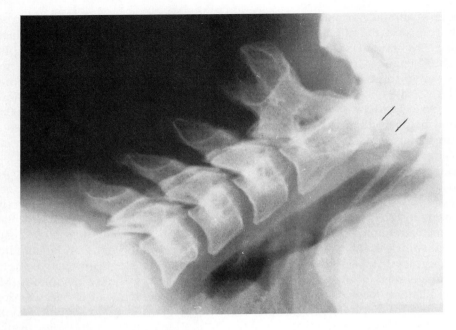

A

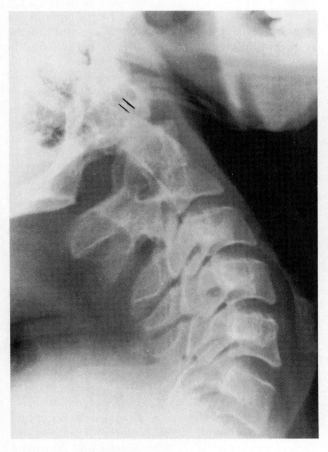

B

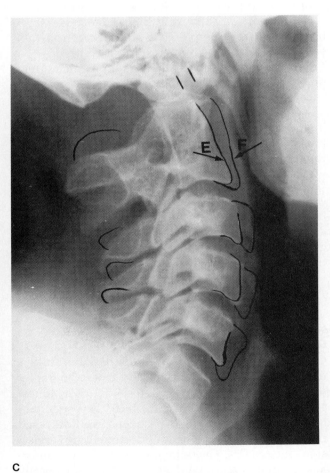

C

Figure 23-5. Compensatory hypermobility of C-1 on C-2 secondary to congenital nonsegmentation of C2–3 and occipitalization of C-1. Movement at C1–2 is increased, as evidenced by the 6.5 mm anteroposterior translation between full flexion and full extension (**A** and **B**). Compare to neutral posture (**C**).

are based on successive superimposition of the vertebral segments in flexion and extension films over the neutral lateral film. The lowest visible vertebra is aligned on the films and the motion of the immediately cephalic vertebra is measured. Subsequent superimposition of each visible vertebra to include C-1 is performed, providing an assessment of the motion at each motion segment. A clear template can be used to simplify this process

Studies attempting to quantify normal ranges of motion as seen on radiographs (Bakke, 1931; Buetti-Bauml, 1954; DeSeze et al., 1951; Penning, 1960) have demonstrated a wide range of normal for each level. Functional examination of the cervical spine is valuable in demonstrating gross hypo- and hypermobility.

Goel et al. (1986) studied the in vitro kinematics of normal, injured, and stabilized cervical spines. Following injury to the capsular ligaments at a single level in the lower cervical spine, the segmental motion increased significantly at the segment immediately superior to the injured level. This seems to contradict the generally held concept that ligamentous disruption tends to produce hypermobility at the level directly affected. Although similar findings have not been documented, the possible implications with regard to treatment of the acutely traumatized neck are obvious.

In general, the greatest amount of flexion and extension in the cervical spine occur at C4–5 and C5–6, and the least at C1–2 and C2–3 or at C7–T1 (Colachis and Strohm, 1965). Penning (1978) emphasized the variability in normal motion, stating that in any given position, the posterior arch of C-1 lies ''somewhere between occiput and spinous process of C-2, and not necessarily halfway between.'' Penning indicated the need for further studies directed at identifying differences in range of motion across age categories and at correlating abnormalities on flexion/extension films with the clinical presentation.

Lumbar Spine Biomechanics

Static Biomechanical Analysis of the Lumbar Spine

Sagittal Alignment. Like the cervical spine, the normal configuration of the lumbar spine is lordotic. The lordosis may be measured by application of Cobb's method using L-1 and L-5 or S-1 as the end vertebrae (Fig. 23–6). Measurements made on upright versus recumbent lateral films do not appear to vary significantly (Saraste et al., 1985). The magnitude of the ''average'' lumbar lordosis in an asymptomatic population has been reported as 42° (Farfan et al., 1972), 64–70° (Pelker and Gage, 1982), 50°

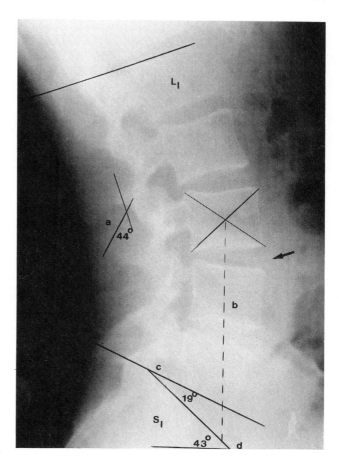

Figure 23-6. Normal lateral lumbar spine. The lumbar lordosis measured from L-1 to L-5 (*a*) is 44°. Ferguson's gravity line (*b*) intersects the anterior one fourth of the sacral base. The apex of the lordotic curve (arrow) lies at L3–4. The lumbosacral disc angle (*c*) measures 19°. The sacral base angle (*d*) measures 43°.

(Stagnara et al., 1980), and 30° or 45° (depending on whether L-5 or S-1 was used as the lower end vertebra) (Ferdnand and Fox, 1985).

Ferdnand and Fox (1985) have suggested that the lumbar lordosis must be less than 23° or more than 68° before it is considered to be hypo- or hyperlordotic. We support the use of a broad range of normal, because the clinical significance of alterations in the lumbar lordosis has not been established (Ferdnand & Fox, 1985; Hansson et al., 1985; Magora, 1975; Magora and Schwartz, 1978; Splithof, 1953, Torgeson and Dotter, 1965). It is known that the degree of lordosis is a principal factor in the conversion of hip extensor power to axial rotation necessary for bipedal ambulation (Lovett, 1903), but quantitative studies as to how altered lumbar lordosis may affect gait have not been forthcoming.

A second parameter in the lumbar spine is Ferguson's sacral base angle. This angle is formed by a line drawn parallel to the sacral base, forming an angle with a horizontal line drawn parallel to the inferior border of the radiograph (Ferguson, 1949; Yochum and Rowe, 1987) (see Fig. 23–7). Again, a wide range of normal with an average of approximately 40° and variation of 8 to 12° in upright versus recumbent posture occurs (Hellems and Keats, 1971). There appears to be a strong correlation between the magnitude of the sacral base angle and the lumbar lordosis (During et al., 1985). Some have considered alterations in the sacral base angle as a cause of mechanical low back pain resulting from altered shear and compressive forces on the lumbosacral junction (Adams and Hutton, 1980; Ferguson, 1949; Jayson, 1983). Unfortunately, as with lumbar lordosis, debate exists over the clinical significance of such alterations (Splithof, 1953; von Lackum, 1924; Yochum and Rowe, 1987).

The lumbar gravity line (Ferguson's gravitational line) provides an estimate of the position of maximum weight bearing in the lumbar spine, analogous to the cervical gravity line already described.

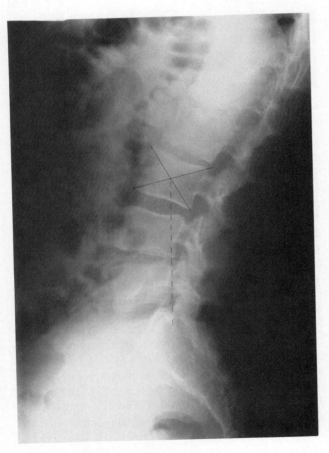

Figure 23–7. An example of swayback posture with posterior shift in lumbar weight bearing (*broken line*), extension in the lower lumbar spine, hypolordosis above L-3, and lowering of the lordotic apex to L-5.

A line extended vertically from the precise center of the L-3 body should lie near the anterior aspect of the sacral base, but no more than 10 mm anterior to it (see Fig. 23–7) (Ferguson, 1934, 1949). An anterior shift in this line has been implicated in the production of increased shear stresses on the lumbosacral disc (Ferguson, 1949). A posterior shift has been considered a cause of mechanical low back pain resulting from increased weight bearing on the posterior joints (Adams and Hutton, 1980, 1982) and possibly an increased potential for spondylolysis (Jayson, 1983; Yochum and Rowe, 1987).

A posterior shift in weight bearing is one component of a commonly encountered constellation of radiographic signs collectively termed a *swayback*. The other three components are (1) relative extension at L-4 and L-5 (which is primarily responsible for the posteriorly shifted weight bearing), (2) relative hypolordosis from L-3 cephalad, and (3) a caudal shift in the lordotic apex from its normal position at L3–4 (Fig. 23–7). Other means of evaluating static biomechanics of the lumbar spine include measurements of the lumbar intervertebral disc angles (Banks, 1983; Busche-McGregor et al., 1981); measurement of the lumbosacral disc angle (Banks, 1983; Ferguson, 1949); assessment of static vertebral malpositions (Yochum and Rowe, 1987); MacNab's line (MacNab, 1977) and Hadley's ''S'' curve (Hadley, 1951, 1981) for evaluating disrelationships of the facet joints; assessment of the level of the intercristal line of the pelvis for locating the lower lumbar motion segment (Fig. 23–8), theoretically at the level of greatest biomechanical stress (MacGibbon and Farfan, 1979); methods of identifying spondylolisthesis (Capener, 1932; Garland and Thomas, 1946; Myerding, 1932; Ullmann, 1924); and methods for evaluating lumbar spine instability (Dupuis et al., 1985; Morgan and King, 1957; van Akkerveeken et al., 1979).

Although more will be said shortly regarding lumbar spinal instability, space does not permit further discussion of these other methods of assessing static lateral lumbar spinal biomechanics. An excellent detailed description may be found in the comprehensive text by Yochum and Rowe (1987).

Coronal Alignment. Assessment of static coronal lumbar biomechanics begins with postural examination of the spine and bony pelvis for evidence of a lower extremity deficiency (anisomelia). This will manifest as a discrepancy in the femoral head heights on a well-positioned upright film of the lumbar spine and pelvis taken with the knees fully extended. This produces secondary pelvic unleveling which should be accompanied by a mild lumbar convexity toward the side of the short leg (Beal, 1950;

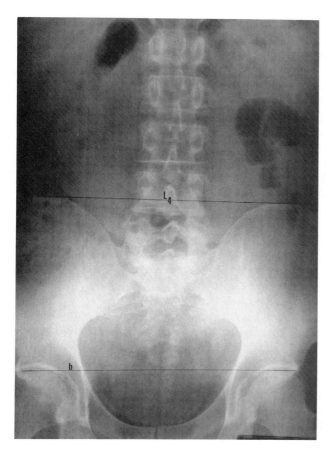

Figure 23–8. Normal anteroposterior lumbar film shows a level pelvis with the intercristal line intersecting L-4. There is no apparent lateral deviation or rotation in the lumbar spine. When the femoral heads are visible, their heights should be compared to rule out a lower extremity deficiency, which may result in pelvic unleveling.

Friberg, 1983, 1985; Ingelmark and Lindstrom, 1963). Normal coupled vertebral body rotation posteriorly on the side of the convexity (spinous processes deviate into the concavity) is also present (Fig. 23–9) (Friberg, 1983, 1985; Lovett, 1903; White and Panjabi, 1978). As for any spinal rotation, semiquantitative (Bunnell, 1985; Coetsier et al., 1977; Drerup, 1985; Mehta, 1973; Nash and Moe, 1969; Stokes et al., 1987) or even quantitative (Matteri et al., 1976) measurement of this rotation may be made by evaluating migration of the pedicle shadows from their normal sites.

A lumbar convexity secondary to pelvic unleveling related to a short leg has been termed a *postural pelvic tilt* or *compensatory scoliosis* (Froning and Frohman, 1968) because it compensates for the pelvic unleveling, bringing the thoracic spine back over the center of the pelvis. These curves are originally nonstructural and nonprogressive (Beal, 1950; Friberg,

1983, 1985; Ingelmark and Lindstrom, 1963; James, 1976; Moll et al., 1972) but may become structural over time (Giles, 1976; Giles and Taylor, 1981, 1982; Morscher, 1977) and have been identified as a source of low back, hip, or leg pain (Beal, 1950; Botte, 1981; Dickson et al., 1980; Friberg, 1985; Giles and Taylor, 1981; Rothenberg, 1988; Rush and Steiner, 1946; Scheller, 1964).

The clinical and radiographic features of lumbar scoliosis associated with anisomelia have been extensively reviewed (Dickson et al., 1980; Giles and Taylor, 1981; Friberg, 1983, 1985, 1987; Ingelmark and Lindstrom, 1963; Papaioannou et al., 1982). Pelvic tilt scoliosis secondary to a leg length deficiency is a common clinical entity often unrecognized on physical examination. Careful observation of plain film radiographs of the lumbar spine and pelvis will often reveal this frequent source of back pain (Clarke, 1972; Fisk and Baigent, 1975; Friberg, 1983, 1985, 1987; Giles and Taylor, 1981). There is an ac-

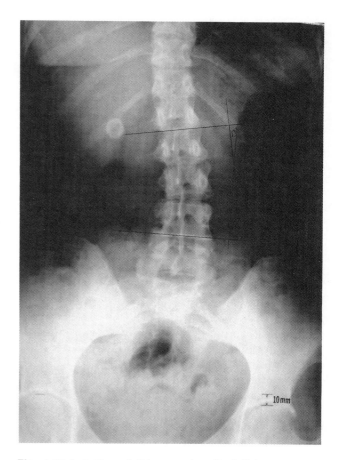

Figure 23–9. A 10-mm left lower extremity deficiency produces moderate pelvic unleveling (low on the left) and a properly compensating mild left lumbar scoliosis with left posterior vertebral rotation.

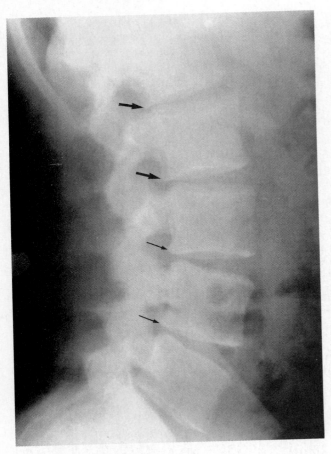

Figure 23–10. Minimal retrolisthesis is present at L-3 on L-4 and L-4 on L-5 (*small arrows*), producing a subtle disruption of George's posterior body line. This should be distinguished from the "false retrolisthesis" seen at L-1 on L-2 (*large arrows*). Rotation of the upper lumbar spine during positioning combined with the normally concave posterior vertebral body contour in this region produces the obvious double cortical margin that causes this false impression of retrolisthesis.

ceptable ± 3-mm error in measuring differences in the femoral head heights (Clarke, 1972; Giles and Taylor, 1981; Rothenberg, 1988). By comparison, clinical evaluation for an anatomically short leg carries an error of ± 12 to 23 mm (Rothenberg, 1988). Orthoroentgenography of the lower extremity to quantify leg length discrepancy is generally reserved for symptomatic patients with differences in leg length of more than 2.5 cm, when surgical correction is contemplated (Hughes and Hogue, 1977).

Caution should be used when interpreting apparent biomechanical abnormalities as seen on x-rays in the light of the clinical findings. The adage that "The physician treats the patient, not the x-rays" is never so true as when discussing biomechanics. The shortcomings of plain film examinations, including the effects of often subtle alterations

in patient positioning (Fig. 23–10), radiographic magnification and distortion, and the inherently low inter- and intraobserver reliability in identifying such biochemical faults, challenge the significance of radiographic biomechanical findings (Frymoyer et al., 1986; Phillips, 1980; Phillips et al., 1986). Even if accurate assessment is assumed, there is poor correlation between static plain film findings in the lumbar spine and the clinical presentation (During et al., 1985; Frymoyer et al., 1984; Liang and Komaroff, 1982; Nachemson, 1976; Phillips et al., 1986; Waddell, 1982). As a rather amusing reminder that biomechanical changes do not necessarily imply a source of back pain, a study by Hrubec and Nashold (1975) showed a positive association between optimal posture and herniated intervertebral discs.

Kinematic Studies of the Lumbar Spine

The kinematics of the lumbar spine are complex and cannot be exhaustively discussed within the confines of this chapter. The aim here is therefore to present the most salient points with references provided that expound on these issues.

Previous workers have described plain film findings in lumbar disc herniation (Begg and Falconer, 1949), and as late as 1981, attempts to correlate plain film findings with disc herniations were being made (Weitz, 1981). However, the acutely symptomatic low back behaves in much the same way regardless of the site of pain origin or the type of lesion. There may be an antalgic scoliosis or lateral list of the trunk, generally thought to be a functional deviation that disappears on recumbency, by suspension from a bar, or by relief of symptoms through SMT (McKenzie, 1981; Porter and Miller, 1986). Antalgic posture was originally thought to be related to the position of the painful lesion (Dandy, 1941; Duncan and Hoen, 1942; Falconer et al., 1948; Hadley, 1949, 1964; White and Panjabi, 1978) and could be instrumental in the diagnosis of lumbar disc herniation from plain films (Begg and Falconer, 1949; Bianco, 1968; van Damme et al., 1979). Antalgia may actually be dependent on hand and leg dominance (Porter and Miller, 1986) or on psoas spasm (Grieve, 1983). With the advent of CT and MRI scanning, some lesions recognized as causes of pain can be directly visualized, often eliminating much speculation regarding diagnosis and treatment. More accurate imaging may diminish the diagnostic significance of postural alterations on plain films of the acute low back.

The effects of trauma (Holdsworth, 1963; Markolf and Morris, 1974; Panjabi et al., 1984a; Roaf, 1960), degenerative disease (Dupuis et al., 1985; Feffer et al., 1985; Freiberg, 1948; Freiberg and Hirsch,

1949; Frymoyer and Krag, 1986; Knuttson, 1944; Lipson and Muir, 1981; Seligman et al., 1984; Stagnara et al., 1980; van Akkerveeken et al., 1979), surgery (Froning and Frohman, 1968; Goel et al., 1986), and anatomic variations (Ferguson, 1934; Hibbs and Swift, 1929) on the motion and stability of the lumbar spine have been extensively reviewed. Just as in the cervical spine, it is important to identify lumbar spine instability. Regardless of its etiology, the presence of instability may contraindicate SMT.

Functional lumbar radiographs can be useful in the initial evaluation of instability, which may be implicated in as many as 20 to 30% of all cases of low back pain (Pope and Panjabi, 1985). Spinal movement is complex, with motion in a given direction always accompanied by at least two other motions (Pope et al., 1977). Thorough evaluation of lumbar spine instability requires clinical studies and application of techniques beyond single-plane radiography (Bergmark, 1989; Hilton et al., 1979; Pearcy, 1985; Pearcy et al., 1985). A universally accepted definition of spinal instability and its clinical implications has yet to be agreed on (Dorr et al., 1982; Farfan and Gracovetsky, 1984; Frymoyer and Selby, 1985; Frymoyer and Krag, 1986; Nachemson, 1985). In general, however, radiographic instability is present when the degree of intervertebral anteroposterior translation is increased with or without an increased flexion-extension motion. In addition, it is anteroposterior translation that constitutes the perceived abnormality. This is presumed to be caused by

plastic as opposed to elastic holding element deformation under load.

A popular method among many workers of determining instability has been to calculate the instantaneous centers of rotation (ICR) for a series of parts of the total tilting range between two adjacent vertebrae (Gertzbein et al., 1985; Gonan et al., 1982; Panjabi et al., 1984a,b; Pearcy and Bogduk, 1988; Seligman et al., 1984; Tanz, 1953) (Fig. 23–11). In unstable segments where there is significant translation, the centers are widely scattered on the radiograph, whereas normally they are confined to an area not much larger than the disc space (Fig. 23–12). This and a number of other techniques based on x-ray marking have been used in research settings; however, the standardization needed to achieve reliability denies them, for the present, to clinical practice.

Despite the inadequacies of plain film radiographs in assessing lumbar spine instability, it may be useful to review the associated findings. They are as follows: (1) anterolisthesis of greater than 3 mm in flexion, (2) asymmetry and disc space collapse between flexion and extension, (3) retrolisthesis in extension (Fletcher, 1947; Frymoyer and Krag, 1986; Melamed and Ansfield, 1947; Morgan and King, 1957), (4) hypermobility of the motion segment (motion greater than 90th percentile for a person of the given age and sex) (Aho et al., 1955a, 1955; Allbrook, 1957), (5) the presence of traction spurs at the suspect level (Frymoyer and Krag, 1986; MacNab, 1971),

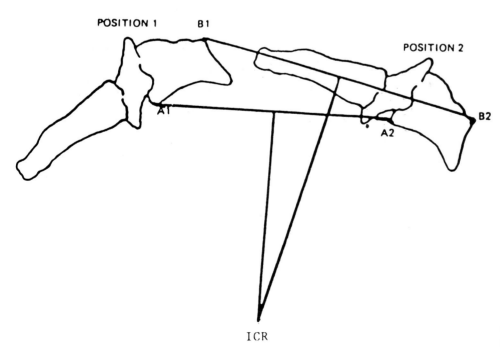

Figure 23–11. Derivation of instantaneous center of rotation (ICR). The ICR is derived as the intersection of the perpendicular bisections of lines joining points marked on the same anatomic coordinates in two positions in a rotational motion sequence. ICR determinations for a series of such increments will demonstrate to what degree translation accompanies rotation. The measurement is very error prone for small rotations. Consequently, translation without rotation cannot be measured by this index.

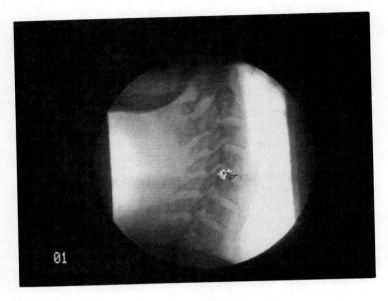

A

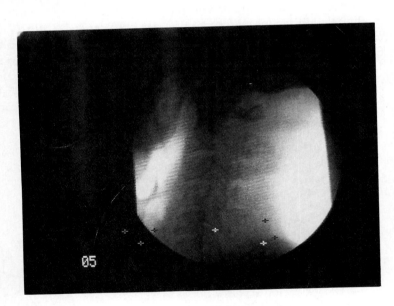

Figure 23-12. (A) Lateral cervical digital video-fluoroscopic (DVF) image showing small cluster of ICRs in a stable C4–5 motion segment and **(B)** widely dispersed ICRs in an injured C4–5 motion segment.

B

and (6) nonrotational shearing in side bending. The combination of a number of these plain film findings may allow a presumptive diagnosis of instability.

As a final note regarding instability, there has been some debate as to whether spondylolisthesis is typically associated with an unstable low back. The current thought is that although degenerative spondylolisthesis is often accompanied by instability (Dupuis et al., 1985; Feffer et al., 1985) lytic spondylolisthesis generally is not (Pearcy and Shepherd, 1985). Thus, although some have advocated prophylactic fusion for spondylolisthesis (Lettin, 1967), this appears to be unnecessary in many cases (Pearcy and Shepherd, 1985; Wiltse and Hutchinson, 1964).

Flexion/extension and lateral bending studies of

the lumbar spine have attempted to quantify normal and abnormal motion (Aho et al., 1955a; Begg and Falconer, 1949; Charnley, 1951; Dimnet et al., 1978; Gianturco, 1944; Hasner et al., 1952; Hoag et al., 1962; Jirout, 1956; Keessen et al., 1984; Pennal et al., 1972; Rosenberg, 1955; Tanz, 1953). As in the cervical spine, the technical difficulties in accurate quantification have been recognized, as has the lack of correlation with clinical findings (Hanley et al., 1976; Pennal et al., 1972). It appears that, at present, little specific information not found on clinical examination will be provided by bending studies of the lumbar spine in most instances (Quinnell and Stockdale, 1983). The primary exception is in the demonstration of instability, for which flexion/extension studies may be very useful

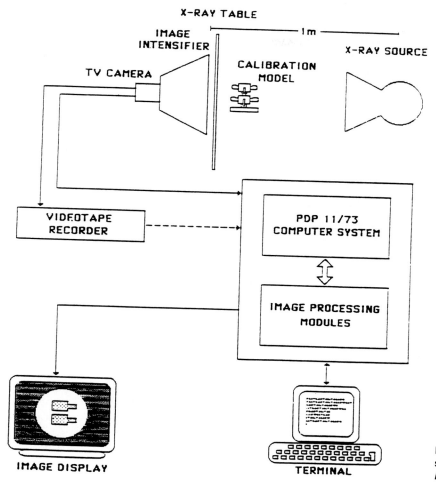

Figure 23-13. Diagram of prototype DVF system. (*Reproduced by kind permission of Butterworth Scientific.*)

(Dupuis et al., 1985; Feffer et al., 1985; Froning and Frohman, 1968; Goel et al., 1986; Holdsworth, 1963; Markolf and Morris, 1974; Roaf, 1960).

Digital Videofluoroscopy

Digital videofluoroscopy (DVF) is a new technique that has been developed in an attempt to overcome the considerable difficulties associated with quantifying the kinematics of the spinal motion segment. The technique involves interfacing an image processing computer with an x-ray image intensifier (Fig. 23-13) and using frame-grabbing techniques to digitize a series of images from a TV sequence of spinal motion. Coordinates can then be electronically placed on vertebral landmarks (Fig. 23-14) and the intersegmental geometry calculated on-line.

An outgrowth of recent advances in the design of image intensifiers and computers, DVF has both strengths and weaknesses. In principle, it suffers the

same limitations as plain x-ray marking, in which calculations from imprecisely placed coordinates can reduce the accuracy of the measurement so much as to render it meaningless. Rigorous calibration, therefore, has been necessary to bring the technique into use (Breen et al., 1988a,b, 1989a,b, 1990c,d; Breen and Allen, 1989, 1990; Humphreys et al., 1990). These studies have shown that it is possible to measure intervertebral angles in the cervical and lumbar spines with an error of between 1 and 2°. Although, as in the example shown in Figure 23–15, this allows intersegmental motion to be analyzed in great detail, it can be applied only when the increments of motion are greater than the errors in measuring them. This would therefore preclude measurement of side bending at L-5–S-1 or at occiput–C-1. Nevertheless, it does open the way for much greater understanding of the significance of paradoxical motion at other levels and in other directions.

Digital videofluoroscopy is particularly well suited to the detection of segmental instability. This

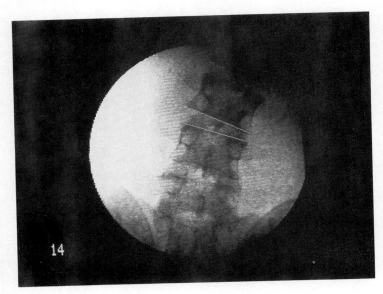

Figure 23–14. Anteroposterior lumbar–pelvic DVF image marked to determine the L3–4 intervertebral angle at one instant in a motion sequence.

can be displayed as large ICRs referred to above. As the entry dosage required to obtain a full motion sequence is considerably less than that needed for a conventional x-ray of the same part, clinical ICR studies may become much more accessible. Once again, however, there are limitations. As can be seen in the example in Figure 23–16, although the precision in these measurements is good, such precision

requires a tilt through at least 5° to sustain it (Breen et al., 1990a,b,c,d; Pearcy and Bogduk, 1988); otherwise other indices must be used.

Despite its expense, digital imaging holds out a good deal of promise for the analysis of spinal mechanics. The facility already available to synchronously pulse x-ray tubes with image intensifiers promises even greater reductions in x-ray dosage,

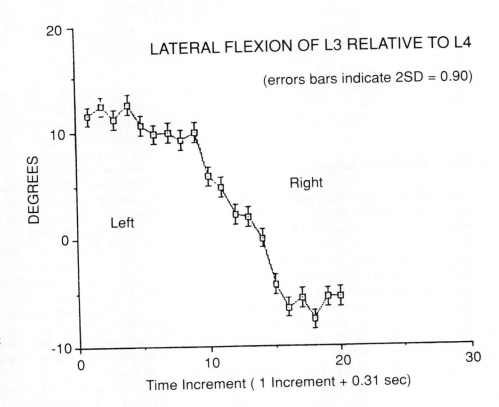

Figure 23–15. Increments in an L3–4 sidebending sequence in a 24-year-old male subject. Radiation entry dosage for this sequence was 15 mGy, which compares favorably with a single plain anteroposterior lumbopelvic x-ray. Error bars represent ± 2SD of the largest discrepancy determined from a calibration model that incorporated soft tissue degradation and coupled motion.

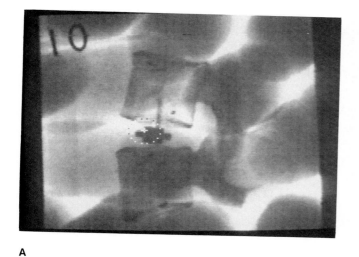

A

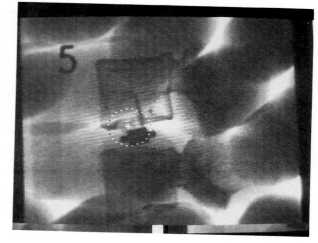

B

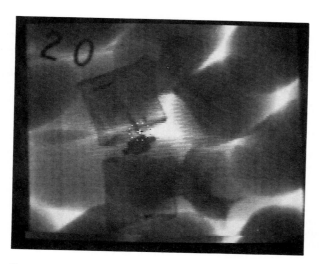

C

Figure 23–16. Digital images of a DVF calibration model in the lateral projection. Ellipses represent 95% confidence levels for accurately computing ICRs for (**A**) 5°, (**B**) 10° and (**C**) 20° rotational increments.

and high-speed parallel processing would assist in the transition to three-dimensional analysis. MRI could eventually replace x-rays in this technique, albeit for the foreseeable future only in relation to the cervical spine, owing to the constraints of the body coils in imaging the lumbar spine. The recent development of sophisticated open-gantry MRI scanners may eventually eliminate these contraints as well.

Conclusion

Understanding of the utility and limitations of spinal imaging techniques in the assessment of spinal biomechanics is gradually increasing, just as the ap-

plication of SMT continues to evolve and mature. More sophisticated research methods have increased our comprehension of the complexities of the spinal motor unit and the postural and kinematic changes in the spine. These techniques may be impractical in the clinical setting, but they provide more precise interpretation of the readily available methods of spinal imaging used in clinical practice.

Though the tenet that structure determines function often appears to be true, the many exceptions of apparently normal function in the context of abnormal structure should caution against overgeneralization (Collis and Ponsetti, 1969; Dieck, 1985; Ginsburg et al., 1979; Hult, 1954a,b; Nachemson, 1968; Weinstein et al., 1981). There is much to consider in attempting to determine what constitutes a truly "optimum spine" (Gracovetsky and Farfan, 1986) if, indeed, such an entity exists.

References

Adams MA and Hutton WC. The effect of posture on the role of the joints in resisting intervertebral compressive force. *J Bone Joint Surg [Br]* 1980;62:358.

Adams MA and Hutton WC. Mechanical factors in the etiology of low back pain. Orthopedics, 1982;5:1461.

Aho A, Vertiainen O, and Salo O. Segmentary mobility of the lumbar spine in anteroposterior flexion. *Ann Med Intern Fenn* 1955a;44:275.

Aho A, Vartiainen O, and Salo O. Segmentary anteroposterior mobility of the cervical spine. *Ann Med Intern Fenn* 1955b;44:287–299.

Allbrook D. Movements of the lumbar spine column. *J Bone Joint Surg [Br]* 1957;39:339.

Arlen A. Methods of measurement of statics and dynamics of the cervical vertebrae in the sagittal plane. *Manual Med* 1978;16:25–32.

Bakke S. Rontgenologische Beobachtungen uber die Bewegungen der Halswirbelsaule. *Acta Radiol (Suppl)* 1931;13.

Banks SD. The use of spinographic parameters in the differential diagnosis of lumbar facet and disc syndromes. *J Manipulative Physiol Ther* 1983;6:113.

Beal MC. The review of the short-leg problem. *J Am Osteopath Assoc* 1950;50:109–121.

Beatson TR. Fractures and dislocations of the cervical spine. *J Bone Joint Surg [Br]* 1963;45:21–35.

Begg AC and Falconer MA. Plain radiography in intraspinal protrusion of lumbar intervertebral discs: A correlation with operative findings. *Br J Surg* 1949;36:225–239.

Benson DR, Schultz AB, and Dewald RL. Roentgenographic evaluation of vertebral rotation. *J Bone Joint Surg [Am]* 1976;58:1125–1129.

Bergmark A. Stability of the lumbar spine: A study in mechanical engineering. *Acta Orthop Scand (Suppl)* 1989;60(230).

Bhalla SK and Simmons EH. Normal ranges of intervertebral joint motion of the cervical spine. *Can J Surg* 1969;12:181–187.

Bianco AJ. Low back pain and sciatica: Diagnosis and indications for treatment. *J Bone Joint Surg [Am]* 1968;50:170–181.

Bohrer SP, Klein A, and Martin W III. "V"-shaped pre-dens space. *Skel Radiol* 1985;14:111.

Borden AGB, Rechtman AM, and Gershon-Cohen J. The normal cervical lordosis. *Radiology* 1960;74:806.

Botte RR. An interpretation of the pronation syndrome and foot types of patients with low back pain. *J Am Podiatry Assoc* 1981;71:243–253.

Bradford DS, Lonstein JE, Ogilvie JW, and Winter RB. *Moe's Textbook of Scoliosis and Other Spinal Deformities*, 2nd ed. Philadelphia: WB Saunders; 1987.

Brav EA. Voluntary dislocation of the neck. Unilateral rotatory subluxation of the atlas. *Am J Surg* 1936;32:144–149.

Breen AC and Allen R. Spine kinematics: A digital videofluoroscopic technique. *J Biomed Eng* 1989;11:224–228.

Breen AC and Allen R. The digital videofluoroscopic assessment of spine kinematics. In *Proceedings of the Foundation for Chiropractic Education and Research 1990 International Conference on Spinal Manipulation*, Washington, DC, May 1990.

Breen AC, Allen R, and Morris A. An image processing method for spine kinematics—Preliminary studies. *Clin Biomech* 1988a;3:5–10.

Breen AC, Allen R, and Morris A. Spine kinematics: A computer/intensifier method. In *Proceedings of the IEEE Engineering in Medicine and Biology Society's 10th Annual International Conference*, New Orleans, Nov. 1988b.

Breen AC, Allen R, and Morris A. A videofluoroscopic technique for spine kinematics. *J Med Eng Technol* 1989a;13(1/2):109–113.

Breen AC, Allen R, and Morris A. Image presentations for spinal kinematic analysis using digital videofluoroscopy. In *Proceedings of the Third International Conference on Image Processing and Its Applications*. Institution of Electrical Engineers, University of Warwick, July 1989b.

Breen, AC, Humphreys K, and Rice S, et al. The analysis of spine kinematics using digital videofluoroscopy. In *Proceedings of the European Society of Biomechanics 7th Meeting, Aarhus, Denmark*, July 1990c.

Breen AC, Rice S, Osborne A, and Allen R. The analysis of the stability of the cervical and lumbar spines using digital videofluoroscopy. In *Proceedings of the 6th IMEKO Conference on Measurement in Clinical Medicine and 8th Hungarian Conference on Biomedical Engineering*, Sopron, Hungary, August 1990d.

Brown RH, Burstein AH, Nash CL, and Schock CC. Spinal analysis using three-dimensional radiographic technique. *J Biomech* 1976;9:355–365.

Buetti-Bauml C. Funktionelle Rontgenddiagnostik der Halswirbelsaule. Thieme: Stuttgart, Fortschritte auf dem Gebiete der Roentgenstrahlen Vereinigt mit Roentgenpraxis. Erganzungsband 70, 1954.

Bunnell WP. Vertebral rotation—A simple method of measurement in routine radiographs. *Orthop Trans* 1985;9:114.

Buonocore E, Hartman JT, and Nelson CL. Cineradiograms of the cervical spine in diagnosis of soft-tissue injuries. *JAMA* 1966;198:143–147.

Busche-McGregor M, Naimen J, and Grice AS. Analysis of the lumbar lordosis in an asymptomatic population of young adults. *J Can Chiropractic Assoc* 1981;25:58.

Capener N. Spondylolisthesis. *Br J Surg* 1932;19:374.

Cattell HS and Filzer DL. Pseudo-subluxation and other normal variations in the cervical spine in children. A study of one hundred and sixty children. *J Bone Joint Surg [Am]* 1965;47:1295.

Charnley J. Orthopaedic signs in the diagnosis of disc protrusion. *Lancet* Jan 27, 1951;186–192.

Clark CR, Goel VK, Galles K, and Liu YK. *Kinematics of the Occipito-atlanto-axial Complex*. Presented at the annual meeting of the Cervical Spine Research Society, Palm Beach, Florida, 1986.

Clarke GR. Unequal leg length: An accurate method of detection and some clinical results. *Rheum Phys Med* 1972;11:385–390.

Coetsier M, Vercauteren M, and Moerman P. A new radiographic method for measuring vertebral rotation in scoliosis. *Acta Orthop Belg* 1977;43:598–605.

Colachis SC and Strohm BR. Radiographic studies of cervical spine motion in normal subjects: Flexion and hyperextension. *Arch Phys Med Rehab* Nov 1965;753–760.

Collis DR and Ponsetti IV. Long-term follow-up of patients with idiopathic scoliosis not treated surgically. *J Bone Joint Surg [Am]* 1969;51:425–445.

Dandy WE. Concealed ruptured intervertebral discs: A plea for the elimination of contrast mediums in diagnosis. *JAMA* 1941;117:821–823.

Davis AG. Injuries of the cervical spine. *JAMA* 1945;127:149–156.

DeSeze C, Dijan A, and Abdelmoula M. Radiologique de la dynamique cervicale dans le plain sagittal. (Une contribution radiophysiologique a' l'etude pathogenique des artheoses cervicales). *Rev Rhumatisme* 1951;18:37–46.

Dickson R, Stamper P, Sharp A-M, and Harker P. School screening for scoliosis: Cohort study of clinical course. *Br Med J* 1980;281:265–267.

Dieck GS. An epidemiologic study of the relationship between postural asymmetry in the teen years and subsequent back and neck pain. *Spine* 1985;10:872–877.

Dimnet J, Fischer LP, Gonon G, and Carret JP. Radiographic studies of lateral flexion in the lumbar spine. *J Biomech* 1978;11:143–150.

Dimnet J, Pasquet A, Krag MH, and Panjabi MM. Cervical spine motion in the sagittal plane: Kinematics and geometric parameters. *J Biomech* 1982;15:959–969.

Dorr LD, Harvey JP, and Nickel VL. Clinical review of the early stability of spine injuries. *Spine* 1982;7:545–550.

Drerup BJ. Improvements in measuring vertebral rotation from the projection of the pedicles. *J Biomech* 1985;18:369–378.

Duncan W and Hoen TI. A new approach to the diagnosis of herniation of the intervertebral disc. *Surg Gynecol Obstet* 1942;75:257–267.

Dunsker SB, Colley DP, and Mayfield FH. Kinematics of the cervical spine. *Clin Neurosurg* 1978;25:174–183.

Dupuis PR, Yong-Hing K, Cassidy JD, and Kirkaldy-Willis WH. Radiologic diagnosis of degenerative lumbar spinal instability. *Spine* 1985;10:262.

During J. Goudfrooij H, and Keessen W, et al. Toward standards for posture: Postural characteristics of the lower back system in normal and pathologic conditions. *Spine* 1985;10:83–87.

Dvorak J. *CT-Functional Diagnostics of the Rotatory Instability of the Upper Cervical Spine*. Presented at the annual meeting of the Cervical Spine Research Society, Cambridge, Mass, 1985.

Dvorak J, Hayek J, and Zehnder R. CT-functional diagnostics of the rotatory instability of the upper cervical spine. Part 2. An evaluation on healthy adults and patients with suspected instability. *Spine* 1987a;12:726–731.

Dvorak J, Panjabi M, Gerber M, and Wichmann W. CT-functional diagnostics of the rotatory instability of the upper cervical spine. Part 1. An experimental study on cadavers. *Spine* 1987b;12: 197–205.

Falconer MA, McGeorge M, and Begg AC. Surgery of lumbar intervertebral disc protrusion: Study of principles and results based upon 100 consecutive cases submitted to operations. *Br J Surg* 1948;1:225–249.

Farfan HF and Gracovetsky S. The nature of instability. *Spine* 1984;9:714–719.

Farfan HF, Huberdeau RM, and Dubow HI. Lumbar intervertebral disc degeneration. *J Bone Joint Surg [Am]* 1972;54:492–509.

Feffer HL, Wiesel SW, Cuckler JM, and Rothman RH. Degenerative spondylolisthesis: To fuse or not to fuse. *Spine* 1985;10: 287–289.

Ferdnand R and Fox DE. Evaluation of lumbar lordosis: A prospective and retrospective study. *Spine* 1985;10:799–803.

Ferguson AB. The clinical and roentgenographic interpretation of lumbosacral anomalies. *Radiology* 1934;22:548.

Ferguson AB. *Roentgen Diagnosis of Extremities and Spine*. New York: Paul B Hoeber; 1949.

Fielding JW. Cineroentgenography of the normal cervical spine. *J Bone Joint Surg [Am]* 1957;39:1280–1288.

Fielding JW. Cineradiography. *J Bone Joint Surg [Am]* 1963;45:1543.

Fielding JW. Normal and selected abnormal motion of the cervical spine from second to seventh cervical vertebra based on cineroentgenography. *J Bone Joint Surg [Am]* 1964;46:1779–1781.

Fielding JW. Atlanto-axial rotatory fixation. *J Bone Joint Surg [Am]* 1977;59:37–44.

Fineman S, Borrelli FJ, and Rubinstein BM, et al. The cervical spine: Transformation of the normal lordotic pattern into a linear pattern in the neutral posture. A roentgenographic depiction. *J Bone Joint Surg [Am]* 1963;45:1179.

Fisk JW and Baigent ML. Clinical and radiological assessment of leg length. *NZ Med J* 1975;81:477–480.

Fletcher GH. Backward displacement of fifth lumbar vertebra

in degenerative disc disease. *J Bone Joint Surg [Am]* 1947;29: 1019–1026.

Fox MG and Young OG. Placement of the gravitational line in antero-posterior standing posture. *Res Quart* 1954;25:277.

Freiberg S. Anatomical studies on lumbar disc degeneration. *Acta Orthop Scand* 1948;17:224.

Freiberg S and Hirsch G. Anatomical and clinical studies on lumbar disc degeneration. *Acta Orthop Scand* 1949;19:222.

Friberg O. Clinical symptoms and biomechanics of lumbar spine and hip joints in leg length inequality. *Spine* 1983;8:643–651.

Friberg O. Biomechanical significance of the correct length of lower limb prostheses: A clinical and radiological study. *Prosth Orthot Int* 1985;8:124–129.

Friberg O. The statics of postural tilt scoliosis: A radiographic study on 288 consecutive chronic LBP patients. *Clin Biomech* 1987;2:211–219.

Froning EC and Frohman B. Motion of the lumbosacral spine after laminectomy and spine fusion. *J Bone Joint Surg [Am]* 1968;50:897–917.

Frymoyer JW, Frymoyer WW, Wilder DG, and Pope MH. The mechanical and kinematic analysis of the lumbar spine in normal living human subjects in vivo. *J Biomech* 1979a;12:165–172.

Frymoyer JW, Hanley EN, and Howe J, et al. A comparison of radiographic findings in fusion and nonfusion patients ten or more years following lumbar disc surgery. *Spine* 1979b;4:435–440.

Frymoyer JW and Krag MH. Spinal stability and instability: Definitions, classifications, and general principles of management. In *The Unstable Spine*. Orlando, Fla: Grune & Stratton; 1986.

Frymoyer JW, Newberg A, and Pope MH, et al. Spine radiographs in patients with low-back pain. *J Bone Joint Surg [Am]* 1984;66:1048–1055.

Frymoyer JW, Phillips RB, Newberg AH, and MacPherson BV. A comparative analysis of the interpretations of lumbar spinal radiographs by chiropractors and medical doctors. *Spine* 1986;11:1020–1023.

Frymoyer JW and Selby DK. Segmental instability: Rationale for treatment. *Spine* 1985;10:280–286.

Garber JN. Abnormalities of the atlas and axis vertebrae—Congential and traumatic. *J Bone Joint Surg [Am]* 1964;46:1782.

Garland LH and Thomas SF. Spondylolisthesis. Criteria for more accurate diagnosis of true anterior slip of the involved vertebral segment. *Am J Roentgenol* 1946;55:275.

Gehweiler JA, Osborne RL Jr, and Becker RF. *The Radiology of Vertebral Trauma*. Philadelphia: WB Saunders; 1980.

George AW. A method for more accurate study of injuries to the atlas and axis. *Boston Med Surg J* 1919;181:13.

Gertzbein SD, Seligman J, Holtby K, et al. Centrode patterns and segmental instability in degenerative disc disease. *Spine* 1985;4:257–261.

Gianturco C. Roentgen analysis of motion of lower lumbar vertebrae in normal individuals and in patients with low back pain. *Am J Roentgenol* 1944;52:261.

Giles LG. Leg length inequality associated with low back pain. *J Can Chiropractic Assoc* 1976;20:25–32.

Giles LG and Taylor JR. Low back pain associated with leg length inequality. *Spine* 1981;6:510–521.

Giles LG and Taylor JR. Lumbar spine structural changes associated with leg length inequality. *Spine* 1982;7:159–162.

Ginsburg HH, Goldstein LA, Robinson SC, et al. Back pain in post-operative idiopathic scoliosis: Long-term follow-up study. *Spine* 1979;4:518.

Goel VK, Nishiyama K, Weinstein JN, and Liu YK. Mechanical properties of lumbar spinal motion segments as affected by partial disc removal. *Spine* 1986;11:1008–1012.

Gofman JW and O'Connor E. *X-rays: Health Effects of Common Exams*. San Francisco: Sierra Club Books; 1985.

Gonan GP, Dimnet J, and Carret JP, et al. Utilite de l'analyse cinematique de radiographies dynamiques dans le diagnostic de certaines affections de la colonne lumbaire. *Acta Orthop Belg* 1982;48(4):589–629.

Gracovetsky S and Farfan H. The optimum spine. *Spine* 1986;11:543–573.

Grieve GP. Treating backache: A topical comment. *Physiotherapy* 1983;69:316.

Hadley LA. Construction of the intervertebral foramen: A cause of nerve root pressure. *JAMA* 1949;140:473–475.

Hadley LA. Intervertebral joint subluxation, bony impingement, and foraminal encroachment, with nerve root changes. *Am J Roentgenol* 1951;65:377.

Hadley LA. *Roentgenographic Studies of the Spine.* Springfield, Ill: CC Thomas; 1964.

Hadley LA. *Anatomico-roentgenographic Studies of the Spine,* 5th ed. Springfield, Ill: CC Thomas; 1981.

Hanley EN Jr, Matteri RE, and Frymoyer JW. Accurate roentgenographic determination of lumbar flexion-extension. *Clin Orthop Relat Res* 1976;115:145–148.

Hansson T, Bigos S, and Beecher P, et al. The lumbar lordosis in acute and chronic low back pain. *Spine* 1985;10:154.

Harris JH Jr. *The Radiology of Acute Cervical Spine Trauma.* Baltimore, Md:Williams & Wilkins; 1978.

Harrison RB. et al. Pseudo-subluxation of the axis in young adults. *J Can Assoc Radiol* 1980;31:176.

Hasner E, Schalimtzek M, and Snorrason E. Roentgenological examination of the function of the lumbar spine. *Acta Radiol Scand* 1952;37:141–149.

Hellems HK and Keats TE. Measurement of the normal lumbosacral angle. *Am J Roentgenol* 1971;113:642.

Hibbs RA and Swift WE. Development abnormalities at the lumbosacral juncture causing pain and disability: Report of 147 patients treated by spine fusion operation. *Surg Gynecol Obstet* 1929;48:604–612.

Hilton RC, Ball J, and Benn RT. In-vitro mobility of the lumbar spine. *Ann Rheum Dis* 1979;38:378–383.

Hinck VC and Hopkins CE. Measurement of the atlanto-dental interval in the adult. *Am J Roentgenol* 1960;84:945.

Hoag JM, Kosok M, and Moser JR. Kinematic analysis and classification of vertebral motion. *J Am Osteopath Assoc* 1962;59:899–982.

Hohl M and Baker HH. The atlanto-axial joint. *J Bone Joint Surg* [*Am*] 1964;46:1739–1752.

Holdsworth FW. Fractures, dislocations and fracture-dislocations of the spine. *J Bone Joint Surg* [*Br*] 1963;45:6–20.

Howe JW. Observations from cineroentgenological studies of the spinal column. *J Am Chiropractic Assoc* 1970;7:65–70.

Howe JW. Cineradiographic evaluation of normal and abnormal cervical spine function. *J Clin Chiropractic* 1974;4:42–54.

Hrubec Z and Nashold BS. Epidemiology of lumbar disc lesions in the military in World War II. *Am J Epidemiol* 1975;102:366–376.

Hughes JL and Hogue RE. Basic rehabilitation principles of persons with leg length discrepancy: An overview. In Hungerford DS, ed. *Progress in Orthopaedic Surgery.* vol. 1: *Leg Length Discrepancy: The Injured Knee.* New York: Springer-Verlag; 1977.

Hult L. The Munkfors investigation. *Acta Orthop Scand* (*Suppl*) 1954a;16.

Hult L. Cervical, dorsal and lumbar spinal syndromes. *Acta Orthop Scand* (*Suppl*) 1954b;17.

Humphreys K, Breen A, and Saxton D. Incremental lumbar spine motion in the coronal plane: An observer variation study using digital videofluoroscopy. Submitted to E.J.C., January 1990.

Ingelmark BE and Lindstrom J. Asymmetries of the lower extremities and pelvis and their relations to lumbar scoliosis. *Acta Morphol Scand* 1963;5:221–234.

Jackson R. *The Cervical Syndrome,* 4th ed. Springfield, Ill: CC Thomas; 1977.

Jacobson G and Adler D. Examination of the atlanto-axial joint following injury: With particular emphasis on rotational subluxation. *Am J Roentgenol* 1956;76:1081–1094.

Jacobson G and Beeckler HH. Pseudo-subluxation of the axis in children. *Am J Roentgenol* 1959;82:472.

James JIP. *Scoliosis,* 2nd ed. Edinburgh: Churchill Livingstone; 1976.

Jayson MIV. Compression stresses in the posterior elements and pathologic consequences. *Spine* 1983;8:338.

Jirout J. The normal motility of the lumbosacral spine. *Acta Radiol Scand* 1956;42:345–348.

Jirout J. Patterns of changes in the cervical spine on lateroflexion. *Neuroradiology* 1971;2:164–166.

Jirout J. The effects of mobilization of the segmental blockades on the sagittal component of the reaction on lateroflexion of the cervical spine. *Neuroradiology* 1972a;3:210–215.

Jirout J. Motility of the cervical vertebrae in lateral flexion of the head and neck. *Acta Radiol Scand* (*Diagn*) 1972b;13:919–927.

Jirout J. The dynamic dependence of the lower cervical vertebrae on the atlanto-occipital joints. *Neuroradiology* 1974;7:249–252.

Jirout J. Persistence of the synkinetic patterns of the cervical spine. *Neuroradiology* 1979;18:167–171.

Jochumsen OH. The curve of the cervical spine. *ACA J Chiropractic* Aug 1970:S49.

Jones MD. Cineradiographic studies of the collar-immobilized cervical spine. *J Neurosurg* 1960a;17:633–637.

Jones MD. Cineradiographic studies of the normal cervical spine. *Calif Med* 1960b;93:293–296.

Jones MD. Cineroentgenographic studies of patients with cervical spine fusion. *Am J Roentgenol* 1962a;87:1054–1057.

Jones MD. Cervical spine cineradiography after traffic accidents. *AMA Arch Surg* 1962b;85:974–981.

Jones MD. Cineradiographic studies of abnormalities of the high cervical spine. *AMA Arch Surg* 1967;94:206–213.

Juhl JH, Miller SM, and Roberts GW. Roentgenographic variations in the normal cervical spine. *Radiology* 1962;78:591.

Keessen W, During J, and Beeker TW, et al. Recordings of the movement at the intervertebral segment L5–S1: A technique for determination of the movement in the L5–S1 spinal segment by using three specified postural positions. *Spine* 1984;9:83–90.

Knuttson F. The instability associated with disc degeneration in the lumbar spine. *Acta Radiol Scand* 1944;25:593.

Kottke FJ and Mundale MD. Range of mobility of cervical spine. *Arch Phys Med Rehab* 1959;40:379–382.

Lee S. Asymmetry of the odontoid–lateral mass interspaces: A radiographic finding of questionable clinical significance. *Ann Emerg Med* 1986;15:1173–1176.

Lettin AWF. Diagnosis and treatment of lumbar instability. *J Bone Joint Surg* [*Br*] 1967;49:520–529.

Liang M and Komaroff. Roentgenograms in primary care patients with acute low back pain. *Arch Intern Med* 1982;142:1108–1112.

Lipson JL and Muir H. Proteoglycans in experimental intervertebral disc degeneration. *Spine* 1981;6:194–210.

Litterer WE. A history of George's line. *ACA J Chiropractic* Dec 1983;39.

Lovett RW. A contribution to the study of the mechanics of the spine. *Am J Anat* 1903;2:457–462.

MacGibbon B and Farfan H. A radiologic survey of various configurations of the lumbar spine. *Spine* 1979;4:258.

MacNab I. The traction spur: An indicator of segmental instability. *J Bone Joint Surg* [*Am*] 1971;53:663–670.

MacNab I. *Backache.* Baltimore, Md: Williams & Williams; 1977.

Magora A. Investigation of the relation between low back pain and occupation. 7. Neurologic and orthopedic condition. *Scand Rehab Med* 1975;7:146–151.

Magora A and Schwartz A. Relation between the low back pain

syndrome and x-ray findings. *Scand J Rehab Med* 1978;10: 135–145.

Markolf KL and Morris JM. The structural components of intervertebral disc. *J Bone Joint Surg [Am]* 1974;56:675–687.

Matteri RE, Pope MH, and Frymoyer JW. A biplane radiographic method of determining vertebral rotation in postmortem specimens. *Chiropractic Orthop* 1976;116:95–98.

McKenzie RA. The lumbar spine: Mechanical diagnosis and therapy. Waikane, NZ: Spinal Publications; 1981.

McRae DL. Craniovertebral junction. In Newton TH and Potts DG, eds. *Radiology of the Skull and Brain*. St. Louis, Mo: CV Mosby; 1971.

McRae DL and Barnum AS. Occipitalization of the atlas. *Am J Roentgenol* 1953;70:23.

Mehta MH. Radiographic estimation of vertebral rotation in scoliosis. *J Bone Joint Surg [Br]* 1973;55:513–520.

Melamed A and Ansfield DJ. Posterior displacement of lumbar vertebrae: Classification and criteria for diagnosis of true retrodisplacement of lumbar vertebrae. *Am J Roentgenol* 1947;58: 307–328.

Moll JMH, Liyanage SP, and Wright V. An objective clinical method to measure lateral spinal flexion. *Rheum Phys Med* 1972;11:225–239.

Morgan FP and King T. Primary instability of lumbar vertebrae as a common cause of low back pain. *J Bone Joint Surg [Br]* 1957;39:6.

Morscher E. Etiology and pathophysiology of leg length discrepancies. In Hungerford DS, ed. *Progress in Orthopaedic Surgery*. vol. 1. *Leg Length Discrepancy: The Injured Knee*. New York: Springer-Verlag; 1977.

Myerding HW. Spondylolisthesis. *Surg Gynecol Obstet* 1932; 54:371.

Nachemson A. A long-term follow-up study of nontreated scoliosis. *Acta Orthop Scand* 1968;39:466–476.

Nachemson A. The lumbar spine, an orthopedic challenge. *Spine* 1976;1:59–71.

Nachemson A. Lumbar spine instability: A critical update and symposium summary. *Spine* 1985;10:290–291.

Nash C and Moe J. A study of vertebral rotation. *J Bone Joint Surg [Am]* 1969;51:223.

Panjabi MM, Krag MH, and Chung TQ. Effects of disc injury on mechanical behavior of the human spine. *Spine* 1984a;9:707–713.

Panjabi MM, Krag MH, and Dimnet JC, et al. Thoracic spine centres of rotation in the sagittal plane. *Orthop Res* 1984b;1(4): 387–394.

Panjabi MM, Dvoral J, and Duranceau J, et al. Three-dimensional movements of the upper cervical spine. *Spine* 1988;13:726–730.

Papaioannou T, Stokes I, and Kenwright J. Scoliosis associated with limb-length inequality. *J Bone Joint Surg [Am]* 1982;64:59–62.

Partain LC, Price RR, and Patton JA, et al. (eds). *Magnetic Resonance Imaging*, 2nd ed. Philadelphia: WB Saunders; 1988.

Paul LW and Moir WW. Non-pathologic variations in relationship of the upper cervical vertebrae. *Am J Roentgenol* 1949;62:519–524.

Pearcy M. Stereo radiography of lumbar spine motion. *Acta Orthop Scand (Suppl)* 1985;56(212).

Pearcy M, Portek I, and Shepherd J. Three-dimensional x-ray analysis of normal movement in the lumbar spine. *Spine* 1984;9:294–297.

Pearcy M, Portek I, and Shepherd J. The effect of low-back pain on lumbar spinal movements measured by three-dimensional x-ray analysis. *Spine* 1985;10:150–153.

Pearcy M and Shepherd J. Is there instability in spondylolisthesis? *Spine* 1985;10:175–177.

Pearcy MJ and Bogduk N. Instantaneous axes of rotation of the lumbar intervertebral joints. *Spine* 1988;13(9):1033–1041.

Pelker RR and Gage JR. The correlation of idiopathic lumbar scoliosis and lumbar lordosis. *Clin Orthop* 1982;163:199–201.

Pennal GF, Conn GS, and McDonald G, et al. Motion studies of the lumbar spine: A preliminary report. *J Bone Joint Surg [Br]* 1972;54:442–452.

Penning L. *Functioneel rontgenoderzoek Bij degenerative en traumatische afwjkingen der laag-cervicale Bewegingssegmenten*. Thesis, University of Gronikge, The Netherlands; 1960.

Penning L. Normal movements of the cervical spine. *Am J Roentgenol* 1978;130:317.

Penning L and Wilmink JT. Rotation of the cervical spine: A CT study in normal subjects. *Spine* 1987;12:732–738.

Phillips RB. The use of x-rays in spinal manipulative therapy. In *Modern Developments in the Principles and Practice of Chiropractic*. New York: Appleton-Century-Crofts; 1980.

Phillips RB, Frymoyer JW, MacPherson BV, and Newberg AH. Low back pain: A radiographic enigma. *J Manipulative Phys Thera* 1986;9:183–187.

Pope MH, Wilder DG, Matteri RE, and Frymoyer JW. Experimental measurements of vertebral motion under load. *Orthop Clin North Am* 1977;8:155–167.

Pope MH and Panjabi M. Biomechanical definitions of spinal instability. *Spine* 1985;10:255–256.

Porter RW and Miller CG. Back pain and trunk list. *Spine* 1986;11:596–600.

Powers B, Miller MD, and Kramer RS, et al. Traumatic anterior atlanto-occipital dislocation. *Neurosurgery* 1979;4:12.

Quinnell RC and Stockdale HR. Flexion and extension radiography of the lumbar spine: A comparison with lumbar discography. *Clin Radiol* 1983;34:405–411.

Rechtman AM, Borden AGB, and Gershon-Cohen J. The lordotic curve of the cervical spine. *Clin Orthop* 1961;20:208–216.

Reich C and Dvorak J. The functional evaluation of craniocervical ligaments in sidebending using x-rays. *Manual Med* 1986;2:108–113.

Resnick D and Niwayama G. *Diagnosis of Bone and Joint Disorders*, 2nd ed. Philadelphia: WB Saunders; 1988.

Rich EA. Cineroentgenological observations of human systems. *Scientific Yearly, Lincoln College of Chiropractic* 1966;1:1–9.

Roaf R. A study of the mechanics of spinal injuries. *J Bone Joint Surg [Br]* 1960;42:810–823.

Rosenberg P. The "R"-Center Method, a new method for analysing vertebral motion by x-ray. *J Am Osteopath Assoc* 1955;55:103.

Rothenberg RJ. Rheumatic disease aspects of leg length inequality. *Semin Arthritis Rheum* 1988;17:196–205.

Rothman SLG. Personal communication re: Work in progress, 1989.

Rush WA and Steiner A. A study of lower extremity length inequality. *Am J Roentgenol* 1946;55:616–623.

Saraste H, Brostrom L-A, Aparasi T, and Axdorph G. Radiographic measurement of the lumbar spine: A clinical and experimental study in man. *Spine* 1985;10:236–241.

Scheller ML. *Uber den Einfluss der Beinverkurzung auf die Wirbelsaule*. Thesis, Universitat zu Koln, Cologne, West Germany; 1964.

Seligman JV, Gertzbein SD, Tile M, and Kapasouri A. Computer analysis of spinal segment motion in degenerative disc disease with and without axial loading. *Spine* 1984;9:566–573.

Shapiro R and Robinson F. Anomalies of the cranio-vertebral border. *Am J Roentgenol* 1976;127:281.

Splithof CA. Lumbosacral junction. Roentgenographic comparisons of patients with and without backaches. *JAMA* 1953; 152:1610.

Stagnara P, DeMauroy JC, Dran G, et al. Reciprocal angulation of vertebral bodies in a sagittal plane: Approach to refrences for the evaluation of kyphosis and lordosis. *Spine* 1980;5:525–528.

Stokes IAF, Wilder DG, Frymoyer JW, and Pope MH. Assessment of patients with low back pain by biplanar radiographic measurement of intervertebral motion. *Spine* 1981;6:233–240.

Stokes N, Bigelow LC, and Moreland MS. Measurement of axial rotation of vertebrae in scoliosis. *Spine* 1987;11:213–218.

Suss RA, Zimmerman RD, and Leeds NE. Pseudo-spread of the atlas: False sign of Jefferson fracture in young children. *Am J Roentgenol* 1983;140:1079.

Swischuck LE. Anterior displacement of C2 in children. Physiologic or pathologic? *Radiology* 1977;122:759.

Tanz SS. Motion of the lumbar spine: Roentgenologic study. *Am J Roentgenol* 1953;69(3):399–412.

Torgeson WR and Dotter WE. Comparative roentgenographic study of a primitive population with North Americans and North Europeans. *J Bone Joint Surg [Br]* 1965;47:552.

Ullmann HJ. A diagnostic line for determining subluxation of the fifth lumbar vertebra. *Radiology* 1924;2:305.

van Akkerveeken PF, Obrien JP, and Park WM. Experimentally induced hypermobility in the lumbar spine. *Spine* 1979;4:236.

van Damme W, Hessels G, and Verhelst M, et al. Relative efficacy of clinical examination, electromyography, plain film radiology, myelography and lumbar phlebography in the diagnosis of low back pain and sciatica. *Neuroradiology* 1979;18:109–118.

von Lackum HL. The lumbosacral region. An anatomical study and some clinical observations. *JAMA* 1924;82:1109.

Waddell G. An approach to backache. *Br J Hosp Med* Sept 1982:187–219.

Weinstein SL, Zavala DC, and Ponseti IV. Idiopathic scoliosis. Long-term follow-up and prognosis in untreated patients. *J Bone Joint Surg [Am]* 1981;63:702–712.

Weitz EM. The lateral bending sign. *Spine* 1981;6:388–397.

Werne S. Studies in spontaneous atlas dislocation. *Acta Orthop Scand (Suppl)* 1957;23:78.

White AA, Johnson RM, Panjabi M, and Southwick WO. Biomechanical analysis of clinical stability in the cervical spine. *Clin Orthop Relat Res* 1975;109:85–96.

White AA, Southwick WO, and Panjabi MM. Clinical instability in the lower cervical spine. A review of past and current concepts. *Spine* 1976;1:15–27.

White AA and Panjabi MM. *Clinical Biomechanics of the Spine.* Philadelphia: JB Lippincott; 1978.

Wiltse LL and Hutchinson RH. Surgical treatment of spondylolisthesis. *Clin Orthop* 1964;35:116.

Woesner ME and Mittis MG. The evaluation of cervical spine motion below C2: A comparison of cineroentgenographic and conventional roentgenographic methods. *Am J Roentgenol* 1972;115:149–154.

Woodring JH, Selke AC Jr, and Duff DE. Traumatic atlanto-occipital dislocation with survival. *Am J Roentgenol* 1981;137:21.

Wortzman G and Dewar FP. Rotary fixation of the atlanto-axial joint: Rotational atlanto-axial subluxation. *Radiology* 1968;90:479.

Yochum TR and Rowe LJ. Arthritides of the upper cervical complex. In *Aspects of Manipulative Therapy,* 2nd ed. New York: Churchill Livingstone; 1985.

Yochum TR and Rowe LJ. *Essentials of Skeletal Radiology.* Baltimore, Md: Williams & Wilkins; 1987.

IV

Chiropractic Care

Chiropractic care has been intimately associated with the manual skills referred to as the *chiropractic adjustment*. These procedures can be considered a specific form of the more generic term *spinal manipulative therapy*. The care offered by chiropractors, however, has always been more than simple manual adjustment or manipulation. It has included an intimate awareness of the patient's environmental, nutritional, psychologic, and social status. Research by Kane et al. (1974), Cherkin and MacCormack (1989), and Pope et al. (1990) has demonstrated a higher level of patient satisfaction with chiropractors and chiropractic manipulation when compared with standard medical care and other modalities. It is not yet clear whether this relates to the "laying on of hands" chiropractic attitude toward patients or some other, as yet unknown factor. The chiropractic adjustment or manipulation remains, however, the primary therapeutic modality offered by chiropractors. It is the primary skill studied and developed by chiropractic students during their training.

Before studying and offering a treatment modality it is incumbent on a clinician to ensure that the treatment is beneficial. Prior to 1975 when the NINCDS Conference on Spinal Manipulative Therapy was held, chiropractic based its treatment on experience and patient satisfaction. Over the last 10 years, however, there has been rapid growth in the number of research trials and publications studying the effectiveness of manipulation and chiropractic. Chapter 24 by Bronfort reviews this research and places it in perspective. It is clear that more research is necessary. It is also clear, however, that manipulation and chiropractic care have justified their role as legitimate treatment modalities.

The practice of chiropractic has undergone a gradual evolution over the past 95 years, with the development of newer adjusting techniques and the discarding of older, often cruder or rougher techniques. Grice and Vernon in Chapter 25 have reviewed the historic evolution of those techniques and have discussed the contribution of the major chiropractic clinicians and colleges that were responsible for this evolution. They also attempt to classify the numerous chiropractic techniques in a manner that is easily understood and used.

There are numerous techniques that have been named and taught by specific clinicians. To place these multiple techniques in perspective they have been divided into four groups. The high-velocity thrust, reviewed in Chapter 26 by Cleveland, is the technique most commonly associated with chiropractic. This chapter describes the basic principles and presents examples of this form of adjustment. The diversified techniques are the oldest and most widely used. The presentation of these techniques by Gitelman and Fligg in a generic format in Chapter 27 makes both their theoretical and practical value very clear. A wide variety of traction and distraction techniques and specialized adjusting tables have been developed and used by chiropractors for the treatment of patients with intervertebral disc disorders. Cox in Chapter 28 reviews the literature in support of these procedures and presents a number of the most commonly used techniques. Meeker in Chapter 29 reviews the techniques developed by chiropractors when a high-velocity thrust or traction is not indicated. These so-called "non-force" techniques together with the various methods of treating the soft tissue muscular and ligamentous structures are becoming important in chiropractic management of older and sicker patients.

The increasing severity of spine injuries treated by chiropractors often makes it at times impossible to totally resolve all of a patient's symptoms. This has lead to the inclusion of rehabilitation into the practice of chiropractic. Mayer and Polatin in Chapter 30 review the principles of spinal rehabilitation and introduce certain techniques and equipment used for this purpose.

The final three chapters cover an area of increasing concern within the profession. The past decade has seen a gradual increase in the understanding of the indications for chiropractic care. At the same time there is a growing understanding of the contraindications and potential complications of certain chiropractic and manipulation techniques. Dvorak in Chapter 31, together with Kranzlin and Naef from the Swiss Chiropractic Association, has reviewed the potential musculoskeletal complications of manipulation and the conditions under which chiropractors must exercise the greatest care. In Chapter 32 Kleynhans and Terrett review the more serious cerebrovascular complications of manipulation and attempt to lay out basic principles to minimize their occurrence. There is growing pressure on the chiropractic profession to develop a more widely accepted and standardized practice that can be assessed in an unbiased peer review procedure.

The evolution of a chiropractic terminology and the tremendous growth of chiropractic around the world are presented in the appendixes. It is increasingly evident that chiropractic is no longer a North American phenomenon. It has spread to multiple countries as demonstrated in the appendix edited by Tamulaitis and Auerbach and an international list of authors who review this growth in their respective parts of the world. As chiropractic continues to grow we can anticipate further evolution of its science, techniques, and terminology.

Scott Haldeman

References

Cherkin DC and MacCormack FA. Patient evaluations of low back pain care from family physicians and chiropractors. *West J Med* 1989;150:351–355.

Kane RC, Olsen D, and Lymaster C, et al. Manipulating the patient—A comparison of physician and chiropractic care. *Lancet* 1974;1:1333–1336.

Pope R, Phillips B, and McDonald L, et al. A prospective randomized trial of manipulation, corset, massage and transcutaneous muscle stimulation. In *Proceedings, International Society for the Study of the Lumbar Spine,* Boston, June 13–17, 1990.

chapter 24

Effectiveness of Spinal Manipulation and Adjustments

Gert Bronfort

The first section of this chapter discusses why it is of paramount importance that spinal manipulative and adjustive therapy (SMT), like other therapies, be subjected to rigorous scientific scrutiny through clinical research. The basic principles of clinical trials are then introduced to provide a better background for the next section of the chapter, which is a selected review of the literature on the clinical ef-

fectiveness of SMT. The final section is an introduction to critical evaluation of clinical research publications. The ability to critically review journal articles is

Acknowledgements
The assistance of Theresa Gromala, Grace Jacobs, Joseph Keating, William Elkington, Mae Beth Lindstrom, Todd Olson, and Aase Bronfort in critiquing and proofreading this chapter is sincerely acknowledged.

vital to the clinician who wants to draw useful and valid conclusions from the scientific literature. Such conclusions are necessary for subsequent incorporation of the findings into clinical practice to benefit patients.

Importance of Clinical Research

Uncontrolled Clinical Experience

When evaluating the effect of SMT, the clinician must understand the principles of clinical research and how research results may differ from the results observed in clinical practice. Clinical experience of chiropractors is derived primarily from recollection of treatment response in certain patients, anecdotal clinical information from colleagues, and knowledge of the effectiveness of SMT as interpreted from reading the literature.

The treatment of an individual patient in a chiropractic clinic setting in many respects resembles an experiment. If improvement occurs, both patient and chiropractor are likely to conclude that the treatment was effective. This may indeed be the case, but, for a variety of reasons, this conclusion may also be erroneous. Four major factors may contribute to drawing erroneous conclusions from uncontrolled clinical experience:

1. **Spontaneous improvement:** Many of the disorders treated by SMT have a benign course and are often self-limiting. In other words, improvement or recovery will occur even if no treatment is administered. If relapses occur, the patient and doctor often will be motivated by the previously perceived positive outcome to try the same therapy again.
2. **Effective co-intervention:** The clinician may supplement the spinal adjustive therapy with physiotherapeutic modalities, traction, exercise, and ergonomic or nutritional advice. Any observed clinical improvement may be the result of one or several of these other factors. The patient may be receiving other therapy concurrently (e.g., drug therapy), which may account for some or all of the effect. Finally, concurrent nontherapy events (e.g., change in patient's social, psychologic, or work situation) may also affect the clinical condition irrespective of the ongoing therapy.
3. **Clinician bias:** The clinician usually has faith in his or her therapeutic approach and wishes that the patient's condition will improve. This may bias the clinician's observations in favor of the therapy. Also, it often influences the patient's expectations positively. Through a selective, biased memory process, clinicians often have a tendency to base their experience on a limited number of patients remembered especially well for a positive outcome. Because SMT is the primary therapeutic tool for chiropractors (as drug therapy is for most medical doctors) this therapeutic prejudice has a tendency to become deep rooted.
4. **Placebo effect:** The patient's expectation of improvement reinforced by a positive doctor–patient relationship often brings about a therapeutic effect in itself, in the absence of any extra effect of the SMT intervention. This is called a positive placebo effect. Several studies of placebo treatment in a variety of disorders have shown as much as 30 to 40% improvement (Spiro, 1986). This improvement is not merely imaginary or subjective, but is probably brought about by opioid neuropeptide release (Spiro, 1986). There is growing evidence to suggest that such neuroendocrine influences can modulate the function of the immune system (Solomon, 1987). The placebo effect has generally been regarded as a confounding factor to be controlled for or eliminated, but it might be a powerful demonstration of the patient's own healing power that should be included as part of the therapeutic approach. Future research in psycho-neuroimmunology may provide further evidence of these self-healing mechanisms.

Purpose of Clinical Research

One of the main purposes of clinical research is to determine whether study outcomes observed during the course of experimental trials resulted from the therapeutic interventions or must be attributed to other factors such as spontaneous improvement, co-intervention, placebo effect, nontherapy events, chance occurrence, or biased evaluation by the clinician or patient (Haldeman, 1978). In this context, all of these factors are disturbing variables, called *confounding factors*. To help acquire a more objective attitude toward patient care, it is important to control for confounding factors when attempting to study the effectiveness or efficacy of SMT. The placebo effect is a rival explanation in trials of efficacy and must therefore be controlled for, but this is not the case in controlled trials of effectiveness that assess the total beneficial result of a therapeutic intervention.

Principles of Clinical Trials

What do we mean by a clinical trial? The term *trial* indicates that some form of planned experiment has been performed. Trials are usually based on a limited sample of subjects. The purpose of studying the sample is to obtain information on how the administered treatment can be expected to influence the general population of patients who may receive it in the future. Clinical trials typically require two or more groups of subjects to form the basis of reliable treatment comparisons, although it is possible to conduct a trial on a single individual (Keating et al., 1985; Guyatt et al., 1986).

Prospective studies proceed forward in time, whereas descriptive and observational studies may be retrospective. In prospective studies the investigator defines a population sample and usually measures study variables both before and after any outcomes have occurred. Controlling for confounding variables is usually only possible in this type of research design. Diagnostic criteria, definition of the clinical course, and relevant data can be accounted for and documented to a degree that seldom can be done in retrospective investigations.

Retrospective studies, on the other hand, usually involve retrieving case history information gathered over a period from one or more clinicians. As the research question was not known at the time the case histories were taken, important information is often missing, and unknown selection bias may be operating. Consequently, retrospective studies have generally received less credibility and importance.

The essential goals in a controlled trial are to avoid or control for bias and other confounding factors and to secure comparable study groups. To accomplish these goals, it is necessary to assign patients randomly to the study groups. The randomized controlled trial is now considered the gold standard by the scientific community, and is generally the most reliable and valid method for conducting clinical research of therapeutic effectiveness and efficacy (Pocock, 1986).

Selection of Patients

Sampling means selecting a subgroup of a population to represent the whole population. Random sampling involves a random process to guarantee that each person in a population has the same chance of being selected. In contrast, nonrandom sampling is a more practical approach and is often the only type available in most clinical research settings. If random sampling is not feasible, consecutive sampling is often the best choice. With this sampling method every subject meeting the eligibility criteria will be invited to participate in the trial. Finally, convenience sampling uses the patient base that is available to the investigators.

Most trial samples are nonrandomly selected, and are likely to be uncharacteristic, which consti-

tutes a problem when attempting to generalize from study results to a wider population. Sociodemographic characteristics of study subjects usually form a good basis for extrapolation; however, other characteristics of the trial subjects and the intervention used often can be described only to a limited extent. The investigator is therefore always faced with the challenge of avoiding too broad or too narrow generalizations.

Inclusion and Exclusion Criteria

Specific eligibility, or inclusion, criteria serve the purpose of characterizing the subject sample. The type of patients included in the trial must be clearly defined and the study patients must be representative of the subjects who fulfill the inclusion criteria. Presently, no well-defined criteria have been reported capable of objectively identifying the type of patient and complaint likely to respond favorably to SMT, although some degree of success in this respect has been noted by Buerger (1980) in the case of low back pain patients.

One of the important purposes of accurately describing patient demographics and clinical data is to be able later to extrapolate from the study findings to a well-defined population of patients. Exclusion criteria specify who is not being studied and frequently serve the purpose of defining patients who cannot be expected to benefit from the treatment or patients for whom the treatment may be directly contraindicated.

Sample Size

In the planning phase of a trial, it is essential that the investigator determine the number of patients needed. Usually, this number cannot be calculated with any large degree of accuracy, but must be estimated on the basis of how large a treatment difference between the groups is considered of clinical significance and with what degree of certainty one wants to detect such difference. The choice of principal outcome measure is important in this context. Trials using reliable quantitative outcomes, rather than qualitative outcomes, require much smaller sample sizes. In many trials, too small a sample size or inability to recruit the stipulated number of patients has severely jeopardized the validity of the reported results, because the risk of overlooking clinically important therapeutic effects was too high (Freiman et al., 1978). This has also been the case in several controlled trials of SMT (Brunarski, 1984).

Informed Consent

According to the latest Recommendations from the Declaration of Helsinki (Levine and Labacqz, 1984), patients must be fully informed of the research trial plan and of the potential benefits and risks involved in participating. Patients have the right to withdraw at any time and must voluntarily sign a consent form prior to participating in a study.

Random Assignment
Random allocation of patients in controlled clinical trials serves the purpose of chance assignment to each study group. A successful randomization is accomplished if every patient has an equal chance of receiving any of the interventions being studied. Random assignment is required for meeting the assumptions of many statistical tests, and serves to ensure that researcher and patient bias does not influence treatment assignment, and thus study results. When reasonably large samples are used, random assignment of patients to treatment groups tends to create groups that are comparable in baseline variables. It is possible, however, for unbalanced study groups to occur in spite of proper randomization methods (e.g., in the trials by Evans et al., 1978; Rasmussen, 1979; Hoehler et al., 1981; Gibson et al., 1985).

In any randomized trial the goal is that the study groups should be similar in relevant patient characteristics. By use of a stratified randomization procedure (subjects are divided into subgroups according to key characteristics *before* randomization takes place), it is often possible to obtain a higher degree of comparability between the groups, and thus more valid trial conclusions.

Blinding
Elimination of observer, therapist, investigator, and subject bias is an important goal in any trial, particularly in controlled trials. To reduce bias, some measure of blinding must be introduced. Independent observers, that is, clinicians not involved in the treatment phase of the clinical trials, usually examine patients before, during, and after treatment. It is essential that these observers not know the group assignment of subjects. When the patient is unaware of the group that she or he is assigned to, the arrangement is termed a *single-blind study*. A *double-blind study* is the term used if both the researchers/clinicians providing the interventions and the study subjects are not aware of the study group assignment. The term *triple-blind study* is sometimes used to signify that patient, therapist, and observer are unaware of the intervention group assignment.

Control Groups
Ideally, the different study groups should be subjected to interventions that the patients are unable to differentiate. This implies that the same degree of enthusiasm and time commitment must be rendered to patients irrespective of group assignment. The control group may receive a comparable type of intervention or sham procedure (placebo control) to avoid patient bias in the form of therapeutic preference, which may distort trial results. Inclusion of this type of control group has been shown to be possible in several trials on SMT (Hoehler et al., 1981; Waagen et al., 1986; Hadler et al., 1987).

Intervention
Chiropractic spinal adjustment is not a well-defined therapy. Much variation exists in undergraduate and postgraduate training, and presently no controlled studies have been reported that compare one method of chiropractic adjustment with another. It is of extreme importance in trials of SMT to describe the intervention in detail. Most medical trials on SMT have used poorly described, nonspecific, long-lever techniques, and the results of these trials cannot reasonably be extrapolated to patients treated by the specific, short-lever, high-velocity techniques used by most chiropractors. It is the responsibility of the chiropractic profession to investigate this issue, and it is therefore mandatory that chiropractors be involved in the planning and experimental phases of future randomized controlled trials of SMT.

Measuring Outcome
There are presently very few universally accepted methods of recording outcome in SMT trials. In many of the trials so far, there has been little or no scientific justification for the use of the chosen outcome variables, and often the reliability has not been studied. A number of methods that have been shown to be reliable should be considered in future trials, even though their validity in relationship to the biologic effects of SMT has not always been determined. Outcome variables can be divided into two main groups. The first group exemplify patient-rated outcomes: symptomatic relief measured on semiquantitative scales, including visual analog scale (VAS) for pain or disability (Scott and Huskisson, 1976; Million et al., 1982), physical disability scores for low back pain (Fairbank et al., 1980; Roland and Morris, 1983), and questionnaires to evaluate change in general health status, including psychosocial function, activities of daily living, and quality of life (Nelson et al., 1987; Stewart et al., 1989).

In the second group are examples of clinician/observer-rated outcomes: objective measures of spinal biomechanical function, including range of motion (Mayer and Gatchel, 1985; Pearcy, 1986; Triano and Schultz, 1987; Gill et al., 1988) and straight leg raising (SLR) (Fisk, 1979; Lankhorst et al., 1982; Tobis and Hoehler, 1983). Other physiologic measurements can be used as quantitative outcome measures; however, the reliability and, if possible, the validity of the instrumentation used must be documented in each instance.

Other outcome criteria may be used, but are more easily influenced by confounding factors. Some examples are number of days with bed rest, work time loss, and use of analgesic medication. Each of these outcome measures has strengths and weaknesses. It has been shown that the choice of response variable in some cases can make a substantial difference in the reported efficacy of the therapeutic intervention (Howe and Frymoyer, 1985).

Compliance

Investigators always hope for and expect that patients comply with the study protocol (i.e., keep appointments, fill out questionnaires, and avoid nonstudy therapy that may confound study results). In reality, this seldom occurs. Most trials suffer from incomplete data and patient attrition. In some instances involving multiple clinical settings, the compliance of the investigators may be poor, mostly because of unanticipated disruption of the daily clinical routines (Mabeck and Vejlsgaard, 1980; Bronfort, 1989). Such problems can seriously endanger the completion of a trial, or at least put the validity of study results in jeopardy.

Statistical Analysis

Appropriate statistical analysis should be decided in the planning stage of the trial on the basis of design and outcome variables. Preferably, independent statisticians should analyze the original study data. Investigators often fail to follow these rules and choose inappropriate analyses. It has been estimated that in approximately half of the articles published in medical journals, statistical methods are applied incorrectly (Freiman et al., 1978; Glantz, 1980). Several examples of erroneous applications of statistical methods used to analyze data from randomized trials on SMT have been reported (Greenland et al., 1980; Hoehler and Tobis, 1987; Bloch, 1987).

The Null Hypothesis

Statistical tests help to rule out the possibility that differences observed between study groups are due to chance alone. The *null hypothesis* (H_0) states that no true difference exists between study groups. The *alternate hypothesis* (H_a) states that there is a true difference between the groups, and can be accepted only if the null hypothesis is rejected. Inferential statistical tests do not provide evidence of the presence or absence of a cause-and-effect relationship between two events. Instead, they allow an estimation of the probability that a correct decision is being made in

rejecting or not rejecting the null hypothesis. Two types of mistakes or errors can be made:

1. **Falsely rejecting the null hypothesis** (i.e., falsely concluding that a difference exists between study groups), when in fact it is true and should not be rejected, is referred to as a *type I error*. The probability of committing such an error is called *alpha* (α) and is the same as the *p*-value seen in connection with significance testing. The conventional $p \leq 0.05$ means that there is a 5% chance or less of committing a type I error.

2. **Falsely accepting the null hypothesis** (i.e., falsely concluding that no difference exists between study groups), when in fact it is false and should be rejected, is called a *type II error*. The probability of committing such an error is termed *beta* (β). Beta is not a single value like alpha, but is dependent on the magnitude of difference in outcome between study groups.

Statistical Power

Some statistical tests have more statistical power than others. Power is defined simply as percentage chance of rejecting the null hypothesis when it is false and should be rejected: power $= 1 - \beta$. By convention it is recommended that beta should not exceed 0.2, equal to a power 0.8, which means statistically that there is an 80% chance of detecting a certain magnitude of difference, if present, in outcome between study groups.

Small sample sizes are probably the most common reason for type II errors. Outcome measures that have a high degree of variability or are based on nominal or ordinal categories can weaken the statistical power, and can lead to failure to reject a null hypothesis when it should have been rejected.

Additional information on clinical research studies, including the basis for critical evaluation of published research reports, is presented later in this chapter under Guide to Critical Evaluation of Clinical Research Publications.

Review of Clinical Studies of Spinal Manipulation and Adjustment Therapy

This section evaluates the evidence in the clinical research literature regarding the effectiveness/efficacy of SMT in the treatment of a variety of neuromusculoskeletal and other disorders. There have been a number of multidisciplinary conferences on the research status of SMT. The proceedings of the first of these conferences, held in 1975 and sponsored by NINCDS (a subdivision of the National Institutes of Health [USA]), stated that ''specific conclusions cannot be derived from the scientific literature for or against either the efficacy of spinal manipulative therapy or the patho-physiological foundations from which it is derived'' (Goldstein, 1975).

Publications resulting from most of the research conferences have focused on the emerging evidence from randomized trials of the clinical efficacy of SMT, especially for low back pain (LBP) (Buerger and Tobis, 1977; Korr, 1978; Greenman, 1984; Buerger and Greenman, 1985; Winer, 1985; Tobis and Hoehler, 1986). Numerous descriptive studies or clinical series, quasi-experimental trials, and more than 30 randomized controlled clinical trials involving SMT have been published, and are reviewed in this section. Case studies and small case series have not been included. Approximately two thirds of the studies analyze the effect of SMT on LBP, and 15% of the studies analyze cervical pain and headache. The remainder report on other clinical conditions or on physiologic or neurobiologic mechanisms. In a little over half of the descriptive studies, SMT was performed by chiropractors.

Low Back Pain

In the studies selected for this review, an average of 75 to 80% of patients have been reported to be much improved or symptom-free in the investigations done by doctors of chiropractic, medical doctors, and others. These figures are based on a mixed group of LBP patients. When specific reference has been made to chronic LBP and to LBP accompanied by nerve root compression resulting from disc protrusion, the treatment success has been closer to 50% on an average. Table 24–1 reviews descriptive studies of SMT and LBP.

Descriptive studies, including clinical series, are useful in reporting patient demographics and in documenting the clinical course of different disorders treated by SMT. But they suffer from one major shortcoming—lack of control. Studies without proper control cannot ensure that the observed effects result specifically from spinal manipulative intervention, as opposed to therapeutic co-intervention, the placebo effect, or spontaneous recovery. Thus, no firm conclusions can be made on the basis of such studies.

One of the major problems in evaluating the role of SMT in the management of LBP is the highly unpredictable spontaneous course of this disorder. On a yearly basis 5 to 10% of the adult population experiences an acute episode of LBP (Choler et al., 1985). About half of these patients recover and return to work within 1 to 2 weeks. Within 6 weeks, approximately 80% return to work. The remaining 20% still have LBP and they represent a major socioeconomic problem (Nachemson, 1983).

Since the early 1970s more than 25 prospective randomized clinical trials of SMT for LBP have been reported in the literature from many different countries. A summary of these trials, including results and comments, is found in Table 24–2. Most of these trials exhibit one or more of the following limitations:

1. Inclusion–exclusion criteria are either too broadly or too narrowly defined.
2. The outcome measures have poor or uncertain reliability.
3. Most studies on SMT have not controlled for the possible placebo effect of spinal manipulation.
4. The manipulative techniques are generally poorly described and are usually not carried out by a practitioner professionally trained in the art.
5. Many of the trials carry high risk of type II error and sometimes type I error.
6. They often suffer from poor design in both the data collection phase and the analysis phase.
7. Manipulation is often mixed with other treatments (treatment contamination).
8. Poor or inadequate random assignment procedures are seen in several of the studies.
9. Poor patient compliance is also a common feature.

Randomized trials involving SMT have been subject to several extensive reviews (Moritz, 1979; Greenland et al., 1980; Deyo, 1983; Haldeman, 1983; Branson and Buerger, 1984; Brunarski, 1984; Buerger and Greenman, 1985; Winer, 1985; Ottenbacher and DiFabio, 1985; Kukurin, 1985; Tobis and Hohler, 1986; DiFabio, 1986; Curtis, 1987). Conclusions drawn by these reviewers from the two dozen controlled trials on SMT for LBP have not been unanimous. Nevertheless, there is relative agreement that SMT is a fairly safe therapeutic approach that in many cases offers more immediate relief than other forms of conservative therapy. It is generally agreed that long-term benefits of SMT have not yet been conclusively demonstrated. A number of trials have demonstrated improvement in objective measures, including increased spinal mobility and/or straight leg raising (Evans et al., 1978; Jayson et al., 1981; Nwuga, 1982; Tobis and Hoehler, 1986; Waagen et al., 1986).

Only a few randomized trials have evaluated the effectiveness of chiropractic spinal adjustive therapy. In their short-term placebo-controlled trial of chiropractic adjustments for the relief of nonacute LBP, Waagen et al. (1986) concluded that after 2 weeks of therapy the experimental patients had significantly more relief from pain and increase in spinal mobility compared with the control patients. Pain was measured on a visual analog scale, and a global index was used for the objective measurements of change in spinal mobility. Unfortunately, one third of the original sample population dropped out. The authors consider the results preliminary because of the small sample size.

The most recent study of the effectiveness of chiropractic spinal adjustive therapy was reported by Meade et al. (1990), in which chiropractic and outpatient medical hospital treatments in managing LBP of mechanical origin were compared in a randomized clinical trial. The hospital treatment consisted almost exclusively of spinal manipulation and mobilization, carried out by physical therapists. Patients were followed up to 2 years. The main outcome measures were changes in scores of the Oswestry pain/disability questionnaire and tests of straight leg raising and lumbar flexion. The results showed that chiropractic treatment was more effective than hospital outpatient treatment, mainly in patients with chronic or severe LBP. A difference of about 7% points in reduction on the Oswestry Low back disability scale was seen at 2 years. The clinical significance of this difference is uncertain. The superiority of chiropractic treatment became gradually more evident throughout the follow-up period. Data were unavailable for a large percentage of patients at follow-up at 2 years and the chiropractic group received approximately 50% more treatments than the hospital group, rendering study conclusions somewhat uncertain.

Cox and Shreiner (1984) conducted a prospective descriptive study of 576 LBP patients with the participation of 23 chiropractors throughout the United States. This study provided useful preliminary data for assessment of routine chiropractic office diagnoses and treatment for different types of LBP conditions.

A hospital-based interdisciplinary research team in Canada studied the effect of SMT on chronic LBP patients. Cassidy et al. (1985) reported the results of a descriptive, prospective study of 283 patients unresponsive to previous conservative therapy. The treatment outcome was assessed by an independent observer, based on the patients' ratings of pain and physical disability. They found that patients with LBP and/or sciatica *not* extending past the knee responded significantly better than those with distal sciatic radiation of pain. Patients grouped under nerve compression syndromes, including those with nerve root entrapment, and a small select group of

patients with central spinal stenosis had a lower improvement rate. These researchers noted that in their experience anything less than 2 weeks of daily manipulation is inadequate for chronic back pain patients. No control group was employed, so definite conclusions regarding effectiveness cannot be made; however, spontaneous improvement seems to be an unlikely explanation for the positive treatment outcome.

Since 1940, more than 20 studies of workers' compensation patients receiving chiropractic care have been reported (Johnson et al., 1985). Most of these studies (e.g., Bergemann and Cichoke, 1980; Wolk, 1988; Johnson et al., 1989), and also prospective studies from general practice (Dillon, 1981; Bronfort, 1986), have suggested that the chiropractic management of LBP is superior to the medical approach, in terms of limiting patient work time loss and lowering treatment cost. All of these studies are nonrandomized and most of them retrospective in design, resulting in uncertain patient group comparability, precluding any definite conclusions. Table 24–3 reviews 14 nonrandomized comparative studies.

Lumbar Disc Herniation

Several studies of patients with clinical signs of nerve root compression resulting from disc herniation have reported reasonably successful outcome after SMT. Mathews and Yates (1969) reported reduction of disc herniations (verified by epidurographic contrast studies) in five patients. In two other studies of disc herniation and SMT (Wilson and Ilfield, 1952; Chrisman et al., 1964) employing myelography, changes could not be demonstrated despite evidence of symptomatic relief. Three different randomized trials, conducted by Siehl et al. (1971), Nwuga (1982), and Mathews et al. (1987), suggest that spinal manipulation in the hands of osteopaths and medical doctors may be of benefit, although the evidence is by no means conclusive. Nuclear magnetic resonance imaging (MRI) of the spine (and soon MRI spectroscopy) makes it possible to identify small morphological and pathophysiological changes in the vicinity of the intervertebral disc and the nerve roots. Future studies may explore the possible correlation between clinical findings and MRI changes in patients undergoing SMT.

Cervical Pain, Headache, and Thoracic Pain

Success rates similar to those of the descriptive studies of LBP have been reported in the clinical series involving SMT for cervical pain, headache, and other spine-related syndromes (Table 24–4). Since 1977 at least seven randomized clinical trials on cervical pain and/or headache have been conducted.

TABLE 24–1. AN ANNOTATED LIST OF DESCRIPTIVE STUDIES[a] OF SPINAL MANIPULATIVE THERAPY (SMT) AND LOW BACK PAIN (LBP).

Author and Year	Setting	Entry Criteria	Duration	Total Number of Subjects	Design	Average Number of SMT TX	Follow-Up Period	Successful Outcome	Comments
Riches, 1930	Hospital	LBP	A/C	75	R	1–2	Varies	75%	[33–92% depending on diagnosis], general anesthesia, SMT
Henderson, 1952	Hospital	LBP disc protrusion	A/C	68	R	?	>18m	74%	[20% in patients with root tension signs]
Wilson and Ilfeld, 1952	Hospital	Lumb disc herniation	?	18	P	1	0	17%	17% had temporary relief, but no myelographic change
Mensor, 1955	Hospital	LBP/disc protrusion	?	205	R	1–2	Varies (22m)	54%	General anesthesia, SMT-MD
Bremner, 1958	Hospital	Lumboscral strain	C	250	?	1	2w?	87%	General anesthesia, SMT + physiotherapy
Parsons and Cummings, 1958	MD pp	LBP/disc syndrome	A/C	2,000	R	2–3	?	75%	[Patients with root signs had one half as good response]
Bremner and Simpson, 1959	Hospital	LBP	C	150	?	1	4w	87%	1 SMT -TX + physiotherapy + exercise
Bosshard, 1961	DC pp	LBP/sciatica	A/C	44	R	7	0	90%	
Gray, 1967	Hospital	Lumb IVD syndrome	C	10	?	1	?	50%	[General anesthesia, SMT + traction]
Droz, 1969	DC pp	Sciatica	A/C	83	R	?	?	53%	No relapse in 5y [14% symptom-free, 36% intermittent LBP]
Warr et al., 1972	Hospital	LBP/sciatica	C	500	R	1	6m	63%	[No relapse in 6m], general anesthesia, SMT-MD + epidural injection
Tufvesson et al., 1976	MD indust clinic	LBP	C	34	R	?	0	76%	
Shanghai Institute et al., 1977	Hospital	LBP/disc protrusion	C	86	R	?	20m	85%	7% relapse, general anesthesia, SMT-MD
Breen, 1977	24 DCs pp	LBP	A/C	1,598	R	7	Varies	44%	44% had lasting results, 32% temporary improvement, randomly selected patients
Potter, 1977	DC pp	LBP	C	744	R	5	?	71%	[38–94% depending on duration and neurologic signs]
Cassidy et al., 1978	DC pp	LBP spondylolisthesis	C	17	?	10 (2w)	3m	82%	
Heyse-Moore, 1978	Hospital	LBP/sciatica	A/C	38	R	1	1y	50%	[SMT-MD] sciatic stretch under general anesthesia
Valentini, 1981	DC pp	LBP disc syndrome	A	194	R	7	6m	88%	Post-TX; 10% of patients had relapse within 6m
Hoehler and Tobis, 1982	Hospital	LBP	?	27	P	?	0	73%	[SLR post-TX increase] reliability of SLR reported
Banks, 1983[b]	DC pp	LBP facet + IVD syndrome	?	13	P	?	0		Post-TX lumbar disc angle change to values similar to 10 normal controls
Cox et al., 1983	DC pp	LBP ± leg pain	A/C	100	P	16	<6m	71%	[Cox distract + acupressure]
Cox and Shreiner, 1984	23 DCs pp	LBP	?	576	P	19	Varies	75%	TX response of different types of LBP reported

Key: MD = medical doctor, DC = doctor of chiropractic, DO = osteopathic doctor, PT = physiotherapist, A = acute, C = chronic, pp = private practice, d = day, w = week, m = month, y = year, R = retrospective, P = prospective, ? = information not available, TX = treatment.
[a]Unless specified in the comments, there was no blinding of patients and observers. No reliability of outcome measure was reported. And no control group was employed.
[b]Quasi-experimental study

Continues

TABLE 24–1. AN ANNOTATED LIST OF DESCRIPTIVE STUDIES[a] OF SPINAL MANIPULATIVE THERAPY (SMT) AND LOW BACK PAIN (LBP). (*Continued*)

Author and Year	Setting	Entry Criteria	Duration	Total Number of Subjects	Design	Average Number of SMT TX	Follow-Up Period	Successful Outcome	Comments
Fonti and Lynch, 1984	DCs pp	LBP/sciatica	A/C	3,136	R	30	1y	85%	
Salvi et al., 1984	DC pp	LBP/sciatica	?	184	?	20	0	69%	
Kirkaldy-Willis and Cassidy, 1985	Hospital DC	Severe LBP/leg pain	C	283	P	10–15	16m	81% - 48% -	In referred pain syndromes In nerve root compression syndromes
Sheladia and Johnston, 1986	DC college	LBP	?	465	R	?	?	79%	(SMT-DC + physiotherapy + nutritional advice)
Kuo and Loh, 1987	Hospital	LBP/disc protrusion	?	517	R	?	Var	84%	14% had relapses
Mierau et al., 1987	Hosp/DC	LBP/spondylolisthe-sis	C	25	P	7	16m	80%	Observer-blinded study

Most of these studies have addressed only short-term effects. In almost all of the studies SMT has been shown to have some value (Table 24–5). Parker et al. (1978) studied chronic migraine in a randomized trial in which one group received general cervical spine mobilization from physiotherapists/medical doctors, the second group received spinal manipulation from physiotherapists/medical doctors, whereas the third group underwent chiropractic adjustive therapy. At trial completion after 6 months the patients treated by doctors of chiropractic had the greatest reduction in symptoms, with pain statistically significantly reduced compared with the two other therapies. After 20 months of follow-up all three groups had improved further. Leboeuf et al. (1987) showed, in a controlled trial, that by adding soft tissue massage to the chiropractic adjustive therapy, patients suffering from chronic strain of the upper extremity seemed to respond better.

Hypertension

Studies of the effect of SMT on arterial blood pressure have shown equivocal results. Some investigators have reported short-term posttreatment decrease in blood pressure after spinal adjustive therapy (Fischera and Celander, 1969; McNight and DeBoer, 1988; Yates et al., 1988), but others (Wagnon et al., 1988) have not been able to duplicate these findings. The most rigorous controlled trial (Morgan et al., 1985) with a follow-up period of 4 months demonstrated no clinically significant change in blood pressure in either the SMT or the placebo (sham-SMT) group.

Spinal Electromyography

England and Deibert (1972), Grice and Tschumi (1985), Shambaugh (1987), and Ellestad et al. (1988) reported decrease in paraspinal muscle activity after SMT, but because of methodological problems and/or small sample sizes involved, these studies at best provide preliminary evidence.

Pain Tolerance and Neuropeptides

Increase in paraspinal pain tolerance was demonstrated as a result of a single chiropractic adjustment in a controlled trial involving 50 healthy males (Terrett and Vernon, 1984). Changes in circulating neuropeptides immediately after chiropractic adjustments have been studied in three randomized clinical trials. Vernon et al. (1986) reported a small (8%) increase in plasma levels of β-endorphins, but Christian et al. (1988) in a similar trial, and Sanders et al. (1990), did not observe any changes.

Pulmonary Dysfunction

Miller (1975) studied chronic obstructive lung disease treated with SMT in a controlled trial and, as in three studies of asthma and chiropractic treatment (Hviid, 1978; Jamison et al., 1986; Nilsson and Christiansen, 1988), a large percentage of patients reported subjective improvement. Except in the preliminary study by Hviid (1978) that suggested that some patients with asthma may improve their peak flow rate and vital capacity, no studies have demonstrated definite objective lung function improvement in patients treated by SMT.

Infantile Colic

In an uncontrolled prospective clinical series involving 316 infants suffering from nonspecific colic, more

TABLE 24–2. AN ANNOTATED LIST OF RANDOMIZED CLINICAL TRIALS OF SPINAL MANIPULATIVE THERAPY (SMT) AND LOW BACK PAIN (LBP).

Author and Year		Setting	Entry Criteria	Duration	Total Number of Subjects	Degree of Group Comparability	Sampling	Study Groups	Average Number of SMT TX
Siehl et al.	1971	Hospital	LBP Disc herniation	?	47	?	CS	G1: Conservative care + SMT-DO, $n=21$ G2: Conservative Care, $n=7$ G3: Disc surgery, $n=19$	?
Glover et al.	1974	Industrial medical center	LBP unilateral hyperesthesia	Acute + subacute	84	Adequate	CS	G1: 1 SMT-MD + 4 daily sessions of detuned diathermy, $n=43$ G2: 5 daily sessions of detuned diathermy (placebo), $n=41$	1
Doran and Newell	1975	Seven hospitals	LBP	A/C	456	Adequate	CS	G1: SMT-MD, $n=68$ G2: Physiotherapy, $n=67$ G3: Corset, $n=61$ G4: Analgesic + bed rest, $n=58$	6
Bergquist-Ullman and Larsson	1977	Industrial medical center	LBP	<3m, median 9d	217	Adequate	CS	G1: SMT-PT, $n=68$ G2: Back school 3h, $n=70$ G3: Low-intensity heat, $n=79$ (placebo)	4
Evans et al.	1978	Hospital	LBP	>3w	32	Inadequate	?	G1: SMT-MD/analgesics, $n=17$ G2: Analgesics/SMT-MD, $n=15$	3
Sims-Williams et al.	1978	Hospital PT clinic	LBP	75% >1m	94	Adequate	CV	G1: SMT-PT + mobilization + traction, $n=43$ G2: Heat (PT), $n=44$	<14
Rasmussen	1979	Hospital	LBP Males	<3w	24	Inadequate	CV	G1: SMT-MD/PT, $n=12$ G2: Short-wave diathermy, $n=12$	6
Sims-Williams et al.	1979	Hospital PT clinic	LBP	90% >1m	94	Adequate	CV	G1: SMT-PT + mobilization + traction, $n=48$ G2: Heat (PT), $n=44$	<14
Coxhead et al.	1981	Eight hospitals	LBP/sciatica	Mostly chronic	322	Adequate	CV	16 different combinations of: G1: Traction G2: SMT-PT G3: exercise G4: corset	?
Hoehler et al.	1981	Hospital outpatient	LBP	A/C	95	Uncertain	CS	G1: SMT-MD, $n=56$ G2: Soft tissue massage, $n=39$	?
Zylbergold and Piper	1981	Hospital outpatient	LBP	?	28	Adequate	CV	G1: Heat + flexion exercise, $n=10$ G2: Heat + SMT-PT, $n=8$ G3: Ergonomic instruction, $n=10$	8
Farrell and Twomey	1982	Two PT clinics	LBP	<3w	48	Adequate	CS	G1: Passive mobilization/SMT-PT, $n=24$ G2: Diathermy + exercise + ergonomic instruction, $n=24$	4
Nwuga	1982	University hospital	LBP/disc herniation	<2w	51 females	Adequate	?	G1: Heat + low-intensity exercise, $n=25$ G2: Oscillatory SMT-?, $n=26$	?

Follow-Up Period	Subject Blinding	Observer Blinding	Outcome Reliability Reported	Main Outcome Measures	Results	Comments[a]
12m	No	No	No	Electromyography	14% of G1, 0% of G2, and 47% of G3 showed electromyographic improvement. Clinical improvement similar in G1 and G2 but inferior to G3	SMT performed under general anesthesia; no statistics. Inadequate patient description
1m	No	Yes	No	Patient rated pain relief	SMT superior immediately post-TX in patients with duration < 7d, **SS** Similar improvement in G1 and G2 after 3d and 7d	Inadequate patient description. Trial on effect of a single manipulation
12m	No	No	No	Patient rated improvement on ordinal scale	Authors: No important group difference at any time; reanalyzed by Greenland et al.—SMT superior to corset at 3w, **SS**, but not at later assessments	15% dropouts (not analyzed). SMT inadequately described. Faulty statistics: Loss of power
1y	No	?	No	Symptom duration. Sick leave. Relapses	G1 and G2: shorter symptom duration than G3, **SS** G2: shortest duration of sick leave, **SS** Equal numbers of relapses in 1y in all three groups	Inappropriate statistics; reanalysis not possible
6w	No	Yes	Yes	Pain score. Lumbar flexion. Flexion/extension radiographs	Temporary decrease in pain + increased lumbar flexion during SMT phase **SS**; responders were older and had later debut of LBP, **SS**; no change in functional radiographs [Roberts et al., 1978]	Crossover trial. Inappropriate statistics. Reliability of functional radiographic exam not reported
12m	No	Yes	No	Patient rated improvement. Physical disability. Pain, SLR, lumbar ROM	G1 patients rated improvements higher and physical disability lower than G2 at 1m, **SS**, and at 3m, **NS**; increased SLR at 1m **SS** in G1. No difference between groups at 12m	A study of GP-MD patients. SMT-PT only a small part of G1 therapy
12m	No	No	No	MD rated improvement	92% of SMT group versus 25% of G2 were symptom-free after 2w, **SS** Increased lumbar flexion only in SMT group, **SS**	Inadequate information about patients, outcome, and follow-up. Bias likely
12m	No	Yes	No	Patient rated improvement. Physical disability. Lumbar ROM, SLR	No important clinical difference between groups at any time except at 1y follow-up, where G2 had better back status [**SS**] than G1	A study of GP-MD hospital referrals
1m (16m)	No	No	No	Patient rated pain VAS. Patient rated improvement on trichotomous scale. Work time loss	At 4w 78% of patients reported improvement and equal amount of time loss irrespective of TX; least pain in SMT group, **SS** Combining TXs superior to single-treatment approach, **SS**	No reported data on 16m follow-up
3w	Yes	Yes	No	Pain + physical disability + SLR	SMT group had less pain, disability, and increased SLR compared to G2 after the first TX, **SS**, and less pain 3w after discharge, **SS**	39% of patients lost to follow-up (no worst/best case analysis performed); patients not able to distinguish between the two TXs
0	No	?	No	Patient rated pain. ROM. Functional activity	More pain reduction, increased lumbar flexion, and functional activity in SMT group after 1m, when compared with the two other groups, **NS**	Inadequate info about SMT and its use in trial. Low statistical power
0	No	Yes	Yes	Number of days to reach "symptom-free" status. Lumbar ROM	SMT group required fewer days and TXs to reach "symptom-free" status, **SS** 91% of all patients recovered within 4w. No difference in pain between groups after 3w	Difference in group demographics compensated for through statistical analysis
0	No	Yes	No	Spinal ROM. SLR	SMT superior **SS** to heat + exercise in increasing ROM and SLR at 6w	Inadequate randomization. Pain not evaluated

[Continues]

TABLE 24-2. AN ANNOTATED LIST OF RANDOMIZED CLINICAL TRIALS OF SPINAL MANIPULATIVE THERAPY (SMT) AND LOW BACK PAIN (LBP) *(Continued)*.

Author and Year		Setting	Entry Criteria	Duration	Total Number of Subjects	Degree of Group Comparability	Sampling	Study Groups	Average Number of SMT TX
Godfrey et al.	1984	Hospital	LBP	Acute <2w	90	Adequate	U	G1: Soft tissue massage + SMT-MD/DC, n=48 G2: Min mass + low elstim, n=42	4
Gibson et al.	1985	Hospital outpatient	LBP	C	109	Uncertain	CV	G1: SMT-DO, n=41 G2: Diathermy active, n=34 G3: Detuned diathermy, n=34	4
Waterworth and Hunter	1985	Private practice MD	LBP	Acute	108	Adequate	CS	G1: Anti-inflammatory drug, n=36 G2: Heat + exercise, n=34 G3: SMT-PT and/or Mckenzie exercise, n=38	<10
Arkuszewski	1986	Hospital clinic	LBP/sciatica	C	100	Adequate	CS	G1: Drugs, physiotherapy, + SMT-MD, n=50 G2: Drugs, physiotherapy, n=50	6
Waagen et al.	1986	Chiropractic college clinic	LBP	>3w	29	Adequate	CS	G1: SMT-DC, n=11 G2: Sham SMT-DC, n=18	5
Hadler et al.	1987	Hospital	LBP	<1m	54	Adequate	CV	G1: Mobilization-MD, n=28 G2: SMT-MD, n=26	1
Mathews et al.	1987	Hospital	LBP ± sciatica	<3m	291	Adequate	CS	G1: SMT-PT, n=165 G2: Heat, n=126	<10
Ongley et al.	1987	Hospital clinic	LBP without TX response	>1y	81	Adequate	U	G1: Forceful SMT-MD + 6 "proliferant" injections, n=40 G2: Sham SMT-MD + 6 placebo injections, n=41	1
Postacchini et al.	1988	University clinic	LBP with/ without radiation	A/C	398	Adequate	CV	G1: SMT-DC?, n=87 G2: Drug, n=81 G3: Massage + diathermy, n=78 G4: Bed rest, n=29 G5: Back school, n=50 G6: Placebo ointment, n=72	11–17
Kinalski et al.	1989	Hospital	LBP	?	111	?	?	G1: SMT-MD, n=61 G2: G2: Heat + traction + exercise?, n=50	? 2–16 days
MacDonald and Bell	1990	Group practice— MD	LBP	14–28 days	95	Adequate	CS	G1: SMT-DO + LBP prophylaxis, n=49 G2: LBP prophylaxis, n=46	5
Meade et al.	1990	Multisite hospital outpatient and private practicing DCs	LBP	A/C	741	Adequate	CS	G1: Hospital SMT-PT, n=357 G2: SMT-DC, n=384	6 9

*Key: MD = medical doctor, DC = doctor of chiropractic, DO = osteopathic doctor, PT = physiotherapist, A = acute, C = chronic, d = day, w = week, m = month, y = year, CS = consecutive, CV = convenience, U = unselective, G1 = group 1, G2 = group 2, G3 = group 3, P = partially, TX = treatment, ROM = range of motion, ? = information not available, **SS** = statistical significance, **NS** = no statistical significance, CS = consecutive, CV = convenience, S = selective, U = unselective.*
[a]*Unless specified in the comments, there was no blinding of patients and observers. No reliability of outcome measure was reported. And no control group was employed.*

Follow-Up Period	Subject Blinding	Observer Blinding	Outcome Reliability Reported	Main Outcome Measures	Results	Comments
0	No	Yes	No	Global index of patient rated pain and activity impairment	Authors: No group difference. Both groups improved rapidly in 2–3w. Reanalysis by Hoehler et al. (1987): G1 superior to G2 at 3w, **SS**	Faulty statistics: loss of power
12w	P	Yes	No	Patient rated pain (VAS) Lumbar flexion	Similar improvement rate (pain and lumbar flexion) in all three groups at 2w, 4w, and 12w	
0	No	No	No	Work time loss Pain Spinal ROM	All three groups showed similar improvement after 4d and 12d of therapy	Number of SMT sessions uncertain. Efficacy of SMT not directly assessed
6m	No	No	No	Global index: posture, gait, pain, ROM, neurologic exam	G1: Better global score than G2 (**SS**) at 1m and 6m	Inadequate randomization
2w	Yes	Yes	P	Global index of spinal ROM and SLR Patient rated pain VAS	The SMT group had more pain reduction post-TX and at 2w than controls, **SS**. Global index improved significantly at 2w compared to controls, **SS**	33% dropout (no analysis). Results are considered preliminary by authors
2w	Yes	Yes	Yes	Roland Morris LBP questionnaire	Patients with LBP duration of 2–4w at entry improved faster and to a greater degree with SMT than with mobilization, **SS**	Study examines efficacy of a single SMT maneuver
1y	No	Yes	No	6-point patient rated pain score	Faster + greater rate of recovery in SMT group at 2w in patients with decreased SLR, **SS**. No difference in relapse rate between groups at 1y	18% dropouts
6m	Yes	Yes	P	LBP disability scale (Roland) VAS pain scale	G1 >40% better than G2 on both main outcomes at 1m (**SS**), 3m (**SS**), and 6m (**SS**)	Efficacy of SMT not addressed directly
2m and 6m	No		No	Global score of: Patient rated pain, functional disability, trunk muscle function, Finger-Floor Distance, and SLR	SMT superior at 3w in acute patients with/without radiation, **SS**. Back school superior at 6m in chronic patients without radiation, **SS**	SMT not described; statistical method for multiple group comparisons inappropriate; uncertain observer blinding; bias possible.
0	No		No	Trunk muscle strength Observer rated pain	Similar decrease in pain but shorter treatment time in G1	Inadequate information about patients, numbers, and nature of G2 treatments and outcome endpoint; no statistical analysis reported; bias likely
0	No		No	Patient reported recovery and disability score	SMT superior 1–2 w after TX start in patients with 14–28d of LBP duration, **NS**. No difference at 4w	LBP duration of subgroups not comparable at baseline between TX groups; small sample sizes; low statistical power
2y	No		No	Oswestry disability score Lumbar ROM	7% points lower disability in G2 at 6m, 12m, and 24m, **SS**	G2 had 50% more treatments than G1. Uncertain clinical significance of 7% points

Key: MD = medical doctor, DC = doctor of chiropractic, DO = osteopathic doctor, PT = physiotherapist, A = acute, C = chronic, d = day, w = week, m = month, y = year, CS = consecutive, CV = convenience, U = unselective, G1 = group 1, G2 = group 2, G3 = group 3, P = partially, TX = treatment, ROM = range of motion, ? = information not available, **SS** = statistical significance, **NS** = no statistical significance, CS = consecutive, CV = convenience, S = selective, U = unselective.

[a]Unless specified in the comments, there was no blinding of patients and observers. No reliability of outcome measure was reported. And no control group was employed.

TABLE 24-3. NONRANDOMIZED COMPARATIVE STUDIES[a] OF LOW BACK PAIN (LBP) INVOLVING SPINAL MANIPULATIVE THERAPY (SMT).

Author and Year	Setting	Entry Criteria	Duration	Total Number of Subjects	Design	Sampling	Study Groups
Coyer and Curwen, 1955	Hospital	LBP	A	152	P	U	G1: SMT-MD, $n=76$ G2: Bed rest, $n=60$ analgesia + pillow
Chrisman et al., 1964	Hospital	LBP/sciatica Disc herniation No TX response	C	61	P	CS	G1: SMT-MD, $n=29$ + general anesthesia G2: Control, $n=22$
Edwards, 1969	Hospital/PT	LBP/sciatica	A	184	P	S	G1: Heat, massage, exercise, $n=92$ G2: SMT-MD, $n=92$
Mathews and Yates, 1969	Hospital	LBP Disc herniation	A	10	P	?	G1: SMT-MD, $n=5$ G2: Sham SMT, $n=5$
Kane et al., 1974	DCs + MDs PP	Cervical and LBP injury Workers' comp	?	232	R	U	G1: MD, $n=110$ G2: DC, $n=122$
Fisk, 1979	MD PP	Unilateral LBP Decreased straight leg raise (SLR)	A	20	P	S	G1: SMT-MD, $n=10$, LBP G2: SMT-MD, $n=10$, normal controls
Durrington, 1979	DCs + MDs pp	LBP + cervical pain	?	100	R	U	G1: SMT-DC, $n=50$ G2: TX-MD, $n=50$
Bergemann and Cichoke, 1980	MDs + DCs pp	LBP injury Workers' comp	A	227	R	U	G1: TX-MD, $n=114$ G2: SMT-DC, $n=113$
Dillon, 1981	MD + DC pp	LBP injuries	?	32	P	CV	G1: MD, $n=15$ G2: DC, $n=17$
Lewith and Turner, 1982	MD pp	LBP	A	66	R	U	G1: SMT-MD, $n=21$ G2: Rest + analgesia, $n=45$
Bronfort, 1986	10 DCs + 1 MD pp	LBP	A/C	298	P	CS	259 DC patients were compared with 78 MD patients from separate study
Meade et al., 1986[b]	Hospital/DC	LBP	A/C	50	P	CS	G1: SMT-DC, $n=23$ G2: Back school, exercise + SMT-MD, $n=27$
Wolk, 1988	MDs + DCs + DOs	LBP injuries Workers' Comp closed cases	?	10,652	R	U	G1: MD patients, $n=9362$ G2: DC patients, $n=1297$ G3: DO patients, $n=257$
Cherkin and MacCormack, 1989	MDs + DCs	LBP	A/C	457	R	U	G1: MD patients, $n=215$ G2: DC patients, $n=242$

Key :MD = medical doctor, DC = doctor of chiropractic, DO = osteopathic doctor, PT = physiotherapist, pp = private practice, d = day, w = week, m = month, y = year, A = acute, C = chronic, R = retrospective, P = prospective, ? = information not available, CS = consecutive, CV = convenience, S = selective, U = unselective, G1 = group 1, G2 = group 2, G3 = group 3, TX = treatment, pp = private practice.

[a] Unless specified in the comments, there was no blinding of patients or observers, and no reliability of outcome measure was reported.

[b] Randomized clinical trial (pilot/feasibility study)

than 90% improved and 60% became asymptomatic according to diaries kept by the parents (Klougart et al., 1989). The results were obtained within a 2-week period after an average of three chiropractic spinal adjustments, and seem more favorable than the expected natural course of this disorder.

Nocturnal Enuresis

In a prospective clinical study of 171 children with enuresis receiving chiropractic spinal adjustments, Leboeuf et al. (1991) reported that after a 2-week baseline period, the median frequency of wet nights per week dropped from 5.6 to 4 over an average of eight treatments. In 25% of the children a substantial reduction in bed wetting frequency was reported. No control group was employed.

Guide to Critical Evaluation of Clinical Research Publications

Most clinical research articles use a conventional publication format. The format includes an abstract, introduction, material and methods section, results section, discussion, conclusion or summary, and references. From these sections, the critical reader can

Average Number of SMT TXs	Follow-up Period	Results	Comments
?	0	Symptom-free at 1w, G1: 50% G2: 27% Symptom-free at 6w, G1: 88% G2: 72%	12% G2 dropouts No statistical analysis
1	5–10m	G1: 51% success, no change in myelograms, 33% discectomy G2: "Most did poorly," 73% discectomy	Patients without positive myelogram did best; group comparability uncertain
6	0	Sastisfactory results: G1: 67%, G2: 87% G2 had half the number of TXs of G1	Group comparability uncertain Patients with radiating leg pain had response rate similar to that of patients without
?	0	Symptomatic improvement and contrast defect reduction (epidurography) in all G1 patients	Group comparability uncertain
13	< 1y	Similar improvement in functional status in both groups; highest patient satisfaction with DCs; DC patients had more visits but shorter TX duration	
1	0	G1: Reduced hamstring tension G2: No tension reduction	Inadequate group comparability Observer blinded; SLR reliability reported
10	< 1y	Similar improvement rate in both groups; DC patients less depressed and socially limited compared with MD patients; DC TX cost five times more than medical TX	Group comparability acceptable
11	1y	DC patients had about half the work time loss and cost compared with MD patients	Group comparability uncertain
?	?	Substantial less work time loss and TX cost in DC group compared with MD group	Group comparability uncertain
?	1y	G1 had half the number of sick leave days in 1y compared with G2	Group comparability uncertain
9	1y	DC patients had less work time loss and fewer bed rest days than MD patients in 1y 75% success rate in DC patients at 1, 3, 6, and 12m	Comparison of two different studies with same design; DC patients had poorer prognosis at baseline than MD patients; no conclusions on effectiveness possible
?	6m		Results not disclosed Large-scale trial feasible
?	1y	DO and DC care more cost-effective than MD care	Uncertain group comparability on type and severity of low back injury
	8m	Patient reported "very satisfied with care": G1: 22%, G2: 66%	DC patients had a longer previous history of LBP; otherwise acceptable group comparability

expect to learn what questions were asked, how the author sought answers, what was found, and what the author's conclusions were. The Key to Critical Evaluation of Clinical Journal Articles (Box 24–1) provides relevant questions for each section of the report.

Abstract

The abstract is a concise paragraph (or two) preceding the research article. It summarizes the purpose, methods, results, conclusion, and clinical relevance of the study. The abstract does not provide all the details of the study. *Conclusions presented in the abstract should not be accepted before critically reading the entire article.* The abstract should assist the reader in answering the question, Is this article of clinical interest to me?

Introduction

The introduction usually contains four major elements: (1) identification of a research question, (2) literature review, (3) study purpose; and (4) study design. The introduction should clearly define the significance (clinical, social, financial) of the problem the author(s) plans to investigate. The literature review should provide an adequate background to es-

TABLE 24–4. AN ANNOTATED LIST OF DESCRIPTIVE CLINICAL STUDIES[a] OF SPINAL MANIPULATIVE THERAPY (SMT) ON PATIENTS WITH CERVICAL PAIN, HEADACHE, AND OTHER SPINAL RELATED DISORDERS.

Author and Year	Setting	Entry Criteria	Duration	Total Number of Subjects	Design	Average Number of SMT TXs	Follow-up Period	Successful Outcome	Comments
Rosendahl, 1963	MD pp	Cervical + thoracic pain	C	276	R	4	?	69% 80%	[Cervical cases] [Thoracic cases]
Bechgaard, 1966	Hospital	Cervical, thoracic, lumbar pain	A/C	807	R	2	1y	64%	Best response in posttraumatic headache
Wilson, 1967	MD pp	Spinal pain	A/C	50	R	2	0	82%	
Livingston, 1969	MD pp	Cervical, thoracic, lumbar pain	A/C	60	P	3	1y	87%	38% of patients relapsed within 1y
Fisk, 1971	MD pp	Cervical, thoracic, lumbar pain	A/C	327	R	2	<1y	95%	32% of patients relapsed within 1y
Hviid, 1971	DC pp	Spinal symptoms	?	92	P	5	0	78%	78% of patients obtained 15–20° increased cervical rotation approaching ROM of 100 normal controls
Lewit, 1971	Hospital	Cervicogenic headache	?	134	R	?	?		SMT effective in large majority of cases, most of which were posttraumatic
Orpwood Price, 1971	MD pp	Spinal pain	A/C	195	R	4	0	75–85%	75–85% recovered in 4w, SMT-MD + local anesthesia
England and Deibert, 1972	DO college	Thoracic pain	C	10	P	1	0	90%	90% of patients had decreased paraspinal EMG activity post-TX
Wing and Hargrave-Wilson, 1974	MD pp	Cervical pain + vertigo	?	80	P	?	0	89%	(73% had improved nystagmograms) TX: SMT-MD + collar
Stokke, 1977	DC pp	Spinal pain syndromes	A/C	787	R	5	18m	78%	23% relapsed within 18m
Wight, 1978	DCs pp	Migraine	C	87	R	?	2y	75%	(52% fewer episodes at 2y follow-up)
Vernon, 1982	DC college	Headache	C	33	R/P	12	0	84%	84% had reduction in headache frequency
Leach, 1983	DC pp	Abnormal cervical curve	?	35	R	?	0		Improvement of cervical curve in SMT patients compared with six controls
Carrick, 1983	DC pp	Cervical radicolopathy	?	50	P	?	0	88%	
Luisetto et al., 1984	DC pp	Cervical syndromes	?	11	P	10	0		All patients had increased calcitonin levels post-TX No change in β-endorphins
Droz and Crot, 1985	DC pp	Occ. headache	?	332	R	9	Varies	93%	
Grice and Tschumi, 1985	DC pp	Spinal dysfunction	?	26	P	?	0	96%	96% improved ROM post-TX (functional radiography)
Shambaugh, 1987	DC college	Spinal dysfunction	?	20	P	1	0	25%	25% reduced spinal EMG activity and side-to-side imbalance in SMT group; no change in control group, $n=14$
Turk and Ratcolb, 1987	Hospital	Cervicogenic headache	C	100	R	6	6m	75%	75% had much less headache Post-TX, 65% after 6m
Jamison et al., 1986	DC college	Intrinsic asthma	C	18	P	7	5w		All patients satisfied with care; no improvement in respiratory function
Nilsson and Christiansen, 1988	DC pp	Asthma	A/C	79	R	?	0	62%	Improved patients had lower age at debut
Stodolny and Chmielewski, 1989	MD	Cervical migraine	C	31	P	1–2	0		Headache disappeared in 32% of patients Neck pain disappeared in 23% of patients Dizziness disappeared in 58% of patients

Key: MD = medical doctor, DC = doctor of chiropractic, DO = osteopathic doctor, PT = physiotherapist, pp = private practice, d = day, w = week, m = month, y = year, TX = treatment, A = acute, C = chronic, ? = iinformation not available.
[a]*Unless specified in the comments there was no blinding of patients and observers. No reliability of outcome measure was reported. And no control group was employed.*

tablish the necessity and relevance of conducting the study. Often a reader can assess the comprehensiveness of this literature review by noting the number and quality of references. Peer-reviewed journals as references hold more credibility in the scientific community than trade or professional journals. The process of peer review means that a group of colleagues reviewed the article for scientific merit. In their judgment the article has attained a certain standard and is worthy of scientific publication. One should also note that sparseness of the literature may indicate that little research has been done in the area of interest.

BOX 24–1. KEY TO CRITICAL EVALUATION OF CLINICAL JOURNAL ARTICLES.

Abstract
- Study relevance?

Introduction
- Does the literature review provide adequate background?
- Is the purpose clearly defined?

Material and Methods

Design
- Is the study design descriptive, correlational, or inferential/explanatory?

Subject selection
- What were the criteria for inclusion and exclusion?
- How were the subjects sampled?
- Was random allocation used?
- Were subjects adequately described?
- Was blinding used?
- If a group comparison study was conducted, were groups really comparable?

Intervention
- Was the intervention adequately described?

Outcome measures
- Were the reliability and validity of the outcome measures reported?
- Were baseline measurements made?

Results

Reported data
- Are all relevant clinical outcomes presented?
- Are ranges and confidence limits of the data presented?

Dropouts
- Were all subjects that entered the study accounted for at study completion?
- Was a worst or best case analysis performed?

Statistics
- Were the outcome variables measured on quantitative or qualitative scales?
- Have appropriate statistical tests been used?
- Are the prerequisites of the statistical tests fulfilled?
- What was the statistical power of the study?
- Are the results statistically significant?
- Are the results clinically significant?

Discussion and Conclusion
- Are the results discussed adequately in relation to other relevant studies?
- Are study weaknesses discussed?
- Are confounding factors and sources of bias identified?
- Are suggestions for further research made?
- Are the conclusions valid?
- Can the study results be extrapolated to a larger population of patients?

Material and Methods

The materials and methods section explains exactly how the study was done. It should provide enough details to allow other investigators to duplicate the study if they desired to do so. A critical reader should attempt to determine what research design and type of research the investigators have used, which to a large degree determines the type of statistical analysis used and the generalizability of study results.

Design

Descriptive Study Design. The simplest *descriptive study design* is a case report, which reports an interesting or unusual manifestation of a clinical syndrome or outcome of a therapeutic intervention. Such reports may point to possible risks or benefits of a particular diagnostic procedure or therapeutic method, sometimes leading to further investigations that result in change of clinical practice.

Clinical series, which are studies of a well-defined group of patients, can be very useful in reporting the clinical course of different syndromes under therapeutic intervention, especially if done prospectively.

Literature reviews summarize and analyze a group of research reports. This type of descriptive study, if done in an unbiased fashion, can summarize the current state of knowledge and help formulate relevant new research questions.

The major limitation of descriptive studies is that they do not permit inferences about the effectiveness of a therapeutic method because they lack use of control groups.

Correlational Design. The degree of association between clinical variables is examined in correlational designs. For example, do static or functional x-ray findings correlate with patient symptomatology? When looking for associations between clinical variables, it is very important to keep in mind that this type of research does not permit causal inferences.

Test–retest reliability studies of clinical instruments is a common type of *correlational research*. An instrument in this context is defined as a method of measuring clinical change, and can be anything from a measuring tape to a questionnaire. Intra- and inter-observer agreement studies of spinal range of motion or spinal motion palpation are examples of correlational studies.

Inferential or Explanatory Design. The third major group of research designs if the *inferential or explanatory design*, which can be further divided into observational, quasi-experimental, and experimental designs. Comparison is the main purpose of inferential studies.

In observational studies, the emphasis is on ob-

TABLE 24–5. AN ANNOTATED LIST OF RANDOMIZED CLINICAL TRIALS OF SPINAL MANIPULATIVE THERAPY (SMT) AND CERVICAL PAIN AND HEADACHE.

Author and Year	Setting	Entry Criteria	Duration	Total Number of Subjects	Degree of Group Comparability	Sampling	Study Groups	Average Number of SMT TXs
Bitterli et al., 1977	Hospital clinic	Cervicogenic headache	C	30	?	CV	G1: Mobilization MD, $n=10$ G2: SMT-MD, $n=10$ G3: 3w waiting list control, then SMT-MD, $n=10$	3–4
Kogstad et al., 1978	Hospital	Cervicobrachialgia	>3w	50	Adequate	CS	G1: SMT-MD + heat + massage, $n=13$ G2: Heat + massage + traction + exercise, $n=21$ G3: Placebo drug, $n=16$	8
Parker et al., 1978	Multidiscipli-nary	Migraine	C	85	Adequate	CV	G1: SMT-DC, $n=30$ G2: SMT-PT/MD, $n=27$ G3: Cervical mobilization PT/MD, $n=28$	8
Hoyt et al., 1979	DO hospital	Headache	C	22	?	?	G1: Massage + SMT-DO, $n=10$ G2: Palpatory exam, $n=6$ G3: 10-minute rest, $n=6$	1
Brodin, 1982	Hospital	Cervical pain	A/C	63	Adequate	CV	G1: Analgesics, $n=23$ G2: Analgesia, light massage, "cervical school," $n=17$ G3: = G2 + passive, SMT-PT, $n=23$	9
Sloop et al., 1982	Hospital	Cervical pain	C	39	Adequate	CV	G1: Amnesic dose diazepam + SMT-MD, $n=21$ G2: Amnesic dose diazepam, no TX, $n=18$	1
Howe et al., 1983	Private practice, two MDs	Cervicobrachial pain	Recent onset	52	Adequate	CS	G1: SMT-MD, $n=26$ G2: No TX, $n=26$	1

Key: MD = medical doctor, DC = doctor of chiropractic, DO = osteopathic doctor, PT = physiotherapist, A = acute, C = chronic, G1 = group 1, G2 = group 2, G3 = gorup 3, d = day, w = week, m = month, y = year, CV = convenience, CS = consecutive, ? = information not available, **SS** = statistical significance, **NS** = no statistical significance, P = partially, TX = treatment.

serving the spontaneous course of health phenomena in an attempt to determine the etiology and predisposing factors of different clinical disorders. Gehlbach (1982) provides definitions and discussion of the different types of observational studies.

Studies with *quasi-experimental design* usually involve group comparisons and often contain extraneous factors or variables that are not easily controlled for by the design. Frequently, interventions are not delivered in a blinded manner, or randomization of subjects is not performed. This immediately raises the question of comparability of the study groups. Differences seen between subjects may not result from the intervention but from uncontrolled, external factors (confounding variables). This type of research is often performed in clinical practice, where fully controlled experiments are not feasible. A variety of such quasi-experimental designs exist (Campbell and Stanley, 1966).

Time series studies, including single-case designs, provide an opportunity for the practicing clinician to contribute to the clinical knowledge base and help formulate pertinent research questions that can be addressed in more rigorous and intensive experimental investigations. Time series studies may be useful in evaluating individual patients both for routine documentation of treatment effectiveness and in quality assurance studies. This type of design can be used in the individual clinical setting without seriously disrupting clinical routine (Kazdin, 1982; Keating et al., 1985).

The *experimental design* considered to be the optimal standard in experimental clinical research is the randomized clinical trial (RCT). In the classical sense, it is a prospective study that serves the purpose of comparing one treatment with a placebo treatment under controlled conditions. Experimental therapy usually does not benefit every patient randomly assigned it. If a relevant RCT with sufficient statistical power has generated a negative result, at least some patients will usually benefit from the experimental therapy. The clinicians are therefore faced with uncertainty when they try to practice according to scientific standards. They cannot neces-

Follow-Up Period	Subject Blinding	Observer Blinding	Outcome Reliability Reported	Main Outcome Measures	Results	Comments
3m	P	Yes	No	Patient rated pain VAS	Pain reduction at 3w: G1:35%, G2:56%, G3:25%, **NS**; all three groups equal at 3m	Inadequate patient description Randomization method uncertain Low statistical power
18m	No	No	No	MD/patient rated improvement on dichotomous scale	Improved patients at 5w: G1:92%, G2:81%, G3:50%, **SS** Improved patients at 18m: G1:84%, G2:80%, G3:53%, **NS**	Low statistical power; outcome measure and randomization method inadequately described
20m	No	Yes	Yes	Episode frequency + duration, disability Pain	After 6m DC group had an average reduction of 34% in symptom outcomes compared to 9% in G2 and 22% in G3, **NS** At 6m G1 reported about 30% more pain reduction than G2 and G3, **SS**	At 20m follow-up further reduction in migraine attacks was noted in all three groups G1: 21%, G2: 20%, G3: 10%; Low statistical power. [Parker et al., 1980]
0	No	Yes	P	Headache severity Frontalis m. EMG	Most decrease in headache severity in SMT group, **SS**, but no EMG change	Inadequate subject description High-risk of type I and II errors Randomization method uncertain
1w	P	No	No	Patient rated pain Cervical ROM	No/slight pain 1w post-TX: G1:61%, G2:59%, G3:84%, **SS**; G3 larger post-TX ROM than G1 and G2, **SS**	Statistical method not reported
12w	Yes	Yes	P	Patient rated pain VAS Patient rated improvement on dichotomous scale	Patients reporting improvement at 3w: G1:57%, G2:28%, **NS** VAS improvement: G1:18%, G2:5%, **NS**	Partly a crossover design Low statistical power
3w	No	Yes	Yes	Goniometry Pain	G1 less pain than G2 post-TX, **SS**, and after 1w, **NS**, and 3w, **NS**; cervical rotatation increased in G1, **SS**, at 1w and 3w	Pain measured on dichotomous scale: low statistical power

sarily trust their own clinical experience, but neither can they always rely on a large-scale RCT for definitive treatment recommendations for the individual patient. Future RCTs that include repeated measurements during the course of treatment using the principles of time series design can provide a more detailed analysis of the response pattern of individual patients.

Subject Selection

Inclusion and exclusion criteria for entry into a study must be clearly defined, and the subject material should be selected in a random fashion on a consecutive basis to establish the best basis for extrapolating results. Often this principle is not adhered to or is not possible for practical reasons. If one suspects that patients were selected without adhering to strict eligibility criteria, the validity of the study results is reduced.

In comparative trials, adequate *group comparability* regarding patient characteristics such as age, gender, and duration and severity of the disorder being studied is essential. The subjects must be de-

scribed in sufficient detail to allow the reader to evaluate the degree of this comparability. Outcome differences between study groups can then be caused by the therapeutic intervention, but may also be the result of confounding variables, selection bias, or chance difference. If potential confounding variables are detected, the investigators are obliged to take them into consideration in the analysis phase with the statistical technique known as adjustment of data (Rimm et al., 1980). In performing such an adjustment, the investigators separate into groups those who possess the same levels of confounding variables, and then compare to see if the outcome differences persist. For example, gender can be a confounding variable. More advanced statistical techniques known as multiple regression are available for adjusting more than one variable (factor) at a time.

Intervention

Therapeutic interventions should be adequately described in terms of type, frequency and length, interval between treatments, and specific details of the therapeutic procedure.

Outcome Measures

The *reliability and validity* of instruments (e.g., questionnaires, range of motion tests) used in the study must be reported by the investigator even if they have been determined by previous researchers. It is always pertinent to document that the instruments have been used reliably in the present study. Reliability of a test or instrument refers to the reproducibility of its results at different points in time or by different observers or raters. The validity of a test or instrument is the degree to which the test really measures the phenomenon of interest. For example, does spinal motion palpation accurately determine intersegmental biomechanical dysfunction?

The comparison of study groups at trial completion is a central issue in any experimental clinical research study. It is important for the investigators to perform baseline measurements of the major response variables before the therapeutic intervention is introduced. This allows for more accurate evaluation of study group comparability. Often two or three such measurements are needed.

Results

Reported Data. All relevant clinical outcomes should be reported, not only those that fit the author's hypothesis. To fully evaluate the results, the raw data must be reported. This seldom happens, partly because space constraints in journals will not allow it. At the very least, ranges and confidence limits of the data should be presented. These concepts are briefly defined in the statistics section below.

Dropouts. Often, a substantial amount of study data is missing, or patients may have dropped out of the study. This problem must be addressed by the author. In group comparison trials, a critical approach is to conduct a "worst and best case" analysis, that is, to arbitrarily assign a bad outcome to all missing members of the groups and subsequently assign a successful outcome to the missing group, and then reanalyze the group difference under both conditions. This test can potentially change the study conclusions completely.

Statistics

Unfortunately, errors in experimental design and misuse of elementary statistical techniques such as the *t*-test and χ^2 test occur in a large percentage of clinical studies (Freiman et al., 1978). These errors may lead investigators to faulty conclusions regarding the effectiveness of a treatment or clinical procedure. Accepting such conclusions at face value, just

because they have appeared in reputable journals, can be a serious mistake. This section discusses the most common statistical concepts and tests used in clinical studies, for the purpose of facilitating critical interpretation of the clinical trials reported in the literature. Several texts are available that introduce statistics in an easily understandable fashion (Rimm et al., 1980; Leaverton, 1986; Norman and Streiner, 1986; Elston and Johnson, 1987).

Variables. Any clinical measurement of an individual, such as age, sex, height, or range of motion of a joint, is referred to as a variable. There may be only one variable, but usually there are several in any study. Variables that are under the control of the investigators, and in clinical trials often the therapeutic interventions themselves, are termed *independent variables*. *Dependent* or *response variables* are measured as results or outcomes of the experiment.

Variables have different characteristics, and different statistical methods must be applied when analyzing them. Variables are either qualitative/categorical or quantitative/numerical. A qualitative variable can be on either an ordinal scale or a nominal scale. A nominal variable is simply a named category. A particularly common sort is a binary or dichotomous variable where the response is one of two alternatives, for example, male/female or positive/negative outcome. An ordinal variable is a set of ordered or ranked categories, for example, a subjective rating of outcome, such as symptom-free, much better, somewhat better, no better, or worse. Although a relationship exists between individual grades, nothing is implied about how much that difference is. Ordinal variables can be semiquantitative in nature. An example is pain rating on a visual analog scale.

The pure quantitative variable consists of actual measurements on individuals. A quantitative variable is either discrete or continuous. The value of a discrete variable is usually a whole number, such as number of headache episodes per week. A measurement on a continuous numerical scale is called a continuous variable. Examples are height, weight, age, blood pressure, and temperature.

Types of Statistics. It is important to have a basic understanding of descriptive, correlational, and inferential statistics to be able to critically evaluate the clinical literature. A few of the most important concepts are discussed in this section.

DESCRIPTIVE STATISTICS. The mean, median, and mode are used to describe the central tendency of observations in a study group. The *mean* is the sum of observations divided by the number of observations taken. If the data are not normally distributed or represent ordinal or nominal scale measurements, it is more appropriate to describe the frequency distributions in terms of the *median,* which is the middle observation from a data set dividing the values into two equal halves, or the *mode,* which is the most frequently occurring observation.

To describe the measure of variability, *standard deviation (SD)* and *standard error of the mean (SE)* are used. Experimental data are often summarized as mean ± SD or mean ± SE. If the data are normally distributed, they will form a nearly symmetric bell-shaped curve. The mean ± 1 SD then roughly defines 68%, and the mean ± 2 SD roughly 95%, of the observations under the curve, thus characterizing the variability of the data. Many authors, however, fail to summarize their data with SD; instead they use SE. SE measures the precision with which the sample mean estimates the true population mean. The likely reason that SE is used so much is that it yields a smaller value than the SD; thus it gives the impression of less variability. It is very important not to confuse the two.

Percentile ranges are used for nonnormally distributed continuous data and ordinal data. The location of the 0th and 100th percentiles describes or defines the total range of sample observations; most commonly, the 5th and 95th percentiles are used to characterize the dispersion or spread of the data.

Although significance tests provide the strength of evidence for a difference between two treatments, confidence limits offer an estimate of the magnitude of this difference. The confidence interval (CI) for a percentage frequency in a sample defines the range within which the population percentage frequency lies. The CI for a percentage frequency and for a mean should not be confused. The 95% CI of a mean defines a range within which we can be 95% certain that the true (population) mean lies.

CORRELATIONAL STATISTICS. Correlation characterizes the existence of a relationship (association) between variables (Table 24–6). Although there may be many reasons for a relationship, cause and effect cannot be inferred from correlational statistics. The degree of correlation is expressed as a correlation coefficient (r) and has a range of from + 1.0 (perfect positive corre-

lation) through − 1.0 (perfect negative correlation). Different ranges of r values indicate different degrees of correlational reproducibility: 0–0.25, poor; 0.25–0.50, fair; 0.50–0.75, moderate; and 0.75–1.0, good to excellent. In addition to the direction of and magnitude of r, it is possible to test whether the r value is of statistical significance.

Confidence in research results comes from the assurance that findings reported by investigators have been shown to be reliable and valid. Because the various types of errors discussed earlier have a strong influence on the degree of accuracy of the data, reliability analysis becomes very important, and is usually performed by using one of the tests listed in Table 24–7.

INFERENTIAL STATISTICS. The most common inferential statistical tests in clinical research are the *t*-test, the chi square (χ^2) test, and analysis of variance (Table 24–8). Most studies involve a comparison of two groups or samples. The *t*-test is used to compute the probability of being wrong (the *p*-value) when claiming that the mean values of two groups are different.

The level of significance of a test is a statement about the probability of a difference between groups occurring by chance. A 5% level of significance ($p \leq 0.05$) means that the observed difference would occur by chance fewer than one out of 20 times. By convention, if the *p*-value falls at or below 0.05 the results are considered statistically significant.

But are statistically significant study results necessarily of clinical significance? If large groups of subjects are used in a research study, very small outcome differences may result in statistical significance. If small groups of individuals are studied, a very large, absolute outcome difference between study groups must exist before it can reach statistical significance. Thus, statistically significant outcome differences seen in large group experiments might be too small to be of clinical interest, whereas large differences that are statistically insignificant in small group studies may be both clinically and statistically significant when reduplicated on a larger scale.

TABLE 24–6. CORRELATIONAL STATISTICAL ANALYSIS OF GROUP RELATIONSHIPS: COMMONLY USED TESTS.

	One Continuous Variable	Two or More Continuous Variables	One Ordinal Variable
One continuous variable	Pearson's r [a] simple regression	Multiple correlation R [a] multiple regression	
Two or more continuous variables		Canonical correlation	
One ordinal variable	Spearman's ρ [rho] Kendall's τ [tau]		Spearman's ρ [rho] Kendall's τ [tau]

[a]*Simple statistical regression is used to predict one variable from another variable; similarly, multiple regression is used to predict one variable from two or more other variables.*

TABLE 24–7. COMMONLY USED STATISTICAL TESTS OF RELIABILITY AND VALIDITY.

	One Rater	Two or More Raters
One quantitative variable, two measurements	Pearson's r Coefficient of variation (CV%) Interclass correlation coefficient (ICC)	ICC
One quantitative variable, three or more measurements	ICC CV%	ICC
One ordinal variable, two measurements	Spearman's ρ (rho)	Kendall's W
One nominal variable, two or more classifications (usually dichotomous)	κ (kappa)	κ (kappa)

The t-test is frequently used to test the differences among more than two groups by comparing all possible pairs of means with t-tests. This practice is nearly always inappropriate, because the true probability of falsely concluding that there is a significant difference (say at the 5% level) increases with the number of tests performed (Godfrey, 1985). In such cases the true p value may be estimated by multiplying the average of the reported p values by the number of conducted t tests.

When three or more groups of subjects are being compared on the basis of one quantitative outcome variable, analysis of variance (ANOVA) should be employed. ANOVA is a statistical method that measures the ratio of the "between"-group variability to the "within"-group variability. By calculating the overall differences between the group parameters, it is determined whether any differences between/within groups are larger than can be accounted for by chance alone.

Chi square (χ^2) is by far the most commonly used nonparametric test of significance, but should be applied only to data derived from independent samples. The chi square test is not appropriate to use with ordinal or continuous data because it is insensitive to quantification of data and could very easily re-

TABLE 24—8. INFERENTIAL STATISTICAL ANALYSIS OF GROUP DIFFERENCES: COMMON PARAMETRIC AND NONPARAMETRIC TESTS.

		Two Independent Groups, One Factor[a]	Three or More Independent Groups, One Factor	Two or More Independent Groups, Two or More Factors	Two Matched (Related) Groups or repeated measures on same group	Three or More Matched (Related) Groups or repeated measures on groups
Univariate analysis (one dependent variable)						
One quantitative[b] dependent variable	**P**	t test[c]	One-way ANOVA[c]	Factorial ANOVA[c]	Paired t test	Repeated-measures ANOVA
One ordinal (ranked) dependent variable	**N**	Mann–Whitney test	Kruskal–Wallis (one-way ANOVA)		Wilcoxon signed rank test	Friedman's test
One nominal dependent variable	**N**	Fisher's exact[d] χ^2	χ^2		McNemar test	Cochran Q test
Multivariate analysis (two or more dependent variables)						
Two or more quantitative dependent variables	**P**	Hotelling T^{2c}[e] discriminant function analysis	MANOVA[c] discriminant function analysis			

Key: P = parametric tests. Used with quantitative data sets derived from normal distributions with homogeneity of variance. **N** = nonparametric tests. Used when assumptions for parametric tests cannot be met.
[a] Factor is equal to an independent variable (in clinical trials, often the intervention itself).
[b] Quantitative variables represent data on continuous and discrete scales. Although controversial among statisticians, semiquantitative ordinal scale data (e.g., visual analog scale ratings) can also be analyzed with parametric tests (Hoehler and Tobis, 1987).
[c] Assumptions: (1) Homogeneous variances in each group. (2) Approximately normally distributed data sets. (3) "Quantitative data."
[d] Assumption: Use χ^2 if none of the expected values are less than 5; otherwise, Fisher's exact test is indicated.
[e] If T^2 or MANOVA is significant, discriminant function analysis can be used to indicate which dependent variables are most important in accounting for the group differences.

sult in overlooking a real difference. This mistake has been made in several controlled trials on spinal manipulation (Greenland et al., 1980).

Data Analysis. *Primary analysis* is the original analysis of data as they are commonly reported by investigators in original research reports. *Secondary analysis* is reanalysis of original published data, often using more appropriate statistical techniques for assessing the original research question. This type of analysis may sometimes yield conclusions that differ from those of the original authors, as in the case of several studies of SMT (Greenland et al., 1980).

Finally, *meta-analysis* is a comparison and summation of findings from different studies using a statistical approach. Frequently, it is not possible to draw valid conclusions from qualitative literature reviews because of the lack of comparability and equivocal results of the studies under review. Such reviews are also subject to potential biases by the reviewer. In essence, meta-analysis regards the findings from one study as a data point, and calculates an index known as the effect size that quantifies how different two groups are with respect to the dependent outcome variable. Findings from multiple studies on the same topic can therefore be combined and treated statistically.

Discussion and Conclusion

The discussion section of an article should elaborate on the method and the results and place these into clinical perspective. Studies done in the same or related areas by other investigators should be brought into the discussion. The reasons for discrepancies in study results should be analyzed. On the basis of this discussion, recommendations for relevant future research should be made. All studies have weaknesses. In well-designed, well-conducted, and well-reported studies, the authors themselves will identify the limitations and not leave it up to the reader.

After scrutinizing the different parts of a research report the reader should be in a better position to determine whether the investigators were able to arrive at valid study conclusions. During the design and analysis phase, did the investigators succeed in adequately controlling for the confounding elements always present in research? Campbell and Stanley (1966) elaborate on the many factors that can threaten study validity and the basis for extrapolating results to the general population.

Several references have been made to investigator bias and patient bias, but publication bias and reader bias must also be taken into account. If a trial fails to show efficacy of the therapy, the investigators may not want to publish their results. Or, if the investigators submit their study findings for publica-

tion, many clinical and scientific journals may choose not to publish what may appear to be irrelevant clinical information. Therefore, the general tendency is for a higher percentage of trials with positive outcome to be published (Pocock, 1986). Owen (1982) describes numerous types of reader bias. Some of these biases are prejudices for or against certain therapeutic approaches, investigators, research institutions, and/or journals. All of these factors are likely to influence the reader in the interpretation process.

Further help in critical evaluation of the clinical research literature is provided by, e.g., Cuddy et al. (1983), Gehlbach (1982), and Payton (1988).

Conclusion

Conclusions drawn by reviewers of trials on SMT have not been unanimous. Nevertheless, there appears to be consensus that SMT is a therapeutic approach that in many cases offers more immediate pain relief to patients with spinal-related disorders than other forms of conservative therapy, particularly so in the case of LBP. It is generally agreed that long-term benefits of SMT have not yet been convincingly demonstrated. A number of trials have demonstrated improvement in objective measures, including increased spinal mobility and/or straight leg raising. There are currently no published randomized trials to suggest that SMT is efficacious in the treatment of visceral disorders.

Many chiropractors are of the opinion that SMT is valuable in preventing recurrences of neuromusculoskeletal disorders. Although difficult to design and conduct, future studies need to address the prophylactic value of SMT, as there is as yet no scientific evidence to support it. A multitude of unanswered research questions regarding SMT remain. Future clinical research efforts need to address in which type of disorders, at which stage of these disorders, and with which frequency of application, SMT is likely to be beneficial. Different SMT techniques need to be compared in controlled trials. Does SMT have a role to play in the treatment of certain visceral disorders? Very little is known about the neurobiologic and biomechanical mechanisms involved in SMT. As many of the conditions traditionally treated with SMT, for example, low back pain, are multifactorial disorders, it seems relevant to investigate the effectiveness of SMT in combination with other conservative therapeutic approaches that have been shown to have beneficial effect (e.g., certain back school, exercise, and functional restoration programs).

To provide high quality health care, it is essential that the clinician understand basic research principles and is able to critically evaluate the clinical research literature.

References

Arkuszewski Z. The efficacy of manual treatment in low back pain: A clinical trial. *Manual Med* 1986;2:68–71.

Banks SD. Lumbar facet syndrome: Spinographic assessment of treatment by spinal manipulative therapy. *J Manipulative Physiol Ther* 1983;6:175–180.

Bechgaard P. Late post traumatic headache and manipulation. *Br Med J*, June 1966:1419.

Bergemann BW and Cichoke AJ. Cost effectiveness of medical vs. chiropractic treatment of low-back injuries. *J Manipulative Physiol Ther* 1980;3:143–147.

Bergquist-Ullman M and Larsson U. Acute low back pain in industry. A controlled prospective study with special reference to therapy and confounding factors. *Acta Orthop Scand* 1977;suppl 170:11–117.

Bitterli J et al. Zur Objektivierung der manualtherapeutischen Beeinflussbarkeit des spondylogenen Kopfschmerzes [Objective criteria for the evaluation of chiropractic treatment of spondylotic headaches]. *Nervenarzt* 1977;48;259–262.

Bloch R. Methodology in clinical back pain trials. *Spine* 1987; 12:430–432.

Bosshard R. The treatment of acute lumbago and sciatica. *Ann Swiss Chiropractic Assoc* 1961;2:51–61.

Branson MH and Buerger AA. Randomized clinical trials in the validation of cervical and lumbar manipulation. In Greenman PE, ed. *Concepts and Mechanisms of Neuromuscular Functions*. New York: Springer-Verlag; 1984:90–105.

Breen AC. Chiropractors and the treatment of back pain. *Rheumatol Rehab* 1977;16:46–53.

Bremner RA. Manipulation in the management of chronic low backache due to "lumbosacral strain." *Lancet*, Jan 1958:20–21.

Bremner RA and Simpson M. Management of chronic lumbosacral strain. *Lancet*, Nov 1959:949–950.

Brodin H. Cervical pain and mobilization. *Manuelle Med* 1982;20:90–94.

Bronfort G. Chiropractic treatment of low back pain. A prospective survey. *J Manipulative Physiol Ther* 1986;9:99–113.

Bronfort G. Chiropractic versus general medical treatment of low back pain: a small scale controlled clinical trial. *Am J Chiropractic Medicine* 1989;2:145–150.

Brunarski DJ. Clinical trials of spinal manipulation: A critical appraisal and review of the literature. *J Manipulative Physiol Ther* 1984;7:243–249.

Buerger AA. A controlled trial of rotational manipulation in low back pain. *Manuelle Med* 1980;2:17–26.

Buerger AA and Greenman PE. *Empirical Approaches to the Validation of Spinal Manipulation*. Springfield, Ill: CC Thomas; 1985.

Buerger AA and Tobis JS. *Approaches to the Validation of Manipulation Therapy*. Springfield, Ill: CC Thomas; 1977.

Campbell DT and Stanley JC. *Experimental and Quasi-experimental Designs for Research*. Chicago: Rand McNally; 1966.

Carrick FR. Cervical radiculopathy: The diagnosis and treatment of pathomechanics in the cervical spine. *J Manipulative Physiol Ther* 1983;6:129–137.

Cassidy JD et al. Spinal manipulation for the treatment of chronic low-back and leg pain: An observational study. In Buerger AA and Greenman PE eds. *Empirical Approaches to the Validation of Spinal Manipulation*. Springfield, Ill: CC Thomas;1985:119–148.

Cassidy JD et al. Manipulative management of back pain in patients with spondylolisthesis. *J Can Chiropractic Assoc*, Mar 1978:15–20.

Cherkin DC and MacCormack FA. Patient evaluations of low back pain care from family physicians and chiropractors. *West J Med* 1989;150:351–355.

Choler U et al. *Ont i ryggen-forsog med vardsprogram for patienter med lumbale smerttilstand* [Study of Low Back Patients]. SPRI-Rapport 188/85. Stockholm: Socialstyrelsen; 1985.

Chrisman OD et al. A study of the results following rotatory manipulation in the lumbar intervertebral disc syndrome. *J Bone Joint Surg* [Am] 1964;46:517–524.

Christian GF et al. Immunoreactive ACTH, beta-endorphin, and cortisol levels in plasma following spinal manipulative therapy. *Spine* 1988;13:1411–1417.

Cox JM and Shreiner S. Chiropractic manipulation in low back pain and sciatica: Statistical data on the diagnosis, treatment and response of 576 consecutive cases. *J Manipulative Physiol Ther* 1984;7:1–11.

Cox JM et al. Chiropractic statistical survey of 100 consecutive low back pain patients. *J Manipulative Physiol Ther* 1983;6:117–128.

Coxhead CE et al. Multicentre trial of physiotherapy in the management of sciatic symptoms. *Lancet* 1981;1:1065–1068.

Coyer AB and Curwen IHM. Low back pain treated by manipulation: a controlled series. *Br Med J* Mar 1955:705–707.

Cuddy PG et al. Evaluating the medical literature, Parts I–III. *Ann Emerg Med* 1983;12:549–55, 610–620, 679–686.

Curtis P. Spinal manipulation: Does it work? *Spine, State of the Art Reviews*, Occupational Back Pain, 1987;2:31–44.

Deyo RA. Conservative therapy for low back pain. Distinguishing useful from useless therapy. *JAMA* 1983;250:1057–1062.

DiFabio RP. Clinical assessment of manipulation and mobilization of the lumbar spine. A critical review of the literature. *Phys Ther* 1986;66:51–54.

Dillon R. A comparative study of the treatment of lower back pain by chiropractors and medical physicians in terms of work time loss and treatment cost. *ACA J Chiropractic* 1981;12:18–21.

Doran DM and Newell DJ. Manipulation in treatment of low back pain: A multicentre study. *Br Med J* 1975;2:161–164.

Droz JM. Frequency and causes of recurrence of sciatica. *Ann Swiss Chiropractic Assoc* 1969;4:69–77.

Droz JM and Crot F. Occipital headaches. *Ann Swiss Chiropractic Assoc* 1985;8:127–135.

Durrington L et al. A comparison of spinal manipulation by medical practitioners and chiropractors. *Aust J Soc Issues* 1979;14:126–133.

Edwards BC. Low back pain and pain resulting from lumbar spine conditions. A comparison of treatment results. *Aust J Physiother* 1969;15:104–110.

Ellestad SM et al. Electromyographic and skin responses to osteopathic manipulative treatment for low back pain. *J Am Osteopath Assoc* 1988;88:991–997.

Elston RC and Johnson WD. *Essentials of Biostatistics*. Philadelphia: FA Davis; 1987.

England RW and Deibert PW. Electromyographic studies. Part I. Consideration in the evaluation of osteopathic therapy. *J Am Osteopath Assoc* 1972;72:221–223.

Evans DP et al. Lumbar spinal manipulation on trial. *Rheumatol Rehab* 1978;17:46–53.

Fairbank JCT et al. The Oswestry low back pain questionnaire. *Physiotherapy* 1980;66:271–273.

Farrell JP and Twomey LT. Acute low back pain. Comparison of two conservative treatment approaches. *Med J Aust* 1982;1:160–164.

Fichera AP and Celander DR. Effect of osteopathic manipulative therapy on autonomic tone as evidenced by blood pressure changes and activity of the fibrinolytic system. *J Am Osteopath Assoc* 1969;68:1036–1038.

Fisk JW. Manipulation in general practice. *NZ Med J* 1971;74:172–175.

Fisk JW. A controlled trial of manipulation in a selected group of patients with low back pain favoring one side. *NZ Med J* 1979;90:288–291.

Fonti S and Lynch M. Etiopathogenesis of lumbosciatalgia due to disc disease. Chiropractic treatment (statistics on 3,136 patients). In Mazzarelli JP, ed. *Chiropractic Interprofessional Research*. Torino, Italy: Edizioni Minerva Medica;1983/1984:53–57.

Freiman JA et al. The importance of beta, the type II error and sample size in the design and interpretation of the randomized control trial. *N Engl J Med* 1978;299:690–694.

Gehlback SH. *Interpreting the Medical Literature: Practical Epidemiology for Clinicians.* Macmillan Publishing Company, 1988.

Gibson T et al. Controlled comparison of short-wave diathermy treatment with osteopathic treatment in non-specific low back pain. *Lancet* 1985;1:1258–1261.

Gill K et al. Repeatability of four clinical methods for assessment of lumbar spinal motion. *Spine* 1988;13:50–53.

Glantz SA. Biostatistics: How to detect, correct and prevent errors in the medical literature. *Circulation* 1980;61-1-7.

Glover JR et al. Back pain: A randomized clinical trial of rotational manipulation of the trunk. *Br J Ind Med* 1974;31:59–64.

Godfrey CM et al. A randomized trial of manipulation for low-back pain in a medical setting. *Spine* 1984;9:301–304.

Godfrey K. Statistics in practice: Comparing the means of several groups. *N Engl J Med* 1985;313:1450–1456.

Goldstein M. *The Research Status of Spinal Manipulative Therapy.* NINCDS Monograph No. 15. Bethesda: DHEW; 1975.

Gray FJ. Combination of traction and manipulation for the lumbar disc syndrome. *Med J Aust* 1967;13:958–961.

Greenland S et al. Controlled trials of manipulation: A review and a proposal. *J Occup Med* 1980;22:670–676.

Greenman PE. *Concepts and Mechanisms of Neuromuscular Functions.* New York: Springer-Verlag; 1984.

Grice AS and Tschumi PC. Pre- and postmanipulation lateral bending radiographic study and relation to muscle function of the low back. *Ann Swiss Chiropractic Assoc* 1985;8:149–165.

Guyatt G et al. Determining optimal therapy—Randomized trials in individual patients. *N Engl J Med* 1986;314:889–892.

Hadler NM et al. A benefit of spinal manipulation as adjunctive therapy for acute low-back pain: A stratified controlled trial. *Spine* 1987;12:702–706.

Haldeman S. Basic principles in establishing a chiropractic clinical trial. *ACA J Chiropractic,* May 1978; 33–37.

Haldeman S. Spinal manipulative therapy: A status report. *Clin Orthop* 1983;179:62–70.

Henderson RS. The treatment of lumbar intervertebral disc protrusion. An assessment of conservative measures. *Br Med J,* Sept 13, 1952:597–598.

Heyse-Moore GH. A rational approach to the use of epidural medication in the treatment of sciatic pain. *Acta Orthop Scand* 1978;49:366–370.

Hoehler FK and Tobis JS. Low back pain and its treatment by spinal manipulation: Measures of flexibility and asymmetry. *Rheumatol Rehab* 1982;21:21–26.

Hoehler FK and Tobis JS. Appropriate statistical methods for clinical trials of spinal manipulation. *Spine* 1987;12:409–411.

Hoehler FK et al. Spinal manipulation for low back pain. *JAMA* 1981;245:1835–1838.

Howe DH et al. Manipulation of the cervical spine. A pilot study. *J R Coll Gen Pract* 1983;33:574–579.

Howe J and Frymoyer JW. The effect of questionnaire design on the determination of end results in lumbar spinal surgery. *Spine* 1985;10:804–805.

Hoyt WH et al. Osteopathic manipulation in the treatment of muscle-contraction headache. *J Am Osteopath Assoc* 1979;78:322–325.

Hutton SR. Combination of traction and manipulation in the lumbar disc syndrome. *Med J Aust,* June 1967:1196.

Hviid C. A comparison of the effect of chiropractic treatment on respiratory function in patients with respiratory distress symptoms and patients without. *Bull Eur Chiropractic Union* 1978;26:17–34.

Hviid H. The influence of the chiropractic treatment on the rotary mobility of the cervical spine–A kinesiometric and statistical study. *Ann Swiss Chiropractic Assoc* 1971;5:31–44.

Jamison JR et al. Asthma in a chiropractic clinic: A pilot study. *J Aust Chiropractic Assoc* 1986;16:137–143.

Jayson MIV et al. Mobilization and manipulation for low-back pain. *Spine* 1981;6:409–416.

Johnson MR et al. Treatment and cost of back or neck injury—A literature review. *Res Forum* 1985;1:68–78.

Johnson MR et al. A comparison of chiropractic, medical and osteopathic care for work-related sprains and strains. *J Manipulative Physiol Ther* 1989;12:335–344.

Kane RL et al. Manipulating the patient. A comparison of the effectiveness of physician and chiropractor care. *Lancet,* June 1974:1333–1336.

Kazdin AE. *Single-Case Research Designs. Methods for Clinical and Applied Settings.* New York: Oxford University Press; 1982.

Keating JC et al. Toward an experimental chiropractic: Time-series designs. *J Manipulative Physiol Ther* 1985;8:229–238.

Kinalski R et al. The comparison of the results of manual therapy versus physiotherapy methods used in treatment of patients with low back syndromes. *Manual Med* 1989;4:44–46.

Kirkaldy-Willis WH and Cassidy JD. Spinal manipulation in the treatment of low-back pain. *Can Fam Physician* 1985;31:535–540.

Klougart N et al. Infantile colic treated by chiropractors: A prospective study of 316 cases. *J Manipulative Physiol Ther* 1989;12:281–288.

Kogstad OA et al. Cervicobrachialgia. A controlled trial with conventional therapy and manipulation. *Tidsskr Nor Laegeforen* 1978;98:845–848.

Korr IM. *The Neurobiologic Mechanisms in Manipulative Therapy.* New York: Plenum Press; 1978.

Kukurin GW. Chiropractic and spinal manipulative therapy: A critical review of the literature. *ACA J Chiropractic* 1985;19:41–49.

Kuo PP and Loh Z. Treatment of lumbar intervertebral disc protrusions by manipulation. *Clin Orthop* 1987;215:47–55.

Lankhorst GF et al. Objectivity and repeatability of measurements in low back pain. *Scand J Rehab Med* 1982;14:21–26.

Leach RA. An evaluation of the effect of chiropractic manipulative therapy on hypolordosis of the cervical spine. *J Manipulative Physiol Ther* 1983;6:17–23.

Leaverton PE. *A Review of Biostatistics. A Program for Self-Instruction.* Boston: Little, Brown; 1986.

Leboeuf C et al. Chiropractic treatment of repetitive strain injuries. A preliminary prospective outcome study of SMT versus SMT combined with massage. *J Aust Chiropractic Assoc* 1987;17:11–14.

Leboeuf C et al. Chiropractic care of children with nocturnal enuresis: A prospective outcome study. *J Manipulative Physiol Ther* 1991;14:110–115.

Levine JL and Lebacqz K. Ethical considerations in clinical trials. In Abrams N and Buckner MD, eds. *Medical Ethics. A Clinical Textbook and Reference for the Health Care Professions.* Cambridge, Mass: MIT Press; 1984.

Lewit K. Ligament pain and anteflexion headache. *Eur Neurol* 1971;5:365–378.

Lewith GT and Turner GMT. Retrospective analysis of the management of acute low back pain. *Practitioner* 1982;226:1614–1618.

Livingston M. Spinal manipulation: A one year follow-up study. *Can Fam Physician,* July 1969:35–38.

Luisetto G et al. Plasma levels of beta-endorphin and calcitonin before and after manipulative treatment of patients with cervical arthrosis and Barre's syndrome. In Mazzarelli JP, ed. *Chi4prac-*

tic Interprofessional Research. Torino, Italy: Edizioni Minerva Medica; 1983/1984:47–52.

Mabeck CE and Vejlsgaard R. Multipractice studies: Significance of the information given to participating doctors. *J R Coll Gen Pract* 1980;30(214):283–284.

MacDonald RS and Bell CMJ. An open controlled assessment of osteopathic manipulation in nonspecific low-back pain. *Spine* 1990;15:364–370.

Mathews JA and Yates DAH. Reduction of lumbar disc prolapse by manipulation. *Br Med J* 1969;3:696–697.

Mathews JA et al. Back pain and sciatica: Controlled trials of manipulation, traction, sclerosant and epidural injections. *Br J Rheumatol* 1987;26:416–423.

Mayer TG and Gatchel RJ. Objective assessment of spine function following industrial injury: A prospective study with comparison group and one-year follow-up. *Spine* 1985;10:482–493.

McKnight ME and DeBoer KF. Preliminary study of blood pressure changes in normotensive subjects undergoing chiropractic care. *J Manipulative Physiol Ther* 1988;11:261–266.

Meade TW et al. Comparison of chiropractic and hospital outpatient management of low back pain: A feasibility study. *J Epidemiol Community Health* 1986;40:12–17.

Meade TW et al. Low back pain of mechanical origin: Randomized comparison of chiropractic and hospital outpatient treatment. *Br Med J* 1990;300:1431–1437.

Mensor MC. Non-operative treatment including manipulation for lumbar intervertebral disc syndrome. *J Bone Joint Surg [Am]* 1955;37:925–936.

Mierau D et al. A comparison of the effectiveness of spinal manipulative therapy for low back pain patients with and without spondylolisthesis. *J Manipulative Physiol Ther* 1987;10:49–55.

Miller WD. Treatment of visceral disorders by manipulative therapy. In Goldstein M, ed. *NINCDS Monograph.* Bethesda, Md: DHEW; 1975:295–301. The Research Status of Spinal Manipulative Therapy.

Million R et al. Assessment of the progress of the back-pain patient. *Spine* 1982;7:204–212.

Morgan JP et al. A controlled trial of spinal manipulation in the management of hypertension. *J Am Osteopath Assoc* 1985; 85:308–313.

Moritz U. Evaluation of manipulation and other manual therapy. Criteria for measuring the effect of treatment. *Scand J Rehab Med* 1979;11:173–179.

Nachemson A. Work for all: For those with low back pain as well. *Clin Orthop* 1983;179:77–85.

Nelson K et al. Assessment of function in routine clinical practice: Description of the coop chart method and preliminary findings. *J Chron Dis* 1987;40:55S–63S.

Nilsson N and Christiansen B. Prognostic factors in bronchial asthma in chiropractic practice. *J Aust Chiropractic Assoc* 1988;18:85–87.

Norman GR and Streiner DL. *PDQ Statistics.* Philadelphia: BC Decker Inc; 1986.

Nwuga VCB. Relative therapeutic efficacy of vertebral manipulation and conventional treatment in back pain management. *Am J Phys Med* 1982;61:273–278.

Ongley MJ et al. A new approach to the treatment of chronic low back pain. *Lancet* 1987;2:143–146.

Orpwood Price DI. Manipulative methods for treating locomotor pain in general practice. *J R Coll Gen Pract* 1971;21:214–220.

Ottenbacher K and DiFabio RP. Efficacy of spinal manipulation/mobilization therapy: A meta-analysis. *Spine* 1985;10: 833–837.

Owen R. Reader bias. *JAMA* 1982;247:233–234.

Parker GB et al. A controlled trial of cervical manipulation for migraine. *Aust NZ J Med* 1978;8:589–593.

Parker GB et al. Why does migraine improve during a clinical trial? Further results from a trial of cervical manipulation for migraine. *Aust NZ J Med* 1980;10:192–198.

Parson WB and Cummings JDA. Manipulation in back pain. *Can Med Assoc J* 1958;79:103–109.

Payton OD. *Research: The Validation of Clinical Practice.* Philadelphia: FA Davis; 1988.

Pearcy M. Measurement of back and spinal mobility. *Clin Biomech* 1986;1:44–51.

Pocock SJ. *Clinical Trials. A Practical Approach.* Chichester, England: Wiley; 1986.

Postacchini F et al. Efficacy of various forms of conservative treatment in low back pain. A comparative study. *Neuro-Orthopedics* 1988;6:28–35.

Potter GE. A study of 744 cases of neck and back pain treated with spinal manipulation. *J Can Chiropractic Assoc,* Dec 1977:154–156.

Rasmussen GG. Manipulation in treatment of low back pain. A randomized clinical trial. *Manuelle Med* 1979;1:8–10.

Riches EW. End results in manipulation of the back. *Lancet* 1930;1:957–959.

Rimm AA et al. *Basic Statistics in Medicine and Epidemiology.* New York: Appleton-Century-Crofts; 1980.

Roberts GM et al. Lumbar spinal manipulation on trial. Part II. Radiological assessment. *Rheumatol Rehab* 1978;17:54–59.

Roland M and Morris R. A study of the natural history of low back pain, Parts I & II. *Spine* 1983;8:141–150.

Rosendahl B. Manipulationsbehandling av cervikal- och thorakalcolumna [Manipulative therapy of the cervical and thoracic spine]. *Nord Med* 1963;69:681–684.

Salvi S et al. Clinical evaluation of chiropractic treatment of lumbosciatica. In Mazzarelli JP, ed. *Chiropractic Interprofessional Research.* Torino, Italy: Edizioni Minerva Medica; 1983/1984: 121–124.

Sanders GE et al. Chiropractic adjustive manipulation on subjects with acute low back pain: Visual analog pain scores and plasma beta-endorphin levels. *J Manipulative Physiol Ther* 1990;13: 391–395.

Scott J and Huskisson EC. Graphic representation of pain. *Pain* 1976;2:175–184.

Shambaugh P. Changes in electrical activity in muscles resulting from chiropractic adjustment: A pilot study. *J Manipulative Physiol Ther* 1987;10:300–303.

Shanghai Institute et al. Manipulation in lumbar intervertebral disc protrusion. *Chin Med J* 1977;3:31–36.

Sheladia VL and Johnston DA. Efficacy of various chiropractic treatments, age distribution and incidence of accident- and non-accident-caused low back pain in male and female patients. *J Manipulative Physiol Ther* 1986;9:243–247.

Siehl D et al. Manipulation of the lumbar spine with the patient under general anesthesia: An evaluation by EMG and clinical–neurologic examination of its use for lumbar nerve root compression. *J Am Osteopath Assoc* 1971;70:433–441.

Sims-Williams H et al. Controlled trial of mobilization and manipulation for patients with low back pain in general practice. *Br Med J* 1978;2:1338–1340.

Sims-Williams H et al. Controlled trial of mobilization and manipulation for low back pain: Hospital patients. *Br Med J* 1979;2: 1318–1320.

Sloop PR et al. Manipulation for chronic neck pain. A double-blind controlled study. *Spine* 1982;7:532–535.

Solomon GF. Psychoneuroimmunology: Interactions between central nervous system and immune system. *J Neurosci Res* 1987;18:1–9.

Spiro HM. *Doctors, Patients and Placebos.* New Haven, Conn: Yale University Press; 1986.

Stewart AL et al. Functional status and well-being of patients with chronic conditions. Results from the medical outcomes study. *JAMA* 1989;262:907–913.

Stodolny J and Chmielewski H. Manual therapy in the treatment of patients with cervical migraine. *Manual Med* 1989;4:49–51.

Stokke O. *Statistikk om Kiropraktikk [Statistics on Chiropractic]*. Oslo, Norway: Universitets-forlaget; 1977.

Terrett ACJ and Vernon H. Manipulation and pain tolerance: A controlled study of the effect of spinal manipulation on paraspinal cutaneous pain tolerance levels. *Am J Phys Med* 1984;63:217–225.

Tobis JS and Hoehler FK. Musculoskeletal manipulation in the treatment of low back pain. *Bull NY Acad Med* 1983;59:660–668.

Tobis JS and Hoehler F. *Musculoskeletal Manipulation. Evaluation of the Scientific Evidence*. Springfield, Ill: CC Thomas; 1986.

Triano JJ and Schultz AB. Correlation of objective measure of trunk motion and muscle function with low back disability rating. *Spine* 1987;12:561–565.

Tufvesson B et al. Strack- och manipulationsbehandling av landryggen [Traction and manipulation of the low back]. *Lakartidningen* 1976;73:1088–1090.

Turk Z and Ratkolb O. Mobilization of the cervical spine in chronic headaches. *Manual Med* 1987;3:15–17.

Valentini E. Acute lumbar disc syndromes under chiropractic care. A two year statistical study. *Ann Swiss Chiropractic Assoc* 1981; 7:67–83.

Vernon H. Chiropractic manipulative therapy in the treatment of headaches: A retrospective and prospective study. *J Manipulative Physiol Ther* 1982;5:109–112.

Vernon HT et al. Spinal manipulation and beta-endorphin: A controlled study of the effect of a spinal manipulation on plasma beta-endorphin levels in normal males. *J Manipulative Physiol Ther* 1986;9:115–123.

Waagen GN et al. Short-term trial of chiropractic treatment for the relief of chronic low back pain. *Manual Med* 1986;2:63–67.

Wagnon RJ et al. Serum aldosterone changes after specific chiropractic manipulation. *Am J Chiropractic Med* 1988;1:66–70.

Warr AC et al. Chronic lumbosciatic syndrome treated by epidural injection and manipulation. *Practitioner* 1972;209:53–59.

Waterworth RF and Hunter IA. An open study of diflunisal, conservative and manipulative therapy in the management of acute mechanical low back pain. *NZ Med J* 1985;98:372–375.

Wight JS. Migraine: A statistical analysis of chiropractic treatment. *ACA J Chiropractic* 1978; 15:28–32.

Wilson DG. Results of manipulation in general practice. *Proc R Soc Med* 1967;60:971–972.

Wilson JN and Ilfeld FW. Manipulation of the herniated intervertebral disc. *Am J Surg*, Feb 1952:173–175.

Winer CER. A survey of controlled clinical trials of spinal manipulation. In *Aspects of Manipulative Therapy*. New York: Churchill Livingstone; 1985:97–108.

Wing LW and Hargrave-Wilson W. Cervical vertigo. *Aust NZ J Surg* 1974;44:275–277.

Wolk S. *An Analysis of Florida Worker's Compensation Medical and Indemnity Claims for Back-Related Injuries*. Arlington, Va: Foundation Chiro Ed & Research; 1988:1–29.

Yates RG et al. Effects of chiropractic treatment on blood pressure and anxiety: A randomized, controlled trial. *J Manipulative Physiol Ther* 1988;11:484–488.

Zylbergold RS and Piper MC. Lumbar disc disease: Comparative analysis of physical therapy treatments. *Arch Phys Med Rehab* 1981;62:176–179.

chapter 25

Basic Principles in the Performance of Chiropractic Adjusting: Historical Review, Classification, and Objectives

Adrian Grice
Howard Vernon

This chapter presents a brief historical overview of the development of chiropractic procedures and concepts, and then discusses the characteristics and classification of the adjustment and paratherapeutic procedures.

Evolution of Adjustment Technique

The first chiropractic adjustment delivered by Palmer on Harvey Lilliard has been described and even debated by many authors and has assumed a mythical status in chiropractic literature. Such debate and discussion were characteristic of the emerging chiropractic profession and began early in the development of adjustive procedures and paratherapeutic chiropractic procedures.

In the early 1900s, a number of techniques rapidly developed, coupled with the emergence of strongly principled belief systems. Stephenson (1927) was one of the first authors to categorize the early development of techniques into four biomechanical descriptors: (1) the shove, (2) the push–pull, (3) the recoil, and (4) the toggle recoil. Along with biomechanical advancements in spinal corrective methods came theoretic concepts that altered the application of chiropractic treatment and often established the basis for the formation of a new school. These early schools initiated slightly different philosophical explanations and methodologies of application of therapy.

The Palmer School of Chiropractic

The first school of chiropractic was initiated by D. D. Palmer who taught his son B. J. Palmer and others his early adjustive procedures and the principles of practice as he saw them. The Palmer Infirmary and Chiropractic Institute was founded in the late 1890s. Later, B. J. Palmer took over the clinic and changed the institute in 1904 to the Palmer School of Chiropractic. It was incorporated in 1905 as an educational institute in Davenport, Iowa, where an organized curriculum in chiropractic began (Dye, 1939).

The first Palmer school of teaching developed the concept that the adjustment replaced displaced vertebrae and, therefore, treated disease by relieving impingement on nerves. D. D. Palmer (1910) stated that "the first chiropractic adjustment was given to Harvey Lillard in September 1895"; he further stated that with this incident an "important question was answered by the discovery that displaced (subluxated) vertebrae impinged nerves, which are tubular cords of the same substances as that which composes the brain and spinal cord and where functions are to convey impulses and symptoms to and from nerve centers. This pressure caused by projections modifies the force of Innate's desire; therefore, disease is but aberrated impulse, increase or decrease from that which is normal."

D. D. Palmer (1910) described disease as "nothing more or less than functions performed in either a too great or too little degree." Health was described as functions "performed in a normal or a natural amount as desired by Innate." His theory was that "pressure on nerves causes irritation and tension with deranged function as a result." Practice was therefore formulated simply: locate the subluxated vertebra, adjust it, and thereby correct the cause of disease and allow the self-healing (Innate) to restore the body to health. D. D. Palmer, along with B. J. Palmer, emphasized that a vertebra was subluxated by static malposition of the vertebral body and that palpation was one of the most important examinations used to diagnose these abnormalities, which both Palmers felt were quite common.

B. J. Palmer (1908-1911) developed the "Meric System" of adjusting. Anatomic charts showing the spinal level of the autonomic nerve distribution to each organ were used to explain chiropractic results. It was clearly postulated that adjustments of subluxated vertebrae corrected organ function in the re-

lated vertemere. Clinical results and the observation that subluxations did occur in the spinal levels related to the dysfunctional organs confirmed this hypothesis to the satisfaction of chiropractic clinicians. Spinal analysis used not only palpation but also nerve tracing, i.e., increased areas of skin temperature in relation to the subluxation. At first, both D. D. Palmer and B. J. Palmer felt that only five to six vertebrae should be adjusted in the entire spine (Dye, 1939). In 1910, the concept of the Major (spinal subluxation) and Minor (spinal subluxation) was developed and, with it, the number of adjustments to be given was reduced to major areas or two or three areas in the whole spine.

B. J. Palmer's influence and writing in 1908-1911 was significant. He developed the recoil adjustment, which he felt was superior to the slower lunge thrust more commonly in use at that time, and was the first to use spinal x-ray for diagnosis at Palmer School of Chiropractic. His text, *An Exposition of Old Moves* (Palmer, 1911-1916) reviewed a number of full-spine adjustments. The "Palmer recoil adjustment" was, in his view, superior because he reasoned that the effect of the adjustment was "a combination of that external force and the internal innate recoil force within the patient." His theory was that innate intelligence, or the body, in the final analysis "set the bone," not the doctor; therefore, it was important to "set the bone" in motion and allow the body to recoil and establish the final position (Palmer, 1908-1911). Further emphasis was thus placed on the body's ability to self-regulate and heal. Dye points out that other factors were involved in the development and exclusive use of the recoil; probably most important was that this procedure was less painful than the stiff arm thrust on the unpadded bench that caused patients to tense their muscles and resist. In this new procedure, the doctor's muscles and the patient's muscles were completely relaxed prior to the thrust. The recoil adjustment also allowed a setup and contact that took into consideration the direction of the thrust and the position of the displaced vertebra more precisely than the stiff arm adjustment, which by some was delivered straightforwardly or directly anterior (Dye, 1939).

In Volume III of B. J. Palmer's *Science of Chiropractic*, compiled in 1908-1911, careful studies were made of numerous anatomic specimens. As a result, palpation techniques were modified and refined. Lines of drive and positioning for adjustments of cervical, thoracic, and lumbar regions were developed, most of which were based primarily on the recoil adjustment. This adjustment used the utmost care for line of drive and patient position in its setup. Little or no prestress force was used, and speed of the thrust and rapid release were considered important. Prior to the thrust, the patient's position was neutral, that is, with the passive range of motion taken out of the segment involved. The thrust on the lumbar and thoracic regions was often a triceps thrust combined with a body drop. The knee–chest position was used for lumbar adjustments. The adjustment was applied on the basis of the Meric System, using the concepts of Majors and Minors. Static palpation and specific listings were given to vertebrae; and soft tissue palpation for sensitivity, pain or tenderness, and skin temperature change (''hot box'') was used in clinical diagnosis. The last test was called nerve tracing, and complex patterns were traced and related to subluxations (Palmer, 1911).

Nerve tracing originated with D. D. Palmer, who thought that the nerves exerted a calorific effect through which they heated the body. B. J. Palmer and others developed (1) examination techniques called nerve tracings, (2) palpation of skin temperature for ''hot boxes,'' and (3) palpation for taut and tender fibers, all of which were related to spinal subluxation. To improve diagnosis, B. J. Palmer invented the neurocalometer around 1924–1925 to more accurately measure skin temperature changes. This device was considered essential in diagnosis and assessment of a patient's progress.

Common clinical experience and theoretical and philosophical reasoning indicated to B. J. Palmer that the atlas was the most frequently subluxated region and the most important area with respect to clinical results. In searching for mechanisms to explain clinical results and to support philosophical beliefs, B. J. Palmer reasoned that cord pressure or traction was important in the ''dis-ease'' process. As all nerves pass through the atlas, and because his investigations with instrumentation and dissection convinced him that this was the level at which the greatest nerve pressure could be applied, he refined the recoil to the ''hole-in-one'' atlas recoil technique, which was used to adjust mainly the atlas and on occasion the axis. B. J. Palmer introduced the ''hole-in-one'' technique at Lyceum in 1930 (Dye, 1939).

The American School of Chiropractic

The American School of Chiropractic, founded and headed by Smith, Langworthy, and Paxson, who wrote the text *Modernized Chiropractic* (1906), suggested that naprapathy formed one of the roots of chiropractic. These authors and teachers discussed several concepts related to the subluxation. Vertebral joints were seen to have a range or field of motion as well as a normal axis of motion. They pictured the subluxation as a wheel whose hub was off-center. Thus, as early as 1906 the important concept of vertebral dynamics was born. Diagnoses included static palpation, early motion evaluation, inspection, gait analysis, and nerve tracing.

Smith et al. (1906) set forward the concepts necessary for proper chiropractic practice: (1) a correct philosophy, (2) well-developed technique, (3) a dependable system of diagnosis, and (4) a reliable and extensive system of care. Further development of short-lever techniques occurred, using, as levers, the spinous process, the transverse process, or the ribs, with double and single contacts: in addition, two-person techniques and strap fixing to provide traction and stabilization to ease the application of adjustive techniques were developed. Traction was seen as an adjunct to chiropractic treatment, and traction treatment tables were introduced separately and as part of the adjustment table with both steady and intermittent applications. Procedures were taken from other sources, e.g., lay Bohemian methods and osteopathic methods. Examples of these expanded procedures include the strap thrust technique for ribs and the long-lever techniques for lumbars. Treatment was still based on a static listing; however, restoration of movement and consideration of the forces (muscles) involved became part of the diagnosis. Techniques were demonstrated for peripheral joints as well, particularly for the rib cage and foot (Smith et al., 1906). Treatment took into consideration muscle forces, other anatomic structures, and overall body posture.

These authors made a distinction between three forms of adjustive thrust: (1) fast delivery, rapid release; (2) fast delivery, slow release; (3) slow delivery or pressure thrusts.

Overall, the body was seen as a vital machine, self-healing and self-regulatory. Less emphasis was placed on disease or conditions; more emphasis was placed on normal bony alignment, joint motion, soft tissue function, and the self-regulatory systems of the body.

The National College of Chiropractic

In 1906 the National College of Chiropractic was in operation. This school eventually also taught drugless therapy methods with electrotherapy, hydrotherapy, muscle techniques, massage, as well as the use of remedies both internally and externally applied. These contrasting principles of practice formed the foundation for the ''mixer/straight'' dichotomy in clinical chiropractic.

Forster (1915), a graduate of the National College in Chicago, presented ten characteristics of spinal subluxation: pain, thickening and tenderness of nerves, temperature change, disturbed function, contracted ligaments, reduced mobility, change in anatomic structures related to the spine, and vertebral malalignments were included in the list. Diagnosis of the subluxation was accomplished by inspection, palpation, and x-ray.

The classification of adjustments by Forster (1915) included cervical adjustments—rotary, lateral, superior–inferior, compression, scoliotic, and anterior (15 adjustments); dorsal adjustments—posterior, kyphotic, lordotic, scoliotic compression, superior–inferior, lateral, and rotary (39 adjustments); lumbar adjustments—posterior, kyphotic, lordotic, scoliotic, compression superior–inferior, anterior (L-5), and rotary (26 adjustments).

The Howard System

The Howard System (Howard, ca. 1920), based on Dr. John Howard's lectures at the National School of Chiropractic, is a broad system of chiropractic practice. This system focused on the nervous system but recognized environmental and hereditary factors as well. Diagnosis was basically by static alignment, but spinal movement was also considered, as were structural deficits, such as scoliosis and joint pathology. Adjustments, along with massage techniques, stripping, vibrating, and so forth, were made not only for biomechanical faults but also for diseases. Mobilization and exercise procedures for disc therapy, diet, and mental or suggestive therapy were presented. These broader drugless methods had their origin much earlier in chiropractic (McNamara, 1913).

Arnholz (1949) presented further ideas on the treatment of the spastic muscle using pressure, stripping techniques, and muscle manipulative procedures. These were taught secondary to adjustive techniques and were further systematized by Nimmo (1957, 1963).

The Carver College of Chiropractic

In 1907, the Carver College of Chiropractic was established, and many new adjustive procedures and treatments were taught. Carver (1909) classified sources of stimulation, motor reaction, and occlusion of nerves as articular, ossific, skeletal tissue, visceral tissue, lacerational, contusional, disintegrational, and enlargement. The last two classifications dealt with chemical causes and inflammatory causes of nerve interference. Adjustive procedures and treatments were developed for peripheral joints, muscles, fascia, ligaments, and visceral organs. Carver developed the concept that normal body function of neuromusculoskeletal structures related to health, and abnormality, particularly functional abnormality, of these structures, local or general, related to disease. Carver recognized physical, chemical, and mental causes of abnormal function, and therefore disease. He presented the art of adjustment as producing a "shocklike" effect on the nervous system similar to many other "shocks," thus expanding the explanation of how the nervous system was affected not only by pressure or irritation of nerve structures but also by reflex activity. (D. D. Palmer's "too much or too little" concept was thus expanded.) Carver's (1915) text systematically presented adjustments of all skeletal joints, viscera, and soft tissue, and included massage techniques. He considered the body as a whole, suggesting that the musculoskeletal system was in fact a coordinated system and that the therapist should approach the total body as an integrated system. He therefore taught that diet, footwear, clothing, posture, exercise, emotions, and other factors were important in chiropractic practice.

His treatment emphasized adjustive procedures, which included short-lever techniques using the spinous process and transverse process as levers, long-lever techniques for muscles, lumbar spine, and pelvis, as well as visceral adjustments and peripheral joint adjustments. Carver (1921–1924) promoted various spinal adjustments. Cervical adjustments included the prone Carver occipital lift for C0–C1-2 modified for lower cervicals; prone, supine, and lateral cervical adjustments; and prone, supine, and sitting cervical rotational adjustments. In the thoracic region, not only was the thumb move taught, but also thrusts to relax the musculature, recoil adjustments, and a saddle-back two-hand adjustment to assist in correction of lordosis. Carver felt that in a scoliosis or lordosis a key vertebral unit was present in the curve and a specific adjustment could correct this curvature. The lumbar spine was adjusted as a unit with prone adjustments. The same position for the sacrum and pelvis was used. A pelvic roll or cushion was employed to enhance and facilitate the adjustment. Particular emphasis was placed on a concept of normal compensation of the spine in the form of four opposite rotational scolioses. The neurologic relationship of musculoskeletal function (Meric System) formed the basis for spinal vertebral adjustment in the treatment of many named diseases.

The Carver school developed many areas of specialization and, because it was concerned with the whole system, general health suggestions became important. Views on personal and public sanitation, hygiene, housing, safety, protection of air, and water, ventilation, heating, lighting, fumigation methods, disinfection, special care of the sick, foods and food toxins, vitamins and minerals, and exercise were presented in *Hygiene and Pediatrics* (Craven, 1924) along with special adjustive procedures for infants as well as procedures for specific problems. Under Carver, chiropractic emphasized the total person's health, the body's recuperative powers, and the role of the musculoskeletal systems in health and disease.

DeJarnette

DeJarnette (1938) emphasized "the disease of abnormal posture," extending Carver's views that related normal structure to normal function. Examination of the patient was expanded to include individual joint testing and the relationship between muscles, ligamentous holding elements, and pain. DeJarnette understood subluxation to be an effect as well as a cause. He believed that imbalance of muscles caused bony malalignment, which in turn could be caused by metabolic changes, congestion, and spinal nerve pressure. Diseases of the viscera were seen to produce muscular joint changes in the corresponding dermatome and myotome. Thus, muscle spasm and vertebral subluxation are seen to be both cause and effect.

DeJarnette (1937) discussed the fact that nerves could inhibit as well as stimulate, and emphasized that muscle function was influenced by mechanical, chemical, electrical, and thermal factors. He made what was, to some at that time a heretical statement: ''We do not believe that the subluxation of the vertebrae or vertebra are always the primary cause of disease.'' He stated that the ''muscular system, due to abnormal fatigue or muscle tension, is the primary cause of disease.'' DeJarnette thought that the spinal roots, through congestion, overexcitement, or excessive stimulation, produced muscle hypertension. Spinal adjustments, massage, heat, and other modalities were therefore considered beneficial. The thrust was seen to reduce muscle spasm and stimulate or inhibit the nervous system. Through clinical observations and on the basis of anatomic relationships, DeJarnette developed many reflex pressure techniques and interrelated points to treat pain and spasm. The occipital and sacroiliac regions became the main focus. He developed his own reflex techniques to correct pelvic distortions. In his assessment, postural analysis (plumbline) and leg length evaluation were the most important diagnostic criteria in selecting and monitoring the effect of the adjustive procedures.

The Development of Diversified Techniques

Janse, Hauser, and Wells (1947) wrote an extensive review called *Chiropractic Principles and Techniques*, in which they attempted to establish the anatomic, physiologic, neurologic, and physical bases for chiropractic practice. Factors in disease other than the nervous system were recognized but the unique ability of the body to avoid some illnesses or to recover from others was seen as an integrated function of the nervous system. As nervous system function was viewed to be altered by skeletal dysfunction, the underlying cause of disease was seen to be neuromusculoskeletal dysfunction.

Subluxation was viewed as a vertebra relatively fixed in abnormal position, no longer functioning in normal movements of the spine. Chronicity of a subluxation was seen to be related to the holding elements—muscles, ligaments, and discs. The intervertebral foramina were viewed as the important location of interference to nerves, blood vessels, and lymphatic vessels. Subluxation and/or impingement caused increased activity or irritability or a decrease in nerve activity. Increase in motor response was thought to be responsible for increased tone or muscle tension related to a subluxation; however, increased muscle tone was also seen as being a result of the sensory input for all types of stimuli, e.g., physical, mental, or chemical.

Janse et al. (1947) clearly stated that subluxation was an important cause of disease but qualified it by commenting that the concept ''that the subluxation of vertebra is the one and only cause of disease is incorrect.'' They recognized other factors, such as environmental influences, but stated that a subluxation could be the direct or indirect cause of some diseases, a predisposing factor in other diseases, and an inducing or perpetuating factor in still others. The neural mechanisms that were disturbed in a subluxation were those of the normal afferent input or normal efferent motor output; therefore, treatment was directed toward correcting and reestablishing this reflex balance. Thus, there was a definite shift in emphasis from subluxation as the only cause of disease, to subluxation as the most important factor in regulation of the body. Examination took into consideration body posture, static alignment, motion in relationship to the spine and vertebral segments, organ function, and nerve supply (as an extension of the Meric System), muscle tension, ligament and disc contractures, and sensory changes, including tenderness, pain, and temperature.

Three main areas of spinal diagnosis were presented: (1) Inspection included posture and gait with plumbline analysis and spinal movement. (2) Palpation included temperature change, muscle and ligament change, sensory changes, skin changes, osseous landmarks, and nerve tracing through skin sensitivity. (3) X-ray included pathology, anatomic variation, and x-ray marking for subluxation. Treatment was directed toward normalizing osseous structure and soft tissues including muscles, ligaments, and discs. The thrust given was modified according to need—slow pressure, dynamic, or rhythmic. More than 117 procedures were presented including spinal adjustments, peripheral joint adjustments, and sinus and organ techniques. These techniques, with only slight modifications, continue to be used by the majority of chiropractors and often are referred to as ''diversified techniques.'' This term seems to have originated from the opinion that the specific recoil or toggle technique developed and emphasized by B. J. Palmer and adopted by many practitioners was too restrictive for general practice. Diversified technique allowed a broad, total body approach based on an anatomic–physiological understanding and was not usually connected to a system or individual. Diversified techniques often became the core techniques taught at various chiropractic schools.

Named specific techniques or technique systems, often taught on a postgraduate basis by field practitioners or groups not necessarily connected directly with any chiropractic school, also formed an important part of the historical development of chiropractic techniques as practiced today. Many stimulatory, vibratory, and percussion reflex procedures and light pressure techniques are used adjunctive to or in place of the adjustment; some may have originated with the spondylotherapy taught by Gregory and Palmer (Gregory, 1912), or with the light mechanical technique (Logan basic technique) developed by H. B. Logan and presented by his son (Logan, 1950). Traction procedures, both manual and mechanical, have been part of the chiropractic adjustive approach since 1906. Beatty (1939), who developed and presented Carver's work, outlined two such traction procedures, 1) incline plane and 2) extension swing traction, which were used during or after an adjustment procedure to enhance the effectiveness of treatment. The Cox–McManis, Leander, Hill, and Anatomotor equipment represent a few of the traction or continuous passive motion devices available today.

In retrospect, one can see that the first school of chiropractic, that of Palmer, focused on a disease-related system; adjustments were located by palpation, temperature (''hot box''), nerve tracing, and occasionally x-ray, and symptoms were correlated to these findings by the Meric System of nerve distribution. Carver developed a holistic approach to health and disease, emphasizing total body analysis based on postural, static, and functional analysis including the Meric System of symptom/organ function. DeJarnette emphasized structure and function of the nerve and muscle systems, deemphasized subluxation as the single cause of disease, and developed reflex neurological methods of treatment and diagnosis as well as biomechanical postural analysis on which to apply adjustive techniques.

Classification of Adjustment and Paraphysiologic Manipulation

The term *spinal manipulative therapy* (SMT) has gradually grown to represent all manipulative techniques applied to vertebral and nonvertebral joints. Distinctions between mobilization, articulation, manipulation, and adjustive procedures have been made and, in some circles, are still felt to be important.

Manipulation was defined, at the second NINCDS conference, as ''the application of accurately determined and specifically directed manual forces to the body'' (Korr, 1978). The American Chiropractic Association's Council on Technique (1988) adopted the definition of manipulation as proposed by Haldeman (1980) and Ward (1981), i.e., ''the therapeutic application of manual force. Spinal manipulative therapy broadly defined includes all procedures where the hands are used to mobilize, adjust, manipulate, apply traction, massage, stimulate or otherwise influence the spine and paraspinal tissues with the aim of influencing the patient's health.'' This definition is very general and broad and seems to comprise most of the procedures related to SMT.

Mobilization and articulation are somewhat similar and can be defined as methods of purposefully moving the joint or articulation through its ranges of active and passive motion. The ACA's definition of mobilization is the process of making a fixed part movable, a form of manipulation applied within the physiologic passive range of joint motion and characterized by nonthrust passive joint manipulation. The adjustment that has been characteristic of the chiropractic profession since its inception may be defined as a passive, carefully regulated thrust or force delivered with controlled speed depth, and magnitude to articulations at or near the end of the passive or physiologic range of motion, but not exceeding the anatomic limits of motion, often accompanied by joint ''crack'' or vacuum phenomenon and the resultant physiologic responses (Sandoz, 1976; Grice, 1979). ACA states that the chiropractic adjustment is a specific form of direct articular manipulation using either long- or short-lever techniques with specific contacts and is characterized by a dynamic thrust of controlled velocity, amplitude, and direction.

These definitions, although helpful, do not, in the strict sense, define all procedures related to adjustive techniques in chiropractic. Probably the most widely accepted characteristics of the adjustive thrust are (1) a controlled force delivered with high velocity, (2) a line of drive or specific direction, and (3) regulated depth and magnitude that are delivered through a specific contact using muscle power, body weight, or a mechanical apparatus.

Accurate control of the depth, direction, speed, amplitude, and magnitude requires a great degree of skill. The field of spinal manipulation is still largely a clinical art form in which classification, research, and interprofessional or intraprofessional discussion have been difficult. Therefore, many forms and systems of therapy have developed. Various classifications have been presented by Haldeman (1978), Buerger (1984), Ward and Sprafka (1981), Mannington (1985), Grice (1979), Grieve (1981), and Peterson (1988). The classification discussed here and shown in Table 25–1, when coupled with the characteristics and an understanding of what one is trying to achieve, should be useful to the practitioner.

TABLE 25-1.   CLASSIFICATION OF SPINAL MANIPULATION

Adjustive and manipulative techniques
    Short-lever techniques
    Long-lever techniques
    Nonthrust procedures
        Nonforce
        Mobilization
Physiologic therapeutics
    Manual techniques
        Muscle techniques
        Reflex techniques
    Nonmanual techniques
        Exercise
        Mechanotherapy

Adjustive and Manipulative Techniques

These techniques include short-lever techniques, long-lever techniques, and nonthrust procedures. General characteristics of adjustive and manipulative techniques include the following:

1. The contact is usually specific on a leverage advantage point on the motion segment, e.g., over the vertebral TVP, the spinous process, the articular pillar, or the mammillary process.
2. The thrust is given in a specific direction, depth, and magnitude to effect mobilization in a specific range of motion or direction of motion, effect alignment of the vertebral or stretch or compress specific soft tissue-holding elements, restore character of motion, or alter reflex mechanisms in that area.
3. The contact may include little or no prestressed force or sufficient prestress loading to take out joint laxity. This loading may be compressive (e.g., thoracic or spine), distractive (e.g., cervical spine), or rotational (e.g., lumbar spine).
4. The patient may be in a neutral posture or may be positioned so as to take out much of the active and/or passive motion. In fact, when the art of adjusting is carefully analyzed, the most efficient, most easily tolerated procedures combine directed movements and prestressing phenomenon, such that the motion segment is not taken to its extreme of motion in any given direction, but rather a main direction is used to take out part of the active motion and a coupled motion takes out the passive movement. First, rotation or lateral flexion is established; then a secondary coupled motion is introduced to focus the force. Finally, dis-

traction or compression is used to preload the segment or further focus the force so that a minimal thrust can be instituted to move the joint to its physiologic limits and create the joint separation ("joint crack") that is often desired for many adjustive procedures (Sandoz, 1976).

5. The direction of the thrust takes into consideration the plane of the articular facets as well as the other joint structures. The most efficient and most easily tolerated direction is along the plane of the facets or in a direction that would separate or open the facet joints.
6. Short-lever techniques usually utilize triceps thrusts, the shoulder drop, finger/wrist pressure, or a combination of these (Grice, 1979).

Some of these techniques are directional pressure techniques or very mild thrusting procedures designed to produce directional or positional change with mild impact or continuous pressure. The attempt in the adjustive procedure is to initiate little or no reflex contraction response or resistance of the patient's musculature. Other procedures use a high-velocity thrust with a very controlled amplitude, often thought to produce maximum neurologic response and minimal restrictive or reactive muscular response. Short-lever techniques often use less overall force and amplitude than do long-lever techniques, and often the most effective procedures require a good deal of practice to develop a controlled high-velocity, short-amplitude thrusting technique. The recoil procedure emphasizes fast release, using the triceps muscles to deliver the force and the relaxed stretch response of the biceps to generate the recoil (Fig. 25–1). Other thrust procedures using a shoulder or body drop may incorporate a slower release of adjustive force but with control; these can still prove to be comfortable yet achieve greater force (Fig. 25–2). Occasionally, the thrust is delivered fast and released slowly e.g., the kneeling Gonstead adjustment (Fig. 25–3), which is thought to produce a greater effect on ligamentous and discal elements.

Clinical skill is required to regulate the force of the thrust and respond to the clinical requirements of patients at various ages or with various clinical deficits and pathologic or congenital abnormalities.

Common mistakes made by students and novice adjusters include release of preloading prior to the thrust; slow thrust because preload force has taken away the adjuster's control or muscle power; thrust given with too great a magnitude or depth, causing stress and discomfort or damaging soft tis-

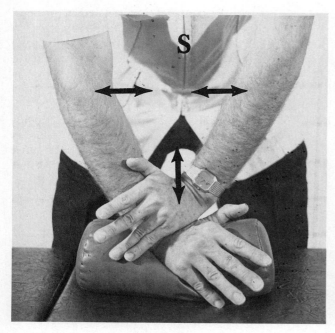
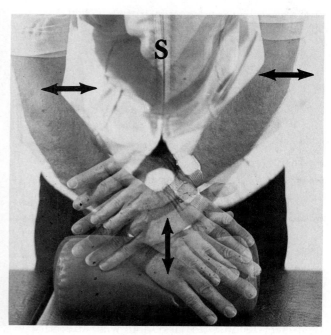

A   B

Figure 25–1. (A) Recoil position: hands are dorsiflexed and arched; triceps are simultaneously contracted; body is kept stable (S); line of drive is established from episternal notch through hand contact to vantage contact on the patient. **(B)** Recoil thrust; controlled sharp contraction until both arms reach full extension; results in biceps recoil; no prestress is used. Variation of contact using thumb is often used on upper cervicals.

sue-holding elements; and lack of control of muscle strength and body weight, resulting in lack of overall force.

Short-Lever Techniques. Short-lever techniques are commonly used on the extremities, and a direct contact is taken on the segment involved. Various contacts are used. The indifferent hand may reinforce the contact, as in adjustments of, for example, the carpals, tarsals, or knee joints. One hand may stabilize the joint while the second hand produces distraction, as in digital adjustments. One hand may produce distraction while the adjustive hand produces a rotation or lateral flexion thrust, e.g., elbow, knee, shoulder, or hip adjusting. Extremity techniques may or may not use prestressed procedures. Usually, however, distraction is used to separate the joint surfaces. The procedure may be a single thrust or may be multiple gross vibratory techniques to free the joint, stretch the holding elements, or break down adhesions.

NEUTRAL-POSITION SHORT-LEVER THRUST. In one of the most common procedures, called the "toggle recoil" (Fig. 25–4), a sharp contraction of the triceps is produced using a specific contact and a coupled leverage system with both arms. The patient is positioned in a fully relaxed posture and no prestressing of the joint is affected. The thrust is delivered in a specific direction and is characteristically a high-

velocity, short-amplitude thrust. Often a drop mechanism on the table is used to facilitate the procedure. The "joint crack" usually does not occur with this procedure. Low amplitude and rapid release are also characteristic. Side posture is used for upper cervical vertebrae; prone posture for dorsal vertebrae, the ribs, lumbar vertebrae, and the pelvis. Sometimes kneeling postures (see Fig. 25–3) are used. The toggle recoil is only occasionally used for extremity adjusting.

PRESTRESSED DIRECTIONAL THRUST. Another common procedure of adjusting with a short-lever technique uses a specific contact but develops force with a shoulder drop, body drop, or combination (Fig. 25–5). In this procedure, a recoil is not used, and the contact may be a single contact with the indifferent hand reinforcing the contact or with the indifferent hand taking a second leverage position, crossed the bilateral thrust used in thoracic or rib adjusting. Typically, a prestressed technique or preloading is used to facilitate the procedure. The adjustment is usually of high velocity and low amplitude, and postthrust release may be rapid or slow.

PASSIVE MOTION DIRECTIONAL THRUST. In this short-lever technique used for the cervical spine, the patient may be supine or sitting (Fig. 25–6). A specific contact is taken, most commonly on the cervical spi-

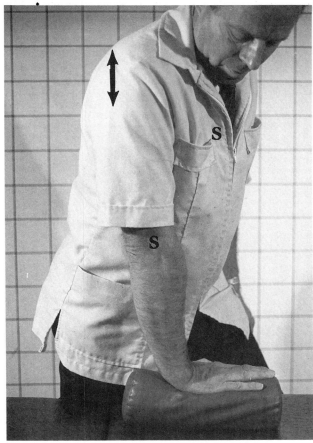

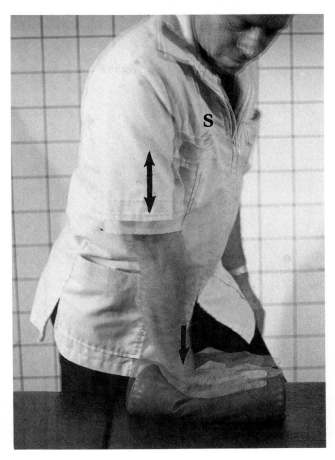

A   **B**

Figure 25-2A. Shoulder drop: body is stationary; arm is straight; line of drive is along the line of the arm; doctor's cuff is close to point of contact for strength of thrust. **B.** Shoulder drop: body is stable, shoulder is depressed sharply on the trunk using pectorals and latissimus dorsi (Continued next page).

nous, articular pillar, or transverse process, and the indifferent hand cradles the head, helping to focus the force and produce traction to facilitate the adjustment. This adjustment is given with high velocity, short amplitude, and rapid or slow release.

Long-Lever Techniques. A long-lever technique may use a specific or general primary contact on the body part but the second contact is remote from the segment, forming a broad or long leverage system of forces.

NONSPECIFIC ADJUSTING. Some consider this nomenclature a misnomer, as the definition of an adjustment might include the concept of a specific contact, focus, or purpose in the adjustment; however, nonspecific thrusts are occasionally used regionally in the lumbar or thoracic spine and less frequently in the cervical region. This procedure is indicated to free general fixations or general muscular spasms, such as those seen in spinal curvatures. In the lumbar region the contacts may be on the shoulder and pelvis, and, with rotation, force is distributed throughout the lumbar spine. In the thoracic or cervical regions, long-lever techniques use broad contacts and torsional, rotational, or lateral flexion methods of developing force that is distributed throughout a number of segments.

COMBINED LONG-LEVER–SPECIFIC CONTACT PROCEDURES. These are more frequently used procedures. A long lever produces the necessary leverage, but a specific contact is employed, similar to short-lever techniques (Fig. 25–7). By incorporating specific short-lever contacts within long-lever positioning and by directly focusing the force on a specific segment or joint, the general leverage technique becomes quite specific and more efficient. Specific facets can be released within the motion segment and each facet can be released individually (Johnston, 1976).

Nonthrust Procedures

NONFORCE TECHNIQUES. Pressure or directional force procedures using the hand or fingers to reposition motion segments or stretch soft tissue are used in cases

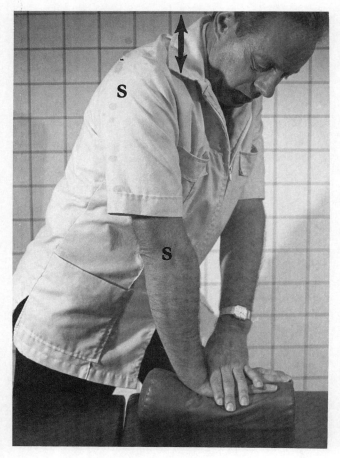

C

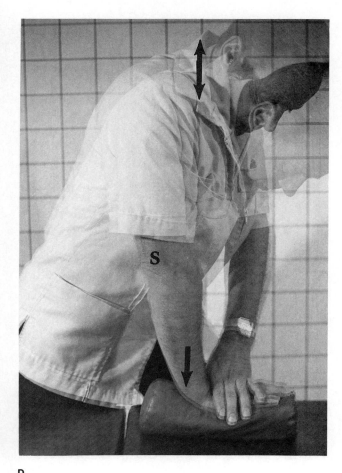

D

Figure 25-2 Continued, **C.** Body drop: generates greater force; the shoulder is kept stable; indifferent hand may reinforce the contact, arm is kept straight; body is accelerated onto the shoulder. **D.** Body drop: doctor's body mass is rocked over contact point, then accelerated within the shoulders. The force is delivered through body–shoulder–arm to the contact point. Arm is kept stable (S). Maneuver is often combined with shoulder drop to produce a forceful kinetic chain.

in which adjustive thrusts are contraindicated or in patients for whom these techniques, such as micromanipulation or Morrison technique, are most effective.

MOBILIZATION TECHNIQUES. Directional mobilizations using repetitive movements are procedures that stress joints in a specific direction to increase mobility and stretch holding elements. The joint is forced through its active and passive ranges of motion while challenging end range of motion by slow or rapid rhythmic movements. Usually, the type of joint separation that involves a ''joint crack'' is not included. General mobilization of a joint in all ranges of motion is often employed in peripheral joint therapy, for example, shoulder or hip joint, where the purpose is to stretch the holding elements: the extrinsic factors (muscular elements) and the intrinsic factors (ligamentous or discal elements).

Physiological Therapeutics

Physiological therapeutics include manual techniques, for example, massage, stripping, trigger-point therapy, and acupressure; and nonmanual techniques, such as exercise and mechanotherapy.

Manual Techniques

MUSCLE TECHNIQUES. Massage techniques of effluerage, petrassage, taponage, friction, and stroking are used to relax muscles, reduce spasm, and increase blood flow. These procedures are parachiropractic techniques and are used as adjuncts to chiropractic procedures.

Stripping techniques are similar, in their effect and application, to massage. Lubricating creams may or may not be used. The focus is usually on the belly of the muscle, at the trigger point, or at the most contracted region of the muscle.

REFLEX TECHNIQUES. Trigger-point therapy seeks to relieve pain, relax muscles, and increase blood flow.

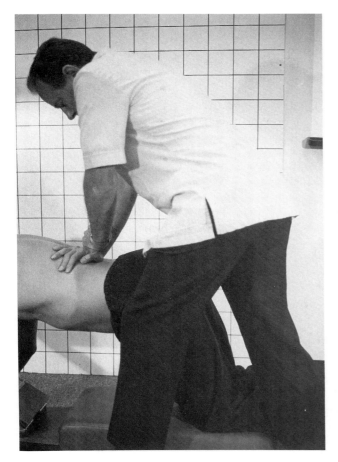

Figure 25–3. Knee–chest lumbar adjustment (Gonstead adjustment). Thrust is triceps, shoulder, body drop, or combination. Line of drive is straight through or in headward direction from episternal notch through contact point. Indifferent hand reinforces contact point—spinous process, mammillary process. Doctor's weight is balanced equally on feet close to contact point.

Acupressure is similar to trigger-point therapy and purports to have some of the reflex effects related to acupuncture. Percussion or spondylotherapy is used to stimulate reflex responses to help in pain control, alter reflex responses through the autonomic system, relax muscle tension, and increase blood flow regulation. Proprioceptive neuromuscular facilitation (PNF) is used to increase joint motion and relax muscle contraction. Systematic sports stretching (SSS) is similar. Reciprocal innervation techniques use muscle contraction and stretching to reflexly relax the antagonist muscles and enhance the range of motion. Muscle energy techniques or muscle facilitation is used to increase joint motion and decrease muscle spasm. Lewit (1986) reviews these techniques and suggests some new modifications (postisometric relaxation).

Nonmanual Techniques

EXERCISE. Active exercise is used to increase muscle tone, strengthen and balance muscle action, increase blood flow, reciprocally relax antagonist muscles, and restore muscle patterns. Stretching exercise is used to relax muscles, reduce unnecessary muscle tone, increase joint mobility, and restore optimal neurologic patterning.

MECHANOTHERAPY. Traction procedures include static or intermittent and continuous motion traction procedures and are used to increase joint motion, relax musculature, and increase circulation. They are also purported to have specific effects on discs and other soft tissue elements. Locomotor motor apparatus and exercise equipment, such as soft carpet walkers, normal walkers, Cybex units, and other exercise apparatus, are designed to improve muscle function and facilitate the locomotor system. Other general appliances include heel or shoe lifts, special corrective orthotics, braces, corsets, collars, and peripheral

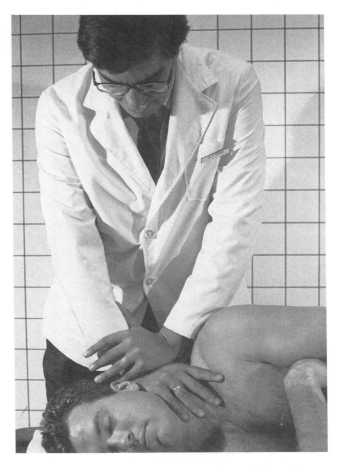

Figure 25–4. Short-lever technique: toggle recoil. Uses drop headpiece mechanism. Patient is in neutral relaxed position; no prestress force is required.

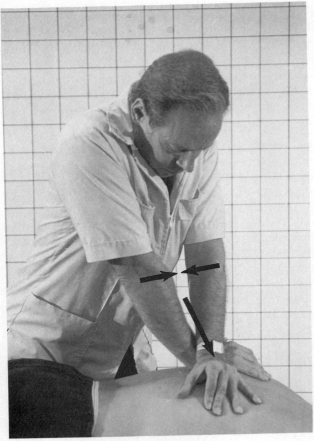

Figure 25–5. Prestressed directional thrust. Force is developed by shoulder drop, body drop, or both; prestress force is in the direction of the thrust; takes out skin slack and much of the tissue elasticity. Indifferent hand may form counterforce (crossed bilateral) or may reinforce adjusting hand.

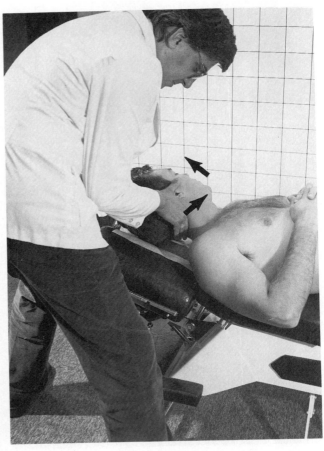

Figure 25–6. Short-lever technique: passive motion directional thrust. Rotation—cervical primary ROM rotation; mild lateral flexion to focus force; distraction prestress force, particularly with indifferent hand which allows ease of correction. Thrust is generated mainly by pectoral muscles or, if only mild force is necessary, with forearm abductors.

supports, all of which have the purpose of enhancing or supporting locomotor activity.

Objectives of a Spinal Adjustment

This section addresses the question "what is one trying to achieve by a spinal adjustment?" A number of different themes are discussed that, taken together, help to build our understanding of the objectives of an adjustment. Guidelines are presented that define the approaches used by most chiropractors and other practitioners of manipulation to rationalize the daily clinical application of spinal adjustments to benefit their patients' health.

There is a difference between the "objectives" and the "mechanisms of action" of an adjustment. The former are clinician directed; the latter are scientifically validated constructs of cause-and-effect relationships between a therapeutic action and the set of

effects of a treatment. Ideally, the question of what we are trying to achieve by an adjustment would be answered by invoking a list of "mechanisms of action" of this treatment and by citing the activation of these mechanisms as the therapeutic objective.

Unfortunately, far more is speculated than is truly and scientifically known about the effects or mechanisms of action of a manipulation or adjustment. Clinicians often have the same clinical objectives but may select various adjustive techniques or use various clinical models to achieve these objectives.

"Objectives" of adjustment constitute a set of target behaviors and clinical decision-making principles that are shared by like-minded practitioners and derive their validity from the empirical discipline of clinical practice as opposed, exclusively, to the experimental discipline of research. Examination of the objectives and the models of clinical practice facilitates a better understanding of the similarities and differences in chiropractic (Table 25–2).

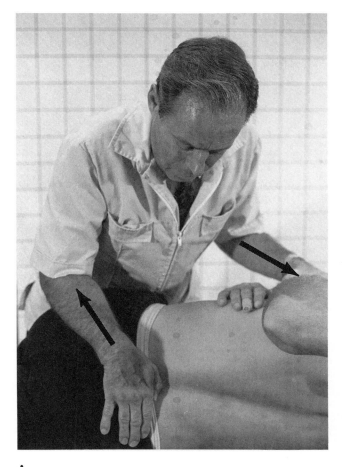
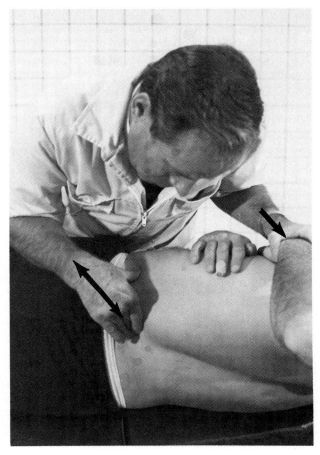

A   **B**

Figure 25–7. Long-lever technique: lumbar or pelvic adjustments. **(A)** Contacts use body torsion, lateral flexion, flexion or extension with general contacts, and prestress in the direction of the thrust and in an opposed direction; shoulder drop or body drop as well as muscle force provides the force. **(B)** Short-lever contact is often noticed within long-lever positioning to focus the force of the adjustment.

Static Model Versus Dynamic Model

There has occurred in chiropractic what could arguably be referred to as a paradigm shift in the approach to viewing the objectives of an adjustment. The original paradigm could be described as a static model, emphasizing spinal alignment and the influence of structure on function. Although concepts of

TABLE 25–2.   MODELS OF OBJECTIVES OF AN ADJUSTMENT

1. Static model versus dynamic model
2. Lesion model
3. Mechanical model versus neurologic
4. Anatomic model
5. Systems model
6. Physiologic model
7. Pathologic model
8. Health model

spinal dynamics have early origins, this simpler static model, coupled with its relationship to neural function, formed the dominant clinical model in the early development of chiropractic. The newer concept is a dynamic model that emphasizes movement-related disorders of the spinal structures, their effects on related function of musculoskeletal structures, and their relationship to neurohumoral and circulatory systems. As such, the objectives of an adjustment can be described in terms that apply to the older static model or to the newer dynamic model.

Lesion Model

One cannot understand what one is "trying to achieve with an adjustment without considering the object of the adjustment," which Haldeman (1983), in a marvelous tautology, described as "the manipulable lesion." In other words, with a pathological perspective, one cannot understand the nature of a treatment unless one first understands the disorder for which the treatment is given. This lesion or disorder could affect the spinal motion segments and has, in the pathological sense, been described as a "derangement of function." Numerous authors, using a variety of names, have described these lesions, some of which have literally attained the status of an icon within each of the professional disciplines (Brantingham, 1985): subluxation, fixation (chiropractic), osteopathic lesion (osteopathy), joint dysfunction (medical or manual therapists), hypomobility (all groups), blockage (German manual medicine), and functional disorders/derangements (all groups).

Mechanical Model Versus Neurological Models

The archetypical configuration of the spine in chiropractic thinking weds the spinal column with the spinal cord (i.e., the nervous system). This unified construct gives rise to two interdependent clinical domains—the mechanical and the neurologic. The objectives of an adjustment can be described in mechanical terms: realignment of joint surfaces, increase in joint mobility (reduction of fixation or "blockage"), reduction of muscle spasm, and so forth. On the other hand, the objective of an adjustment can be described in neurological terms; reduction of nerve pressure; reduction of pain; alteration, stimulation, or inhibition of reflex pathways; or alteration of neurohumoral responses. Korr (1978) subdivided the neurologic domain into two basic areas: impulse-based, related to the reflex disturbances associated with spinal lesions; and non-impulse-based, related largely to the deleterious effects of compression on nerves associated with the spinal lesion.

Anatomic Model

The anatomic model (Table 25–3) evaluates the body system on a gross postural basis, taking into consideration the body and the individual as a totality and the musculoskeletal system as an adaptive whole, as well as on a spinal level. The spine, in turn, is evaluated on the basis of a number of subdivisions.

1. The multisegmental component refers to the larger regions of the spine, e.g., cervical, dorsal, and lumbar, or rib cage, pelvis, and so forth, and takes into consideration adaptive curves and responses involving numbers of muscle groups (extrinsic factors) and the fascial structures that influence an area of the spine, e.g., the lumbar–dorsal fascia.

2. The intersegmental component refers to the three-joint vertebral complex, including the

TABLE 25–3. ANATOMIC MODEL

Multisegmental
Intersegmental
Infrasegmental
Intrasegmental

anterior division of the motion segment (vertebral centrum, endplates, discs, and the associated ligaments) and the posterior division (articulations, capsules, and ligaments)—the intrinsic factors—as well as the short segmental muscles or long muscles that may have segmental influence—the extrinsic factors.

3. The infrasegmental component refers to the foraminal environs including the nerve roots, dorsal root ganglion, mixed spinal nerve, sympathetic rami and ganglionic chain, recurrent meningeal nerve, and foraminal arteries and veins.

4. The intrasegmental component refers to the spinal cord and its primary receptor and effector neuronal pools, i.e., the dorsal horn (particularly the termination zones of afferents subserving pain and proprioception), the motor horn, the intermedial lateral horn cells from T-1 to T-12, the interneuronal pathways, and the longitudinal pathways.

In this anatomic model, the objectives of manipulation relate to target changes in each of these anatomic subcomponents, separately and interdependently.

Systems Model

A systems approach (Table 25–4) can be used to frame the various objectives of an adjustment. In an anatomic model, the locomotor system can be viewed as a whole, and a hierarchy of subsystems can be explored ranging from the macro level to the micro level of organization.

Objectives for an adjustment are contingent on the specific system under consideration. At the locomotor level, a host of abnormalities of the total motor system, such as short leg, pelvic obliquity, and increased spinal curvature, may form part of the functional disturbances that ultimately target themselves at one focal lesion or symptom complex (the object of

TABLE 25–4. SYSTEMS MODEL

Segmental level
Regional level
Locomotor level

clinical concern by the doctor and patient). As such, a multidimensional perspective on the motor system is required so that the objectives of manipulation can be understood.

Adjustment of a single spinal segment when it attains the status of lesion may be done to achieve very different objectives when manifest within the context of the regional system or the locomotor system.

Physiological Model

The physiological model (Table 25–5) has three major components: regulatory, functional, and psychosocial.

1. The regulatory component refers to changes in regulatory effect mediated by the neurohormonal system as the objective of manipulation-induced effects.
2. The functional model involves behavioral changes induced by a manipulation, such as less pain, less anxiety, improvements in posture, and improvement in the dynamic behaviors of the locomotor system (gait, bending, twisting).
3. The psychosocial model includes objectives related to the whole person: less illness behavior, return to normal activities of daily living, and so forth.

Pathological Model

The pathological model concerns itself with recognition of pathogenic process, limitations of tissue adaptability, and contraindications to adjustive procedures. Spinal subluxation and joint dysfunction are viewed as resulting from as well as contributing to the pathogenic process. Treatment may address itself to the pathogenesis or to the symptoms or dysfunction related to the pathology.

Wellness Model

Beyond the pathological model lies the controversial area of wellness with its implications that adjustments may improve general wellness and that the chiropractic approach to patient care may enhance wellness. This exciting but largely untested area may well define the challenges to chiropractic in the next century.

Health Model

At the most complex level, the adjustment and the total chiropractic approach to the patient are seen to have an overall therapeutic affect and to have the potential for improving the total health of the patient. This health model includes a number of models of care: (1) the anatomic model, in that structure is related to function; (2) the physiological model, in that function is related to structure; (3) the pathological model, which recognizes limitations of tissue response and contraindications to certain therapies; (4) the illness model, which seeks to modify illness behavior; and (5) the wellness model, which recognizes multicausal factors in health and disease and seeks to improve total body health.

Conclusion

This chapter has presented a historical review of the development of adjustive procedures, outlined a variety of techniques of mobilization, manipulation, and adjustment; and described a variety of objectives of these treatments. Although there are variations, a central theme runs through virtually all of chiropractic practice and all of the various technique systems. This theme can be described as the "chiropractic clinical paradigm" and is proposed to consist of the following:

1. A common approach to the musculoskeletal system that seeks to identify and characterize derangements of structure and function of the various parts, units, subsystems, and totality of the body
2. A sense that the various subunits of the locomotor system are integrated functionally into a structural totality—a Gestalt of structural holism
3. A *materiae chiropracticae* that consists of a large number and variety of somatic therapies and treatments—some organized into systematic models, others part of an eclectic armamentarium of techniques—all of which purport to normalize the function of the musculoskeletal system
4. A consensus that the objectives of these various treatments involve changes not only in the musculoskeletal system, but in the nervous system, certainly at the level of peripheral receptors and spinal cord segmental and local reflex centers and possibly at more central levels. (These objectives involve physiological effects that have been observed empirically and are receiving experimental attention with emerging support for some.)
5. A belief that these physiological effects have an impact on the health of the whole person

TABLE 25–5. PHYSIOLOGICAL MODEL

Regulatory model
Functional model
Psychosocial model

and, as such, should be part of health enhancement care

6. An awareness of the whole person who suffers with the clinical effects of structural and functional derangement. (This has translated itself into a clinical approach in which the techniques of treatment are applied in a regimen of care, not just as modalities of physical intervention.)

The chiropractic clinical paradigm is applied in a healing encounter that emphasizes attention to illness behavior and the physiological needs of the patient, involvement of the patient in his or her own recovery toward functional independence, a concern for long-term rehabilitation (often stated as a concern for the cause of the problem not only its symptoms), and finally a keen interest in prevention and the promotion of healthy lifestyles and wellness.

References

Arnholz W. *The Adjustment of Spastic Muscle*. California, 1949.

Beatty HG. *Anatomical Adjustive Technic*. Denver, Colo: 1939.

Brantingham JW. A survey of literature regarding the behaviour, pathology, etiology and nomenclature of the chiropractic lesion. *ACA J Chiropractic* 1985;19: .

Buerger AA. A non-reductant taxonomy of spinal manipulative techniques suitable for physiological explanation. *Manual Med* 1984;1: .

Carver W. *Carver's Chiropractic Analysis of Chiropractic Principles*, vols. 1 and 2. Oklahoma: 1909.

Carver W. *Carver's Chiropractic Analysis of Chiropractic Principles*, vols 1 and 2. Oklahoma: 1915.

Carver W. *Carver's Chiropractic Analysis*, vols. 1 and 2. Semco Color Press; 1921.

Craven J. *Chiropractic Hygiene and Pediatrics*. Iowa: Hammond Press/WB Conkey Co; 1924.

DeJarnette B. *Spinal Distortions*. Nebraska, 1938.

Dye AA. *The Evolution of Chiropractic—Its Discovery and Development*. Dye, Pa: 1939.

Forster A. *Principles and Practice of Chiropractic*. Chicago: National Publishing Assoc; 1915.

Gregory AA. *Spinal Treatment*. The Palmer–Gregory College; 1912.

Grice AS. *A Biomedical Approach to Cervical and Dorsal Adjusting: Modern Developments in Principles and Practice of Chiropractic*. New York: Appleton-Century-Crofts; 1979.

Grieve GP. *Common Vertebral Joint Problems*. New York: Churchill Livingston; 1981.

Haldeman S. The clinical basis for discussion of mechanics of manipulative therapy. In Korr I, ed. *The Neurobiological Mechanisms in Manipulative Therapy*. New York: Plenum Press; 1978.

Haldeman S. Spinal manipulative therapy in the management of low back pain. In BE Finneson, ed. *Low Back Pain*.

Haldeman S. Spinal manipulative therapy: A status report. *Clin Ortho*. 1983: 179.

Homewood AE. *The Neurodynamics of the Vertebral Subluxation*. Toronto: 1962.

Howard JFA. *Encyclopedia of Chiropractic*, vols. I–III. Chicago: National School of Chiropractic; ca. 1920.

Janse J, Houser RH, and Wells BF. *Chiropractic Principles and Technic*. Chicago: National College of Chiropractic; 1947.

Johnston RJ. Selective adjustments of articular components within a single joint. *J Can Chiropractic Assoc* 1976; 20(4).

Korr I. Objectives and hypotheses in the design of the workshop. In Korr I. ed. *The Neurobiological Mechanisms in Manipulative Therapy*. New York: Plenum Press; 1978.

Lewit K. Postisometric relaxation in combination with other methods of muscle facilitation and inhibition. *Manual Med* 1986; 2.

Logan HB and Murray, eds. *Textbook of Logan Basic Methods*. St. Louis, Mo: 1950.

Nimmo RL. Receptor, effector and tonus. A new approach. Newsletter The Receptor Texas Vol 1 No 1 1957.

Nimmo RL. *The Receptor Tonus Method*, self-published notes; 1963.

Mannington JV. *Glossary of Terms for the Chiropractic Student*. Canadian Memorial Chiropractic College; 1985.

McNamara PE. *Chiropractic—Other Drugless Healing Methods with Criticism of the Practice of Medicine*. Davenport, Iowa: Universal Chiropractic College; 1913.

Palmer DD. *The Science, Art and Philosophy of Chiropractic*. Portland, Oreg: Portland Printing House Company; 1910.

Palmer BJ. *The Philosophy and Principles of Chiropractic Adjustments*. Davenport, Iowa: Palmer School of Chiropractic; 1908–1911.

Palmer BJ. *An Exposition of Old Moves*. Davenport, Iowa: Palmer School of Chiropractic; 1911–1916.

Palmer BJ. *The Philosophy, Science and Art of Chiropractic Nerve Tracing*. Davenport, Iowa: Palmer School of Chiropractic; 1911.

Peterson DH. Chiropractic terminology—A report. Panel of Advisors ACA Council of Technic. *ACA J Chiropractic* 1988: Oct.

Sandoz R. Some physical mechanisms and effects of spinal adjustment. *Ann Swiss Chiropractic Assoc* 1976;6.

Smith OG, Langworthy SM, and Paxson MC. *Modernized Chiropractic*. Iowa: Laurance Press; 1906.

Stephenson RW. *Chiropractic Textbook*. Stephenson, Iowa, 1927.

Ward R and Sprafka S. Glossary of osteopathic terminology. *J Am Osteopath Assoc* 1981;80(8).

The High-Velocity Thrust Adjustment

Carl S. Cleveland, III

The fundamental concept of chiropractic encompasses the hypothesis that vertebral subluxations, or biomechanical impairments of the musculoskeletal system may cause disturbances in neural mechanisms resulting in functional irregularities that may lead to pathophysiological and pathological change.

The chiropractic subluxation or manually diagnosed entity to which spinal manipulative therapy or adjustment is to be directed has been identified through chiropractic, osteopathic, and medical literature by a variety of terms including *manipulable spinal lesion* (Haldeman, 1983); *vertebral subluxation* (Palmer, 1908–1911; Cleveland, 1951; Homewood, 1963; Reinert, 1983); *osteopathic lesion* (Kimberly, 1979; Stoddard, 1980; Denslow, 1975); *somatic spinal complex* (Walton, 1970); *vertebral fixation* (Gillet and

Liekens, 1973); *vertebral blockage* (Lewit, 1985); *somatic joint dysfunction* (Mennell, 1960); *spatially and functionally abnormal position of an axial skeletal part* (Dvorak and Dvorak, 1984/1988); and *vertebral subluxation complex* (Schafer and Faye, 1989). The characteristics of the manipulable lesion have been described by Haldeman (1983) to include (1) vertebral malposition, (2) abnormal vertebral motion, (3) abnormal joint play or end feel, (4) soft tissue abnormalities, and (5) muscle contraction or imbalance. Additionally, Haldeman presents a sixth characteristic termed *response to treatment*, stating that "the criteria for determining whether a manipulable lesion caused a patient's symptoms depend on the patient's response to treatment."

An early conceptualization relating to the intent

of vertebral adjustment was restoration of the normal articular position of contiguous vertebral structures (Palmer, 1920; Dye, 1939/1969; Cleveland, 1951; Kirk, 1978; Grove, 1979; Barge, 1982 a,b). There is growing consensus within the profession that the effect of spinal manipulative therapy or vertebral adjustment should be expanded to include a dynamic component of freeing restricted articular movement and restoring normal joint function (Buerger and Tobis, 1977; Lewit, 1985; Schafer and Faye, 1989; Bourdillon, 1970/1987; Paris, 1983; Dvorak and Dvorak, 1984/1988). The current view of vertebral subluxation has emerged as a complex clinical entity (Schafer and Faye, 1989) comprising neuropathophysiological, kinesiopathological, myopathological, histopathological, and biochemical components. The chiropractic clinical approach is based on the rationale that such subluxations may be manually corrected by the application of the manipulative or adjustive thrust.

Terminology

Static and Dynamic Descriptions

As various techniques of spinal manipulation or adjustment have evolved throughout the years, there have been extreme variations within the profession with respect to terminology or descriptive listings related to vertebral subluxation. Charts of illustrations of static listings and dynamic listings of vertebral subluxation are provided in Figures 26–1 and 26–2. Terminology is being developed by the Technique Council of the American Chiropractors Association (Peterson, 1988) with the intent of addressing interrelationship of static descriptions of vertebral subluxation listings, which designate spatial orientation of one vertebra in relation to the adjacent segment, and kinetic descriptions of subluxation listings, designating abnormal movement characteristics of one vertebra in relationship to subadjacent segments (see Appendix B).

Vertebral Adjustment

Haldeman defines spinal manipulative therapy as "all procedures where the hands are used to mobilize, adjust, stimulate or otherwise influence the spinal and paraspinal tissues with the aim of influencing the patient's health." Confusion exists concerning the terms *manipulation, mobilization,* and *adjustment.* Certain authors in chiropractic (Barge, 1982a,b; Gonstead, 1980) identify the term *manipulation* with nonspecific, long-lever, manual therapy and reserve the term *adjustment* for short-lever, direct articular contact applied to specific vertebral segments. Schneider et al. (1988), a Swiss medical physician, recognizes the variation in meaning in different countries,

stating that in the United States manipulation is a general term referring to "any therapeutic procedure in which the hands are used to treat the patient," and that mobilization is known as "soft tissue and articular type of treatment, including muscle energy techniques." According to Schneider, European practitioners describe manipulation as "high-velocity, low-amplitude thrust," and mobilization is used to refer to "various types of articular mobilization without thrusting force." Schafer and Faye (1989) use the terms *manipulation* and *adjustment* as synonymous for the application of a specifically directed, dynamic thrust to a vertebra, and the term *mobilization* to identify nonspecific manual therapy. General mobilization has been proposed to relax the patient prior to the administration of specific adjustment.

Schafer and Faye describe the purpose of specific adjusting as "to deliver an adjustment to a specific vertebra to alter specific symptomatology. The bio-mechanical objective of specific chiropractic adjustments is to restore motion through the active, passive, and paraphysiological range of motion." Further, "the application of any clinical procedure without consideration of the cause and effect anticipated is not within the confines of scientific chiropractic."

There are not many studies comparing the effects of specific adjusting versus general manipulation; however, Luttges and Cleveland (1982) evaluated the effects of specific adjusting versus general manipulation on nervous system function as determined by qualified performance of motor and sensory tasks. They defined the terms *adjustment* and *manipulation* as follows:

- *Adjustment:* "the process of manually contacting a subluxated vertebra as directly as possible on a specific point and thrusting in a specific direction toward correction of the subluxation."
- *Manipulation:* "the use of a non-specific manipulative action, traction or thrust to the body in an attempt to correct the subluxated vertebra without contacting the subluxated vertebra directly."

In the experiment, patients randomly assigned to a group receiving specific chiropractic adjustment demonstrated enhanced motor and sensory function in terms of their performance on a force estimation test and a two-point discrimination evaluation when compared with patients randomly assigned to either the general manipulative therapy group or the nontreatment group. Patient evaluation was performed on the affected (symptomatic) and unaffected (asymptomatic) limbs.

	ACA Advisory panel adopted Winter 1988 (Medicare) (Vertebral body reference)	Palmer Gonstead (Spinous process reference)	National (Vertebral body reference)
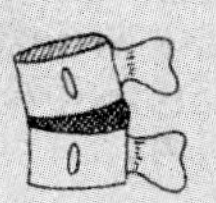	Flexion malposition (F)	None	Anterior inferior (AI)
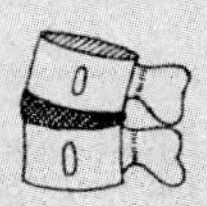	Extension malposition (E)	Posterior inferior (PI)	Posterior inferior (PI)
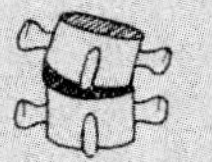	Right lateral flexion malposition (RLF)	None	Right inferior RI
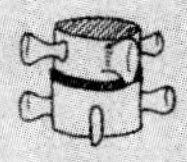	Left rotational malposition (LR)	Posterior spinous right (PR)	Left posterior (LP)
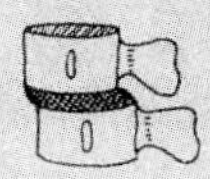	Anterolisthesis (A)	None	Anterior (A)
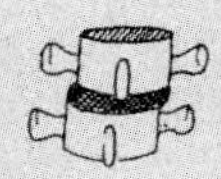	Right laterolisthesis (L)	None	Right laterolisthesis (RL)
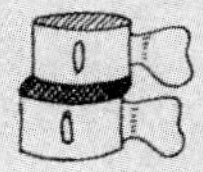	Retrolisthesis (R)	Posterior (P)	Posterior (P)
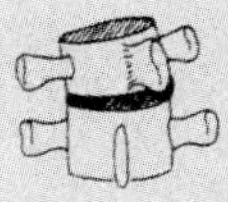	Left rotational malposition (LR) Left lateral flexion malposition (LLF)	Posterior right superior spinous (PRS)	Left posterior inferior (LPI)
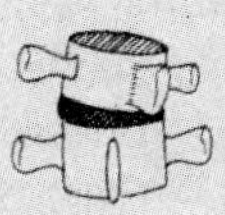	Left Rotational malposition (LR) Right lateral flexion malposition (RLF)	Posterior right inferior spinous (PRI)	Left posterior superior (LPS)
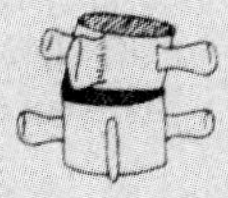	Right rotational malposition (RR) Right lateral flexion malposition (RLF)	Posterior left superior spinous (PLS)	Right posterior inferior (RPI)
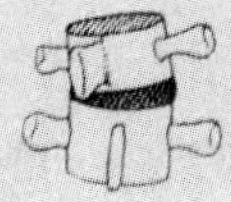	Right rotational malposition Left lateral flexion	Posterior left inferior spinous (PLI)	Right posterior superior (RPS)

Figure 26–1. Comparative chart of static listing system. (*Reproduced with permission of ACA Council on Technique, 1988; K. Edwards, artist.*)

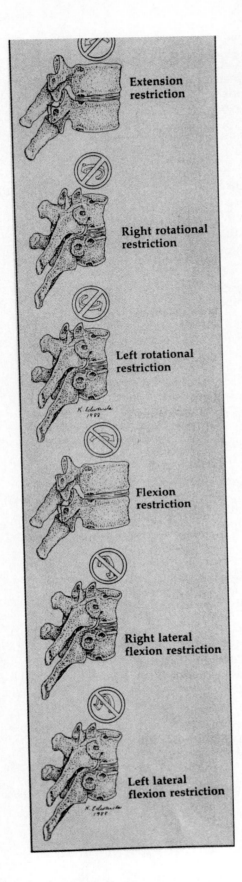

Figure 26-2. Dynamic listing system. (*Reproduced with permission of ACA Council on Technique, 1988; K. Edwards, artist.*)

The Dynamic Thrust

A forceful dynamic thrust has been described as part of the application of spinal manipulative therapy from the time of ancient Greece (Lomax, 1975; Smithson, 1988), as identified by Withington's (1959) English translation of the writings of Hippocrates circa 400 BC, who recommended that with the patient lying prone on a wooden bed, combined extension and pressure be exerted on the patient's spine. ''The physician, or an assistant who is strong and not untrained, should put the palm of hand on the hump, and the palm of the other hand on that, to reduce it forcibly, taking into consideration whether the reduction should naturally be made straight downwards or towards the head or towards the hip.'' Reference in this ancient writing to the hand positioning and consideration for directing the force downwards or towards the head or the hip, are basic components of toggle type thrusts and angle of drive (direction of thrust) which may be found in chiropractic technique textbooks.

In terms of chiropractic procedure, the most commonly used method is the specific short-lever, high-velocity spinal adjustment. To a lesser extent the long-lever manipulation may also be used. The chiropractic adjustment has traditionally been characterized by a dynamic thrust, described as a quick, small-amplitude, high-velocity thrust delivered to a single vertebral process with a specific line of direction (Grecco, 1953; Janse, 1975, 1976). The osseous levers consist of spinous, transverse, or mammillary processes, the lamina, articular pillars, and the iliac and ischial spines of the innominate bone (DeGiacomo, 1981; Christensen, 1984; Thompson, 1987). Examples of dynamic thrusts include the following:

1. Torsional or leverage techniques incorporating long levers
2. Straight-arm body drop procedures
   a. Double-arm body drop—body thrust
   b. Single-hand body drop—shoulder thrust
3. Impulse-type thrusts
4. Toggle thrusts—specific short-lever techniques
   a. Toggle recoil
   b. Toggle and hold
   c. Toggle with torque

Leverage-type moves or thrusts refer to utilization of counterpressure or contralateral stabilization. The counterpressure is used to balance the force of the adjustive thrust. Schafer and Faye (1989) indicate that the leverage move is used to prevent loss of the applied force and to concentrate the force at the directed point of contact.

The *straight-arm body drop procedure* (Stephenson, 1927; Beatty, 1983; Schafer and Faye, 1989) is accomplished by using the weight of the trunk as the force of the adjustive thrust. With the adjustor's trunk weight centered over the contact hands (contact hand in single-hand body drop) and with the elbows straight, the trunk is raised between the shoulders using straight arms. The trunk is then dropped between the shoulders with a short sharp impulse, thus transmitting the force of the momentum through the arms to the contact point.

To apply *impulse-type thrusts,* the adjustor positions the hands with a preset tension in the direction of the impulse. The impulse-type thrust is a high-velocity, low-depth thrust and is described by Faye and Schafer (1989) as a fast or spasmodic muscular contraction from the diaphragm, as in coughing or spitting. According to Beatty (1983), ''every muscle of the body suddenly cooperates for the administration of force in a given direction.''

The term *toggle thrust* derives from the toggle joint relationship of the hingelike function of the practitioner's elbows combined with the two crossed hands (crossed pisiform contact) applied to the patient's spine. A toggle joint is defined as an elbowlike joint composed of two arms positioned so that a force applied to their hinge to straighten them produces an outward force at the ends. With a toggle thrust, the two hands are appropriately positioned, one on the other, with specific vertebral contact on osseous levers and with the elbows in a relaxed position. The practitioner quickly and simultaneously contracts both triceps and anconei muscles, and both pectoralis muscles. The result is a sudden dynamic thrust with the force directed to the specific point of crossed hands. The adjustive thrust is the creation of an invasive force met by the resistance force of the patient's body, producing a concussion of forces. Recognizing that multiple segments are affected by the force of an adjustive thrust, the purpose of such a maneuver is to provide specifically directed, high-velocity, short-amplitude, forceful motion that is maximized at specific articular components of a vertebral segment.

Toggle recoil with torque is described by Stephenson (1927/1948) as a light twist applied at the contact point formed when one elbow moves toward, and the other away, from the adjustor as the elbows are straightened during the toggle thrust. This was considered by Stephenson to be a most efficient approach to adjusting atlas subluxations.

To develop the necessary skill in spinal adjustive technique the student of chiropractic must study static and kinetic palpation, and practice adjusting exercises to perfect psychomotor skills required for development of proper hand positioning. The student must demonstrate the ability to execute toggle recoil and impulse thrusts required for an effective dynamic force adjustment. Mastery of these psychomotor skills is fundamental and prerequisite to the study of adjusting technique. To the casual observer, procedures of the skilled manipulator appear simple (Paris, 1983). Control of the adjustive thrust demands much discipline and skill, requiring hours of practice to become proficient in manipulative therapy (Dvorak and Dvorak, 1984/1988; Maigne, 1972/1979). Kirkaldy-Willis and Cassidy (1988) feel that those practitioners with a special interest in spinal manipulative therapy should not only read the books on the subject but also be prepared to complete a full apprenticeship with one or more skilled practitioners before embarking on this method of treatment.

Early Chiropractic Technique Systems

Although there is variation among chiropractic techniques, certain long-standing fundamental principles are basic to all dynamic force technique systems. Adaptation around these fundamental principles must be amended to the size, strength, and level of skill of the doctor, as well as the age, health status, and pain tolerance of the patient (Schafer and Faye, 1989).

One of the first technique systems to be developed around basic principles of spinal biomechanics is the toggle recoil, meric recoil or, full-spine specific technique. This technique system, developed by D. D. Palmer and B. J. Palmer, served as an early foundation from which a variety of techniques popular in the profession today have evolved. Today's typical practitioner most probably uses certain fundamentals of this system in conjunction with a variety of diversified technique procedures. Initially, the toggle recoil technique system provided for placement of the patient prone on a padded table with adjustable sections for abdominal suspension of the patient. Rigid rules were adopted that prescribed the position of the patient and the specific stance of the doctor that provided the maximum efficiency of the dynamic adjustive thrust in a posterior-to-anterior direction in a plane parallel to the vertebral bodies or articular facets; a simultaneous objective was the maximum comfort and relaxation of the patient. This technique system, as other early adjusting procedures, evolved from the concept that the purpose of a chiropractic adjustment was the restoration of a subluxated vertebra to its normal position (Stephenson, 1927). Vertebral subluxation was viewed as a misalignment or malpositioning of vertebral segments and thus was generally described in reference to a static (positional) listing system. Stephenson (1927) identified the "listing" as a description of the direction in which a vertebra has moved from its normal position and represented such by the initial letters of directions used in nomenclature for anatomic position. For example, PRS indicated that the vertebra had subluxated toward the posterior on the right side and superiorly. Stephenson described the "line of drive," also called direction of thrust, as the direction of movement necessary to restore the vertebra to normal positional alignment, that is, the direction opposite the "listing." The listings of subluxation in this technique are described using a spinous process reference system as in the Palmer–Gonstead listings, with the added component described as "body subluxation," which in this technique system is equivalent to the term "laterolisthesis" in the static listing system chart (see Fig. 26–1). The term body subluxation, also called rotational subluxation, in this instance, refers to a classification of subluxation in which the centrum or body of the vertebra has moved either right or left relative to the body of the vertebra above and the body of the vertebra below. Rotation is considered to be around a vertical axis posterior to the centrum in the area of the zygapophysis (Stephenson, 1927). Figures 26–1 and 26–2 may be used as comparative charts for cross-referencing technique listing systems.

Contemporary description of vertebral subluxation may involve either loss of proper motion (dynamics) or loss of position (statics) of a vertebral articulation and allows for the potential of a combination of improper motion and improper position of the intervertebral motor unit (Grice, 1980; Haldeman, 1983). The biomechanical foundation of the toggle recoil technique system places emphasis on direction of thrust in relation to the plane of the articulation of the vertebral joints and specificity of vertebral contact. For this reason the fundamentals of this early technique system may be adapted to address either the static or dynamic components of subluxation and provide the student an excellent introduction to technique.

Full-Spine Specific/Meric Recoil Technique

The following description of procedures related to full-spine specific adjusting (toggle recoil technique) represents an abridged overview of the fundamentals of one of the early specific adjusting systems. In this technique system, the patient is positioned prone on the adjusting table and toggle recoil–type dynamic thrusts are specifically applied to vertebral segments associated with manifestations characteristic of vertebral subluxation. At one point in the development of chiropractic, a technique of this type was used by a large portion if not the majority of practitioners (Dye, 1939/1969), and has served as a foundation from which other techniques in use today have evolved.

Early in the evolution of the art and science of chiropractic, members of the profession observed patterns of clinical associations between vertebral subluxation at specific levels of the spine and symptoms in organs or areas within the segmental distribution of nerves. On the basis of these clinical manifestations, B. J. Palmer, assisted by James C. Wishert, developed a concept of clinical analysis, the meric system (Dye, 1939/1969; Leach, 1986). The term *mere* denotes a part or segment. In view of the utilization of toggle recoil technique in conjunction with the system of ''meric analysis'' of clinical relationships and symptomatology, the term *meric recoil technique* is therefore also used to identify this technique system. The meric analysis of symptomatology has been used in conjunction with a variety of diversified technique systems in addition to toggle recoil.

The description that follows is by no means inclusive, but represents an introduction to the concepts related to a specific toggle recoil technique, a full-spine technique, and is adapted from the writings of Stephenson (1927) and Cleveland (1951) and from interviews of C. S. Cleveland, Jr.

Patient Positioning

With a patient positioned prone on the adjusting table, the patient's face is turned toward the side of laterality of subluxation for posterior and lateral subluxations. Such patient positioning provides for the application of tension to ligamentous fibers, removing slack from the joint prior to the execution of the adjustive thrust. It brings into prominence the point of contact of osseous structure on the vertebra, allowing the delivery of a posterior-to-anterior thrust with intent to influence the laterality and posteriority of subluxation. Such patient positioning provides for formation of an open wedge anteriorly between the vertebral bodies and the disc space, and thus allows the thrust to be directed from posterior to anterior into the open side of the wedge (Kirk, 1978). When laterality is not a factor, as in a posterior subluxation, the patient's face is straight down and the doctor may stand on either side of the table to deliver the thrust.

Doctor's Standing Position

The adjustive thrust is executed parallel to the plane of the disc space (Gonstead, 1980; Cleveland, 1951). To accomplish this goal, the doctor assumes a standing position that provides for an efficient adjustive thrust in line with the plane of the vertebral body. When making contact on the spinous process in the thoracic and lumbar area, the adjuster stands on the side of spinous laterality of subluxation from the second thoracic downward inclusive (Fig. 26–3) and opposite the side of spinous laterality of the subluxation from T-1 upward inclusively (Fig. 26–4). For subluxations identified to be straight posterior with no laterality, the doctor may stand on either side. In

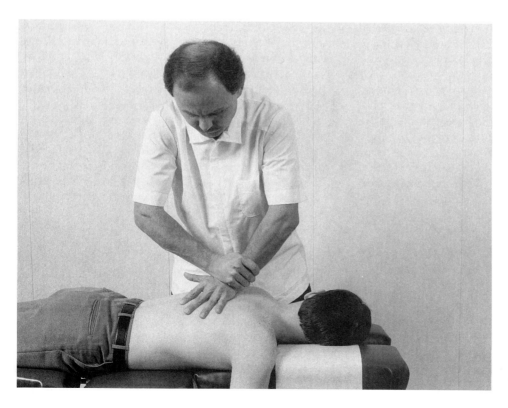

Figure 26-3. Positioning for adjustment of sixth thoracic spinous left.

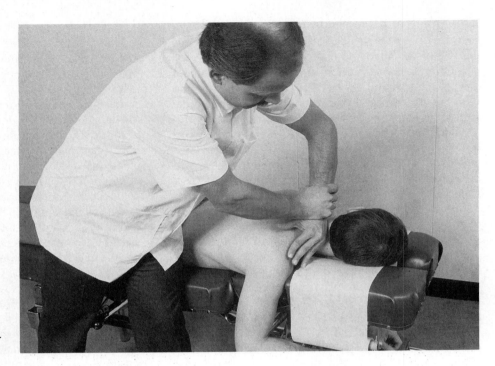

Figure 26-4. Positioning for adjustment of third cervical spinous left.

making contact on the lamina, transverse process, or articular pillar, as in body subluxations (laterolisthesis) combined with rotational malposition in the thoracic or lumbar area, the adjuster stands on the side opposite vertebral body laterality of subluxation from the sixth cervical downward inclusive and on the side of body laterality (laterolisthesis) from the fifth cervical upward inclusive.

The adjuster assumes a standing position facing the table, with feet positioned at a right angle in relation to the patient's spine when making adjustments with the spinous process contact in the region from T-2 through the sacrum (see Fig. 26–3). For atlas contacts and cervical spinous process contacts of C-2 through C-5, the adjuster stands opposite the side of spinous laterality, backing up while facing the head of the table (see Fig. 26–4). For spinous process contacts on the sixth cervical, seventh cervical, and first thoracic vertebrae, the adjuster backs up to the table and faces the foot of the table (Fig. 26–5). With the adjuster in the appropriate standing position, he or she may then proceed to position the hands and make osseous contact to achieve the appropriate direction of thrust in relation to the articulations to be adjusted.

Direction of Thrust

For posterior and lateral subluxations, the direction of thrust or line of drive is a right angle to the slope of the patient's spine (Gonstead, 1980; Cleveland, 1951). For superior or flexion malposition subluxations and for inferior or extension malposition subluxations, the line of drive should be a 45° angle from the superior (cephalic) or inferior (caudal), respectively.

Adjustment of Articulations of Atlas

Atlas subluxations are divided into two general categories that consider functional or positional disrelationships of the atlanto-occipital articulation and the atlantoaxial articulation. A variety of authors have developed complex systems of analysis and listings of atlanto-occipital and atlantoaxial subluxations, as well as complex procedures for adjusting these articulations. (Palmer College of Chiropractic, 1981; Pettibon, 1976; Gonstead, 1980).

Adjustment of the atlas with the patient positioned in the prone position on a standard Hylo table is demonstrated in Figure 26–6. The patient's face is turned toward the side of laterality to remove the ligamentous slack within the articulation and to bring the osseous point of contact into an uppermost position in relation to the doctor.

As an example, with an atlas subluxated left, or with restricted motion on the left, the patient's face is turned to the left with the doctor in a standing position along the right side of the patient, backing up to the table and facing the head of the table. The atlas does not subluxate directly posterior in relation to the axis because the odontoaxial articulation limits posterior movement, except in the case of fracture of the odontoid process. Proponents of the recoil technique maintained that the atlas shifts to the right or,

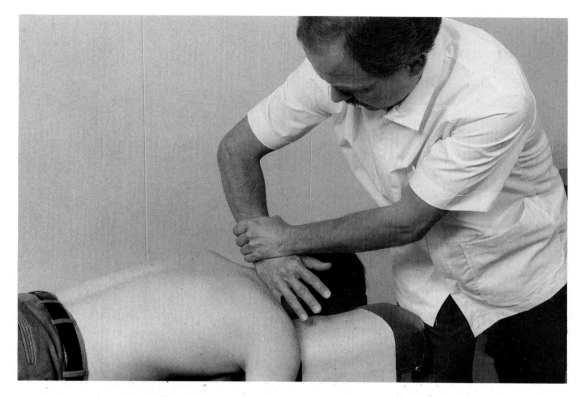

Figure 26-5. Positioning for adjustment of sixth cervical spinous left.

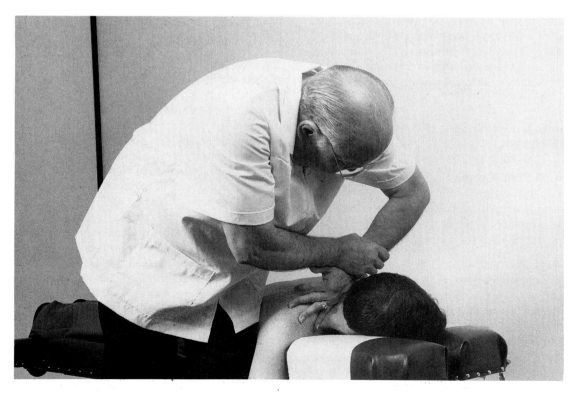

Figure 26-6. Positioning for adjustment of atlas posterior and left.

conversely, to the left, and pivots around the odontoid process to the posterior on the side to which it subluxates; therefore, the bony ring and the transverse processes gave the appearance of moving posterior on the side of laterality of subluxation. The point of contact in this example is the posterior arch of the atlas on the left side. A nail point two contact is placed on this posterior arch with a forceful adjustive thrust directed at right angles to the slope of the spine. Subluxations with listing identifying superiority or inferiority with respect to this articulation may be addressed by directing the line of drive cephalad or caudad. In atlas listings involving subluxation directly right or left, the patient's face is turned toward the side of restricted motion, or laterality of subluxation. A nail point one contact point is applied to the tip of the transverse process. The line of drive is directed lengthwise through the opposite transverse of the atlas. For subluxations to the right or left combined with unilateral anterior rotation, the contact point is on the side of laterality of the transverse process with the contact on the anterior portion of the transverse process, with line of drive directed slightly posterior.

Side-posture adjusting was introduced by Carver as early as 1908; however, it was during the mid-1930s that the side-posture technique was made popular by Palmer (Wells, 1987). Side-posture patient positioning and adjustment of the atlas using the Thompson–Williams drop table equipment are demonstrated in Figure 26–7. Toggle thrusts involving torque, or corkscrew-type movements, may be incorporated to bring about motion in the joint as it relates to particular relationships of the condyles of the occiput (Palmer College of Chiropractic, 1981).

Adjustment Using Spinous Process Contact

Axis Through Fifth Cervical

From the axis to the fifth cervical inclusive, the doctor stands on the side opposite the subluxation, backing up alongside the trunk of the patient, the adjuster facing the head of the table (see Fig. 26–4).

EXAMPLE: AXIS POSTERIOR LEFT [AxPL]. The doctor stands alongside the patient's thoracic region on the right side of the patient, backing up to the table while facing the head of the table. The patient's head is turned to the left, toward the side of laterality of subluxation listing. The doctor palpates with the right hand to locate the spinous process of the axis. A nail point two contact (halfway between the pisiform bone and metacarpal phalangeal joint) is placed under the spinous process (inferior to the spinous).

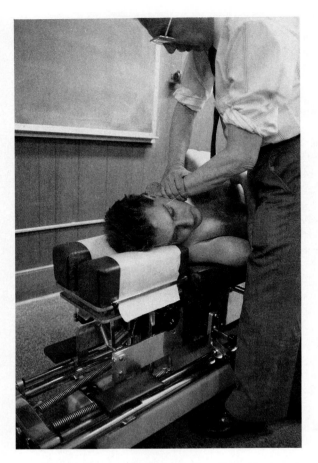

Figure 26–7. Side-posture positioning for atlas adjustment using current-technology Thompson–Williams drop table.

The extreme tip of the palpating index finger is placed slightly under the tip of the spinous process to be adjusted. The index finger of the palpating hand serves as a guide to locate the specific contact point. With the hammer arm tucked close to her or his body, the doctor grasps the wrist of the contact nail hand (contact hand). The doctor relaxes the upper arms completely. When the patient relaxes, a quick dynamic recoil thrust is delivered at right angles to the slope of the neck.

For an opposite listing as on an axis posterior right (AxPR), the procedure is as described above, except in a contralateral manner. The third, fourth, and fifth cervicals are similarly adjusted, considering the varying slopes of the back and the direction of line of drive at right angle to the slope of the neck.

It is important to note that from the axis to the fifth cervical inclusive, the line of drive of the dynamic thrust must be in line with the upward and oblique slope of the articulating processes of this region of the spine. The thrust must be directed in such a way that it does not jam together the articulating processes.

Sixth Cervical, Seventh Cervical, and First Thoracic

The doctor stands at the head of the table on the side opposite the laterality of subluxation listing, backing up and facing the foot of the table. The patient's head faces the side of spinous laterality of subluxation.

EXAMPLE: SEVENTH CERVICAL POSTERIOR RIGHT. Standing on the left side of the patient at the head of the table, the doctor backs up facing the foot of the table. The doctor palpates with the right hand, locating the tip of the seventh cervical spinous process. A nail point two contact is made with the left hand. The wrist of the contact hand is grasped with the hammer hand, and with the contact on the extreme tip of the spinous process, the doctor proceeds with a toggle recoil thrust at right angle to the slope toward the inferior.

If the sixth cervical, seventh cervical, or first thoracic is posterior and left, the same procedure is followed on the opposite side with the opposite hands. Figure 26–5 demonstrates standing position for adjustment of a sixth cervical, spinous left subluxation.

Second Thoracic Through Fifth Lumbar

In posterior and lateral spinous subluxations from the second thoracic to fifth lumbar inclusive, the doctor stands on the side of the laterality. In posterior and lateral subluxations in this region the doctor stands facing the adjusting table. For a posterior right superior (PRS) subluxation, the doctor stands at a 45° angle to the superior of the point of contact and thrusts anterior and inferiorly. For a posterior left superior (PLS) or posterior left inferior (PLI) subluxation, the doctor stands on the left side and steps to the superior or inferior at 45° angles as indicated by the listing.

Adjustment Using Lamina or Articular Pillar Contact (Body Subluxations—Laterolisthesis)

Axis Through Fifth Cervical

The patient's face is turned toward the side of laterality of subluxation. The doctor stands facing the patient on the side of laterality of subluxation, making a pisiform contact on the lamina pedicle junction of the vertebra in question. A dynamic thrust is directed anteriorly and somewhat superiorly. A thrust with the line of drive slightly superior is necessary in adjusting the axis and third, fourth, and fifth cervi-

cals because of the slope of the articulating processes.

Sixth Cervical, Seventh Cervical, and First Thoracic

Standing on the side opposite the body subluxation (laterolisthesis), the doctor makes a pisiform contact on the lamina pedicle junction. The line of drive and thrust are calculated with consideration given to the varying slopes of the articulating processes.

Second Thoracic Through Fifth Lumbar

Thoracic Laterolisthesis. To correct laterolisthesis of vertebral bodies in the thoracics, lamina contacts are used. Transverse process contacts may be used in the thoracic region except for T-11 and T-12, where such processes are rudimentary and may be absent entirely.

EXAMPLE: SEVENTH THORACIC PL BODY RIGHT [RIGHT LATEROLISTHESIS]. Such a listing may also be termed seventh thoracic body retrolisthesis with left rotational malposition and right laterolisthesis using the Medicare Listings (see Fig. 26–1 and 26–2). The doctor stands on the left side of the patient. To locate the lamina in the thoracic region, he or she palpates the spinous process and transverse process of the vertebra to be adjusted. The point between these two osseous processes approximates the lamina of the vertebra in question. It must be recognized that ordinarily the fifth through ninth thoracic spinous processes slope most obliquely downward and the eleventh and twelfth thoracic transverse processes are rudimentary. These anatomic factors must be considered in location of lamina contacts in a thoracic adjustment.

After calculation of the proper line of drive and adoption of the proper standing position, the doctor attains the proper hand position for toggle thrust by placing the pisiform bone of the nail or contact hand on the lamina, ensuring the fingers of the contact nail hand are spread and straight with the hand positioned in a high arch to provide stable contact. The wrist of the contact hand is grasped loosely with the hammer hand, ensuring that the adjuster's elbows and shoulders are in the same plane as the patient's spine. While maintaining the nail hand arch contact by contraction of the forearm muscles the adjuster should relax the muscles of the upper arms, then proceed with a quick dynamic thrust, contracting the biceps, anconei, and pectorals, driving from posterior to anterior.

The first through fourth thoracics are adjusted similarly except that the spinous process in this region of the spine slopes less obliquely downward and there is a shorter distance between the tips of the spinous process and the transverse processes of a given vertebra, which must be considered in locating the area of the lamina between these two osseous reference points. For left laterolisthesis or body subluxations, the procedure described is followed for the seventh thoracic subluxated posterior left, vertebral body right. On the opposite side of the patient the opposite hand positioning is used.

Lumbar Laterolisthesis.

In view of the thin and bladelike transverse processes of the lumbar vertebra, it is recommended that only lamina contacts or mammillary contacts used.

EXAMPLE: SECOND LUMBAR BODY RIGHT [RIGHT LATEROLISTHESIS]. Standing on the left side of the patient, the doctor makes a nail point one contact on the lamina or mammillary process on the right side of the vertebra. The line of drive at right angles to the slope of the spine is calculated. The doctor relaxes the upper arm muscles, taking care not to lose vertebral contact. After the patient completely relaxes, the dynamic thrust is executed from posterior to anterior. Certain authors (Grice, 1980; Cleveland, 1951) describe toggle recoil–type thrusts in this area of the spine; others describe toggle and hold (Gonstead, 1980; Barge, 1982b).

Lumbosacral and Sacroiliac Adjustment

Static listings related to the sacrum may be identified as base posterior, left base posterior, right base posterior, and apex posterior.

For base posterior a flat arch, nail point one contact is made on the second tubercle of the sacrum, with the dynamic thrust directed at right angles to the slope of the back. For sacral apex posterior, the posterior-to-anterior thrust is made with the contact on the fourth tubercle of the sacrum, taking care not to be in contact with the sacral hiatus or the segments of the coccyx. For a left sacral base posterior subluxation, the doctor stands opposite the side of laterality of subluxation (on the right side of the patient). The contact point is $\frac{1}{2}$ to $\frac{3}{4}$ inch to the left of the second sacral tubercle. Opposite positioning would occur in adjustment of a right base posterior.

For adjustments related to the sacroiliac joint, the adjuster may contact the posterosuperior spine of the ilium. Detailed techniques and procedures of analysis for adjusting the sacroiliac articulations have been developed by Gonstead (1980), and Gillet and Liekens (1973).

Evolution of Chiropractic Adjusting Tables

As procedures for high velocity technique became refined, and as various diversified procedures were incorporated into chiropractic practice, the chiropractic adjusting table evolved to accommodate the patient positioning, the doctor's standing position, and the direction and type of adjustive thrust. The adjusting table and related equipment has been modified and adapted in response to the needs of the practitioner.

According to Dye (1939), Palmer School graduate of 1912, the earliest of D. D. Palmer's chiropractic adjustments were given with the patient lying prone on the floor, face downward, the patient's nose pointing directly to the floor. The force was directed with a straight or stiff arm with no concern for laterally, inferiorly, or superiorly directed thrusts. Later adjustments were given on tables.

Early Tables

Dye describes the earliest adjusting table as a flat, one-piece table, much like a workman's bench, but with the surface of the bench approximately knee high. They were usually made out of plain oak or pine wood; a leather cover was tacked over the table, and there was no felt or hair padding underneath. The patient would lie on the table face downward, with nose and chin pointed into the table. With a straight anterior shove on a subluxated vertebra, the patient's face and nose were pushed abruptly into the table. This type of table and patient positioning created extreme discomfort and often resulted in nosebleeds from thrusts applied to the patient's cervical region.

D. D. Palmer's initial intent was to reduce or adjust the subluxation by the application of great force and weight, forcibly thrusting or pushing the subluxated vertebra straight anterior into normal relationship with adjacent vertebra. The weight of the upper part of the chiropractor's body, arms and shoulders, was often supplemented by additional bags of sand of varying size and weight, which were placed over the adjustor's shoulders. Adjustments using such technique produced great discomfort and pain to the patient.

An attempt to improve the table provided for a sloping board positioned at the forward end of the table projecting downward at approximately a 45° angle. The patient would be placed in a prone position, with the head and neck bent downward over the angled board. This table provided for greater ease of adjustment and required less force on the part of the adjuster; however, with the nose and chin pointing into the board, the patient continued to suffer pain and nosebleeds (Dye, 1939).

As chiropractic evolved as a science, pioneers broadened their technical procedures to include adjustments of various regions of the spine. Because of the contour of the human body, provision had to be made in the table to permit delivery of an adjustment with as little physical discomfort to the patient as possible, and with greater ease and facility on the part of the chiropractor. To enhance patient comfort for adjustments to the thoracic region, pads or pillows were placed under the upper chest; however, these pads or soft pillows were considered to impair the effectiveness of the adjustment.

With the objectives of lessening the pain and discomfort to the patient and increasing the efficiency of the adjustment through greater patient relaxation, it was determined that raising the forward end of the table, using hard pillows or pads, and applying the thrust to the cervical region, turning the patient's face to the right or to the left, were useful.

At the beginning of the 1900s, the typical chiropractic office included a flat, one-piece adjusting table supplemented by pillows or pads to elevate the patient's chest and hips. This provided for a limited degree of suspension of the patient's abdomen and lower chest. As techniques expanded beyond a straight posterior-to-anterior adjustment, they took into consideration factors requiring dynamic thrusts directed laterally, superiorly, and inferiorly. It was determined that the lower chest and abdomen of the patient should be elevated above the flat, one-piece table to avoid injury resulting from heavy stiff-arm adjusting procedures. Firm pillows were placed under the upper chest and pelvic regions, leaving the abdomen and lower thorax completely suspended in midair. Such abdominal suspension provided greater separation of the vertebral bodies anteriorly. The patient's sensation of suspension, however, caused the patient to tense muscles, interfering with the chiropractor's efficiency in delivering the thrust of the adjustment.

About 1905, the flat, one-piece table was replaced by a two-piece table. The front part of the table had an upward slant and the lower table consisted of a short flat bench (Fig. 26–8). The forward table was narrowed at the lower end, permitting the patient's arms to drop and allowing the shoulders to rest flat on the table surface. The higher end of the table was broadened outward and padded with hair or felt. This forward table supported the patient's body and the upper edge of the sternum as the upper thoracics and cervicals were being adjusted. The rear of the two-piece table supported the lower part of the body from the hips. With this table, the patient's body between the sternum and the lower abdomen or hips was suspended in midair. Early writings of Stephenson describe such positioning in which the patient is "placed upon two benches with the dorsal and lumbar regions bulging over a gap between two benches. The superior end of the rear bench comes across the thighs a few inches just below the hip joints. The inferior end of the front bench comes across the chest on a line between the axillae. This gives two fixed points for dorsal or lumbar adjustments with the body swinging fully." In the lower piece, a portion of the table surface was cut out to avoid injury to the male genitalia.

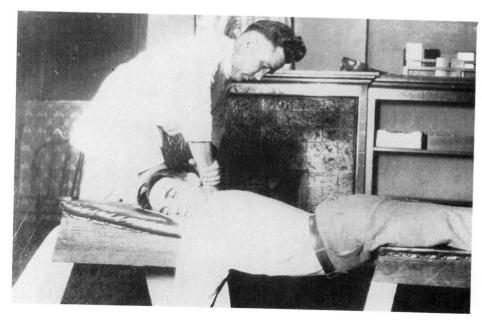

Figure 26–8. Early two-piece adjusting table developed to allow for suspension of abdomen, circa 1922.

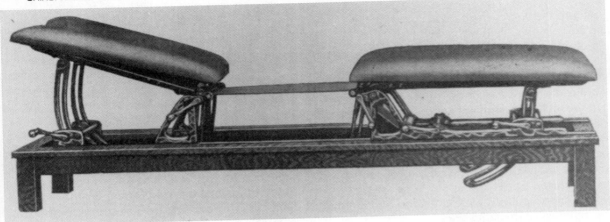

Figure 26–9. Adjustable two-piece table with cloth abdominal support band.

Patients continued to tense their bodies as a result of the feeling of suspension, particularly when the lower thoracics or lumbars were being adjusted. Beginning in 1911, a middle table with soft padding was used. Variation included a wide belt or cloth support between the two-piece tables to overcome the patients' tendency to stiffen up when suspended between the two-piece adjusting table. About 1912 to 1914 a hinged, tablelike support was attached to the rear of the headpiece with a spring attachment, which provided the patient a semblance of support to the upper abdomen. However, the rebound of this attachment during a forceful thrust often resulted in a slap to the patient's abdomen from this abdominal support.

The two-piece table was gradually replaced by a table in which the front piece and rear piece were movable and glided in a raillike motion at the base on the floor (Fig. 26–9; note the wide cloth band to provide a semblance of abdominal support). These tables were made with the forward part divided into two sections or with a deep slot through the greater part of the center to allow the patient's face to be directed straight downward, with the patient's nose and chin in this slot. Promotional materials identify Adams Manufacturing Company, manufacturers of suitcases and office tables, as "the designer and builder of the first table used in the practice of Chiropractic" (Fig. 26–10).

Hylo Tables

After an adjustment, it was desirable for the patient to be able to arise from the adjusting table with little strain or exertion so as not to undo the effects of the adjustment. A precursor of what was later identified by the term *Hylo table* used levers on an adjustable base at the most caudal portion of the table. This allowed the entire structure to be raised from a horizontal position to a nearly 90° angle. With the table in the raised position, the patient would be able to step onto the footplate of the table; the table would then be lowered by the chiropractor to a level approximately 18 inches parallel to the floor, thus positioning the patient for the chiropractic adjusting procedures. Following the adjustment, the table and patient would be elevated, and the patient could step directly off, without the twisting or turning previously required when arising from the stationary-type adjusting tables.

Early tables of this type developed in 1910 by Bert Clayton of Davenport, Iowa, were elevated by compressed air or manually through a series of springs and levers allowing the doctor to raise or lower the table. These tables had immediate appeal to the profession (Dye, 1939). Advertisements promoted the Palmer Hylo Table IV (Fig. 26–11), approximate shipping weight 200 pounds, which could be purchased from the Palmer School with abdominal support for $80 or without abdominal support for

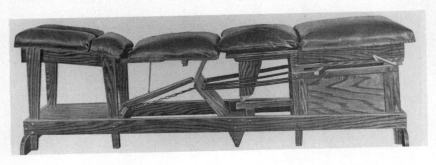

Figure 26–10. Adam's wooden table, circa 1910.

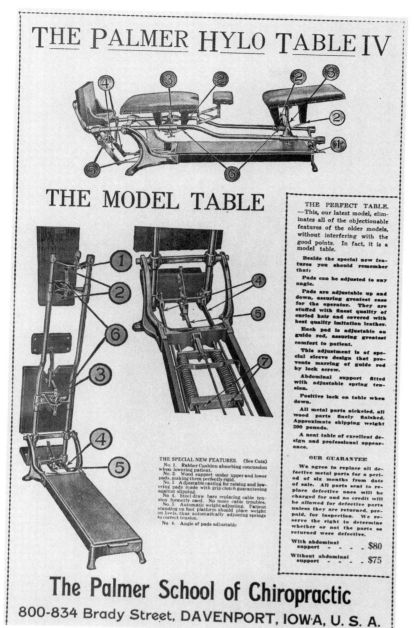

Figure 26–11. Palmer Hylo Table IV, circa 1920.

$75. Evins and Styles (Wells, 1987) developed a mechanical table that was raised and lowered by means of springs and was adjustable according to the patient's weight and height. Early promotional materials for the Styles Hylo tables (Fig. 26–12 and 26–13) stated that the table ''Can be adjusted according to the length of the patient. Easily changed to suit individual curvatures and for various adjustic moves. No twisting, straining, or wrenching. Patients return to standing position without any effort on their part and without the slightest jar.'' These tables incorporated modified screen door coil springs. As many as 30 springs were required in the early hylo table to provide adequate tension. Tables developed later

used three or four heavy garage door–type springs to assist in table elevation.

In 1923 Williams patented the first Zenith Hylo table. Such tables provided a headpiece, chestpiece, and movable abdominal support that could be guided cephalad or caudad along rails attached to a common base. Williams Manufacturing Company was founded in Moline, Illinois, by W. G. Williams, D.C., in 1916 and appears to be the oldest of the current manufacturers of chiropractic tables serving the profession today (Wells, 1987).

As techniques in chiropractic changed, other adjusting tables evolved. As early as 1925, electrical tables were introduced into the profession (Williams

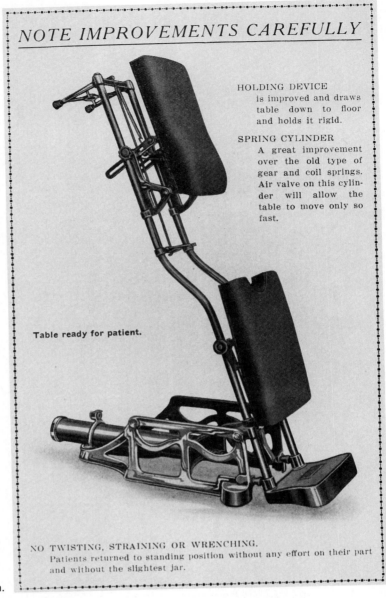

NOTE IMPROVEMENTS CAREFULLY

HOLDING DEVICE
is improved and draws table down to floor and holds it rigid.

SPRING CYLINDER
A great improvement over the old type of gear and coil springs. Air valve on this cylinder will allow the table to move only so fast.

Table ready for patient.

NO TWISTING, STRAINING OR WRENCHING.
Patients returned to standing position without any effort on their part and without the slightest jar.

Figure 26–12. Styles Hylo Table, upright position.

Manufacturing, 1988). The Palmer-Evins Hylo Table (Fig. 26–14) was constructed as a spring lift table that could be converted to a motor lift. Promotional materials indicated that the motorized conversion may "easily be installed by your local electrician or mechanic." The first electric-powered Zenith Hylo became available in 1940.

Knee–Chest Table

Stephenson (1927) described knee-posture positioning in which the patient kneels on a pad, bends forward, and places the head and shoulders on the forward bench of the two-piece table. The patient's thighs positioned approximately perpendicular to the floor give support to the lower end of the spine.

The weight of the head and chest is supported on the forward bench. The knees were positioned forward for adjusting the cervicals and upper thoracics and positioned backward for adjusting the lumbars and sacrum. According to Stephenson, "the correct placement of the knees can be ascertained by placing the palpating hand on the back at the location of the subluxated vertebrae and then move the patient's knees forward or backward until the back muscles are relaxed at that place." Stephenson considered the flexing of the thighs as providing "the best possible relaxed posture." He did not consider knee posture good for adjusting the sacrum and ilium. In 1937 the knee–chest table appeared with the announcement of the "B.J.–Zenith Special Kneeling Posture

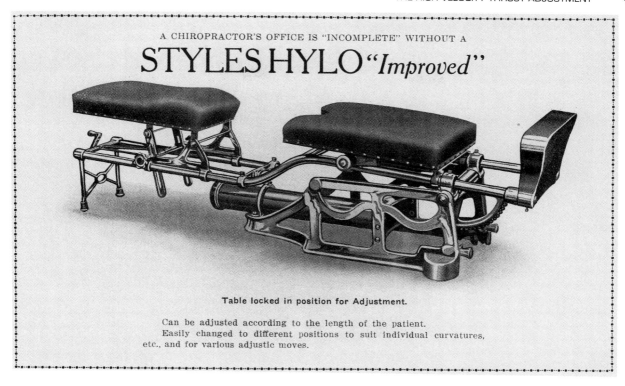

Figure 26–13. Styles Hylo Table, lowered position.

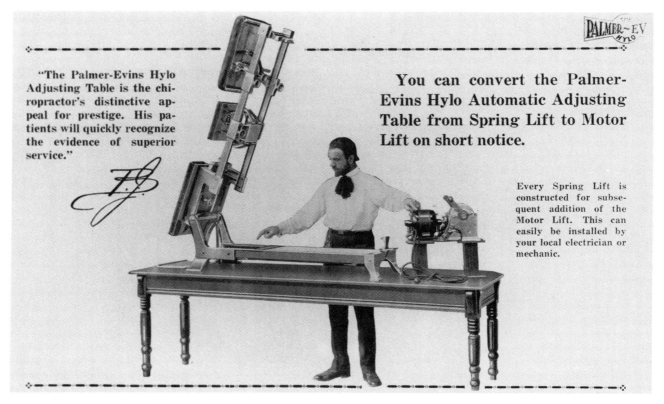

Figure 26–14. Palmer–Evins Hylo Table, circa 1925.

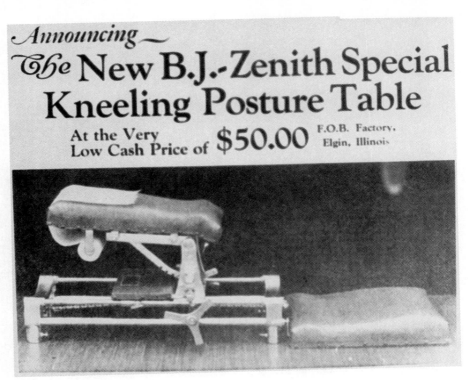

Figure 26–15. Kneeling-posture table, circa 1927.

Table, cash price $50.00, F.O.B., Factory, Elgin, Illinois'' (Fig. 26–15). The modern version of the knee–chest table (Fig. 26–16) along with the cervical chair and pelvic bench was made popular by Gonstead (1980).

Side-Posture Table

The side-posture table was introduced by Carver as early as 1908; however, not until 1935 was it announced that this table was being incorporated into

the Palmer Hole-in-One technique (Wells, 1987). Stationary side-posture tables could be ordered through the Palmer School for the cash price of ''$55.00, F.O.B., Factory, Elgin, Illinois'' (Fig. 26–17). In 1952, J. Clay Thompson introduced the side-posture drop-headpiece mechanical table.

Drop Tables

A table incorporating separate drop-piece mechanisms for the head, thoracic, lumbar, and pelvic sup-

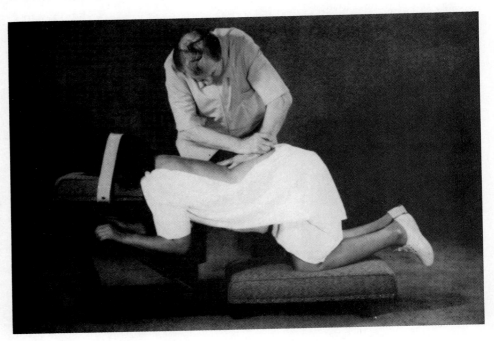

Figure 26–16. Patient positioning on a Gonstead knee–chest table.

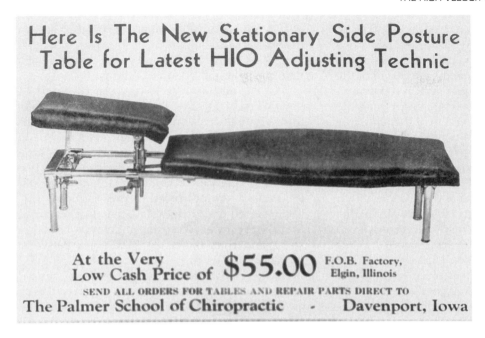

Here Is The New Stationary Side Posture
Table for Latest HIO Adjusting Technic

At the Very
Low Cash Price of $55.00 F.O.B. Factory,
Elgin, Illinois

SEND ALL ORDERS FOR TABLES AND REPAIR PARTS DIRECT TO

The Palmer School of Chiropractic - Davenport, Iowa

Figure 26–17. Side-posture
table, circa 1935.

ports was first introduced to the profession in London, during the 1958 European Chiropractic Union convention. The drop-piece was developed with the intent to lessen patient pain during an adjustment and to reduce the concussion of force experienced by the adjuster. The practitioner thus suffered less fatigue. Each drop-piece support would allow approximately $\frac{3}{8}$-inch downward movement toward the floor as the dynamic thrust was applied (see Fig. 26–7).

Early drop tables involved a pedal-activated tension mechanism with a magnetic catch to hold the drop-piece in the cocked position prior to application of the dynamic thrust. Wells described modifications to the table, including a metal catch bar that pivoted to allow for variable tension by having less of the bar come in contact with the magnet. Later, a spring tension ballbearing mechanism was incorporated, allowing variation in the force required to overcome the cocked position setting. Spring tensioned roller bearings were later incorporated to provide smoother release. Pneumatic cocking mechanisms

are in use today. In a personal interview, Thompson stated that the tension required to activate the drop-piece was set according to the patient's weight and a dynamic thrust of approximately 3 pounds of applied weight was required to activate the drop-piece.

McManis Table

Certain tables in use today originated within the osteopathic profession and were marketed to a variety of health-care practitioners. McManis, an osteopath, patented a table in 1909 that was later called the McManis table (Fig. 26–18). McManis had set out to design a multipurpose table that could serve as a surgery table, an ear/nose/throat examination chair, a gynecologic examination table, and a manipulation table. A modern version of this table used by chiropractors for lumbar distraction was made popular within the chiropractic profession by Cox. In the McManis table, a universal joint provided for multidirectional movements of the spine and sacroiliac joints, allowing flexion, extension, and rotation, in addition to axial traction.

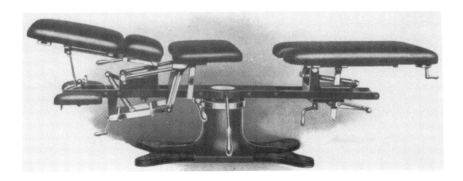

Figure 26–18. McManis multipurpose
table, circa 1927.

Distraction Tables

Flexion distraction tables provide for patient positioning that stabilizes the torso from the area of the midlumbar spine upward and allows pivoting of the thoracolumbar and sacral areas through movement of the caudal portion of the table, which supports the pelvis and legs. A motorized version of the table was developed by Cox in 1976; however, Cox discontinued production because he preferred manual control of the manipulative procedure. In 1981, Leander Eckard produced a motorized distraction table combining the flexion table for spinal distraction with a segmented full-spine adjusting table. An adjustable abdominal suspension mechanism allows positioning of the patient to provide for the lordotic lumbar curve. Such positioning allows separation of the lumbar disc spaces and produces an opening of the disc space wedge anteriorly. This has been proposed by Eckard to enhance the disc distraction process.

Traction Tables

The Pandiculator Company (1913) produced an axial traction table followed by the Cropp "all-in-one" Master Service Device (Fig. 26–19) around 1925, patented by David Bertram Cropp and marketed to doctors of medicine, osteopathy, chiropractic, naturopathy, napropathy, and mechanotherapy. The Cropp table was promoted as a tension therapy device combined with "an examination and adjusting table for physicians of all schools." Donahoe, an osteopath, commenced production in 1937 of an intersegmental traction table and established the Spinalator Company (Wells, 1987).

Table Pads

Beatty, as early as 1939, described the use of a "pelvic roll," a cushionlike firm pillow approximately 16 inches long and 7 inches in diameter, placed under the pelvis just caudal to the anterior superior iliac spines for facilitation of adjustment below the upper thoracics. This was considered to relax the dorsal musculature and release pressure on the stomach area when the thrust was given. Beatty also proposed utilization of a small roll positioned to raise the ankles to assist in relaxation of the back musculature. Ankle supports or foot rests are available on many adjusting tables in use today.

L. F. and Berniece Widmoyer, founders of Re-Lax-O Products, Inc., 1944, developed a table pad that served to cushion the chest area to maintain the "normal dorsal curve for easier adjustment and patient comfort." Initially, these pads fit over an existing table and created a thoracic hump, which became known as the "dorsal roll." Later, standard stationary tables were produced incorporating all the pad features. It should be noted that utilization of the dorsal roll produced posterior arching of the thoracic spine and thus increased separation between the thoracic spinous processes, facilitating palpation of the area. Such positioning, however, tended to wedge the thoracic disc spaces anteriorly. Thrust directed anterior with the patient arched over the dorsal roll tended to wedge the vertebral bodies anteriorly, resulting in an unwanted force on the anterior aspect of the thoracic spine.

DeJarnette developed a system in which padded "blocks, wedges, sternal rolls and pelvic boards," were used on the adjusting table to position the patient and apply corrective force to the patient's body. Beginning in 1965, this equipment was manufactured by Steffensmeier, founder of Lloyd Table Company.

As chiropractic technique and related procedures continue to evolve, chiropractic adjusting tables will be adapted to meet the needs of the profession. A variety of adjusting tables and related equipment is available to the profession today. A description of the present technology is beyond the scope of this chapter.

Conclusion

Various authors in medicine, osteopathy, chiropractic, and physiotherapy have independently observed and described the clinical biomechanical entity, re-

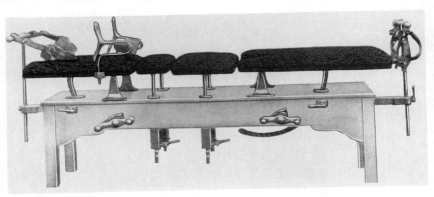

Figure 26–19. Cropp "all-in-one" axial traction table, circa 1925.

ferred to as somatic joint dysfunction, spinal lesion, or subluxation, which is responsive to spinal manipulative therapy or spinal adjustment (Mennell, 1930; Cleveland, 1951; Mitchell, 1973; Buerger, 1977; Fisk, 1977; Nachemson, 1979; Gitelman, 1980). Wide variation exists in nomenclature identifying this manually diagnosed entity. Standardization of nomenclature may lead to enhanced interdisciplinary communication and facilitate research related to the assessment of spinal manipulative therapy. Commonality exists between disciplines, however, when one considers the observed physical findings and descriptive clinical characteristics associated with the manipulable spinal lesion.

The relationship between spinal biomechanical instability, spinal curvature, restricted spinal motion, or palpable soft tissue changes at specific spinal levels has been associated with clinical findings in tissues or organs within the segmental distribution of nerves associated with lesions at specific segmental spinal levels (Winsor, 1922; Davis, 1947; DePalma, 1970; Jackson, 1973; Inman, 1973; Gunn, 1976; Hadley, 1977; Latan, 1979; Greenman, 1989). Correlation of sympathetic segmental dysfunction with biomechanical derangements of the spine has been proposed by various health care practitioners (Gregory, 1969; Braaf, 1973; Janse, 1975; Hildebrandt, 1978; Korr, 1981; Tilley, 1987; Wislowska, 1989). The concept of biomechanical impairments at specific segmental levels of the spine being a potential indicator of the disease process has been described by Korr (1955), Denslow (1975), Walton (1970) and Lewit (1985). The chiropractic profession's early recognition of the vulnerability of the segmental nervous system to somatic insult is reflected in the association of early chiropractic technique systems with the clinical concept of meric analysis. Such analysis associated vertebral subluxation and its influence on segmentally mediated changes within dermatomes, myotomes, and autonomic nervous system pathways (Firth, 1921; Forster, 1923; Craven, 1924; Biron, 1939; Cleveland, 1951). According to the Report of the Commission of Inquiry into Chiropractic, New Zealand (1979), ''In a limited number of cases where there are organic and/or visceral symptoms, chiropractic treatment may provide relief, but this is unpredictable, and in such cases the patient should be under concurrent medical care if that is practicable.'' Further investigation of the somato-visceral reflex relationships and the manipulable spinal lesion is required.

A central element common to health disciplines incorporating use of spinal manipulative therapy is the application of motion to the involved spinal articular segment. Such application may range from traction, mobilization, non-specific long-lever manipulation, or to specific short-lever, high velocity spinal adjustment. It is the short-lever high velocity thrust adjustment that is most commonly associated with chiropractic practice, although more generalized procedures may also be used. Preliminary study suggests (Luttges, 1982) that specifically directed short-lever high velocity thrust adjustment results in enhanced motor and sensory function as demonstrated by accuracy of patient performance on two-point discrimination and force estimation testing, and lesser accuracy in subjects receiving long-lever non-specific manipulation when compared to a non-treatment group. The comparative effectiveness of various technique procedures requires further investigation.

The control and delivery of the adjustive thrust demands much discipline and skill, and requires intensive training. Specific procedures for patient positioning and doctor standing positioning have developed to provide patient relaxation and comfort and to enhance the doctor's technique of application of motion through controlled dynamic thrusts directed to specific articular structures. A description of one of the early technique systems, Full Spine Specific Technique, also termed Toggle or Meric Recoil Technique, has been provided in this chapter. Chiropractic adjusting tables and related equipment evolved in relation to the changing technique procedures, and will continue to be modified in response to the needs of the practitioner.

As conservative management of back pain and spinal-related conditions gains importance within mainstream health care (Deyo, 1983), and as trends toward increased medical referral of back pain patients to chiropractors progresses (Cherkin, 1989), opportunities for interdisciplinary research into spinal manipulative technique and the chiropractic adjustment can be expected to increase.

References

Barge FH. *Chiropractic Technic: Tortipelvis,* vol. I. Davenport, Iowa: FH Barge; 1976, 4th ed 1982(b).

Barge FH. *Chiropractic Technic: Scoliosis,* vol. III. Davenport, Iowa: FH Barge; 1981; 2nd printing 1982., 1982(a).

Beatty HG. *Anatomical Adjustive Technic.* Expanded & enlarged by AE Homewood. Fort Worth, Tex: Parker Chiropractic Research Foundation; 1983.

Biron WA et al. *Chiropractic Principles and Technique.* Chicago: National College of Chiropractic; 1939.

Bourdillon JF and Day FA. *Spinal Manipulation.* London: William Heinemann Medical Books; Norwalk, Conn: Appleton & Lange; 1970 4th ed 1987.

Braaf MM and Rosner S. Trauma of cervical spine as cause of chronic headache. *J Trauma* 1973;15(5):441–446.

Buerger AA and Tobis JS. *Approaches to the Validation of Manipulation Therapy.* Springfield, Ill: CC Thomas; 1977.

Cassidy JD and Kirkaldy-Davis WH. Manipulation. In *Managing Low Back Pain.* New York: Churchill Livingstone; 1988: vol. IV, pp. 125–135.

Christensen DC. *Clinical Chiropractic Biomechanics.* Dubuque, Iowa: Educational Division Foot Levelers, Inc; 1984.

Cleveland CS. *Chiropractic Principles and Practice—Outline.* Kansas City, Mo: CS Cleveland, Sr; 1951.

Commission of Inquiry Into Chiropractic. *Chiropractic in New Zealand.* Wellington, NZ: The Government Printer; 1979. Report, Davenport, Iowa: Palmer College of Chiropractic; n.d.

Craven JH, *A Text-Book [sic] on Hygiene and Pediatrics.* Davenport, Iowa: John H. Craven; 1924.

Davis D. Spinal nerve root pain (radiculitis) simulating coronary occlusion: A common syndrome. *Am Heart J* 1947.

DeGiacomo FP. *Textbook of Chiropractic Technique.* Plainview, NY: LSR Learning Associates, Inc.; 1981.

Denslow JS. Pathophysiologic evidence for the osteopathic lesion, data on what is known, what is not known, and what is controversial. In *The Research Status of Spinal Manipulative Therapy,* NINCDS Monograph 15. Bethesda, Md: U.S. Department of Health, Education, & Welfare; 1975:227–234.

DePalma AF and Rothman RH. *The Intervertebral Disc.* Philadelphia: WB Saunders; 1970.

Deyo, RA. Conservative therapy for low back pain—Distinguishing useful from useless therapy. *JAMA* 1983;250:1057–1062.

Dvorak J and Dvorak V. *Manual Medicine: Diagnostics.* Gilliar WG and Greenman PE, transl. and eds. Stuttgart: George Thieme Verlag; 1984/1988.

Dye, AA. *The Evolution of Chiropractic.* 1939. Richmond Hall, NY: Richmond Hill; 1939/1969.

Firth JN. *A Text-book [sic] on Chiropractic Symptomatology.* Davenport, Iowa: JN Firth; 1921.

Fisk JW. *a Practical Guide to Management of the Painful Neck and Back.* Springfield, Ill: CC Thomas; 1977.

Forster AL. *Principles and Practice of Chiropractic.* Chicago: National Publishing Assoc; 1923.

Gillet H and Liekens M. *Belgian Chiropractic Research Notes.* Brussels: Gillet & Liekens; 1973.

Gitelman R. A chiropractic approach to biomechanical disorders of the lumbar spine. In Haldeman S, ed. *Modern Developments in the Principles and Practice of Chiropractic.* New York: Appleton-Century-Crofts; 1980; ch. 14.

Gonstead, CS. In W. Herbst, *Gonstead Chiropractic Science & Art.* USA: SCH-CHI Publications; 1980.

Grecco MA. *Chiropractic Technic Illustrated.* New York: Jarl; 1953.

Greenman, P. *Principles of Manual Medicine.* Baltimore: Williams and Wilkins, 1989.

Gregory R. The ASC and leg imbalance. *NUCCA News* 1969; 7(7):1–2.

Grice AS. A biomechanical approach to cervical and dorsal adjusting. Ch. XV in *Modern Developments in the Principles and Practice of Chiropractic.* New York: Appleton-Century-Crofts; 1980.

Grove AB. *Chiropractic Technique: A Procedure of Adjusting.* Madison, Wisc: S. Krauss; 1979.

Gunn CC and Milbrandt WE. Tennis elbow and the cervical spine. *Can Med Assoc J* 1976;114:803–809.

Hadley LA. *Anatomico-Roentgenographic Studies of the Spine.* Springfield, Ill: CC Thomas; 1977.

Haldeman S. Spinal manipulative therapy and spinal adjustments. In *A Comprehensive Interdisciplinary Approach to the Management of Spinal Disorders.* Las Vegas, Nev: 1980 Haldeman Interprofessional Conference on the Spine; 1980a.

Haldeman S. Spinal manipulative therapy in the management of low back pain. In Finneson B. E. ed. *Low Back Pain,* 2nd ed. Philadelphia/Toronto: JB Lippincott; 1980b.

Haldeman, S. Spinal manipulation therapy: A status report. In *Clinical Orthopaedics and Related Research.* Philadelphia: JP Lippincott; 1983: vol. IV, pp. 116–124.

Hildebrandt RW. The scope of chiropractic as a clinical science and art: An introductory review of concepts. *JMPT* 1978;1(1):7–17.

Hippocrates. *Hippocrates,* vol. III. Withington ET, transl. vol. III. Cambridge: Harvard University Press; 1959.

Homewood AE. *The Neurodynamics of the Vertebral Subluxation.* Ontario: Chiropractic Publishers; 1963.

Inman OB, editor-in-chief. *Basic Chiropractic Procedural Manual.* Des Moines, Iowa: American Chiropractic Association; 1973.

Jackson R. *The Cervical Syndrome,* 3rd ed. Springfield, Ill: CC Thomas; 1976.

Janse J. History of the development of chiropractic concepts: Chiropractic terminology. In *NINCDS Monograph 15.* Bethesda, Md: U.S. Department of Health, Education, and Welfare; 1975.

Janse, J. *Principles and Practices of Chiropractic.* Lombard, Ill: National College of Chiropractic; 1976.

Kimberly E. *Outline of Osteopathic Manipulative Procedures.* Kirksville: Kirksville College of Osteopathic Medicine; 1979.

Kirk CR et al, eds. *States Manual of Spinal, Pelvic, and Extravertebral Technic.* JMPT 1978;1(1):7–17.

Kirkaldy-Willis WH. *Managing Low Back Pain,* 2nd ed. New York: Churchill Livingstone; 1988.

Korr IM. The concept of facilitation and its origins. *J Am Osteopath Assoc* 1955;54: 265–268.

Korr IM. The spinal cord as organizer of disease processes. IV. Axonal transport and neurotrophic function in relation to somatic dysfunction. *J Osteopath Soc* 1981;80(7)451–459.

Latan ML. Spinal maneuver eases chronic pain. *Med Tribune,* Jan. 3, 1979;20(1)

Leach RA. *The Chiropractic Theories: A Synopsis of Scientific Research.* Williams and Wilkins, 1986.

Lewit K. *Manipulative Therapy and Rehabilitation of the Locomotor System.* Stoneham, Mass: Butterworth; 1985.

Lomax E. Manipulative therapy: A historical perspective from ancient times to the modern era. In *NINCDS Monograph 15.* Bethesda, Md: U.S. Department of Health, Education, and Welfare; 1975:11–17.

Luttges MW and Cleveland CS III. Spinal correction effects on motor and sensory functions. In Mazzarelli JP, ed. *Chiropractic Interprofessional Research* (based on proceedings of the World Chiropractic Conference, Venice). Torino, Italy: Edigioni Minerva Medica; 1982.

Maigne R (transl. and ed.) and Liberson WT. *Orthopedic Medicine: A New Approach to Vertebral Manipulations.* Springfield, Ill: CC. Thomas; 1972, 3rd printing, 1979.

Mennell J. Manipulative therapy for low back pain. In Monica JJ et al., eds. *Advances in Pain Research and Therapy.* New York: Raven Press, 1979:685–96. Report in *A Comprehensive Interdisciplinary Approach to the Management of Spinal Disorders* (S. Haldeman, ed.). Las Vegas, Nev. The 1980 Haldeman Interprofessional Conference on the Spine, 1980.

Mennell J McM. *Back Pain—Diagnosis and Treatment Using Manipulative Therapy.* Boston: Little, Brown; 1960.

Mitchell FL. Introduction to chiropractic treatment. In *An Evaluation and Treatment Manual of Osteopathic Manipulative Procedures.* Kansas City, Mo: Kansas City Institute for Osteopathic Principles; 1973.

Nachemson A. A critical look at the treatment for low back pain. *Scand J Rehab Med* 1979;11:143–147.

Nicholas AS et al. A somatic component of myocardial infarction. *Br Med J,* July 6, 1985, vol. 291.

NINCDS *The Research Status of Spinal Manipulative Therapy,* Monograph 15. Bethesda, Md: U.S. Department of Health, Education, and Welfare; 1975.

Palmer BJ. *The Philosophy and Principles of Chiropractic Adjustments.* Davenport, Iowa BJ Palmer; 1908–1911.

Palmer BJ. *A Text Book [sic] on the Palmer Technique of Chiropractic.* Davenport, Iowa: BJ Palmer; 1920.

Palmer College of Chiropractic. *Adjusting Technique Manual.* Davenport, Iowa: Palmer College of Chiropractic; 1981.

Paris SV. Spinal manipulative therapy. In *Clinical Orthopaedics and Related Research*. Philadelphia: JB Lippincott Company; 1983: vol. 4, pp. 107–114.

Peterson DH (chairman). Chiropractic terminology: A report. *ACA J Chiropractic*, Sept 1988, pp. 46–57; Oct 1988, pp. 57–76.

Pettibon BR. *Biomechanical and Bioengineering of the Cervical Spine and X-Ray Analysis and Instrument Adjusting*. Davenport, Iowa: Pettibon & Associates; 1976.

Reinert OC. *Fundamentals of Chiropractic Techniques and Practice Procedures*. Chesterfield, Mo: Marian Press; 1962/1983.

Schafer RC and Faye LJ. *Motion Palpation and Chiropractic Technic*. Huntington Beach, Calif: Motion Palpation Institute; 1989.

Schneider W et al. *Manual Medicine: Therapy* (Gilliar WG and Greenman PE, transl. and eds.). Stuttgart/New York: George Thieme Verlag; 1988.

Smithson DJ. Manipulation from antiquity to the fifth century. *Digest Chiropractic Econ*, Nov–Dec 1988, pp. 17–18.

Stephenson, RW. *The Art of Chiropractic*. U.S.A.: RW Stephenson; 1927.

Stephenson RW. *Chiropractic Textbook*. Davenport, Iowa: Palmer School of Chiropractic; 1927/1948.

Stoddard A. *Manual of Osteopathic Technique*. London: Hutchinson; 1959. 3rd ed 1980.

Thompson JC. *Thompson Technique Reference Manual*. 1984. U.S.A.: Williams Manufacturing; 1984, Rpt. 1987.

Tilley RM. The physiologic basis of manipulative medicine. *Manual Med* 1987;3:57–62.

Walton WJ. *Textbook of Osteopathic Diagnosis and Technique Procedures*. St. Louis, Mo: Matthews Book Co; 1970.

Wells D. From workbench to high tech: The evaluation of the adjustment table. *Chiropractic History* 1987;7(2):35–39.

Winsor H. *Sympathetic Segmental Disturbances II*. Haverford, Pa: Henry Winsor; 1922.

Wislowska, M. A study of the contribution of pain to rotation of vertebra in the etiology and pathogenesis of lateral spinal curvature. *Manual Medicine* 1989;4:161–165.

chapter 27

Diversified Technique

Ronald Gitelman
Bruce Fligg

It has been said that all techniques are good and all techniques are bad. The question is, When to use which one and on whom? This is still the credo of the practitioner who practices diversified technique, which has maintained its eclectic approach to the management of functional disorders of the locomotor apparatus.

Over the years, many technique systems have been developed in chiropractic, osteopathy, physiotherapy, orthopaedics, and other disciplines. Many of these techniques are held in common by each discipline, primarily because they are extremely useful and they consistently show good results; an example is the classic lumbar roll. These systems have created different approaches to the analysis and application of many of the old standard techniques. A number of individualized techniques and methods have also been developed and taught within the profession. Unfortunately, as a result, these approaches have systematized, categorized, embalmed, and reduced information and have then been referred to as unique techniques. Too frequently, these methods have been based on the biased and dogmatic approach of single individuals who have systemized and then promoted a technique as their own, leading to polarization within the profession. Few of these system techniques take into account the many facets of standardized examination procedures, pathomechanics, and the pathogenic process as it relates

to the locomotor apparatus. Unlike the system technique approaches, diversified technique is applied after a detailed consultation documenting symptomatology and taking into account age, sex, lifestyle, occupation, and nature of the injury, and with appreciation of the fact that the patient is in the midst of an ongoing process. Therefore, the diversified approach attempts to apply the most ideal technique within the context of the reality of the clinical picture.

History of Diversified Technique

The origin of the label diversified technique is unclear but the concepts of this approach are not new in chiropractic. Currently, two chiropractic colleges offer technique courses labeled "diversified technique," and one textbook is referred to as a textbook on diversified technique (Rheinhard, 1962, 1983). Dye (1939), in his textbook, uses the word "*diversified*" very loosely to describe the situation that existed in the first two decades of chiropractic.

Initially, chiropractic adjustments were given in a shotgun approach to correct subluxations of the spine; that is, any vertebra that was deemed to have been misaligned was manipulated. In 1910, B. J. Palmer developed the meric system of full-spine adjustment. This meric approach correlated the various system diseases with spinal subluxations. A maximum of six adjustments were given at any one treatment. In 1915, B. J. Palmer developed the "major–minor" approach to adjustment of subluxations. The major subluxations were identified and a maximum of three adjustments were given, directed mostly toward the upper cervical region (C1–2). Still pursuing the one-cause-of disease, he developed, the hole-in-one technique, in the early 1920s which was a specialized upper cervical recoil adjustment. B. J. then developed the neurocalometer from 1924 to 1928 to isolate the upper cervical subluxation. It was during this period (1905–1928) that the more reductionistic B. J. Palmer became, the more determined other chiropractors and chiropractic colleges were to be diversified in their approach.

W. H. Carver (1909), referred to as the constructor, was a Palmer graduate of the early 1900s who established the Carver Chiropractic College in Oklahoma in 1906. Carver, along with many others, developed a much broader scope of chiropractic, including electrotherapy, osteopathic, naturopathic, extremity, and other techniques. This diversified approach can therefore be attributed to chiropractors such as Carver and others who were opposed to B. J. Palmer's reductionistic approach.

In contrast to B. J. Palmer's "hole-in-one" approach and the diversified approach, other chiropractors were developing their own technique systems. These system techniques emerged largely in the 1930s and 1940s and chiropractors would often align themselves with a specific technique system. Parts of the rationale and teaching of these systems have subsequently been incorporated into the diversified approach.

The criteria originally used by the diversified approach for adjustment selection were based on a static model of joint alignment. The main diagnostic tools for this decision-making process were static palpation, x-ray, postural analysis, and in some cases the neurocalometer. Biomechanical concepts were added by Illi (1951), Janse et al. (1947), Grecco (1953), Gillet and Liekens (1953), Beatty (1939), Homewood (1979), and States (1965). With the addition of the biomechanical model, motion palpation was developed and added to the armament of diagnostic tools. The manipulative procedures took on a more specific approach. For example, there was less long-lever action, and more short-lever action, and the angle of the thrust was more consistent with the planes of the joints, the axis of rotation, and the direction of muscle and ligament fibers. The diversified approach also included orthopaedic and neurologic examinations. This permitted testing of gross ranges of motion, integrity of various structural and supporting elements, neurological manifestations of the subluxation, a primary pathology other than a subluxation, for example, multiple sclerosis and spinal cord tumor. This can be seen in more recent publications by Grice (1977, 1980), Gitelman (1980), Cassidy (1976), and Sandoz (1965, 1976).

The incorporation of other technique systems, or of any technique, has had to pass the scrutiny of the diversified rationale, which is based on sound neurobiomechanical–orthopaedic principles.

Principles of Diversified Technique

Recent rapid growth of the science of biomechanics and development of motion palpation have allowed the diversified practitioner to more effectively assess the structures of the human body. They have also added to the understanding of posture and gait, which has helped to clarify many of the movement patterns of patients. The key to diversified technique has always been the importance of (1) the specific diagnosis of the active lesion and (2) the structural environment of that lesion within the patient, realizing that an individual patient is subject to external stresses from the environment, lifestyle, occupation, and so forth that play vital roles in the patient's neurobiomechanical adaptive mechanism.

Many techniques have been developed relative to the dynamic and physiological activity of muscles and in response to the relationship between joint and muscle dysfunction. It is important to realize that there is no clear dichotomy between these two and there has been confusion over therapeutic approaches and differential diagnosis, often to the point where emphasis is placed on joint dysfunction and the muscular component is ignored. The diversified approach attempts to correlate appropriate adjustive spinal manipulative procedure with joint dysfunction while taking into consideration the additional factors of muscle dysfunction. It maintains that muscle dysfunction is important whether it is the primary factor in either the segmental or overall abnormal movement pattern that has stressed the area to the point of being symptomatic, or it is secondary to the joint dysfunction. The therapeutic approach therefore involves techniques that not only influence the musculature but also facilitate the manipulation. It should also include principles of rehabilitative therapy (exercise programs, reeducation of the patient with respect to occupation and lifestyle). This holistic approach is entrenched in the current wellness concepts of health care and plays a critical role in the treatment of the patient's condition. Emphasis on biomechanics and postural hygiene rounds out the approach taken by the practitioner of diversified technique.

Application of Diversified Technique

General Considerations

A description of the standardized methods of examination is beyond the scope of this chapter. The patient is first evaluated using an integrated approach, before any specific method or technique of treatment is begun. This approach requires (1) diagnosis of the lesion or the discrete focus of pathomechanical behavior with its local tissue responses, (2) assessment of the spacial ecology or broader status of the statics and dynamics of the locomotor system, (3) awareness of the temporal factors involved in the disease process, and (4) ability to determine where the patient's condition is in the midst of an ongoing process. The practitioner of diversified technique also considers the developmental factors leading to the spinal lesion and the adaptive mechanisms that the body has undergone in response to the symptomatic lesion. All these considerations are made prior to selecting an approach to treatment and rehabilitation.

Several factors must be considered with any manipulation: positioning of the patient, positioning of the therapist, identification of the articular dysfunction to be corrected, and direction of the thrust or mobilization required.

Once the slack has been taken up, the practitioner gently springs the joint to its end position in an attempt to mobilize that joint. If so indicated, the adjuster may simply carry the force to this degree. If, however, the preference is to gap the joint (perform an adjustment) then a thrust is made from this end position using a high-velocity, low-amplitude, specifically directed force. Each of the manipulations described in this chapter can be applied as a mobilization or an adjustment. In each case, appropriate pretreatment preparation of the patient using soft tissue massage, reflex techniques, trigger points, and so forth may be necessary.

There are two therapeutic objectives of spinal manipulative therapy. One is biomechanical and the other is neurologic and/or reflex. Similar to the dichotomy of muscles and joints it is also difficult to separate the biomechanical from the reflex mechanisms. When manipulation of a joint is successful, the neurologic ramifications are very far-reaching, including the effect on segmental innervation of that level. Similarly, a practitioner cannot apply reflex techniques to muscles without affecting the dynamics of movement and, hence, the biomechanics of the joints.

Many specific and systemic reflexes can be used by the practitioner. These include the facilitation of muscles in a specific pattern related to inspiration and expiration of the patient, to the direction in which the eyes move, or to the positioning of the head. Also, specific techniques are used for the treatment of individual myofascial pain patterns, the so-called trigger-point therapies. As most practitioners of diversified technique use a broad spectrum of treatment approaches it is not uncommon for physiologic therapeutic methods, including thermal therapy, cryotherapy, and various forms of electrotherapy, to be applied. These are used not only in the traditional therapeutic sense (i.e., the way a physiotherapist would apply them to a lesion), but to influence the neurophysiological reflex and biomechanical component of the active lesion as related the manipulative procedure.

The Cervical Spine

There are more reported cases of side effects resulting from manipulation of the cervical region (usually vascular insults to the vertebrobasilar arteries) than from manipulation of any other area of the body (Kleynhams, 1980; Gotlieb 1985). Therefore, the chiropractor's clinical decision-making process in the application of cervical adjustment is being challenged.

Upper Cervical Spine The greatest challenge to the diversified technique practitioner lies in the upper cervical region. The most confusing question that arises is, When to adjust the occiput versus the atlas or axis? The answer is based on principles of biomechanics blended with an understanding of the neurologic and orthopaedic aspects of the chiropractic sciences. For example, major consideration in performing an occipital adjustment would be a flexion-extension subluxation fixation, as opposed to an atlas adjustment that is used for correcting a rotary subluxation fixation. It is well documented that the main motion of the occiput is flexion–extension, and the main motion of the atlas is rotation. Also, these motions are usually coupled with secondary motions involving lateral flexion. It is this coupled motion that makes the discrete difference to the primary adjustment and/or mobilization procedures. The following adjustment procedures will help demonstrate these principles: splenius capitus occipital, semispinalis capitus occipital, and rotary atlas.

The upper cervical region is noted for its vascular sensitivities and, although numerous tests are helpful in determining whether manipulative procedures are appropriate (without provoking vertebrobasilar artery compromise), they are not completely foolproof. Therefore, in questionable instances the treatment regimen should begin with mobilization techniques. These are discussed here as premanipulative procedures and also as a means of testing the patient's tolerance to upper cervical region manipulation.

MOBILIZATION TECHNIQUES. The figure-eight mobilization procedure for the upper cervical region is extremely beneficial for producing flexion–extension with elements of rotation and lateral flexion for the following patients: those for whom there is concern about vertebrobasilar insufficiency, patients with inflammatory conditions of the upper cervical regions resulting from trauma and/or arthritis, geriatric patients in whom the chronicity of the condition inhibits the ability of the practitioner to position the patient's head and neck for an adjustment procedure, and for apprehensive patients who are unable to allow their muscles to relax sufficiently for an adjustment procedure.

The occipital flexion with traction technique (Fig. 27–1) is extremely beneficial for mobilization in the sagittal plane producing flexion. This procedure also helps stretch the smaller suboccipital muscles, such as the rectus capitus posticus major and minor, and the larger supporting muscles of the occiput and cervical spine (i.e., the semispinalis capitus). The rotation mobilization procedure can be applied with ei-

ther long- or short-lever emphasis. The long-lever procedure uses a contact on the occiput, whereas in the short-lever procedure a specific rotary mobilization force is applied to the posterior arch of the atlas. In each case, the emphasis is on long-axis traction followed by graded oscillations of rotation. Any traction procedure can be facilitated by the patient's exhaling.

MANIPULATIVE TECHNIQUES. Splenius capitus occipital adjustment (Fig. 24–2) is applied when there is a loss of occipital flexion coupled with rotation and extension. This adjustment resembles closely an older adjustment described by States (1968), called the "posterior occiput adjustment" which was used to correct for a rotary fixation (posterior) of the occiput on the atlas. It has been demonstrated that there are smaller amounts of rotation of the occiput on the atlas compared with atlas rotation and compared with the amount of flexion–extension of the occiput. Therefore, a posterior occiput adjustment would presumably produce rotation of the atlas on the axis. The splenius capitus adjustment for the occiput, however, incorporates the primary fixation of flexion with rotation and lateral flexion.

Semispinalis capitus occipital adjustment (Fig. 27–3) resembles closely an older adjustment described by States (1968) called "the lateral occiput adjustment." Similar to the posterior occiput adjustment in its correction for rotation, it has been demonstrated that, like rotation, there are smaller

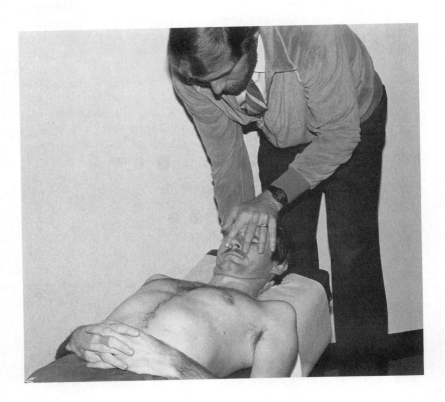

Figure 27–1. Occipital flexion with traction mobilization: flexion component. It is important to produce traction at this point to stretch the posterior muscular component.

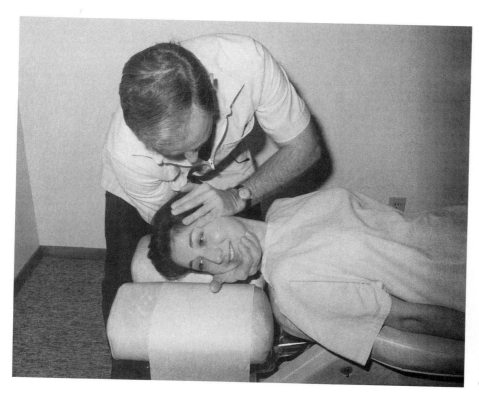

Figure 27-2. Splenius capitus occipital adjustment. The articulation and splenius capitus muscle on the up side are affected. The forearm provides the necessary fulcrum for lateral flexion in this procedure.

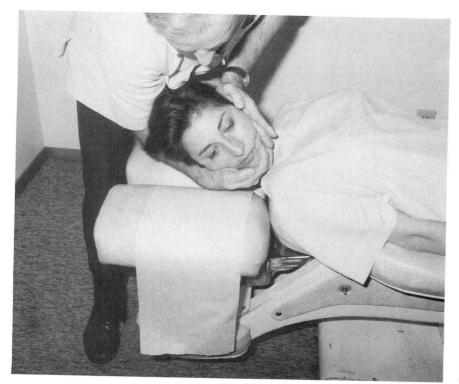

Figure 27-3. Semispinalis capitus occipital adjustment. The articulation and semispinalis muscle on the down side are affected. The forearm assists the contact hand on the mastoid to produce traction and lateral flexion of the occiput at the same time, thus maintaining occipital flexion.

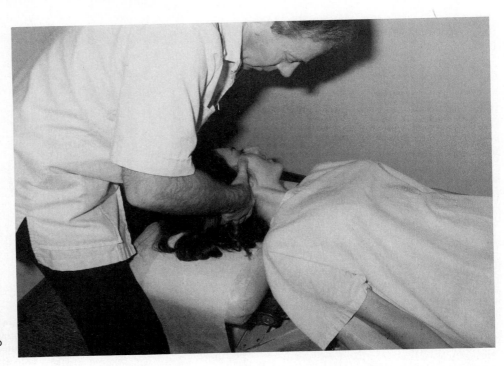

Figure 27-4. Rotary atlas adjustment: rotary atlas with lateral flexion applied superior to inferior.

amounts of lateral flexion of the occiput on the atlas when compared with flexion–extension of the occiput on the atlas. The semispinalis capitus is one of the major muscular forces acting on the occiput and when it becomes overdominant as a postural stabilizing muscle of the upper cervical, cervical-thoracic region, it produces extension with smaller amounts of lateral flexion of the occiput. It is felt that the occiput rarely subluxates/fixates in a pure lateral flexion manner. Similar to the older lateral occiput adjustment, lateral flexion is incorporated into this procedure; however, long-axis traction with emphasis on occipital flexion during the thrusting procedure makes this procedure more specific for the correction of this type of subluxation/fixation complex.

Rotary atlas adjustment (Fig. 27–4) corrects for a subluxation/fixation of the atlas on the axis. As demonstrated by Illi (1951), the atlas undergoes coupled motions of lateral flexion with shifting. Therefore, to determine the specific type of rotary atlas correction necessary, a number of motion palpation procedures can be performed. For example, a rotary procedure can include a lateral flexion component directed from inferior to superior, as in the case when a rotary subluxation/fixation of the atlas originates from the lower cervical region. This procedure can also be applied with a lateral flexion component directed superior to inferior in cases in which the occiput becomes primary in influencing the rotary subluxation/fixation of atlas. Another critical distinguishing component of this procedure is how far into the range of cervical motion should the ''setup'' take. For example, if the fixation is felt within the first 50° of cervical

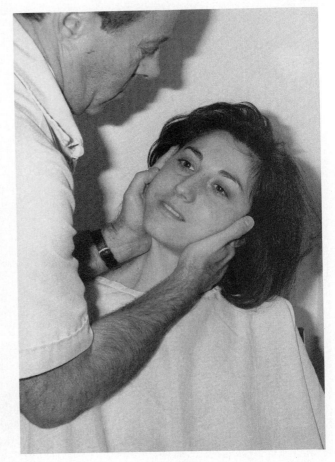

Figure 27-5. Scalenus anticus adjustment. The contact point is over the anterior tubercle of the involved vertebra. Traction is applied longitudinally to stretch the muscular component.

rotation yet the patient's capability is still within a 90° range of motion, then it is not practical to take a full range of preloading (to the full 90°) prior to manipulation of the atlas. This type of premanipulative loading is most likely to produce multiple segment releases, especially in the C4–5–6 area. Care must be taken to ensure that the patient's neck is rotated to the point of fixation with adequate traction and end-joint loading at that point.

Lower Cervical Spine. To demonstrate how the diversified principle applies to the lower cervical spine, two mobilization and five manipulative procedures that can be used to correct a rotary cervical fixation are considered: (1) anterior scalenus, (2) supine rotary cervical, (3) sitting cervical, (4) prone cervical, and (5) supine finger push. Each of these adjustments corrects for a rotary fixation component, taking into account a different second component of this type of fixation.

MOBILIZATION TECHNIQUES. An excellent mobilization technique for the lower cervical spine is a figure-eight mobilization similar to that applied to the occiput. A very specific contact is taken on the articular pillar of the desired segment to be mobilized, and a mobilizing force in a figure-eight movement helps accomplish mobilization in all planes of motion. The static joint challenge motion palpation procedures are also excellent mobilization techniques in which each segment can be mobilized using an oscillation of eight to ten times. For example, if rotation mobilization is desired, then a finger contact is made on the

articular pillar on the involved segment. The segment is then challenged in rotation and is enhanced by a small amount of rotation of the overall head and neck. Here an oscillation of eight to ten times is performed with increasing amplitude at the desired segment.

The long-lever mobilization technique involves a general hand contact over the region of cervical restriction, and a general stretching and mobilization in rotation are applied again in increasing amplitudes of oscillations anywhere up to eight times.

MANIPULATIVE TECHNIQUES. Scalenus anticus adjustment (Fig. 27–5) was first described by Grice (1977), and is applied when the fixation component of rotation as determined by motion palpation has a loss of the anterior-to-posterior component of rotation. As anterior compartment (thoracic outlet) syndromes often occur when the scalenus anticus muscle is hypertonic, resulting in this fixation, this is the most direct approach to correcting this type of fixation.

Supine rotary cervical adjustment (Fig. 27–6) is the most frequently used technique and corrects for the posterior-to-anterior component of the fixation as identified by motion palpation. This procedure can be applied either in a passive state, which affects mostly joint receptors, or with a slight amount of traction, which then involves the muscle receptors as well (i.e., splenius cervicis).

Sitting cervical adjustment (Fig. 27–7) is best applied to fixations in which there is an involvement of

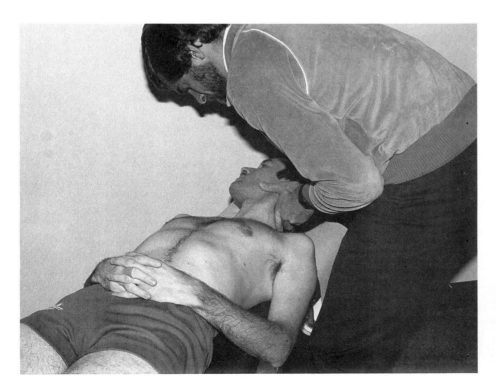

Figure 27-6. Rotary cervical adjustment: the rotary component applied with traction. It should be noted that the amount of rotation is to the point of fixation, not to the full range of the patient's cervical motion.

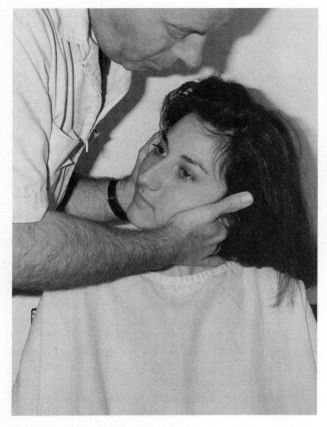

Figure 27-7. Sitting cervical adjustment. It should be noted that the best way to produce traction of the levator scapula is to have the patient sit on his or her hands during the adjustment.

the levator scapula muscle as indicated by motion palpation. The advantage of the sitting cervical adjustment is in the ability to traction and stretch the supporting muscles and at the same time correct for joint dysfunction.

Prone cervical adjustment (Fig. 27-8) is best applied to posterior–anterior rotary fixations (as indicated by motion palpation) of the lower cervical (C5-6) region and in individuals who have short, thick necks (e.g., football players). This procedure allows the practitioner to focus on the fixated segment while the table and headpiece support the patient's body and head weight.

The supine, finger-push adjustment (Fig. 27-9) is most suitably applied to rotary fixations in which the goal is a corrective thrust through the posterior elements (facets) while simultaneously minimizing rotational forces through the anterior component (disc). This is necessary in cases of cervical spondylosis in which a rotary cervical contact using the articular pillar would produce excessive rotary forces through the anterior component and possibly aggravate the patient's condition. The fingertip-push adjustment contacting the spinous process focuses most of the rotary thrust through the facets. The muscular implication often associated with this type of fixation can be rectus capitus posticus major affecting C-2, semispinalis cervicis affecting C2-4, or splenius capitus affecting C5-6-7.

Each of these manipulations can be applied before or after treatment has been directed toward the

Figure 27-8. Prone cervical adjustment. It is important with this procedure to produce traction with the indifferent hand. The angle of thrust is cephalad to comply with the angle of the facets.

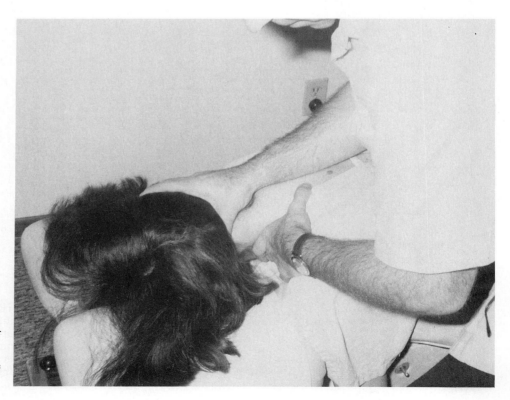

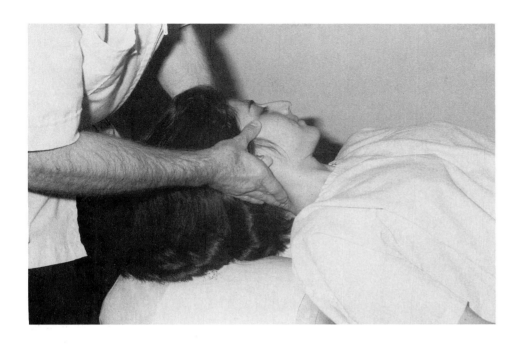

Figure 27–9. Finger-push adjustment. The thrust is applied caudally and medially against the spinous of C-2 in the same direction as the rectus capitus posticus major.

soft tissue component, i.e., trigger-point therapy and/or electrotherapy.

For example, if motion palpation determines there is a large muscular component to the fixation and digital palpation reveals active myofascial trigger points, it is appropriate to address the muscular component via massage techniques and/or modality application prior to the manipulative procedure. In the case of a rotary cervical with involvement of the levator scapula muscle, then these techniques should be directed toward relaxing the levator scapula muscle before the adjustive procedure is performed. In a patient who presents with a headache syndrome involving upper cervical fixation with active trigger points and muscular hypertonicity of the splenius capitus, it is appropriate to address the muscular component via trigger-point therapy and/or modality application to the soft tissue component prior to the manipulative procedure. It is also appropriate, if these muscular imbalances are due to or aggravated by poor postural habits, that the patient be advised in the correction of these habits and supported by a home program of exercises.

In dealing with adjustive procedures of the cervical spine, there often is a level of apprehension in the patient that inhibits the ability of the practitioner to perform these techniques. There are numerous methods that will enhance the patient's cooperation, and allow the practitioner to adjust the patient's neck with minimal resistance. The practitioner can ask the patient (1) to look in the direction of head rotation; (2) to coordinate breathing, i.e., to exhale just prior to the adjustive procedure; and (3) to alternate the wiggling of fingers and toes, i.e., right fingers, left toes, and so forth.

The Thoracic-Rib Region

Too frequently, the approach taken for manipulation of the thoracic-rib region is reductionistic. This is a result of the seemingly low priority this region is often given. It is often treated by general mobilization techniques, which can lead to chronic recurring midthoracic pain syndromes. Therefore, a clinician must have the ability to ''split hairs'' in the selection of the manipulation technique.

MOBILIZATION TECHNIQUES. Techniques for mobilization of the thoracic spine are equally important to those for the cervical and lumbo pelvic regions. Under certain conditions (e.g., geriatric patients, pregnant women, patients with breast sensitivities or rib sensitivities) patients cannot tolerate the adjustive thrusting. Mobilization techniques can take the form of static joint challenge motion procedures with graded oscillations of eight to ten times in the direction of fixation. They can be done while the patient is seated (Fig. 27–10) with the practitioner seated behind. The mobilization produces directional forces in rotation, lateral flexion, extension, and flexion of all areas of the thoracic-rib region.

MANIPULATIVE TECHNIQUES. Four adjustments can be applied to the thoracic region to correct for a rotation subluxation/fixation: (1) cross-bilateral adjustment, (2) hypothenar lateral spinous adjustment, (3) anterior thoracic with rotation adjustment, and (4) lateral recumbent rib adjustment.

Cross-bilateral technique is one of the manipulation procedures most frequently applied to the thoracic region. Numerous modifications of this adjustment exist; the basic cross-bilateral used for correcting a midthoracic rotation fixation/subluxation is reviewed here. The main indicator for a cross-bilateral is a loss of the rotational component of movement as indicated by motion palpation. Muscular implications are those that attach to the transverse processes, such as longissimus and iliocostalis thoracis. The adjustment (Fig. 27–11) is applied posterior to anterior in line with the facet angle of the thoracic vertebrae and the kyphosis of the thoracic region. A common modification of this adjustment is to include lateral flexion where the adjusting arm is angled inferior to superior and the indifferent hand superior to inferior on the opposite side. This modification has a torquing component to it to achieve a lateral flexion component during the rotational correction.

Hypothenar lateral spinous technique is used more frequently when the following muscular components are involved: spinalis thoracis, semispinalis thoracis, and superior and inferior serratus posterior. It is applied when motion palpation indicates a loss of the normal coupled rotation during lateral flexion. Often this rotational fixation is associated with flexion or extension. Therefore, the hypothenar lateral spinous thrust is angled either superior to inferior, lateral to medial, or inferior to superior, lateral to medial, respectively; however, in midthoracic situations the thrust is usually lateral to medial (Fig. 27–12).

Anterior thoracic with rotation adjustment is an excellent adjustment to correct for an extension malposition, flexion fixation. In many circumstances, such as with spinalis thoracis involvement, there is a loss of the normal thoracic kyphosis; therefore, a

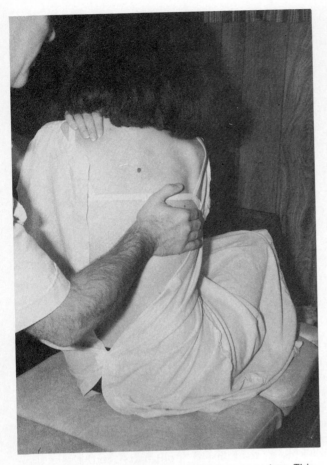

Figure 27–10. Seated thoracic mobilization procedure. This procedure demonstrates rotation mobilization of the mid-thoracic region.

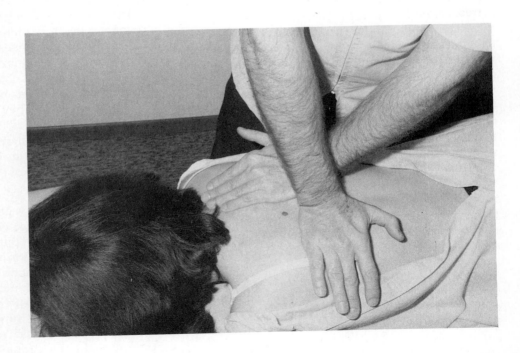

Figure 27–11. Cross-bilateral adjustment: the lateral flexion component with rotation.

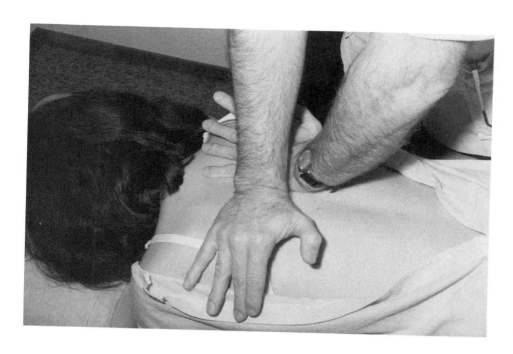

Figure 27-12. Hypothenar lateral spinous adjustment with a cephalad component.

compressive force type of manipulative procedure is not indicated. The extension malposition and the need to correct for flexion are the primary concerns; however, rotation is frequently involved. The contact hand is usually placed below the involved segment while the patient is rolled down over the fulcrum, maintaining a flexed posture. To enhance a rotational correction component to this, the contact hand is placed slightly lateral (from transverse process to spinous process) and the patient is rotated and rolled over the hand. The force of the hand on the transverse process produces a counterrotation correction while producing flexion (Fig. 27-13).

Lateral recumbent rib adjustment is used when patients have sensitivities to compression and therefore prone posterior-to-anterior manipulative procedures are not indicated, i.e., cross-bilateral using the nonarticulating tubercle of the involved rib. This is most frequently seen in pregnant patients during the midtrimester and last trimester. A more desirable posture is the lateral recumbent position. The contact hand is on the nonarticulating tubercle of the involved rib and the manipulative procedure is performed with the patient exhaling (Fig. 27-14).

It should be noted that the thoracic region is a common site of chronic myofascial pain syndromes and therefore there is a need to direct treatment to the soft tissue component via massage therapies, i.e., trigger-point therapy, petrissage, and/or modality applications. It is also important to address postural concerns: whether they be in an anteroposterior plane (hyperkyphosis or hypokyphosis) or in the frontal plane (S or C curves). This may require teach-

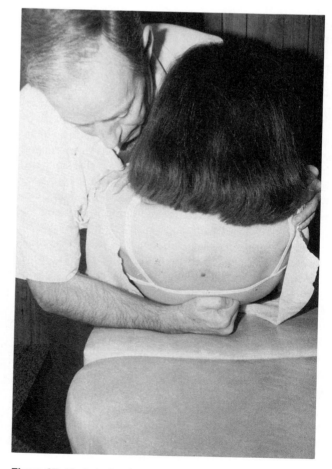

Figure 27-13. Anterior thoracic adjustment with rotation. Observe that the patient is rotated over the contact hand to produce rotation during the procedure.

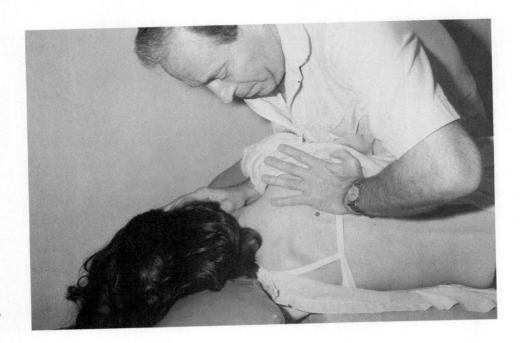

Figure 27–14. Lateral recumbent rib adjustment, with a cephalad component to correct for a caliper-open, bucket-handle-down subluxation.

ing the patient appropriate exercises to enhance the function of the region and therefore the effects of the manipulation-mobilization procedures.

The Pelvis and Lumbar Spine

Pelvis. The examination establishes the biomechanical relationships of the pelvis and the muscles that affect the sacroiliac joint. Combinations of sacroiliac fixations are commonly seen, such as bilateral upper joint fixations in many cases of increased lumbar lordosis with anterior tipping of the sacrum. Upper joint fixation on one side and lower joint fixation on the other are also quite common when fixations occur in the oblique axis of motion of the sacrum. This pattern of fixation is often seen as the pelvic response to a leg deficiency. It is also possible for the sacrum to look posterior in an upper joint (flexion) fixation; however, this does not usually occur. Often, a complete fixation of one sacroiliac joint is seen when both the upper and lower aspects of the joint are fixed; this produces a hypermotoricity of the opposite sacroiliac joint. As a point of interest, hypermobile sacroiliac joints are nearly always palpated statically as a flexion distortion.

MOBILIZATION TECHNIQUE. Mobilization of a typical upper joint fixation may be accomplished in the prone position with a contact at the superior aspect of the posterior superior iliac spine. Force is directed laterally toward the foot. With the other hand contacting the inferior aspects of the sacrum on the same side force is directed toward the head and anteriorly (Fig. 27–15). A springing action is used and a shallow

thrust, if desired, may be given equally with each hand. Increased leverage may be gained by use of a Dutchman's roll or a pelvic block (DeJarnette, 1967; Gravel, 1966). If more force is required, then the leg in extension may be used as a long lever in either the prone or side-posture position (Fig. 27–16). The state of the lumbar spine must be a major consideration when use of the last two techniques is considered as they do produce hyperextension of the lumbar spine. Similar mobilizing techniques can be used for the typical extension fixation (Figs. 27–17 and 27–18). The practitioner can mobilize in the seated position by forcing flexion of the thigh toward the middle of the chest when sitting behind the patient (Fig. 27–19) (Gillet and Liekens, 1969).

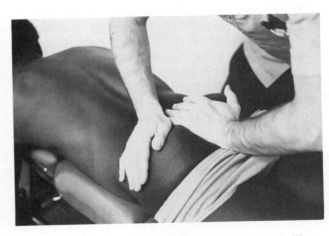

Figure 27–15. Technique for mobilizing an upper sacroiliac joint flexion fixation of the sacroiliac joint.

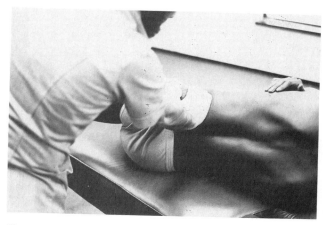

Figure 27-16. Mobilization of upper sacroiliac joint using the extended leg as a long lever.

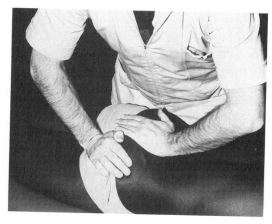

Figure 27-17. Technique for mobilizing a lower sacroiliac joint or correcting an extension fixation of the sacroiliac joint.

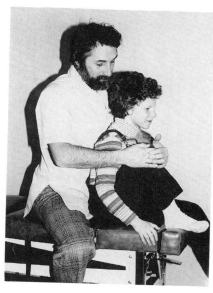

Figure 27-19. Technique for mobilizing the sacroiliac joint in the sitting position.

Stoddard (1959) described the leg-tug method in which the leg on the side of flexion is tractioned at an angle of approximately 45° (Fig. 27-20) and the long-leg side or the side of supposed extension is tractioned at approximately 10° (Fig. 27-21). These maneuvers are carried out individually. Another dynamic myofascial maneuver would be to carry the knee on the flexed side up toward the chest. As external rotation of the hip occurs, the lower leg is carried inward. In this way, the entire leg is then extended (Fig. 27-22). This is done on side of the short leg. To complement this maneuver, the musculature of the hip on the long-leg side is passively stretched by internally rotating the femur on the side

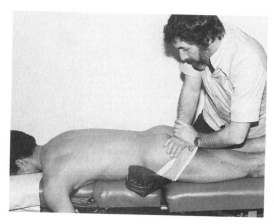

Figure 27-18. Technique for mobilizing a lower sacroiliac joint or correcting an extension fixation of the sacroiliac joint.

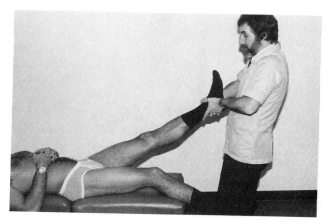

Figure 27-20. Leg-tug method of sacroiliac joint mobilization. The leg on the side of sacroiliac flexion is tractioned at 45°.

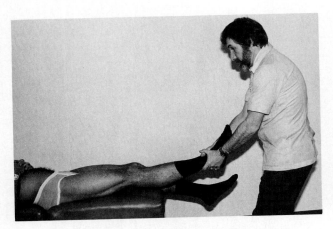

Figure 27–21. Leg-tug method of sacroiliac joint mobilization. The leg on the side of the sacroiliac extension is tractioned at 10°.

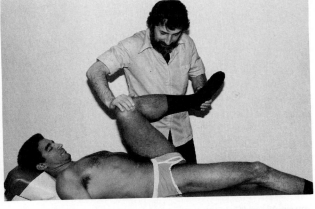

Figure 27–23. Technique for mobilizing the sacroiliac joint with the hip and knee flexed (see text). Technique for lower sacroiliac joint mobilization.

of thigh flexion as the leg is extended (Fig. 27–23). This is repeated two to five times.

There are various myofascial techniques specifically directed toward individual muscles and muscle groups, such as, the piriformis, the psoas major, the hamstrings, and the adductors and abductors of the hip. These techniques are described in Chapter 29.

MANIPULATIVE TECHNIQUES. Perhaps the most frequently used manipulation, and often the manipulation of choice, for a typical upper sacroiliac joint fixation (flexion) is performed in the side-posture position with the fixed innominate upward. The patient is positioned by having him or her hold the side of the table with the superior hand. The lower arm is tractioned under the patient. The patient therefore remains with the superior shoulder up, thus pre-

venting undue lumbar spinal torsion (Fig. 27–24). The lower leg is slightly bent to allow the lumbar lordosis to achieve a neutral position. The upper leg is drawn up approximately 75° and the foot is placed comfortably into the popliteal space of the lower leg. The pelvis is now perpendicular to the table. The contacts are made by the manipulator on the deltoid with one hand and on the superior aspects of the posterior superior iliac spine with a pisiform contact with the other hand. Traction is applied on the long lever of the leg by the thigh of the manipulator and a headward force is exerted on the deltoid (Fig. 27–25). As the patient relaxes with a deep breath, traction is taken up. Two or three breaths can be used to increase traction to paraphysiologic limits. An impulse is delivered in the direction of the line of the superior femur while the upper hand stabilizes the trunk of

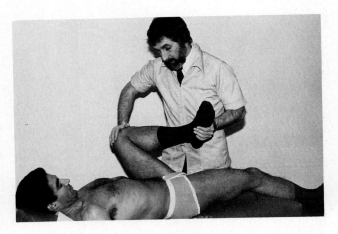

Figure 27–22. Techniques for mobilizing the sacroiliac joint with the hip and knee flexed (see text). Technique for upper sacroiliac joint mobilization.

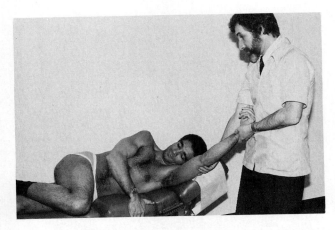

Figure 27–24. Technique for adjusting an upper joint flexion fixation of the sacroiliac joint. In preparation for this adjustment, the inferior arm is tractioned beneath the patient, who grips the side of the table with the superior hand.

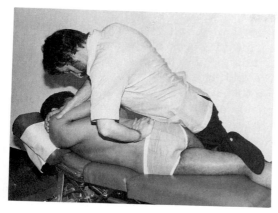

Figure 27–25. Technique for adjusting an upper joint of flexion fixation of the sacroiliac joint on the left. The adjustive thrust is given in 10° direction cephalad and toward the floor.

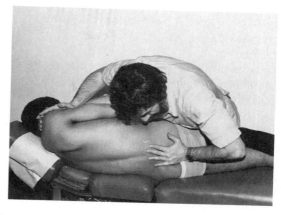

Figure 27–27. Alternate contact points and direction of thrust for adjusting the various sacroiliac fixations. The same contact point and direction of thrust as in Figure 27–26, but with the fixed sacroiliac joint placed inferior.

the body. Manipulation of this same distortion in an inferior position of the sacrum can be achieved with a contact on the inferior aspect of the sacrum and a corrective thrust given in a straight headward direction (Fig. 27–26). This same sacral contact on the lower side of the apex can be used if the flexed sacroiliac is on the down side (Fig. 27–27). In commonly encountered upper joint fixation on one side and lower joint fixation on the other, the upper joint fixation angle of the sacrum below is taken. The thrust is delivered in an arching motion headward and laterally as if to come over the buttock (Fig. 27–28). The best way to correct a posterior sacrum on the down side is contact on the posterior of the sacrum on the down side with the thrust perpendicular to the floor.

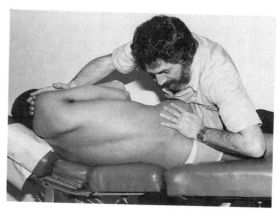

Figure 27–28. Alternate contact point and direction of thrust for adjusting the various sacroiliac fixations. Technique for adjusting a combination right upper sacroiliac fixation and left lower sacroiliac fixation. An arching motion is used during the thrust.

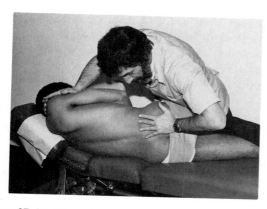

Figure 27–26. Alternate contact points and direction of thrust for adjusting the various sacroiliac fixations. Contact on the inferior aspect of the sacrum with thrust along the axis of the body for an upper joint fixation of the sacroiliac joint.

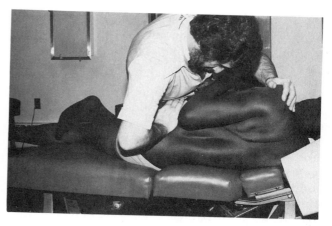

Figure 27–29. Techniques for adjusting a lower joint extension fixation of the sacroiliac joint. The contact point is taken on the posterior aspect of the sacrum and the thrust is directed perpendicular to the sacroiliac joint.

This also has the effect of gaping the lumbosacral facet on that side (Fig. 27–29).

The manipulation of choice for a lower joint or extension fixation is accomplished by placing the fixated sacroiliac joint up and preparing the patient in a way similar to that described for an upper joint fixation. In this situation, however, the upper leg is flexed past 90° to take advantage of the force applied to the pelvis by the hamstring muscles. The slack is taken up by moving the clinician's leg against the superior leg of the patient during exhalation. The contact hands are placed on the ischial tuberosity and the deltoid. The adjustive thrust is directed toward the midpoint between the patient's lower shoulder and chin. The extension fixation may also be adjusted by making direct contact on the posterior sacrum and using a thrust directed perpendicular to the sacroiliac joint toward the adjuster (see Fig. 27–29). Alternately, a closed-fist contact may be used in an attempt to draw the sacrum inferiorly. After manipulation of the pelvis, reexamination of the patient should reveal an immediate change in the movement palpation tests. Reassessment of the remaining muscular components will direct the clinician to the next procedure.

Lumbar Spine

MOBILIZATION TECHNIQUES. Mobilization techniques may be directed toward individual motion segments or muscles that have a multisegmental effect. The individual motion segments can merely be toggled in a rhythmic fashion in a variety of directions or a specific contact can be made, the position required for the manipulative reduction assumed, and passive stretch applied in a rhythmic manner without a thrust. For the multisegmental musculature (sacrospinalis, quadratus lumborum, and so forth), passive stretching or neuromuscular facilitative techniques can be used. The traction and distraction techniques, using the chiromanus and Leander and Hill tables, may be effective.

MANIPULATIVE TECHNIQUES. All adjustive procedures require the proper positioning of the patient, a specific contact on the spine, and the removal of joint slack to the point at which a controlled dynamic impulse can accomplish a specific movement of an articulation. Correction of a type 4 L4–5 fixation (Gitelman, 1980) determined by movement palpation will serve as an example of how this is accomplished. In this situation, the vertebral body has rotated to the right and a multifidus muscle contraction exists on the left. There is failure of the disc to form a wedge on the right side on lateral bending to that side. The facet on the left is fixed in extension. To correct this problem, the patient is placed in the side-posture position with the left side up. The adjuster places his or her fingers at the L3–4 interspace and rotates the lower shoulder girdle around the long axis of the body. The adjuster should now be able to appreciate the progressive rotation and blocking that are occurring down through the spine. The patient's hands are placed comfortably on the anterior aspect of the opposite shoulder. The right leg is flexed slightly to reduce the lordosis of the lumbar spine. This causes a slight gaping of the facets which, in turn, assists in the restoration of intersegmental flexion. The upper leg is flexed to the point at which the palpating finger can feel movement at the L5–S1 interspace. The upper leg is now rotated toward the floor until rotation of the pelvis and lower lumbar spine can be appreciated at the level of L4–5. The patient is stabilized in his or her longitudinal axis around the contact point at L4–5. Any increase in pressure through either of the long levers (the shoulders or the leg) will produce stress at the L4–5 segment. Contact is now taken with the reinforced index finger on the lateral aspects of the spinous process of L-4. Additional slack may be taken up at this time by having the patient take a deep breath. On expiration, a gentle stress on both long levers will take the articulation to be manipulated into the paraphysiologic range. At the moment of maximal relaxation (end of expiration) a thrust is delivered in such a way as to dynamically separate the attachments of the involved multifidus contraction. This is done by thrusting toward the floor and slightly headward. This should cause a gaping of the upper facet and create a negative pressure within the disc. At the same time the multifidus muscle on the left is subject to a dynamic stretching force. This adjustment is aimed at reinstating the normal motoricity of the L4–5 motion segments by specifically applying a force in all directions in which motion was compromised, that is, rotation, lateral bending, and flexion (Fig. 27–30).

A number of variations in the application of the thrust can be made. A light thrust on the shoulder can produce greater isolation of rotation in this distortion (Sandoz, 1965). Additional kyphosis can be introduced by increasing thigh flexion to facilitate the restoration of intersegmental flexion. If more force is required, a pisiform contact or a reinforced double-spinous push (Fig. 27–31) can be used by threading the clinician's arm through the flexed elbow of the patient and taking a contact on the lateral aspect of the spinous process. When there is a specific discal component to the fixation motion segment, excess axial torsion should be avoided to minimize the stress on an already compromised annulus.

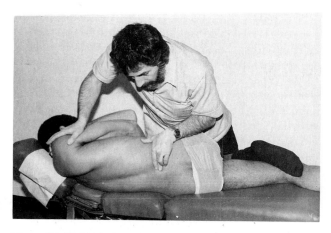

Figure 27–30. Technique for adjusting a type 4 L4–5 fixation using a single-spinous push (see text).

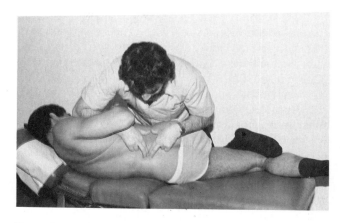

Figure 27–32. Alternate method of adjusting the lumbar spine: the double-spinous hook technique.

Correction of the same fixation can be accomplished from the opposite side using a hook contact on the spinous processes (Fig. 27–32) or a mammillary contact (Fig. 27–33). In this case, the patient is placed on the opposite side with the fixation down. The procedure is less effective, as one is forced to depend on the passive introduction of one or more of the compromised coupled motions to achieve reduction of the fixation. Given these limitations, however, certain clinical situations make this technique the adjustment of choice, especially when rotation to the left in the side-posture position is not tolerated by the patient.

The sacrospinalis stretch technique is, in fact, a reverse lumbar roll in which the specific contact made by the adjuster is at the lateral aspect of the spinous process and an assisted thrust is given headward and anteriorly by the other hand (Fig. 27–34). The application of a voluntary isometric contraction

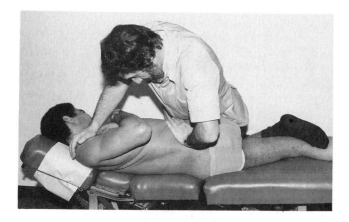

Figure 27–33. Alternate method of adjusting the lumbar spine: the mammillary process rotary adjustment.

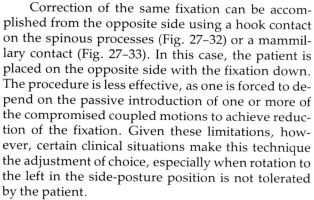

Figure 27–31. Technique for adjusting the lumbar spine using a reinforced double-spinous push.

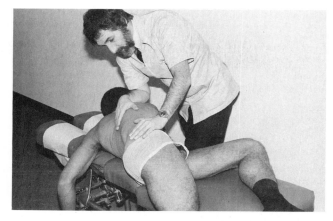

Figure 27–34. Alternate method of adjusting the lumbar spine: the sacrospinalis stretch adjustment.

by the patient against resistance allows the adjuster to take up additional slack when the patient relaxes. If this is repeated two or three times, the adjustment may be facilitated and hence made more effective (Gaymans, 1973).

Each of the adjustments aimed at stretching the sacrospinalis, quadratus lumborum, or multifidus muscles may be accomplished in the seated position with the patient either straddling the treatment table or using a safety belt tightened across his or her thighs to provide stabilization. Some of the earliest adjustments were given in the prone position with a thrust on either the spinous process or mammillary process, with the thrust usually directed headward or straight through to the floor. The lower vertebra of the fixation segment is the one that is contacted and mobilized in this adjustment. This adjustment can be more effective when the pelvic section of a multi-segmental adjustment is of greater use for general mobilization, as a high-force thrust in this position can be uncomfortable to the patient.

The late Dr. Clarence Gonstead developed a sophisticated variation of this type of adjustment in which the patient is positioned on a specifically designed lumbar knee–posture bench (Fig. 27–35). The same type of prone manipulation may be accomplished using traction–distraction tables or the drop centerpiece in the open position (Schafer and Faye, 1989).

Manipulative techniques directed toward specific levels of disc pathology deserve special attention as there is always a degree of risk; however, in conjunction with rest and adjunctive therapies, manipulations may be given to other areas of the spine. Reflex and myofascial techniques may be applied as long as further torsional insult does not occur at the

level of the lesion. Passive traction and distraction maneuvers may also be helpful. It should be pointed out that with a true sequestration or herniation of the disc, surgical intervention may be necessary.

In intervertebral disc syndromes unaccompanied by herniation or sequestration, the following manipulative procedures represent a rational approach. Sandoz (1971) and Matthews and Yates (1969) have described the effect of helicoid traction previously demonstrated by LeVernieux (1960). This adjustment is accomplished in the side-posture position, similar to the classical lumbar roll. A mammillary contact on the lower segment of the fixation complex is made and used to resist a thrust to the shoulder directed headward and posteriorly. This adjustment is an attempt to produce negative intradiscal pressure by gaping the disc. Bonyon (1967) and Grice (1979) described an adjustive maneuver designed to cause closure of the disc on the superior side while opening the wedge disc on the inferior side. This adjustment avoids rotational strain. The patient is placed in the side–posture position with both the pelvis and trunk elevated either by pillows or by adjustment of the treatment table. A double mammillary or finger-push contact is taken and the thrust is directed to the floor to open the lower facet and gap the disc on the lower side. The aim of this adjustment is to produce negative intradiscal pressure in the hope of reducing the incarcerated nuclear material in radial annular tears. Reduction may conceivably also occur where nuclear material has fractured through the end plate. It is possible that an adjustment may result from the shifting of a sequestrated piece of discal material to a more innocuous location. Before-and-after studies have shown that even when the pain is reduced, the protrusion remains (Quan et al., 1989; Kou and Loh, 1987). In these cases, another explanation must be offered. Either the neurologic picture with changed proprioceptive input has altered, a reduction of a local inflammatory response has occurred, or the associated dysfunction has been reversed.

Conclusion

The responsible practitioner of diversified technique follows up treatment with appropriate exercises. These exercises are designed to maintain the mobility introduced into the fixated joint and also to assist the body in developing more appropriate movement patterns. The patient must also be instructed in proper biomechanical behavior and encouraged to practice good postural hygiene.

As new information develops in the fields of biomechanics, kinesiology, bioengineering, neuro-

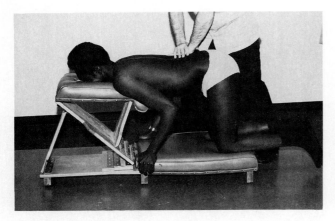

Figure 27–35. Alternate method of adjusting the lumbar spine: the anterior-to-posterior adjustment in the kneeling position.

physiology, clinical studies, etc., the diversified techniques can be expected to change as well for any technique or methodology in the clinical sciences should be ever evolving.

References

Beatty AG. *Anatomic Adjustive Technique*. Denver, Colo;1939.

Bonyon J. Lumbar instability. *Postgraduate Seminar at the Canadian Memorial Chiropractic College*. 1967.

Cassidy JD. Reotoenological examination of the functional mechanics of the lumbar spine in lateral flexion. *JCCA* 1976;20(2):13.

DeJarnette MB. Sacro-occipital technic. Unpublished notes, 1967.

Dye AA. *The Evolution of Chiropractic*. Philadelphia, 1939.

Gaymans F. Neue mobilisations prinzipien und techniken an der wirbelsaule. *Manual Med* 1973;11:35.

Gillet H and Liekens M. A further study of spinal fixations. *Ann Swiss Chiropractic Assoc* 1969;4:41.

Gillet H and Liekens M. Belgium chiropractic research notes, 1953.

Gitelman R. A chiropractic approach to biomechanical disorders of the lumbar spine. In Haldman S, ed. *Modern Developments in the Principles and Practices of Chiropractic*. New York: Appleton-Century-Croft; 1980.

Gotlieb AC. A selected annotated bibliography of the core biomedical literature pertaining to stroke cervical spine manipulation and head/neck movement. *JCCA* 1985;29(2):80–89.

Gravel P and Gravel AL. *Integrated Chiropractic Methods*. Montreal; 1966.

Grice AS. Scalenus anticus syndrom: Diagnosis and Chiropractic adjustive proceedure. *JCCA* 1977:5.

Grice AS. Radiographic biomechanical and clinical factors in lumbar lateral flexion. *JMPT, 2*, 1979.

Grice AS. A Biomechanical Approach to Cervical and Dorsal Adjusting. In Haldeman S, ed. *Modern Developments in the Principles and Practices of Chiropractic*. New York: Appleton-Century-Croft; 1980.

Grecco MA. *Chiropractic Technique Illustrated*. New York: Jarl; 1953.

Homewood AE. *The Neurodynamics of the Vertebral Subluxation*, 3rd ed. St. Petersburg, Fla. 1979.

Illi FW. The vertebral column, life-line of the body. Chicago, 1951.

Janse J, Houser RH, and Wells BF. *Chiropractic Principles and Techniques*. Chicago, 1947.

LeVernieux J. *Les traction vertebrales l'expansion*. Paris, 1960.

Kleynlams AM. Complications of and Contraindications to spinal manipulative therapy. In Haldman S, ed. *Modern Development in the Principles and Practices of Chiropractic*. New York: Appleton-Century-Croft; 1980.

Kou PP and Loh Z. Treatment of lumbar intervertebral disc protrusion by manipulation. *Clin Orthop* 1987;215:47–55.

Matthews JA and Yates EAH. Reduction of lumbar disc prolapse by manipulation. *Br Med J* 1969;3:392.

Quan JA, Cassidy JD, O'Conner SM, and Kirkaldy-Willis WH. Lumbar intervertebral disc herniation: Treatment by rotational manipulation. *J Manipulative Phys Ther* 1989:12(3):220–226.

Rheinhard O. *Chiropractic Procedure and Practice*, 1962.

Rheinhard O. *Fundamentals of Chiropractic Techniques and Practice Procedures*. Chestenfield, 1983.

Sandoz R. Technique and interpretation of the functional radiography of the lumbar spine. *Ann Swiss Chiropractic Assoc* 1965;3:66.

Sandoz R. Newer trends in the pathogenesis of spinal disorders. *Ann Swiss Chiropr Assoc* 1971;5:93.

Sandoz R. Some physical measurements and effects of spinal adjustments. *Ann Swiss Chiropractic Assoc* 1976;6:92.

Schafer RC and Faye LJ. *Motion Palpation and Chiropractic Technique*. Huntington Beach, Calif: Motion Palpation Institute; 1989: 235.

States AZ. *Spinal and Pelvic Techniques*. Illinois, 1965.

chapter 28

Traction and Distraction Techniques

James M. Cox

Traction is not a new or novel adjunct to spinal manipulation. It was described in the works of Hippocrates (Peltier, 1968) and by a French surgeon in the 15th century (Paré, 1582). Figure 28–1 shows Hippocrates applying combined traction and spinal manipulation (Galenius, 1625; Avicenna, 1650). In another primitive form of traction, the patient was fastened in an inverted position to a ladderlike frame that was repeatedly dropped from a gallows to the ground, producing axial spinal traction as the patient's relatively free trunk and head created a tractive force for the spine. This procedure was termed *succussion* (Coplans, 1978).

This chapter discusses the use of traction forces applied to the spine by the following methods: (1) externally by the use of tractive weights as a mechanical load, (2) through use of the patient's body weight as the force load, (3) through muscle power of the patient applied to a static restraint, (4) controlled passive distraction and manipulation to a spe-cific spinal level by a clinician using a treatment instrument. Such forces may be applied horizontally or vertically and in constant or intermittent duration.

Traction Versus Distraction

Traction in this setting refers to unassisted multilevel traction force applied to the spine. Distraction, on the other hand, is a doctor-controlled tractive force applied to a specific level of the spine with or without articular facet adjustments.

Traction is applied for immobilization or pain relief (Kekosz et al., 1986). Immobilization by cervical or lumbopelvic traction ensures that the spine is held in a restful position. Pain relief is attained by applying sufficient traction force to effect a change in the articular and soft tissue structures, such as separation of intervertebral disc spaces. Scientific validation of the efficacy of this treatment modality is

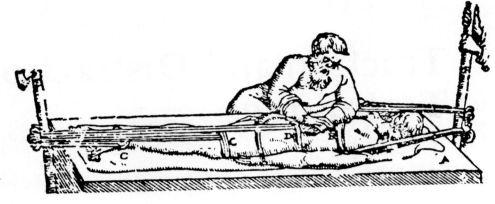

Figure 28–1. Hippocrates applying a spinal adjustment.

scant, but considerable empirical benefit has been observed.

In principle, application of static or intermittent forces to a nonuniform structure such as the spine results in the weakest joints receiving the greatest tractive stretch, primarily in two ways. First, in a comparison of cervical and lumbar spine strength, application of tractive force to the full spine results in the exertion of greater forces on the smaller cervical segments. Second, unstable segments receive greater stress than stable segments. Thus, there is a danger of inflicting greater stress to an already hypermobile unstable segment, while failing to produce motion at a hypomobile site.

Principles of Traction and Distraction

The effects of differing traction forces on the intervertebral disc spaces have been measured by a number of investigators. A tractive force of 730 pounds produces an increase of 2 mm at the L3–4 level. A force of 200 pounds produces a temporary widening of the intervertebral spaces on the ventral and dorsal aspects amounting to 1 mm (de Seze and Levernieux, 1951a). A force of 100 to 200 pounds applied for 30 minutes results in an increase of 2.5 mm in each lumbar vertebral space (Neuwirth et al., 1952; Cyriax, 1959). A tractive force of 300 pounds applied for 5 minutes causes the L3–L4, L4–L5, and L5–S1 disc spaces to increase in vertical height by 1.3, 1.5, and 2.6 mm, respectively (Lehmann and Brunner, 1958). The intradiscal spaces have been measured by a computerized d-mac Pencil Follower while 600 to 800 N (134 to 178 pounds) of tractive force was applied with a lumbopelvic harness. Table 28–1 shows the increase in ventral and dorsal distances during traction in patients with and without back pain. On average, the dorsal distance increased by 18%, and the ventral distance by 8%, from rest following the

application of a distractive force. No difference was seen between patients and healthy subjects. These changes reflected an alteration in the shape of the disc and were always accompanied by a decrease in the lordosis during traction (Lind, 1973). Cervical traction appears to require forces from 35 to 45 pounds, and lumbar traction forces of 75 to 100 pounds, to be effective (Judovich 1952, 1954; Judovich and Nobel, 1957).

Pelvic traction in conjunction with bed rest has been used with a traction apparatus arranged to create increased lumbar flexion. This position is reported to promote distraction of the posterior elements of the lumbar spine, reducing tensile stress on the annulus fibrosus and widening the intervertebral foraminal apertures at the lower two interspaces to allow increased sagittal diameter to the vertebral canal. Nerve root compression at these levels may be relieved by altering the position of the lumbar spine in this manner (Finneson, 1973).

Sustained lumbar traction, using a load of 9 kg for 30 minutes, results in the greatest vertebral separation in those specimens with wide disc spaces and the least vertebral separation where there is evidence of disc degeneration (Twomey, 1987).

In a postmortem study of specimens with all muscle tissue removed, a force of 9 kg was sufficient to bring about a 1.5-mm separation between adjacent lumbar vertebrae. Radiographic studies indicated separation between vertebrae to range between 0.4 and 2.0 mm on traction with forces of up to 55 kg (de Seze and Levernieux, 1951a).

Traction basically has four capabilities: (1) distraction of the vertebral bodies with enlargement of the intervertebral space, producing a suction effect; (2) stretching of muscles, with the tautening of the posterior longitudinal ligament exerting a centripetal force on the adjacent annulus fibrosus; (3) separation of the apophyseal joints; and (4) enlargement of the foramina (McElhannon, 1985).

The rule of three must be adhered to; that is, the

TABLE 28–1. PERCENTAGE CHANGES IN VENTRAL AND DORSAL DISTANCES IN THE INTERVERTEBRAL SPACES DURING TRACTION IN SUBJECTS WITH AND WITHOUT A HISTORY OF LOW BACK PAIN

Intervertebral space	Change in the distance (%)							
	Film 2		Film 3		Film 4		Film 5	
History of low back pain								
Ventral distances [210]								
Th 12/1	+ 2.7	[4]a	−19.0	[4]	−27.6	[5]	−20.0	[5]
L 1/2	− 8.7	[12]	− 5.8	[11]	− 8.9	[12]	−11.3	[12]
L 2/3	− 1.5	[12]	− 5.9	[12]	− 5.2	[12]	−12.0	[12]
L 3/4	− 0.8	[12]	− 1.6	[12]	− 9.6	[12]	−12.2	[12]
L 4/5	− 7.3	[9]	− 4.2	[11]	− 1.8	[10]	− 9.6	[10]
L 5/S 1	+14.2	[2]	+ 5.3	[2]	− 6.3	[3]	−13.5	[2]
Dorsal distances [208]								
Th 12/1	− 5.4	[6]	+27.3	[5]	+25.3	[5]	+30.4	[3]
L 1/2	− 2.3	[12]	+19.0	[11]	+20.2	[11]	+26.8	[11]
L 2/3	+11.0	[12]	+10.4	[11]	+22.3	[10]	+20.7	[12]
L 3/4	+18.6	[12]	+22.7	[12]	+23.1	[12]	+15.4	[12]
L 4/5	+17.6	[10]	+20.7	[9]	+19.8	[10]	+31.3	[10]
L 5/S 1	−11.7	[3]	+20.8	[3]	+ 8.3	[3]	−14.2	[3]
No history of low back pain								
Ventral distances [108]								
Th 12/1	−21.6	[4]	−19.3	[4]	−30.8	[4]	−30.1	[4]
L 1/2	+ 2.9	[6]	− 0.3	[6]	− 2.6	[6]	− 2.1	[5]
L 2/3	− 7.4	[6]	− 3.6	[6]	− 6.6	[6]	−16.1	[6]
L 3/4	− 4.2	[6]	− 2.1	[6]	− 8.7	[6]	−15.6	[6]
L 4/5	− 0.4	[5]	+ 2.6	[5]	− 9.5	[5]	−16.3	[2]
L 5/S 1	− 8.7	[1]	+ 6.4	[1]	+ 4.7	[1]	− 3.8	[1]
Dorsal distances [111]								
Th 12/1	+ 4.4	[4]	+27.6	[5]	+18.0	[3]	+29.7	[4]
L 1/2	+ 3.7	[6]	+ 7.6	[6]	+10.8	[6]	+ 9.5	[6]
L 2/3	+18.3	[6]	+16.0	[6]	+29.0	[6]	+ 9.5	[6]
L 3/4	+12.9	[6]	+19.3	[6]	+22.4	[6]	+33.8	[6]
L 4/5	+30.2	[5]	+ 7.0	[5]	+30.0	[5]	+23.7	[6]
L 5/S 1	− 0.2	[1]	− 6.2	[1]	− 4.9	[1]	+ 3.8	[4]
							+ 0.2	[1]

a Values are means for the respective number of distances, which are given in parentheses.
From Lind G. Auto-traction treatment of low back pain and sciatica. Thesis. University of Linkoping; 1973.

patient must receive traction 3 consecutive days (McElhannon, 1985). The first time the patient is placed in traction, he or she may experience some side effects, such as increased radicular pain or increased soreness. On the second and third days, the patient should have accommodated to the traction; however, the patient must understand that some reaction is expected from the first traction treatment and it is important that she or he receive traction 3 days in a row, then three times weekly, until the desired result is obtained.

For distraction of the lumbar spine, the pelvis must be lifted and the lordotic curve must be flattened to distract the vertebrae. Static traction should be used for the first three treatments. After the first three visits, when the muscles and ligaments have adapted to the pull, intermittent or kinetic traction should be used. Traction should be held for 30 seconds and then released for 10 seconds. Static traction is the preferred method for severe muscle spasm and for a hot disc with acute radiculitis. After the spasm

and radiculitis start to subside, kinetic traction can be safely used.

Traction in various forms is frequently used in the treatment of patients with low back pain and/or sciatica. In spite of extensive literature on the subject, there seems to be no agreement as to what effects traction has, either physically on the spine or clinically on pain.

Traction is reported to have three beneficial effects (Cyriax, 1984):

1. *Suction:* A subatmospheric pressure is induced when the bones move apart, with a centripetal effect on the contents.
2. *Distraction:* The increase in distance between the articular edges may disengage a protrusion that was too large to shift during mere avoidance of compression during recumbency. X-rays have shown an increase in width of the joint of up to 2.5 mm.

3. *Ligamentous tautening:* Separation of the vertebrae tautens the posterior longitudinal ligament, which then exerts centripetal force on a central protrusion.

Further discussion by Cyriax (1984) on the use of traction in the flexion, extension, or plain distractive modes includes the following:

1. If extension is pain-free and flexion hurts, traction will be comfortable if given in slight extension.
2. If both (or neither) flexion and extension are painful, distraction of the joints with the articular surfaces parallel may be attempted.
3. When extension is painful and flexion is pain-free, the distraction should fall mainly on the posterior part of the joint. The lumbar spine needs to be in a slight degree of flexion to achieve this.

Gravity Lumbar Reduction

The Gravity Lumbar Reduction Therapy Program (GLRTP) developed at the Sister Kenny Institute has been of particular value in managing three entities (Kirkaldy-Willis, 1983):

1. Disc "bulging" that produces distention of the annulus and posterior longitudinal ligament. This entity results in pain by stimulating branches of the sinuvertebral nerve. A dorsal ramus pain syndrome typically referred to the low back, hips, and knees is produced. Pain is rarely referred as far as the ankles.
2. A herniated disc in which nuclear material extends beyond the annulus but is contained by the posterior longitudinal ligament (sometimes called a "roof disc"). Compression of a spinal nerve either exiting or traversing the interspace produces sciatic pain that radiates to the toes and feet and the neurologic findings that are associated with this compression.
3. A herniated disc in which nuclear material extends beyond the annulus and is beginning to erode through the posterior longitudinal ligament but has not yet become a free protrusion.

Experience has shown that when herniated disc material extrudes past the posterior longitudinal ligament (free protrusion) or migrates into the spinal canal (sequestered fragment), the application of gravity traction accentuates pain and neurologic def-

icit rather than alleviating it. This phenomenon occurs during the first few days of treatment and is most important to document because it signals the need to discontinue the GLRTP and consider more aggressive treatment modalities such as chemonucleolysis and surgery.

The clinical rationale for the use of continuous gravity traction therapy is based on the relief of nerve root pressure both during the procedures and for a considerable time after, the relief of muscle spasm, and, possibly, its effects on the intervertebral disc and apophyseal joints.

It has also been suggested that traction as therapy exerts a beneficial effect on some patients by its stretching influence on the mechanoreceptors present in the discs, ligaments, and apophyseal joints, or by a direct mechanical effect on the richly innervated apophyseal joints. In this last regard, it is possible that traction achieves its effect by releasing an entrapped interarticular meniscus or fold of capsule or synovial membrane that may block apophyseal joint movement.

Gravity traction on 20 chronic low-back-pain sufferers showed that distraction of the lower lumbar intervertebral spaces resulted in increased spacing (range 0.3–4.0 mm) in all cases (Gianakopoulos, 1985). Not only did the patients note substantial relief, but the effects of distraction were confirmed radiographically.

Cervical Spine Traction

The optimal angle of tractive force in the cervical spine is 20° to 25° of forward neck flexion (Kekosz et al., 1986). This is most comfortable and allows the intervertebral foramina to increase in vertical and sagittal diameter and also decreases intrafacetal pressure by opening the facet joint spaces. Five to ten pounds of weight should be used initially. This is increased to patient tolerance during the next two or three sessions until the effective weight of 15 to 20 pounds (not to exceed 35 pounds) is reached. A tractive weight of 30 pounds for 7 seconds produces posterior separation of the cervical vertebrae (Colachis and Strohm, 1965, 1966). This appears to be the least weight and duration that effectively separate the vertebrae. Longer time can aggravate rather than relieve pain. The greatest separation of the cervical vertebrae occurs at a flexion angle of 24°, and the amount of separation of the vertebrae is as great at 30 pounds as at 50 pounds of tractive weight when this 24° angle is maintained. Distractive forces of one third of the body weight have produced 1 to 2 mm of separation of cervical vertebrae (Schlicke et al., in press).

Tractive weight of 40 to 60 pounds for 20 minutes results in a 3.4-mm increase in height in the cervical spine (Lawson and Godfrey, 1968). Application of 260 pounds to the cervical spine results in a 2-mm increase in disc space at C6–C7 (de Seze and Levernieux, 1951b). Traction of 45 to 100 pounds applied to 63 patients with cervical spine complaints resulting from osteoarthritis resulted in an increased interspinous spacing of 10.9 to 6.5 mm along the posterior margins and 2.8 mm along the anterior margins of the vertebral bodies (McFarland and Krusen, 1943). Application of tractive forces of 30 and 50 pounds for 7, 30, and 60 seconds caused the space between the posterior margins of the vertebral bodies to increase in every case, the effect being greater with 50 than with 30 pounds (Colachis and Strohm, 1965). The anterior bodies did not open consecutively in every case. The posterior body spaces increased five times as much in vertical dimension as did the anterior interbody disc spaces.

Cervical traction may be applied with the patient either sitting or supine. There are advantages and disadvantages to each method. Most authors prefer the supine posture for traction application (Colachis and Strohm, 1965; Cox, 1985; Deets et al., 1977). Temporomandibular joint (TMJ) pressure, however, can be a problem in the use of cervical traction. Walker (1986) described the Goodley system of supine cervical traction, which prevents pressure on the TMJ while allowing the application of tractive force to specific intervertebral restrictions to mobilize specific cervical segments.

When cervical traction is applied in the sitting patient, less stability is provided to the cervical spine than when the patient is supine. If this system is found helpful by the patient, home units may be used for 15- to 20-minute sessions.

When traction is applied to the cervical spine with the patient sitting or standing with the arms hanging, more discomfort is felt, as the cervical nerve roots are extended farther in this posture. The direction of pull in cervical traction should be in a flexed position of about 45°, which gives the greatest relaxation. Traction for correction of increased lordosis of the cervical sagittal curve is ineffective. Such traction would narrow the intervertebral foramina while increasing tension on the anterior neck muscles (Kramer, 1981).

The lumbar spine has very similar problems in allowing hyperflexion or extension during treatment. Extension of the lumbar spine causes protrusion of the intervertebral discs with dorsal displacement of the cauda equina roots. It also decreases the length of the spinal canal and forces an increase in the cross-sectional diameter of the cauda equina roots (Breig, 1960). Lordosis increases in extension movement to cause blockage of the cauda equina, while flexion permits contrast medium on myelographic study to pass through the blocked area

(Ehni, 1965). Therefore, both the cervical spine and the lumbar spine should be tractioned in the flexion mode to allow maximum sagittal diameter of the vertebral canal and to avoid instituting stenosis that would adversely affect the clinical outcome.

A series of treatments can be given daily for 7 to 10 days or three times a week for 3 to 4 weeks. If relief is not attained in this time, traction should be discontinued (Hinterbuchner, 1985). Cervical traction application is initiated with 5 to 10 pounds, and is increased on successive visits to a maximum of 35 pounds. An average weight of 15 to 20 pounds should restrict adverse side effects.

Thoracic Spine Traction

Thoracic spine traction is less frequently successful than lumbar or cervical spine traction, but it can be exactly applied as in the other spinal areas. Upper thoracic traction is applied by having the patient lie on his or her back with a cervical halter in place and a pelvic belt attached to a stabilizing resistance at the foot of the couch. Lower thoracic spine traction is applied by using a thoracic belt to apply cephalad traction and a pelvic belt to stabilize the spine during traction. The indications for thoracic traction are generalized thoracic spine pain as is commonly found in degenerative disc disease. In thoracic nerve root pain, Maitland (1977) feels that traction is the treatment of choice. A friction-free couch is required for this treatment. Distraction application to specific thoracic levels is shown later in this chapter in Figure 28–10.

Lumbar Spine Distraction and Traction

Lumbar spine distraction may be applied in the supine, prone, or inclined posture. Supine distraction requires an effective tractive force of about 35% to 50% body weight and is applied either by weights and a pulley system or by a motorized device (Basmajian, 1985). Ten percent of the body weight is the optimal force used in pelvic distraction (Coplans, 1978). A pelvic harness is used to provide the tractive force. The caudal section of the table should be movable and the head section stationary to afford anchoring of the thoracic spine with a thoracic harness while the lumbar force is applied. The patient lies in the semi-Fowler position with the hips flexed 70° so that lumbar flexion can be provided. This opens the intervertebral foraminae, reduces facet interarticular compressive force, and provides patient comfort (Cailliet, 1981).

A thoracic belt is attached to a stabilizing bar at

the head of the treatment table and a pelvic harness is used to exert caudal distraction on the lumbar spine as weight is added to the spine at the caudal end of the couch (Maitland, 1977). A friction-free couch is best and the tractive force is initiated with 13 kg for up to 10 minutes.

To separate the L4–5 disc space 1.5 mm, 730 pounds is needed, whereas 810 pounds is required to gain a 2-mm separation at the L3–4 level (de Seze and Levernieux, 1951b). Frazer (1954) found the same disc increases at 300 to 400 pounds of tractive force; however, 100 to 200 pounds for $\frac{1}{2}$ to 1 hour is reported to achieve the same result (Cyriax 1984).

Techniques of Spinal Traction and Distraction

STATIC TRACTION. Shorter periods of traction with higher weights are applied for a few minutes to 30 minutes. Split tables are most effective and reduce friction.

MANUAL DISTRACTION. Here the doctor applies the force in a controlled fashion. This can be done by hand or with a movable sectioned manipulation table that allows all ranges of motion to be applied to a specific joint. Stoddard (1961) stressed that a physician who applies manipulation manually develops a keen sense of tissue tension compared with a physician who does not manipulate.

CONSTANT CONTINUOUS TRACTION. Low weights are used over a long period, up to several hours. The main objective is to attain a restful and sustained position of the spine.

INTERMITTENT TRACTION. Either manual or mechanized methods may be used. Tractive force is applied and withdrawn in relatively short periods. Coplans (1978) uses 12 rhythmic distractions per minute in intermittent distraction. The knees and hips are supported in flexion to abolish lordosis and increase the efficiency of traction. A 30- to 40-kg intermittent pull is used for 10 minutes.

GRAVITY TRACTION. Gravity traction is applied either by inversion hanging from gravity boots, by flexion at the waist, or by means of a chest harness. This last system, called gravity lumbar reduction (Burton, 1980), has been found to handle 70% of patients with protruding lumbar discs without surgical reduction. It is also used for lumbosacral strain, mechanical back syndromes, spondylolisthesis, scoliosis, lateral recess stenosis, and postsurgical management of patients with residual pain. Approximately 5% of patients cannot tolerate distractive manipulation (Burton, 1980; Cox, 1985).

COX DISTRACTION MANIPULATION. Manual controlled distraction is applied to the intervertebral disc space and articular facets with the patient positioned on a table designed for its application and described later in Figures 28–5 and 28–6. Under distraction, the facet articulations are manipulated throughout their physiologic ranges of motions.

Comparison of Static, Intermittent, and Manual Traction

Static traction, intermittent traction, manual traction, and no traction were compared in 100 consenting patients with cervical spine disorders. The patients, all of similar age, sex, diagnosis, and chronicity, were randomly assigned to a treatment type, and scheduled for two visits weekly over a 6-week period. Intermittent traction patients performed significantly better than those assigned to no traction or static traction care in terms of pain, flexion, and rotation movements (Zylbergold and Piper, 1985).

On the other hand, Jette et al. (1985) looked at muscle relaxation of the cervical spine during 20 minutes of intermittent supine cervical traction by reading electromyographic recordings of the upper trapezius muscle. No significant change in myoelectric activity was found during the administration of traction, and thus it was concluded that supine traction did not produce cervical muscle relaxation.

Stoddard (1954) recommends the use of sustained traction at an average weight of 35 pounds with about 30° of flexion of the cervical spine when the patient's symptoms are very severe. For less severe symptoms he recommends intermittent traction at an average effective pull of 35 pounds. He feels that less than 30 pounds is ineffective, whereas more than pounds 40 irritates nerve roots. He stresses that the patient must be relaxed and comfortable, and have confidence in and an understanding of the procedure. He places ankle cuffs on the patient for stability during traction and makes sure that the patient suffers no jaw or teeth pain. The tractive force is started and ended gradually, with no jerky movements. He starts with a force of 20 to 25 pounds and increases the weight to patient tolerance.

Indications for Spinal Traction or Distraction

Intervertebral Disc Herniation with Disc Protrusion
When disc protrusion is treated with distraction, the time of spinal traction application should be short. Intradiscal pressure drops under traction. This decrease in pressure needs to be maintained only for a short period as osmotic forces will soon equalize

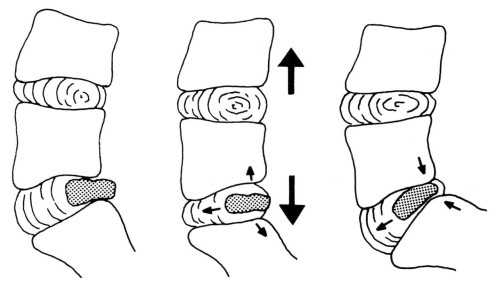

Figure 28-2. Return of a disc protrusion during traction. Besides traction, a slight kyphosis is necessary. It is obtained in the back rest position. (*Reproduced, with permission, from Kramer 1981, p. 165*).

pressure with that of the surrounding tissue. When this equalization occurs, the suction effect is diminished or lost and the continuation of distraction might have a detrimental effect. When treatment time was kept under 10 minutes, and sustained treatments under 8 minutes, this adverse change was not observed (Saunders, 1983). The effective treatment time ranges from a few days to 2 weeks (Coplans, 1978), and each treatment session should be followed by the use of a well-fitted lumbar support before weight bearing is allowed. Kramer (1981) feels it is important to increase the disc space in the treatment of disc disease. Figures 28–2 and 28–3 show the positive and negative results of distraction on an intervertebral disc protrusion. There are five goals in applying traction to the disc spaces:

1. Widening of the intervertebral foramen
2. Widening of the disc space
3. Traction of the paravertebral muscles and ligaments
4. Correction of vertebral joint deformities
5. Increase in volume of disc tissue

The kyphotic posture created by traction is thought to allow a decrease in nerve root pressure by improving blood flow through the valveless veins of the spine and absorbing edema fluids. Further, by reducing intradiscal pressure, the protruded disc may tend to return to its original location. Elongation of paravertebral muscles and ligaments may relieve spasm and pressure on nerves and blood vessels.

The most important factor in traction is its ability

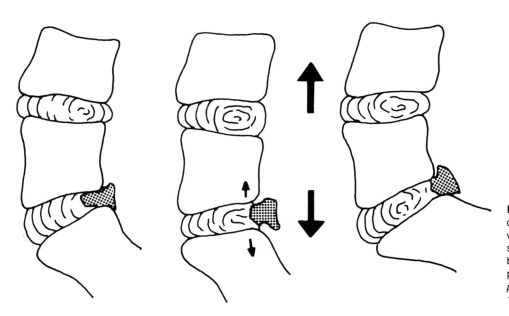

Figure 28-3. Increase in pain during traction. The prolapse, which is kept in its original position by the vertebral border, becomes dislocated further posteriorly. (*Reproduced, with permission, from Kramer, 1981, p. 168*).

to lower intradiscal pressure and facilitate normalization of the disc fragment (Kramer, 1981). Such traction may be applied by having the patient hang from the "chinning bar," by long-time traction with small weights, by short-time traction with large forces, or by intermittent traction at regular intervals. A traction girdle can also be used in applying pelvic traction for this purpose.

Extension may be used in conjunction with distractive reduction of the disc lesion (McKenzie, 1981). Following reduction of the disc herniation, extension exercises are used to maintain the correction. This is felt to maintain the nucleus pulposus within the disc space while healing of the annular fibers

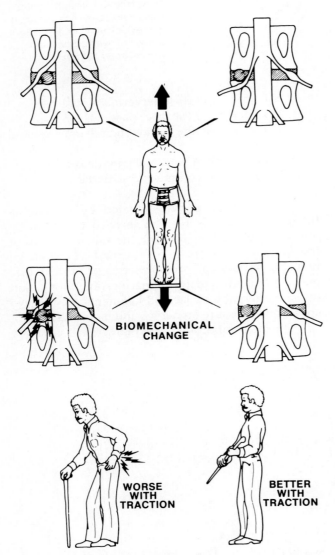

Figure 28–4. This is a hypothetical explanation of why some patients may respond well to traction, and others may respond with more pain. When the disc is in the axilla of the nerve root, axial traction may irritate the problem. (*Reproduced, with permission, from White AA and Panjabi MM.*) *Clinical Biomechanics of the Spine.* Philadelphia: JB Lippincott; 1978:313.

takes place (Kapandji, 1974; Cyriax, 1950; Gupta and Ramarao, 1978; Morris et al., 1961).

Figure 28–4 shows the potential benefits and dangers of treating various types of disc lesions with traction. Pelvic sustained traction can aggravate medial disc protrusions and relieve lateral disc protrusions.

Facet Subluxation Complexes

Distraction can be used as the initial manipulative treatment in (1) degenerative disc disease, (2) facet hyperextension subluxation with facet telescoping of the superior facet of the inferior vertebra into the foramen, (3) stenosis in which the lateral recess is narrowing by hypertrophic facet arthrosis, (4) spondylolisthesis, (5) transitional segment, (6) and retrolisthesis subluxation. After distraction or traction, the vertical height and sagittal diameter of the intervertebral foramina are increased. In this positions, the other motions of the facet joints, namely, lateral flexion, circumduction, rotation, and extension, can be applied. Application of distraction of the facet joints first will allow the other facet motions to be carried out without danger of inflicting lateral recess stenosis through telescoping of the superior facet of the inferior vertebra upward and anteriorly into the foramen.

Other Conditions

Spinal traction and distraction may also be used in failure of rotational manipulation to relieve pain (Cyriax, 1984); postsurgical return of pain or failure to gain surgical relief (Cyriax, 1984); degenerative disc disease, with or without nerve root irritation (Kekosz et al., 1986); relaxation of paravertebral muscles; and increase in vertical and sagittal diameters of the intervertebral foramina to reduce nerve root compression forces.

Contraindications to Spinal Traction

History and physical examination are paramount before any treatment program, including traction, is instituted. Diagnostic imaging involving plain film radiographs or more detailed studies such as magnetic resonance imaging and computed tomography may be included. Any acute trauma to soft tissue should not be tractioned as this may result in further tearing and bleeding of torn or strained muscles or ligaments. Plain film radiographs should be taken following cervical injury to rule out fracture of the odontoid process or atlas ring. In this situation, traction in an office setting is not indicated, although treatment in a hospital setting may be necessary.

Conditions not to be tractioned include tumor (primary or metastatic), infection (spondylitis or osteomyelitis), and signs of vertebrobasilar or carotid artery spasm or ischemia. The course and anatomic location of the vertebral artery make it susceptible to mechanical trauma. Three possible sites of compression have been located: (1) the intervertebral foramina above C5–6, (2) the atlantoaxial joint, and (3) the occipitoatlantal joint (Schneider and Schemm, 1961). Reduced vertebral artery flow has been demonstrated in cadavers when the head is hyperextended and tilted to the opposite side, even by maneuvers well within the physiologic range of movement. The vertebral arteries are often of unequal size, the left being larger in 51% of patients, the right in 41% (Tissington and Bammer, 1957; Toole and Tucker, 1960; Stopford, 1916). The posterior inferior cerebellar artery on the occluded vessel side is particularly vulnerable to ischemia in these circumstances (Parkin et al., 1978).

Patients with signs of instability, as in rheumatoid arthritis of the upper cervical spine, should not be tractioned. For pregnant women, tractive manipulation can be applied to the lumbar spine with the woman lying in the side posture. This technique is shown later in this chapter in Figure 28–9.

Persons with the following disorders also should not be tractioned:

- Acute sprains and stains
- Claustrophobia from being placed in ankle cuffs or a pelvic harness
- Aortic aneurysm
- Vascular insufficiency of the lower extremities
- Temporomandibular disease, which could be aggravated by cervical traction (Special harnesses, which avoid pressure on the jaw, are available.)
- Advanced cardiovascular disease, including uncontrolled hypertension
- Large disc prolapses causing cauda equina syndrome
- Lumbago with severe pain on movement (Cyriax, 1984)
- Osteoporosis

Testing Patient Tolerance to Distraction Application

Distraction testing is done prior to submitting the patient to treatment with the following concepts in mind:

1. If a decrease in pain is demonstrated on distraction, treatment should be instituted. Usually pain will change in character, and a lateral extremity pain will become a central type of low back pain. A sharp lancinating

pain may become a dull ache. A patient with night pain may find he or she is able to sleep through the night. Full leg pain may become localized to the buttocks. There may be both a decrease in and a change in distribution of pain.

2. Increased pain from traction may occur when shearing forces influence a displaced fragment and dislocate it posteriorly into the vertebral canal (see Fig. 28–3); when a prolapse is still within the boundaries of the vertebral margins but during traction becomes displaced into the spinal canal; or when traction is applied to adhesions around the nerve root or in the spinal canal.

3. Increased pain after long periods of relaxation, as when sleeping at night, is thought to be caused by an increase in the disc volume from imbibition of fluids at rest. In these circumstances, distraction and traction should not be used, as these could possibly allow increased intradiscal pressure to force protruded disc material into a sequestration.

4. Hypermobile segments or muscle insufficiency findings are a contraindication to tractive force.

The following testing is used to identify the patient's resistance or acceptance of distraction when treating the lumbar spine. With the patient lying prone on the table, a thenar contact using the doctor's hand is made on the spinous process from the first through the fifth lumbar vertebrae while the caudal section of the table is gently flexed caudally by no more than 1 to 2 inches (Fig. 28–5). No cuffs are placed on the patient during testing; rather, the weight of the patient's pelvis and lower extremities is the only distractive force used as the caudal section is distracted downward. If this amount of distraction causes patient pain, the cuffs should not be placed and use of this distraction technique should be avoided. In the case of acute low back pain, it may be hours or days before the patient will tolerate any distractive treatment. Occasionally, a patient will not be able to tolerate the distractive force at all. It is necessary to repeatedly test the patient's ability to withstand distraction until there is no adverse reaction. If no pain is felt using the patient's weight as the tractive force, the doctor should proceed to test right and left spinal distractive tolerance of the facet joints. This is achieved by grasping first the right ankle and tractioning the right facets as contact is made with the doctor's hand over the right facet joints; this is repeated on the left side. In this way both central and lateral distractive tolerance to traction is tested prior

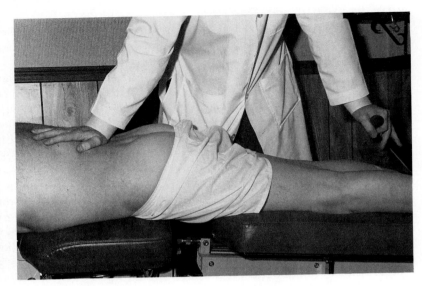

Figure 28–5. Testing patient tolerance to distraction without the ankle cuffs applied. Contact on the spinous process of the lumbar vertebral segment is made while applying cephalad pressure to stabilize the vertebral segment. The caudal section is distracted downward 1 to 2 inches while the patient is observed for pain or muscle spasm.

to application of the cuffs. If the patient feels no pain, the cuffs are applied as shown in Figure 28–6.

The adjuster should never distract downward more than 2 inches with the caudal section of the table in treating the lower lumbar spine; however, as distraction is applied to the thoracic and upper lumbar spine, more than 2 inches of tractive force is needed as the force is dissipated over a longer section of the spine.

Distraction should not be used where a fully sequestered disc fragment is causing sciatica (Charnley, 1955); however, patients with true sciatica may

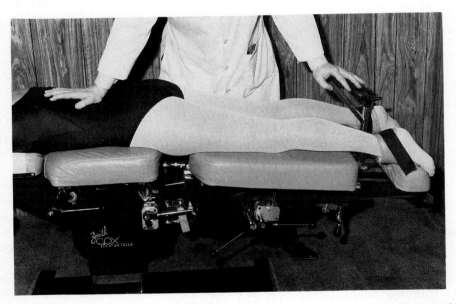

Figure 28–6. Flexion distraction is applied to the lumbar segment to be distracted by contacting the spinous process above the segment with the thenar process of the treatment hand. The caudal section of the table is flexed until tautness of the interspinous space occurs and motion is felt between the adjacent vertebrae. This necessitates 1 to 2 inches of downward distractive force with the caudal table section. This maneuver is repeated three times, each for 20 seconds. For non–disc protrusion conditions, flexion distraction is performed until the spinous processes are felt to separate and then the other motions of lateral flexion, circumduction, extension, and rotation are performed at each facet level.

improve with distraction, depending on the location of the fragment (see Fig. 28–4) (Hood and Chrisman, 1967).

Clinical Studies on Lumbar Distraction and Traction

After reviewing 30,000 patients under traction, Neugebauer (1976) cites three potential therapeutic effects of distraction: (1) the disc is reestablished, (2) the intervertebral foramina are enlarged, and (3) stretching of the anterior and posterior longitudinal ligaments brings the vertebrae back into normal position. Sustained lumbar traction of 120 pounds is reported to reduce the defect in myelographic contrast, as the protrusion appears to be sucked back into the intervertebral disc space (Mathews and Yates, 1974). Reduction of the protruded nucleus pulposus, approximation of the fissure in the annulus fibrosus, and attainment of normal alignment of the articular facets by manipulation have been reported by Tien-You (1976). Similarly, Mathews (1975) reported a series of epidurograms showing flattening of a protrusion after manipulation, accompanied by relief of all symptoms and signs. Additional case studies are presented by Tkachenko (1973) who reported that 10 cases of acute slipped disc were successfully reset by manipulation. Similarly, Pomosov (1976) documented that two doctors had achieved reduction of slipped discs in patients under anesthesia using a rotation traction maneuver. Variation in traction technique is reported by Sharubina (1973), who treated slipped discs in a 37°C pool with a 6- to 32-kg weight. Of the 281 patients treated, 4 became worse, 20% considerably improved, and 79% improved. Similar results were reported by Li (1977) in 74 cases of displaced disc treated by suspended traction manipulation.

Kessler (1979) states that management in the acute stage of disc prolapse should include bed rest with short periods of ambulation; avoidance of positions or activities that may increase intradiscal pressure, especially sitting, forward bending, and valsalva maneuver; relaxation of reflex muscle splinting; and specific segmental distraction techniques.

Herniation of a nucleus pulposus causing nerve compression can heal spontaneously provided low intradiscal pressure can be maintained for 3 months. Clinical experience shows that it takes approximately 3 months until a patient can carry out the activities of daily living without danger of recurrence (Hirschberg, 1974).

Traction stretches the back so that vertebrae are pulled away from each other, and roentgenographic studies have suggested that spinal traction is capable of distracting vertebrae and diminishing disc protrusion in patients with herniated discs (Deyo, 1983).

The Cottrell 90/90 Backtrac System works by flattening the lumbar spine and reducing the lumbar curve. It simply and effectively achieves anterior pelvic tilt. This tends to elongate the lumbar intervertebral disc spaces, which reduces pressure on the disc. It is indicated for the treatment of muscle spasms, overstretched or torn ligaments, back sprains and strains, and some facet syndrome patients. It is also suitable for pregnant or obese patients (Lossing, 1983).

The pressure in the third lumbar discs, in vivo, during active and passive traction, has been measured. It has been found that pressure always increases during active traction. Physically, if the purpose of spinal traction is to reduce pressures within the disc and/or to open up the disc space, then traction has to be administered in a way that allows the trunk muscles to relax. Passive traction over a long period might accomplish that (Andersson et al., 1983).

Clinical and computed tomography (CT) scan changes during autotraction treatment in 17 patients with lumbago–sciatica were studied by Natchev and Valentino (1984). Although the treatment produced excellent results in most patients, the follow-up CT scans revealed no improvement in most. They concluded that the size and shape of the disc protrusion as seen on a CT scan have little correlation with the neurologic deficits and pain experienced by the patient. Natchev and Valentino felt that autotraction's success is related more to stimulation of a neurologic mechanism that inhibits pain than to mechanical reduction of the disc. Vertebral separation can be measured on lateral roentgenograms, both before and after inversion, by outlining the margins of the intervertebral bodies anteriorly and posteriorly and determining the greatest vertical heights of the intervertebral foramina. Mean anterior separation is significant at all levels except L3–4. Mean posterior separation is significant at all levels except L1–2 and L5–S1. If the increases in intervertebral dimension play a role in the relief of low-back syndrome, then gravity-facilitated traction may be an effective modality in the treatment of this condition.

Patients with lower back pain and sciatica were myelographically examined before traction by Gillstrom et al. (1985a) to establish the existence and size of any herniation. Within 2 to 6 months of the traction treatment, the patients were clinically reexamined and myelography was repeated. The size and shape of the herniation before and after traction were compared on the myelograms. The size and location of the disc herniation were the same before and after autotraction despite marked clinical relief of pain. Similarly, Chrisman et al. (1964) could not demonstrate any change in CSF in 27 patients who had positive myelograms prior to manipulation. They found that patients with negative myelograms responded better to manipulation than patients with positive myelograms.

In a second study by Gillstrom et al. (1985b), a special distraction table was placed into a computed tomography unit to measure the intervertebral disc space opening during autotraction. The L4–5 and L5–S1 disc spaces were studied for configuration change during administration of the tractive force to 4 patients with lumbago and sciatica, and before and after administration to 21 others. None of the patients showed any difference in the disc herniation even though good clinical relief was attained. On the other hand, thermography studies on 49 sciatic patients before and after autotraction treatment and at 1-year follow-up showed that 79% of patients improved with distraction (Gillstrom and Ehrnberg, 1985).

Manual traction and autotraction were described by Ljunggren et al. (1984) as being equally effective in the treatment of 49 patients with prolapsed intervertebral discs in a hospital setting. Treatment lasted 1 week and was administered by the same therapist. Follow-up occurred at 1 and 2 weeks and 3 months by a blinded assessment. At the end of 2 years there had been no recurrence of symptoms, and one fourth of the patients had avoided surgery. Manual traction was preferred over autotraction.

Pal et al. (1986) carried out a controlled trial of continuous lumbar traction in the treatment of back pain and sciatica. They showed similar improvements in both the treated group (weighted traction) and the control group (simulated traction). The findings of this study have brought into question the justification of admitting patients with back pain into hospitals for purposes of traction alone.

Manipulation Versus Traction in Sciatica

Manipulation is indicated when, first, there is a history of sudden onset of low back pain, and, second, physical examination discloses a partial articular pattern and the pain is increased by side flexion away from the painful side (i.e., small axillary displacement). If side flexion toward the painful side (i.e., large displacement lateral to the nerve root) increases the pain, the manipulation cannot be expected to be as effective. Manipulation works best for a small, hard displacement in the intervertebral joint. In this situation, the patient should leave the office symptom-free.

Traction is indicated when there is a history of gradual onset of low back pain (i.e., soft disc, as it takes time for the nucleus to infiltrate the fissures of the annulus. This semigelatinous infiltration cannot be manipulated back in place, and distraction is needed to create a negative intradiscal pressure, theoretically to suck the nuclear material back into the interstices of the annulus fibrosus. After 2 weeks of therapy, reduction of the herniated disc is usually complete (Quellette, 1987).

Lumbar Distractive Manipulation

Distraction manipulation for low back pain can increase the intervertebral disc height to remove annular distortion in the pain-sensitive peripheral annular fibers; allow the nucleus pulposus to assume its central position within the annulus fibrosus and relieve irritation of the pain-sensitive annular peripheral fibers; restore the vertebral zygopophyseal joints to their physiologic relationships of motion; and improve posture and locomotion while relieving pain, improving body function, and creating a state of well-being (Cox, 1985).

Some common conditions treated with lumbar distractive manipulation are degenerative disc disease, spondylolisthesis, facet subluxation syndrome, disc protrusion with radiculopathy, scoliosis, and some stenotic conditions. Treatment by flexion distraction to the lumbar spine is shown in Figures 28–7 to 28–9. Figure 28–7 shows the instrument used for the application of the technique of distraction. Figure 28–6, presented previously, shows the application of distraction. The patient lies prone on the instrument and the ankles are placed in the ankle cuffs. The patient's ability to tolerate this form of manipulation is tested as described previously. The doctor's thenar aspect of the treating hand contacts the spinous process above the disc or facet articulation to be distracted. This spinous contact is held in place by a cephalad pressure as the caudal section of the table is opened in distraction by pressing downward with the assist handle as shown in Figure 28–6. When this downward force is applied, the caudal section is depressed until a tautening of all tissues under the spinous process contact is felt. From this point of tautness, the caudal section is not depressed downward more than 2 inches. In the case of a patient with an intervertebral disc protrusion, three 20-second sessions of traction are applied to the intervertebral disc interspace. During each 20-second session, the adjuster exerts a milking action, or push–pull pumping action, on the disc space by

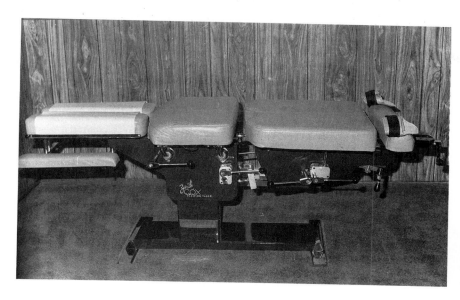

Figure 28-7. The Zenith Cox distraction instrument. The table shown is the product of research design between the author and the Williams Manufacturing Company, Inc., of Elgin, Illinois.

gently moving the caudal section up and down five or six times during the 20 seconds of distraction. The thrust of the downward effort is from the point of tautness to about 1 or 2 inches of downward effort with the caudal section of the instrument. This allows a gentle oscillation of the disc space as opposed to just holding a sustained traction for the 20-second period.

Figure 28–8 shows the use of lateral flexion with flexion distraction. This procedure is used in patients who have no sciatica but merely facet syndrome or degenerative disc disease.

Figure 28–9 shows the patient lying on the side during application of flexion distraction. This procedure is used in patients whose pain is too great to allow them to lie prone. The disc protrusion or facet articulations to be distracted are placed over the pivot opening of the instrument with the patient's pelvis on the caudal table section. The spinous processes above and below the disc or facets are held and used to direct the tractive force in lateral flexion movement of the instrument.

Cervical Distractive Manipulation

Figure 28–10 shows the stabilization of the spinous process with the dorsal web of the doctor's thumb and index finger as distraction is applied by the actual contact as shown in Figure 28–11.

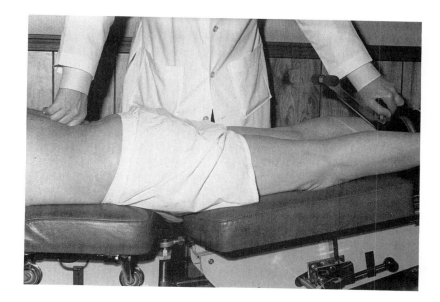

Figure 28-8. Lateral flexion is shown being applied to the vertebral facet joints following flexion distraction.

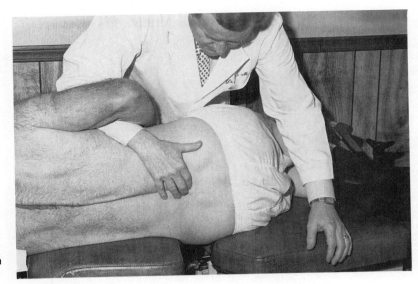

Figure 28-9. Flexion distraction application with the patient lying on the side.

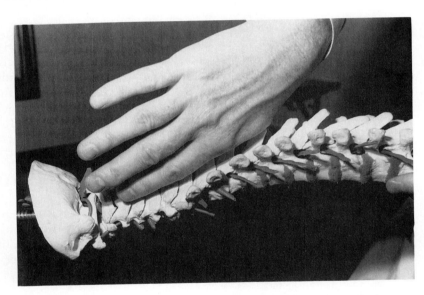

Figure 28-10. The spinous processes of the cervical or upper thoracic vertebrae are held by the web between the index and thumb as flexion distraction is applied to the lower cervical or upper thoracic spines.

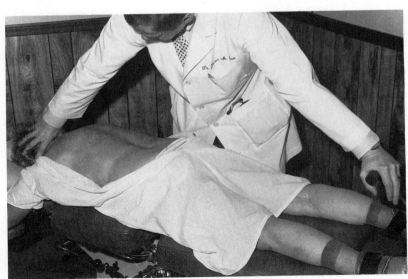

Figure 28-11. Application of distraction to the cervical spine. The tractive force is used to gently separate the posterior arch of the cervical segments, stretch ligaments and muscles, and relieve tension and nerve root irritation.

Conclusion

Traction and distraction are felt to relieve back pain and muscle spasm by effecting changes in the articular and soft tissue structures of the vertebral functional spinal units. Various authors are cited who have demonstrated increases in the intervertebral spaces with tractive force.

Chiropractic adjustments can be performed while distraction is applied to the functional spinal units. Such tractive posturing is felt to reduce stenosis by flattening lordosis, increasing disc height, widening the intervertebral foramina and apophyseal joint spaces, and reducing disc herniation, while stretching lumbar ligaments and muscles to restore normal excitatory reflex response. Traction applied in slight flexion posture affords the greatest relief of discal, facetal, and ligamentous induced stenosis (Onel et al., 1989; Penning and Wilmink, 1987; Epstein et al., 1987; Adams and Hutton, 1988; Dai Liyang et al., 1989; Stephens and O'Brien, 1986; Schonstrom et al., 1989; Vanharanta et al., 1989; Zusman, 1988; Zusman et al., 1989).

Reduction of stenotic factors increases physiological facet joint motion and restores range of facet movement with reduced chance of nerve root compression in the vertebral canal or intervertebral foramina through further stenosis inflicted by the facet, disc, or ligamentous compression. This in turn is felt to reduce iatrogenic side effects during adjustive procedures while affording relief of facet subluxation, disc herniation, and hypertrophic ligamentous stenosis.

References

Adams MA and Hutton WC. Mechanics of the intervertebral disc. In Ghosh P, ed. *The Biology of the Intervertebral Disc*, vol. 1 (1). Boca Raton, FL: CRC Press; 1988.

Andersson GBJ, Schultz AB, and Nachemson AL. Intervertebral disc pressures during traction. *Scand J Rehab Med (Suppl)* 1983;9:88–91.

Avicenna, cited by Gotfredsen E. *Medicinens Historie, Copenhagen* 1650:94–95.

Basmajian JV. *Manipulation, Traction and Massage*, 3rd ed. Baltimore, Md: Williams & Wilkins; 1985.

Breig A. *Biomechanics of the Central Nervous System: Some Basic Normal and Pathologic Phenomena*. Chicago: Year Book; 1960.

Burton CV. The Sister Kenny Institute, Gravity Lumbar Reduction Therapy Program. In *Low Back Pain*, 2nd ed. Philadelphia: JB Lippincott; 1980.

Cailliet R. *Low Back Pain Syndrome*, 3rd ed. Philadelphia: FA Davis; 1981.

Charnley J. Acute lumbago and sciatica. *Br Med J* 1955;1:344.

Chrisman OD, Mittnach T, Snook GA: A study of the results following rotatory manipulation in the lumbar intervertebral disc syndrome. *J Bone Joint Surg [Am]* 1964;46:517–524.

Colachis SC and Strohm BR. A study of tractive forces and angle of pull on vertebral inter-spaces in the cervical spine. *Arch Phys Med Rehab* 1965;46:820–830.

Colachis SC and Strohm BR. Effect of duration of intermittent cervical traction on vertebral separation. *Arch Phys Med Rehab* 1966;47:353.

Coplans CW. The conservative treatment of low back pain. In *Disorders of the Lumbar Spine*. Philadelphia/Toronto: JB Lippincott; 1978.

Cox JM. *Low Back Pain, Mechanism, Diagnosis, Treatment*. Baltimore, Md: Williams & Wilkins; 1985.

Crue BL. Importance of flexion in cervical traction for radiculitis. *US Armed Forces Med J* 1957;8:374.

Cyriax J. The treatment of lumbar disc lesions. *Br Med J* 1950; 2:1434.

Cyriax J. *Textbook of Orthopaedic Medicine*. London: Bailliere, Tindall & Cassell; 1959.

Cyriax J. Traction couch for reduction of nuclear protrusion. In Cyriax J, ed. *Textbook of Orthopaedic Medicine*, 11th ed. London: Bailliere, Tindall, Cassell; 1984: vol. 2, pp. 164–170.

Dai Liyang MD, Yinkan XU, Wenming Z, and Zhihua Z. The effect of flexion-extension motion of the lumbar spine on the capacity of the spinal canal: An experimental study. *Spine* 1989;14(5):523.

Deets D, Hands KL, and Hopp SS. Cervical traction: A comparison of sitting and supine positions. *Phys Ther* 1977;57: 255–261.

de Seze S and Levernieux J. Les tractions vertebrales: Premieres etudes experimentales et resultats therapeutiques d'apres une experience de quatre annees. *Semin Hop Paris* 1951a;27:2085–2104.

de Seze S and Levernieux J. Pratique rhumatologie des tractions vertebrales. *Semin Hop Paris* 1951b;27:2105.

Deyo RA. Conservative therapy for low back pain—Distinguishing useful from useless therapy. *JAMA* 1983;250(8):1058, 1059.

Ehni G. Spondylotic cauda equina radiculopathy. *Texas J Med* 1965;61:746.

Epstein N, Hyman R, Epstein J, and Rosenthal A. Technical note: Dynamic MRI scanning of the cervical spine. *Spine* 1987; 13(8):937–940.

Finneson BE. *Low Back Pain*. Philadelphia/Toronto: JB Lippincott; 1973:169.

Frazer EH. The use of traction in backache. *Med J Aust* 1954;41:694.

Galenius C. Opera, Bd IV (Venetia, cited by Brockbank and Griffiths) 1625. De Locis Affectis Libre 1, Kap 6 (cited by Ligeras).

Gianakopoulos G, Waylonis GW, and Grant PA, et al. Inversion devices: Their role in producing lumbar distraction. *Arch Phys Med Rehab* 1985;66:100–102.

Gillstrom P and Ehrnberg A. Long-term results of autotraction in the treatment of lumbago and sciatica. An attempt to correlate clinical results with objective parameters. *Arch Orthop Trauma Surg* 1985;104(5):294–298.

Gillstrom P, Erickson K, and Hindmarsh T. Autotraction in lumbar disc herniation. A myelographic study before and after treatment. *Arch Orthop Trauma Surg* 1985a;104(4):207–210.

Gillstrom P, Ericson K, and Hindmarsh T. Computed tomography examination of the influence of autotraction on herniation of the lumbar disc. *Arch Orthop Trauma Surg* 1985b;104(5):289–293.

Grieve GP. Thoracic Traction. In *Modern Manual Therapy of the Vertebral Column*. London: Churchill Livingstone; 1986.

Gupta R and Ramarao S. Epidurography in reduction of lumbar disc prolapse by traction. *Arch Phys Med Rehab* 1978;59:322.

Hinterbuchner C. Traction. In *Manipulation, Traction and Massage*, 3rd ed. Baltimore, Md: Williams & Wilkins; 1985:172–200.

Hirschberg GG. Treating lumbar disc lesion by prolonged continuous reduction of intradiscal pressure. *Tex Med* 1974;70:35–41.

Hood LB and Chrisman D. Intermittent Pelvic Traction in the Treatment of the Ruptured Intervertebral Disc. *J Am Phys Ther Assoc* 1967;48:21.

Jette DU, Falkel JE, and Trombly C. Effect of intermittent, supine cervical traction on the myoelectric activity of the upper trapezius muscle in subjects with neck pain. *Phys Ther* 1985; 65(8):1173–1176.

Judovich BD. Herniated cervical disc—A new form of traction therapy. *Am J Surg* 1952;84:646.

Judovich BD. Lumbar traction therapy and dissipated force factors. *Lancet* 1954;74:411.

Judovich BD and Nobel GR. Traction therapy, a study of resistance forces. *A J Surg* 1957;93:108.

Kapandji I. *The Physiology of the Joints*, vol. 3, 3rd ed. London: Churchill Livingstone; 1974.

Kekosz VN, Hibert L, and Tepperman PS. Cervical and Lumbopelvic Traction. *Postgrad Med* 1986;80(8):187–194.

Kessler RM. Acute symptomatic disc prolapse. *Phys Ther* 1979;59(8).

Kirkaldy-Willis WH. *Managing Low Back Pain*. London: Churchill Livingstone; 1983:193.

Kramer J. *Intervertebral Disc Diseases, Causes, Diagnosis, Treatment, and Prophylaxis*. Chicago: Year Book; 1981: vol. 89, pp. 164–168.

Lawson GA and Godfrey CM. A Report on Studies of Spinal Traction in the Treatment of Burns. *Ann Surg* 1968;168:981.

Lehmann JF and Brunner GD. A Device for the Application of Heavy Lumbar Traction: Its Mechanical Effects. *Arch Phys Med Rehab* 1958;39:696–700.

Li T-M. Vertical Suspension Traction with Manipulation in Lumbar Intervertebral Disc Protrusion. *Chin Med J* 1977;3(6):407–412.

Lind G. *Auto-traction Treatment of Low Back Pin and Sciatica*. Thesis, University of Linkoping; 1973.

Ljunggren AE, Weber H, and Larsen S. Autotraction versus manual traction in patients with prolapsed lumbar intervertebral discs. *Scand J Rehab Med* 1984;16(3):117–124.

Lossing W. Low back pain and the Cottrell 90/90 Backtrac System. *Orthotics Prosthetics* 1983;37(2).

Macnab I. *Backache*. Baltimore, Md: Williams & Wilkins; 1977:183.

Maitland GD. Techniques of mobilization. In *Vertebral Manipulation*, 4th ed. London: Butterworths; 1977.

Mathews J. Symposium on Lumbar Intervertebral Disc Lesions. *J Rheum Rehab* 1975;14:160.

Mathews JA and Yates DAH. Treatment of sciatica. *Lancet*, Mar 2, 1974.

McElhannon JE. Council on Chiropractic Physiological Therapeutics: Traction, a protocol. *ACA J*, Oct 1985, p. 82.

McFarland JW and Krusen FH. Use of the Sayre head sling in osteoarthritis of cervical portion of spinal column. *Arch Phys Ther* 1943;24:263.

McKenzie R. *The Lumbar Spine*. Waikanae, New Zealand: Spinal Publications; 1981.

Morris J, Lucas M, and Bresler M. Role of the trunk in stability of the spine. *J Bone Joint Surg [Am]* 1961;43:327.

Natchev E and Valentino V. Low back pain and disc hernia observation during auto-traction treatment. *Manual Med* 1984;1: 39–42.

Neugebauer J. Die Wiederaufrichtung Der Bandscheibe Durch Dekompression. *J Med Welt Bd* 1976;27:19.

Neuwirth E, Hilde, W, and Campbell R. Tables for vertebral elongation in the treatment of sciatica. *Arch Phys Med* 1952;33: 455–460.

Onel D, Tuzlaci M, Sari H, and Demir K. Computed tomographic investigation of the effect of traction on lumbar disc herniations. *Spine* 1989;14(1):82–90.

Pal B, Mangion P, Hossain MA, and Diffey BL. A controlled trial of continuous lumbar traction in the treatment of back pain and sciatica. *Br J Rheumatol* 1986;25:181.

Paré A. Apera. Paris 1582;15:440.

Parkin PJ, Wallis WE, and Wilson JL. Vertebral artery occlusion following manipulation of the neck. *NZ Med J* 1978;88:441–443.

Peltier LF. A brief history of traction. *J Bone Joint Surg [AM]* 1968;50(8):1603–1607.

Penning L and Wilmink JT. Posture-dependent bilateral compression of L4 on L5 nerve roots in facet hypertrophy: A dynamic CT–myelographic study. *Spine* 1987;12(5):488.

Pomosov DV. Treatment of slipped discs by a closed reduction method. *Voen Med Izh* July 1976, p. 7.

Quellette JP. Low back pain: An orthopedic medicine approach. *Can Fam Physician* March 1987;33:693–694.

Saunders HD. Use of spinal traction in the treatment of neck and back conditions. *Clin Orthop Relat Res* 1983;179:31–36.

Schlicke L et al. A quantitative study of vertebral displacement in the normal cervical spine under axial load. In press.

Schneider RC and Schemm GW. Vertebral artery insufficiency in acute and chronic spinal trauma. *J Neurosurg* 1961;18:348–360.

Schonstrom N, Lindahl S, Willen J, and Hansson T. Dynamic changes in the dimensions of the lumbar spinal canal: An experimental study in vitro. *J Orthop Res* 1989;7:115–121.

Sharubina JY. Effectiveness of using medical gymnastics together with traction in a swimming pool in the overall treatment of discogenic radiculitis. *Vopr Kurortol Fizioter Lech Fiz Dult* Nov/Dec 1973;38.

Stephens MM and O'Brien JP. The morphological changes in the lumbar intervertebral foramina in normal and abnormal motion segments after distraction. *Ann R Coll Surg Engl* 1986;68(4):229.

Stoddard A. Traction of cervical nerve root irritation. *Physiotherapy* 1954;40:48–49.

Stoddard A. *Manual of Osteopathic Technic*. London: Medical Publications; 1961:236–243.

Stopford JSB. The arteries of the pons and medulla oblongata. *J Anat Lond* 1916;50:131–164.

Tien-You F. Lumbar intervertebral disc protrusion, new method of management and its theoretical basis. *Chin Med J* 1976;2(3):183–194.

Tissington Tatlow WF and Bammer HG. Syndrome of vertebral artery compression. *Neurology, Minneapolis* 1957;7:331–340.

Tkachenko SS. Closed one stage reduction of acute prolapse of the intervertebral disc. *Orthop Travmatol Protez*, Aug 1973;34

Toole JF and Tucker SH. Influence of head position upon cerebral circulation. *Arch Neurol* 1960;2:616–623.

Twomey LT. Sustained lumbar traction. An experimental study of long spine segments. *Spine* 1987;10(2):146–149.

Vanharanta H, Ohnmeiss D, and Stith W, et al. Effect of repeated trunk extension and flexion movements as seen by CT/discography. North American Spine Society Third Annual Meeting held at Colorado Springs, Colorado, July 24–27, 1988. *J Bone Joint Surg*, Spring 1989, p. 26.

Walker GL. Goodley polyaxial cervical traction—A new approach to a traditional treatment. *Phys Ther* 1986;66(8):1255–1259.

Zusman M. Prolonged relief from articular soft tissue pain with passive joint movement. *J Manual Med* 1988;3:100–102.

Zusman M, Edwards BC, and Donaghy A. Investigation of a proposed mechanism for the relief of spinal pain with passive joint movement. *J Manual Med* 1989;4:58–61.

Zylbergold RS and Piper MC. Cervical spine disorders. A comparison of three types of traction. *Spine* 1985;10(10):867–871.

Soft Tissue and Nonforce Techniques

William C. Meeker

- **RATIONALE FOR SOFT TISSUE TECHNIQUES**
- **DESCRIPTIVE CHARACTERISTICS OF SOFT TISSUE TECHNIQUES**
- **DIAGNOSIS IN SOFT TISSUE AND NONFORCE TECHNIQUES**
  Palpation
  Posture
  Muscle Testing
  Range-of-Motion Testing
- **SOFT TISSUE TECHNIQUES**
  Myofascial Pain (Trigger-Point) Syndrome
  Massage
  Chapman's Reflexes
  Neurovascular Reflexes
  Acupuncture
  Craniosacral Therapy
  Logan Basic Technique
  Active Muscular Relaxation Techniques
  Sacro-occipital Technique
  Applied Kinesiology
- **RELATIONSHIP BETWEEN TENDER SITES AND REFLEX POINTS**
- **NONFORCE TECHNIQUES**
  Atlas-Specific Adjustive Techniques
  Activator Technique
- **MECHANISMS OF SOFT TISSUE TECHNIQUES**
  Mechanical Effects
  Neurophysiological Effects
  Psychological Effects
- **ACKNOWLEDGMENTS**
- **REFERENCES**

Chiropractic soft tissue techniques are those physical methods applied to muscles, ligaments, tendons, fascia, and other connective tissues with the goal of therapeutically affecting the body. Nonforce techniques may be defined as very light force methods sometimes applied to the soft tissues but most often to the bony parts of the spine and pelvis with the goal of improving the health of the patient.

Although soft tissues can be broadly defined as all nonbony parts of the human body, this chapter limits its discussion to those techniques most used by chiropractors, especially those that affect spinal functions.

Conceptually, chiropractic soft tissue and nonforce techniques should not be seen as simply a set of manual maneuvers to be applied in a "cookbook" fashion to every patient who walks through the door. A technique also includes the process of obtaining accurate clinical observations before drawing any diagnostic conclusions. The actual manual maneuver is only part of a chiropractic technique.

Rationale for Soft Tissue Techniques

In the course of touching their patients, chiropractors, like other manual therapists, often observed that certain anatomic sites in the soft tissues seemed more tender than others. The pain and tenderness generated by pressing in a certain place appeared to be the cause of, or have a relationship to the patient's chief complaint. After these areas were pressed, massaged, adjusted, or otherwise stimulated, the patient often remarked on an improvement in the condition. This has been the genesis of most soft tissue techniques. Explanations about the physiological mechanisms have usually arisen after the clinical observations were made.

Acknowledgments

The assistance of Arden Lawson, D.C., for background research, and Tom Milus, D.C., and Wendy Toomey, M.A., for the illustrations is greatfully acknowledged.

Many chiropractors believe that patients sometimes recover more quickly and fully if various therapeutic methods are used in addition to traditional spinal adjustments. Although not a chiropractor, Korr (1976) articulates ideas that profoundly mirror chiropractic's traditional emphasis on the nervous system:

> The spinal cord is the keyboard on which the brain plays when it calls for activity or change in activity. But each "key" in the console sounds, not an individual "tone" such as the contraction or a particular group of muscle fibers, but a whole "melody" of activity, even a "symphony" of motion. In other words, built into the cord is a large repertoire of patterns of activity, each involving the complex, harmonious, delicately balanced orchestration of the contractions and relaxations of many muscles. The brain "thinks" in terms of whole motions, not individual muscles. It calls selectively, for the preprogrammed patterns in the cord and brain stem, modifying them in countless ways and combining them in an infinite variety of still more complex patterns. Each activity is also subject to further modulation, refinement, and adjustment by the afferent feedback continually streaming in from the participating muscles, tendons and joints.

Grieve (1981) puts the same idea in a more prosaic form:

> Much abnormality presenting, apparently simply as joint pain, may be the expression of a comprehensive underlying imbalance of the whole musculoskeletal system, i.e., articulation, ligaments, muscles, fascial planes and intermuscular septa, tendons and aponeuroses, together with defective neuromuscular control and co-ordination in the form of abnormal patterns of afferent and efferent neuron traffic.

Janda (1986, 1988) and Lewit (1985) have popularized their concepts of "functional pathology of the motor system." From their point of view, joint dysfunctions occur as consequences of faulty motion patterns that may have their etiology in any tissue. The neuromuscular system acts as a magnifier and, through aberrant compensatory reflex physiology, may allow joint dysfunctions to persist. The initial injury may have been to a joint or other structure, or the damage may be related to poor posture or other unhealthy habits (e.g., smoking is related to back pain). Logically then, they incorporate soft tissue as well as joint manipulations into treatment plans.

The rationale underlying most soft tissue techniques is holistic and is explained by the complex and intricate nature of the physiological interrelationships between all body systems.

Descriptive Characteristics of Soft Tissue Techniques

Many characteristics must be considered in the delivery of soft tissue and nonforce techniques to a human being (Table 29–1). As in any manual skill, proper knowledge, practice, and clinical experience are necessary before all characteristics can be smoothly integrated. The final result is truly a skillful art in which chiropractors take justified pride.

The patient's position may be prone, supine, sitting, standing, or other, depending on the problem and the physical technique to be applied. The position and posture of the doctor likewise must be tailored to the specific situation at hand. Size, strength, training, and skill level of the doctor require additional variations in position and posture relative to the patient. The age of the patient, general level of health, and the severity of the complaint must be considered. The patient may be passive throughout the procedure or actively involved, for example, in contracting certain muscles. Thus, two doctors might handle the same patient in very different ways.

In manipulation of soft tissues a variety of manual contacts can be used, for example, fingertips, thumbs, "pisiform" contacts, elbows, and knuckles. Authorities on different techniques of manipulation recommend different contact points depending on their experience and preference.

The way in which a force is applied to the soft tissues also varies widely (Table 29–2). This is related to the patient and doctor characteristics mentioned earlier and the physiologic models on which the technique is based. Characteristics include the direction, amplitude, frequency, velocity, acceleration, and duration of applied force. Pressure may be cyclic or sustained. Some approaches, for example, require single, high-velocity, low-amplitude thrusts similar to joint

TABLE 29–1. DESCRIPTIVE CHARACTERISTICS OF SOFT TISSUE TECHNIQUES

Patient's position and posture
Doctor's position and posture
Size of doctor versus patient
Doctor's strength and coordination
Patient's strength and coordination
Doctor's skill level and experience
Patient active or patient passive
Severity of patient's complaint
Patient's general health
Patient's age

TABLE 29-2. COMPONENTS OF SOFT TISSUE AND NONFORCE MANEUVERS

Anatomic sites of application
Direction of force
Amplitude of force
Frequency of force
Velocity of force
Duration of force

TABLE 29-3. ABNORMAL PALPATORY FINDINGS

Tenderness
Indurations
Edema
Skin texture changes
Skin temperature changes
Muscle hypertonicity
Joint hypermobility or hypomobility

adjustments. Most however indicate low-velocity application of forces or a steady application of pressure over a period of several seconds to minutes.

Forces may be applied at right angles to the long axis of a muscle to cause a lateral stretch, in the direction of the long axis to cause a longitudinal stretch, or in both long-axis directions to cause a separation of the origin and insertion of the muscle. Deep (heavy) point pressure may be applied near connective tissue attachments or to the muscle belly if indicated.

Frequency of sessions with the doctor over the course of care varies considerably in practice as does the actual length of each session. Professionwide agreement on standards of practice for various soft tissue and nonforce approaches is virtually nonexistent at this time.

Diagnosis in Soft Tissue and Nonforce Techniques

The clinical indication for using soft tissue and nonforce techniques is the diagnosis of lesions or dysfunctions that are treatable by these methods. Soft tissue lesion diagnosis is, or course, highly related to the physiological model on which the technique is based. For example, trigger-point techniques are based on a pathological model of muscle dysfunction (myofascitis), acupuncture is performed on active acupuncture points and meridians, and adjustment of an atlas vertebra with a nonforce technique is based on spinal misalignment factors measured on cervical radiographs.

The type of diagnosis also varies considerably with the presumed specificity of the technique favored by the practitioner. For example, general massage may be prescribed in the absence of a specific diagnosis for its general relaxing and soothing effects. On the other hand, various reflex and trigger-point techniques generally require precise localization of the tender site contributing to the clinical picture, as well as consideration of any modifiable risk factors, such as poor posture, lack of exercise, repetitive work tasks, and poor nutrition.

Palpation

Palpation of the soft tissues remains the primary diagnostic procedure today as it has for centuries. It is usually done with the fingertips, the pads of the fingers, the palm, and the ventral surface of the hands. Palpation yields a great deal of clinical information. Abnormal findings may include skin texture changes, indurations, temperature changes, tenderness to pressure, edema, muscle spasm, and hypomobility of joints (Table 29–3). The skin of the patient may also be pinched or rolled to assess mobility and uncover tender areas (Figure 29–1). A great deal of experience and training are required before this firm yet sensitive sense of touch is developed. One experimental study using a mechanical palpation simulator found significant differences between experienced and inexperienced therapists (Evans, 1986).

Skillful palpation is an efficient clinical tool because lesions found with the hands can be treated in most techniques by the same or a similar palpatory maneuver at the same time. The diagnostic and therapeutic components overlap to a great degree. The feedback immediately available after a manual treatment gives the doctor and patient a clear indication of success (or lack of it) in a close and supportive relationship.

The reliability of palpation is currently under rigorous scrutiny by the research communities of the several professions that use palpatory diagnosis heavily (Evans, 1986; Keating, 1989; Johnston, 1982). Most of the studies concentrating on palpation of joint dysfunctions have found statistically significant but clinically low levels of agreement. Whether these findings can be extrapolated to palpation of soft tissues is relatively unknown. Some investigators using algometers to quantify tenderness in the soft tissues have reported good reliability (Reeves et al., 1986).

Posture

Postural assessment has long been associated with chiropractic (Jenness, 1975). It provides another means of assessing the soft tissues if one assumes that asymmetrical muscle function or fascial contractures cause postural abnormalities. Various instruments exist that help to quantify posture but very few have been subjected to rigorous testing (Vernon, 1983).

Also under the rubric of posture is the attention given to assessments of leg length. Unequal lower-extremity length is probably associated with back

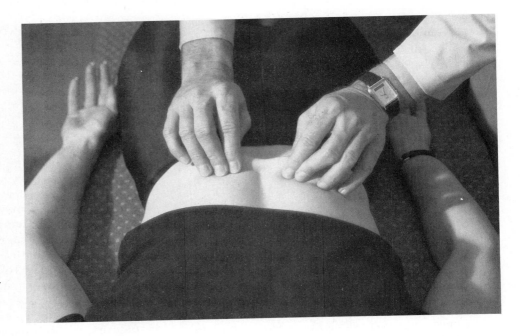

Figure 29–1. Rolling the skin between the thumb and fingers can uncover areas of increased tenderness and variations in subdermal tissues said to be indicative of a soft tissue lesion.

pain (Giles, 1981) and is often said to be related to functional distortions of the pelvic or spinal musculature. Short leg determinations used in several techniques provide many chiropractors with the clinical information they need to make treatment decisions (Triano, 1980).

Muscle Testing

Assessment of muscle function for strength and quality of contraction is a standard test of the motor system. Manual muscle testing is popular and, indeed, forms the basis of several techniques used by chiropractors (Fig. 29–2). Abnormal patterns of weak and strong muscles may lead to undue wear and tear and predispose to injury. Weak muscles are often associated with myofascial trigger points and other painful complaints (Mayer and Gatchel, 1988). A technological explosion in the past few years has given clinicians many sophisticated muscle testing instruments, yet their clinical utility is still controversial.

Range-of-Motion Testing

Assessing the range of limb and trunk motion is still considered to be one of the most objective ways to judge disability of the motor system and is a standard part of the chiropractor's diagnostic procedures. Voluminous research in this area has not necessarily led to a

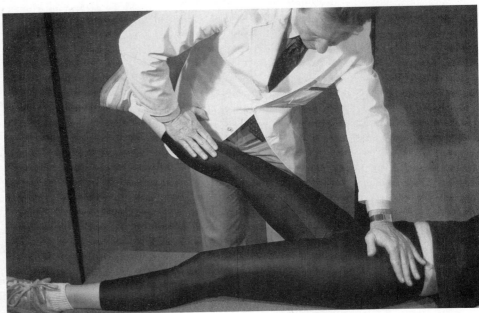

Figure 29–2. The strength of the hip flexors, primarily the psoas muscle in this case, can be assessed manually by stabilizing the pelvis with one hand and applying pressure with the other while the patient attempts to flex and adduct the leg.

full understanding of the relationship between hypomobility and painful syndromes, nor to an understanding of the chiropractic subluxation complex. Nevertheless, range-of-motion testing seems to be an indispensable part of the clinical exam (Fig. 29–3). Spinal manipulation has been demonstrated to cause an increase in motion in the cervical spine (Jirout, 1972; Hviid, 1971; Nansel et al., 1989) and to affect certain kinematic findings in the lumbar spine. Soft tissue manipulative techniques are said to result in increased motion because of relaxation of hypertonic muscles (Travell and Simons, 1983; Lewit, 1985; Janda, 1978).

Soft Tissue Techniques

Myofascial Pain (Trigger-Point) Syndrome

One of the best documented and accepted models of soft tissue dysfunction and treatment is referred to as the "myofascial pain syndrome." The genesis of this model in the scientific literature is often traced to the work of Dr. Janet Travell in the late 1940s (Travell and Rinzler, 1952), but it is probable that the same painful abnormalities of soft tissues have been noted by chiropractors before formal recognition in the scientific literature. Chiropractors have long been taught to palpate for "taut and tender" fibers. Traditional so-called "nerve tracing" is probably based on the same clinical findings. Vannerson and Nimmo (1973) have published and taught seminars for many

years describing their "receptor tonus" technique, which relies on palpation and treatment of tender points in muscles by digital compression.

The myofascial syndrome has as its primary diagnostic component the existence of tender, palpable "nodules" within the soft tissues that when pressed on or otherwise stimulated cause a marked pain response by the patient. Often the pain can be referred to a different site. These "trigger points" appear to be the cause of the patient's condition because when they are treated by a variety of physical methods, the patient seems to improve.

Over the years, patterns of trigger-point findings have emerged that appear somewhat consistent from complaint to complaint and patient to patient. Travell and Simons (1983) have produced impressive illustrations of locations of trigger points and their referred pain patterns. They also distinguish single-muscle syndromes from a more systemic condition known as fibrositis/fibromyalgia (Simons and Travell, 1989).

In general, treatment of trigger points consists mostly of direct stimulation by some physical means, stretching of the involved muscle, and rehabilitation of the function of the anatomic area by exercise and other environmental interventions (e.g., an improved desk chair). Occasionally, nutritional and endocrine disorders are simultaneously addressed. Medical physicians often use needling techniques.

The most common treatment in chiropractic practice is direct digital "ischemic compression" of the tender nodules. Thumbs, elbows, fingers, and

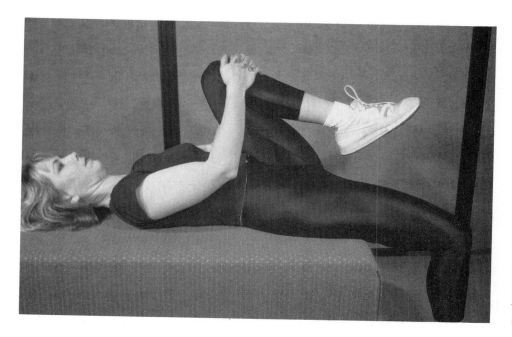

Figure 29–3. Tight hip flexors may be assessed by having the patient hold one flexed hip and knee while allowing the other leg to extend to its natural length. Inability of the extended leg to touch the table or to go into slight extension is said to indicate tightness. This subject demonstrates a normal range of hip extension.

even wooden dowel rods are used. The pressure is held steadily to the patient's tolerance directly on the trigger point for a period that varies from 7 seconds to several minutes (Fig. 29–4). Another method, popularized by Travell and Simons (1983), is called "spray and stretch." The skin overlying the affected muscle is sprayed with ethyl chloride or water to induce rapid cooling and neurological distraction. Immediately thereafter, the muscle is gently passively stretched to the patient's tolerance. Artificial warming by hot pack or other physical therapy modality is often recommended. After treatment, specific exercises designed to stretch the tight muscles and strengthen the weak muscles are prescribed.

Despite almost unanimous agreement among practitioners who use their hands to treat patients, the myofascial model of soft tissue dysfunction is still a matter of some controversy. There is no con-

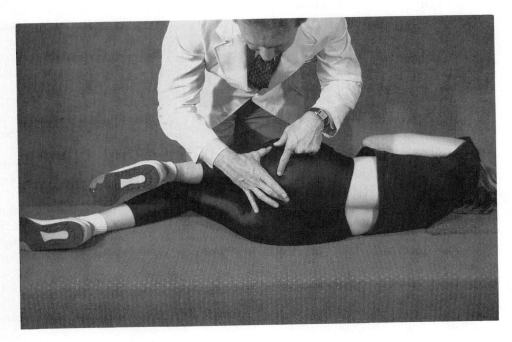

A

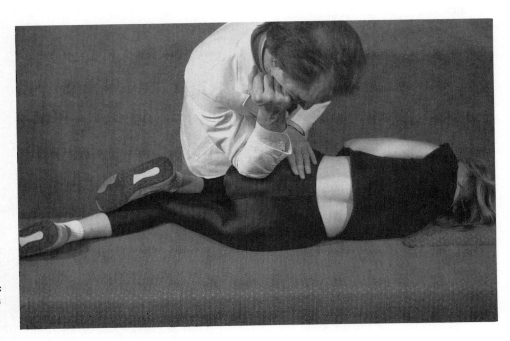

Figure 29–4. Trigger points located in the piriformis muscle (**A**) may be treated by ischemic compression with the doctor's elbow, with the patient in a side-lying position (**B**).

B

sensus about the physiologic nature of the tender, palpable nodules that are so clinically apparent to the chiropractor and patient (Awad, 1973; Travell and Simons, 1983).

Massage

Soft tissue manipulation by traditional forms of massage is a time-honored type of manual care often associated with chiropractors. There are various techniques of massage, many of them named after their originators. As with chiropractic adjustive techniques, origins are sometimes obscure, but it is clear that massage has been a part of manual therapy from time before recorded history. A fascinating account is presented by Kamenetz (1985). Books by Tappan (1980) and Wood and Becker (1981) and a classic work on ''connective tissue massage'' by Ebner (1962) are very useful sources of information.

Massage is usually applied for its general relaxing and inhibitory effects on large muscular portions of the body. It is generally thought massage strokes help to ''flush'' blood and lymph from a muscle, thus increasing exchange of nutrients (Wakim, 1985). Massage may be prescribed alone or in conjunction with other manual care, for example, as with strokes applied to the shoulder and upper thoracic region to loosen and relax it prior to a more specific chiropractic adjustment.

Four basic massage strokes are usually described (Hofkosh, 1985). Effleurage refers to application of long, gentle, slow strokes to the skin without attempting to move deep muscle masses. They are usually applied longitudinally to muscle fibers in a headward direction. Deep effleurage may passively stretch the soft tissues. Petrissage is a slightly more vigorous set of strokes attempting to lift, separate, and squeeze the tissues below the hand. Friction massage, popularized by Cyriax (1978), is the use of the fingertips or the heel of the hand to press on and move tissues under the skin. Small circular or transverse movements are used around joint surfaces, at musculotendinous junctions, and where tendons and ligaments insert into bone. Friction massage is designed to soften fibrosed tissue and break adhesions that may be limiting motion and causing pain. Tapotement is rarely used. It may be described as the application of a series of light to heavy blows to the soft tissue in a rapid fashion. It has a stimulating effect. Vibration delivered with the hands, or more effectively with a machine, may also be considered a form of tapotement.

Chapman's Reflexes

Chapman's reflexes have been incorporated into several chiropractic techniques, notably applied kinesiology and sacro-occipital technique. Discovered by Frank Chapman (Chaitow, 1987), they are described as very tender points located on the anterior and posterior of the body usually in the midline between the intercostal spaces and just lateral to the spinous processes of vertebrae. Diagnosis and treatment are by palpation and rotatory digital pressure. The tender points hypothetically reflect sluggish or blocked lymphatic flow, which can be removed by treatment of the reflex points. The nature of the relationship between the reflex point and lymph is obscure.

Neurovascular Reflexes

Terence Bennett (Martin, 1977) described points on the cranium and body that he felt reflected the vascular condition of organs and other structures. Some chiropractors believe that light manual stimulation of these ''neurovascular reflexes'' can strengthen specific muscles. As with Chapman's reflexes, that nature of the relationship between the tender neurovascular point and the cardiovascular system is still to be elucidated.

Acupuncture

Volumes have been written from both Eastern and Western perspectives on the clinical use of acupuncture concepts. Many chiropractors practice acupressure or electroacupuncture in which traditional acupuncture points are treated to alleviate the patient's complaints. The points are organized along meridians that, in traditional Chinese medicine carry *chi*, the life force that innervates the body. Theoretically, blockage or other dysfunction in the meridian network causes a departure from health. The applied kinesiology technique has been noted for incorporating acupuncture into its clinical procedures (Walther, 1988). The text by Mann (1987) is highly regarded in the West.

Craniosacral Therapy

Several chiropractic techniques incorporate craniosacral concepts. The most noted are the sacro-occipital technique (DeJarnette, 1984) and applied kinesiology (Walther, 1988). The origins of craniosacral therapy are in some dispute (Cottam, 1981). Embraced by some chiropractors and many traditionally oriented osteopaths, the technique is based on the existence of an inherent rhythmic pulsation that reflects the circulation of cerebrospinal fluid from the brain to the sacral spinal column. In this model, immobility or asymmetric mobility of the cranial bones and the sacrum in response to the circulatory pulsations is a treatable dysfunction. Treatment consists of palpating, holding, and applying specific forces to bones, joints, and soft tissues of the cranium and the pelvis, especially the sacrum. Upledger and

Vredevoogd (1983) have described these concepts in great detail.

Logan Basic Technique

The Logan system, originated by Hugh Logan (1956), was one of the first biomechanical models of the spine and pelvis. The Logan basic technique is not exclusively a soft tissue technique. Nevertheless, it shares many characteristics. The most important maneuver, known as the basic adjustment, is made with the thumb pressed lightly close to the sacrotuberous ligament in an attempt to influence the position of the sacrum. The pressure may be maintained for as long as 15 minutes. Other maneuvers are also applied along with more traditional spinal adjustments.

Active Muscular Relaxation Techniques

Active muscular relaxation techniques have been developed by many individuals and have many names. Some of the more famous include proprioceptive neuromuscular facilitation (PNF), muscle energy procedures, and post-isometric relaxation. In these techniques, the patient is required to contract muscles isometrically or isokinetically against the holding force of the doctor's hands (Liebenson, 1989; Goodridge, 1981). The primary goal is to induce muscular relaxation. Very specific positioning is necessary to put the involved hypertonic or shortened muscle at the correct angle of stretch (Fig. 29–5). The methods are popular for myofascial syndrome and have been discussed in the osteopathic (Greenman, 1989), physical therapy (Grieve, 1988), and chiro-

practic (Liebenson, 1989) professions. Lewit and Simons (1984), in a clinical trial, demonstrated apparent clinical benefits. Some of the advantages of muscular relaxation techniques over generally more forceful joint manipulations are patient acceptance, and possibly, safety.

Sacro-occipital Technique

Sacro-occipital technique (SOT) was developed by Major B. DeJarnette. In this approach, which incorporates many treatment concepts from diverse sources, the pelvis and sacrum are very important. Through a variety of postural, muscular, and neurologic tests, patients are placed into one of three categories of pelvic dysfunction. The signature treatment method consists of the use of padded wedges placed strategically to reposition the pelvis as the patient lies prone or supine (Fig. 29–6). Traditional adjustments, reflex-point therapy, and cranial manipulations are also incorporated (DeJarnette, 1984).

Applied Kinesiology

Traced to George Goodheart, applied kinesiology is difficult to characterize briefly. Proponents have eclectically incorporated many concepts into the diagnostic and treatment methods (Walther, 1988). The common denominator, however, is reliance on manual muscle testing as the primary decision-making tool. In this model, muscle weakness is taken as a sign of many types of somatic and visceral dysfunctions. Some are said to be directly related to the spine and may be handled by traditional adjustments; others are related to visceral pathophysiology,

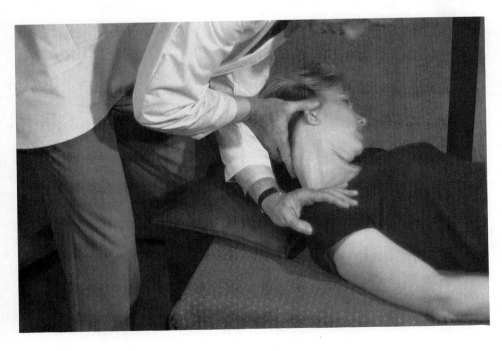

Figure 29–5. Pain and spasm in the levator scapulae may be treated by post-isometric relaxation technique. The patient laterally bends, flexes, and rotates the head away from the painful side as the doctor stabilizes the position. The patient is then instructed to gently push posteriorly against resistance for 7 to 10 seconds. The process may be repeated several times before full range of motion is obtained.

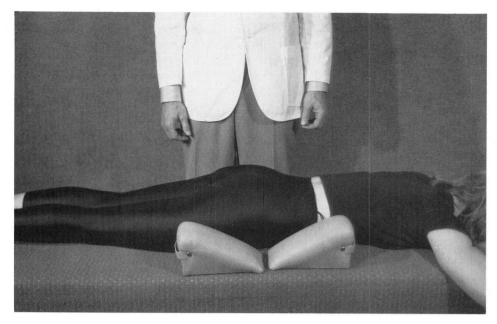

A

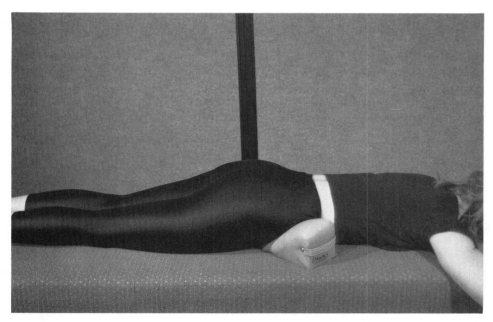

B

Figure 29-6. In the sacro-occipital technique, triangular-shaped wedges (**A**) placed under the pelvis (**B**) are said to reposition structures and normalize neuromusculoskeletal function.

nutritional deficiencies, craniosacral dysfunctions, and blocked meridian systems. Strengthening of a weak muscle is considered to indicate successful treatment.

Relationship Between Tender Sites and Reflex Points

One of the most fascinating controversies in the literature today is the nature and significance of clinically noted tender areas in the somatic tissues of the body.

Empirically, many clinicians have observed and mapped the distribution of tender points in their patients. Many different explanatory mechanisms have been proposed and yet it is logical that there are common threads.

For example, Melzack (1977) and MacDonald (1989) note the very high correlation between trigger-point patterns and maps of traditional acupuncture points. Liu et al. (1975) notes significant similarities between trigger points and muscle motor points. The reflexes of Bennett, which are theoretically related to vascular responses, and Chapman's reflexes, said to be related to lymph flow, also share many of the same clinical characteristics with trigger points and acupuncture points, namely, similar anatomic distribution and tenderness that responds to physical treatment of some sort.

Treatment of trigger points, acupuncture points, and other "reflex points" takes many forms including manual methods of manipulation, mechanically induced vibration, various physical therapy modalities, acupuncture with needles, and numerous types of electrical stimulation. In a review of 24 controlled studies (Reichmanis and Becker, 1977), 17 demonstrated significant analgesic effects with manual or electrical stimulation. Others (Melnick, 1954; Simons and Travell, 1989) report that pain and some symptoms in visceral disease also respond to the same methods.

According to Melzack (1989), the common denominator is explained by hyperstimulation of afferent nerve fibers. In this model, the sensation of pain is mediated by brainstem mechanisms that exert descending inhibitory control over neural transmission through the dorsal horns. This may explain why a variety of peripheral stimulation methods have similar symptom-reducing effects. There is some evidence that stimulation of precise points as required by traditional methods may not be necessary, at least for pain reduction (Gaw et al., 1975; Lewit, 1979). The effects of acupuncture may also be increasingly explainable by our developing knowledge of neuroendocrine functions (Han and Terenius, 1982).

Nevertheless, Simons and Travell (1989) and Chaitow (1987) do not accept the conclusion that acupuncture points, other reflex points, and trigger points represent the same physiologic phenomenon and can be treated by the same approach. Further research in the clinical realm and in elucidating the underlying physiology is needed.

Nonforce Techniques

A variety of chiropractic techniques may be conceptualized under the "nonforce" heading. In reality, these techniques do deliver forces to the body (primarily the spine and pelvis), but these forces tend to be very light.

Atlas-Specific Adjustive Techniques

Atlas-specific adjustive techniques include many upper cervical techniques. All are based on ideas popularized originally by B. J. Palmer (1934) with his hole-in-one (HIO) technique. In fact, Palmer probably borrowed the idea from Wernsing (Harrison Chiropractic Seminars Inc, 1981). Today, chiropractors

may choose several variations on the theme, e.g., Grostic, NUCCA, Blair, Mears, spinal biomechanics, spinal biophysics, and atlas orthogonality.

In this model, misalignments of the atlas vertebra in relation to the occiput and the axis vertebra are supremely important (Gregory, 1987). The rationale is based on the complex anatomy and physiology of the upper cervical area. It is presumed that a misaligned atlas can have serious deleterious effects on the neurophysiology of the spinal cord as it exits from the foramen magnum that can logically be expected to manifest in distal problems (Grostic, 1988). The *Upper Cervical Monograph*, published by the National Upper Cervical Association (NACCA), has printed interesting papers supporting these concepts.

In most approaches, carefully positioned radiographs of the upper cervical spine are obtained to visualize the structures in three planes. The radiographs are marked and measured to yield "misalignment factors," primarily of the atlas vertebra, which are then said to be reduced by a specific adjustment. In some cases, postadjustment radiographs are taken to ensure that a correct adjustment has been delivered. At least one uncontrolled study has indicated differences in alignment of the atlas vertebra after a course of adjustive care (Grostic and DeBoer, 1982).

The differences between the various upper cervical techniques are in the details of the radiographic marking procedures and in the types of adjustments recommended. The traditional adjustment is delivered by hand, usually with a pisiform contact on the skin overlying the transverse process of the atlas vertebra (Grostic, 1946; Gregory, 1971). The actual adjustment maneuver requires prolonged training and practice. Machines that deliver a force to the atlas via a small metal stylus are used in some approaches (Pettibon, 1968; Harrison, 1981; Sweat, 1983). The stylus is positioned to reverse the "misalignment factors" obtained from the radiographs.

Activator Technique

The activator technique is based on the work of Arlan Fuhr and his colleagues (Activator Methods, 1985). In this approach a small spring-loaded adjusting instrument (Fig. 29–7) is used to deliver a small measurable force (Smith et al., 1989). Subluxations of the axial skeleton are sought by their putative effects on "functional leg lengths." Through observation of leg lengths and notation of changes after a series of physical maneuvers by the doctor and patient, the locations of vertebral dysfunction are determined. Application of the activator instrument is then said to reduce or eliminate the subluxations. The forces in this technique are generally applied to the processes of the spinal vertebrae and bony prominences of the pelvis and it therefore should not be considered a soft tissue technique.

Mechanisms of Soft Tissue Techniques

Soft tissue techniques probably affect the body (1) by direct mechanical stimulation of tissues; (2) through neurologic consequences, which may be local, distal, or reflex in nature, and (3) through the psyche. These are discussed very briefly below. More detailed discussions may be found elsewhere in this book and the references.

Mechanical Effects

Application of forces to the soft tissues of the body results in local mechanical deformation. Hypothetically, several physiologic consequences are possible. These are not materially different from the effects of joint manipulation and may be conceptualized as occurring on some sort of physiologic continuum. Manipulations have been said to break adhesions, soften scar, increase local blood flow, "pump" areas of fluids and metabolites, stretch, compress, increase lymph flow, reduce edema, and increase range of motion.

Neurophysiological Effects

It is assumed, largely on the basis of decades of empirical clinical experience, that the local mechanical effects of soft tissue manipulations must have more profound physiologic effects on the body. Gillette (1987) describes the presence of numerous types of nerves and receptors in the soft tissues that are potentially able to react to an externally applied force. Stimulation of these peripheral mechanoreceptors, proprioceptors, and nociceptors probably modulates complex spinal reflex pathways (Wyke, 1985).

Many technique approaches rely on putative reflex patterns to make diagnostic and treatment decisions. The regular appearance of "trigger points" as mapped by Travell and Simons supports such concepts. Also, the presence of somato-somatic and somato-visceral reflexes has been demonstrated under experimental conditions (Koizumi, 1978; Beal, 1985). Nevertheless, regardless of the logic of the models that practitioners use to support their techniques, the neurophysiological effects of soft tissue manipulations still are largely experimentally unexplored.

Psychological Effects

Many detractors of the chiropractic profession say that going to a chiropractor is no better than receiving a placebo treatment. This is meant to be, and is often perceived as, a negative comment in explaining positive clinical benefits. Although it is undoubtedly true that there is a powerful component of chiropractic care that is mediated through rather unknown psychological mechanisms, that is hardly a condemnation of spinal adjustments or soft tissue techniques. Quite the contrary, the effect of simply touching patients as a way to gain trust, inspire confidence, and convey caring has always been an artful component of the healing process. In this age of technological and mechanical marvels with empha-

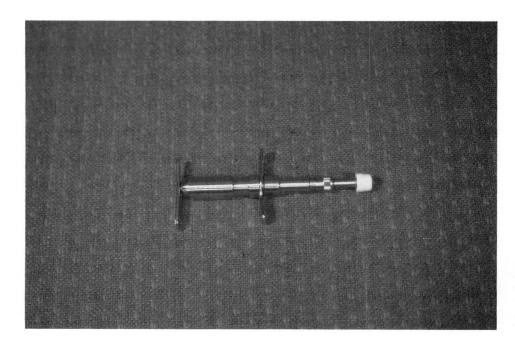

Figure 29–7. The spring-loaded, hand-held adjusting instrument (activator) used in the activator technique. The amount of force delivered via the stylus can be varied.

sis on cold logic and deduction, the injection of warmth and empathy demonstrated by skillful and confident touching is a welcome characteristic in a doctor. Chiropractors enjoy an enviable reputation in this area (Coulehan, 1985; Cherkin and MacCornack, 1989) that cannot be ignored.

References

Activator Methods Chiropractic Technique Siminar Workbook. Willmar, Minn: Activator Methods Inc.; 1985.

Awad EA. Interstitial myofibrositis: Hypothesis of the mechanism. *Arch Phys Med Rehab* 1973;54:449–453.

Beal MC. Viscerosomatic reflexes: A review. *J Am Osteopath Assoc* 1985;85(12):786–801.

Chaitow L. Soft-tissue manipulation. Wellingborough, Northamptonshire, England: Thorsons Publishing Group; 1987.

Cherkin DC and MacCornack FA. Patient evaluations of low back pain care from family physicians and chiropractors. *West J Med* 1989;150(3):351–355.

Cottam C. The roots of cranial manipulation: Nephi Cottam and ''craniopathy.'' *Chiropractic Hist* 1981;1:31–35.

Coulehan JL. Chiropractic and the clinical art. *Soc Sci Med* 1985;21(4):383–390.

Cyriax J. *Textbook of Orthopaedic Medicine*, 7th ed. London: Bailliere Tindall; 1978.

DeJarnette MB. *Sacro Occipital Technic.* Nebraska City, Neb: privately published; 1984.

Ebner M. *Connective Tissue Massage, Theory and Therapeutic Application.* Baltimore, Md: Williams and Wilkins; 1962.

Evans DH. The reliability of assessment parameters; Accuracy and palpation technique. In Grieve GP, ed. *Modern Manual Therapy of the Vertebral Column.* Edinburgh: Churchill-Livingstone; 1986.

Gaw AC, Chang LW, and Shaw LC. Efficacy of acupuncture on osteoarthritic pain. *N Engl J Med* 1975;293:345–378.

Giles LGF and Taylor JR. Low back pain associated with leg length inequality. *Spine* 1981;6(5):510–517.

Gillette RG. A speculative argument for the coactivation of diverse somatic receptor populations by forceful chiropractic adjustments: A review of the neurophysiological literature. *Manual Med* 1987;3:1–14.

Goodridge JP. Muscle energy technique: Definition, explanation, methods of procedure. *J Am Osteopath Assoc* 1981;81:249–259.

Greenman PE. *Principles of Manual Medicine.* Baltimore, Md: Williams & Wilkins; 1989.

Gregory R. *Manual of Upper Cervical Analysis.* Monroe, Mich: National Upper Cervical Chiropractic Association; 1971.

Gregory RR. The C1 subluxation syndrome. *Upper Cervical Monogr* 1987;4(3):6–11.

Grieve GP. *Common Vertebral Joint Problems.* London: Churchill Livingstone; 1981.

Grieve GP. *Common Vertebral Joint Problems.* 2nd ed. London: Churchill Livingstone; 1988.

Grostic JF. *Grostic Procedure Seminar Notes.* Ann Arbor, Michigan; 1946.

Grostic JD. Dentate ligament-cord distortion hypothesis. *Chiropractic Res J* 1988;1(1):47–55.

Grostic JD and DeBoer K. Roentgenographic measurement of atlas laterality and rotation: A retrospective pre- and post-manipulation study. *J Manipulative Physiol Ther* 1982;5:63–71.

Han JS and Terenius L. Neurochemical basis of acupuncture analgesia. *Annu Rev Pharmacol Toxicol* 1982;22:193–220.

Harrison Chiropractic Seminars Inc. *Chiropractic Biophysics, Phase I.* Privately published; 1981.

Hofkosh JM. Classical massage. In Basmajian TC, ed. *Manipula-*

tion, Traction and Massage, 3rd ed. Baltimore, Md: Williams & Wilkins; 1985.

Hviid H. The influence of chiropractic treatment on the rotatory mobility of the cervical spine—a kinesiometric and statistical study. *Ann Swiss Chiropractors Assoc* 1971;5:31–39.

Janda V. Muscles, central nervous system regulation, and back problems. In Korr IM, ed. *The Neurobiologic Mechanisms in Manipulative Therapy.* New York: Plenum Press; 1978.

Janda V. Muscle weakness and inhibition (pseudoparesis) in back pain syndromes. In Grieve GP, ed. *Modern Manual Therapy of the Vertebral Column,* Edinburgh: Churchill Livingstone; 1986.

Janda V. Muscles and cervicogenic pain syndromes. In Grant R, ed. *Physical Therapy of the Cervical and Thoracic Spine.* New York: Churchill-Livingstone; 1988.

Jenness M. The role of thermography and postural measurement in structural diagnosis. In Goldstein M, ed. *The Research Status of Spinal Manipulative Therapy.* NINCDS Monograph 15. Washington DC: US Department of Health Education and Welfare; 1975.

Jirout J. The effect of mobilization of the segmental blockade on the sagittal component of the reaction on lateral flexion of the cervical spine. *Neuroradiology* 1972;3:210–214.

Johnston WL, Elkiss ML, Marino RJ, and Blum GA. Passive gross motion testing, Part II: A study of interexaminer agreement. *J Am Osteopath Assoc* 1982;81:304–308.

Kamenetz HL. History of massage. In Basmajian JV, ed. *Manipulation, Traction, and Massage*, 3rd ed. Baltimore, Md: Williams & Wilkins; 1985.

Keating JC. Inter-examiner reliability of motion palpation of the lumbar spine: A review of quantitative literature. *Am J Chiropractic Med* 1989;2(3):107–110.

Koizumi K. Autonomic system reactions caused by excitation of somatic afferents: Study of cutaneo-intestinal reflex. In Korr I, ed. *The Neurobiologic Mechanisms in Manipulative Therapy.* New York: Plenum Press; 1978.

Korr I. The spinal cord as organizer of disease processes: Some preliminary perspectives. *J Am Osteopath Assoc* 1976;76:35–45.

Lewit K. The needle effect in the relief of myfascial pain. *Pain* 1979;6:83–90.

Lewit K. *Manipulative Therapy in Rehabilitation of the Motor System.* London: Butterworths; 1985.

Lewit K and Simons DG. Myofascial pain: Relief by postisometric relaxation. *Arch Phys Med Rehab* 1984;65:452–456.

Liebenson C. Active muscular activation techniques. Part II. Clinical application. *J Manip Physiol Ther* 1990;13:2–6.

Liu YK, Varela M, and Oswald R. The correspondence between some motor points and acupuncture loci. *Am J Clin Med* 1975;3:347–358.

Logan VF. *Logan Basic Methods.* St Louis Mo: Logan College of Chiropractic; 1956.

Macdonald AJR. Acupuncture analgesia and therapy. In Wall PD and Melzack P, eds. *Textbook of Pain,* 2nd ed. Edinburgh: Churchill Livingstone; 1989.

Mann F. *Textbook of Acupuncture.* London:: Heinemann Medical; 1987.

Martin R. *Dynamics of Correction of Abnormal Function.* Sierre Madre, Calif: privately published; 1977.

Mayer TG and Gatchel RJ. *Functional Restoration for Spinal Disorders: The Sports Medicine Approach.* Philadelphia: Lea & Febiger; 1988.

Melnick J. Treatment of trigger mechanisms in gastrointestinal disease. *New York State J Med* 1954;54:1324–1330.

Melzack R. Folk medicine and the sensory modulation of pain. In Wall PD and Melzack R, eds. *Textbook of Pain,* 2nd ed. Edinburgh: Churchill Livingstone; 1989.

Melzack R, Stillwell DM, and Fox EJ. Trigger points and acupuncture points of pain: Correlations and implications. *Pain* 1977;3:3–23.

Nansel D, Cremata E, Carlson J, and Szlazak M. Effect of unilateral spinal adjustments on goniometrically-assessed cervical lateral-flexion end-range asymmetries in otherwise asymptomatic subjects. *J Manipulative Physiol Ther* 1989;12(6):419–427.

Palmer BJ. *The Subluxation Specific—The Adjustment Specific.* Davenport, Iowa: Palmer School of Chiropractic; 1934.

Pettibon B. *Pettibon Method of Cervical X-Ray Analysis and Instrument Adjusting.* Tacoma, Wash: privately published; 1968.

Reeves JL, Jaeger B, and Graff-Redford SB. Reliability of the pressure algometer as a measure of myfascial trigger point sensitivity. *Pain* 1986;24:313–321.

Reichmanis M and Becker RO. Relief of experimentally induced pain by stimulation at acupuncture loci. *Comp Med East West* 1977;5:281–288.

Simons DG and Travell JG. Myofascial pain syndromes. In Wall PD and Melzack R, eds. *Textbook of Pain,* 2nd ed. Edinburgh: Churchill Livingstone; 1989.

Smith DB, Fuhr AW, and Davis BP. Skin accelerometer displacement and relative bone movement of adjacent vertebrae in response to chiropractic percussion thrusts. *J Manipulative Physiol Ther* 1989;12(1):26–37.

Sweat RW. Atlas orthogonality. *Today's Chiropractic* 1983;12(2):10–14.

Tappan FN. *Healing Massage Techniques.* Reston, Va: Reston Publishing; 1980.

Travell J and Rinzler SH. The myofascial genesis of pain. *Postgrad Med* 1952;11:425–434.

Travell JG and Simons DG. *Myofascial Pain and Dysfunction, the Trigger Point Manual.* Baltimore, Md: Williams & Wilkins; 1983.

Triano JJ. The use of instrumentation and laboratory examination procedures by the chiropractor. In Haldeman S, ed. *Modern Developments in the Principles and Practice of Chiropractic.* New York: Appleton-Century-Crofts; 1980.

Upledger JE and Vredevoogd JD. *Craniosacral Therapy.* Chicago: Eastland Press; 1983.

Vannerson JF and Nimmo RL. Specificity and the law of facilitation in the nervous system. *Am Chiropractic Assoc Chiropractic* 1973;10(VII):s78.

Vernon H. An assessment of the intra- and inter-reliability of the posturometer. *J Manipulative Physiol Ther* 1983;6(2):57–60.

Wakim KG. Physiologic effects of massage. In Basmajian JV, ed. *Manipulation, Traction and Massage,* 3rd ed. Baltimore, Md: Williams & Wilkins; 1985.

Walther DS. *Applied Kinesiology Synopsis.* Pueblo, Colo: Systems DC; 1988.

Wood EC and Becker PD. *Beards's Massage,* 3rd. ed. Philadelphia: WB Saunders; 1981.

Wyke B. Articular neurology and manipulative therapy. In Glasgow E, Twomey L, Scull E, et al., eds. *Aspects of Manipulative Therapy.* Edinburgh: Churchill Livingstone; 1985.

chapter 30

Spinal Rehabilitation

Tom Mayer
Peter Polatin

Rehabilitation of the low-back-pain patient must be distinguished from acute conservative care. As used in this classification, acute care relates to treatment of an acute "episode" of low back pain or the immediate sequelae of invasive treatment or other posttraumatic injury. A reasonable time interval for a course of conservative care should not be longer than 6 months, and often considerably less. After surgical treatment and a period of tissue healing, some variation may be expected depending on the type of surgical procedure performed. Based on the level of soft tissue disruption, number of levels treated, and type of fusion attempted, the implementation of post-surgical rehabilitation may last anywhere from 2 weeks to 6 months. Conservative care can be considered to occur during the period of tissue healing. Rehabilitation care, by contrast, occurs *after tissue healing* and is terminated by *maximum medical recovery*. The period of rehabilitation treatment is thus more open-ended and requires greater judgment on the part of the clinician.

The period of rehabilitative care involves several concepts not generally considered as part of conservative care. The first of these is the concept of *deconditioning*. From a physical point of view, disuse and immobilization lead to many deleterious effects on joint mobility, muscle strength, endurance, and soft tissue homeostasis. A corollary to this problem is the lack of visual feedback to complex spinal structures, necessitating *quantification of function* not specifically required in extremity rehabilitation.

The second major issue involves *psychosocial* and *socioeconomic* factors in disability that often accompanies chronic and postoperative low back pain. *Disability* refers to the inability to perform all of the usual functions of daily living, and is frequently linked to prolonged episodes of severe low back pain. Various treatment interventions are designed to cope with the psychosocial and socioeconomic factors involved in total or partial disability. *Psychosocial assessment* is often necessary to identify those factors and guide treatment. In addition to psychosocial problems originating because of persistent pain and disability, latent psychopathology may also be activated by these issues. As such, psychiatric interventions, use of psychotropic drugs, detoxification from narcotic and tranquilizer habituation, and other items may prove necessary.

Finally, not infrequently, individual modalities alone are insufficient to deal with chronic dysfunction, and programmatic care delivered by an interdisciplinary team may prove necessary. Such approaches will be considered separately.

Importance of Measurement to Spine Rehabilitation

Consciously and unconsciously, measurement is a part of all of our activities of daily living. We regularly use our senses to determine temperature, distance, size, or texture of objects. In many cases, a fairly qualitative evaluation will suffice, usually because there is no visual or tactile limitation on frequent repeated assessment of the object we are interested in, such as observing a moving vehicle in traffic or placing food in our mouths. In some cases, however, greater precision is necessary, usually occurring when the object at hand is *not* amenable to regular visual inspection. In these cases, a quantitative assessment is usually accompanied by knowledge of a range of normal values (obtained by testing many ''normal'' subjects). Variation from a mean score in a patient is then used as a mechanism for evaluating the presence of disease or dysfunction or the return to an improved state from an abnormal one. The spinal anatomy does not lend itself easily to visual or tactile examination, and thus demands indirect, quantitative measurement to describe its performance.

Musculoskeletal clinicians are somewhat spoiled by visual access to most parts of our organ system. We have not had to develop the discipline of our hematologist and cardiologist brethren who must rely on indirect measurements (such as blood component, heart rate, and blood pressure) to diagnose abnormalities. Although quantitative measures of joint motion or muscle strength have been available for many years, all too often a hasty qualitative assessment is substituted for the quantitative one. The novice physician or therapist soon learns that quantitative measurements are time consuming and generally unnecessary for routine clinical practice. We ''eyeball'' the comparison between motion of both knees and the size of a quadriceps (often without even using a tape measure), reserving the use of a goniometer or isokinetic testing device for special occasions when an evaluation specifies quantification.

In the spinal anatomy, the small, inaccessible, three-joint complexes stacked on each other do not lend themselves to easy inspection. Intersegmental spine movement is difficult to measure even with biplanar x-ray devices. Multiple small muscles interdigitate over variable numbers of segments, and ligamentous structures may share surprising amounts of load and certain joint positions. Moreover, bilateral comparisons are difficult! Until recently, no valid indirect measurement methods to assess spine function were available, producing ignorance of pathologic processes in the vast majority of cases of spine dysfunction not resolving spontaneously. Currently, however, though absence of direct visualization methodology persists, novel technology for assessing spine function has become part of clinical routine. Yet, many clinicians persist in ignoring or refusing to use such technology. In so doing, therapeutic errors are encouraged, outcomes remain unevaluated, and fringe/fad treatments are perpetuated.

We must recognize our weaker clinical areas before we can expect to move forward! In the case of diagnosis of spinal disorders, lack of recognition of the deconditioning syndrome has adversely affected our therapeutics. Many individuals currently embracing ''work hardening'' (often as fervently as they embraced ''pain management'' previously) continued to do so with eclectic therapies applied uniformly to all patients, rather than individualized on the basis of functional testing. Surgical treatment is performed on only 2 to 3% of patients with spinal disorders. Nevertheless, surgeons will search diligently for that small percentage with a wide variety of expensive and sophisticated diagnostic tools (computed tomography scan, magnetic resonance imaging, electromyography, myelography, etc.). A structural diagnosis, when made, may lead to the ability to correct an anatomic aberration, such as a prolapsed disc. For the remaining 97% of the back-injured population, spontaneous recovery may account for many successful outcomes; however, a substantial percentage of patients, perhaps as high as 30 to 40%, will show some evidence of disuse and deconditioning, making them candidates for physical retraining once the functional deficits are identified. Without quantification, the deficits are simply not recognizable, leading to inevitable over- or underutilization of therapeutic services. This observation is not merely true for spinal disorders, nor has it escaped the attention of health-care planners. Medicare requires periodic testing to document progress in other areas of rehabilitation. It is likely that similar rules will ultimately apply to treatment of spinal problems, once their necessity becomes more generally perceived.

Designing Efficient Spinal Measurement

The term *deconditioning syndrome* has been applied to the cumulative disuse changes produced in the chronically disabled patient suffering from spinal dysfunction. It is initially produced by the immobilization and inactivity attendant on injury. It is supplemented by disruption of spinal soft tissue and scarring resulting from a surgical approach or repetitive microtrauma. As pain perception is enhanced, learned protective mechanisms lead to a vicious cycle of inactivity and disuse. As physical capacity decreases, the likelihood of fresh sprains/strains to unprotected joints, muscles, ligaments, and discs increases. These inevitable alterations of pain and function are perceived by the patient as a "recurrence" or "reinjury."

In assessing spine function, we have drawn from experience with the extremities in identifying elements of performance that are of value in characterizing extremity physiologic "functional units." Such factors as range of motion, strength, neurological status, endurance combined with whole-body aerobic capacity and activities of daily living measurements are some of the major factors traditionally assessed.

Unfortunately, evaluation of extremity neurologic function (straight leg raising, lower-extremity strength, sensation and reflexes in dermatomal/myotomal patterns) is still viewed by the majority of clinicians as the ideal spine functional evaluation. In view of the aforementioned, we must now recognize that this is simply another test to find the 2 to 3% of patients requiring surgical intervention. As tests of spine function, these neurologic characteristics may be irrelevant for several reasons. First, they are a measure of acute change when noted in relation to surgical pathology. In the chronic situation, persistence of neurological changes generally reflects epidural fibrosis or other permanent, noncorrectable anatomic abnormalities. In addition, the neurologic deficits, though emanating from spinal structures, are perceived by the patient as *extremity abnormalities* producing pain, sensory changes, and weakness of arms/legs. Once appropriate surgical decompression has been achieved, rehabilitative treatment of a "drop foot" is focused on bracing, mobilizing, and strengthening the foot and ankle, not on retraining the spinal elements. In sum, what the clinician currently views as standard "objective" functional tests may provide inadequate information regarding spinal deconditioning.

Isometric lifting tests have been used to "measure back strength" (Chaffin et al., 1978; Kishino et al., 1985). Although principles require that the force of an isometric test is transmitted through the body from hands to foot/floor contact, the spine can often be placed in such a position that virtually no spinal muscular strength is required to support the load (Keeley et al., 1986). This exemplifies the first criterion for any functional evaluation: the test must be *relevant* to the physiology being measured. If isolated spinal muscular strength is what one wishes to assess, then measures of trunk torques in flexion/extension, rotation, or lateral bend, not whole-body tasks such as lifting, must be sought.

A second critical principle of measurement is the need to know the *validity* and *responsibility* of the measurement. Validity refers to the accuracy of the test device itself; reproducibility refers to the ability of the test (device *plus* subject) to give a repeatable and precise measure of a clinical variable. A valid test is not necessarily reproducible and vice versa. An invalid test is simply useless, but an irreproducible test may reflect actual clinical reality (such as comparing intersubject body weight or changes in spinal mobility before and after exercise in the same individual). As in these examples, reproducibility problems can often be corrected by restructuring the test protocol.

Once a functional test has been found to be valid, reproducible, and relevant, an *effort factor* must be defined. Without the ability to identify suboptimal effort, invalid low readings may be accepted as true physical deficits. While suboptimal effort may reflect a clinical abnormality (such as low motivation, pain, fear of injury, or a personality disorder leading to conscious malingering), the clinician must be able to assess whether she or he is dealing with a true physical deficit or not.

Finally, a *normative database* must be compiled on a large sample to permit comparisons to be drawn to a patient population. Degree of deviation from "normal'' may significantly affect treatment protocols. Although much more should be said about measurement criteria, it is most important to select the optimal measurement device in the first place, to avoid the onerous task of repetitively collecting normative data (Keeley et al., 1986; Kishino et al., 1985; Mayer and Gatchel, 1988; Mayer et al., 1984, 1985b, c, 1987; Smith et al., 1985).

Quantified functional evaluations currently available for the lumbar spine include inclinometric range of motion (Keeley et al., 1986; Mayer et al., 1984, 1987), trunk strength (Mayer, 1986; Mayer et al., 1985b,c; Smith et al., 1985), aerobic capacity (Chaffin et al., 1978; Mayer et al., 1988a,b, 1990; Mayer and Gatchel, 1988; Troup et al., 1987), and standardized task performance capacity (Mayer, 1985). It is beyond the scope of this chapter to discuss these measurements in detail. The highest-cost devices are those used for assessing isokinetic strength and lifting capacity. Isokinetics has the advantage of providing a measurement of dynamic performance with methodology that ''locks in'' the speed and acceleration variables so that they become known quantities. Then, torque and force become the only independent variables, making calculation of both inter- and intraindividual differences relatively easy. Other dependent variables, such as work and power, can be derived from curves produced on an isokinetic device. On the other hand, when these variables are *not* stabilized, reproducing a test can become merely a computer fabrication. We had the privilege of working with the original Cybex prototypes (Lumex, Ronkonkoma, New York) to develop many of the trunk strength testing concepts. Other manufacturers also produce isokinetic trunk strength testing equipment. They include Lido (Loredan, Inc., Davis, California), Kin-Com (Chatteck Corp., Chattanooga, Tennessee), and Biodex (Biodex Co., Shirley, New York). Other functional measurements (such as ROM) can, however, be performed with equipment that is considerably less costly.

Specific Measurement Protocols

A variety of standardized testing and measurement protocols exist that are useful in establishing a baseline of information on the deconditioned patient. These tests can then be used to monitor the degree of improvement over the course of conservative conditioning.

Some procedures in widespread use have been shown to be of little value because of problems with reliability and validity. The following review provides a summary of various testing procedures and comments on their clinical utility.

Although most chiropractors do not have the more sophisticated and advanced technologies available within the private practice setting, an understanding of what is available and what measurements are appropriate will serve to assist the chiropractor in clinical decision making and/or referral.

Range-of-Motion Measures

Goniometric Measurement. The patient stands vertically erect in a neutral position and then bends in coronal and sagittal planes with knees locked. One arm on the goniometer is postured in the vertical position while the upper arm is aimed along the spine. This technique measures a compound motion that does not specifically reflect true lumbar motion. Additionally, there are problems with interrater reliability and lack of an effort assessment in the test.

''Fingertip to Floor''. Only sagittal flexion is assessed, the distance between the fingertips and the floor being measured on maximum forward flexion. There is intertest and interrater variability, and no effort assessment is included.

Schöber Technique. This technique measures from the middle of a line connecting dimples of Venus to 5 cm below and 10 cm above in the midline, recording the actual distraction between the most superior and inferior points on forward flexion. There is some variability, depending on the anatomic differences in the dimples. Additionally, there is no hip measurement, and the entire lumbar segment is not measured.

Spondylometer. In this protractor-type measurement of thoracolumbar spine mobility between C-7 and the sacrum, there is variability, which some motion artifact, no effort factor, and somewhat cumbersome methodology.

Flexicurve. A draftsman's device is made to conform to the patient's spine, and then transferred to paper where tangents are constructed. The methodology is somewhat cumbersome, with continuous movement not monitored, and no effort factor is assessed; however, it does separate hip motion from spine motion.

Inclinometers. An inclinometer is placed over L-1 to measure maximum lumbar flexion/extension, and a second inclinometer is used or a repeat reading is made with the first over the sacrum to separate hip motion, thereby deriving true lumbar motion by subtracting the sacral reading from the L-1 reading. Though somewhat cumbersome on initial use, proficiency develops rapidly, and newer technology makes this technique even easier with a computerized inclinometer (EDI-320). There is minimal variability and good interrater reliability. True lumbar motion is derived from the compound motion of hips and spine, effort is delineated, and spinal motion pattern is assessable as normal or abnormal.

Radiologic Evaluation

FLEXION/EXTENSION X-RAY. This technique is subject to too much error, secondary to position and variations of lateral bend or torsion. Additionally, it exposes the patient to x-ray.

STEREO RADIOGRAPHY. Simultaneous x-ray exposure of the lumbar spine in a fixed position is achieved by one of several techniques. Micromotion between exposures makes x-ray landmarks difficult to reproduce. Additionally, x-ray exposure and cumbersome equipment are required.

VECTOR STEREOGRAPHY. An electromechanical device is required, with three-dimensional measurement through movement of a pointer over the spine whose position is constantly computed from a fixed base. There is variation as a result of movement artifact, sometimes requiring a stabilizing frame. It is a cumbersome technique and there is no assessment of effort.

Optical Methods. There are a number of techniques using photography, with skin marker, often supplemented by film or video tape; however, there is limited accuracy, secondary to the questionable relationship between the skin marking and the underlying spinal segment. Additionally, the methods tend to be expensive and cumbersome, and effort is not assessed.

Trunk Strength Testing

Emerging technology has provided a number of accurate assessment devices for this purpose. These devices must actually measure the functional capacity of the lumbopelvic unit and therefore appropriate isolation of the segment is necessary.

Isometric Technology. The maximal force a muscle can generate in contraction is measured. Isometric technology is felt by some investigators to be more accurate than other technologies. Trunk extensor strength, with good pelvic stabilization, is assessed by the Med X. Training may also be done on this unit.

Isokinetic Technology. Trunk flexion and extension torque with the speed kept constant are measured. It can generate peak torque as well as a specific curve shape, from which average points curve, maximum points curve, best work repetition curve, and power numbers may be derived. Additionally, one may derive an effort factor through "average

points variance" and fatigue and recovery ratios indicative of endurance and recovery after a specific work task. Available devices providing these types of measurements include Cybex TEF unit (Fig. 30–1), Cybex torso rotation unit, Kin-Com device, BioDex Back attachment, and Lido back tester.

Isodynamic Technology. The torques and position changes occurring about multiple centers are measured. This is essentially an electronically monitored hydraulic system, permitting no motion until a preselected minimum torque is produced after which the acceleration and velocity increase in proportion to the degree to which a torque exceeds the preset minimum. As torque varies, acceleration and velocity also vary independently. Currently the only available device using this technology is the isotechnology B-200.

Lift Testing

Isotonic Testing. In isoinertial testing, or "lifting under load," which the velocity is not controlled,

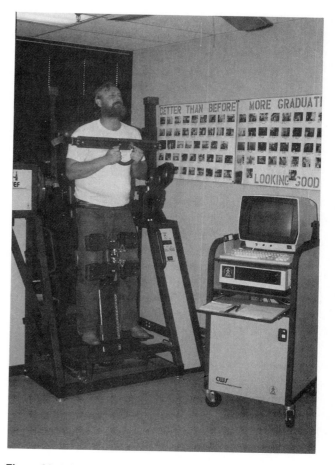

Figure 30–1. Isokinetic trunk extension/flexion device for dedicated sagittal trunk strength testing by Cybex. Note that the need to place the axis of motion in close proximity to L5–S1 prevents simultaneous multiplanar measurements.

but the mass is held constant or progressed. The endpoint of the test is determined by subject's self-report of maximum capability, discomfort, or perception of pending injury ("psychophysical test"), or by the subject's reaching target heart rate (aerobic test). The Progressive Isoinertial Lifting Evaluation (PILE) offers a standardized protocol with a normative database to assess this capability in an individual (Fig. 30–2) (Mayer et al., 1988a,b, 1990). Another assessment method uses the West 2, testing over preset ranges (Fig. 30–3). Loredan has a lift unit about to be released, described as having isoinertial as well as isokinetic capability.

Isometric Testing. Distance is kept constant, so that force is measured directly, with no actual movement of the lever arm, so that velocity is "zero." Several pieces of equipment use this technology: the Dynodex ISTU and the Cybex Liftask.

Isokinetic Testing. Velocity is kept constant, and distance is limited to a range, so that force may be

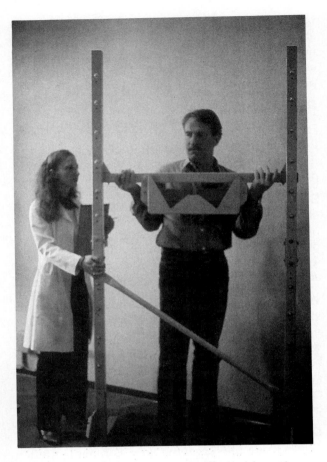

Figure 30-3. Individual training on the West equipment, which permits isoinertial lifting on a sturdy steel frame over limited ranges of motion for both testing and training.

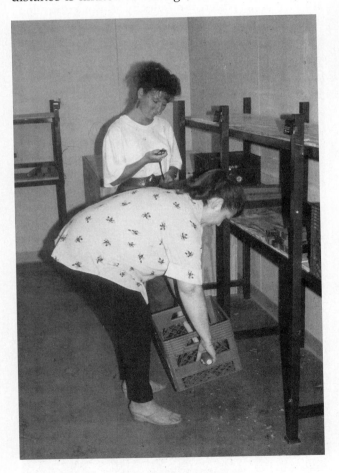

Figure 30-2. The equipment for the progressive isoinertial lifting evaluation (PILE), which involves a simple and inexpensive lifting technique, can be placed in any office, and comprises shelves (30 and 54 inches high) with milk cartons and bricks.

studied dynamically. Ergonomic and anthropometric protocols are available. Effort is assessable through average points variance as in isokinetic strength testing. Assessment devices include the Cybex Liftask and the soon-to-be-available Lido Lift. Both of these units are also capable of alternative protocols (see above) (Fig. 30–4).

Aerobic Capacity Testing

The following is not intended to be a comprehensive review of stress testing, but rather a brief overview of different approaches.

Single-Load Tests. These protocols are simple and require no specialized equipment, but are limited in that heart rate and blood pressure are not recorded during the testing, and thus no measurements are available to evaluate the percentage of maximal work. They are suitable for a "fitness screen" in a healthy population.

MASTER'S STEPS TEST. The Master's Steps test is of historic interest only. The subjects walk repeatedly

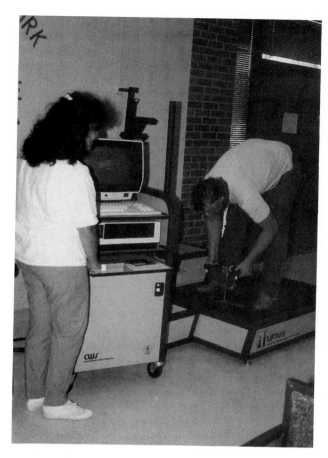

Figure 30-4. Isokinetic lifting device by Cybex, also capable of performing isometric lifts.

up and over a three-step standardized device (Master's Steps) for a prescribed number of ascents, to be completed in $1\frac{1}{2}$ or 3 minutes based on a normative table for sex, age, and weight. Blood pressure and pulse are recorded at the end of the test, and the work per minute is derived.

HARVARD STEP TEST. The patient is asked to step up and down on a 20-inch platform 20 times a minute for 5 minutes. The pulse is counted from 1 to $1\frac{1}{2}$ minutes after the test, 2 to $2\frac{1}{2}$ minutes, and 3 to $3\frac{1}{2}$ minutes. The score is obtained by dividing the duration of exercise in seconds, multiplied by 100, by twice the sum of the pulse counts during the recovery period. The scores are normalized as follows: below 55 = poor, 55–64 = low average, 65–70 = high average, 80–89 = good, above 90 = excellent.

600-YARD RUN/WALK. The subject is required to cover 600 yards in the shortest possible time, interspersing running and walking, if he or she wishes. There are norms based on time for completion. Results have been found to correlate with those obtained on incremental cycle ergometry in one study comparing the two methods.

12-MINUTE TEST. The subject is asked to cover as much distance as possible during a 12-minute period by running or walking. There is a normative database, and correlation with intermittent incremental treadmill testing has been found in one study comparing the two methods.

Treadmill Tests. Treadmill tests are advantageous in that the speed and grade of walking may be adjusted to the agility of the subject. A major disadvantage is the bulk and cost of the equipment involved; however, there is a wide clinical range of experience. A number of different standardized protocols are available, in which speed and/or grade per interval are varied or progressed according to the specific protocol. Examples are the Bruce, the modified Astrand, the Ellestad, the Naughton, and the Balke protocols, generating maximal VO_2. These results may be 5 to 11% higher than results on cycle ergometry, but maximal heart rates are similar. Electrocardiograms may be monitored throughout the testing. Several treadmills are available.

Bicycle Ergometry Tests. The use of a stationary bicycle makes electrocardiographic and blood pressure recordings easier. Additionally, body weight becomes less influential and less anxiety is generated in the subject than on the treadmill. Protocols may be intermittent or continuous, involving a progressively increasing work load that is easily calibrated in watts or kilogram-meters. The subject's weight or fitness has less influence on work load on the bike than on the treadmill. Nomograms are available, based on body weight, in which maximum VO_2 can be derived from the work load, with an accuracy of 10%. A number of stationary bicycles suitable for this testing are available.

Arm Ergometry. The protocol is similar to bicycle ergometry testing, and may be used as a primary aerobic fitness test if there is lower-extremity dysfunction; however, arm cycling does not stress the cardiovascular and respiratory systems as much as bicycle or treadmill testing and is more reflective of upper body conditioning. There are several commercially available devices.

Barriers to Functional Recovery

A multitude of psychosocial and socioeconomic problems may confront the patient recovering from a spinal disorder, particularly if disability from a productive lifestyle is associated with the back pain. The patient's inability to see a ''light at the end of the tunnel'' may produce a severe situational depression often associated with anxiety and agitation. The back injury itself may be a sign of emotional conflicts involving rebellion against authority or job dissatisfaction (Bigos et al., 1986a,b; Spengler et al., 1986). Personality changes may be manifested in anger, hostility, and noncompliance directed at the therapeutic team. Minor head injuries, organic brain dysfunction from age, alcohol, or drugs, or limited intelligence may produce cognitive disorders that make patients difficult to manage and refractory to education. A variety of personality disorders, such as sociopathy, may also complicate treatment (Gatchel et al., 1986a,b; Mayer and Gatchel, 1988; Mayer et al., 1987; Ward, 1986).

Many chronic spinal disorders exist within a ''disability system.'' Worker's compensation laws were initially devised to protect workers' income and provide timely medical benefits following industrial accidents. Employers ultimately agreed to this because of a compensatory benefit: in return for providing these worker rights, they were absolved of certain consequences of negligence, generally including cost-capped liability for any injury, no matter how severe, and set by state statute. As in any compromise situation, certain disincentives to rational behavior may emerge. One outcome of a guaranteed paycheck while temporary total disability persists is that there may be no clear incentive to an early return to work.

A casual approach to surgical decision making and rehabilitation may lead to further deconditioning, both mental and physical, thus making ultimate recovery more problematic. Complicating matters even further is the observation that *no group* (other than the employer) has verifiable financial incentive to return patients to productivity as soon as possible. In consequence, an odd assortment of health professionals, attorneys, insurance companies, and vocational rehabilitation specialists may be minimally motivated to combat foot-dragging on the disability issue. Altering the contingencies may correct some of the problems; however, this assumes that the present system has not already evolved to a near-perfect balance of interests, or that legislators will respond to changes in outlook regarding optimal patient care.

Psychological Assessment of the Patient's Barriers

Early efforts to distinguish between ''functional'' and ''organic'' low back pain did not meet with success. The complex nature of chronic pain makes it difficult to clearly categorize component factors as purely physical or purely psychological. Instead, chronic pain must be understood as an interactive, psychophysiological behavior pattern where the physical and the psychological constantly overlap and intertwine. The focus of psychological evaluation of the low-back-pain patient therefore must shift away from ''functional'' versus ''organic'' distinctions to the identification of important psychological characteristics of each individual. These characteristics will obviously impact an individual's disability and his or her response to treatment efforts. Identification of such characteristics will facilitate treatment planning and assist with the prediction of treatment outcome. What follows below is a brief review of extant procedures for the comprehensive psychological assessment of low-back-pain patients.

The aforementioned assessment procedures are intended to be a representative rather than an exhaustive list of techniques available for the psychological evaluation of low-back-pain patients. The primary purpose of the psychological evaluation is not to identify malingering but to identify important psychological characteristics that may contribute to treatment efforts. A comprehensive psychological evaluation best reveals a patient's personality and emotional resources to treatment personnel so they can make appropriate treatment decisions.

Psychologic Tests

Self-Report Assessment of Pain and Disability

QUANTIFIED PAIN DRAWING. The pain drawing provides a nonverbal assessment tool of pain location, severity, and subjective characteristics (Mooney et al., 1976). Patients are encouraged to freely display all of their pain and rate its intensity on a 10-cm line. Scoring uses an overlay that reliably quantifies pain by dividing the human drawing into a series of boxes, yielding scores for trunk, extremity, and ''outside-the-body'' pain. This last dimension is useful for identifying pain magnifiers, as well as for suggesting the possibility of somatic delusions in rare cases. Such a pain drawing provides an easy and reliable method for documentation of changing pain perception on repeated measures in response to treatment.

MILLION VISUAL ANALOG SCALE. This analog scale consists of 15 questions relating to perceptions of pain and disability. Responses are recorded by placing a mark on a 10-cm line that represents an index of severity. Scores are easily obtained using a ruler or grid. This scale is particularly useful because of its nonverbal form of expression, and its ease of administration and reproducibility make it ideal for monitoring progress through repeated administrations.

Extremely exaggerated responses that do not correlate with clinical assessment may also indicate the need for further, in-depth psychological evaluation.

Personality Measures

MINNESOTA MULTIPHASIC PERSONAL INVENTORY. The Minnesota Multiphasic Personal Inventory (MMPI) is one of the oldest and most frequently used indices of psychologic functioning. Its first three clinical scales, Hypochondriasis (Hs), Depression (D), and Hysteria (Hy), provide valuable information when evaluating the patient with chronic low back pain. (CLBP). Relative elevations of these three clinical scales can alert the clinician to the possibility of important problems such as symptom magnification, poor insight into emotions, and defenses based on denial and somatization tendencies. Many ancillary scales have been developed within the MMPI that also provide specific information pertinent to CLBP treatment. Notable among these are the McAndrew (Mac) and Ego Strength (Es) scales. The Mac scale helps to identify patients with alcoholic or drug-dependent personality types, which may assist the treatment team in preventing drug abuse before habituation actually occurs. The Es scale is designed to identify those individuals with limited emotional resources who might lack the motivation and personal responsibility to adequately benefit from an intensive treatment regimen.

BECK DEPRESSION INVENTORY. The Beck Depression Inventory (BDI) consists of 21 items pertaining to symptoms of depression such as sleep disturbance, sexual dysfunction, weight change, and anhedonia (Fig. 30–5). It is very brief and easy to complete, and it has a cumulative scoring system that takes less than 1 minute to complete. The BDI is designed to identify cognitive factors of depression and, along with the Hamilton Rating Scale for Depression mentioned earlier, can provide the clinician with valuable information about the existence and severity of depression in the CLBP patient (Beck et al., 1988; Polatin, 1990; Polatin et al., 1989; Ward, 1986). The BDI's ease of administration makes it easy to use on repeated visits, offering the clinician a relatively simple means of following depressive symptoms and treatment progress.

SYMPTOM CHECKLIST-90. The Symptom Checklist-90 (SCL-90) is a 90-item self-report inventory of psychologic symptoms. Patients are asked to self-report on a 0–4 scoring dimension the severity of various symptoms as they might apply to themselves at the present time. Scoring yields totals for nine primary symptom dimensions and three global indices of psychological distress. The SCL-90 is brief and easily administered and typically produces minimal problems with patient compliance. Results provide the clinician with valuable clinical information about symptom patterns that are currently present and may provide a useful indirect assessment of personality type and how individual patients may respond to treatment efforts.

Other Psychological Tests

TRAIL MAKING TEST. This is a global screening instrument for potential neuropsychological dysfunction. Organic brain dysfunction secondary to drug or alcohol abuse and head injury may accompany persistent low-back-pain symptoms and are surprisingly common when cervical and postconcussive syndromes accompany low-back-pain symptoms. The presence of any unusual or bizarre behaviors should alert the clinician to use this screening instrument. Should any subtle abnormalities be discovered, a

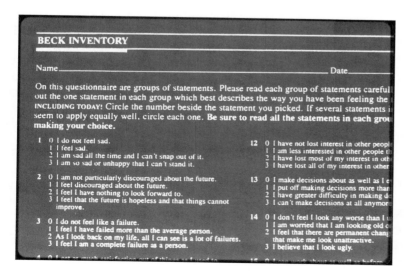

Figure 30–5. Part of the Beck Depression Inventory test filled out by patients each time a Quantitative Functional Evaluation (QFE) is performed at the Productive Rehabilitation Institute of Dallas for Ergonomics.

more extensive neuropsychological evaluation is warranted.

WECHSLER ADULT INTELLIGENCE SCALE—REVISED. A comprehensive intelligence test such as the Wechsler Adult Intelligence Scale—Revised (WAIS-R) should be administered when there is question about whether a patient has adequate intellectual resources to participate in and understand his or her treatment. WAIS-R results inform treatment personnel about the level of integration of information that can be expected from patients. Results are further useful in corroborating subtle neuropsychological findings demonstrated elsewhere and in providing further illustrative information pertaining to coping styles and basic psychological functioning.

Interview Procedures

Clinical Interview. The sine qua non of any comprehensive assessment effort, the clinical interview provides the clinician with firsthand evidence of an individual's psychological functioning. The interview is structured to address the critical psychosocial factors associated with low back pain, including potential signs of depression, individual and family history of substance abuse, history of head injury, or other impairment of function.

Hamilton Rating Scale for Depression. The Hamilton Rating Scale for Depression (HRSD) provides 21 symptom classifications typically associated with depression and scoring ranges for each symptom. The clinician is asked to make an assessment on each classification using the scoring anchors that are provided. No specific questions are provided to elicit the symptomatic information. This is incorporated within the clinician interview; the clinician uses the symptom classifications to guide inquiries and acquire accurate and reliable information pertaining to both qualitative and quantitative aspects of depression.

Spinal Rehabilitation Treatment

After a thorough assessment of the complex low-back-pain patient, the clinician has a variety of options available. Approaches range from passive pain control modalities to active exercise, conditioning, and work simulation approaches. Current interest in back school and rehabilitation has seen the development of multidisciplinary rehabilitation centers where a full range of services are available.

Usually the private practitioner does not have direct access to the large amount of equipment, staff resources, and expertise available in better rehabilitation clinics. Referral for evaluation and care of chronic and serious posttraumatic low-back-pain patients may be indicated in certain cases.

The following sections outline several major components of spinal rehabilitation. In addition to a description of each approach, guidelines are provided for times required to produce optimal effects, what kinds of treatment frequencies should be employed, and durations of care that should be anticipated. The time intervals refer to the onset of rehabilitation care, not the onset of the pain episode or surgical intervention. These guidelines are intended to provide the reader with baselines for comparison and by no means replace competent clinical judgment that is required to tailor care to the individual patient's circumstances.

Individual Modalities

Passive Approaches. Passive modalities are thought to be of minimal value in rehabilitative care; however, as part of a progressive program, they may be useful for pain control. Reactivation may produce pain from remobilization of stiff joints and weak muscles. For this reason, modalities of greatest usefulness may include those that produce no heat and involve minimal rest. Passive mobilization and manipulation, passive assisted exercise, contract–relax procedures, as well as various electrical muscle stimulation modalities and cryotherapy are examples of treatment that may be used as passive modalities. For a more detailed description of passive modality options, see Lee (1990).

Time to produce effect	1 or 2 treatments
Frequency of treatment	Occasionally only
Optimum duration	Early rehabilitation only (1–2 months)
Maximum duration	Unspecified (sporadic use only)

Education. Education may take many forms in rehabilitative care and is a critical modality. It generally is considerably more comprehensive, global, and individualized than the typical "back school" used in conservative care. It may be presented in individual or group didactic sessions concerning such issues as reconditioning, functional assessment, disability, stress, social productivity, and pain control. Certain specific educational programs may be particularly useful in dealing with disabled low-back-pain patients undergoing rehabilitative care as follows.

SMOKING CESSATION PROGRAMS. Smoking, particularly in large amounts, may have deleterious effects on circulation and healing of tissues. Smoking may be used as a self-defeating tool for patient attempts to control stress and anxiety. As such, programs to address smoking cessation may be particularly effective as part of rehabilitative care.

DRUG DETOXIFICATION PROGRAMS. Our society has become progressively more accepting of mind-altering substances in daily life. Use of drugs may contribute to industrial accidents, and to the disability that accompanies such accidents. Drug education and detoxification efforts may be useful for the responsible patient who accepts the relationship between drugs and disability.

NUTRITIONAL/OBESITY PROGRAMS. Weight gain accompanying inactivity and depression is common in patients requiring rehabilitative care for low back pain. Both primary and secondary obesity interferes with efforts to recondition and reestablish fitness. Patients embarking on rehabilitative care may be motivated to comply with a variety of dietary and nutritional instruction programs. In addition, certain ingested food and substances may be harmful, whereas other naturally occurring substances may be useful, for the rehabilitation process. Nutritional education for the individual of normal weight should be included.

EDUCATION DURATION. The wide variety of educational programs related to low-back-pain rehabilitation makes a general duration statement difficult to formulate. The following is intended only as a guideline.

Time to produce effect	3–4 treatments
Frequency of treatment	Variable
Optimum duration	Throughout rehabilitative care
Maximum duration	Until maximum medical recovery

Medications. Because back pain is usually mechanical in nature, medications specific for pain control customarily play a secondary role. Medications generally considered useful for conservative care may be contraindicated in rehabilitative care.

NARCOTICS. The action of narcotics is central, affecting pain perception rather than the peripheral pain process itself. Over time, multiple deleterious effects have been documented, including heightened pain sensitivity, psychological and physical dependence, social alienation, and loss of initiative. Inadvertent iatrogenic drug dependence (occasionally potentiated by alcohol or street drug use) is a difficult problem for providers of rehabilitative care and their patients. In general, these medications should be used only on a sporadic basis for acute pain flares, and for brief periods with careful attention to habituation potential.

MINOR TRANQUILIZERS. So-called ''muscle relaxants'' may have a beneficial effect on acute low back pain; however, their action is central and long-term effects include physical and psychological dependence, development of tolerance, and depression. In rehabilitative care, they may occasionally be used to control symptoms of anxiety, but more appropriate medications are usually available. Psychopharmacologic consultation may be necessary to define most appropriate uses and duration for these medications.

NONSTEROIDAL ANTI-INFLAMMATORY DRUGS. The anti-inflammatory medications are probably the most useful medication in both acute and chronic low back pain. In mild cases, they may be the only drug required for analgesia. There are several classes of nonsteroidal anti-inflammatory drugs (NSAIDs) and the response of the individual patient to a specific medication is unpredictable. For this reason, a range of NSAIDs may be tried in each case, with the most effective preparation demonstrating the fewest side effects being continued. Acetaminophen and acetylsalicylic acid are also common nonsteroidal medications. Only the latter has a major anti-inflammatory effect, but both are common and self-administered nonnarcotic analgesics.

ANTIDEPRESSANTS. Depression is a common fellow traveler of chronic disabling low back pain. Occasionally, depressive episodes have been preexisting, or the depression is partly produced by excessive or prolonged use of centrally acting narcotics and tranquilizers. After appropriate detoxification, selection of the most useful antidepressant medication can be made, based on assessment of vegetative signs by use of various measurement instruments (BDI, HRSD, RIDS, etc.). As significant side effects may occur, the treating physician must have a thorough understanding of these medications. Small doses of tricyclic antidepressants have gained popularity in the management of some chronic fibromyalgia syndromes. They may have some value in reducing sleep disturbances secondary to myofascial pain.

OTHER PSYCHOTROPIC MEDICATIONS. Other psychiatric difficulties may arise when chronic disabling back pain is combined with underlying psychosis or personality disorders that have remained latent until development of the chronic pain syndrome. Identification of such underlying problems may occur only during an ineffective course of treatment after careful attention to the response to psychosocial modalities. Psychiatric or psychopharmacologic consultation may be necessary to identify appropriate major tranquilizers, anxiolytics, antidepressants, or combinations thereof to provide the patient an optimum opportunity for recovery.

Reactivation and Reconditioning. *Reactivation* implies returning the patient to a higher level of activity than was previously used during the disabling episode. This may be entirely nonspecific, including resumption of activities such as walking, sitting, or riding a stationary bicycle. *Reconditioning* is considered to be more specific, involving mobilization, strength training, and endurance/agility training of the injured body parts. Reconditioning should generally be performed only after quantified functional assessment identifies the degree and location of substantial deficits.

Time to produce effect	1–4 weeks
Frequency of treatment	2–7 times weekly (often with multiple sessions)
Optimum duration	6–8 weeks
Maximum duration	3–4 months

Reconditioning and reactivation programs are generally intended as training programs also. It is only during the educational phase that supervision is necessary. Unsupervised maintenance programs typically follow medical treatment for an indefinite period using either home or fitness center devices. Occasional reevaluations and supervised "refresher courses" may prove desirable for optimum care.

WorkSimulation. Simulated activities of daily living, including those generally performed in the workplace, are an important component of rehabilitative care. Appropriate utilization of this modality requires a job analysis to identify fundamental tasks to be simulated, as well as functional assessment to identify substantial performance deficits in the patient. Only with appropriate assessment can effective treatment be individualized. Supervisors must also be aware of issues of occupational competence such as attitude, efficiency, and tardiness. Vocational planning skills must be available to the medical care providers in addition to the ability to simulate functional tasks. Communication and coordination between the employer, patient, and clinicians is essential for optimum success.

Time to produce effect	1–4 weeks
Frequency of treatment	2–7 times weekly (often with multiple sessions)
Optimum duration	6–8 weeks
Maximum duration	3–4 months

Maintenance skills for work simulation treatment involve actual performance of activities of daily living, including gainful employment. Until return to productivity in some capacity is achieved, or the individual retires to a full and functional life, work simulation goals have not been met. Work capacity evaluation (e.g., quantitative functional evaluation prior to return to gainful employment) may be useful to the patient and employer.

Psychosocial Interventions. Psychosocial interventions have a major role to play in rehabilitative care of low back pain. These interventions may include the following.

INDIVIDUAL COUNSELING. This modality may be used best to deal with *barriers to functional recovery* identified through psychosocial assessment. A variety of such barriers related to the response to disability and/or preexisting psychopathology may have to be dealt with in an educational, problem-solving, and/or crisis-intervention mode. Psychotherapists skilled in promoting independence and return to activity are preferred.

GROUP THERAPY. Disabled individuals frequently become fearful, socially alienated, and lacking in confidence and self-esteem. As such, appropriately directed group sessions may lead to a sharing of solutions from one patient to the next that can be more effective than didactic sessions or individual counseling.

STRESS MANAGEMENT. Stress, anxiety, and depression often accompany each other when pain is unresolved after tissue healing. The "pain–spasm–pain" cycle is adversely modified by fear, stress, and tension. Biofeedback and other training methods may teach control of stress effects if used in an appropriate training session.

PSYCHOSOCIAL TREATMENT DURATION. The pitfall of any psychologic treatment is that it may become dependency producing and exacerbate the fundamental difficulties it is designed to redress. As such, caution must be taken to use psychosocial interventions in a *crisis-intervention* model, rather than as long-term psychotherapy. Patients are provided education and training to achieve certain goals in a set period. If severe underlying psychopathology is discovered, longer-term treatment may be provided; however, a line should clearly be drawn between problems related to low back pain and latent or preexisting psychopathology. Existence of the latter should not delay definition of maximum medical recovery in a specific case. The following are duration statements for all psychosocial interventions in general, though a wide range is anticipated.

Time to produce effect	2–4 weeks
Frequency of treatment	2–6 times weekly (multiple sessions maybe necessary)
Optimum duration	6–8 weeks
Maximum duration	3–4 months

Interdisciplinary Modalities

This section reviews programs involving a grouping of modalities, often under the control of an interdisciplinary team of therapists and/or physicians. In general, such programs are more comprehensive, time consuming, and costly, and are therefore appropriate for patients with greater levels of disability, deconditioning, and psychosocial involvement. Potential for abuse with such programs may make it necessary to justify them with outcome measurement.

Work Hardening Programs. Work hardening programs are generally more comprehensive than the work simulation modality. They are intended primarily for patients in a relatively early stage following tissue injury or repair, and who have only minor degrees of psychosocial involvement. Modalities customarily used in work hardening programs include education, reconditioning, and work simulation. Work hardening programs may involve some degree of quantitative functional evaluation, but such use may vary with the severity of disability treated by the facility. Physical and/or occupational therapists may be involved in such treatment, with or without the assistance of vocational professionals. Detailed job analysis may be offered as a service.

This type of outpatient treatment should be restricted to patients who respond in a reasonably short period. For patients showing early physical deconditioning (2–4 months after injury) or after postoperative healing (1–3 months) such programs may be effective for the majority of patients. Identification of severe barriers to functional recovery should lead the therapist to consider a more comprehensive program.

Time to produce effect	2–4 weeks
Frequency of treatment	2–5 times weekly
Optimum duration	4–6 weeks
Maximum duration	2–3 months

Functional Restoration Programs. Functional restoration programs are characterized by use of all of the identified modalities *except* passive modalities. Functional restoration is intended for patients with both physical deconditioning and significant psychosocial and socioeconomic involvement. The term *restoration* (as opposed to reactivation) is used to

connote the fact that extensive supervision, training, coaching, and education are necessary to deal effectively with this most severely disabled patient population. The interdisciplinary team must consist of physicians *and* therapists working in a structured environment with appropriate preprogram, intensive follow-up, and patient tracking phases clearly delineated to achieve maximum benefit. *Outcome monitoring* and *sequential quantitative functional evaluation* are integral parts of the program. In many circumstances, work hardening programs should be attempted first in the interest of lowering costs; however, for chronically disabled patients with substantial barriers to recovery, and with no remaining reasonable surgical alternative, primarily functional restoration programs should be used (Kohles et al., 1990; Mayer and Gatchel, 1988; Mayer et al., 1985a, 1987).

Time to produce effect	4–6 weeks
Frequently of treatment	2–6 times weekly (often with multiple sessions depending on program phase)
Optimum duration	6–12 weeks
Maximum duration	4 months (excluding patient tracking phase)

Pain Clinics. Pain clinics have been the traditional rehabilitation program for chronically disabled back-pain patients. They have used psychological assessment and behavior modification techniques as their primary modalities. There is less agreement and standardization on the other modalities used, which may vary from extensive use of passive modalities (including injections) to use of gentle exercise, medications, reconditioning, and work simulation. In general, pain clinics are strongest in dealing with psychosocial issues, including drug dependence, high levels of stress and anxiety, and preexisting or latent psychopathology; however, lack of standardization of methods and terminology prevents clear delineation of programmatic definitions from generic terminology used by practitioners of this widespread treatment.

Time to produce effect	4–8 weeks
Frequency of treatment	2–6 times weekly (multiple sessions maybe necessary)
Optimum duration	6–12 weeks
Maximum duration	4 months

Vocational Rehabilitation

Vocational rehabilitation is really a separate form of treatment that is often considered ''nonmedical.'' It is usually initiated once maximum medical recovery has been achieved and has traditionally been handled by professionals in state or private agencies making decisions on vocational issues based on prior medical reports. More recently, however, there has been a blurring of distinctions, with some aspects of vocational rehabilitation gradually being integrated into rehabilitative care for low back pain. Several types of work hardening programs are currently based on vocational rehabilitation models and use individuals trained only in vocational rehabilitation, while aspects of this modality have been integrated into other categories of group programs. Once reconditioning and work simulation have identified the highest functional level for a patient, vocational decisions (e.g., job modification, job change, retraining, education) can be made without the need for extensive bureaucratic delay. The future will probably see a gradual integration of work hardening/functional restoration and vocational rehabilitation functions. At this point, vocational rehabilitation remains as a posttreatment alternative in most cases.

Conclusion

This chapter has emphasized the importance of measurement of physical capacity in devising a treatment program. Quantification of function through indirect means is the only objective route available to document progress in a treatment program, inform the patient and clinician of physical deficits and the effect of treatment, identify effort, and provide objective work evaluation information. Ultimately, after appropriately validated prospective studies documenting their predictive value, such functional tests (or subsets) may be used for worker selection in such areas as preemployment screening or placement activities. If used fairly and scientifically, such techniques may offer the opportunity of better matching the work force to the task, combined with modifying the task to suit the average worker. Significant implications for disability/impairment evaluation are also inherent in functional quantitative measurements. By using such measurements, rehabilitation programs can document specific functional restoration outcomes. These programs typically employ a team approach that can provide optimum therapeutics. Costs rise as more intensive treatment is provided, but with appropriate selection and effective application of early conservative care, the cost/benefit ratio for such therapy will remain low. In this way, the "sports medicine" approach to functional restoration addresses the critical personal societal issues facing the conservative care practitioner in dealing with the chronically disabled patient with structurally irremediable spinal disorders.

References

Beck A, Steer R, and Garbin W. Psychometric properties of the Beck Depression Inventory: Twenty-five years of evaluation. *Clin Psychol Rev* 1988;8:77–100.

Bigos S, Spengler D, and Martin N, et al. Back injuries in industry: A retrospective study. II. Injury factors. *Spine* 1986a;11:246–251.

Bigos S, Spengler D, and Martin N, et al. Back injuries in industry: A retrospective study. III. Employee-related factors. *Spine* 1986b;11:252–256.

Chaffin D, Herrin G, and Keyserling W. Pre-employment strength testing: An updated position. *J Occup Med* 1978;20:403–408.

Gatchel R, Mayer T, and Capra P, et al. Millon Behavioral Health Inventory: Its utility in patients with low back pain. *Arch Phys Med Rehab* 1986a;67:878–882.

Gatchel R, Mayer T, and Capra P, et al. Quantification of lumbar function. Part 6: The use of psychological measurements in guiding physical functional restoration. *Spine* 1986b;11:36–42.

Keeley J, Mayer T, and Cox R, et al. Quantification of lumbar function. Part 5: Reliability of range of motion measures in the sagittal plane and an *in vivo* torso rotation measurement technique. *Spine* 1986;11:31–35.

Kishino N, Mayer T, and Gatchel R, et al. Quantification of lumbar function. Part 4: Isometric and isokinetic lifting simulation in normal subjects and low back dysfunction patients. *Spine* 1985;10:921–927.

Kohles S, Barnes D, Gatchel R, and Mayer T. Improved physical performance outcomes following functional restoration treatment in patients with chronic low back pain: Early versus recent training results. *Spine* 1990;15:1321–1324.

Lee C, ed. *Conservative Care for Low Back Pain*. Park Ridge, Ill: Diagnostics and Therapeutics Committee, North American Spine Society; 1990.

Mayer T. Using physical measurement to assess low back pain. *J Musculoskel Med* 1985;2:44–59.

Mayer T. Physical assessment of the postoperative patient in failed back surgery. In White A, ed. *State-of-the-Art Reviews*. Philadelphia: Hanley & Belfus; 1986:93–101.

Mayer T, Barnes D, and Kishino N, et al. Progressive isoinertial lifting evaluation. I. A standardized protocol and normative database. *Spine* 1988a;13:993–997.

Mayer T, Barnes D, and Nichols G, et al. Progressive isoinertial lifting evaluation. II. A comparison with isokinetic lifting in a disabled chronic low-back pain industrial population. *Spine* 1988b;13:998–1002.

Mayer T and Gatchel R. *Functional Restoration for Spinal Disorders: The Sports Medicine Approach*. Philadelphia: Lea & Febiger; 1988.

Mayer T, Gatchel R, and Barnes D, et al. Progressive isoinertial lifting evaluation: Erratum notice. *Spine* 1990;15:5.

Mayer T, Gatchel R, and Kishino N, et al. Objective assessment of spine function following industrial injury: A prospective study with comparison group and one-year follow-up: 1985 Volvo Award in Clinical Sciences. *Spine* 1985a;10:482–493.

Mayer T, Gatchel R, and Mayer H, et al. A prospective two-year study of functional restoration in industrial low back injury: An objective assessment procedure. *JAMA* 1987;258:1763–1767.

Mayer T, Smith S, Keeley J, and Mooney V. Quantification of lumbar function. Part 2: Sagittal plane trunk strength in chronic low back pain patients. *Spine* 1985b;10:765–772.

Mayer T, Smith S, and Kondraske G, et al. Quantification of lumbar function. Part 3: Preliminary data on isokinetic torso rotation testing with myoelectric spectral analysis in normal and low back pain subjects. *Spine* 1985c;10:912–920.

Mayer T, Tencer A, Kristoferon S, and Mooney V. Use of noninvasive techniques for quantification of spinal range-of-motion in normal subjects and chronic low back dysfunction patients. *Spine* 1984;9:588–595.

Mooney V, Cairns D, and Robertson J. A system for evaluating and treating chronic back disability. *West J Med* 1976;124:370–376.

Polatin P. Functional restoration for the chronically disabled low back pain patient. *J Musculoskel Med* 1990;7:17–39.

Polatin P, Gatchel R, and Barnes D, et al. A psychosociomedical prediction model of response to treatment by chronically disabled workers with back pain. *Spine* 1989;14:956–961.

Smith S, Mayer T, Gatchel R, and Becker T. Quantification of lum-

bar function. Part 1: Isometric and multi-speed isokinetic trunk strength measures in sagittal and axial planes in normal subject patients. *Spine* 1985;10:757–764.

Spengler D, Bigos S, and Martin N, et al. Back injuries in industry. A retrospective study. I. Overview and cost analysis. *Spine* 1986;11:241–245.

Troup J, Foreman T, Baxter C, and Brown D. The perception of back pain and the role of psychophysical tests of lifting capacity: 1987 Volvo Award in Clinical Sciences. *Spine* 1987;7:645–657.

Ward N. 1986 Volvo Award in Clinical Sciences: Tricyclic antidepressants for chronic low-back pain: Mechanisms of action and predictors of response. *Spine* 1986;11:661–665.

chapter **31**

Musculoskeletal Complications

Jiri Dvorák
Peter Kränzlin
Daniel Mühlemann
Beat Wälchli

Ethical and legal concerns necessitate that for every health care procedure, whether purely diagnostic or therapeutic, serious consideration be given to possible or actual complications. Common, well-accepted terminology and prospective studies among the chiropractic and medical professions are necessary to reach this goal.

Data on the frequency of side effects or complications associated with new drugs or surgical techniques must be known before widespread use. Complications from manual therapeutic interventions have only been reported individually or sometimes together in a series (Wolff, 1972, 1978; Krueger and Okazaki, 1980; Lädermann, 1981; Dvorák and Orelli, 1982, 1985; Bayerl et al., 1985; Gotlib and Thiel, 1985). The frequency of complications resulting from a specific technique, however, has not been determined. During the past 70 years of chiropractic in Switzerland, no prospective studies have been undertaken concerning the complication rate of chiropractic manipulative therapy. This is due partly to the different interpretations of the term _complication_ and lack of consensus on what is an acceptable reaction to a manipulation and what is a complication.

In view of the increased interest in and use of spinal manipulation among different professional groups, such as chiropractors, osteopaths, physicians, and physiotherapists, it is necessary to be aware of the relative risks of the various methods and techniques. This information is important also for medicolegal reasons.

Definitions and Terminology

The terms complication and adverse effect are rather unclear and diffuse. When applied to chiropractic manipulative treatment, they are frequently subject to misunderstandings and misinterpretations. Strictly speaking, the so-called complication or adverse effect of a chiropractic manipulation covers the entire spectrum, from the moment when a certain complaint is activated by a manipulation, to the moment when it causes an irreversible problem.

In daily practice, as well as for statistical recording purposes (prospective studies), it seems appropriate to accept the current terms as generic, and at the same time to define and designate a more precise subclassification system. Clear and precise terminology is an indispensable tool for the recording and interpretation of clinical data.

Assuming that every adverse effect of a manipulation causes a certain clinical deficit that has an onset at a certain time and lasts a certain time, one may deduce that the so-called complication implies *a chronological and a clinical criterion*. Based on this con-

cept, the current terms complication or adverse effect are subclassified into four categories (Fig. 31–1).

1. Adequate reaction
2. Exceeding reaction
3. Reversible complication
4. Irreversible complication.

Adequate Reaction

Any kind of spinal manipulation may cause transient discomfort to the patient, usually showing spontaneous remission within hours but that can last up to 2 days. The patient may register an activation of the primary complaint, there may be regional soreness in the area of manipulation, and lightheadedness or general tiredness are often noted.

In the case of an adequate reaction, the discomfort of the patient is purely subjective, the patient's working ability is not influenced by the discomfort (Fig. 31–2).

Definition. The clinical criterion of an adequate reaction is subjective discomfort of the patient, not influencing his or her working ability.

The chronological criterion of an adequate reaction is onset appearing within the first 6 to 12 hours with spontaneous remission completed at the latest 2 days after the manipulation.

Exceeding Reaction

Less frequently, one finds strong and more or less unexpected reactions to spinal manipulations in which the spontaneous remission exceeds 2 days.

Acute lumbago may turn into a radiculopathy, a chronic cervicalgia may turn into an acute cervical syndrome, or a radicular irritation syndrome may be considerably worsened. In the case of an exceeding

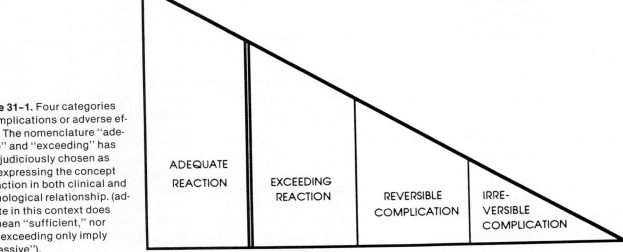

Figure 31–1. Four categories of complications or adverse effects. The nomenclature "adequate" and "exceeding" has been judiciously chosen as best expressing the concept of reaction in both clinical and chronological relationship. (adequate in this context does not mean "sufficient," nor does exceeding only imply "excessive").

ADEQUATE REACTION

EXCEEDING REACTION

REVERSIBLE COMPLICATION

IRRE-VERSIBLE COMPLICATION

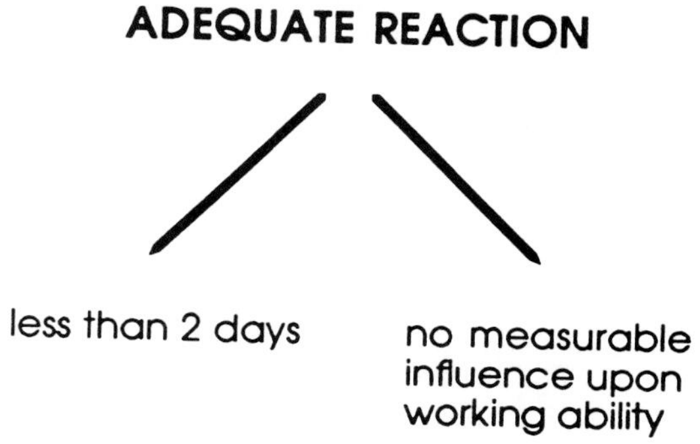

ADEQUATE REACTION

less than 2 days   no measurable influence upon working ability

Figure 31-2. Adequate reaction.

reaction, an examination will find definite, objective, clinical evidence proving the stated discomfort of the patient. The subsequent loss of function reduces the patient's working ability for a certain period (Fig. 31–3).

Definition. The clinical criterion of an exceeding reaction is objective worsening of the preexisting state, with decreased work capacity.

The chronological criterion is onset within the first 6 to 12 hours, with spontaneous remission exceeding 2 days.

Reversible Complication

For whatever reason, a spinal manipulation may cause an unforeseen worsening of the status quo that requires immediate revision of the therapeutic approach. Eventually, additional diagnostic procedures and other therapeutic measures may be necessary.

Examples of reversible complications include: a sternoclavicular joint may luxate ventrally, ribs may fracture, a disc protrusion may turn into a prolapse, a sequestered disc may be luxated, or a vertebral artery irritation may cause transient ischemia to the brainstem.

Depending on the specific lesion, the onset of a reversible complication may be insidious or sudden. In some cases, it may suffice to refrain from further manipulations. Other cases may require immediate hospitalization (Fig. 31–4).

EXCEEDING REACTION

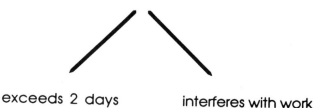

exceeds 2 days   interferes with work

Figure 31-3. Exceeding reaction.

REVERSIBLE COMPLICATION

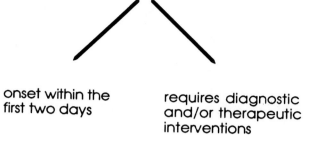

onset within the first two days   requires diagnostic and/or therapeutic interventions

Figure 31-4. Reversible complication.

Definition. The clinical criterion of a reversible complication is a clear organic lesion that requires special diagnostic and/or therapeutic interventions; nevertheless, the "restitutio ad integrum" is maintained.

The chronological criterion is immediate or insidious onset within the first 2 days.

Irreversible Complication

Historically, discussions about irreversible complications after spinal manipulations have filled many chapters in different journals and books. However, in relation to the number of manipulations performed, such irreversible complications are still an extremely rare event.

In a retrospective survey in Switzerland (Swiss Chiropractors Association, 1989), the irreversible damages caused by spinal manipulation in the past decades covered the spectrum from drop-foot and Wallenberg syndrome to paraplegia and tetraplegia. In these cases, the manipulation caused permanent tissue damage and subsequent permanent loss of function (Fig. 31–5).

Definition. The clinical criterion of an irreversible complication is irreversible tissue damage caused by a manipulation, with the subsequent disablement of the patient.

The chronological criterion is immediate or insidious onset within the first 2 days.

Frequency of Complications

A survey among the members of the Swiss Medical Society for Manual Medicine was undertaken to obtain more precise data about morbidity and mortality rates (Dabbert et al., 1970; Dvorák and Orelli, 1982, 1985; Cellerier and Georget, 1984). The study included 203 physicians: 128 general practitioners, 28

IRREVERSIBLE COMPLICATION

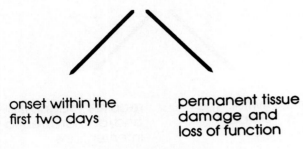

onset within the
first two days

permanent tissue
damage and
loss of function

Figure 31-5. Irreversible complication.

rheumatologists, 21 internists, 14 orthopedic surgeons, 11 surgeons, and 1 neurologist.

On average, the physicians had practiced manual therapy for 8.1 years and had been trained by the official educational program of the Swiss Medical Association. These 203 physicians carried out a total of 214,163 manual treatments per year, which makes an average of 5.2 manipulations per day. Manipulations to the cervical spine (135,307) were performed (3.3 manipulations daily per physician). The total number of manipulations was extrapolated by multiplying the number of manipulations per year times the number of years each physician had manipulated. According to this calculation a total of 2,268,000 manipulations (with 1,535,000 manipulations of the cervical spine) were performed (Fig. 31–6). The returned questionnaires indicated 1408 complications, 1255 of which were due to manipulation of the cervical spine and 153 to the lumbar spine.

Complications of Manipulation of the Cervical Spine

The most frequent side effect associated with manipulation of the cervical spine was vertigo or asystematic dizziness (1218 cases). Ten patients showed diminished consciousness and 12 patients had a total loss of consciousness lasting from several seconds to 5 minutes. Four patients developed additional neurological symptoms after a brief loss of consciousness. Eleven patients had neurological disturbances, with paresthesias and reflex changes that resembled radicular syndromes in spinal segments (C-6, C-7, and C-8 (Fig. 31–7). These patients had been treated by rotatory manipulation of the lower cervical spine. The radicular deficit was temporary in all cases, and surgical intervention was not necessary. Precise analysis of the cause was not possible as at the time of the study neuroradiological imaging (CT, MRI) was not routine.

Complications of Manipulation of the Lumbar Spine

Complications after manipulation of the lumbar spine are not as frequent as those of the cervical spine. Most often, forceful long-lever rotational manipulations led to complications.

In 140 cases the pain was perceived to be worse than before manipulation. Nine patients demonstrated radicular deficits (absent reflexes, sensory changes). Three patients underwent surgery due to acute radicular symptoms, and one patient was operated on because of development of a cauda equina syndrome (Fig. 31–8). There was complete recovery of the neurological deficit after surgery.

From this survey, a minimal cervical spine manipulation complication rate of 1 per 41,500 manipulations was observed. Severe neurological complications were encountered at a ratio of 1 per 383,750 manipulation procedures. The procedures applied at the time of this study were high velocity thrust techniques. Neurological complications with radicular deficits occurred in 1 per 174,000 manipulations of

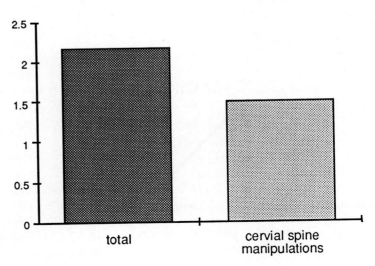

Figure 31-6. Number of manipulations performed during the period 1948–1980 by 203 members of the Swiss Society for Manual Medicine.

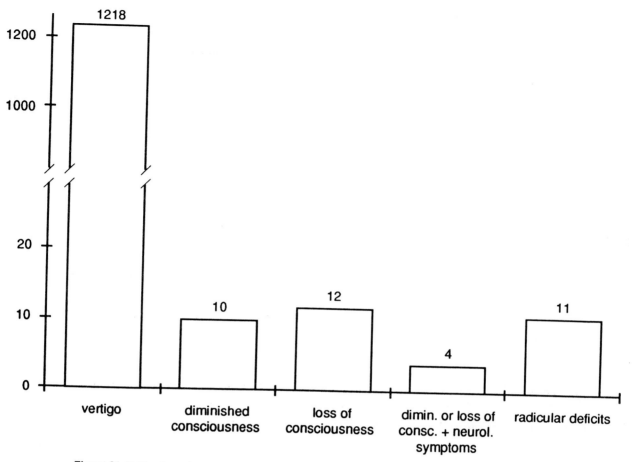

Figure 31-7. Number of recorded cervical spine complications in 1.53 million manipulations.

the lumbar spine. Out of 565,000 manipulations performed, only one led to an acute radicular syndrome with progressive neurological deficit.

Patient Response as a Guide to Routine Procedures

Treatment should always be guided by the response of the patient. In the case of manipulation, the following are recommended actions according to different responses of a patient:

1. The patient feels improvement after treatment:
   Treatment is repeated until the patient is symptom-free or until the treatment goal is attained.
2. The patient's symptoms are exacerbated hours after treatment but show remission the day after treatment (adequate reaction):
   Continue treatment regimen.
3. The patient's symptoms are exacerbated immediately after treatment:

The patient should be reassured.
Gentle traction of the treated spinal segments and massage of the paravertebral muscles.
Cryotherapy and other THE-(thermo-, hydro-, electrotherapy) modalities,
Reevaluation of the previous findings.
Detailed documentation of the physical findings, including neurological assessment and history.

4. Progressive worsening of symptoms over days, weeks, or months (exceeding reaction):
   Reevaluation of the previous diagnostic findings.
   Change of technique or change of therapeutical approach
   Referral: neurological, rheumatological, or orthopedic consultations may become necessary and should not be postponed.
5. In case of severe neurological complications, for example, progressive paresis (reversible or irreversible complication):
   Immediate hospitalization.

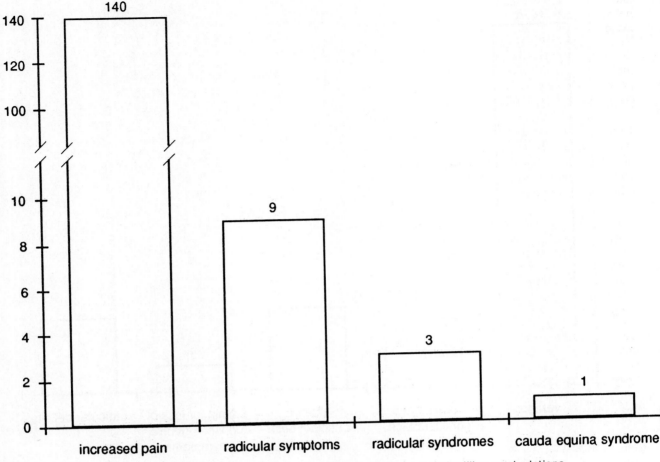

Figure 31–8. Number of recorded lumbar spine complications in 2.26 million manipulations.

Complete documentation of history, incident, and findings.
6. The patient shows neither improvement nor worsening of the initial symptoms after several (9 to 10) treatments:
Reevaluation of the previous diagnostic findings.
Change of technique or change of therapeutic approach
Consideration of the patient's psychosocial situation.

Pathoclinical Predispositions to Complications

The complications discussed in this section were reported to us in a retrospective survey initiated in the summer of 1989 (Swiss Chiropractic Association, 1989). Most complications are associated with eight clinical predispositions:

1. Inflammation/infection
2. Degeneration
3. Neoplasm
4. Intoxication
5. Metabolic disturbances
6. Congenital malformations
7. Trauma
8. Psychogenic disturbances/neurovegetative lability
9. No predisposition

Inflammation and Infection

Acute inflammatory processes in joints are a contraindication for manipulative procedures. The resulting complication of a manipulation can be a prolongation of the symptoms and a delay in the healing process at the acute stage of the inflammation.

Example 1. A 27-year-old man suffering from pain in the sacroiliac region (that later was diagnosed to be due to ankylosing spondylitis) was manipulated in the acute stage of the disease at the left sacroiliac joint. Exacerbation of pain, difficulties in walking, and a protracted healing process led to further investigations. Laboratory tests and x-rays were not conclusive. A bone scan finally revealed increased activity at the left sacroiliac joint that, together with a positive HLA B 27 test, confirmed the suspected diagnosis of ankylosing spondylitis. Because special diagnostic and therapeutic measures were required to relieve the patient from the pain, the complication has to be classified as a reversible complication.

Inflammatory or infectious processes in the vicinity of the area to be manipulated can also pose the risk of complication, although there may be no direct connection between manipulation and complication as in the following case:

Example 2. A 71-year-old man, complaining of acute cervical pain, consulted a chiropractor. Physical examination was unremarkable and plain film x-rays showed severe degenerative changes of the cervical spine. Twelve hours after a cervical manipulation, the patient developed a tetraplegia and was hospitalized. A CT scan showed no signs of cervical cord compression. Laboratory tests revealed an urinary tract infection (*Staphylococcus aureus*). Suspected diagnosis was a spinalis anterior syndrome due to cervical manipulation. After 7 days in hospital, the patient died. Autopsy revealed a subdural abscess at level C4-5.

Degeneration

Manipulative procedures directed at a degenerated three-joint complex of the spinal unit may cause the following complications:

- Iatrogenic torticollis
- Iatrogenic lumbago
- Radiculopathies (in the lumbar and the cervical spine)

Reactive torticollis and reactive lumbago are examples of an exceeding reaction. In all these cases, the complication exceeded 2 days, but no special diagnostic or therapeutic measures were required to relieve the patients from the adverse symptomatology.

Radiculopathies are complications classified as reversible or irreversible, depending on the outcome. In almost all reported cases, disc surgery had to be carried out. In our classification, these complications are considered reversible because there is no permanent loss of function after surgery.

Example 3. A 44-year-old man with acute lumbar pain consulted a chiropractor. History and physical examination were at best cursory and led to the diagnosis of an acute lumbovertebral syn-

drome. Manipulation in side posture position at the L-5 level exacerbated the condition. A short time after the manipulation, the pain worsened and neurological compression signs appeared. Further repeated manipulations caused the necessity of immediate surgery with removal of the herniated intervertebral disc.

Example 4. A 57-year-old man with pain and weakness in the right anterior thigh consulted an unspecified primary contact physician who manipulated in side posture position at an unspecified level. Immediately after the procedure, the patient was paralyzed in both lower extremities. A myelogram revealed a massive prolapse at level L3-4 with compression of the cauda equina. The paraparesis did not regress, which makes this case one of the few severe irreversible complications.

Radiculopathies of the cervical spine showed a clinical progression different from the lumbar spine. Surgery was never necessary, but some of the patients had to be hospitalized. Except for one case, the complications can be classified as reversible. The case of the irreversible complication showed permanent paralysis of the upper extremity muscles.

Example 5. A 39-year-old woman made a somersault and experienced mild cervical pain immediately afterward. Shortly after consultation of and unspecified treatment by a physical therapist, the patient started to develop motor weakness in her left arm (wrist extensors and triceps brachii) as well as to complain of some pain in the lateral aspects of arm and forearm. A CT scan revealed a herniated disc at the C6-7 level. Full remission of pain and weakness after 5 months of conservative therapy (manual traction, electrotherapy, stabilization exercises).

Example 6. A 52-year-old man hit his head on an iron bar and experienced severe neck pain immediately afterward. He consulted a chiropractor who examined and diagnosed a mild cervical ligamentous sprain resulting from this whiplash injury. Numerous treatments (electrotherapy and rotary manipulations) aggravated the condition such that hospitalization was necessary. At this point, the patient demonstrated paresis of the arm abductors and elbow flexors on the right side while the pain was intolerable. Pain persisted for several months and the patient's paresis was permanent.

Neoplasm

Two cases of irreversible complications due to spinal cord compression in patients with metastasis of the thoracic and cervical spine are documented. In one case, permanent paraplegia resulted from manipulation of a lower thoracic vertebra with metastasis, in the other case manipulation of an affected cervical vertebra caused permanent tetraplegia.

> Example 7. A woman, age not documented, suffered from neck pain and sought unspecified professional help. Plain film x-rays revealed degenerative changes throughout the cervical spine but destructive osseous lesions at cervical vertebrae 4 and 5 (later found to be a local metastasis of breast cancer) went unremarked by the practitioner. Immediately after cervical manipulation, tetraparesis developed. Neurosurgical decompression brought partial remission only.

> Example 8. An elderly man suffering from acute thoracolumbar pain consulted a chiropractor who, after unspecified diagnostic procedures, manipulated the thoracolumbar region. Bony metastasis of a prostatic carcinoma in the upper lumbar spine was present. Paraplegia, permanent even after surgical decompression, occurred within minutes.

Intoxication
No complications documented.

Metabolic Disturbances
Complications reported in this survey were limited to fractures of ribs due to osteoporosis (steroid induced, high turnover osteoporosis, postmenopausal, senile). Rib fractures in most cases are documented in elderly female patients with radiologic signs of osteoporosis who happened to consult a relatively inexperienced chiropractor. These complications are classified as reversible, as no permanent tissue damage or loss of function results.

> Example 10. A man, in his fifties, on long-term steroid therapy for myasthenia gravis, regularly sought chiropractic care for different aches and pains. During treatment of his lumbar spine in side posture, he experienced severe pain in his thorax and later on had difficulty breathing. X-rays revealed an incomplete fracture of a rib.

Congenital Malformation
Headaches due to an anomaly in the upper cervical region may be exacerbated by upper cervical manipulation.

> Example 11. A 32-year-old woman suffering from migraine and tension headaches consulted a chiropractor. Physical examination was unremarkable, no x-rays were taken before treatment. Manipulation of the upper cervical spine caused immediate and severe exacerbation of the headaches. X-rays revealed aplasia of the posterior arch of the atlas with a unilateral free segment paramedially. The reactive headache was self-limiting within a few days and therefore is considered to be an exceeding reaction.

Strangulation of preexisting umbilical and inguinal hernias after manipulation made emergency surgery necessary. In both cases, a congenital weakening of the abdominal wall was the common reason for the hernias to occur.

> Example 12. A man in his fifties with a preexisting inguinal hernia consulted a chiropractor because of low back pain. After manipulation of the lumbar spine in side posture, he experienced acute pain in his left groin. Emergency surgery of the hernia was too late to prevent massive necrosis of the intestinal loop of the strangulated hernia, the patient died a few days later.

> Example 13. In a similar case with a preexisting umbilical hernia, the patient recovered completely after surgery of the strangulated hernia, this recovery making it a reversible complication.

Trauma
Several cases of exacerbation after cervical manipulation of recent whiplash injuries have been reported. The cases observed often show a considerable delay in healing because of exacerbation of pain and symptoms. These exacerbations are classified as exceeding reactions or reversible complications, depending on the outcome.

> Example 14. A 29-year-old woman consulted a chiropractor 2 days after an automobile rear-end collision. Physical examination and plain film as well as functional x-rays of the cervical spine showed no signs of instability. Several cervical manipulations in the acute stage of the injury exacerbated the condition. Reevaluation by functional CT scan revealed rotatory instability of the atlantoaxial joint. Rest, immobilization, and passive physical therapy improved the condition.

Psychogenic Disturbances/ Neurovegetative Lability
Loss of consciousness and hysterical reactions were the complications observed. Two cases are documented in which the patient lost consciousness for a few seconds after manipulation of the cervical spine. An overreaction of the autonomic nervous system was the reason for the exceeding reaction in example 15. A psychotic predisposition provoked the complication in example 16.

Example 15. A 14-year-old girl consulted a chiropractor because of tension headaches and dizziness. Physical examination and x-rays were unremarkable. Only 2 hours after rotatory manipulation of the lower cervical spine, the patient lost consciousness while in school and was hospitalized and regained consciousness shortly thereafter. Detailed history revealed that the patient had often fainted in stressful situations before.

Example 16. A 45-year-old woman consulted a chiropractor because of panvertebral complaints. She fell into stupor immediately after manipulation of the cervical spine. The patient had to be referred to the local hospital for neurological evaluation where the diagnosis of hysteria was established.

No Predisposition

Manipulative maneuvers that cause a complication in the apparent absence of a pathoclinical predisposition must be attributed to the so-called "inherent risk" (Fig. 31–9). Fractures or sprains of ribs, as well as surgical subluxations of the sternoclavicular joints are reversible complications that fit into this category. Surgical subluxations of the sternoclavicular joints in this study occurred only in patients whose lumbar spine was manipulated in the side-posture position. The same is true for sprains of ribs. These complications depend on the technique of the manipulative maneuver.

Contraindications for Spinal Manipulative Therapy

Inflammation and Infection

Rheumatoid Arthritis and Instability or Acute Inflammation. Systemic inflammatory disease, especially rheumatoid arthritis (RA), commonly affects the spine (the cervical spine is involved in approximately 25 to 40% of patients with RA) (47, 48). Osteoarthrosis and instability due to rheumatoid arthritis of the upper cervical spine (Dvorák et al., 1989) are contraindications to rotatory high-velocity thrust

techniques. Axial traction in patients with primary affection of the intervertebral joints may be beneficial.

Example 17. A 64-year-old woman with atlantoaxial subluxation due to rheumatoid arthritis. The atlanto-odontoid interspace was increased in flexion up to 17 mm. In neutral position, the interspace was 0 mm. MRI showed inflammatory tissue behind the odontoid process leading to compression of spinal cord during flexion (Dvorák et al., 1989). Contraindication for manipulation (Fig. 31–10).

In the chronic stage of the disease, mobilization (without impulse) combined with neuromuscular therapies (static stretch [SS], contract-relax [CR], contract–relax–antagonist contract [CRAC] may improve range of motion and reduce the patient's symptoms. Careful and regular functional evaluation, neurological assessment, and radiologic controls are necessary.

Ankylosing Spondylitis. In the acute inflammatory state, mobilization or manipulation may increase pain and is, therefore, contraindicated, while neuromuscular therapy using reciprocal inhibition of the antagonists (CR techniques) may help to relax the secondary paravertebral muscle spasm. In the absence of clinical signs of acute inflammation, mobilization exercises, especially those using direct muscle force of agonists (CRAC techniques), are helpful in specific home exercise programs. The use of postisometric relaxation (CR) Janda, 1979; Lewit, 1987; Schneider et al., 1989) is of benefit when restriction of movement is due to muscular imbalances of the paravertebral muscles. Manipulation is contraindicated in spinal areas adjacent to areas of bony hypertrophy (compensatory hypermobility). This is true for hyperostotic spondylosis as well as psoriatic arthropathy.

Degeneration

Degenerative Joint Disease (DJD). Osteoarthrosis and spondylosis are indications for manual ther-

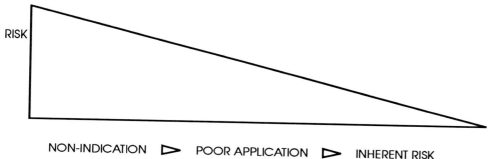

Figure 31-9. Causes of complications.

RISK

NON-INDICATION ▷ POOR APPLICATION ▷ INHERENT RISK

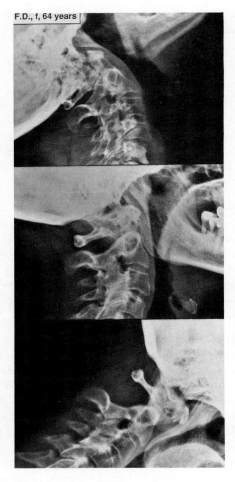

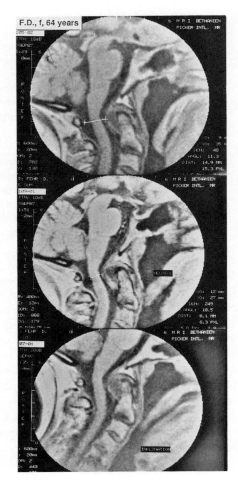

Figure 31–10.   A   **B**

apy. Mobilization without impulse, neuromuscular therapy, and muscular rehabilitation rather than rotatory manipulations should be applied. Manipulation may aggravate the pain in the affected segments. In such cases, careful radiologic evaluation should take place to avoid inappropriate applications of manipulation. Cases with marked osteoarthrosis of the intervertebral joints, especially in the cervical spine, may not benefit from manipulation.

> Example 18. A 54-year-old man, therapy-resistant, left-sided cervicobrachialgia, and paraesthesias in C-7 dermatome on the right side. The plain radiographs in side and oblique views presented marked degenerative changes in the lower cervical spine with narrowing of the intervertebral foramen C6-7. The CT scan documented the narrowing of the intervertebral canal at C6-7 due to hypertrophy of the uncovertebral joints. Manual therapy was not of much benefit to this patient. Surgical intervention was necessary. (See Fig. 31–11 A and B.)

Patients with traumatically induced atlantoaxial and atlanto-occipital osteoarthrosis may benefit from mobilization, axial traction, and muscular rehabilitation. These segments may only be manipulated after careful evaluation of their integrity and stability.

> Example 19. A 23-year-old woman, 12 years after severe trauma of the cervical spine due to a car accident, suffering from motion-induced suboccipital pain. The plain lateral and anteroposterior radiographs documented the atlantoaxial posttraumatic left-sided osteoarthrosis (narrowing of the atlantoaxial joint base, osteophytes). High velocity thrust was counterproductive, axial traction relieved the pain temporarily. (See Fig. 31–12.)

Calcification of ligaments, especially of the upper cervical spine, either due to trauma or degenerative disease (for example, ossification of the posterior longitudinal ligament) are contraindications for ma-

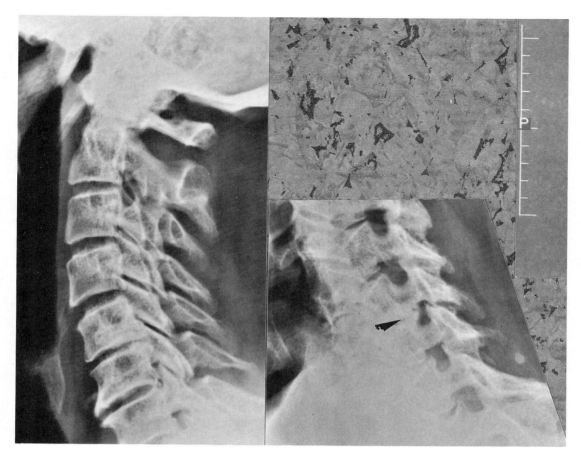

Figure 31–11A.

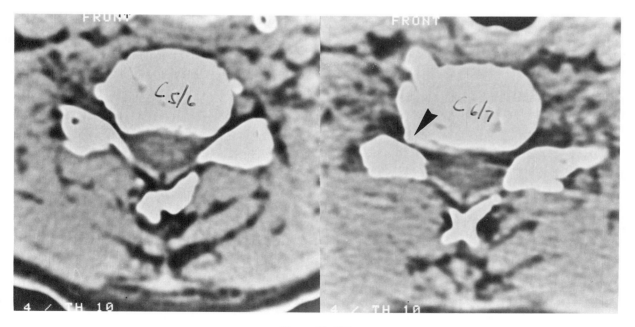

Figure 31–11B.

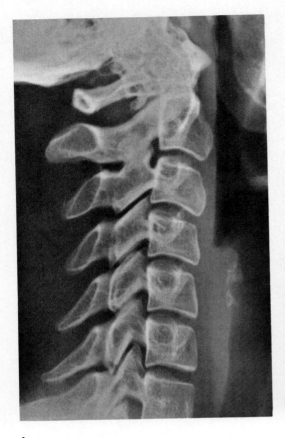

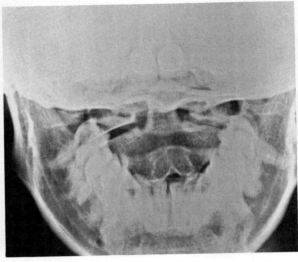

A

B

Figure 31–12.

nipulation and mobilization. Axial traction and neuromuscular therapy can be useful.

> Example 20. A 52-year-old man, 20 years after trauma of the cervical spine, suffering from motion-induced suboccipital pain. Mobilization or manipulation caused pain exacerbation. The plain lateral view radiographs were more or less normal, the axial CT scan demonstrated a complete, most probably posttraumatic calcification of the left alar ligament. Mobilization or manipulation were not indicated. (See Fig. 31–13.)

Degenerative disorders of the lumbar spine may benefit from manipulation, and complications are extremely rare. The temporary pain reduction after manipulation may encourage the low back pain patient to start a rehabilitation program.

Degenerative disorders with hypertrophy of the intervertebral joints and hypertrophy of the flaval ligaments are common causes of motion-induced spinal stenosis. These patients usually do not benefit from repeated manipulations.

Progressive osteoarthrosis of the sacroiliac joints leading to spontaneous fusion is a contraindication for repeated manipulations, if they increase the pain. The CT scan is a superior examining technique in identifying the degree of degenerative changes in the sacroiliac joint.

> Example 21. A 60-year-old man suffering over 30 years of severe pain in the lumbosacral junction without radicular signs. The CT scan demonstrated a complete ankylosis of both sacroiliac joints. Over a period of 30 years, the patient had been manipulated many times by chiropractors and physicians, without any marked benefit. After complete fusion of the sacroiliac joint, the patient reported spontaneous relief of the motion induced pain. (See Fig. 31–14.)

Discopathies. In the acute phase of cervical spine disc herniation with neurological deficit, manipulation and mobilization of the affected segments are

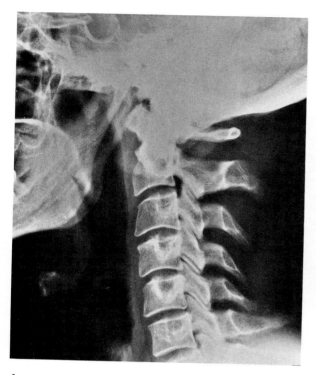

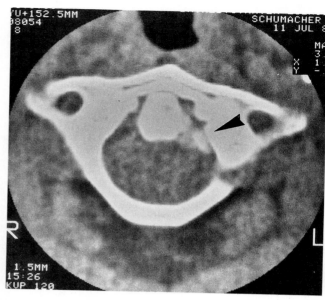

B

A

Figure 31-13.

contraindicated as there is a high risk of spinal cord compression due to a massive prolapse. In the chronic stage, manipulation may be attempted once recovery of the neurological deficits have occurred.

If surgery is not indicated, mobilization using CR techniques (neuromuscular therapy, type III (Schneider et al., 1989) may be of value even in the acute stage. However treatment should concentrate on immobilization and pain relief. Neuromuscular techniques that avoid excessive forces on the injured disc should be used later (Schneider et al., 1989).

MRI and neurophysiological evaluation are often necessary to determine the disc pathology.

Example 22. A 55-year-old woman, progressive spastic tetraparesis, severe neck pain, increased

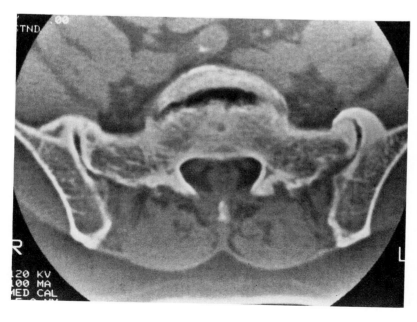

Figure 31-14.

jerk reflexes, positive Babinski signs on both sides. MRI showed a large disc herniation C4-5 with compression from anterior of the spinal cord. The motor evoked potentials showed a delay of the central motor latency to the abductor digiti minimi muscle of 9.5 msec and to the extensor digitorum brevis muscle of 18.8 msec. Mobilization and manipulation are contraindicated. Surgical revision was necessary because of the progressive neurological signs. (See Fig. 31–15.)

Disk herniations of the thoracic spine are rare, but can lead to dramatic symptoms and progressive neurological deficit due to the relative narrowing of

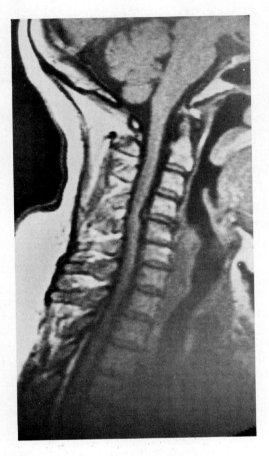

A

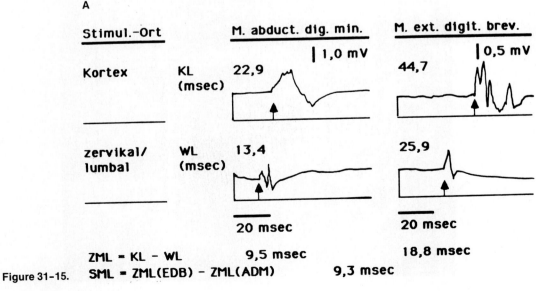

Figure 31–15.

B

the thoracic spinal canal. Manipulation is strictly contraindicated with thoracic disc protrusion or herniation that compresses the spinal cord. In such cases, MRI is the appropriate diagnostic technique.

> Example 23. A 42-year-old woman, acute spastic paraparesis with increased jerk reflexes, positive Babinski sign, severe midthoracic pain. MRI showed a large disc herniation at the T6-7 level. Marked compression of the spinal cord. Emergency surgery was necessary. Mobilization, manipulation, or any kind of conservative treatment in such a situation is absolutely contraindicated. (See Fig. 31–16.)

In acute lumbar disc herniation the presence of radicular signs and symptoms indicating nerve root compression, manipulation is inappropriate. Manipulation is not contraindicated in the case of a mere radicular irritation syndrome (irritation vs compression!). If manipulation is attempted, the following criteria should be fulfilled:

- Failure of other treatment modalities
- Surgery or chemonucleolysis are for one reason or another not indicated
- Relatively pain-free positioning
- Successful probative manipulation
- The patient is informed about the increased risk of this therapeutic procedure.

Neuromuscular therapy type II (CR techniques) or mobilization using reciprocal inhibition of the antagonists (CRAC techniques) are often the only treatments possible in the acute phase. These techniques, combined with procedures that utilize manual axial traction of the lumbar spine can be beneficial in cases with disc protrusion, and help initiate muscular rehabilitation by temporarily or even permanently relieving pain and other symptoms. Surgery is indicated or should at least be recommended to the patient if progressive neurological deficits occur (for example, progressive paresis) and neuroradiologic imaging procedures (MRI, CT scan, myelo-CT) demonstrate nerve root compression.

> Example 24. A 57-year-old woman, chronic right-sided sciatica, without neurological deficits, severe low back pain. The myelogram showed a compression of S-1 root right, the myelo-CT presented a large disc herniation L5-S1 on the right side. Surgical revision was necessary with successful results. (See Fig. 31–17.)

Neoplasm

Primary and secondary tumors of the spinal column and neural structures are contraindications for any kind of manipulative therapy. Manipulation can lead to fractures or dislocations of vertebrae and acute compression syndromes of the spinal cord or nerve roots.

> Example 25. A 39-year-old man, constant pain in the lumbosacral junction. The lateral radiographs showed a spondylolisthesis grade 1 with bilateral spondylolyses. As the pain was atypical, and not motion induced, a CT scan had been performed. Osteolysis of the vertebral body L-5 was observed

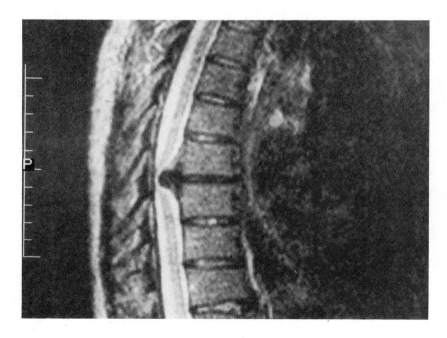

Figure 31–16.

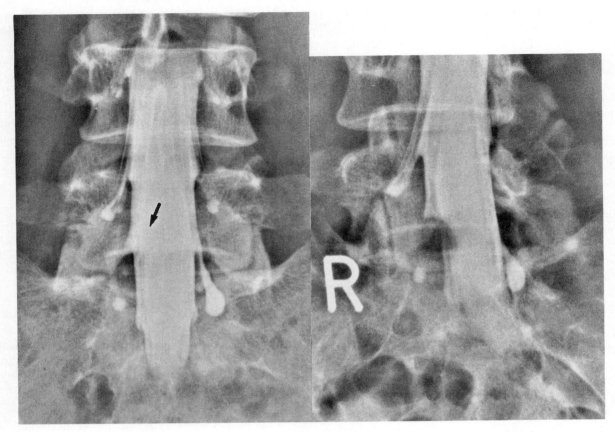

A

Figure 31–17A.

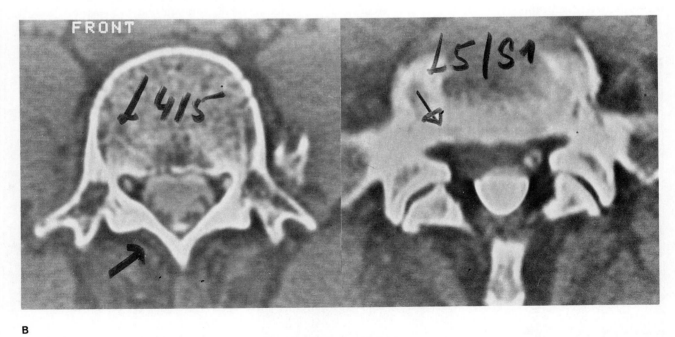

B

Figure 31–17B.

most probably causing the constant local pain. Mobilization and manipulation are contraindicated. (See Fig. 31–18.)

Intoxication

No cases documented.

Metabolic Disturbances

Osteoporosis appears on x-ray as decreased density, but only the presence of pathological fractures confirms the diagnosis. Recently, quantitative computerized tomography has been used to obtain more precise graduations of bone density.

Mobilization and manipulation of fresh pathological fractures are contraindicated. Pathological fracture may be induced by forced manipulation. Medical treatment such as calcium–fluoride substitution and analgesics, passive physical therapy procedures, and supports are the treatments of choice, at least in the acute fracture situation. In the chronic state, after bone mineral content has been restored, mobilization and neuromuscular therapies may be helpful for the initiation of postural physical therapy and training exercises. Here, manipulation is a relative indication.

Congenital Malformations

Exact functional and functional radiologic assessment is necessary to detect hypermobility or instability of a particular spinal region. In such cases, mobilization techniques are not indicated. Occasionally, mobilization or manipulation may be of benefit in the acute segmental or regional motion restriction state. The therapeutic modality of choice is neuromuscular therapy, using the reciprocal inhibition, which should be supplemented by a stabilizing exercise training program.

Manipulation is unlikely to reduce spondylolisthesis, but commonly the neighboring segments and/or sacroiliac joints can be treated successfully by manipulation or mobilization. Utilizing direct muscle force of the agonists may help in starting home exercise programs.

Progressive spondylolisthesis with clinical signs and symptoms indicating radicular compression are contraindications for manipulative treatment, as the symptoms are likely to be exacerbated.

Trauma

The term trauma is used here to describe tissue damage caused by unexpected external mechanical forces exerted on the spine (macrotrauma). This contrasts with trauma induced, for example, by lifting or brisk, uncontrolled movements (microtrauma).

In the acute phase after trauma of the spine, manipulation may not be indicated. After severe cervical spine injuries, commonly described as whiplash, injuries, therapeutic stabilization (immobilization) with a soft or hard collar is often more appropriate. Manipulation of the traumatized region might be counterproductive during the first 4 weeks after trauma. After hyperflexion–hyperextension injuries of the cervical spine, the majority of the patients recover completely (Dvorak and Orelli, 1982; Dvorák et al., 1989), while about 25% continue to suffer from symptoms for many years.

In the subacute and chronic stages after injury, manipulation and neuromuscular therapies are useful if bony lesions, such as fractures of the articular or uncovertebral processes or malformations are excluded.

> Example 26. A 47-year-old man fell on his head from a bicycle. Cervicobrachialgia left with motion-induced paraesthesias in the C-7 dermatome on the left. Mobilization immediately after trauma was performed by a physiotherapist. The lateral x-rays did not show any bony lesions. The oblique view showed a slight asymmetry of the left superior articular process of C-7. The IVF C6-7 was not markedly narrowed. Mobilization caused increased pain and paraesthesias. CT scan presented a fracture of the articular and transverse process C-7 left. The mobilization was inappropriately performed. (See Fig. 31–19.)

> Example 27. A 20-year-old man fell from a horse. Suffering from motion-induced pain. On the plain lateral x-rays, the instable fracture of the odontoid process was overlooked. Mobilization was performed by a physiotherapist; after each treatment the patient reported increased pain. Three weeks later the functional x-rays (actively performed) showed an unstable fracture of the odontoid process. The missed diagnosis could have caused disastrous complications if manipulation had been performed. Surgical fusion, using transarticular screws between the axis and the atlas was performed. (See Fig. 31–20.)

> Example 28. A 27-year-old woman with chronic suboccipital neck pain over months due to soft-tissue injury of the cervical spine after rear-end car collision. The CT scans (including reconstruction) presented a hypoplasia of the atlas (anterior portion), the functional CT scans did not demonstrate rotatory instability. Surgical fusion was not necessary, but mobilization or manipulation were not justified in such a case. (See Fig. 31–21.)

> Example 29. A 13-year-old girl fell from a horse. Motion-induced suboccipital pain, positive L'hermitte sign. The anteroposterior x-ray showed an os odontoideum. The actively performed flexion x-ray demonstrated atlantoaxial instability with

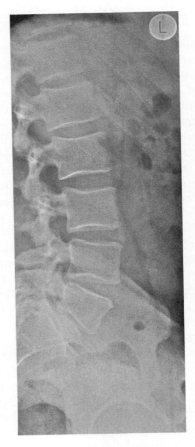

A

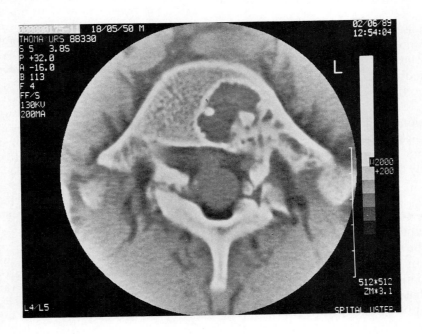

Figure 31–18.

B

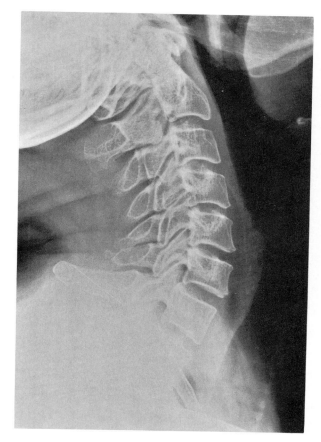

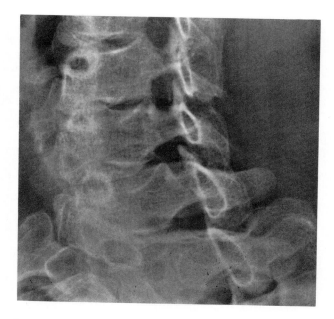

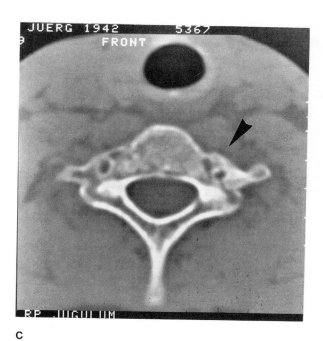

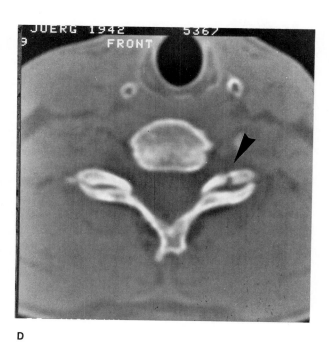

Figure 31–19.

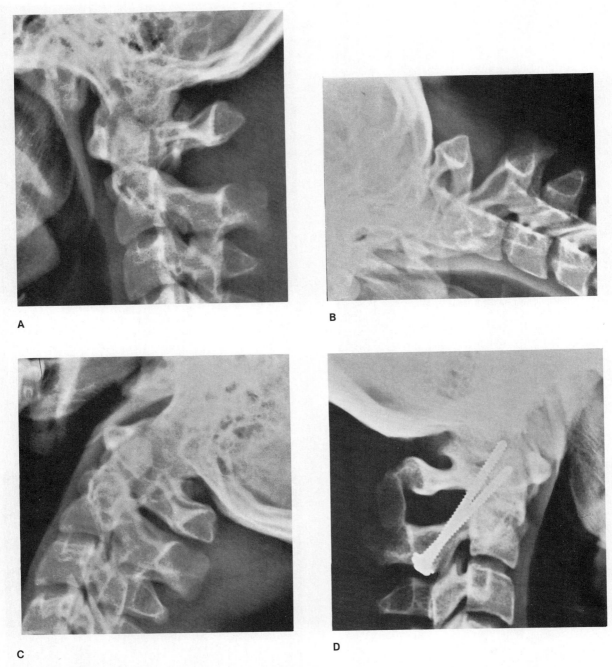

Figure 31-20.

anterior gliding of the atlas, most probably together with the os odontoideum. This situation presented a contraindication for mobilization or manipulation. Due to recurrent neurological symptoms, surgical fusion was necessary. (See Fig. 31–22.)

Diagnosis of the bony lesions, using only plain radiographs (anteroposterior, lateral, and oblique views) is not always satisfactory. CT scan, including two-dimensional or even three-dimensional reconstructions, may be helpful. Fractures are contraindications for manipulation. After consolidation of the lesion, mobilization and neuromuscular therapies may be helpful to restore range of motion and to reduce pain.

After trauma, patients may present with soft-tissue injuries causing instability or hypermobility that may be more or less obvious. If hypermobilities or instabilities are confirmed by functional x-rays

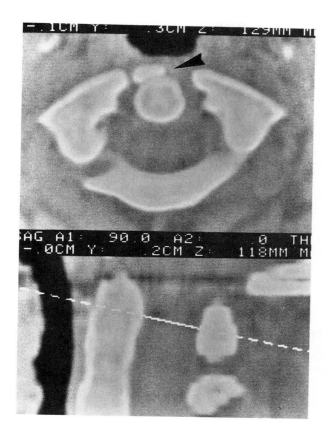

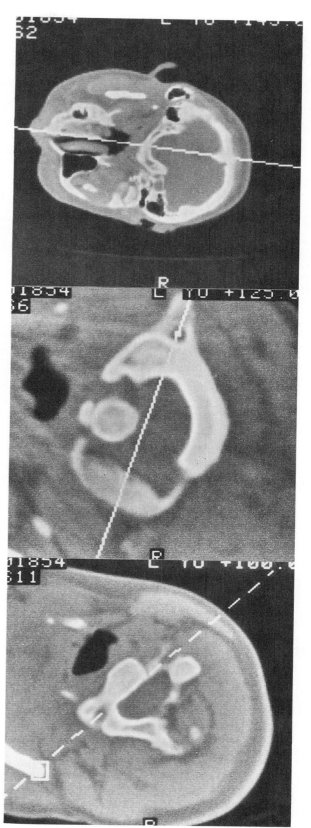

Figure 31–21.

B

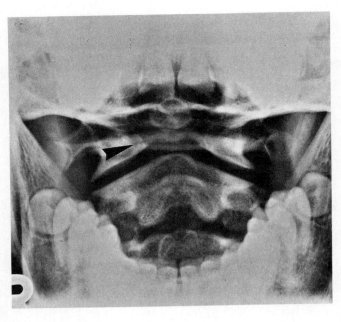

A

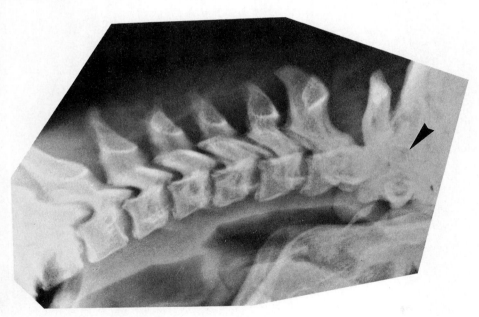

Figure 31–22.

B

(Dvorák et al., 1987, 1988) (including functional CT scans to diagnose a rotatory instability of the upper cervical spine), manipulation is also contraindicated. Traumatic lesion of the alar and transverse ligaments can easily be overlooked on plain radiographs.

Example 30. A 58-year-old man fell from a tree on his head. Motion-induced suboccipital pain, no neurological symptoms or signs. In the neutral and lateral x-rays an atlanto-odontoid interspace of 4 mm, increasing to 6 mm in flexion, was measured. The most probable cause of such atlantoax-

ial instabilities is the rupture of the transverse ligament. Functional CT scans were normal, documenting the intact alar ligament. Mobilization and manipulation are contraindicated. The severe pain was the main reason for surgical fusion C1-2. (See Fig. 31–23.)

Neurological deficits after cervical spine trauma require delay of manual treatment. Neuroradiological imaging (including MRI) and neurophysiological assessment (including sensory and motor-evoked potentials) may be helpful in establishing the cause of the symptoms.

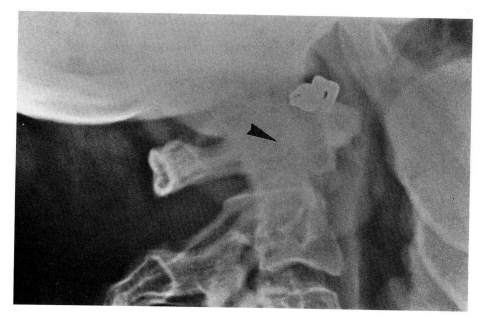

A

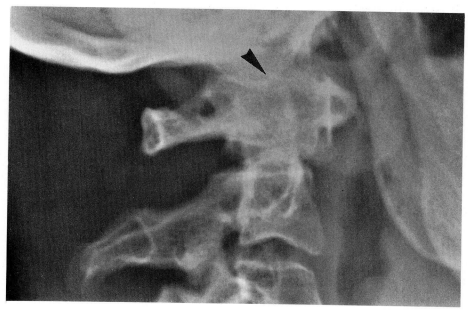

B

Figure 31-23 A and B.
(*Continues.*)

Direct and indirect trauma of the thoracic and lumbar spine leading to functional disorders is less common. Again, in the acute stage, bed rest for 1 to 2 days is preferable until the diagnosis is established. Traumatically induced disc protrusions or disc herniations, instability, and bony lesions with neurological symptoms and signs indicating radicular involvement should be considered contraindications for manual therapy using high-velocity rotational thrust techniques at the lumbar spine. Techniques applying axial traction, however, are indicated.

The sacroiliac joint may already show degenerative changes in the third and fourth decade (Boven and Cassidy, 1981), and commonly causes local and referred pain that is not reduced by bed rest (Benecke and Rudolf, 1985). Direct trauma can cause a minor dis-

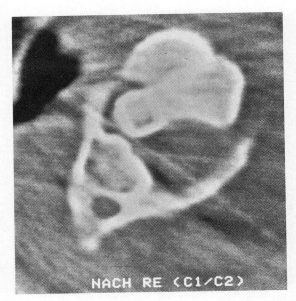
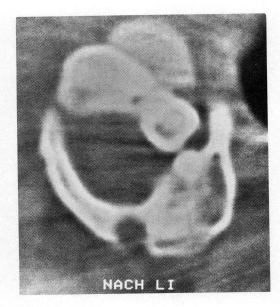

NACH RE (C1/C2)

NACH LI

C

Figure 31–23, *Continued,* **C.**

placement within the sacroiliac joint. In such cases, manipulation might correct the position of the articular surfaces and consequently reduce pain.

Psychogenic Disturbances/ Neurovegetative Lability

Patients with psychogenic disorders must be carefully evaluated by a interdisciplinary team including psychologists and psychiatrists. The indication for manipulation should be based on reproducible findings, indicating a dysfunction of the spine. These patients tend to develop a tendency for "addiction to manipulation" and force the therapist to perform manipulation, even if the results are only temporary. Regular manipulation over weeks and months may be counterproductive.

Technical Causes of Complications

In chiropractic practice, complications due to poor application of a manipulative maneuver are far less frequent than those due to failure of recognition of nonindications. However, we have observed that the application of some maneuvers seems to increase the risk of complications. These maneuvers are usually rotational, nonrecoil, less specific in contact, and do not use drop pieces (Fig. 31–24). Therefore, four basic aspects of the spinal manipulative maneuver have to be considered:

1. Technique
   Direction of thrust
   Force
   Amplitude
   Speed
2. Contact
3. Maneuver applied
4. Positioning of the patient

Upper Cervical Region

Apart from vertebrobasilar incidents, problems commonly seen are transient vertigo, lightheadedness, nausea, dizziness, or loss of consciousness, which are all exceeding reactions. They seem to occur independently of the technique applied. In our experience, however, forceful rotatory techniques as well as neglecting to take the joint to full tension augment the risk of such complications.

Lower Cervical Region

Severe complications, such as herniated discs that cause nerve root entrapment or spinal cord compression, often seem to be a result of neglected or inadequate diagnostic measures and are most likely to occur when rotatory techniques are applied.

Thoracic Region

Anteroposterior techniques, when used at the thoracic spine of the osteoporotic patient theoretically could be risky, because the force transmitted to the spine of the patient is difficult to control. Despite this potential danger, the technique seems to be commonly applied also to the osteoporotic patient; as a result, rib fractures or sprains are possible.

Posteroanterior manipulations at the thoracic

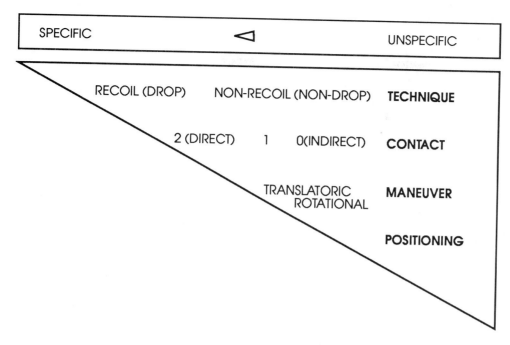

Figure 31-24. The four technical aspects of manipulative maneuvers.

spine are safer in these cases, especially when equipment with drop-pieces is used. Specific contacts are possible and the forces applied are more easily controlled.

Lumbar Region

The techniques used at the lumbar spine are fairly uniform: side-posture, posteroanterior, or anteroposterior techniques with or without drop-piece. Positioning of the patient and the contact of the treating hand for the manipulative maneuver seem to be important. In general, rotatory maneuvers seem to be the riskier choice, as torque generated at the spine is directly proportional to the risk of complications, such as sprains of ribs, luxations of the sternoclavicular joints, and sequestrations of the intervertebral discs.

Review of the Literature

This literature review is based on a Medline search in which all journals indexed in the *Index Medicus* are accessible, executed in August 1989. The search is cumulative, the oldest sources dating back to 1966, with quoted material going back to the early 1900s.

The search yielded 40 sources, of which we reviewed 32. Eight were not available or not translatable. The majority of these 32 articles are case reports. Literature reviews were published mostly after 1984. References (926) are contained in the material.

Articles of the "warning or deterring type"

were prevalent in the 1960s and early 1970s. Some of these are very adamant about manipulative therapy in general and specifically so about chiropractic and its proponents. With few exceptions, they contain case studies that are rarely adequately documented. The article "Spinal Manipulation Causing Injury" by Michael C.P. Livingstone (1971) may illustrate this general tendency. The author examined 672 patients for whom spinal manipulation was considered as a form of therapy. One hundred seventy-two visited chiropractors, 11 saw osteopaths, and 6 received manipulative treatment by MDs or PTs. Twelve of the 172 patients treated by chiropractors received an injury. Six cases are described, cases 1 and 3 are exemplary:

Case 1 (May, 1966). A 31 year-old mechanic had visited a chiropractor 2 years previously for back pain. He stated that he lay on a table and the chiropractor stood on a high stool and jumped on his back with both knees. He suffered extreme pain directly following this and was unable to work for 2 weeks. Since that time he had suffered intermittent back pain radiating into the back of the left thigh and calf, and weakness of the legs. He lived in the outlying country and sought no further treatment from any source.

Case 3 (July, 1967). An 82 year-old retired druggist complained of low back pain for 12 months and numbness of the right leg for 2 months. Lumbar spine roentgenograms at Peace Arch hospital (August 30, 1966) were within normal limits. His

TABLE 31-1. COMPLICATIONS FOUND IN REVIEW OF LITERATURE IN RELATION TO THE PREDISPOSITION

Predisposition	Complication (C)	# of C	Literature
Inflammation/Infection	None documented	0	
Degeneration		26	
Lumbar disc herniation	Radiculopathy and cauda equina syndrome	19	Austin, 1985; Dabbert et al., 1970; Foreman and Croft, 1988; Grenman, 1989; Grieve, 1981; Lewit, 1987; Rageot 1968; Schmitt, 1988
	Root compression	11	Foreman and Croft, 1988; Schmitt, 1988
	Cauda equina syndrome	2	Foreman and Croft, 1988; Greenman, 1989; Lewit, 1987; Rageot, 1968; Schmitt, 1988
	Paraparesis	2	Grieve, 1981; Austin 1985
	Paraplegia [15 more cases when manipulated under general anesthesia]		Dabbert et al., 1970; Greenman, 1989
Thoracic disc herniation	Spinal cord injuries	2	Austin, 1985; Krueger and Okazaki, 1980
Cervical disc herniation and osteoarthrosis	Spinal cord injuries where of tetraplegia	3	5	Greenman, 1989; Janda, 1979; Rana, 1989; Seiler et al., 1937; Greenman, 1989; Janda, 1979; Rana, 1989
Neoplasm	Fractures	5	Austin, 1985; Kewalramani et al., 1982; Livingstone, 1971; Schmitt, 1988
	Axis due to spondylosis carcinomatosa	1	Schmitt, 1988
	Thoracic vertebra due to metastasis	1	Bayerl et al., 1985
	Lumbar vertebra due to		
	Multiple myeloma	2	Austin, 1985; Livingstone, 1971
	Metastasis	1	Austin, 1985
Intoxication	None documented	0	
Metabolic disturbances	Hemorrhage due to anticoagulants resulting in paraplegia	1	Dabbert et al., 1970
Congenital malformations	Dissecting aneurysms	5	Bonard and Ragli, 1979; Cellerier and Georget, 1984; Kornberg, 1988; Mas et al., 1989; Schmitt, 1988
	Vertebral artery	4	
	Lumbar artery	1	Kornberg, 1988
	Hypoplasia or aplasia of one or both vertebral arteries	Unknown	
	Osteogenesis imperfecta		
	Paraparesis	1	Ziv et al., 1983
Trauma	Dissecting aneurysm of the internal carotid artery	1	Bonard and Regli, 1979
Psychogenic disturbances/neuro-vegetative lability	Cardiac arrest	1	Gorman, 1978
No predisposition or predisposition unknown		71	Bayerl et al., 1985
	Dislocation of atlas	1	
	Fracture of cervical vertebra	2	Kawalramani et al, 1982
	Upper plexus paresis	1	Bayerl et al.,. 1985
	Axillary nerve paresis	3	Bayerl et al., 1985; Hensell, 1976
	Cervical spinal cord injury	1	Bonard and Regli, 1979
	Infarction of cerebral tissue due to diminished blood supply by the vertebrobasilar artery system	65	Bayerl et al., 1985; Bonard and Regli, 1979; Brownson et al., 1986; Cellerier and Georget, 1984; Dahl et al., 1982; Kewalramani et al., 1982; Lanska, 1987; Nick et al., 1967; Nielsen, 1984; Nyberg-Hansen et al., 1978; Rageot, 1968; Schmitt, 1988
	Sensorineural hearing loss	1	Brownson et al., 1986
	Internuclear ophthalmoplegia	1	Bonard and Regli, 1979

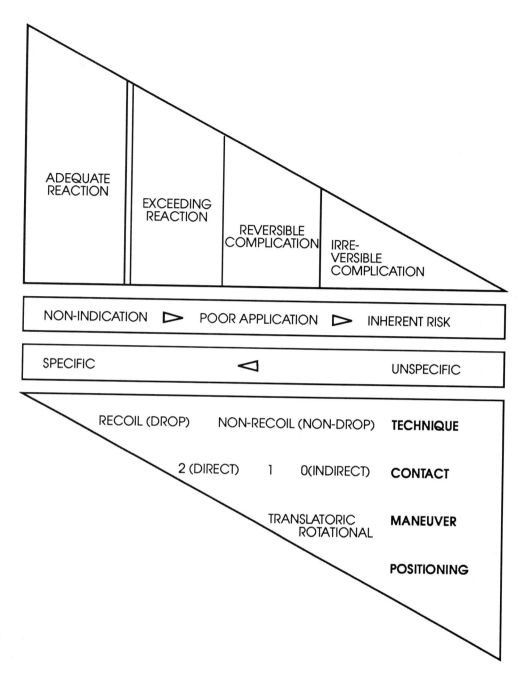

Figure 31-25. Summary of complications.

back pain was unrelieved by bed rest. He received chiropractic treatment in June and July, 1967. This consisted of forceful direct pressure on his lumbar spine while he lay prone. "He was pretty rough on me," described this tough old British Columbian pioneer. The pain was unchanged, but the leg numbness increased.

Another interesting observation is that most material published in the 1960s originated in France; the 1970s were dominated by English-speaking authors; whereas in the eighties, the German-speaking countries seem to have published more extensively.

We have compiled all the complications and adverse effects, be they documented or just quoted in the 32 articles reviewed. They are categorized according to nine predispositions under the assumption that a predisposition has the potential to lead to certain complications given the right circumstances and environment. The data are presented in Table 31–1.

Conclusion

At the present time, the terms complication and adverse effect have not been adequately defined. To facilitate communication, these terms must be considered as generic only; four graduations have been created and defined in this paper: adequate reaction, exceeding reaction, reversible complication, and irreversible complication.

The most frequent cause of complications is perceived to be the failure or negligence to recognize or respect nonindications. Certain pathoclinical predispositions must be considered nonindications for spinal manipulative therapy.

Spinal manipulation, if specifically and judiciously applied, is a safe procedure. Technical aspects in relation to the risk of complication are secondary, but must nevertheless be considered when choosing the type of maneuver to be applied (Fig. 31–25).

References

Albertini VA, et al. *Gutachten über die chiropraktik*, Zürich: Orell Füssl, Verlag 1937;92.

Austin RT *Pathological vertebral fractures after spinal manipulation Br Med J* 1987;291 (6502):1114–1115.

Bayerl JR, et al. Nebenwirkungen und kontraindikationen der manuellen therapie im bereich der halswirbelsäule. *Nervenarzt* 1985;56:194–199.

Benecke D, and Rudolf T. Zur Problematik des ISG Syndroms. Manuelle Therapie beim ISG Syndrom: Eine Pilotstudie. Diss med, Bern

Bonard M and Regli F. Complications neurologiques des manipulations cervicales. *Rev Med Suisse Romande*, 1979;99:319–320.

Boven V and JD Cassidy. Macroscopic and microscopic anatomy of the sacroiliac joint from embryonic life until the eighth decade. *Spine* 1981;6:820–8274.

Brownson RJ et al. Sudden sensorineural hearing loss following manipulation of the cervical spine. *Laryngoscope* 1986;96:166–170.

Bureau of Legal Medicine and Legislation of the American Medical Association. Die Chiropraktik im gerichtlichen Kreuzverhör. Autorisierte Übersetzung der Gesellschaft der Ärzte des Kantons Zürich; 1963.

Cellerier P, and Georget AM. Dissection des artères vertebrales après manipulation du rachis cervical. *J Radil* 1984;65:191–196.

Dabbert O, et al. Spinal meningeal hematoma, warfarin therapy, and chiropractic adjustment. *JAMA* 1970;214:2058.

Dahl A, et al. Cerebrovaskulaere komplikasjoner til manipulasjonsbehandling av nakken. *Tidsskr Nor Laegeforen* 1982; 102:155–157.

Dan NG, and Saccasan PA. Serious complications of lumbar spinal manipulation. *Med J Aust* 1983;2:672–673.

Dvorák J, and Dvorak V. *Manual Medicine Diagnostics*. New York: Thieme Medical Publishers Inc.; 1990.

Dvorák J, Fröhlich D, and Penning L. et al. Functional radiographic diagnosis of the cervical spine: flexion/extension. *Spine* 1988;13:748–755.

Dvorák J, Valach L, Schmid S. Cervical spine injuries in Switzerland. *J Manual Medicine* 1989;4:7–16.

Dvorák J, Grob D, and Baumgartner H, et al. Functional evaluation of the spinal cord by magnetic resonance imaging in patients with rheumatoid arthritis and insability of upper cervical spine. *Spine* 1989;14:1057–1064.

Dvorák J, Hayek J, and Zehnder R. CT-functional diagnostics of the rotatory instability of the upper cervical spine. part 2. an evaluation on healthy adults and patients with suspected instability. *Spine* 1987;12:726–731.

Dvorák J, and v. Orelli F. How dangerous is manipulation to the cervical spine? case report and results of a survey. *Manual Medicine* 1985;2:1–4.

Dvorák J, and v. Orelli F. Wie häufig sind Komplikationen nach Manipulation der Halswirbelsäule? Fallbericht und Ergebnisse einer Umfrage. Schweiz. Rundschau f. Med. (Praxis) 1982; 71:64–69.

Dvorák, J. Manual medicine in the United States and Europe in the year 1982. *Manual Medicine* 1983;1:3–9.

Foreman SM, and Croft AC. *Whiplash Injuries. The Cervical Acceleration/Deceleration Syndrome*. Baltimore: 1988. Williams and Wilkins.

Fraser DM. Neck manipulation as a cause of stroke (letter). *Stroke* 1982;13:260–261.

Galinaro P, and Cartesegna M. Three cases of lumbar disc rupture and one of cauda equina associated with spinal manipulation (chiropaxis). *Lancet* 1983;1:411.

Gorman, RF. Cardiac arrest after cervical spine manipulation. *Med J Aust* 1978;2:169–170.

Gotlib A, and Thiel H. A selected annotated Bibliography of the core biomedical literature pertaining to stroke, cervical spine, manipulation and head-neck movement. *J Can Chirop Ass* 1985; 29:80–89.

Greenman P. Principles of manual medicine. Baltimore: Williams & Willkins: 47–48, 99–100.

Grieve G. Common vertebral joint problems. New York: Churchill Livingston: 465–467.

Haldemann S. Personal communication; 1990.

Hensell V. Neurologische Schäden nach Repositions-Massnahmen an der Wirbelsäule. *Med Welt* 1976;27:656–658.

Hooper J. Low back pain and manipulation. Paraparesis after treatment of low back pain by physical methods. *Med J Aust* 1973;549–551.

Janda V. Muskelfunktionsdiagnostik. Fischer, Leuven 1979.

Kaltenborn FM. Manuell Mobilisering av Ryggraden. Kap. 8: Kontraindikasjoner, Olaf Norlis Bokhandel, Oslo: 78–80.

Kewalramani LS, et al. Myelopathy following cervical spine manipulation. *Am J Phys Med* 1982;61:165–175.

Kornberg E. Lumbar artery aneurysm with acute aortic occlusion resulting from chiropractic manipulation. *Surgery* 1988;103: 122–124.

Krueger RK, and Okazaki H. Vertebral-basial distribution infarction following chiropractic cervical manipulation. *Mayo Clin Proc* 1980; 55:322–332.

Lädermann JP. Accidents of spinal manipulation. *Annals of the Swiss Chiropractors' Association* 1981; Vol. VII: 161–208.

Lanska DJ. Thoracic disc herniation associated with chiropractic spinal manipulation (letter). *Arch Neurol* 1987;44:996–997.

Lewit K. *Manuelle Medizin*, 5th ed, München: Urban und Schwarzenberg; 1987.

Livingstone MCP. Spinal manipulation causing injury, a three year study. *Clin-Orthop* 1971;81:82–86.

Malmivaara A, and Pohjola R. Cauda equina syndrome caused by chiropraxis on a patient previously free of lumbar symptoms. *Lancet* 1982; 2:986–987.

Mas JL, et al. Dissecting aneurysm of the vertebral artery and cervical manipulation. *Neurology* 1989;39:512–515.

Mühlemann D. Erarbeitung der gelenkfunktion, indikation und technik. In vonOw, and D, G. Hüni eds. *Muskuläre Rehabilitation*, Erlangen: Perimed Verlagsgesellschaft; 1987.

Mühlemann D, and Zahnd F. Segmental hypermobility, accepted for publication, 1988.

Nick J, et al. Incidents et accidents neurologiques dus aux manipulations cervicales (à propos de trois observations). Paris: BUll Mem Soc Med Hop; 1967;118:435–440.

Nielsen AA. Cerebrovaskuære insulter forarsaget af manipulation of columna cervicalis. *Læger* 1984;146:3267–3270.

Nyberg-Hansen, R., et al. Brainstem lesion with coma for five years following manipulation of the cervical spine. *J Neurol* 1978;218:97–105.

Pellici PM, et al. A prospective study of the progression of rheumatoid arthritis of the cervical spine. *J Bone Joint Surg* 1981;63:342–350.

Rageot E. Les accidents et incidents des manipulations vertebrales. *Cah Coll Med Hop* 1968;9:1149–1154.

Rana NA. Natural history of atlanto-axial subluxation in rheumatoid arthritis. *Spine* 1989;14:1054–1056.

Richard J. Disc rupture with cauda equina syndrome after chiropractic adjustment. *NY State J Med* 1967;67:2496–2498.

Rinsky LA, et al. A cervical spinal cord injury following chiropractic manipulation. *Paraplegia* 1976;13:223–227.

Seiler F, et al. Die Chiropraktik, ihr Wesen, ihre Erfolge und Gefahren. 30-31, Paul Haupt Verlag, Bern, Leipzig.

Schmitt HP. Manuelle Therapie der Halswirbelsäule. *Manuelle Medizin* 1978;4:71–77.

Schmitt HP, and Wolf HD. Memorandum zur Verhütung von Zwischenfällen bei gezielter Handgriff-Therapie an der

Halswirbelsäule. DGMM 1979.

Schmitt HP. Risiken und Komplikationen der Manualtherapie aus neuropathologischer Sicht. *Nervenarzt* 1988;59:32–35.

Schneider W, et al. *Manuelle Medizin, Therapie,* 2nd ed. New York: Thieme Verlag: 1989:17–21.

Stoddard A. *Manual of Osteopathic Practice.* London: Hutchinson & Co; 179, 279–280.

Swiss Chiropractic Association. Examining Catalogue for the Intercantonal Examination, 1989.

Thierry-Mieg J. Techniques de manipulations vertebrales utilisées dans le traitemant des sciatiques par hernie discale. indications, contre-indications et accidents. *Sem Ther* 1966;42:376–379.

Werne S. Studies in spontaneous atlas dislocations. *Acta Orthopaedica Scandinavica Supplementum* Copenhagen: *Munksgaard;* No. XXIII.

Wolff HD. Zervikaler Bandscheibenvorfall nach ''chiropraktischer'' behandlung. *Manuelle Medizin* 1972;10:124–127.

Wolff HD. Komplikationen bei Manueller Therapie der Halswirbelsäule. *Manuelle Medizin* 1978;16:77–81.

Wolff HD. Kontra-Indikationen gezielter Handgrifftherapie an der Wirbelsäule. *Manuelle Medizin* 1980;18:39–49.

Ziv I., et al. Paraplegia in osteogenesis imperfecta. *J Bone Joint Surg* 1983;65:184–185.

chapter **32**

Cerebrovascular Complications of Manipulation

Allan G.J. Terrett
Andries M. Kleynhans

The first mention of manipulative iatrogenesis appears to have been in 1871 when Wharton Hood wrote: '' . . . serious and often fatal results have occurred in the practice of all bone setters'' (Hood, 1871). However, the first case of manipulative iatrogenesis was not described for another 36 years until 1907 (Roberts, 1907). The first vascular accident after manipulation was reported in 1934 in the case of Foster v Thornton (_Foster_ v _Thornton,_ 1934). Critics of manipulative therapy emphasize the possibility of serious injury, especially of the brainstem, due to arterial trauma after cervical manipulation. It has required only the very rare reporting of these accidents to malign a therapeutic procedure that, in experienced hands, gives beneficial results with few adverse side effects.

Vascular accidents are responsible for the major criticism of spinal manipulative therapy (SMT). It should be the primary objective of those who manipulate to take all available steps to minimize the occurrence of these accidents. A rationale for the prevention of complications from SMT may be based on an understanding of:

- The causes of reported complications from SMT
- The contraindications to SMT
- Diagnostic assessment of patients before SMT
- Avoiding certain therapies in patients thought to be at risk
- Avoiding those techniques that appear to carry the greatest risk

Acknowledgments
Thanks are expressed to Drs. Glynn Till, Michael Webb, Peter Bryner, and Mr. Ian Hansen for helpful comments in the preparation of this paper. For translations of articles in French, German, and Norwegian, thanks are expressed to Mrs. Melitta Davidson, and Drs. Daniel Danuser, and John and Charlotte Leboeuf. For help with literature searches, thanks are expressed to Michael Gavin, Sue Crocker, Deirdre Gillespie, and Annabelle McCooke of Phillip Institute of Technology Library. For the artwork, thanks are expressed to Cathie Allan, Phillip Institute of Technology Media Production and Services Department.

Incidence of Cerebrovascular Injury

In estimating incidence, it should be recognized that the actual incidence can be expected to be higher than the reported incidence. Grieve (1986) suggests an analogy to motor vehicle accidents in which the number of people injured according to reports in the press in no way gives any indication of the true incidence of people injured. The following comments from various authors on the incidence of complications from SMT reveal that the injuries are not common, but the estimated incidence is increasing as the subject is being better investigated.

Maigne (1972) suggests "there is probably less than one death of this nature out of several tens-of-millions of manipulations." Cyriax (1978) states " . . . this risk works out to about one in ten million manipulations, and is no argument against manipulative reduction in suitable cases." Hosek et al. (1981) suggest " . . . we may form a conservative likelihood esti-

mator by looking at the ratio of vertebrobasilar injuries to adjustments performed. This ratio would be 100 injuries per 100 million adjustments . . . about one in one million." Gutmann (1983) concludes "there are 2–3 serious incidents involving the vertebrobasilar system occurring in 1 million manipulations to the upper cervical spine." Dvorák and Orelli (1985) state that "following an inquiry amongst members of the Swiss Medical Group for Manual Medicine, it was calculated that there were slight neurological complications in one in 40,000; and one important complication in 400,000 cervical manipulations."

Case Analysis

This section examines 126 accidents described in various publications listed in the references, which occurred over 55 years (1934–1987). Fig. 32–1 shows the age distribution curve of the patients, while Tables 32–1 and 32–2 tabulate the practitioner involved and the sequellae. Of the 126 cases reviewed, 63 were women, 50 were men, and gender was unknown in 13.

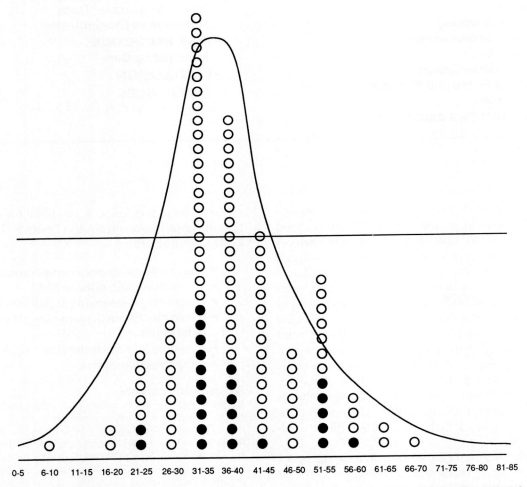

Figure 32–1. Age distribution of 113 vascular accidents after manipulation (age not known in 13 cases, 4 died, 6 survived, 3 outcome unknown). Curve represents an age analysis of 6187 consecutive patient visits to a chiropractor's office. *Solid line* = 10%.

TABLE 32-1. ANALYSIS OF 126 CASES OF VERTEBROBASILAR ACCIDENTS FOLLOWING MANIPULATION

Manipulator	# Cases	# Died	Outcome Unknown
Chiropractor	79	14	4
Medical	18	8	
Osteopath	9	2	
Naturopath[a]	4	2	
Physiotherapist	2		
Kinesitherapist	1		1
Wife	1	1	
Self	1		1
Unknown	11	2	
Total	126	29	6

[a]Includes one German Heilpraktiker.

This does not necessarily indicate a sex predilection to post-SMT vertebrobasilar incidents, because most epidemiological studies of chiropractic practices demonstrate a slight preponderance of female patients.

The age distribution when reported for mortality was: women 20 to 66 years (average 38.1 years); men 7 to 55 years (average 40.1 years). There have been many assumptions made as to the significance of the age of the victims, and the presence or absence of degenerative osseous or vascular changes. Ladermann (1981) mentions that the average age is too young for gross anatomicopathological alteration to be the cause, and implies that the middle-age group is predisposed to accidents because of a phase of joint instability occurring during middle life. The risk decreases with aging as arthrosis restores stability. Taylor (1981) suggested that most risks of this nature are expected to be found in the elderly, where degenerated arterial vertebralis can be the genesis of many symptoms where advanced spondylitic and arteriosclerotic changes have taken place. The age distribution curve in Figure 32–1 appears to contradict this.

TABLE 32-2. SEQUELAE OF 126 CASES OF VASCULAR POST-SMT ACCIDENTS

Sequela	N
Death	29
Tetraplegia[a]	7
Neurological deficit	38
Intellectual/memory deficit	2
Almost complete recovery	12
Complete recovery	12
Residual deafness	3
Barre-Lioeu syndrome	1
Hearing loss and tinnitus	2
Hearing loss and nystagmus	1
Hearing loss and residual facial paresis	1
Homonymous hemianopia	1
Unknown, but survived 30 years	1
Unknown	16

[a] Two cases of tetraplegia are included in the "death" group and 1 case is included in the complete recovery group.

While at first glance there does appear to be a predilection for manipulative accidents in the 30 to 45-year age group, closer examination does not reveal a greater risk in any one age range. The increased number of accidents reported in the 30 to 45-year age group appears simply to be a reflection of the age group most likely to seek the services of a practitioner of manual therapy. Therefore, factors such as a patient's age and the presence or absence of degenerative osseous or vascular changes do not appear to be important in assessing a patient's risk of manipulative iatrogenesis (Terrett, 1987a).

Mechanisms of Cerebrovascular Injury

Clinical Anatomy

The vertebral artery arises from the subclavian artery and then enters the vertebral foramen of the sixth cervical transverse process. From here it courses upward, encased by the bony rings formed by the transverse foramina (Fig. 32–2). On exiting the foramen in the axis vertebra, the artery abandons its almost vertical course to pass upward and laterally to reach the foramen of the atlas transverse process.

After emerging from the transverse foramen of the atlas, the vertebral artery proceeds posteriorly and medially around the lateral mass of the atlas, to pass via a groove in the posterior arch of the atlas, between the atlanto-occipital joint capsule anteriorly and the posterior atlanto-occipital membrane posteriorly (Fig. 32–3). It then passes through the foramen magnum and at the lower border of the pons it unites with the vertebral artery of the opposite side to form the basilar artery. The basilar artery passes up the anterior surface of the brainstem, divides, and becomes the posterior cerebral arteries. The posterior inferior cerebellar arteries (PICA), the largest branches off the vertebral arteries, leave the vertebral arteries just before their joining each other. The PICA run a tor-

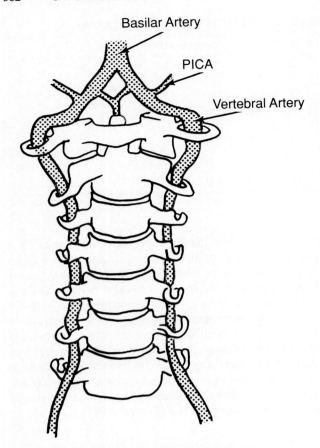

Figure 32-2. Relationship of the vertebral artery to the cervical spine. PICA = posterior inferior cerebellar artery.

tuous course along the lateral part of the medulla, to which they are the main blood supply.

Clinical Biomechanics

Rotation of the cervical spine to the extent of 45 to 50 degrees occurs chiefly at the atlantoaxial joint. This is about half of total cervical spine rotation (Selecki, 1969). Reduction of vertebral artery flow due to cervical spine rotation has been well documented (de-Kleyn, 1927, 1933; Elkin and Harris, 1946; Biemond, 1951; Falconer, 1951; Tissington Tatlow and Bammer, 1957; Toole and Tucker, 1960; Brown and Tatlow, 1963; Faris et al., 1963; Hadesty et al., 1963; Scatliff et al., 1967; Selecki, 1969; Andersson et al., 1970; Barton and Margolis, 1975; Grossman and Davies, 1982; Yang et al., 1985).

deKleyn and co-workers (1927, 1933) were the first to postulate that decreased flow, or even cessation of flow, through one vertebral artery might occur when the head is turned (Fig. 32-4). To test their theory they perfused the vertebral arteries of cadavers and discovered that when the head was turned to one side and extended slightly, flow through the contralateral vertebral artery ceased, and that the brainstem then depended on blood flow from the other vertebral artery. They suggested that the atlantoaxial joint was the most probable site of vessel compression.

In 1960, Toole and Tucker (1960) cannulated the major neck vessels in 20 cadavers aged newborn to

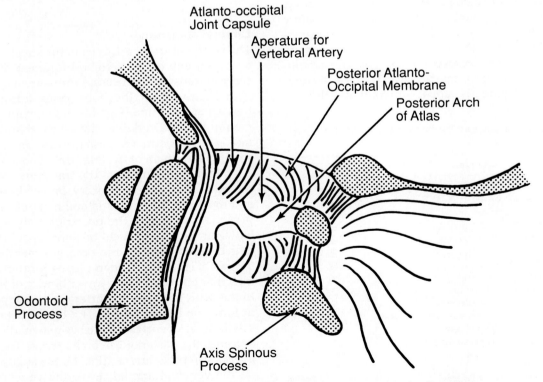

Figure 32-3. Craniovertebral region, viewing laterally from a midsagittal position.

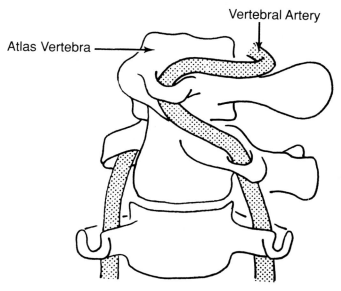

Vertebral Artery

Atlas Vertebra

Figure 32–4. Stretch applied to vertebral artery between atlas and axis vertebrae with contralateral cervical rotation.

78 years within 24 hours of death to study the effect of various head positions on water flow. Flow could be reduced by more than 90% by movements well within the normal range of head motion (Table 32–3). Rotation produced the greatest alteration in flow. Interference with the arterial circulation was more often contralateral to the direction of rotation. Extension alone did not significantly affect the flow, but when rotation was combined with extension, flow in both arteries was affected equally often. They found that rotation to the right occluded the vertebral arter-

ies in 11 cases and the carotid arteries in 8. The same rotation combined with left lateral flexion resulted in no cases of vertebral artery occlusion and only one case of carotid artery occlusion. Left lateral flexion resulted in three cases of vertebral artery occlusion and none of the carotid arteries. These results suggest that lateral flexion causes less stress to the vertebral arteries than does rotation.

Brown and Tatlow (1963) in postmortem angiographic studies found complete occlusion of the contralateral vertebral artery in 17 of 41 cases (41.5%) during neck rotation and extension. During normal daily activities the blood flow in the vertebral arteries fluctuates (Bakay and Sweet, 1953), but symptoms do not occur in healthy individuals due to adequate circulation from the opposite vertebral artery. After invivo occlusion of one vertebral artery proximal to the PICA, Bakay and Sweet (1953), were unable to demonstrate any significant reduction in ipsilateral vertebral and PICA pressure. Further evidence that mere occlusion of one vertebral artery does not usually produce symptoms was evidenced when Falconer (1951) and Elkin and Harris (1946), reported on 11 patients with either intracranial aneurysms or arteriovenous fistulas treated by ligation of one vertebral artery, resulting in only one complication, a Horner's syndrome. Grossman and Davies (1982) described a case demonstrated angiographically of a 19-year-old man in whom 60 degrees of rotation to the right completely occluded the vertebral artery at C1-2, yet the patient was totally asymptomatic.

Occlusion of one vertebral artery does not nec-

TABLE 32–3. OCCLUSION OF ARTERIAL FLOW BY HEAD MOVEMENT IN 20 CASES

1. Rotation < 45 degrees		
	Right Rotation	*Left Rotation*
Left vertebral artery	7 cases [35%]	4 cases [20%]
Right vertebral artery	4 cases [20%]	9 cases [45%]
Left carotid artery	—	5 cases [25%]
Right carotid artery	8 cases [40%]	1 case [5%]
2. Lateral flexion < 30 degrees		
	Right Lateral Flexion	*Left Lateral Flexion*
Left vertebral artery	—	2 cases [10%]
Right vertebral artery	1 case [5%]	1 case [15%]
Left carotid artery	—	—
Right carotid artery	—	—
3. Combined Rotation and Contralateral Flexion		
	Right Rotation	*Left Rotation*
Left vertebral artery	—	
Right vertebral artery		not
Left carotid artery	1 case [5%]	recorded
Right carotid artery	—	

Based on a study of 20 cadavers by Toole JF and Tucker SK. Influence of head position upon cerebral circulation. Arch. Neurol 1960; 2:616–23.

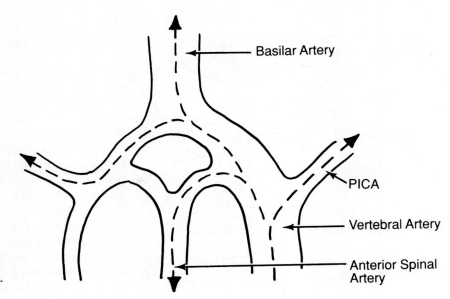

Figure 32–5. Vertebrobasilar blood flow with a stenotic left vertebral artery. PICA = posterior inferior cerebellar artery.

essarily reduce the arterial supply to the posterior fossa via the basilar or posterior cerebellar arteries (Fig. 32–5). It is quite common for one vertebral artery to be much larger than the other, the right usually being the smaller in a significant number of cases. In a study of 180 cadavers (Stopford, 1916), vertebral arteries of unequal size were found in 92% of cases. When one artery is significantly smaller, or if the vertebral artery terminates in the PICA, then occlusion of the larger dominant artery embarrasses blood supply to the brainstem (Husni and Storer, 1966; Andersson et al., 1970; Barton and Margolis, 1975; Fast et al., 1987; Sherman et al., 1987). Support for this is found in Husni and Storer's (1967) study of 23 patients with vertebrovasilar insufficiency induced by occlusion of one vertebral artery through cervical spine rotation. The vertebral artery opposite to the side of rotation was hypoplastic in 22 and narrowed at its origin in one. Hence, it appears that compression of a vertebral artery from rotational occlusion will induce symptoms only if flow in the contralateral vertebral artery is already compromised.

There have been a number of cases where sustained head position during normal activities has produced brainstem ischemic accidents in the absence of SMT (Table 32–4).

Injury Sites

Injury to the vertebral arteries can occur anywhere along their path, by stretching, shearing, or crushing. Various authors postulate that there are eight potential sites in the cervical spine at which arterial structures can be compressed or injured by spinal movement.

1. Between C1-2 transverse processes. The vertebral arteries are relatively fixed at the C-1 and C-2 transverse foramina. Rotation, therefore, tends to produce stretching of the vertebral artery at this site (see Fig 32–4).
2. At the level C2-3 due to compression of the vertebral artery by the superior articular facet of C-3 on the ipsilateral side to head rotation (Brownson et al., 1986) (Fig. 32–6).
3. By the C-1 transverse process compressing the internal carotid artery (Beatty, 1977; Boldrey et al., 1956).

TABLE 32–4. NONMANIPULATIVE VASCULAR ACCIDENTS ASSOCIATED WITH HEAD ROTATION AND/OR EXTENSION

Precipitating Factor	Reported By
Calesthenics	Nagler, 1973
Yoga	Hanus et al., 1977; Nagler, 1973
Turning the head while driving a vehicle	Easton and Sherman, 1977; Sherman et al., 1981; Yang et al., 1985
Overhead work	Okawara and Nibblelink, 1974
Star gazing	Barty, 1983
Archery	Sorenson, 1978
Swimming	Tramo et al., 1985
Neck position while sleeping	Hope et al., 1983
Childbirth	Yates, 1959
Emergency resuscitation	Saternus and Fuchs, 1982
Neck extension for a bleeding nose	Fogelholm and Karli, 1975
Head extension during radiography	Fogelholm and Karli, 1975

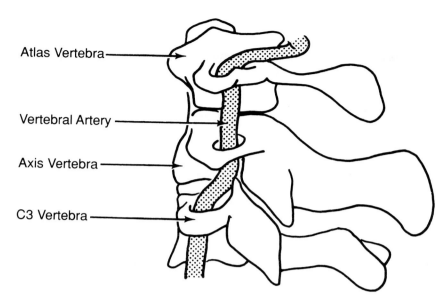

Atlas Vertebra

Vertebral Artery

Axis Vertebra

C3 Vertebra

Figure 32-6. Compression of the vertebral artery by the superior articular facet of C–3 on ipsilateral cervical rotation.

4. At the C4-5 or C5-6, levels due to osteoarthrosis of the uncovertebral joints, which can displace the artery anteriorly and laterally. Compression of the artery is ipsilateral to the side of head rotation (Hutchinson and Yates, 1956; Tissington and Tatlow et al., 1957; Friedenberg et al., 1959; Hardin et al., 1960; Sheehan et al., 1960; Keggi et al., 1966; Fields, 1974; Jackson, 1977; Pasztor, 1978). Fast et al. (1987) described a subintimal tear at the C4–5 level, but this occurred in a 27-year-old woman and osteoarthritic change is unlikely to be the cause.

5. Through compression before entering the C-6 transverse process, by traction over a prominent longus colli muscle (Andersson et al., 1970), or by tissue communicating between the longus colli and scalenus anticus muscles (Husni et al., 1966).

6. By constriction of the vertebral artery by the ventral ramus of the second cervical nerve during head rotation (Tomita et al., 1987).

7. At the atlanto-occipital aperture, on extension (Kleynhans, 1980):
   i. compression between the posterior arch of atlas, and the rim of the foramen magnum, or
   ii. folding of the atlanto-occipital joint capsule (anteriorly), and the atlanto-occipital membrane (posteriorly) (see Fig. 32–3).

8. Through compression by the obliquus capitis inferior muscle or intertransversarius muscle between the two transverse foramina of the C-1 and C-2. The artery can be compressed by either of these muscles between the C-1 and C-2 (Okawara and Nibblelink, 1974).

Although it is theoretically possible that the vertebral artery could be compressed or damaged at all of the above sites as a result of manipulation, such has not been reported at sites 6 to 8, and only one case is known to have occurred at each of sites 4 and 5 (Fast et al., 1987).

Occlusion of the vertebral arteries by lower cervical osteophytes has been reported with rotation of the neck, but has not been considered to be responsible for accidents from SMT. Hardin et al. (1960), described a case of rotation-induced ischemia, in which occlusion was due to an osteophyte between C5–6, and was relieved by surgical removal. Only one case of internal carotid artery injury due to manipulation has been reported (Beatty, 1977). Due to its rarity relative to other more common etiologies, it will not be discussed further in this chapter.

In conclusion, therefore, it appears that it is rotation, either with or without extension, that is mainly responsible for manipulative iatrogenesis. Rotation appears to affect the vertebral arteries mainly in the upper cervical spine. It is important to note that, in most cases, lateral flexion of the neck apparently has little effect on vertebral artery blood flow (Toole and Tucker, 1960; refer to Table 32–1). This should be considered when a rationale for the application of SMT to the upper cervical spine is developed.

Arterial Wall Trauma

The mechanism of injury to the nervous system from a vertebrobasilar accident is brainstem ischemia, which may be due to:

1. Trauma to the arterial wall producing vasospasm, or
2. Trauma to the arterial wall producing damage to the arterial wall.

In trauma to the arterial wall producing vaso-spasm, thrombus formation is dictated by Virchow's triad: (1) change in vessel wall; (2) change in blood flow; and (3) change in blood constituents.

Neck rotation causes the artery to be momentarily compressed or stretched, which may result in spasm (Smith and Estridge, 1962). This may persist only for a short period and produce only temporary symptoms. However, even after the removal of the irritant, the constriction of the vessel may persist with reduction in the blood supply to the irrigated parts, or stagnation of the blood flow within the involved vessel even in the absence of vessel wall injury. The finding of thrombus in the distal vertebrobasilar system (Pratt-Thomas and Berger, 1947; Ford and Clark, 1956; Schwarz et al., 1956; Okawara and Nibblelink, 1974) suggests that the vertebral arteries can be sufficiently compromised (stasis) to initiate a propagating thrombus and subsequent embolism (Kunkle et al., 1952; Grossman and Davies, 1982). Propagation of a thrombus distal to ligation of the vertebral artery has been documented (French and Haines, 1950).

In trauma to the arterial wall producing damage symptoms are due to one of the following mechanisms:

1. Intimal tear. Exposure to the subendothelial tissue leads to the cascade mechanism, resulting in clot formation (thrombosis). Following clotting, the vessel may undergo repair with no further symptoms or it may go into spasm and progress through the changes described above (Fig. 32–7).
2. Intimal tear with embolic formation. If the thrombus extends into the lumen, the blood flow may "break off" part and form an embolus (Fig. 32–8).
3. Vessel wall dissection with subintimal hematoma. Intimal dissection, subintimal hemorrhage, or hematoma may result in exposing the subendothelial tissue and lead to activation of the cascade mechanism, resulting in thrombosis and occlusion of the vessel (Fig. 32–9); or the dissection propagates distally to occlude the PICA (Fig. 32–10).
4. Perivascular bleeding. Blood may break into

Direction of flow

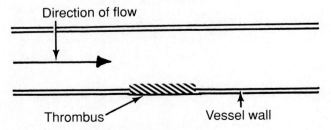

Figure 32–7. Intimal tear.

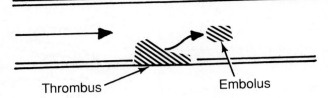

Figure 32–8. Intimal tear with embolic formation.

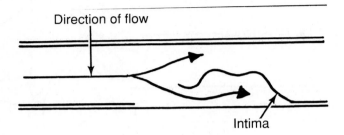

Figure 32–9. Vessel wall dissection.

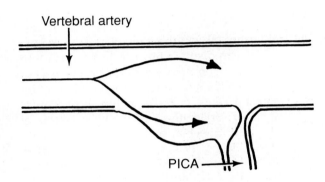

Figure 32–10. Distal propagation occluding the PICA.

the surrounding soft tissue and produce external compression of the vessel resulting in either occlusion of the lumen or turbulence. This turbulence may initiate thrombus formation (Fig. 32–11).

Onset of Signs and Symptoms

The time between the application of SMT and the onset of symptoms and signs can vary from immediately to several days later. The interval is probably related to the mechanism of injury. When ischemia is due to vasoconstriction or embolism, symptoms would be expected immediately, whereas those due to thrombus formation resulting from a vessel wall dissection may only become symptomatic after some time.

A review of cases drawn from the references in this paper revealed 60 in which the time between manipulation and onset of symptoms was given. Analysis showed that:

1. 80% of symptoms arose within the first hour, usually immediately.

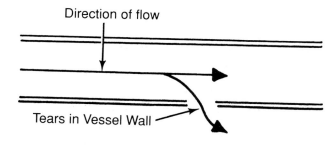

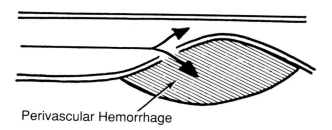

Figure 32-11. Vessel occlusion due to perivascular bleeding.

2. 12% occurred within 1 to 16 hours.
3. 8% occurred during 24 to 48 hours.

Signs and symptoms of brainstem ischemia produced by manipulation usually occur immediately and should be recognized by the practitioner. These include:

1. Dizziness/vertigo (or lightheadedness)
2. Loss of consciousness (syncope, stupor, or coma)
3. Visual problems (diplopia, amaurosis fugax)
4. Nausea and/or vomiting
5. Walking difficulties/incoordination of the extremities/ataxia (falling to one side)
6. Numbness on one side of the body
7. Tinnitus
8. Speech problems, for example, dysarthria
9. Nystagmus

An understanding of the mechanisms involved in the production of ischemic symptoms clearly indicates why the spine should not be remanipulated if signs and symptoms develop after manipulation. There is nothing to be gained by continuing to traumatize an artery already undergoing pathological change. It can only be expected to aggravate the problem.

Syndromes

Postmanipulative symptoms from vascular injury usually result from trauma to the vertebral artery, with resultant ischemia to the brainstem. In many,

these symptoms are transient and rapidly resolved, or there is minimal residual neurological deficit. When serious residual effects occur, the symptoms usually conform to occlusion of the PICA producing the dorsolateral (retro-olivary) medullary syndrome of Wallenberg, or occlusion of the basilar artery, producing the ''locked-in'' syndrome.

The dorsolateral medullary (retro-olivary) syndrome of Wallenberg (Patten, 1977) is usually produced by occlusion of the PICA, but can also be produced by occlusion of the parent vertebral artery (syndrome of Babinski Nageotte). The signs and symptoms are due to the destruction of the nuclei and pathways located in the dorsolateral medulla oblongata (Fig. 32-12). The following structures are involved:

1. Inferior cerebellar peduncle, producing asynergia (ataxia) and hypotonia on the side of lesion
2. Descending spinal tract and nucleus of cranial nerve V, producing loss of pain and temperature on the ipsilateral side of the face and loss of the corneal reflex
3. Ascending lateral spinothalamic tract, producing a loss of pain and temperature on the contralateral trunk and limbs. Involvement of this tract and the trigeminal nerve tract results in an alternating analgesia (Fig. 32-13).
4. Descending sympathetic tract, which results in an ipsilateral Horner's syndrome.
5. Lower vertibular nuclei, producing nystagmus, vertigo, nausea, and/or vomiting
6. Nucleus ambiguous of the glossopharyngeal and vagus nerves, which results in hoarseness, dysphagia, or intractable hiccups.

The acute signs usually disappear within several weeks. Most patients have a significant degree of recovery but often experience residual neurological deficits.

The locked-in syndrome, or cerebromedullospinal disconnection syndrome, (Latchaw et al., 1974; Lyness and Wagman, 1974; Schellhas et al., 1980; Plum and Posner, 1982; Horn, 1983) is produced by occlusion of the midbasilar artery (Fig. 32-14). It was first reported in the medical literature by Plum and Posner (1966) and described as a condition of total consciousness, with or without impaired sensation, and no voluntary movement except vertical eye movement and convergence—''a corpse with living eyes.'' These patients are conscious, paralyzed mutes. It is interesting to read a description of this syndrome, written in 1844 by Alexander Dumas, in the person of M. Noitier de Villafort in the novel *The Count of Monte Cristo* (Dumas, 1844).

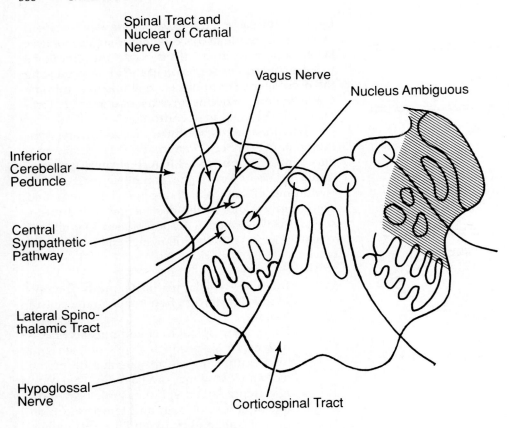

Spinal Tract and Nuclear of Cranial Nerve V

Vagus Nerve

Nucleus Ambiguous

Inferior Cerebellar Peduncle

Central Sympathetic Pathway

Lateral Spino-thalamic Tract

Hypoglossal Nerve

Corticospinal Tract

Figure 32–12. Cross section of the medulla oblongata. *Hatching* indicates area involved in Wallenberg syndrome.

Interference to basilar artery blood flow in the region of the midpons produces bilateral ventral pontine infarction that effectively transects the brainstem at the midpons region (Fig. 32–15). This manifests as:

1. Consciousness is retained because the reticular formation of the midbrain and rostral pons is unaffected, and the electroencephalogram is normal or near normal.
2. Movement of the body is eliminated because the corticospinal tracts are destroyed, with resultant decerebrate rigidity.
3. The nuclei of cranial nerves V to XII are destroyed resulting in their paralysis. The oculomotor nucleus is above the infarcted area, but is paralyzed because its caudal connections to the para-abducens nucleus in the pons and the medial longitudinal fasciculus (MLF) lie in the infarcted region.
4. The sensations carried in the medial lemniscus are lost, but cutaneous sensation may be grossly intact because the lateral spinothalamic tract may be spared due to its lateral position in the brainstem.
5. The patient can still hear because the auditory nerves ascend the brainstem lateral to the infarcted area.
6. The cranial nerve IV nucleus and the supe-

rior colliculus of the quadrigeminal plate are spared, and therefore, the patient is still capable of convergence and upward gaze of the eyes. Using these eye movements, the patient is able to communicate using a code.

This lesion transects the lower ventral pons and is compatible with long-term survival because the medullary vital centers automatically maintain respiratory and cardiovascular function.

Risk Factors and Testing

The most important risk factors to identify in the history are vertigo or ischemic attacks. When present, the questioning should focus on the aggravating factors, such as neck position. It does not appear that any of the other factors (Table 32–5), either alone or in combination, specifically increase susceptibility, as vascular injury does not appear to be related specifically to any age group or sex (Terrett, 1987a). It would be imprudent, however, to totally ignore the presence of one or more significant factors that indicate possible predisposition to accidents.

Screening Procedure
A four-step screening procedure developed by George et al. (1981), includes:

1. Case history
2. Blood pressure measurement
3. Neck auscultation
4. Functional vascular tests

Each of these is briefly described with reference to difficulties with predictability.

Case History

PRESENTING COMPLAINT. A review of the major complaints of patients who subsequently suffered a manipulation-induced vertebrobasilar accident (Table 32–6) reveals little that could alert the astute practitioner as to the impending accident. Most patients presenting with symptoms, such as dizziness, in association with cervical musculoskeletal complaints respond well to SMT.

TRANSIENT ISCHEMIC ATTACKS [TIAs]. When a review of systems reveals transient ischemic symptoms, it strongly suggests the necessity for medical referral and for the exclusion of SMT. If the patient suffers from carotid TIAs including amaurosis fugax (tran-

sient unilateral loss of vision), medical referral is imperative as patients may suffer a complete stroke after only a few episodes (10% in the first 6 months, then 6% a year). Patients with vertebrobasilar TIAs have many attacks before they suffer a stroke (Weiner, 1981). Symptoms due to vertebral artery compromise, such as dizziness, nausea and vomiting, lack of balance, dysarthria, diplopia, dysphagia, and headache, should alert the astute practitioner and may require immediate medical referral (Weiner, 1981).

BRUITS. If, on review of symptoms, a patient states that an audible bruit has developed (which may be associated with symptoms such as headache and neck pain), the patient should not be manipulated, as this may indicate signs of an impending spontaneous dissecting aneurysm (Mas et al., 1985). Medical referral is essential after confirmation.

CONTRACEPTIVES. Women taking oral contraceptives are at a greater risk of vertebrobasilar thrombosis than those not taking contraceptives (Bickerstaff, 1975). However, as the source of the emboli in these cases is not from the vertebral arteries but from the heart or the pulmonary vascular bed (Ask-Upmark

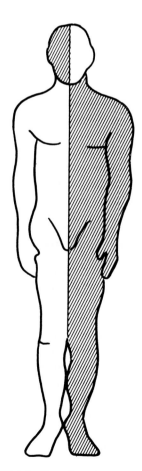

Figure 32–13. Distribution of analgesia (alternating) in Wallenberg syndrome.

TABLE 32–5. PREDISPOSING FACTORS TO VERTEBROBASILAR ISCHEMIA

Osseous factors
    Cervical spine spondylosis
    Osteophytes
    Abnormal bone structure
Injury
    Whiplash
    History of neck sprain
Vascular factors
    History of vertebrobasilar ischemia after head turning or neck extension
    Arteriosclerosis
    Transient ischemic attacks
    Hypertension
    Hypotension
    Cardiovascular disease
    Diabetes
    Medications [e.g., anticoagulants]
Neurological factors
    Headaches
    Visual disorders
    Drop attacks
    Transient weakness in the legs
    Family history of strokes
Women
    Immediately postpartum
    Mid 30s on the pill, especially if a smoker

Adapted from George PE, et al. Identification of the high risk pre-stroke patient. J. Chirop 1981 [Mar]; 15:S26–8; Terrett AGJ. Importance and interpretation of tests designed to predict susceptibility to neurocirculatory accidents from manipulation. J Aust Chiropractors' Assoc 1983 [Aug]; 13[2]:29–34.

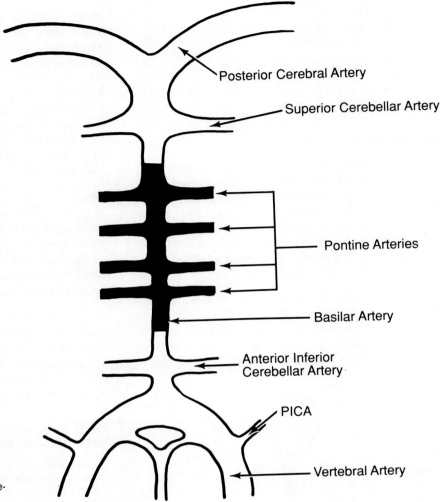

Figure 32–14. Area of the basilar artery (*dark*) involved to produce a "locked-in" syndrome. PICA = posterior inferior cerebellar artery.

and Bickerstaff, 1976), the taking of the contraceptive pill does not predispose to any greater risk of manipulative iatrogenesis.

CIGARETTE SMOKING AND ATHEROSCLEROSIS. Chronic cigarette smoking is known to decrease cerebral artery blood flow in subjects without any other known risk factors for stroke, probably by enhancing cerebral arteriosclerosis (Rogers et al., 1983). In patients with other stroke risk factors, such as hypertension, hyperlipidemia, heart disease, and/or diabetes mellitus, chronic smoking enhances the decrease in cerebral blood flow (Rogers et al., 1983). Although chronic smoking appears to increase the risk of cerebral stroke, it does not appear to increase the risk of vertebrobasilar stroke after SMT; otherwise, such injuries could be expected to be more common in older age groups.

OSTEOARTHRITIS. Osteoarthritis per se does not appear to increase the risk of vertebrobasilar stroke after SMT. If it did then it would be expected that (1) the older age group would be at a significantly greater risk, which they are not (Terrett, 1987a), and (2) osteoarthritis compromise of the vertebral artery would be most likely to occur at the C4-6 spinal levels. Radiographs of elderly patients with a diagnosis of vertebrobasilar insufficiency secondary to cervical spondylosis, when compared to age- and sex-matched controls, failed to demonstrate any difference in the severity of radiographic changes (Adams et al., 1986). "There was no relationship between the extent or severity of radiographic changes and the presence of dizziness, giddiness or falls related to neck movements." It was the investigator's view that radiographs of the cervical spine were of little value, only confirming the high incidence of cervical spondylosis in the elderly (Adams et al., 1986).

In summary, the most important points in the case history appear to be a history of dizziness, nausea, visual disturbances, and/or TIAs after neck rotation and/or extension; or a history of such symptoms after SMT. The importance of asking a person whether turning the neck induces any symptoms was mentioned in one court case as equatable to "if

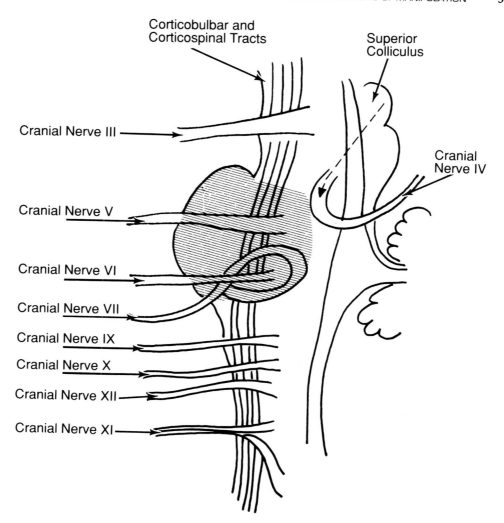

Figure 32–15. Area infarcted (ventral pons) in "locked-in" syndrome.

you are going to give an injection of penicillin you don't do so without asking them if they are allergic to it beforehand'' (Barty, 1983).

Blood Pressure Measurement. The taking of blood pressure bilaterally does not appear to be particularly useful, as the victims are usually young and there is no consistently found hypotension or hypertension among the victims. The taking of blood pressure bilaterally may reveal a subclavian steal syndrome. Although injury after SMT has never been reported to have occurred in any patient suffering from this syndrome, it would appear to be unwise to manipulate the cervical spine of such a patient, as the brainstem is largely dependent on blood flow from only one vertebral artery, and therefore, at greater risk if blood flow is diminished in the normal artery.

Neck Auscultation. Blood flow in the vertebral arteries may be normal in the neutral position, but compromised in the rotated position. It has been suggested (Terrett, 1987b) that if neck vessels are to be auscultated, this should be done in the rotated position. Asymptomatic cervical bruits occur in 4% of the population over age 40 (Chambers and Norris, 1986). Bruits tend to be audible when stenosis reaches about 50%, and they become inaudible if the stenosis exceeds 85 to 95% because of a decrease blood flow (Fields, 1978; Ackerman, 1979; Ginsberg et al., 1979). The reliability of auscultation has been questioned.

Zeigler and co-workers (1971) conducted a study to determine any correlation of bruits with angiographically demonstrated lesions of the carotid arteries. Their conclusion was that the presence of bruits over the carotid artery is a very unreliable indicator of carotid artery disease. Large numbers of stenotic lesions are not detected by ordinary auscultation of the neck. A much smaller number of patients with moderate to loud bruits do not have any demonstrable underlying carotid stenosis or occlusion. Tirone et al. (1978) state that an estimated 65% of

TABLE 32-6. PRESENTING COMPLAINTS OF PATIENTS WHO SUFFERED VERTEBROBASILAR ACCIDENTS

Complaint	Author(s)
Headache	Sherman et al., 1981; Sherman et al., 1987; Zauel and Carlow, 1977; Kanshepolsky et al., 1972; Kunkle et al., 1952; Mueller and Sahs, 1976; Easton and Sherman, 1977; *Foster* v. *Thornton*, 1934; Zimmerman et al., 1978; Krueger and Okazaki, 1980
Neck pain and/or stiffness	Bladin and Merory, 1975; Fritz et al., 1984; Green and Joynt, 1959; Smith and Estridge, 1962; Zak and Carmony, 1984; Braun et al., 1983; Daneshmend et al., 1984; Lennington et al., 1980; Mehalic and Farhat, 1974; Miller and Burton, 1974; Schellhas et al., 1980; Simmons et al., 1982; Wood et al., 1971; Jentzen et al., 1987
Neck and arm pain	Kommerell and Hoyt, 1973
Neck and shoulder pain	Fritz et al., 1984
Headache and neck stiffness and/or pain	Lindy, 1984; Lyness and Wagman, 1974; Mehalic and Farhat, 1974; Parkin et al., 1978; Sherman et al., 1981; *York* v. *Daniels*, 1955; Krueger and Okazaki, 1980
Headache, giddiness, and nausea	Pratt-Thomas and Berger, 1947
Pressure sensation in the back of the neck	Gittinger, 1986
Neck pain and stiffness	Fast et al., 1987; Gorman, 1978
"A catch in the neck"	Krueger and Okazaki, 1980

bruits are associated with stenotic lesions. Increasing prevalence rates of cervical arterial bruits are correlated with increasing age, hypertension, and female gender (Cote and Battista, 1984). In follow-up studies of subjects with asymptomatic bruits, there is a higher risk of death from myocardial infarction, not cerebrovascular disease (Cote and Battista, 1984; Chambers and Norris, 1986).

It must be remembered that the (1) presence of neck bruits is normal in children under age 5 (Demyer, 1980), (2) neck bruits in patients younger than age 40 rarely originate from arterial disease (Chambers and Norris, 1986), and (3) a false-positive bruit may be simply due to compression of a normal artery by a stethoscope bell (Van Allen and Rodnitzky, 1981).

Functional Vascular Tests. There are five variations of the vertebral artery patency tests (Terrett and Webb, 1982; Kleynhans and Terrett, 1985). In all, the patient's head is held for a period in the premanipulative position (e.g., rotation, rotation with extension, and so forth) before thrust and observed for any symptoms and signs of brainstem ischemia. Dizziness is most common and may be unaccompanied by any other symptoms or signs.

Kleynhans and Terrett (1985) consider that the head should be held in the provocative position for up to 40 seconds unless symptoms occur earlier. Personal communication with George (1982) indicated that positive tests will usually appear within 10 seconds (Kleynhans and Terrett, 1985). It has been shown that nystagmus occurring immediately (no latent period) and later decreasing (possibly due to adaptation), is proprioceptive cervical nystagmus. In contrast, nystagmus appearing only after maximal torsion of the neck and a latency period of up to 50 seconds with increasing strength, is vascular cervical nystagmus (Hulse, 1983). If ischemic symptoms do appear, the head should be returned quickly to the neutral position, and any manipulation using that position should be abandoned. It is the authors' practice to hold the patient's head in the premanipulative position on all visits, as it is to be remembered that such accidents do not usually occur on the first visit, but usually by the fifth.

This test, when positive, only indicates that rotation has produced brainstem ischemia, possibly due to either compression of the vertebral artery or vasoconstriction due to irritation of the artery. There are two major problems with the reliability of this procedure as a predictor of vertebrobasilar injury after manipulation:

1. Even if you have a negative test result, an accident may still occur because this test in no way is a predictor as to whether or not a thrust, (which with rotational SMT moves the atlas transverse process further anterior, thereby further stretching the vertebral artery), could damage the vessel wall (See Figure 32-4).

2. There is a problem of false-positive tests (Terrett, 1983), as vertigo and nystagmus of cervical origin are well documented with theories as being related to the stimulation of cervical sympathetics or to cervical muscle and joint receptors (Gayral et al., 1954; Neuwirth, 1955; Weeks and Travell, 1955; Gray, 1956; Stewart, 1962; Biemond, 1969;

Hikosaka and Maeda, 1973; Hinoki and Niki, 1975; Dionne, 1974; deJong, 1977; Maeda, 1979; Liedgren and Odkvist, 1980; Hulse, 1983).

Also, it must be remembered that merely placing the head into the rotated position may induce a stroke (Daneshmend et al., 1984).

Reaction to Manipulation

It has been documented (Terrett, 1987b; Terrett, 1990) that many vertebrobasilar accidents after SMT could have been avoided had the practitioners understood that the symptoms postmanipulation were due to arterial trauma and that further manipulation of an artery already undergoing pathological change would tend to aggravate rather than help the condition.

Symptoms after cervical manipulation, such as fainting and nausea, have been called by Maigne (1972) *sympathetic storms.* Several authors have postulated that irritation of the posterior cervical sympathetic nerves may cause spasm of the vertebrobasilar arteries and their branches (Neuwirth, 1955; Stewart, 1962; Maigne, 1972; Jackson, 1977). Although this is an attractive theory for various head, chest, and arm symptoms, it is not supported by recent research. Bogduk et al. (1981) investigated the neural control of vertebral artery blood flow and found no evidence to support the contention that cervical lesions could affect hindbrain blood flow. They found the vertebral artery blood flow to be profoundly unresponsive to stimulation of any component of the cervical sympathetic system and concluded that the theory that irritation of cervical sympathetic nerves can alter vertebral blood flow is untenable. Therefore, practitioners should be careful before ascribing postmanipulative reactions to sympathetic storms, and be aware that they most likely indicate either alteration of upper cervical proprioceptive input or, more dangerously, brainstem ischemia induced by vascular trauma (Terrett, 1990).

The problem for the practitioner is that dizziness is usually the prominent symptom in both cases and, in the absence of other signs of ischemia, it is not possible to determine the cause. These patients may subsequently respond well to SMT and suffer no ill effect. However, it is suggested that in such cases, because of potentially serious damage, it would be irresponsible to proceed with rotation thrust techniques. It seems to be courting possible disaster, as there are no diagnostic methods available to determine whether the symptoms of ischemia in such cases are due to cervical proprioceptive or sympathetic system stimulation or to arterial vessel wall damage. In these patients other forms of therapy to the upper cervical spine should be used, such as soft tissue therapy, accessory joint play movements, heat, ice, or electrical treatment, with benefit in many instances.

To illustrate that to continue manipulation of the neck after a reaction to previous manipulation or in the presence of signs and symptoms of vertebrobasilar ischemia is irresponsible, 21 detailed case histories have been collected (Terrett, 1990). Of the 21 case histories, 18 were chiropractic, which represents 27% of the documented (not anecdotal) cases (n = 66). Five of these cases died, which represents 38% of the documented cases of death associated with chiropractic (n = 13). Ten cases are discussed briefly below.

Case 1. After a manipulation the patient complained of feeling dizzy. She was again manipulated the following day. The chiropractor took her home in an unconscious state and she died that night (Pratt-Thomas and Berger, 1947; patient #1).

Case 2. The chiropractor manipulated the neck both to the right and to the left. The patient then said several times "I'm falling," but the chiropractor continued to manipulate the neck. The patient died 18 hours later (*York* v. *Daniels*, 1955).

Case 3. After chiropractic treatment the patient felt a sharp discomfort and seconds later intense vertigo and flashes of light all over her visual fields. Within a minute she noted the lower half of her visual fields had "blacked out." She communicated her distress to the practitioner, who, somewhat discomforted by all this, summoned his colleague and he found it all most puzzling and promptly remanipulated the patient's neck. The patient now noted paresthesia in both arms and legs and found her face going numb, especially the right side. Her tongue was clumsy to the extent of rendering her inarticulate and dysphagic. She was dizzy, nauseated, and quite prostrated. She was taken to the hospital. Examination revealed bilateral ptosis, ataxia of the right arm and leg, rotatory nystagmus, and right upgoing plantar response. Angiography revealed a 3- to 4-cm attenuated segment of the right vertebral artery in the C1-2 region. The patient was anticoagulated (Bladin and Merory, 1975).

Case 4. A 7-year-old boy suffered recurrent headaches for 4 months. A course of SMT was initiated. After one treatment session, the child became ill with severe occipital and bifrontal headaches, vomiting, and left facial weakness. A neurologist found no abnormalities the following day. About 2 weeks later, the chiropractor resumed cervical manipulation, which produced severe headaches with intermittent vomiting and diplopia, difficulty with fine movements of left hand (writing), and ataxic gait. Examination revealed a right homonymous superior quadrantanopia, marked right dysmetria, dysdiadochokinesia, an intention tremor, and scanning speech. Diagnosis: traumatic thrombosis of the left vertebral artery with emboli to the basilar, right superior cerebellar and left posterior cerebral arteries (Zimmerman et al., 1978).

Case 5. During the initial treatment, the patient, a 25-year-old man, complained of dizziness. An hour later he was still symptomatic and also complained of headache and nausea. The patient was again manipulated and he suddenly lost consciousness and stopped breathing. The patient died and supportive measures were withdrawn 48 hours later (Krueger and Okazaki, 1980; patient #1).

Case 6. After "gentle" chiropractic manipulation, the patient suffered unsteadiness of gait, numbness on the right side of his face, and feeling "out of control" for a few minutes. One week later, the patient was again treated and several hours later woke with the above symptoms. He returned to bed and awoke the next morning with persistent symptoms. Angiography demonstrated occlusion of the right vertebral artery at C1-2 and a clinical diagnosis of infarction of the right lateral pontomedullary region was made (Braun et al., 1983).

Case 7. A 31-year-old woman developed mild dizziness after SMT. Two days later she was again manipulated with rotation to the right, with extension. Almost immediately she noted instability of gait, a tendency to fall to the right, tinnitus in the right ear, vertigo, and diplopia. A diagnosis of a pontine infarct was made (Fritz et al., 1984).

Case 8. After a rear-end motor vehicle injury, a 34-year-old man suffered persistent headache, dizziness, stiffness and had noted difficulty walking and maintaining balance. He consulted a chiropractor who decided to proceed with SMT, during which he complained of dizziness, nausea, and faintness. Then, he suddenly became unresponsive with stiffening of all extremities and tongue biting. Diagnosis: locked-in syndrome (Horn, 1983).

Case 9. Five years earlier, a 63-year-old hypertensive man had a right-sided cerebral infarct. Four months previously, he had a vertebrobasilar infarct. He consulted a physiotherapist complaining of neck stiffness. SMT consisted of hyperextension and right rotation. He immediately felt dizzy. During the next several hours he developed dysarthria, dysphagia, and paralysis of the left arm and leg. Diagnosis: medullary infarct (Fritz et al., 1984).

Case 10. A 39-year-old man felt dizzy and clammy, and vomited. The following morning a medical practitioner made a house call and prescribed Aspinox and Stemitil and advised him to continue heat treatment and exercise. Later that day, the patient consulted an osteopath, who performed rotatory cervical manipulations with traction. The patient lapsed into a semicomatose state and later

vomited. He was subsequently taken to the hospital, where he died 19 hours later. Diagnosis: cerebellopontine infarction after bilateral dissection of the vertebral arteries (Bolton, 1987).

The injuries and deaths in these cases may well have been avoided had the practitioners concerned simply ceased SMT after the initial symptoms of brainstem ischemia. The actual percentages of chiropractic involvement in these types of cases may well be higher, as the authors in many reports may have failed to identify what type of practitioner carried out the manipulation and whether or not the patient was remanipulated. Another factor that could well reduce the reported prevalence of brainstem ischemia after manipulation is that some cases would seem to be transient and self-remitting.

Risk Reduction

It is apparent that even after performing the relevant case history, physical examination, and vertebrobasilar functional tests, accidents may still occur (Parkin et al., 1978; Lindy, 1984). There is no conclusive, foolproof screening procedure to eliminate patients at risk. Most victims are young, without osseous or vascular pathology, and do not present with vertebrobasilar symptoms. The screening procedures described cannot detect those patients in whom SMT may cause an injury. They give a false sense of security to the practitioner.

Techniques, such as Doppler ultrasound, may be useful in determining the state of arterial blood flow. But all that such a device demonstrates is that there is less flow in an artery (Ginsberg et al., 1979). Fluctuations in vertebral artery blood flow occur continually, without changes to cerebral oxygenation. Such devices, therefore, would appear to be of limited value, for even if there is decreased flow, it cannot predict whether or not a thrust will damage the artery or cause it to go into spasm. Until such time as more reliable screening procedures are developed and readily available, chiropractors can attempt to reduce the incidence of vertebrobasilar ischemia by modifying those techniques that appear to carry the greatest risk.

Of the 126 cases reviewed, the method of manipulation was described in 26 cases. Of these, 81% received neck rotation ("twisted" or "turned") and 19% involved rotation with concomitant longitudinal axis extension ("extended and pulled to the right," "stretch and twist"). It is in the rotated position that the greatest stress to the vertebral artery is imparted. A thrust on the cervical spine to induce further atlantoaxial rotation, which further stretches the artery, therefore, carries the highest risk of causing vascular trauma and should be avoided whenever possible.

The addition of traction to a rotatory manipulation has been considered by some to make the manipulation safer. This is not supported by the study of Brown and Tatlow (1963). Of 41 cadavers (82 vertebral arteries), extension and rotation occluded 5 (6%) vertebral arteries; and when traction was added, another 27 complete occlusions occurred (n = 32) or 39%. All occurred at or above the level of the second cervical vertebrae. None occurred opposite osteophytes and other projections in the midcervical and lower cervical spine.

The authors disagree with Grieve (1986) that this rules out all thrust techniques as dangerous, and that "we should stay our hand until indications for thrust techniques are quite unequivocal." Rotation is the movement most likely to interfere with vertebral artery blood flow, with or without thrust. Lateral flexion has the least effect on blood flow. Therefore, it would appear prudent that those who engage in SMT thrust techniques to the upper cervical spine, use primarily techniques that require either no movement to lock the spinal joints (toggle recoil technique) or that take their tension using lateral flexion (Gonstead, or supine lateral flexion techniques).

Emergency Care

If, even after all precautions have been taken (history, examination, avoiding rotatory-type manipulations), a chiropractor is unfortunate enough to have a patient develop signs of brainstem ischemia (as it may still occur on evaluating cervical range of motion, extension x-rays, or testing for joint end-feel) it would appear advisable to:

1. Cease manipulation: Do not remanipulate the neck. There is nothing to gain from retraumatizing an artery undergoing pathological change, and it may in fact result in disaster.
2. Observe the patient: The symptoms may resolve within a short time.
3. Refer: If the symptoms to not subside, do not panic and remanipulate. If the person's symptoms progress and do not abate, he or she needs to be hospitalized and promptly anticoagulated (Schwarz et al., 1956; Pribek 1963; Latchaw et al., 1974; Easton and Sherman, 1977; Schellhas et al., 1980; Sherman et al., 1981; Brownson et al., 1986; Fast et al., 1987), as this may prevent recurring thromboembolic events. The chiropractor's assistance in describing what happened may be helpful in getting the correct therapy instituted quickly.

Conclusion

This chapter reviewed the mechanisms of vascular injury after SMT to the upper cervical spine. After reviewing the mechanisms and possible predisposing factors, it has been proposed that previously recommended screening procedures are unreliable. Therefore, in the light of the rare disasterous consequences of SMT to the upper cervical spine, until better screening procedures are available, the authors propose that practitioners of SMT alter their techniques to the upper cervical spine to reduce rotation.

After understanding the mechanisms of injury of vascular accidents after upper cervical SMT, practitioners should understand that to further manipulate (traumatize) an artery already undergoing pathological change can only worsen the situation.

References

Ackerman RH. A perspective on noninvasive diagnosis of carotid disease. *Neurology* 1979;29:615–22.

Adams KHR, Yung MW, Lye M, and Whitehouse GH. Are cervical spine radiographs of value in elderly patients with vertebrobasilar insufficiency? *Age and Ageing* 1986;15:57–59.

Andersson R, Carleson R, and Nylen O. Vertebral artery insufficiency and rotational obstruction. *Acta Med Scand* 1970;188:475–477.

Ask-Upmark E, and Bickerstaff ER. Vertebral artery occlusion and oral contraceptives. *Br Med J* 1976;1:487–488.

Attali P. Accidents graves apres une manipulation intempestive par un chiropractor. *Rev Rheum* 1957;24:652.

Bakay L, and Sweet WH. Intra-arterial pressures in the neck and brain. *J Neurosurg* 1953;10:353–359.

Bakewell v Kahle. Medicolegal abstracts. Chiropractors: Rupture of brain tumor following adjustment. *JAMA* 1952;148:699. (See Krueger and Okazaki for discussion of this case 30 years later.)

Barton JW, and Margolis MT. Rotational obstruction of the vertebral artery at the atlantoaxial joint. *Neuroradiol* 1975;9:117–120.

Barty GM. Expert testimony. *Klippel* v *Alchin*. Wagga Wagga, Australia. 12.Aug.1983:33.

Beatty RA. Dissecting hematoma of the internal carotid artery following chiropractic cervical manipulation. *J Trauma* 1977;17(3):248–249.

Bickerstaff ER. *Neurological Complications of Oral Contraceptives.* Oxford Clarendon Press;1975:57–58.

Biemond A. On cervical nystagmus and related disorders. *Brain* 1969;92:437–458.

Biemond A. Thrombosis of the basilar artery and vascularization of the brainstem. *Brain* 1951;74:300.

Bladin PF, and Merory J. Mechanisms in cerebral lesions in trauma to high cervical portion of the vertebral artery—Rotation injury. *Proc Aust Assoc Neurol* 1975;12:35–41.

Bogduk N, Lambert G, and Duckworth JW. The anatomy and physiology of the vertebral nerve in relation to cervical migraine. *Cephalgia* 1981;1:1–14.

Boldrey E, Maass L, and Miller E. The role of atlantoid compression in the etiology of internal carotid thrombosis. *J Neurosurg* 1956;13: 127–139.

Bolton SP. Vascular accidents. *J Australian Chir Asoc* June 1987; 17:75. Case commented on: Terrett AGJ. Vascular accidents. *J Australian Chir Assoc* Sept 1987;17:117.

Boshes LD. Vascular accidents associated with neck manipulations. *JAMA* 1959;171:1602.

Bouchet MM, and Pailler P. Surdite brutale et chiropractie. *Ann Otolaryngol* 1960;77:951–953.

Boudin G, Barbizet J, Pepin B, and Fouet P. Syndrome grave du tronc cerebral apres manipulations cervicales. *Bull Mem Soc Med Hop* 1957;73:562–656.

Braun IF, Pinto RS, and DeFilipp GJ, et al. Brain stem infarction due to chiropractic manipulation of the cervical spine. *Southern Med J* 1983;76:1199–1201.

Brown BSJ, and Tatlow WFT. Radiographic studies of the vertebral arteries in cadavers. *Radiol* 1963;81:80–88.

Brownson RJ, Zollinger WK, Madiera T, and Fell D. Sudden sensorineural hearing loss following manipulation of the cervical spine. *Laryngoscope* 1986;96:166–170.

Carmody E, Buckley P, and Hutchinson M. Basilar artery occlusion following chiropractic cervical manipulation. *Irish Med J* 1987;80:259–260.

Cellerier P, and Georget AM. Dissection des arteres vertebrales apres manipulation du rachis cervical. A propos d'un cas. *J Radiol* 1984;65:191–196.

Chambers BR, and Norris JW. Outcome in patients with asymptomatic neck bruits. *New Eng J Med* 1986;315:860–865.

Cote R, and Battista RN. Asymptomatic cervical bruits. *Can Med Assoc J* 1984;130:997–1000.

Cyriax J. *Textbook of Orthopaedic Medicine*. Vol 1. *Diagnosis of Soft Tissue Lesions*, 7th ed. London: Bailliere Tindall;1978:165.

Dahl A, Bjark P, and Anke I. Cerebrovaskulaere kompliskasjoner til manipulasjonsbehandling av nakken. *Tidsskr Nor Laegeforen* 1982;102:155–157.

Daneshmend TK, Hewer RL, and Bradshaw JR. Acute brain stem stroke during neck manipulation. *Br Med J* 1984;288:189.

Davidson KC, Weiford EC, and Dixon GD. Traumatic vertebral artery pseudoaneurysm following chiropractic manipulation. *Radiology* 1975;115:651–652.

de Jong PTVM. Ataxia and nystagmus induced by injection of local anaesthetic in the neck. *Ann Neurol* 1977;1:240–246.

deKleyn A, and Nieuwenhuyse P. Schwindelanfaelle und Nystagmus bei einer bestimmten Stellung des Kopfes. *Acta Otolaryng* 1927;11:155.

deKleyn A, and Versteegh C. Ueber verschiedene Formen von Menieres Syndrom. *Deutsche Ztschr* 1933;132:157.

Demyer W. *Technique of the Neurologic Examination*, 3rd ed. New York: McGraw-Hill Book Co;1980:9.

Dionne J. Neck torsion nystagmus. *Canad J Otolaryngol* 1974; 3:37–41.

Dumas A. *The Count of Monte Cristo*. Toronto: Bantam Books; 1956:1844, 203–210.

Dunne JW, et al. Dissecting aneurysms of the vertebral arteries following cervical manipulation: A case report. *J Neurol Neurosurg Psychiatry* 1987;50:349–353.

Dvorák J, and Orelli F. How dangerous is manipulation to the cervical spine? *Manual Med* 1985;2:1–4.

Easton JD, and Sherman DG. Cervical manipulation and stroke. *Stroke* Sept–Oct 1977;8:594–597.

Elkin DC, and Harris MH. Arteriovenous aneurysm of the vertebral vessels. Report of ten cases. *Ann Surg* 1946;124:934–949.

Falconer MA. The surgical treatment of bleeding intracranial aneurysms. *J Neurol Neurosurg Psychiatry* 1951;14:153–186.

Faris AA, Poser CM, Wilmore DW, and Agnew CH. Radiologic visualization of neck vessels in healthy men. *Neurol* 1963;13: 386–396.

Fast A, Zinicola DF, and Marin EL. Vertebral artery damage complicating cervical manipulation. *Spine* 1987;12:840–842.

Fields WS. Aortocranial occlusive vascular disease (stroke). *Clinical Symposia* 1974;26:14.

Fields WS. The asymptomatic carotid bruit—Operate or not? *Stroke* 1978;9:269–271.

Fogelholm R, and Karli P. Iatrogenic brainstem infarction. *Eur Neurol* 1975;13: 6–12.

Ford FR. Syncope, vertigo and disturbances of vision resulting from intermittent obstruction of the vertebral arteries due to defect in the odontoid process and excessive mobility of the second cervical vertebra. *Bull John Hopkins Hosp* 1952;91:168–173.

Ford FR, and Clark D. Thrombosis of the basilar artery with softenings in the cerebellum and brain stem due to manipulation of the neck. *Bull John Hopkins Hosp* 1956;98:37–42.

Foster v. *Thornton*. medicolegal abstract. malpractice: death resulting from chiropractic treatment for headache. *JAMA*. 1934; 103:1260.

Malpractice. Cerebral hemorrhage attributed to chiropractic adjustment. *JAMA*. 1935; 105:1714. Malpractice: Death resulting from chiropractic treatment for headache. *JAMA* 1937;109:233–234.

French LA, and Haines GL. Unilateral vertebral artery ligation; report of a case ending fatally with thrombosis of the basilar artery. *J Neurosurg* 1950;7: 156–158.

Friedenberg ZB, Eideken J, Spencer HN, and Tolentino SC. Degenerative changes in the cervical spine. *J Bone Joint Surg* 1959; 41:61–70.

Fritz VU, Maloon A, and Tuch P. Neck manipulation causing stroke. *South African Med J* 1984;66:844–846.

Gayral L, France T, and Neuwirth E. Oto-neuro-ophthalmologic manifestations of cervical origin. Posterior cervical sympathetic syndrome of Barre-Lieou. *New York State J Med* 1954: 1920–1926.

George PE, Silverstein HT, Wallace H, and Marshall M. Identification of the high risk pre-stroke patient. *J Chiropr* 1981;15:S26–28.

Ginsberg MD, Greenwood SA, and Goldberg HI. Noninvasive diagnosis of extracranial cerebrovascular disease. Oculoplethysmography–phonoangiography and directional Doppler ultrasonography. *Neurology* 1979;29:623–631.

Gittinger JW. Occipital infarction following chiropractic cervical manipulation. *J Clinical Neuro-ophthalmology* 1986;6:11–13.

Godlewski S. Dignostic des thromboses vertebro-basilaire. *Assises Med* 1965;23:81–92.

Goodbody RA. Fatal post-traumatic vertebro-basilar ischaemia. *J Clin Pathol* 1976;29:86–87.

Gorman RF. Cardiac arrest after cervical spine mobilization. *Med J Aust* 1978;2:169–170.

Gray LP. Extralabyrinthine vertigo due to cervical muscle lesions. *J Laryngol* 1956;70:352–360.

Green D, and Joynt RJ. Vascular accidents to the brainstem associated with neck manipulations. *JAMA* 1959;170(5):522–524.

Grieve GP. Incidents and accidents of manipulation. In Grieve GP ed. *Modern Manual Therapy of the Vertebral Column*. London: Churchill-Livingstone; 1986;873–884.

Grossman RI, and Davies KR. Positional occlusion of the vertebral artery: A rare cause of embolic stroke. *Neuroradiology* 1982; 23:227–230.

Gutmann G. Verletzungen der arteria vertebralis durch manuelle therapie. *Manuelle Medizin* 1983;21:2–14.

Hanus SH, Homer TD, and Harter DH. Vertebral artery occlusion complicating yoga exercises. *Arch Neurol* 1977;34:574–575.

Hardesty WH, Whitacre WB, and Toole JF, et al. Studies on vertebral artery blood flow in man. *Surg Gynecol Obstet* 1963;662–664.

Hardin CA, Williamson P, and Steegman A. Vertebral artery insufficiency produced by cervical osteoarthritic spurs. *Neurol* 1960;10:855–858.

Hensell V. Neurologische Schaden nach Repositions-massnahmen an der Wirbelsaule. *Med Welt* 1976;27:656–658.

Heyden S. Extra Kraniler thrombotischer Arterienverschlussalsfolge von kopfund halsverletzung. *Mat Med Nordm* 1971; 23:24–32.

Hikosaka O, and Maeda M. Cervical effects on abducens motoneurons and their interaction with the vertibulo-ocular reflex. *Exp Brain Res* 1973;18:512–530.

Hinoki M, and Niki H. Neurological studies in the role of the sympathetic nervous system in the formation of traumatic vertigo of cervical origin. *Acta Otolaryngologica Suppl* 1975;330:185–196.

Hood WP. *On Bone-Setting (so called), and Its Relation to the Treatment of Joints Crippled by Injury Rheumatism, Inflammation.* London: Macmillan;1871:10.

Hope EE, Bodensteiner JB, and Barnes P. Cerebral infarction related to neck position in an adolescent. *Pediatrics* 1983;72:335–337.

Horn SW. The "Locked-In" syndrome following chiropractic manipulation of the cervical spine. *Ann Emerg Med* 1983;12:648–650.

Hosek RS, Schram SB, Silverman H, and Myers JB. Cervical manipulation. *JAMA* 1981;245:922.

Hulse M. Disequilibrium, caused by a functional disturbance of the upper cervical spine. Clinical aspects and differential diagnosis. *Man Med* 1983;1:18–23.

Husni EA, Bell HS, and Storer J. Mechanical occlusion of the vertebral artery. A new clinical concept. *JAMA* 1966;196:101–104.

Husni EA, and Storer J. The syndrome of mechanical occlusion of the vertebral artery: Further observations. *Angiol* 1967;18:106–116.

Hutchinson EC, and Yates PO. Cervical portion of the vertebral artery: Clinicopathological study. *Brain* 1956;79:319–331.

Jackson R. *The Cervical Syndrome*, 4th ed. Springfield: Thomas; 1977:245–246.

Janzen-Humburg R. Schleudertrauma der halswirbelsaule, neurologische probleme. Langenbecks. *Arch Klin Chir* 1966; 316:461–469.

Jentzen JM, Amatuzio J, and Peterson GF. Complications of cervical manipulation: A case report of fatal brainstem infarct with review of the mechanisms and predisposing factors. *J Forensic Sci.* 1987;32:1089–1094.

John Bell. Buried alive. *New Idea* Aug 29, 1987;21.

Kanshepolsky J, Danielson H, and Flynn RE. Vertebral artery insufficiency and cerebellar infarct due to manipulation of the neck. *Bull LA Neurol Soc* 1972;37:62–66.

Katirji MB, Reinmuth OM, and Latchaw RE. Stroke due to vertebral artery injury. *Arch Neurol* 1985;42:242–248.

Keggi KJ, Granger DP, and Southwick WO. Vertebral artery insufficiency secondary to trauma and osteoarthritis of the cervical spine. *Yale J Biol Med* 1966;38:471–478.

Kipp W. Todlicher Hirnstamminfarkt nach HWS-Manipulation (dissertation). Tubingen: Eberhard Karls Universtitaet; 1975:39 (quoted by Ladermann).

Kleynhans AM, and Terrett AGJ. The prevention of complications from spinal manipulative therapy. In Glasgow EF, et al., eds. *Aspects of Manipulative Therapy*, 2nd ed. London: Churchill Livingstone; 1985:161–175.

Kommerell G, and Hoyt WF. Lateropulsion of saccadic eye movements. *Arch Neurol* 1973;28:313–338.

Kosoy J, and Glassman AL. Audiovestibular findings with cervical spine trauma (Case #4). *Tex Med* 1974;70:66–71.

Kramer KH. Wallenburg Syndrom nach manuellerBehandlung. *Manuelle Medizin* 1974;12:88–89.

Krueger BR, and Okazaki H. Vertebral-basilar distribution infarction following chiropractic cervical manipulation. *Mayo Clin Proc* 1980;55:322–332.

Kunkle EC, Muller JC, and Odom GL. Traumatic brain-stem thrombosis: Report of a case and analysis of the mechanism of injury. *Ann Int Med* 1952;36:1329–1335.

Ladermann JP. Accidents of spinal manipulations. *Ann Swiss Chiropractors Assoc* 1981;7:161–208.

Latchaw RE, Seeger JF, and Gabrielsen TO. Vertebrobasilar arterial occlusions in children. *Neuroradiology* 1974;8:141–147.

Lennington R, Laster DW, Moody DM, and Ball MR. Traumatic pseudoaneurysm of ascending cervical artery in neurofibromatosis: Complication of chiropractic manipulation. *Am J Neuroradiol* 1980;1:269–270.

Liedgren C, and Odkvist L. The morphological and physiological basis for vertigo of cervical origin. In Claussen C, ed. *Differential Diagnosis of Vertigo.* Proceedings of the 6th scientific meetings of the NES, Finland 1979. New York: Walter de Gruyter; 1980:567–587.

Lindy DR. Patient collapse following cervical manipulation: A case report. *Br Osteopathic J* 1984;16:84–85.

Lorenz R, and Vogelsang HG. Thrombose der arteria basilaris nach chiropraktischen Manipulationen an der Halswirbelsaule. *Deutsche Med Wochenschrift* 1972;97:36–43.

Lyness SS, and Wagman AD. Neurological deficit following cervical manipulation. *Surg Neurol* 1974;2:121–124.

Maeda M. Neck influences on the vestibulo-ocular reflex arc and the vestibulocerebellum. *Prog Brain Res* 1979;50:551–559.

Maigne R. *Orthopedic Medicine. A New Approach to Vertebral Manipulations.* Springfield, Ill: Thomas; 1972:155, 169.

Martin H, and Guiral J. Surdite brusque au cours d'une manipulation vertebrale. *J Franc ORL* 1960;9:177–178.

Mas JL, Goeau C, and Bousser MG, et al. Spontaneous dissecting aneurysms of the internal carotid and vertebral arteries—Two case reports. *Stroke* 1985;16:125–129.

Masson M, and Cambier J. Insuffisance circulatoire vertebrobasilaire. *Presse Medicale* 1962;70:1990–1993.

Mehalic T, and Farhat SM. Vertebral artery injury from chiropractic manipulation of the neck. *Surg Neurol* 1974;2:125–129.

Meyermann R. Moglichkeiten einer schadigung der arteria vertebralis. *Mannuelle Medizin* 1982;20:105–114.

Miglets AS. Discussion in: Brownson RJ, Zollinger WK, Madiera T, Fell D. *Laryngoscope* 1986;96:170.

Miller RG, and Burton R. Stroke following chiropractic manipulation of the spine. *JAMA* 1974;229:189–190.

Mueller S, and Sahs AL. Brain stem dysfunction related to cervical manipulation. *Neurology* 1976;26:547–560.

Nagler W. Vertebral artery obstruction by hyperextension of the neck: Report of three cases. *Arch Phys Med Rehabil* 1973;54:237–240.

Neuwirth E. The vertebral nerve in the posterior cervical syndrome. *New York State J Med* 1955;55:1380.

Nick J, Contamin F, and Nicolle MH, et al. Incidents et accidents neurologiques dus aux manipulations cervicales: A propos de trois observations. *Bull Mem Soc Med Hop* 1967;118:435–440.

Nielsen AA. Cerebrovaskulaere insulter forarsaget af manipulation af columna cervicalis. *Ugeskr Lager* 1984;3267–3270.

Nyberg-Hansen R, Loken AC, and Tenstad O. Brainstem lesion with coma for five years following manipulation of the cervical spine. *J Neurol* 1978;218:97–105.

Okawara S, and Nibblelink D. Vertebral artery occlusion following hyperextension and rotation of the head. *Stroke* 1974;5:640–642.

Pamela F, Beaugerie L, and Couturier M, et al. Syndrome de deefferentiation motrice par thrombose du tronc basilaire apres manipulation vertebrale. *Presse Medicale* 1983;12:1548.

Parkin PJ, Wallis WE, and Wilson JL. Vertebral artery occlusion following manipulation of the neck. *NZ Med J* 1978;88:441–443.

Pasztor E. Decompression of the vertebral artery in cases of cervical spondylosis. *Surg Neurol* 1978;9:371–737.

Patten J. *Neurological Differential Diagnosis.* London: Harold Starke Ltd.; 1977:108–118.

Plum F, and Posner JB. *The Diagnosis of Stupor and Coma*, 3rd ed. Philadelphia: FA Davis Co.; 1982: 9.

Povlsen UJ, Kjaer L, and Arlien-Soborg P. Locked-in syndrome following cervical manipulation. *Acta Neurol Scand* 1987;76:486–488.

Pratt-Thomas HR, and Berger KE. Cerebellar and spinal injuries after chiropractic manipulation. *JAMA* 1947;133:600–603.

Pribek RA. Brainstem vascular accident following neck manipulation. *Wisc Med J* 1963;62:141–143.

Roberts JB. Fracture dislocation of the atlas without symptoms of spinal cord injury. *Ann Surg* 1907;45:632–635.

Roche L, et al. Lesions traumatiques de la colonne cervicale et attaintes de l'artere vertebrale. Responsabilite d'une examen medical. *Ann Med Leg* 1963;43:232–235.

Rogers RL, Meyer JS, and Shaw TG, et al. Cigarette smoking decreases cerebral blood flow suggesting increased risk for stroke. *JAMA* 1983;250:2796–2800.

Saternus KS, and Fuchs V. Is the arteria vertebralis endangered in resuscitation? *Manelle Medizin* 1982;20:101–104.

Scatliff JH, Hyde L, and Gautot HJ. Vertebral artery reflux: a laboratory investigation of the non-obstructive cases of retrograde flow of constant material in the contralateral vertebral artery. *Radiology* 1967;88:64.

Schellhas KP, Latchaw RE, Wendling LR, and Gold LHA. Vertebrobasilar injuries following cervical manipulation. *JAMA* 1980;244:1450–1453.

Schmitt HP, and Tamaska L. Disseziierende Ruptur der arteria vertebralis mit todlichem vertebralis und basilaris-Verschluss. *Z Rechtsmedizin* 1973;73:301–308.

Schmitt HP. Manuelle therapie der halswirbelsaule. *Zeitschrift fur Allgemeinmedizine* 1978;54:467–474.

Schmitt HP. Rupturen und thrombosen der arteria vertebralis nach gedeckten mechanischen insulten. *Schweizer Archiv fur Neurologie Neurochirurgie und Psychiatrie* 1976;119:363–369.

Schwarz GA, Geiger JK, and Spano AV. Posterior inferior cerebellar artery syndrome of Wallenberg after chiropractic manipulation. *Arch Intern Med* 1956;97:352–354.

Selecki BR. The effects of rotation of the atlas on the axis: Experimental work. *Med J Aust* 1969;1012–1015.

Sheehan S, Bauer RB, and Meyer JS. Vertebral artery compression in cervical spondylosis. *Neurology* 1960;10:968–986.

Sherman DG, Hart RG, and Easton JD. Abrupt change in head position and cerebral infarction. *Stroke* 1981;12:2–6.

Sherman MR, Smialek JE, and Zane WE. Pathogenesis of vertebral artery occlusion following cervical spine manipulation. *Arch Pathol Lab Med* 1987;111:851–853.

Simmons KC, Soo YS, Walker G, and Harvey P. Trauma to the vertebral artery related to neck manipulation. *Med J Aust* 1982; 1:187–188.

Smith RA, and Estridge MN. Neurologic complications of head and neck manipulations. *JAMA* 1962;182:528–531.

Sorensen BF. Bow hunter's stroke. *Neurosurg* 1978;2:259–261.

Stewart DY. Current concepts of "Barre Syndrome" or the posterior cervical sympathetic syndrome. *Clin Ortho Rel Res* 1962; 24:40–48.

Stopford JSB. The arteries of the pons and medulla oblongata. *J Anat* 1916;50:131–164.

Taylor HH. Letter to the editor. *J Chiropr* 1981;11–12.

Terrett AGJ, and Webb MN. Vertebrobasilar accidents following cervical spine adjustment/manipulation. *J Aust Chiropractors Assoc* 1982;12:24–27.

Terrett AGJ. Importance and interpretation of tests designed to predict susceptibility to neurocirculatory accidents from manipulation. *J Aust Chiropractors' Assoc* 1983;13:29–34.

Terrett AGJ. Vascular accidents from cervical spine manipulation: Report on 107 cases. *J Aust Chiropractors' Assoc* 1987a; 17:15–24. Reprinted in *J Chirop* 1988;25:63–72.

Terrett AGJ. Vascular accidents from cervical spine manipulation: The mechanisms. *J Australian Chiro Assoc* 1987b; 17:131–144. Reprinted in *J Chiropr* 1988;22:59–74.

Terrett AGJ. It is more important to know when not to adjust. *Chiropractic Technique* 1990;2:1–9.

Tirone ED, Humphries AW, Young JR, and Beven EG. A correlation of neck bruits and arteriosclerotic carotid arteries. *Arch Surg* 1973;107:729–733.

Tissington Tatlow WF, and Bammer HG. Syndrome of vertebral artery compression. *Neurol* 1957;7:331–340.

Tomita K, Tsuchiya H, and Nomura S. Dynamic entrapment of the vertebral artery by the nerve branch: A new etiology for transient cervical vertigo. *Neuro-orthop* 1987;4:36–43.

Toole JF, and Tucker SH. Influence of head position upon cerebral circulation. Studies in blood flow in cadavers. *Arch Neurol* 1960; 2:616–623.

Tramo MJ, Hainline B, and Petito F, et al. Vertebral artery injury and cerebellar stroke while swimming: A case report. *Stroke* 1985;16:1039–1042.

Van Allen MW, and Rodnitsky RL. *Pictorial Manual of Neurologic Tests*, 2nd ed. Chicago: Year Book Medical Pub; 1981:17.

Weeks VD, and Travell J. Postural vertigo due to trigger areas in the sternocleidomastoid muscle. *J Pediatr* 1955;47:315–327.

Weiner HL. Transient ischemic attacks, when do they foreshadow a stroke? *Diagnosis* 1981;51–57.

Weintraub MI. Dormant foramen magnum meningioma "activated" by chiropractic manipulation. *NY State J Med* 1983; 83:1039–1040.

Wood MJ, Lang EK, Faludi HK, and Woolhandler GJ. Traumatic vertebral artery thrombosis. *J Louisiana Med Soc* 1971;123:413–414.

Yang PJ, Latack JT, and Gabrielson TO, et al. Rotational vertebral artery occlusion at C1–C2. *AJNR* 1985;6:98–100.

Yates PO. Birth trauma to the vertebral arteries. *Arch Dis Child* 1959;34:436–441.

York v. Daniels. Medicolegal abstracts. Chiropractors: injury to spinal meninges during adjustments. *JAMA* 1955;159:809.

Zak SM, and Carmody RF. Cerebellar infarction from chiropractic neck manipulation: Case report and review of the literature. *Ariz Med* 1984;41:333–337.

Zauel D, and Carlow TJ. Internuclear ophthalmoplegia following cervical manipulation. *Ann Neurol* 1977;1:308.

Zeigler DK, Zeleli T, Dick A, and Sebaugh JL. Correlation of bruits over the carotid artery with angiographically demonstrated lesions. *Neurology* 1971;21:860–865.

Zimmerman AW, Kumar AJ, Gadoth N, and Hodges FJ. Traumatic vertebrobasilar occlusive disease in childhood. *Neurology* 1978;28:185–188.

Chiropractic Growth Outside North America

Christine M. Tamulaitis
Gary A. Auerbach
Mary Ann Chance
Louis Gaucher-Peslherbe
Reginald V. Engelbrecht
Kazuyoshi Takeyachi

The World Health Organization (WHO) divides the world's nations into six regions: the Americas, Africa, Europe, Eastern Mediterranean, Pacific and Asia. Demographic and ethnic similarities within each region pose similar problems and solutions. As the general health concerns of the world's nations are studied by WHO, the world's chiropractic interests are represented by the World Federation of Chiropractic (WFC), an international body representing all national chiropractic associations.

This appendix contains a brief overview of each country where chiropractic is known to be practiced. They are listed in alphabetical order within each region. Special thanks is given to the *FACTS Bulletin,* a publication of FACTS (the Foundation for the Advancement of Chiropractic Tenets and Science) from which much of this information is made available.

Africa*

Africa is the second largest continent after Asia, covering nearly 12 million square miles, yet there are scarcely 200 chiropractors on the entire continent. There are singular practices in Ethiopia, Kenya, Nigeria and Namibia, some of these being chiropractic practices operated by Christian missionaries. There is relatively scant information about chiropractic in many of these African nations.

The most dramatic inroads in the development of chiropractic legislation have taken place in the southern parts of the continent, in Zimbabwe, Namibia and in South Africa.

*We gratefully acknowledge the assistance provided by Reginald V. Engelbrecht, DC, in the preparation of this section.

Ethiopia

There are two chiropractors in Ethiopia. One is located in the capital city of Addis Ababa. In addition to his private practice, he is an administrator of a redevelopment program for the famine-stricken area. The other chiropractor has a private practice in Nazareth and is also an administrator of a multi-service health center.

Although there is no chiropractic legislation, chiropractic pioneers have practiced in Ethiopia intermittently since the 1950s. The first to do so were Drs. Robert and Hazel Thompson. Through their efforts and with scholarship assistance provided by the Christian Chiropractors' Association, the two Ethiopian citizens, graduates of Palmer College of Chiropractic, have busy practices.

The practice of chiropractic has been tolerated, although since the dethronement of the Salassie regime in 1974, the now ruling communist government has been less tolerant of all nonlegislated professions.

(From information provided by the Rev. Ron Murphy, executive director, Christian Chiropractors' Association.)

Kenya

There are five chiropractors practicing in the capital city of Nairobi: three are African nationals, one is an American, and one is an Asian.

There is no chiropractic law, nor is there a licensing or regulation process. There is little government interference in chiropractic practice. Non-nationals in all professions must obtain a work permit.

Public awareness is scant, though local media coverage of some of the work done by chiropractors has helped spur interest in chiropractic health care.

Scholarship and missionary funding by the Christian Chiropractors' Association has helped place one practitioner in Nairobi.

(From information provided by Lucille Chevrefils, DC, of Nairobi, Kenya, and from the Rev. Ron Murphy of the Christian Chiropractors' Association.)

Nigeria

There is no registration or licensure of chiropractic in Nigeria. Three chiropractors serve a population of 85 million people. Due to the lack of practitioners, chiropractic is not well known here.

In 1983 a study entitled "Chiropractic Overview" was submitted to the Ministry of Health and its Medical Council. There were no public hearings on the report and no action was ever taken. The Medical Council has publicly opposed legalizing all healing arts, including chiropractic. There are many unlicensed, nonmedical healers including acupuncturists, homeopaths, and bonesetters.

One Nigerian who has been successful in gaining employment with a state government office, has been asked to set up a chiropractic department in one of the state hospitals.

(From information provided by Edet Ekwere, DC, of Cross River State, Nigeria.)

Namibia

Namibia was recently declared independent from South Africa; however, chiropractic practice laws in this country were developed under the same laws as in South Africa. One chiropractor is in practice and has actively worked for greater professional parity and to recruit students for enrollment in chiropractic colleges.

Chiropractic has been legally recognized here since 1971. In 1981, the South African Associated Health Service Professional Board was created by statute to regulate chiropractic and homeopathy. It has parity with the Medical Board which governs the practice of medicine.

In 1985, by an act of the South African Parliament, the chiropractic register is now open, after being closed for 14 years.

(From information provided by Athol McLean, DC, of Windhoek, Namibia)

South Africa

The South African Medical and Dental Act was passed in 1928. Because chiropractic was a relatively unknown profession in these early years, chiropractic was not included under this act. Early records indicate that there were four or five chiropractors practicing in South Africa in the early 1900s; all were graduates of North American chiropractic institutions.

By 1960, the profession had grown considerably and chiropractic doctors began to seek legislative recognition. In 1962, a bill to legislate chiropractic was introduced into parliament and a commission of inquiry was appointed to review the request. No chiropractic experts were consulted, nor were any chiropractic institutions visited and the medically oriented commission's report was entirely negative in its findings. The Minister of Health did not act on the commission's recommendations, and tabled the report.

In 1970, another attempt was made to gain chiropractic legislation. Although a new Minister of Health based his findings on the previous report and recommended denial, lobbying, with active support from the profession and patients, resulted in the passing of Act 76 of 1971, better known as the Chiropractors Act.

While the Act granted recognition to qualified chiropractors, it also, in effect, froze the profession by not allowing any additional chiropractors to register and practice in South Africa. The medical and dental associations considered the Act a triumph, for they firmly believed the profession would eventually phase itself out.

The Chiropractic Association of South Africa, while not pleased with some portions of the Act, favored its passage because it granted the profession a degree of legal recognition, and recognized the Chiropractic Association as the official body representing the profession.

Further good resulted from the legislation when the Minister of Health refused to grant the profession any further recognition until it "spoke with one voice". Thus, South African chiropractors, forced to set aside ideological differences united under the banner of the Chiropractic Association of South Africa.

In February 1977, after discussions with the Department of Health, the association was given the task of answering to the negative 1962 Report. The subsequent *Memorandum on the Developments within the Profession* and the *Rebuttal to the 1962 Report* required two years of development and substantial financial commitment on the part of the Chiropractic Association.

In the interim, the chiropractic profession had reached a critical stage: of the 176 chiropractors registered under the Chiropractic Act, only 102 remained in active practice, due in part to retirement or emigration.

In 1980, the Association was granted a meeting with the Minister of Health, during which the Association stressed the importance of legislation enforcing their ethical rules, and of the opening of the register to allow for new, incoming chiropractic doctors. The Minister reviewed the situation sympathetically, and the ethical rules were enforced.

Health disciplines such as homeopathy, osteopathy and naturopathy continue to seek legal recognition. After some debate, the minister proposed the establishment of a council to exercise strict control over various health disciplines not covered under the Medical and Dental Act of 1928. The council was named the South African Associated Health Professions Board, and with its establishment in 1982, chiropractic at last gained statutory recognition. The council is made up of five chiropractors, three homeopaths, two medical practitioners, one osteopath, one naturopath, one legal counsel and one educator—all elected for five-year terms.

In 1984, a delegation of the council toured Europe and the United States and upon their return recommended standards in keeping with the U.S. Council on Chiropractic Education standards for education and licensure.

An Amendment Bill to reopen the chiropractic register was passed on June 7th, 1985, and the profession turned its course towards establishing an associated health profession's educational program in South Africa. After discussions with many Universities and Technikons (Institutes of Technology), the facilities of the Technikon Natal in Durban were selected. An advisory committee made up of representatives of the Technikon, the South African Associated Health Services Profession Board and representatives of the respective health professions met to draw up an instructional program.

In 1987, the proposed curriculum was approved by the Universities and Technikons Advisory Committee and the Health Minister officially approved the training program as part of the National Tertiary Education System, which would entitle the course to government subsidies.

The first course in chiropractic at Technikon Natal commenced on January, 1989. The Technikon Natal is motivated towards increasing the numbers of registered chiropractors in the country and is actively seeking qualified applicants. It is a multiracial facility.

Currently there are 140 registered chiropractic doctors in South Africa, serving a population of 44 million.

(From information provided by Reginald V. Englebrecht, DC.)

Zimbabwe

Chiropractic was introduced to Zimbabwe (formerly the British colony of Rhodesia) when Dr. A. Scott, a Palmer School of Chiropractic graduate, established a practice in 1932. Through the years more chiropractors settled and conducted successful practices in the country. Prior to declaring its independence in 1980, when the state of Zimbabwe was founded, there were 17 chiropractors scattered throughout the country. Since the country's independence, the number of practicing chiropractors has dwindled to five. Drs. Howat and Henderson have practiced in the country since 1938 and 1939 respectively, though Dr. Howat recently emigrated to the United Kingdom.

Chiropractic is recognized in Zimbabwe by an Act of Parliament and is governed by a Chiropractors' Council. The council is made up of three elected chiropractors and two members appointed by the government. The Act allows the chiropractor to manipulate the spine, pelvis or limbs, take x-rays and use modalities normally associated with the profession.

All chiropractors must be registered with the Chiropractors' Council in order to practice in Zimbabwe. A registrant must be a graduate of one of a dozen accredited chiropractic colleges, and be in possession of an American or Canadian state or national board qualification.

The Chiropractors Association of Zimbabwe (formerly of Rhodesia) was formally established in 1969.

Chiropractors use standard techniques, including x-ray and some also use physiotherapy. Most health insurers, including Workmens' Compensation, Medicaid, and the national army and air force, pay for chiropractic services.

Chiropractic is well accepted, but used almost exclusively by the white population. Traditional healers service much of the African population.

(From information provided by the Chiropractors' Association of Zimbabwe.)

EUROPE*

In most European nations, the right to practice a profession is granted under one of two legal environments: those countries governed by common law allow the practice of a profession as long as there is no law against it, while countries governed by Napoleanic Law (or Roman Dutch Law) deems that any professional practice not legislated is, in fact, illegal.

As a general rule, northern European countries

*We gratefully acknowledge the assistance provided by Pierre Louis Gaucher-Peslherbe, DC, PhD, in the preparation of this section.

are governed by common law, while central and southern European countries are legislated by Napoleanic or Roman Dutch Law.

Belgium

The Belgian Chiropractors' Association (BCA) was formed in 1932, and in 1945 it gained legal recognition as a professional association. The association is affiliated with the European Chiropractors' Union, and represents 78 Belgian chiropractors.

Chiropractic is not a registered profession in Belgium. Professions are governed under Napoleonic Code, which states that a profession not legislated is illegal. Further, a 1967 medical bill states that primary health physicians include only medical doctors, dentists and pharmacists. Belgian chiropractors continue to face numerous legal challenges on the basis that chiropractic is an illegal practice of medicine.

The BCA is actively committed to gaining full recognition for chiropractors as primary health care physicians and has undertaken numerous legal challenges on behalf of its members. Since 1973, there has been intermittent interrogation of chiropractors by authorities, resulting in 28 lawsuits filed against chiropractors. With the help of the BCA, the chiropractors have won all of these lawsuits.

Belgian chiropractors are, for the most part, a tolerated illegal profession. They may not take x-rays, but have access to films from some doctors, hospitals, and clinics. They are not included in any national health insurance program, though many private and company insurance plans cover chiropractic health care.

In 1983, the Consumers' Union of Belgium released their findings of a large survey of the population regarding alternative health care. The study found that a large majority had seen a practitioner of alternative health care (chiropractic, acupuncture and homeopathy) and that approximately 28 percent of the population were more satisfied with alternative health care providers than with providers of traditional medicine.

In 1984, the Council of Europe, a bipartisan union of 18 European nations, released the findings of its study "Legal Status of Nonconventional Medicine." The study concluded that compared to other health providers, chiropractic is a well-defined profession; that its standards of training exceed other alternative health care professions and are equivalent qualitatively to medical training.

Twice yearly, the Belgian Chiropractors' Association presents a scientific postgraduate program; attendance is compulsory for all association members.

(From information provided by the Belgian Chiropractors' Association.)

Denmark

The first Danish chiropractor established a practice in Copenhagen in 1920. Five years later, in 1925, the Danish Chiropractors' Association was founded. A lay organization, the Danish Pro Chiropractic Association, was established the same year. The two organizations have collaborated on many fronts, enabling chiropractic to flourish into a highly recognized and growing profession.

Although chiropractic legislation has been requested during the past 50 years, no law exists to protect or restrict the practice of chiropractic; however, the 229 Danish chiropractors practice legally under common law which allows any professional to practice as long as there is no law that prohibits that practice. Also, Danish medical law recognizes the treatment of the sick by persons other than medical doctors.

There are no government requirements for practice. The Danish Chiropractic Association has professional, ethical, and educational requirements for the membership, providing some self-regulation of the profession. For example, one of the association's requirements is for a mandatory six-month internship as a prerequisite to establishing private practice.

In 1970, a government commission to examine chiropractic produced favorable conclusions and chiropractic was included, on a trial basis, in the National Health System. In 1978, the Danish Parliament voted for permanent inclusion in its public insurance law.

Federal reimbursements now provide for partial payment of chiropractic services, contingent upon membership in the Danish Chiropractors' Association. A number of private, union and company insurance plans also reimburse for chiropractic care.

The Danish Chiropractors' Association continues to strive for chiropractic authorization, which would provide for a more equitable reimbursement for chiropractic care.

The Odense University of Denmark has a pre-chiropractic curriculum which has received accreditation from the US Council on Chiropractic Education.

(From information provided by the Danish Chiropractors' Association)

Finland

Twelve chiropractors practice in Finland and are represented by the Finnish Chiropractic Union, established in 1977. While many are US chiropractic college graduates, the last six to enter practice are from the Anglo-European College of Chiropractic. The profession will see greater growth when ten Finnish students at the AECC college return to practice.

There is no chiropractic legislation and no state reimbursement for chiropractic. Chiropractors are but one of many unlicensed health providers and, as such, chiropractors do not face legal challenges. There is one chiropractic x-ray clinic, which is operated by a medical radiologist.

There are many lay manipulators, and because there is no registration of the chiropractic profession, the title ''chiropractor'' is, in many cases, used indiscriminately by unqualified practitioners. Medical doctors, physiotherapists, and naprapaths attend courses on manipulation and use it to some degree in their practices. More than 60 naprapaths practice in Finland. They are well organized, and are close to getting some form of legal recognition. They are already included in the national health insurance program on the condition of a medical referral.

The Finnish Chiropractic Union continues its work to have chiropractors legislated as primary health care providers.

(From information provided by the Finnish Chiropractic Union.)

France

No chiropractic law governs chiropractic practice in France. France is governed under Napoleonic Code, which states that a profession not legislated is illegal. For most of the 300 qualified chiropractors practicing in France this situation has resulted in intermittent harrassment. The lack of legislation has allowed numerous other practitioners to practice manipulation and call themselves chiropractors. As such, more than 600 persons who have not graduated from a chiropractic college also practice as ''chiropractors.''

The French medical community is particularly powerful and has been successful in enacting laws to restrict chiropractors from practice. A 1953 decree recognized chiropractic, but only as a means to ban chiropractors from practicing it. The decree affirms that sciences and therapies must be taught in medical universities in order to gain government recognition. In 1962, the ban was further strengthened by an order of the French Minister of Health, which restricted chiropractic practice to registered doctors of medicine. Due to this combination of legal devices, chiropractors have lost all major court battles. Some chiropractors have recently received fines of 25,000 francs ($8,000 US).

Many French medical doctors have incorporated manipulation into their practices. A three-year, 300-hour degree course in manipulation has been offered to medical doctors since 1982. While there is a national health plan (*securite social*), chiropractors are not reimbursed. Some private insurance companies provide limited reimbursements for care provided by

chiropractors. Manipulation performed by medical doctors is a therapy covered by some insurance companies.

The largest French chiropractic association, with a membership of 150, is the *Association National Francaise de Chiropractic* (ANFC), an affiliate of the European Chiropractors' Union. There are one or two opposition groups having memberships under 50, and defending different aspects of chiropractic philosophy.

The *Institute de Francaise de Chiropractic*, established in 1984, offers a six-year curriculum in chiropractic education leading to a doctorate in chiropractic. The sixth year, a requirement added in October, 1989, includes internship, paid assistantship, and completion of a research paper to be defended before an educational jury. The six-year curriculum includes one-year preparatory program at the *Propedeutique J Janse*. Established in 1979, the preparatory program has been approved by the US Council on Chiropractic Education. Entrance requirements for the French Chiropractic Institute are similar to those required for entrance into CCE-recognized colleges in the United States.

The ANFC continues to work for recognition. The French government has issued statements that it will not consider the recognition of chiropractic as an independent, primary contact profession, until there is an established institute of chiropractic in France. With the French chiropractic institute now firmly established, there is renewed hope for the eventual passage of chiropractic legislation.

While chiropractors are the only group of health providers with extensive education in specific adjusting techniques, bony manipulation is provided by thousands of others. The largest of the groups is the osteopaths, numbering approximately 3000. While an osteopathic diploma requires three years of education, most of the self-proclaimed ''osteopaths'' are physical therapists who have accumulated study in weekend courses in osteopathic techniques.

A second group is the etiopaths, numbering a few hundred. They resemble the osteopaths, but have incorporated many chiropractic techniques into their practice.

A third group is the medical manipulators, who, by virtue of their political power, have been able to claim manipulative practice as their own. Those using manipulation range from practitioners who have read a few books to those who have attended the large numbers of seminars on manipulation.

A fourth group are the traditional bonesetters, known as *rebouteux, rebouteurs* or *rabilleurs*. They are at least as numerous as the chiropractors. They are usually considered as having been born with the ''gift'' of bonesetting.

(From information provided by *Association National Francaise de Chiropractic*.)

Great Britain

Chiropractors in the United Kingdom practice legally under common law. Common law grants chiropractors the right of practice without the statuatory privilege of licensure or registration. Since there is no government mechanism to prove professional and educational qualifications for chiropractic practice, the British Chiropractic Association (BCA) sets its own educational and ethical requirements for membership. The association continues active pursuit of government registration.

Since chiropractic is not a registered health profession, it is not included in the country's National Health Service, a comprehensive social health insurance program which also determines eligibility for federal reimbursement. This exclusion is cause for the vast under-use of chiropractic health care. The only other major health profession excluded from the NHS are osteopaths; they outnumber chiropractors by three to one.

Two related doctor and patient organizations lobby on behalf of the chiropractic profession in Great Britain. The Chiropractic Advancement Association was founded in 1965 to obtain acceptance of chiropractic in the National Health Service and to promote chiropractic career pursuits. The Back Pain Association was founded in 1970 to finance research into the cause, effect, treatment, and prevention of back pain.

The Anglo-European College of Chiropractic (AECC), established in 1965, is located in Bournemouth, a small seaside community outside of London. AECC is partially funded by member national associations of the European Chiropractors' Union. The AECC graduate is granted the Bachelor of Science degree in Chiropractic, equivalent to the doctorate degree in the United States.

British student entrance requirements include three passes at 'A' level, to include biology or zoology, and chemistry; and five 'O' levels to include English and physics. Applicants from the USA and Canada must comply with Council on Chiropractic Education requirements. Countries other than North America must have university entrance standards or their equivalent in science, with studies in biology or zoology, chemistry, and physics.

(From information provided, the British Chiropractic Association.)

Iceland

A native-born Icelander practices in the capital city of Reykjavik. A graduate of the Anglo-European College of Chiropractic in Great Britain, he has practiced here since 1978 under a license issued by the Minister of Health. Icelandic law provides for the issuance of a license to professionals having a bonafide educational degree that certifies expertise in a given field. There is no specific legislation relating to chiropractic.

Use of x-ray is not allowed under the license, though this restriction has not been challenged. High custom tariffs have made it financially infeasible for the chiropractor to purchase x-ray equipment.

Four chiropractors are studying at the Anglo-European College of Chiropractic. It is anticipated that when these students graduate chiropractic legislation will be pursued. Associate practices may also make the purchase of x-ray equipment possible.

(From information provided by Triggui Jonasson, DC of Reykjavik, Iceland.)

Ireland, Republic of

In 1948, an Irish law declared the country a republic rather than a dominion and the Republic of Ireland withdrew from the Commonwealth of Great Britain. The British Parliament recognized both actions in 1949, but reasserted its claim to incorporate the six northeastern counties in the United Kingdom. Those six counties are Northern Ireland.

There are 14 chiropractors in the Irish Republic, about half of which practice in Dublin. There is no chiropractic law, however, chiropractors practice legally, under common law provisions that allow the practice of a profession so long as there is no law against the practice of that profession.

Chiropractors may take their own x-rays, but most use the resources of radiologists and medical doctors. An association representing the interests of all of Ireland's chiropractors is in formation. Some Irish chiropractors are members of the British Chiropractic Association.

There is no federal reimbursement of chiropractic services; only legislated professions are covered under the National Health Insurance plan. Some private insurance programs and group insurance plans reimburse for chiropractic services.

(From information provided by Chiropractic Association of Ireland.)

Italy

The estimated number of chiropractors practicing in Italy is 130; only 10 percent are Italians. Of the 130 DCs, 40 percent are in private practice. The remaining 60 percent are employed in privately owned companies and practice under the responsibility and authorization of specialists in orthopedics. These companies operate within the National Health Service (*Servizio Mutualistico*). The largest of the privately owned clinics is known as the Static Clinics (*Instituto Nazionale Static*), employing about 40 chiropractors.

The main difference between the private and company clinics is that, within the company-owned clinics, patients are first screened by medical specialists then sent for treatment with a prescription to the chiropractor. In privately owned practices, the chiropractor decides whether a patient needs to be treated or not, the type of treatment needed, and the duration.

Italy's Health Ministry has issued qualifications only for foreign chiropractors who work for the private clinics. To qualify, applicants must be graduates of an accredited chiropractic college, and have passed the US National Board Exam. Chiropractors are then authorized to work in a medical center operated in conformity with the rules of the National Health Service, which stipulates that a medical doctor (orthopedist or physiatrist) be the responsible party.

The *Associazione Italiana Chiropractici* (AIC) has 45 members and is a member of the European Chiropractors' Union. Seventy percent of its members are in private practice. Since 1985, AIC members must pass a national chiropractic exam before membership is granted.

The AIC has created a foundation whose purpose is, as stated in its statutes: to create a free university institute for the formation of doctors of chiropractic; to act so the science and art of chiropractic remain an autonomous and distinct profession to the service of humankind; to maintain unchanged the principle of the chiropractic profession, namely that the relationship between structure and function is important to the health of the human being.

(From information provided by Association of Italian Chiropractors.)

Liechtenstein

Chiropractic is fully recognized in Liechtenstein and the one chiropractor in practice holds full professional rights. The chiropractic law allows manipulation of the spine and pelvis, and the use of x-rays for diagnostic purposes. The law does not provide for chiropractors to use physical therapy, though they may prescribe it. Chiropractic procedures are fully covered by most insurances.

Chiropractors wanting to practice in Liechtenstein must be graduates of an accredited chiropractic college, and must have three years' experience in a chiropractic practice. Only Liechtenstein citizens may have a private practice. Non-nationals (in all professions) must work for a Liechtenstein citizen.

(From information provided by Beatrice Mikus, DC)

The Netherlands

Chiropractors have practiced in The Netherlands since 1968. Currently there are 53 chiropractors in practice, represented by the Netherlands Chiropractic Association (NCA), established 15 years ago. Chiropractic is not a registered profession in the Netherlands, though common law allows for any profession to be practiced as long as there is no law legislating against it.

Due to the absence of registration for chiropractors, their title is not protected. Nearly 2000 physical therapists are in practice, most of whom have taken some courses in manipulation and have incorporated it into their practices.

In the absence of a government board to regulate the profession, the NCA has qualifications for membership that has served as self-regulation for the profession. NCA applicants must be citizens of a Common Market country, and be graduates of a college accredited by the US Council on Chiropractic Education, or a reciprocal council. The NCA also requires foreign applicants to take a language proficiency test.

Various insurance companies (private as well as government) reimburse portions of chiropractic fees, with the provision that the practitioner is a NCA member.

The government is now pursuing preparatory studies to evaluate the national health care system. This study will review non-conventional methods of treatment, which includes chiropractic. A government committee several years ago on the importance of "alternative health professions" evaluated chiropractic most favorably, based primarily on educational qualifications.

Health officials have looked at chiropractic even more favorably since the results of a survey conducted by the National Sick Fund revealed the efficiency of chiropractic care. The study advises that chiropractors should be regulated as "primary care providers" (PCP). The survey results were so promising that a more extensive study of chiropractic efficiency has been launched.

The NCA has organized government committees into Switzerland to examine Swiss chiropractic law and see its effect on public health.

(From information provided by the Netherlands Chiropractic Association.)

Norway

Norwegian chiropractors received statuatory recognition on February 18, 1988. There are 120 chiropractors in Norway, and all but a few are members of Norwegian Chiropractors' Association (*Norsk Kiropraktor Forening*).

Under this law, the chiropractors have the right to refer patients to a hospital for x-rays and use other diagnostic imaging procedures.

In 1975, by order of the Norwegian parliament, chiropractic was included in the national health plan; however, coverage is based on a medical referral. The reimbursement is for approximately 25 percent of the cost of the adjustment, limited to ten adjustments annually. X-rays and clinical examination are not included under the reimbursement plan.

The chiropractic profession has widespread public support. A recent survey revealed that 20 percent of the adult population has been treated by a chiropractor. The study also showed that of those patients who had been treated by both a chiropractor and a physical therapist, three to one favored the chiropractor.

Foreigners wishing to practice in Norway should be aware that the existing law requires a ten year residency before application for professional practice can be made.

(From information provided by the Norwegian Chiropractors' Association.)

Portugal

Two chiropractors are in practice in Portugal; one is Portuguese, the other is American. There is no chiropractic legislation. Portugal is governed under Roman Dutch Law, which states that a profession not specifically legislated is illegal. Though the two chiropractors do not have the benefit of legal practice, their practices have not been restricted.

There is no reimbursement for chiropractic services. A work permit, enabling non-nationals to practice a profession, is difficult to obtain.

(From information provided by Lyle W. Grenz, DC of Estoril, Portugal.)

Spain

The first chiropractor practiced in Spain in the mid-1940s. Twenty-two doctors of chiropractic are practicing in Spain; 18 are members of the *Asociacion Espanola de Quiropractica (AEQ)*. The chiropractic association gained legal recognition in 1986 by the Spanish Ministry of the Interior following the approval of its statutes by the Ministry of Health. Of the doctors in practice, 13 are non-Spanish citizens. Two years ago, there were only five chiropractors practicing in Spain.

Chiropractic is not a legally recognized profession in Spain. Contacts to achieve legislation have been established, primarily with the Parliamentary Health Committee, which is expected to review the subject of legislating the profession. The socialist party, which has the majority in Parliament, has shown interest in regulating and legalizing the profession.

Chiropractors, however, do pay the Value Added Tax on the fees they collect, so, from a fiscal point of view, the profession is included among others as a health profession. This also means that patients may deduct their chiropractic expenses from their tax declarations, just as they do for any other medical expenses. Some private health insurances and major business companies cover chiropractic care expenses. Most MDs who are familiar with chiropractic care will refer their patients to chiropractors.

Six Spaniards are studying chiropractic in US chiropractic colleges; among them, four are recipients of full tuition scholarships offered by Palmer College of Chiropractic (Davenport), Life Chiropractic College (Atlanta), and the Cleveland Chiropractic Colleges (Kansas City and Los Angeles). A number of Europeans, mainly French and Danish chiropractors, have expressed an interest in practicing in Spain. The AEQ welcomes interested practitioners but wants to screen applicants in order to verify the qualifications of applicants.

Residents of nations in the European Economic Community need only a residence permit to practice; others need a residence and a work permit. As Spain has a very high unemployment rate, government policy has restricted the number of work permits it will issue. Numerous documents and formalities are necessary and the AEQ assists in advising candidates to deal with these requirements.

The AEQ is developing a quarterly publication on chiropractic for distribution to the general public. It is also attempting to create a national chiropractic board and language proficiency test for new applicants.

There are a small number of practitioners who claim to manipulate the spine, most of these are graduates of two schools in Spain that advertise the instruction of so-called chiropractic techniques in a six-month to one year course.

(From information provided by the Association of Spanish Chiropractors.)

Sweden

The first chiropractor arrived in Sweden in 1920. In 1936 the Swedish Chiropractic Society was established. For years, the numbers of chiropractors in Sweden averaged no more than 30, but in the past few years their numbers increased and Sweden now has 76 chiropractors in practice.

A chiropractic law was passed in June, 1989. The law was a result of a report on alternative medicine, commissioned by Sweden's Health Minister, released in 1988. The Commission proposed registration for chiropractors as independent primary care providers and called for their inclusion into the National Insurance System. The Commission also recommended that people with back problems should consult a doctor of chiropractic. Finally, the Commission concluded that because there were not enough chiropractics to meet the demand, it would recommend the establishment of a chiropractic educational institution in Sweden at a later date.

Chiropractic practice by non-nationals is discouraged by making it difficult to acquire a work permit. Additionally, applicants must show a deposit of $10,000 (US) as a security of independent status. Interested applicants should apply at the Swedish Embassy in their native country.

(From information provided by the Swedish Chiropractic Society.)

Switzerland

While in the early 1900s, pioneering Swiss chiropractic doctors were often persecuted and even imprisoned, today Switzerland has what many consider to be a model chiropractic law. Chiropractic is fully recognized and legislated as a primary health profession: this implies full professional rights in regards to patient management, diagnostic ability, x-rays, physiotherapy, laboratory privileges and insurance coverage. Chiropractic in Switzerland is an independent and specific branch of scientific medicine, as are dentistry, and podiatry.

Chiropractors are represented by the Association of Swiss Chiropractors. Switzerland is a federal state, consisting of 26 cantons. Each canton reserves the right to register health practitioners according to its specific rules. But if, within each canton, a specified number of citizens request a modification of the rules, the modification must be submitted for a vote (referendum). Chiropractic status in many cantons has been achieved because of public involvement.

The first canton to pass a chiropractic law was Lucerne in 1937; the canton last to pass such a law was Berne in 1974. While each canton sets its own qualifications and scope of practice, there is great similarity of chiropractic law in all cantons.

The profession is regulated by the Inter-Canton Chiropractic Commission, a board made up of five chiropractors and five medical doctors of various specialties.

The conditions for chiropractic, set by the Commission, are strict and precise, requiring Swiss nationality, a university entrance examination; a minimum four-year course in a CCE accredited college; a US state board examination; a two-year residency program in a Swiss chiropractic clinic; an intercanto-

nal examination of clinical proficiency; a course of lectures at the *Institut d'Etudes Superierures* (Swiss Chiropractic Training Institute) of the Swiss Chiropractic Association; and a federal examination to gain x-ray privileges.

The above conditions, when completed, results in the grant of a Certificate of Capacity to practice in the country. Lastly, and to keep the right to qualify for insurance coverage privileges, the doctor is required to register at an annual postgraduate course.

While there are a few non-Swiss chiropractors among the 115 chiropractors in the country, required work permits for non-nationals are not readily granted. Non-nationals are also required by law to work under the sponsorship of a Swiss chiropractor for a prescribed period.

Chiropractic is fully integrated into all insurance companies, providing 100 percent recovery of fees to the chiropractor. Chiropractic is included under all accident insurance companies, whether state-owned or private, and under military plans. A recent contract allows the chiropractor to refer patients for physical therapy and laboratory procedures, and for those fees to be paid for. The contract also grants chiropractors the right to treat patients in hospitals.

(From information provided by Association of Swiss Chiropractors.)

West Germany

In West Germany, paramedical health care is authorized by the Health Practitioner (*Heilpraktiker*) statute of 1939. The law permits a broad scope of practice, including chiropractic, homeopathy, naturopathy, acupuncture, and even minor surgery. The law has been criticised for the loosely defined standards under which more than 6,000 health practitioners practice. Medical associations have long opposed the *Heilpraktiker* statute, and the medical code of ethics forbids cooperation with providers covered by the statute.

Chiropractors intending to practice in West Germany must obtain a health practitioner license. Only German citizens may take the license examination.

Chiropractic ''therapy'' can be used without restriction by medical doctors and health practitioners. Many chiropractic courses, varying greatly in quality and character, are offered by medical doctors and chiropractors.

Chiropractic is included in the schedule of tariffs of the medical profession as chiropractic therapeutic treatment. Various national insurance programs, covering 85 percent of the West German population, reimburse only medical doctors. Private insurances and the state subsidy of public servants reimburse the patient for services and fees paid to medical doctors and health practitioners.

The German Chiropractors' Association was founded and legally registered in 1980; there are nine full members and two honorary members.

The use of the DC degree is granted after the Minister of Education reviews the chiropractic institutions' professional education and professional degree program. Three chiropractors who have received recognition of their degrees are graduates of Los Angeles College of Chiropractic and Cleveland College of Chiropractic of Kansas City. Three subsequent applications from three other colleges in Europe, Canada, and the United States were denied. A suit filed against a Minister of Science to force recognition of the Council of Chiropractic of Education as a body sufficient for granting recognition was denied, and the case is on appeal.

(From information provided by German Chiropractors' Association.)

Pacific Region *

Chiropractic was first introduced to the Pacific region in the early 1900s in New Zealand, several years before it reached Australia, Japan, Hong Kong, and other countries in the region.

Since chiropractic education was available only from institutions in North America, there was minimal growth of the profession in the 1920s and 1930s. During the next decade, the profession's growth was arrested altogether because of wartime bans on transpacific travel.

After the war, the numbers of practitioners increased more rapidly as a result of active student recruitment, easier overseas travel, and as Australian training courses in chiropractic emerged. It was not until 1975, however, that education at an internationally acceptable level was available in the southern hemisphere, paving the way for enhanced statutory recognition, self-sustaining growth and independent development of chiropractic in the region.

Australia

The first chiropractor to practice in Australia is widely believed to be Dr. Harold Williams, who set up practice in 1919 in Sydney. Others soon followed and by 1938, 22 chiropractors joined to form the Australian Chiropractors' Association (ACA). In 1943, chiropractors practicing in the territory of Victoria established a separate organization, which united with the ACA in 1961.

*We gratefully acknowledge the assistance provided by Mary Ann Chance, DC, in the preparation of this section.

Growth of the profession was interrupted by World War II, and was re-established by 1949, when chiropractic graduates returning to Australia began recruiting students in earnest. The most dramatic result was in Victoria, where the number of overseas-educated chiropractors increased from seven in 1949 to 40 in 1960.

Meanwhile, another group of practitioners using manipulation were emerging. About the same time as the first chiropractic graduates arrived in Australia, Ernst Kjellberg, a Swedish manipulator who had studied medicine but never completed his degree, set up practice in north Queensland. He attracted patients from all over Australia, and trained scores of apprentices in his methods.

The first formal training institution in Australia incorporating chiropractic subject in its curriculum was the PAX Chiropractic College. Over the next four decades, numerous natural therapy training courses emerged, most teaching some form of manipulative therapy, several including chiropractic courses within their programs, and some issuing diplomas in chiropractic. None, however, approached the standard set by contemporary chiropractic colleges in North America. Only one, the Sydney College of Chiropractic, established in 1959, continues to operate as a chiropractic educational institution.

Graduates of Australian courses and those who had learned chiropractic and other manipulative techniques through apprenticeship or independent study formed various associations, many of which merged during the 1970s under the banner of the United Chiropractors' Association of Australasia.

Regulation of health care services is the responsibility of state and territory governments, thus political legitimation of chiropractic in the eight Australian jurisdictions has followed different patterns.

Until 1946, chiropractors were able to practice as ''unregistered practitioners'' with little hindrance and few significant restrictions. In that year a law came into effect in South Australia requiring any person practicing manipulation to register as a physiotherapist. Chiropractors already in practice in the state were allowed to register, but subsequently only physiotherapy graduates were eligible.

The legislation was eventually repealed and, in 1949, a Chiropractic Act was passed. It contained a definition of chiropractic, and exempted chiropractors from the Medical Practitioners Act 1919–1946 and the Physiotherapy Act 1945–1948, and also allowed the use of x-ray for the purposes of chiropractic diagnosis. Although not a comprehensive piece of legislation, this first chiropractic law secured legal precedents and established the identity of chiropractic in the Australian statutes.

During the 1950s, most other states passed

Physiotherapy Acts. In New South Wales, chiropractors were exempted, and in Western Australia, chiropractic was defined in the Act. Tasmania's Physiotherapy Act of 1951 provided no such concessions, so all chiropractors left the state, which remained without chiropractic services for some three years. The Victorian equivalent, the Masseurs Act of 1958, also had no exemption clause, but no chiropractor was ever charged.

The first chiropractic registration law in Australia was the Western Australian Chiropractors Act, passed in 1964 following recommendations of the 1960–1961 Royal Commission of Inquiry into Matters Relating to Natural Therapists. The Act limits the use of the title "chiropractor" to persons registered as such, but does not restrain persons not so registered from practicing spinal manipulation.

Efforts to achieve similar legislation did not succeed until some 14 years later, after committees appointed by two state parliaments and the federal government (Webb Report) had published their reports.

It was not until 1985 that the practice of chiropractic was regulated by statute in all Australian jurisdictions. All the registration acts prohibit the use of the title "chiropractor" by nonregistered persons, all but Western Australia also regulate the practice of osteopathy, and all except Western Australia and Victoria restrict the practice of chiropractic, osteopathy or spinal manipulation to those registered or specifically exempted (e.g. medical practitioners, physiotherapists). Chiropractic is defined in various ways, or not at all, in the registration acts. The advent of registration arrested the proliferation of inadequately trained and self-proclaimed practitioners who for decades had an adverse effect on the profession's stature.

All Australian jurisdictions accept the Bachelor of Applied Science (Chiropractic) degree granted by the Phillip Institute of Technology (Melbourne) for registration and most also accept the Postgraduate Diploma in Chiropractic from Sydney College of Chiropractic. Acceptance of overseas qualifications differs widely from state to state.

Most jurisdictions include chiropractic in motor accident and workers' compensation plans. In other states, payment for chiropractic services and/or time off work have been dependent upon medical certification of a compensable injury. In Queensland, formal medical referral is required. By the mid-1980s, all states and territories had begun to review the whole system of compensation due to escalating costs and inherent inequities in the system.

Chiropractic is not included in Medicare, a federal government health care scheme which pays for 85 percent of basic medical fees and most public hospital charges.

By the early 1970s, it had become clear that most state governments would be unwilling to register chiropractors if foreign study were the only route to qualification. The Australian Committee on Chiropractic Education and the Australian Chiropractors' Association, conducted separate studies to investigate how a modern chiropractic curriculum could be developed in Australia.

In 1974, one of the proposals of the Victoria branch of the ACA won national support, and in 1975 the International College of Chiropractic was established, supported by teaching services from the Royal Melbourne Institute of Technology. Within the year, Andres Kleynhans, DC, was named Principal, and the college was relocated on the campus of Preston (now Phillip) Institute of Technology, which had agreed to a more comprehensive relationship than could be negotiated through Melbourne Institute.

In 1980, the Bachelor of Applied Science (Chiropractic) program was accredited by the Victoria Institute of Colleges, the state accrediting authority. The following year it received full funding from the Australian government. Subsequently the PIT School of Chiropractic was granted full accreditation by the Australian Council on Chiropractic Education in 1984 and later through reciprocal agreement and joint inspection by the Council on Chiropractic Education of the United States and Canada. Postgraduate fellowship programmes in radiology and chiropractic clinical science have been developed and are approved by the Australian educational council.

Sydney College of Chiropractic, a free-standing private institution, had its origins in the Sydney College of Osteopathy, founded by Alfred Kaufmann. Until the early 1980s it granted diplomas in both osteopathy and chiropractic. The osteopathy diploma is no longer awarded, and entry into the two-year postgraduate diploma course in chiropractic is conditional upon successful completion of the Bachelor of Science program at the University of New South Wales, or its equivalent. The Sydney College "end-on" program was approved in 1981 by the New South Wales Higher Education Board. Sydney College of Chiropractic is now seeking accreditation from the Australasian Council on Chiropractic Education.

In 1989 the Sydney College of Chiropractic agreed to have its chiropractic curriculum adopted into Macquarie University. The new program will become the Centre for Chiropractic Studies within Macquarie University. Sydney College will retain its name under the new arrangement.

The course will award the Masters level degree in chiropractic (MSc. in Chiropractic), equivalent to the doctorate awarded at U.S. chiropractic colleges.

As Macquarie University does not operate a

medical school, chiropractic will be the largest health discipline taught at the University. The Centre for Chiropractic Studies will operate in conjunction with Macquarie University's School of Biological Studies.

Australia's chiropractic register shows 1900 chiropractors practicing in Australia, with New South Wales and Victoria having the greatest concentrations.

(From information provided by Mary Ann Chance, DC, editor, *Journal* of the Australian Chiropractors' Association.)

Guam

Guam is under the jurisdiction of the US Interior Department, and is governed by US constitutional law.

Chiropractic legislation was passed in 1973, under authorization by the Department of Allied Health, and is regulated by the Board of Allied Health Examiners. There is no specific chiropractic law, but the rules and regulations of the examining board govern the parameters of chiropractic scope of practice. The Guam Chiropractic Association, representing the three chiropractors who practice in Guam, are working with appropriate governmental agencies to get a specific chiropractic practice act passed.

Applicants for licensure must be US citizens; be literate in English; be graduates of a fully accredited chiropractic college; have completed a one-year internship; and be at least 21 years of age. Additionally applicants must not have any complaints filed against their previous license. Non-nationals (non-US or Guam citizens) must meet all the above criteria and must also obtain work permits with the US Immigration Department.

Chiropractic services are covered under Workers' Compensation, but it is excluded from all other federal and private insurance plans.

(From information provided by the Guam Chiropractic Association, 1986.)

Hong Kong

Chiropractic was first introduced to Hong Kong by Dr. Molthen, an American citizen and graduate of Palmer School of Chiropractic, who practiced in Hong Kong until his death in 1967. The Hong Kong Chiropractors' Association, founded in 1968, represents the country's 15 chiropractors.

No legislation exists either to restrict or protect the chiropractic profession. Chiropractors are one of many groups of unlicensed health providers who are free to practice as long as they do not use drugs or surgery.

Over the years, the Hong Kong Chiropractors' Association has actively pursued chiropractic legisla-tion to no avail. Organized efforts by the association has sometimes resulted in a backlash of intermittent legal harrassment of chiropractors, including police raids, interrogation, and arrests.

The legal challenges have been made on the basis that doctors of chiropractic are unqualified to call themselves *Ysang*, the term for doctor in the Chinese language. The Medical Registration Ordinance has not issued a definitive legal opinion on this point, but various other legal opinions, including that of the Solicitor-General, have voiced no objection. The title is the common term used for a man of healing and is used by other health professionals, such as doctors of dentistry. The medical profession has adamantly insisted that *Ysang* be used by medical doctors only.

Traditional bonesetters number in the hundreds and are used widely by the Chinese. Hong Kong chiropractors mainly serve the non-Chinese public. Acupuncturists, medical doctors, herbalists, and bonesetters are the country's most used practitioners.

Chiropractors in Hong Kong are distributed around the populous city centers of Kowloon and Hong Kong. Most focus care on the spinal column and pelvis, with very little use of supplemental therapies and modalities. Only medical doctors are licensed to take x-rays, and only radiologists may interpret them. Radiology laboratories provide roentgenological services requested by chiropractors. There is no government compensation for chiropractic, though a few private insurance companies provide limited care reimbursement.

(From information provided by Hong Kong Chiropractors' Association.)

Japan

Chiropractic was first introduced to Japan in 1918 by Saburo Kawaguchi, DC, a graduate of Palmer School of Chiropractic, and one of a dozen American-educated chiropractors practicing in Japan through the 1930s. Since manipulation was a traditional form of therapy, chiropractic was well accepted by the public. Up until 1945, before the end of World War II, nonmedical therapies were governed by local rather than federal authorities. In some jurisdictions, chiropractic was granted licensure by the local police departments, as authorized by the Ministry of Home Affairs.

After World War II, US occupation policy dissolved the Ministry of Home Affairs to form the Ministry of Health and Welfare. Under the new policy, spinal manipulation was banned, along with most other nonmedical healing arts, on the basis that they were unscientific. In 1947, legislation was passed recognizing the most widely practiced nonmedical therapies which included acupuncture, massage, bonesetting and moxibustion.

Five groups of practitioners (spinal manipulators, mechanotherapists, heat, electric and light therapists) not included in the legislation, organized that year to form the Zenkoku Ryojutsushi Kyokai (ZRK) (i.e., All-Japan Natural Therapists Association) for the sole purpose of gaining legislation. Following many years pursuing legislation, a grandfather clause was passed in 1964 granting permission to practice the five therapies, but the legislation did not include any provision for future practitioners.

Chiropractic gained some additional protection under two broad provisions. Article 22 of the Japanese Constitution gives Japanese citizens the right to engage in any occupation provided that it is not detrimental to the public well-being. Then, in 1960, Japan's Supreme Court issued a decision which constitutionally guarantees the right to practice a drugless healing method provided it is harmless, and does not infringe on the scope of a profession already legislated.

In 1968, the first Japanese in 30 years returned from a United States college with a doctorate in chiropractic. Due to favorable legal interpretations that made chiropractic practice legal, numbers of chiropractic graduates returning to Japan to practice increased dramatically.

Nonmedical practitioners, including bonesetters, acupuncturists, and massage therapists, intrigued by chiropractic theory and technique, began to attend the numerous technique seminars taught by US chiropractors visiting Japan. Chiropractic techniques began to overshadow all other therapies, and was practiced by a wide range of skilled and unskilled practitioners. Chiropractic gained significant popularity among the general public, but because of the vast use of the technique by many nonmedical therapists, chiropractic was perceived to be a new technique rather than a professional discipline with its own unique diagnosis and treatment.

In the 1980s, many chiropractic organizations were started, as well as a dozen private chiropractic schools offering training programs of one to three years in duration. With no government control of chiropractic educational standards, Japanese chiropractic schools are far below the international standard.

Legislative efforts continue and the ZRK is pursuing legislation for three separate licenses—chiropractic, light-electricity therapy and mechano-therapy. In 1988, the Ministry of Health sanctioned the Natural Healing Research Foundation, an organization established by the ZRK. This move represents what the profession perceives as the government's willingness to review the issue of nonmedical licenses, which would include chiropractic.

There are widely varying estimates of practitioners practicing what is generally called chiropractic. There are approximately 50 Japanese chiropractors who have chiropractic degrees from accredited chiropractic colleges overseas. There are 800 chiropractic offices listed in the telephone directories of Japan. There is an estimated pool of three to five thousand practitioners of chiropractic who use and advertise chiropractic technique as an adjunct to their practices in acupuncture, bonesetting or other forms of treatment.

There are at least six chiropractic organizations in Japan, many of these organizations are formed to provide technique seminars, rather than serve as professional associations. The Japanese Doctors Chiropractic Association, with a membership under 50, is the only organization restricted to practitioners who are graduates from an accredited chiropractic college. Of the others, the largest is the Japanese Chiropractic Organization, established in 1961. Its membership of 500 includes a few degree-qualified chiropractic doctors, but most of its members are graduates of one of the many sub-standard Japanese schools. Attempts to unify the various organizations have not been successful.

In general, insurance plans do not cover chiropractic unless it is directly for treatments for whiplash resulting from an automobile accident. Chiropractic treatment ranges from Y 3,000 to Y 5,000 (US $23 to $40).

The levels of skill and types of treatment offered under the premise of chiropractic health care varies greatly from practitioner to practitioner. Most practitioners who offer chiropractic as part of their services have a license in another therapy, such as bonesetting, acupuncture, massage, and the like. The use of x-ray is permitted only by medical doctors, but chiropractors are able to refer a patient to an MD for x-rays.

(From information provided by the Japanese Doctors Chiropractic Association, and the Japanese Chiropractic Association.)

Papua New Guinea

One chiropractor practices in New Guinea, jointly sponsored by the Christian Chiropractors' Association and the Wycliff Bible Translators. He has practiced here for four years in a dual role as chiropractic practitioner and active Christian missionary.

He is director of a full-service medical clinic, which includes two medical doctors, four nurses and four physiotherapists.

There is no applicable legislation to either restrict or regulate chiropractic practice.

(From information provided by the Christian Chiropractors' Association.)

New Zealand

The first doctor of chiropractic to establish a practice in New Zealand was Dr. Otterhalt, a graduate of Palmer School of Chiropractic, who began his practice in Dunedin in 1908.

By 1923, there were almost 40 doctors of chiropractic in the country, nearly half of them women. In that year the New Zealand Chiropractors' Association was formed, and it has remained as the singular voice representing the profession.

Statutory recognition of chiropractic was first gained in 1949, when provisions for licensing chiropractors to use x-ray were introduced under the Radioactive Substances Act. The first law to register chiropractic practice was the Chiropractic Act of 1960, administered by the Department of Justice. This has since been replaced by the Chiropractors Act of 1982.

The 1982 Chiropractic Act was precipitated by a private members bill introduced into Parliament in 1975 seeking further recognition of chiropractic, and a petition bearing 94,210 signatures (three percent of the national population), requesting inclusion of chiropractic in the Social Security and Accident Compensation plans. In response, the government appointed a Commission of Inquiry into chiropractic.

The Commission, made up of a professor of law, an educationalist and a professor of chemistry, chose to conduct the inquiry primarily on the basis of evidence given in public, under oath and subject to cross-examination.

Evidence given orally, and in accordance with written submissions filed 30 days beforehand, enabled the principle parties to prepare cross-examination and to allow for collection of technical evidence. Thus tested, much evidence submitted against chiropractic was shown to be without basis in fact. In this respect, the New Zealand Inquiry differed fundamentally from any inquiry into chiropractic before or since, and its findings have had correspondingly more impact and greater value to the chiropractic profession.

When the commission reported its findings in 1979, it made 21 formal recommendations in a number of areas including the regulation of the chiropractic profession and its relationship with other health professions, scope of practice, education, research, access to hospitals, use of the title "doctor" and inclusion under various health compensation programs.

Some recommendations, such as those calling for reforms in licensure laws have been acted upon, while others, such as health and accident compensation benefits for chiropractic without medical referral, have not.

The Chiropractic Board of New Zealand recognizes education degrees offered by the following institutions: the Bachelor of Applied Science (Chiropractic) granted by the Phillip Institute of Technology in Melbourne, Australia and the doctor of chiropractic degree awarded by the Anglo-European College of Chiropractic and 11 North American chiropractic colleges.

In May 1988, there were 235 chiropractors in the official New Zealand register, of whom 132 practice in New Zealand and 103 practice overseas.

Chiropractic health care is covered under Accident Compensation plans, but only with a medical referral. Likewise, some private health insurance policies cover chiropractic care, but usually only upon a medical referral and only for a portion of the total.

All practitioners must apply for an annual Practicing Certificate from the Chiropractic Board of New Zealand. An annual x-ray license, limited to chiropractic diagnosis, is granted, upon medical referral, by the National Radiation Laboratory.

(From information provided by Mary Ann Chance, the editor, *Journal* of the Australian Chiropractors' Association, and the New Zealand Chiropractors' Association.)

Philippines

The first chiropractor to practice in the Philippines was an American graduate of Logan College of Chiropractic, who began his practice in the mid-1970s. Since then, two other chiropractors have opened practice. Only one is a native Filipino, the other has acquired citizenship through marriage.

Manipulation and other nonmedical healing practices have strong historical backgrounds in the Philippines, thus chiropractic is well received by those who are introduced to it. There are hundreds of practitioners known as "hilots" or bonesetters who use manipulative techniques. They are mostly self-trained or have knowledge handed down from elders. The other major health provider is the "herbolerio" (herbalist). Each town may have hundreds of these healers.

There is no legal recognition of chiropractic. There is no government reimbursement for chiropractic services, though a few private insurance companies accept chiropractic claims.

(From information provided by James T. Uy, DC, of Manila, Philippines.)

Singapore

There is no law that governs the practice of chiropractic in Singapore, but work permits (employment passes) have been issued for professional practice. Two chiropractors practice in the only chiropractic clinic in the Republic of Singapore, operated since 1978.

A long an arduous registration procedure can be expected before an employment pass can be issued. Even after it is issued, the Singapore government reserves its right to cancel any pass with 24 hours' notice and without a hearing.

Applications are made to the Ministry of Health and Medical Governing Board. Credentials are submitted to the Immigration Board, where eligibility is determined. A non-native applicant must have the sponsorship of a Singapore citizen to assume liability for the foreigner's conduct, financial solvency and repatriation to home country, if necessary. The sole clinic in Singapore has sponsored several chiropractors to work in its clinic; most are preceptorship doctors who practice for a year or longer before returning to the United States.

There is no federal reimbursement of chiropractic services, but varying levels of reimbursements are available from some private and corporate insurance plans.

A chiropractic association has been legally sanctioned by the Singapore government following 11 years of repeated requests by chiropractors and chiropractic patients.

There are no provisions for licensing or registering health providers other than medical doctors. Chiropractors continue to practice with ''tacit consent'' as long as they abide by the various medical regulations governing professional conduct, i.e., restrictions on advertising.

Traditional healers who use manipulation in their practices are called *sensei*, and number up to one thousand. Their techniques are self-taught and handed down from generation to generation.

(From information provided by Carol Elder-Birnbaum, DC, Singapore.)

South and Central America*

North, Central and South American nations are grouped under one region according to breakdowns as set forth by the World Health Organization; however, due to the relatively large number of chiropractic providers in North America, their status is covered in a separate chapter.

The cohesiveness of the Latin American nations can be grouped together by virtue of their similarities in population densities, language, law, economic and geographical-based interests.

In general, the nations of Central and South America have a low ratio of chiropractic providers to population densities. Lack of chiropractic licensure is evident in all countries but Panama. Though chiropractic is an illegal practice in most countries of this region, chiropractors practice, for the most part, unhampered.

The outlook for the growth of the profession is not assured. Severe devaluations in the currencies of these nations compared to the U.S. dollar have made it nearly impossible for most Latin students to afford the cost of a chiropractic education in the United States. Since there is no chiropractic college based in a Latin American nation, the self-perpetuation of the profession is at risk.

Manipulation is used by many village folk healers in the Central and South American nations, and thus chiropractic health care is well received by those who are introduced to it.

Belize

Two chiropractors practice in Belize. There is no legislation, and Belizian common law has no provisions for licensing any health providers other than medical doctors.

Recent organization by the nation's unlicensed osteopaths to gain legislation may assist chiropractors in gaining the same. An osteopathic school is part of Belize University, and a government task force is planning, as a prelude to granting licensure, to study the education standards of the osteopathic schools in the United States. One of the chiropractors has requested that the task force also study U.S. chiropractic education standards.

The Belizian chiropractors have access to x-ray and laboratory facilities. Professional cooperation is generally good. Reimbursements for chiropractic services are primarily from patients with U.S.-based insurances.

There is no restriction on practice, nor is there any regulation. A small group of Seventh Day Adventists had attempted to relocate their ''quiropractico/naturalista'' school from Guatemala to Belize, but failed. However, several barely-trained to partially-trained students remain, practicing what they profess is ''chiropractic.''

The concept of manipulation is generic to Belizian culture; individuals of diverse cultures and educational backgrounds often refer to their work as

---

*We gratefully acknowledge the assistance provided by Enrique Benet-Canut, DC, president, Latin American Federation, in the preparation of this section.

"chiropractic." Manipulation is practiced by physiotherapists, naprapaths, and massage therapists.

Manipulation is also used by Belizian folk healers, including: *h'men* (Maya); *nointers, trachmoaka* (Mennonite); and *ga supa hati* (Garifuna).

(From information provided by Daniel V. Buffington, DC, of San Ignacio, Belize.)

Bermuda

Bermuda is a British dependency governed by a royal governor and an assembly. The legislative body dates back to 1620, the oldest among all British dependencies. Two chiropractors live in Bermuda; only one is practicing, having done so for the past eight years. Chiropractic is not legislated, though the chiropractor practices under common law interpretation, which states that if there is no legislation prohibiting a profession, then it is legal.

The doctor was granted a work permit from the Minister of Immigration and Labor, assisted by the fact that he is married to a Bermudan. The work permit is issued on an annual basis. Work permits for non-nationals are not usually issued.

Medical cooperation varies from practitioner to practitioner. Chiropractors are not permitted to take x-rays: only hospitals may take x-rays and they will not cooperate with chiropractors.

Chiropractic health care is not a covered service under government insurance plans, but is reimbursable under most private insurance plans.

(From information provided by Dr. Donald Ray, Hamilton, Bermuda.)

Brazil

Four chiropractors practice in Brazil; two in Rio de Janerio, one in Porto Alegre, and one is Sao Paulo. They are represented by the newly formed Chiropractic Association of Brazil.

There is no chiropractic legislation, but one doctor recently won a civil suit that establishes chiropractic as a separate art. There is organization to gain recognition of chiropractic as a primary health care profession.

Chiropractic in Brazil has a long and unusual history. Chiropractic was introduced to Brazil in the 1920s by William F. Fipps, DC. Through 1945, several US chiropractors practiced intermittently in Brazil.

In 1945, a chiropractic course was offered by the Association of Biological Renovation and a group of professionals (chiropractors and professors) from the University of Natural Healing Arts based in Denver, Colorado. The course was offered in Curitibi, in the state of Parana (Brazil) from 1958 through 1964. Twenty-eight persons received a diploma in chiro-

practic and most stayed in the country to practice and did so without restriction.

After a *coup d'etat* in 1964, a military dictatorship was established, and chiropractic practice was severely restricted. In 1972, it was declared an illegal practice of medicine. Because of this action, most of the practitioners either left the country or changed professions.

In 1982, only one chiropractor remained. By 1984, the military government was losing its majority and in 1985 Brazil returned to democratic government. Even so, some fragments of authoritarianism prevailed and the chiropractor was jailed for eight days as a result of a lawsuit filed by the Board of Health.

In February 1986, a judiciary hearing granted the right to practice chiropractic, effective August, 1987. The ruling permits chiropractic practice under supervision of a medical doctor or physiotherapist.

The use of x-ray is authorized for medical doctors only, as are stethoscopes, sphygnomanometers, and electric stimulation.

(From information provided by Chiropractic Association of Brazil.)

Colombia

There are two chiropractors in Colombia. Both practice in the capital city of Bogota. There is no chiropractic law, although chiropractors are registered by the Foreign Offices Department. Work permits to practice in Bogota have been granted without much difficulty.

The two chiropractors do not have x-ray facilities, although radiologists will x-ray upon a chiropractor's prescription.

There is no federal reimbursement of chiropractic services, although chiropractors have been contracted by *Caja de Compensacion*, a subsidiary social security program.

Village healers called *sobanderos* perform some crude forms of manipulation, as do some physical therapists.

There is little hope for the growth of the profession as economic conditions in Colombia make it nearly impossible for Colombian students to afford the cost of a US chiropractic education.

(From information provided by Paulo Arci, DC, of Bogota Colombia, 1988.)

Ecuador

There are eight chiropractors in Ecuador; the majority are not Ecuadorian citizens, but have acquired indefinite resident visas. The first chiropractor began practicing here in the mid-1960s.

Ecuador has no law legislating chiropractic;

however chiropractors practice legally under authorization from the Immigration Department. Work permits are easily issued to persons who can demonstrate that their intended type of work is a technology not taught within the country. Legal fees to acquire the 10-V visa can cost up to $1500 (U.S.).

The Ecuadorian Chiropractic Association continues active pursuit of chiropractic legislation.

Ecuador's Ministry of Health has approved of the premise of chiropractic under the *Instituto Indo-Americano de Medicina Biologico,* an inter-disciplinary organization dedicated to natural healing. It is considered an important first step towards attaining legislation as primary care health providers.

Radiology is a medical specialty, and only radiologists may take x-rays. Local clinics work with chiropractors, as do most other medical specialties. Chiropractors have been granted privileges to admit and treat patients in hospitals.

Private insurance companies cover chiropractic services, reimbursing the patient directly. There is no federal insurance program and chiropractic services are not covered by the military.

Local village healers, administering care primarily to the rural lower classes, are called *salbadores* or *frigadores*. The healers are diminishing in numbers; they use bonesetting and use their hands to cure visceral conditions, reduce fractures and manipulate the articulations of the human frame.

(From information provided by Ecuadorian Chiropractors Association, 1988.)

Guatemala

There are three chiropractors practicing in Guatemala. Even though there is no chiropractic law or registration of chiropractors, chiropractors practice unhampered by legal authorities. The Medical Board has issued a ''letter of trust'' to one of the three chiropractors.

Chiropractors are registered with the Ministry of Finance in order that a patient can be charged and be given a state-approved bill for services.

Despite the lack of government licensure or registration, chiropractic services are reimbursed by nearly all private insurances, military plans, and most U.S. government employee plans.

There are excellent relations with medical doctors, including co-admitting privileges at some hospitals.

Village healers who use bonesetting as one of their techniques are called *curanderos*. Seventh Day Adventist healers who also use bonesetting are called *naturistas*.

(From information provided by Marcos Antonio Torres-Fry, DC, of Guatemala City, Guatemala, 1988.)

Mexico

In 1989 chiropractic became a legislated health profession in Mexico. Before this, the government had provided chiropractors with an intermittent registration process that had allowed legal, but tenuous, practice for the country's 40 chiropractors.

The first chiropractor (Dr. Francisco Montano, Palmer graduate) established a practice in Mexico in 1922. In 1955, the Direction of Professions under the Secretariat of Education registered chiropractors in practice. In 1958, that registration was again closed. In 1975 another registration was opened for new applicants, but this was also closed in 1982 without explanation. The registration process was re-opened in 1988 in a way to allow for a stronger and more permanent registration process.

Mexico is governed under Napoleanic Law which states that a profession not specifically registered is illegal. Of 40 chiropractors practicing in Mexico, five are not registered.

The profession is represented by the *Sociedad Cientifico Quiropractica de Mexico* (SCQM), established in 1984. The Association holds an international, interdisciplinary scientific symposium annually. The Association accepts members only if they are fully qualified doctors of chiropractic, holding a degree from an accredited or widely recognized chiropractic college.

The Association was successful in establishing a regulatory board called *Colegio Profesionistas Cientifica Quiropracticos de Mexico.* This is a collegiate body, authorized by the Direction of Professions in 1988 under exceptional conditions, since it usually requires a profession to have 500 licensed professionals before it will authorize a regulatory board.

Mexico's Chiropractic Association was also successful in gaining official acceptance to work within the *Direccion de Integracion Familiar,* a government social program for infants, children and young adults with neurological problems. The tremendous results with 300–400 patients under chiropractic care was a factor in the government issuing legal professional licenses (*cedula profesional*) to chiropractors in 1988.

Since the positive developments regarding government licensure of chiropractors and their inclusion in social service programs, a number of universities have expressed an interest in incorporating chiropractic as a full career in their curriculum.

There is no federal reimbursement of chiropractic health services, though many private insurance companies reimburse for chiropractic services.

Chiropractic is widely known in Mexico through frequent media coverage, advertising, and patient referrals. Interprofessional cooperation is good, with medical doctors often referring their patients to chiropractors. Few other practitioners practice manipulative techniques. In the countryside, traditional healers use bonesetting techniques and manipulation. They are called *los hueseros* and number in the thousands.

Mexico was once the site of a chiropractic school. In 1927 the first Spanish-language chiropractic institution was established in Mexico City. The Daniel David Palmer Spanish-American School of Chiropractic was operated until 1933, when it closed because of financial difficulties.

The need for a Spanish-language chiropractic college has been addressed continually at regional and international chiropractic conferences. The severe devaluation of Mexico's peso compared to the U.S. dollar has made it virtually impossible for Mexican (and Latin American students, in general) to afford the cost of a chiropractic education in the United States.

In 1988, a regional latin american chiropractic organization was formed, called *La Federation Latinoamerica de Quiropractica, A.C.* Member countries include: Bolivia, Ecuador, Guatemala, Mexico, Panama, Spain (an affiliate member) and Venezuela.

(From information provided by *Sociedad Cientifico Quiropractica de Mexico*.)

Panama

Among all the world's Latin American countries, Mexico and the Republic of Panama are the only two that legislate chiropractic. The five chiropractors practicing in Panama are represented by the Chiropractic Association of Panama, established in 1966.

Panamanian Chiropractic Law, adopted in 1967, grants chiropractors licensure and regulation. The law provides for ''the adjusting, manipulating and treating of the human body,'' and states that chiropractors may ''examine, analyze and diagnose the human body by way of any method physical, chemical, electric or the use of x-ray, and may use any other methods. . . . taught in any recognized chiropractic college.''

To be granted a license, an applicant must be a Panamanian citizen, be a graduate of an accredited chiropractic college, and pass an examination given by Panama's Board of Chiropractic Examiners.

Chiropractic is included in the Technical Council of Public Health, a multidisciplined council, which mandates inclusion of chiropractic services under the federal reimbursement system. Most of the chiropractors work for the social security system, providing chiropractic care as fully recognized, primary care providers. Reimbursements for chiropractic services is almost on par with reimbursements for medical services. A few chiropractors also have private practices.

The public perception of chiropractic continues to grow, as does inter-health professional cooperation.

There are a few local healers who use manipulation, all of them unlicensed. They are called *brujos* (whitchers).

(From information provided by the Chiropractic Association of Panama, 1988.)

Peru

The one chiropractor practicing in Peru is a U.S. citizen, a graduate of Los Angeles College of Chiropractic, and an active member of the Christian Chiropractors' Association. He practices in north central Peru, near the Amazon head waters, administering care to the Indians who live in small villages scattered throughout the dense jungle.

He has operated a fully-equipped chiropractic clinic and first aid center since the mid-1960s. In addition to administering chiropractic care, he attends to snake and insect bites, outbreaks of tropical diseases, dental care, minor surgery and other health problems.

Peru has no chiropractic legislation.

(From information provided by the Rev. Ron Murphy, executive director, Christian Chiropractors' Association, 1989).

Puerto Rico

The Commonwealth of Puerto Rico is a self-governing part of the United States with primarily a Hispanic culture. The commonwealth political status gives the island's citizens virtually the same control over their internal affairs as each of the 50 United States.

A chiropractic law was first passed in 1952. Puerto Rico has one of the lowest densities of chiropractors in the United States; only 27 chiropractors serve more than three million people. The chiropractors are represented by the Chiropractic Association of Puerto Rico.

An applicant for a chiropractic license must be a graduate of a CCE-accredited chiropractic college and pass the Puerto Rico board exam. There are no reciprocity agreements with any other states.

There is federal (Medicare) reimbursement for chiropractic services, but it is limited. A majority of private insurance companies reimburse for a portion of fees for chiropractic care.

(From information provided by Chiropractic Association of Puerto Rico, 1988)

U.S. Virgin Islands

The U.S. Virgin Islands are situated 70 miles from Puerto Rico and include three main islands—St. John, St. Croix and St. Thomas.

Chiropractors were first granted the right to practice in the Virgin Islands in 1978. The judge's ruling was the result of a lawsuit filed by three chiropractors against the Medical Board, which had refused to grant chiropractic licenses. The judge ruled that chiropractors have the proper educational standards and should be licensed. The judges ruling established a chiropractic practice act and a board of chiropractic examiners.

The Chiropractic Practice Act gave chiropractors limited x-ray and laboratory privileges. The examining board was made up of four medical doctors and one chiropractor.

On September 20, 1987 the governor passed a new chiropractic practice act granting chiropractors full x-ray and laboratory privileges. A new chiropractic examining board was created, composed of two MDs, two DCs and one layman. An applicant for the exam must be a graduate of a college with CCE status, and must also have a bachelor's degree.

Of the seven chiropractors living in the Virgin Islands, only three practice year-round.

There is full coverage of chiropractic services under workmen's compensation plans and under government employment plans. There are large numbers of government workers employed in the islands.

Traditional West Indian manipulators, called ''rubbers,'' were at one numerous, but have dwindled to only a few in recent years.

(From information provided by the Virgin Island Chiropractic Association.)

Venezuela

There are nine chiropractors practicing in Venezuela. All are in the capital city of Caracus. While there is no legislation governing chiropractic, the profession is registered by the Minister of Health.

Under Venezuelan law, citizens have the right to practice their profession as long as there is no law that legislates against it; however, a Medical Practice Act states that any health professional not holding a medical degree must practice under medical supervision. The medical law has not been enforced.

Under the registration procedure, chiropractors are allowed to use a variety of therapies and diagnostic tools, including x-ray and physical therapy.

There are good cooperating relationships with medical doctors, though chiropractic health care has minimal recognition among the general public.

Venezuelan chiropractors have been officially sanctioned by the government as Olympic team doctors.

There are no Venezuelan students attending chiropractic colleges because of a devalued currency against the U.S. dollar, which makes a chiropractic education in the United States unaffordable.

Countryside healers called *zobadores* also use manipulation and bonesetting techniques.

(From information provided by Chiropractic Association of Venezuela.)

Eastern Mediterranean

Cyprus

Three chiropractors are in practice in Cyprus. They are represented by the Cyprus Chiropractic Association. There is no chiropractic law.

A formal request for chiropractic legislation was first made to the Medical Services Department of the Ministry of Health in 1977. It ruled that since chiropractors are not considered medical practitioners, the department did not have the authority to create regulations for them.

In 1979, an ammendment to the medical law states that any person diagnosing, treating, or giving advice for any disease of affliction was in violation of the law.

In 1984, another request for legislation was made. After brief study, the Minister of Health ordered the Attorney General to create chiropractic regulation, taking into account chiropractic legislation from around the world. No law has yet been passed.

(From information provided by Cyprus Chiropractic Association, 1985.)

Egypt

There is no chiropractic legislation, though government contacts and research work has been done as a prelude to requesting legislation. Currently, only medical doctors are granted legal status as primary contact providers. One chiropractor had, until recently, practiced here.

In 1982, the International Chiropractors' Association (ICA) initiated discussions with the Egyptian Ministry of Health, the Military Medical Academy, and the Egyptian Orthopedic Association. In 1983, the ICA, and the Cleveland, Life, and Palmer chiropractic colleges completed a three-week research study at three hospital and health clinics under Egypt's National Insurance Authority. This facility serves six million of the nation's laborers. At the facility, the joint chiropractic and medical research team performed double blind studies using chiropractic treatment. The research results were definitive, in the treatment of on-the-job injuries, showing greater effectiveness with chiropractic treatments, as compared to drugs, bed rest, and sham manipulation.

(From information provided by Talaat Ezzeldin, MD, chief orthopedic surgeon, Egyptian Ministry of Health.)

Iran

There are presently five chiropractors practicing in Iran. Four are in Tehran and one is in Shiraz. There is no national association, though the chiropractors meet regularly to discuss matters of mutual concern to the profession.

The chiropractor in Shiraz practices with permission from the Department of Justice. He has the right to x-ray, use modalities, and order laboratory work.

The chiropractors in Tehran have unofficial permission to practice from the Department of Education. Their practices include x-ray, laboratory, physiotherapy, and limited drug prescription (muscle relaxants, vitamin and mineral supplements, pain killers). The unofficial permission to practice is related to favorable results that upper level ministry personnel have had under chiropractic care.

As there is no chiropractic law, there is no licensure requirement. Non-nationals who desire to work in Iran must obtain a work permit from the Department of Immigration.

There are numerous traditional bonesetters in Iran. These practitioners use leg pulling and back twisting, having learned their technique by application and apprenticeship. Bonesetters practice without government restriction. Some of the bonesetters are quite famous nationally.

Chiropractors are perceived to be advanced specialists, partly because chiropractors are educated in the United States, and partly because the numerous patients who have gotten well are apt to tell others of their successful treatment under chiropractic.

Each of the three doctors have extremely busy practices; a waiting list of three months is not uncommon. There is a great need for additional chiropractors.

Many specialties refer to chiropractors, including radiologists, dentists, urologists, gynecologists. Health care specialists of all kind are in short supply, so all health providers use the services of one another.

(From information provided by M. Etminan-Rad, DC, of Tehran, Iran, 1988.)

Israel

Chiropractors in Israel are not licensed. Israel's medical practice act allows the treatment of "defects of the body" by nonmedical practitioners. A nonmedical practitioner may practice unrestricted as long as he does not present himself as a medical doctor or use treatment generally administered by a medical doctor. Because of the lax restrictions, there are dozens of barely-trained practitioners practicing manipulation, some of whom even use the title "chiropractor."

In 1986, the Ministry of Health issued a statement that the chiropractic profession should be licensed. The Israel Chiropractic Society presented a bill based on chiropractic laws in the United States, but no action was taken.

In 1986, the Health Ministry began to issue certificates of recognition to DCs who presented credentials from accredited colleges. The certificate is accompanied by a page of "guidelines," which have been rejected by the Israel Chiropractic Society.

The government has now set up a commission to examine the question of licensing alternative healing methods such as acupuncture, reflexology, Chinese medicine, and chiropractic. Requests from the Israel Chiropractic Society to make a presentation to the commission were resisted until recently. The commission is made up of a Supreme Court judge, a number of MDs, and past Knesset members, about half of whom are chiropractic supporters. Based on the recommendations of the commission, it is possible that some movement toward licensure will be made.

Inclusion in the socialized national health service is not conferred automatically with licensure. The program hires its physicians for a relatively meager salary. Even if chiropractic was included in the national health service, it is probable that few chiropractors would want to participate.

The Israel Chiropractic Society receives numerous requests from chiropractors in the United States who are interested in practicing in Israel. The first deterrent is the lack of licensing laws; the second is the inability to maintain an American standard of living here. Thus, the number of chiropractors has remained relatively constant over the past decade.

A number of Israeli students are studying at chiropractic colleges in the US and England. However, due to economic and political factors, it is impossible to predict how many of these students will return to Israel to practice.

(From information provided by Israel Chiropractic Society.)

Greece

Nine of the ten chiropractors practicing in Greece are located in Athens. Seven of the ten practice with additional degrees (i.e., medicine, physiotherapy), giving them legal protection since there is no chiropractic law, however Greek law, includes the freedom to practice any profession unless it is prohibited by law.

Six of the Greek chiropractors are graduates of Australian chiropractic colleges, three are from US chiropractic colleges, and one is from the European chiropractic college in Great Britain. They are united under the Ellenic Chiropractic Association, an association affiliated with the Ellenic Chiropractic, Naturopathic, and Osteopathic Physicians' Association, a legally sanctioned association.

Much has been written about the use of manipulation by ancient Greek healers. Its use by healers, most notably Aesculapius, and later by Hippocrates, is well documented in ancient literature.

After the decline of Greece, manipulative therapists were not held in as high esteem as before and were called *Practicos Iatros*, which, when translated means "empirical doctor" or "makeshift physician." Greeks associate chiropractic doctors with *Practicos Iatros* because both use manipulation. Greek chiropractors are hampered by the term, and failure to achieve legislative recognition—repeatedly requested since the 1920s—is blamed in part on the association with ancient manipulators.

Chiropractic services are reimbursable under the national health scheme only on the referral of a medical doctor. Chiropractic patients most often are willing to pay themselves, having exhausted efforts to get well under medically covered care. A few private and foreign insurance companies provide partial reimbursement for chiropractic services.

There is good cooperation with various medical specialties, particularly radiologists.

Foreigners wishing to practice chiropractic in Greece must have a work permit, which is issued by the Minister of the Interior, on the condition that a native Greek chiropractor vouch for the applicant's employment.

(From information provided by the Ellenic Chiropractic Association.)

Jordan

Chiropractic was introduced to Jordan in 1979 by its only DC, a Jordanian citizen and a 1978 graduate of Canadian Memorial Chiropractic College. The chiropractor was working at Jordan's King Hussein Medical Centre, a prestigious multispecialty facility, giving him the opportunity to demonstrate the benefits of chiropractic to various high-level individuals including government and medical specialists, and a member of the Royal family. These contacts eventually led the way for official government recognition of chiropractic, achieved in 1987.

Chiropractic is included as one of the main medical and health professions, and is granted full rights as a primary contact health profession. Jordan's Health Supreme Council had first proposed that chiropractic be allowed only under the supervision of a medical doctor. This was rejected by the chiropractor.

In 1988, the Minister of Health visited Canadian Memorial Chiropractic College and upon his return instructed ministry officials to draft regulations to legislate chiropractic as a primary contact provider. Three months later he was replaced by another minister.

The present minister has proposed that chiropractic be registered as a primary contact provider. The scope of practice will include the right to use the title "doctor," full use of diagnostic equipment including x-ray and laboratory, and a treatment regimen that includes the use of physical therapy.

Prerequisites for licensure include Jordanian citizenship, graduation from a recognized and accredited chiropractic college, and at least one year internship in a Jordanian chiropractic clinic. There are presently no provisions for foreign DCs who wish to practice in Jordan.

Interprofessional cooperation is excellent and public awareness of chiropractic is growing rapidly.

(From information provided by Josef Meshki, DC, Amman, Jordan.)

Chiropractic Glossary of Commonly Used Terms

Active Movement. Movement accomplished without outside assistance; the patient moves the joint unassisted (Peterson, 1984).

Adaptation. The adjustment of an organism to its environment (Saunders). A compensatory reaction of the body to a mechanical distortion (LACC).

Adhesion. A fibrous band or structure by which parts adhere abnormally (Saunders).

Adjustment. The chiropractic adjustment is a specific form of direct articular manipulation using either long or short leverage techniques with specific contacts and is characterized by a dynamic thrust of controlled velocity, amplitude, and direction (Janse).

Alignment. To put in a straight line; arrangement of position in a straight line (Houghton Mifflin).

Amplitude. Greatness of size, magnitude, breadth, or range (Houghton Mifflin).

Analysis. Separation into component parts; the act of determining the component parts of a substance (Saunders). Spinal analysis. Examination of the spinal column to determine the relationship of vertebrae to each other and adjacent structures (LACC).

Angiothlipsis. Pressure on an artery, direct or indirect; e.g., in the IVF through pressure generated by a diskopathy, in the foramina transversarii through osteogenic reactions (Houle, 1972).

Anomaly. Congenital or developmental deviation from the normal, standard (Peterson, 1984).

Antagonistic muscles. Muscles or portions of muscles so attached anatomically that when they contract they develop forces that oppose each other (Travell, 1983).

Anterior pelvic tilt. A position of the pelvis in which the vertical plane through the anterior superior iliac spines is anterior to the vertical plane through the symphysis pubes. It is associated with hyperextension of the lumbar spine and flexion at the hip joints (Peterson, 1984).

Anterolisthesis. Anterior translation of the vertebral body (Peterson, 1984).

Arthrosis. Degenerative joint disease of the truly movable joints of the spine or extremities (Yochum, 1984).

Articular strain. The result of forces acting on a joint beyond its capacity to adapt. Refers to stretching of joint components beyond physiological limits causing damage (Ward, 1981).

Asymmetry. Lack or absence of symmetry of position or motion. Dissimilarity in corresponding parts or organs of opposite sides of the body that are normally alike (Saunders).

Axis. A line around which rotatory movement takes place or along which translation occurs. The three-dimensional description of motion of an object with three axes perpendicular to one another. The right handed Cartesian orthogonal system has three axes designated x, y, and z (White, 1978). X axis. It is a line passing horizontally from side to side. May also be referred to as the coronal axis or the frontal axis. Movement around the x axis is said to be in the sagittal plane (White, 1978). Y axis. The y axis is a line perpendicular to the ground. May also be referred to as the vertical axis. Movement around the y axis is said to be in the horizontal or transverse plane (White, 1978). Z axis. The z axis is a line passing horizontally front to back. May also be referred to as the sagittal axis. Movement around the z axis is said to be in the coronal plane (White, 1978).

Axoplasmic flow. The flow of neuroplasm along the axon between synapses and toward and away from end organs (Ward, 1981).

Barrier. Limit of unimpeded motion (Peterson, 1984). Anatomic barrier. The limit of anatomic integrity; the limit of motion imposed by an anatomic structure. Forcing the movement beyond this barrier would produce tissue damage (Griffin, 1973). Elastic barrier (physiologic). The elastic resistance that is felt at the end of the passive range of movement; further motion toward the anatomic barrier may be induced passively (Sandoz).

Biomechanics. The study of structural, functional, and mechanical aspects of human motion. It is concerned mainly with external forces either of a static or dynamic nature dealing with human movements (White, 1978).

Body mechanics. The study of the static and dynamic human body to note the mechanical integration of the parts, and to endeavor to restore and maintain the

Presented by the Terminology Committee of the ACA Council on Technic David H. Peterson, D.C., Chairman body in as nearly as possible normal mechanical condition (LACC).

Bogginess. A tissue texture abnormality characterized principally by a palpable sense of sponginess in the tissue interpreted as resulting from congestion due to increased fluid content (Ward, 1981).

Bucket handle rib motion. Movement of the lower ribs during respiration such that with inhalation the lateral aspect of the rib elevates, resulting in an increase of transverse diameter of the thorax (Ward, 1981).

Caliper rib movement. Movement of lower ribs during respiration such that the rib moves anterior in inhalation (CMCC).

Center of gravity. The point in a body where the body mass is centered (White, 1978).

Chiropractic

Chiropractic practice. Chiropractic is a discipline of the scientific healing arts concerned with the pathogenesis, diagnostic, therapeutics, and prophylaxis of functional disturbances, pathomechanical states, pain syndromes, and neurophysiological effects related to the statics and dynamics of the locomotor system, especially of the spine and pelvis (ECU, 1973).

Chiropractic science. Chiropractic science is concerned with the investigation of the relationship between structure (primarily the spine) and function (primarily the nervous system) of the human body that leads to the restoration and preservation of health (Houle, 1972).

Compensation. Changes in structural relationships to accommodate for foundation disturbance and maintain balance (LACC).

Contact point. The area of the adjustive hand that makes contact with the patient in the delivery of the chiropractic adjustment. There are 12 contact points (ACA, 1987).
Points of contact on the hand
1. Pisiform
2. Hypothenar
3. Metacarpal (knife-edge)
4. Digital
5. Distal interphalangeal (DIP)
6. Proximal interphalangeal (PIP)
7. Metacarpophalangeal (MP or index)
8. Web
9. Thumb
10. Thenar
11. Calcaneal
12. Palmar

Contraction. A shortening or reduction in size; in connection with muscles, contraction implies shortening and/or development of tension (Saunders).

Contracture. A condition of fixed high resistance to passive stretch of a muscle resulting from fibrosis of the tissues supporting the muscle or joint (Saunders).

Coupling. A phenomenon of consistent association of one motion (translation or rotation) about an axis with another motion (translation or rotation) about a second axis. One motion cannot be produced without the other (White, 1978).

Creep. A viscoelastic material deforms with time when it is subjected to a constant, suddenly applied load. This phenomenon is called creep (White, 1978).

Curvature. Deviation from a rectilinear direction (Saunders). An abnormal bending of the spine in any direction away from the natural contour, and involving three or more vertebrae (LACC).

Curve. An anatomical term for a normal bending of the spine in the sagittal plane, e.g., primary dorsal and sacral curves, secondary cervical and lumbar curves (LACC).

Deformation. A change in length or shape (White, 1978).

Degrees of freedom. The number of independent coordinates in a coordinate system required to completely specify the position of an object in space. One degree of freedom is rotation around one axis or translation along one axis. The spine is considered to have 6 degrees of freedom because it has the capability of rotatory movement around three axes as well as translatory movement along three axes (White, 1978).

Diagnosis. The art of distinguishing one disease from another (Saunders). The use of scientific and skillful methods to establish the cause and nature of a person's illness.

Discogenic. Common usage; caused by derangement of an intervertebral disc (Houle, 1972).

Discopathogenic. Abnormal action or function of a disc resulting in a disorder or condition; originating because of disc degeneration (Houle, 1972).

Discopathy. Any pathological changes in a disc (Janse).

Disc herniation. Extrusion of nucleus pulposus into a defect in the annulus fibrosus (Peterson, 1984).

Displacement. State of being removed from normal position; as pertaining to vertebral displacement, it refers to a disrelationship of the vertebrae to its relative structure (LACC).

Distortion. In the body framework, includes any mechanical departure from ideal or normal symmetry (LACC).

Distraction. The movement of two surfaces away from each other (Houghton Mifflin).

Dynamics. A branch of mechanics that consists of the study of the loads and motions of interacting bodies (White, 1978).

Dysarthrosis. The strict meaning of joint motion restriction without the neurological connotations. It refers to kinetics (Houle, 1972).

Dyskinesia. Impairment of the power of voluntary movement, resulting in fragmentary or incomplete movements, aberrant motion (Drum, 1973).

Eccentric work or contraction. Work produced by a muscle when its length is increasing (CMCC).

Effleurage. A form of massage employing slow rhythmic stroking executed with a minimum of force and light pressure (Peterson, 1984).

Elasticity. The property of a material or structure to return to its original form after the removal of the deforming load (White, 1978).

End play (end feel). Discrete, short-range movements of a joint independent of the action of voluntary muscles, determined by springing each vertebrae at the limit of its passive range of motion (Peterson, 1984).

Equilibrium. State of a body at rest in which the sums of all forces and movements are zero (Frankel).

Extension. The separation of two embryologically ventral surfaces; movement away from the fetal position; the return movement from flexion (Peterson, 1984).

Facilitation. An increase in afferent stimuli so that the synaptic threshold is more easily reached; thus, there is increase in the efficacy of subsequent impulses in that pathway or synapse. The consequence of increased efficacy is that continued stimulation produces hyperactive responses (Ward, 1981).

Fibrosis. The formation of fibrous tissue (Saunders).

Fibrositis. Inflammatory hyperplasia of the white fibrous tissue of the body, especially of the muscle sheaths and fascial layers of the locomotor system (Sandoz).

Fixation (dynamic fault). The state whereby articulation has become temporarily immobilized in a position that it may normally occupy during any phase of physiological movement. The immobilization of an articulation in a position of movement when the joint is at rest, or in a position of rest when the joint is in movement (Sandoz).

Flexibility. The ability of a structure to deform under the application of a load (White, 1978).

Flexion. The approximation of two embryologically ventral surfaces; movement toward the fetal position (Peterson, 1984).

Foundation. Any structure that supports or participates in the support of any part of the body framework (LACC).

Friction massage. A form of deep circular or transverse massage where the skin is moved over the subcutaneous tissue (Peterson, 1984).

Functional. (1) Of or pertaining to the function of an organ. Not structural, affecting functions only (Houghton Mifflin). (2) Of, or pertaining to a function; affecting the functions but not the structure (Janse).

Gliding. Movement in which the joint surfaces are flat or only slightly curved and one articulating surface slides on the other (Peterson, 1984).

Gravitational line. A vertical line through the body where body mass is entered. In the theoretical, laterally viewed ideal posture, it starts at the external auditory canal, passes through the lateral head of the humerus at the tip of the shoulder, across the greater trochanter, the lateral condyle of the knee, and slightly anterior to the lateral maleolus (Peterson, 1984).

Health. A state of optimal physical, mental, and social well-being and not merely the absence of disease and infirmity (Saunders).

Homeostasis. (1) Maintenance of static or constant conditions in the internal environment. (2) The level of well-being of an individual maintained by internal environment. (2) The level of well-being of an individual maintained by internal physiologic harmony (Ward, 1981).

Hyper. Beyond excessive (Saunders).

Hypo. Under or deficient (Saunders).

Impinge. To press or encroach upon; to come into close contact; an obstructive lesion causing pressure on a nerve (LACC).

Inhibition. Effect of one neuron on another tending to prevent it from initiating impulses (Kutler, 1976).

Innate. Inborn; hereditary (Saunders).

Innate intelligence. The intrinsic biological ability of a healthy organism to reach physiologically to the changing conditions of the external and internal environment (Janse).

Instability. Quality or condition of being unstable; not firm, fixed or constant (Vear, 1973).

Inversion. A turning inward, inside out, upside down, or other reversal of the normal relation of a part (Saunders). Is often used to describe passive inverted tracation (Peterson, 1984).

Instrumentation. The use of any tool, appliance or apparatus; work performed with instruments (Saunders).

Ischemic compression. Application of progressively stronger painful pressure on a trigger point for the purpose of eliminating the point's tenderness (Travell, 1983).

Isokinetic exercise. Exercise using a constant speed of movement of the body part (Ward, 1981).

Joint dysfunction. Joint mechanics showing area disturbances of function without structural change; subtle joint dysfunctions affecting quality and range of joint motion. They are diagnosed with the aid of motion palpation, and stress and motion radiography investigation (Drum, 1973).

Joint play. Discrete, short-range movements of a joint independent of the action of voluntary muscles, determined by springing each vertebrae in the neutral position (Peterson, 1984).

Kinematics. The division of mechanics that deals with the geometry of the motion of bodies, displacement velocity, and acceleration without taking into account the forces that produce the motion (White, 1978).

Kinesiology. The science or study of movement and the active and passive structures involved (Saunders).

Kinesthesia. The sense by which movement, weight, position, etc., are perceived; commonly used to refer specifically to the perception of changes in the angles of joints (Saunders).

Kinesthetic. Pertaining to kinesthesia (Saunders).

Kinetic chain. A combination of several successively arranged joints constituting a complex unit, as links in a chain (White, 1978). Closed kinetic chain. A system in which motion of one link has determinate relations to every other link in the system (White, 1978). Open kinetic chain. A combination of links in which the terminal joint is free (White, 1978).

Kinetics. A branch of mechanics that studies the relation between the force system acting on a body and the changes it produces in the body motion (White, 1978).

Klapping. Tapotement (clapping, cupping) (Peterson, 1984).

Kneading. A form of massage employing forceful circular and transverse movement of a large raised fold of skin and underlying muscle (Peterson, 1984).

Kyphoscoliosis. Backward and lateral curvature of the spinal column (Saunders).

Kyphosis. Abnormally increased convexity in the curvature of the thoracic spine (Saunders).

Kyphotic. Affected with or pertaining to kyphosis (Saunders).

Lateral flexion. Bending to the side within the coronal plane (Peterson, 1984).

Laterolisthesis. Lateral translatory excursion of the vertebral body (Peterson, 1984).

Lesion. Any pathological or traumatic discontinuity of tissue or loss of function (Saunders).

Lever. A rigid bar moving on a fixed fulcrum (Houghton Mifflin).

Listing (dynamic). Designation of the abnormal movement characteristic of one vertebra in relation to subadjacent segments (Peterson, 1984).
  Dynamic Listing Nomenclature
  1. Flexion restriction
  2. Extension restriction
  3. Lateral flexion restriction (right or left)
  4. Rotational restriction (right or left)

Listing (static). Designation of the spatial orientation of one vertebra in relation to adjacent segments (Peterson, 1984).
  Static Listing Nomenclature
  1. Flexion malposition
  2. Extension malposition

3. Lateral flexion malposition (right or left)
4. Rotational malposition (right or left)
5. Anterolisthesis
6. Retrolisthesis
7. Laterolisthesis

Lordosis. The anterior concavity in the curvature of the lumbar and cervical spine (Saunders).

Lordotic. Anterior spinal curve (ACA, 1987).

Malposition. Abnormal or anomalous position (Houghton Mifflin).
  Static Listing Nomenclature
  1. Flexion malposition
  2. Extension malposition
  3. Lateral flexion malposition (right or left)
  4. Rotational malposition (right or left)
  5. Anterolisthesis
  6. Retrolisthesis
  7. Laterolisthesis

Manipulation. Therapeutic application of manual force (Ward, 1981). Spinal manipulative therapy broadly defined includes all procedures where the hands are used to mobilize, adjust, manipulate, apply traction, massage, stimulate, or otherwise influence the spine and paraspinal tissues with the aim of influencing the patient's health (Haldeman, 1980).

Massage. The systematic therapeutic friction, stroking, and kneading of the body (Saunders). Maneuvers performed by hand on the skin of the patient and through the skin of the patient on the subcutaneous tissue. There may be variables in intensity of pressure exerted, surface area treated, and frequency of application (Sidney, 1960).

Meric System. The treatment of visceral conditions through adjustment of vertebrae at the levels of neuromeric innervation to the organs involved (Janse).

Misalignment. Not in proper alignment (Peterson, 1984).

Mobilization. The process of making a fixed part movable (Saunders). A form of manipulation applied within the physiological passive range of joint motion and is characterized by nonthrust passive joint manipulation (Peterson, 1984).

Motion. The relative displacement with time of a body in space with respect to other bodies or some reference system (White, 1978).

Myofascial syndrome. Pain and/or autonomic phenomena referred from active myofascial trigger points with associated dysfunction. The specific muscle or muscle group that causes the symptoms should be identified (Travell, 1983).

Myofascial trigger point. A hyperirritable spot, usually within a taut band of skeletal muscle or in the muscle's fascia, that is painful on compression and that can give rise to characteristic referred pain, tenderness, and autonomic phenomena. A myofascial trigger point is to be distinguished from cutaneous, ligamentous, periosteal, and nonmuscular fascial trigger points. Types include active, latent, primary, associated, satellite, and secondary (Travell, 1983).

Myofascitis. (1) Inflammation of a muscle and its fascia, particularly of the fascial insertion of muscle to bone. (2) Pain, tenderness, other referred phenomena, and the dysfunction attributed to myofascial trigger points (Travell, 1983).

Myofibrosis. Replacement of muscle tissue by fibrous tissue (Travell, 1983).

Nerve interference. A chiropractic term used to refer to the interruption of normal nerve transmission (nerve energy) (Peterson, 1984).

Nerve transmission. The transmission of information along a nerve cell (Peterson, 1984).

    Impulsed based. Nerve transmission involving the generation and transfer of electrical potentials along a nerve axon (Peterson, 1984).

    Nonimpulsed based. The transfer of chemical messengers along a nerve axon, i.e., axoplasmic flow (Peterson, 1984).

Neurodystrophic. The disease process within a nerve resulting from trauma, circulation disorders, or metabolic diseases, e.g., a neurodystrophic factor (diabetes and pernicious anemia) (Vear, 1973).

Neurogenic. This word is often used to mean originating in nerve tissue; "The cause of the disorder is neurogenic" (Houle, 1972).

Neuropathogenic. A disease within a tissue resulting from abnormal nerve performance, e.g., Barre-Lieou syndrome resulting from neuropathogenic reflexes caused by pathomechanics of the cervical spine (Houle, 1972).

Neuropathy. A general term denoting functional disturbances and/or pathological changes in the peripheral nervous system (Saunders).

Neurophysiological effects. A general term denoting functional or aberrant disturbances of the peripheral or autonomic nervous systems. The term is used to designate nonspecific effects related to (1) motor and sensory functions of the peripheral nervous system; (2) vasomotor activity, secretomotor activity, and motor activity of smooth muscle from the autonomic nervous system, e.g., neck, shoulder, arm syndrome (the extremity becomes cool with increased sweating); (3) trophic activity of both the peripheral and autonomic nervous system, e.g., muscle atrophy in neck, shoulder, arm syndrome (Vear, 1973).

Neurothlipsis. Pressure on a nerve direct or indirect, e.g., in the IVF through congestion of perineural tissues; in the carpal tunnel through direct ligamentous pressure (Houle, 1972).

Nutation. Motion of the sacrum about a coronal axis in which the sacral base moves anteriorly and inferiorly and the tip of the coccyx moves posteriorly and superiorly; nodding, as of the head (Peterson, 1984).

    Counter-nutation. Motion of the sacrum about a coronal axis in which the sacral base moves posteriorly and superiorly and the tip of the coccyx moves anteriorly and inferiorly; nodding, as of the head (Peterson, 1984).

Osteophyte. A degenerative exostosis secondary to musculotendinous stress (Yochum, 1984).

Palpation. (1) The act of feeling with the hands (Saunders). (2) The application of variable manual pressure through the surface of the body for the purpose of determining the shape, size, consistency, position, inherent motility, and health of the tissues beneath (Ward, 1981).

    Motion palpation. Palpatory diagnosis of passive and active segmental joint range of motion (Peterson, 1984).

    Static palpation. Palpatory diagnosis of somatic structures in a neutral static position (Peterson, 1984).

Palpatory diagnosis. The process of palpating the patient to evaluate neuromusculoskeletal and visceral systems (Peterson, 1984).

Palpatory skills. The sensory and tactile skills used in performing a physical examination (Peterson, 1984).

Palpitation. A subjective sensation of an unduly rapid or irregular heart beat (Saunders).

Passive movement. Movement that is carried through by the operator without conscious assistance or resistance of the patient (Peterson, 1984).

Pathomechanical states. Joint pathomechanics with structural changes; those architectural changes are the scars of imbalanced motion and weight bearing, trauma, and biochemical changes associated with aging and deficiency states. These tissue changes may be revealed by static x-ray, biopsy, and definitely diagnosed with surgical exposure; e.g., arthrosis; spondylolisthesis; disc degenerations (Drum, 1973).

Pelvic lateral shift. A movement in the coronal plane of the pelvis in which one anterosuperior spine moves closer to the midline while the opposite anterosuperior spine has moved further away from the midline. It is associated with adduction and abduction of the hip joints (Peterson, 1984).

Pelvic lateral tilt. A position of the pelvis in which it is not level in the horizontal plane, i.e., one anterosuperior iliac spine is higher than the other. It is associated with lateral flexion of the lumbar spine and adduction and abduction of the hip joints (Peterson, 1984).

Pelvic rotation. A position of the pelvis in which one anterosuperior iliac spine is anterior to the other. Pelvic rotation is a rotatory movement around the y or vertical axis (Peterson, 1984).

Pelvic tilt. A deviation of the pelvis in the sagittal plane from neutral position (Peterson, 1984).

Physiological motion. Normal changes in the position of articulating surfaces during the movement of a joint or region (Peterson, 1984).

Plane. A flat surface determined by the position of three points in space (Saunders).

    Coronal plane. Frontal plane (White, 1978).

    Frontal plane. A plane passing longitudinally through the body from one side to the other, and dividing the body into anterior and posterior portions (White, 1978).

    Sagittal plane. A plane passing longitudinally through the body from front to back and dividing it into right and left portions. The median or midsagittal plane divides the body into approximately equal right and left portions (White, 1978).

    Transverse plane. A plane passing horizontally through the body perpendicular to the sagittal and frontal planes, dividing the body into upper and lower portions (White, 1978).

Plastic deformation. A nonrecoverable deformation (Peterson, 1984).

Plasticity. The property of a material to deform permanently when it is loaded beyond its elastic range (White, 1978).

Plumb line. Weighted, true vertical line used for visual comparison with the gravitational line (Peterson, 1984).

Posture. (1) The attitude of the body (Saunders). (2) The relative arrangement of the parts of the body. Good posture is that state of muscular and skeletal balance that protects the supporting structures of the body against injury or progressive deformity irrespective of the attitude (erect, lying, squatting, stooping) in which these structures are working or resting (Krieger, 1952).

Prophylaxis. The branch of applied biology that seeks to reduce or eradicate disease by removing or altering the responsible etiologic factors. The prevention of disease; preventive treatment (Boyd). (1) To prevent occurrence of lesions due to poor postural hygiene, physical fitness, and faulty body mechanics. (2) The prevention of recurrence with follow-up care, e.g., exercise. (3) Many lesions are not curable and become quiescent with treatments; therefore, follow-up care to prevent further pathology, or at least to retard the pathomechanical process, is necessary (Gitelman, 1973).

Proprioception. Sensory perception of movement or position within the body (Saunders).

Range of motion. The range of translation and rotation of a joint for each of its six ranges of freedom (CMCC).

Reciprocal innervation. The inhibition of antagonistic muscles when the agonist is stimulated (Ward, 1981).

Rectilinear motion. Motion in a straight line (Peterson, 1984).

Referred pain. Pain felt in a part other than in which the cause that produced it is situated (Saunders).

Reflex. The result of transforming an ingoing sensory impulse into an outgoing efferent impulse without an act of will (LACC).

Reflex therapy. Treatment that is aimed at stimulating afferent impulses and evoking a given response; i.e., neuromuscular (Janse).

Relaxation. The decrease in stress in a deformed structure with time when the deformation is held constant (White, 1978).

Resilience. The property of returning to the former shape, size, or state after distortion (Saunders).

Restriction. Limitation to movement. Describes the direction of limited movement in subluxated and/or dysfunctional joints (Peterson, 1984).

Retrolisthesis. Posterior translation of the vertebral body (Peterson, 1984).

Roentgenometrics. The direct measurement of structures shown in the roentgenogram/radiograph (Peterson, 1984).

"Rolfing." A 10-hour cycle of deep manual intervention in the soft tissue structure of the body, formerly called structural integration, designed by Ida P. Rolf, Ph.D. Deep effleurage is used to strip tendons and to stretch myofascial tissues to achieve both postural and psychological effects (Ward, 1981). *see* Effleurage.

Ropiness. A tissue texture abnormality (qv) characterized by a cord or string-like feeling (Ward, 1981).

Rotation. Motion of a body around an axis (White, 1978).

Sacroiliac fixation (Sacroiliac joint locking). The absence of normal motion at the sacroiliac joint demonstrable by motion palpation in which the axis of rotation has shifted to either the superior or inferior portion of the sacroiliac joint, or rarely a situation in which there is total joint locking with no axis of rotation (Peterson, 1984).

Sacroiliac extension fixation (AS). A state of the sacroiliac joint in which the posterosuperior iliac spine is fixed in an anterosuperior position with the innominate bone on that side fixed in extension in relation to the sacrum. The axis of rotation then shifts inferior and the superior joint remains mobile (Peterson, 1984).

Sacroiliac flexion fixation (PI). A state of the sacroiliac joint in which the posterosuperior iliac spine is fixed in a posteroinferior position with the innominate bone on that side fixed in flexion in relation to the sacrum. The axis of rotation then shifts superiorly and the inferior joint remains mobile (Peterson, 1984).

Scan. An intermediate screening palpatory examination designed to focus the clinician on regional areas of joint dysfunction (Peterson, 1984).

Scoliosis. An appreciable lateral deviation in the normally straight vertical line of the spine (Saunders).

 Functional scoliosis. Lateral deviation of the spine resulting from poor posture, foundation anomalies, occupational strains, etc., that are still not permanently established (Peterson, 1984).

 Structural scoliosis. Permanent lateral deviation of the spine such that the spine cannot return to a neutral position (Peterson, 1984).

Shear. An applied force that tends to cause an opposite but parallel sliding motion of planes within an object (Saunders).

Short leg. An anatomic, pathological, or functional leg deficiency leading to dysfunction (CMCC).

Side bending. *see* Lateral flexion (Peterson, 1984).

Somatic dysfunction. Impaired or altered function of related components of the somatic (body framework) system: skeletal, arthrodial, and myofascial structures and related vascular, lymphatic, and neural elements (Ward, 1981).

Spinography. Roentgenometrics of the spine (Peterson, 1984).

Spondylitis. Inflammation of the vertebrae (Saunders).

Spondyloarthrosis. Arthrosis of the synovial joints of the spine (Yochum, 1984).

Spondylolisthesis. Anterior slippage of a vertebral body on its caudal fellow (Yochum, 1984).

Spondylosis. An interruption in the pars interarticularis, which may be unilateral or bilateral (Yochum, 1984).

Spondylophytes. Degenerative spur formation arising from the vertebral end plates and usually projecting somewhat horizontally (Yochum, 1984).

Spondylosis. Degenerative joint disease as it affects the vertebral body end plates (Yochum, 1984).

Spondylotherapy. The therapeutic application of percussion or concussion over the vertebrae to elicit reflex responses at the levels of neuromeric innervation to the organ being influenced (Janse).

Sprain. Joint injury in which some of the fibers of a supporting ligament are ruptured but the continuity of the ligament remains intact (Saunders).

Spur. A projecting body as from a bone (Saunders).

Statics. The branch of mechanics that deals with the equilibrium of bodies at rest or in motion with zero acceleration (White, 1978).

Stiffness. A measure of resistance offered to external loads by a specimen or structure as it deforms (White, 1978).

Strain. An overstretching and tearing of musculotendinous tissue (Peterson, 1984).

Stress. The sum of the biological reaction to any adverse stimulus—physical, mental and/or emotional, internal or external—that tends to disturb the organism's homeostasis; should these compensating reactions be inadequate or inappropriate, they may lead to disorders (Ward, 1981).

Stretching. Separation of the origin and insertion of a muscle or attachments of fascia or ligaments by applying a constant pressure lengthening the fibers of muscle or fascia (Ward, 1981).

Stringiness. A palpable tissue texture abnormality characterized by fine or string-like myofascial structures (Ward, 1981).

Subacute. Less than acute, between acute and chronic (Saunders).

Subluxation. Subluxation is an aberrant relationship between two adjacent articular structures that may have functional or pathological sequelae, causing an alteration in the biomechanical and/or neurophysiological reflections of these articular structures, their proximal structures, and/or body systems that may be directly or indirectly affected by them (ACA, 1987).

Symmetry. The similar arrangement in form and relationship of parts around a common axis or on each side of a plane of the body (Saunders).

Syndesmophyte. An osseous excrescence or bony outgrowth from a ligament. Usually projecting vertically in the spine (Saunders).

Tapotement. A tapping or percussing movement in massage; it includes clapping, beating, and punctation (Ward, 1981).

Technique. Any of a number of physical or mechanical chiropractic procedures used in the treatment of patients (Peterson, 1984).

Thrust. The sudden manual application of a controlled directional force upon a suitable part of the patient, the delivery of which effects an adjustment (LACC).

Tonus. The slight continuous contraction of muscle that in skeletal muscles aids in the maintenance of posture (Saunders).

Torsion. A type of load that is applied by a couple of forces (parallel and directed opposite to each other about the axis of a structure) (White, 1978).

Traction. The act of drawing or exerting a pulling force (Saunders).

Translation. Motion of a rigid body in which a straight line in the body always remains parallel to itself (White, 1978).

Trigger point. *see* Myofascial trigger point (Travell, 1983).

Trophic. Of or pertaining to nutrition (Saunders).

Trophic nerve function. Those interactions between nerves and other cells that initiate or control molecular modification in the other cell (Guth, 1969).

Vertebral motion segment. (1) Two adjacent vertebral bodies and the disc between them, the two posterior joints and the ligamentous structures binding the two vertebrae to one another. (2) The consideration of the anatomic and functional relationships of two vertebrae, the mechanical integration of their articular processes and the related musculature, ligaments, and synovial membranes (White, 1978).

Viscoelasticity. The property of a material to show sensitivity to the rate of loading or deformation. Two basic components are viscosity and elasticity (White, 1978).

Viscosity. The property of materials to resist loads that produce shear (Saunders).

REFERENCES

Dorland's Illustrated Medical Dictionary, 26th edition; W.B. Saunders.

American Heritage Dictionary, 2nd edition; Houghton Mifflin.

History of the Development of Chiropractic Concepts; Chiropractic Terminology, Janse, *NINCDS Monograph*, No. 15.

Clinical Biomechanics of the Spine, White and Panjabi; Lippincott, 1978.

Myofascial Pain and Dysfunction, The Trigger Point Manual, Travell and Simons; Williams and Wilkins, 1983.

Western States Chiropractic College Glossary of Chiropractic Terminology, Dave Peterson, 1984.

Canadian Memorial Chiropractic College Glossary of Chiropractic Terminology.

Los Angeles College of Chiropractic, old Principles class notes, author unknown.

Glossary of Osteopathic Terminology, M. Ward, AOA, 1981.

Swiss Annals, Volume VI, 1976, ''Some physical mechanisms and effects of spinal adjustments''; Sandoz.

Basic Biomechanics of the Skeletal System, Frankel and Nordin; Lea and Febiger, 1st edition.

Swiss Annals, Volume VI, 1976, ''Classification of luxations, subluxations and fixations of the cervical spine''; Sandoz.

From Neuron to Brain, A Cellular Approach to the Function of the Nervous System, Kutler and Nicholls; Sinaver Press, 1976.

Low Back Pain, Finneson; Lippincott Co., 2nd edition, 1980; Chapter 7, Haldeman.

Massage, Manipulation and traction, Sidney Licht; Krieger, 1960.

Two In One, A Radiologic Symposium, Yochum, 1984.

Posture and Pain, Kendall and Kendall; Krieger, 1952.

Introduction to the Nervous System, Bullock; Freeman and Company, 1977.

Edgar Houle, 1972.

L. K. Griffin, 1973.

European Chiropractic Union, 1973.

David Drum, 1973.

H. J. Vear, 1973.

Preventive Medicine, William Boyd, 7th edition.

R. Gitelman, 1973.

Houston Conference, 1972.

Indexed Synopsis of ACA Policies on Public Health and Related Matters, 1987 edition, p. 18. (Approved by the House of Delegates, July 1987.)

Guth, L., ''Trophic Effects of Vertebral Neurons,'' *Neuroscience Research Program Bulletin*, Vol. 7 (1969), 1–73.

Index